Elements of Reproduction and Reproductive Diseases of Goats

Elements of Reproduction and Reproductive Diseases of Goats

Edited by

Tanmoy Rana, MVSc, PhD
Assistant Professor, Department of Veterinary Clinical Complex
West Bengal University of Animal & Fishery Sciences
Kolkata, India

WILEY Blackwell

Published by John Wiley & Sons, Inc., Hoboken, New Jersey.
Published simultaneously in Canada.

Library of Congress Cataloging-in-Publication Data Applied for
Hardback ISBN: 9781394189731
ePDF: 9781394190072
ePUB: 9781394190003
oBook: 9781394190089

Cover Design: Wiley
Cover Images: Courtesy of Tanmoy Rana

Set in 9.5/12.5pt STIXTwoText by Straive, Pondicherry, India

Printed in Singapore
M124896_020824

Contents

List of Contributors

Mojetoluwa S. Afolabi
Department of Food and Animal Science
Alabama A&M University, Normal, USA

Akanksha Agnihotri
Department of Veterinary Medicine
College of Veterinary Science and Animal Husbandry
Jabalpur, India

Manoj Kumar Ahirwar
Department of Veterinary Surgery and Radiology
College of Veterinary Science and Animal Husbandry
Jabalpur, India

Allam Lushaikyaa
Faculty of Veterinary Medicine
Ahmadu Bello University
Zaria, Nigeria

Varun Asediya
Animal Nutrition Research Station
Anand Agricultural University
Anand, Gujarat, India

Ashok Ashwini
Department of Veterinary Medicine
Veterinary College
Hassan, India

Ashok Baindha
Post Graduate Institute of Veterinary
Education & Research
Jaipur, India

K. Athira
Department of Veterinary Epidemiology
and Preventive Medicine
College of Veterinary and Animal Sciences
Mannuthy, India

Kolawole Jonathan Bamidele
Faculty of Veterinary Medicine
Ahmadu Bello University
Zaria, Nigeria

Himangshu Baruah
Department of Veterinary Pharmacology and Toxicology
Lakhimpur College of Veterinary Science
Assam Agricultural University
North Lakhimpur, India

Sonam Bhatt
Department of Veterinary Medicine
Bihar Veterinary College, Bihar Animal Sciences University
Patna, India

Suman Biswas
Teaching Veterinary Clinical Complex
Faculty of Veterinary and Animal Sciences
Institute of Agricultural Science
Banaras Hindu University
Mirzapur, India

Antonio Carlos Lopes Câmara
Large Animal Veterinary Teaching Hospital
Universidade de Brasília
Brasília, Brazil

Vipin Chandra
Post Graduate Institute of Veterinary
Education & Research
Jaipur, India

Prakash M. Chauhan
Department of Clinics, College of Veterinary Science
and Animal Husbandry
Kamdhenu University, Sardarkrushinagar
Gujarat, India

Akanksha Choudhary
Post Graduate Institute of Veterinary
Education & Research
Jaipur, India

Bashir Maryam Darma
Veterinary Teaching Hospital
Faculty of Veterinary Medicine
Bayero University
Kano, Nigeria

Bhupamani Das
Department of Clinics
College of Veterinary Science and Animal Husbandry
Kamdhenu University
Sardarkrushinagar, Gujarat, India

Jitumoni Das
Department of Animal Reproduction
Gynaecology and Obstetrics
Lakhimpur College of Veterinary Science
Assam Agricultural University
North Lakhimpur, India

K. Justin Davis
Department of Veterinary Epidemiology
and Preventive Medicine
College of Veterinary and Animal Sciences
Mannuthy, India

Sarita Devi
Department of Medicine
College of Veterinary Science and Animal Husbandry
Kamdhenu University
Sardarkrushinagar, Gujarat, India

Kritika Dhial
Apollo College of Veterinary Medicine
Jaipur, Rajasthan, India

Priyanka Duggal
Department of Veterinary Surgery and Radiology
College of Veterinary Sciences
Lala Lajpat Rai University of Veterinary and
Animal Sciences
Hisar, India

Parimita Dutta
Krishi Vigyan Kendra (KVK)
Tirap, India

Ayyasamy Elango
Department of Veterinary Gynaecology and Obstetrics
Veterinary College and Research Institute
Tamil Nadu Veterinary and Animal Sciences University
Salem, India

Ama Adadzewa Eshun
Department of Food and Animal Science
Alabama A&M University, Normal, USA

Abhijeet Fernandes
Department of Veterinary Gynaecology and Obstetrics
College of Veterinary Science
Guru Angad Dev Veterinary and Animal Sciences University
Bathinda, India

Chetana Gangwar
Animal Physiology and Reproduction Division
ICAR-Central Institute for Research on Goat
Mathura, India

Amaan Ghaazi
Apollo College of Veterinary Medicine
Jaipur, Rajasthan, India

Mohammad M. Islam
Pashupalan Sanshodhan Kendra
Kamdhenu University
Ramna Muvada, Gujarat, India

Manoj Kumar Kalita
Department of Animal Reproduction
Gynaecology and Obstetrics
Lakhimpur College of Veterinary Science
Assam Agricultural University
North Lakhimpur, India

Laishram Sanathoi Khuman
Department of Extension Education
Lakhimpur College of Veterinary Science
Assam Agricultural University
North Lakhimpur, India

Hycinth Ndabatsado Kolo
Department of Animal Health and Production
Federal University of Technology
Minna, Nigeria

Anil Kumar
Department of Veterinary Clinical Complex
Bihar Veterinary College, Bihar Animal Sciences University
Patna, India

Ankesh Kumar
Department of Veterinary Clinical Complex
Bihar Veterinary College, Bihar Animal Sciences University
Patna, India

Gowdaiahnadoddi K. Chetan Kumar
Department of Veterinary Medicine
Veterinary College
Hassan, India

Kaushalendra Kumar
Department of Animal Nutrition
Bihar Veterinary College
Patna, India

Pramod Kumar
Department of Veterinary Physiology and Biochemistry
College of Veterinary Science and Animal Husbandry
Acharya Narendra Deva University of
Agriculture and Technology
Ayodhya, Uttar Pradesh, India

Rajesh Kumar
Department of Veterinary Gynaecology and Obstetrics
College of Veterinary Science and Animal Husbandry
Acharya Narendra Deva University of
Agriculture and Technology
Ayodhya, India

Rohit Kumar
Department of Livestock Production Management
Dr. G.C. Negi College of Veterinary and Animal Sciences
Palampur, India

Sanjay Kumar
Department of Animal Nutrition
Bihar Veterinary College
Patna, India

Rajni Kumari
ICAR-RCER, Patna, India

Neeti Lakhani
Department of Animal Nutrition
College of Veterinary Science
Guru Angad Dev Veterinary and Animal Sciences University
Bathinda, India

Mohan Lal
Post Graduate Institute of Veterinary
Education & Research
Jaipur, India

Mada A. Khumran
Faculty of Veterinary Medicine
Ahmadu Bello University
Zaria, Nigeria

Chinmoy Maji
Division of Animal Health, North 24 Parganas Krishi
Vigyan Kendra, West Bengal University of Animal &
Fishery Sciences, Ashokenagar, West Bengal, India

Kruti Debnath Mandal
Department of Avian Sciences
Faculty of Veterinary & Animal Sciences
West Bengal University of Animal & Fishery Sciences
Nadia, India

Sakthivel Manokaran
Department of Veterinary Gynaecology and Obstetrics
Veterinary College and Research Institute, Tamil Nadu
Veterinary and Animal Sciences University
Salem, India

Varsha Mishra
Department of Veterinary Medicine
College of Veterinary Science and Animal Husbandry
Jabalpur, India

Aliyu Abdullahi Mohammed
Department of Animal Sciences
Usman Danfodio University
Sokoto, Nigeria

Ogunkunle Nathaniel
Department of Food and Animal Science
Alabama A&M University
Normal, USA

Richard Jagatheesan Pitchai Navlon
Veterinary College and Research Institute
Tamil Nadu Veterinary and Animal Sciences University
Theni, India

Pauline Chiezey Ngozi
National Animal Production Research Institute/
Faculty of Veterinary Medicine, Ahmadu Bello University
Zaria, Nigeria

Ram Niwas
Department of Veterinary Surgery and Radiology
College of Veterinary Sciences
Lala Lajpat Rai University of Veterinary
and Animal Sciences
Hisar, India

Adeniyi Njideka
Department of Biological Sciences, Alabama A&M
University, Normal, USA

Padmanath Krishnan
Veterinary Clinical Complex
Veterinary College and Research Institute
Tamil Nadu Veterinary and Animal Sciences University
Theni, India

Chirag P. Parmar
Pashupalan Sanshodhan Kendra
Kamdhenu University
Ramna Muvada, Gujarat, India

Husen R. Parsani
Department of Veterinary Parasitology
College of Veterinary Science and Animal Husbandry
Kamdhenu University
Sardarkrushinagar, Gujarat, India

Kashyap Patel
Department of Medicine
College of Veterinary Science and Animal Husbandry
Kamdhenu University
Sardarkrushinagar, Gujarat, India

Ramesh M. Patel
Department of Clinics
College of Veterinary Science and Animal Health
Kamdhenu University
Sardarkrushinagar, Gujarat, India

Abhishek Pathak
Apollo College of Veterinary Medicine
Jaipur, Rajasthan, India

Salil Kumar Pathak
Department of Veterinary Medicine
College of Veterinary Science and Animal Husbandry
Jabalpur, India

Prerona Patowary
Department of Veterinary Clinical Medicine, Ethics and Jurisprudence, Assam Agricultural University – Goat Research Station, Burnihat, India

Shashi Pradhan
Department of Veterinary Medicine
College of Veterinary Science and Animal Husbandry
Jabalpur, India

Ankit S. Prajapati
Veterinary Clinical Complex (Medicine), College of Veterinary Science and Animal Health, Kamdhenu University, Sardarkrushinagar, Gujarat, India

Ravi D. Prajapati
Department of Veterinary Gynaecology and Obstetrics
College of Veterinary Science and Animal Husbandry
Kamdhenu University
Sardarkrushinagar, India

Aditya Pratap
Department of Veterinary Medicine
College of Veterinary Science and Animal Husbandry
Jabalpur, India

Saahithya Rajamohan
Department of Veterinary Pathology
Veterinary College and Research Institute
Tamil Nadu Veterinary and Animal Sciences University
Salem, India

Ranjani Rajasekaran
Department of Veterinary Microbiology
Veterinary College and Research Institute
Tamil Nadu Veterinary and Animal Sciences University
Theni, India

Nirmal Singh Rajawat
College of Veterinary and Animal Sciences
Rajasthan University of Veterinary and Animal Sciences
Bikaner, India

Ramasamy Rajkumar
Department of Veterinary Gynaecology and Obstetrics
Veterinary College and Research Institute
Tamil Nadu Veterinary and Animal Sciences University
Salem, India

Jeetendra S. Rajoriya
Department of Veterinary Gynaecology and Obstetrics
College of Veterinary Science and Animal Husbandry
Jabalpur, India

Tanmoy Rana
Department of Veterinary Clinical Complex
West Bengal University of Animal and Fishery Sciences
Kolkata, India

Ravi Ranjan
Animal Physiology and Reproduction Division
ICAR-Central Institute for Research on Goat
Mathura, India

Jigar Raval
National Dairy Development Board
Anand, India

Sunant Raval
College of Veterinary Science and Animal Husbandry
Kamdhenu University
Anand, India

Meesam Raza
Department of Livestock Production Management
Dr. G.C. Negi College of Veterinary and Animal Sciences
Palampur, India

Bhavanam Sudhakara Reddy
College of Veterinary Science, Sri Venkateswara
Veterinary University, Proddatur, Andhra Pradesh, India

Peter Ibrahim Rekwot
Faculty of Veterinary Medicine
Ahmadu Bello University
Zaria, Nigeria

Abdul Reshma
Department of Veterinary Gynaecology and Obstetrics
Veterinary College and Research Institute
Tamil Nadu Veterinary and Animal Sciences University
Salem, India

Amitava Roy
Department of Livestock Farm Complex
West Bengal University of Animal & Fishery Sciences
Kolkata, India

Vikas Sachan
Department of Veterinary Gynaecology, DUVASU
Mathura, India

Rayala S. Sagar
Department of Veterinary Medicine
Veterinary College
Hassan, India

Gitesh Saini
Department of Veterinary Gynaecology and Obstetrics
College of Veterinary Science
Guru Angad Dev Veterinary and Animal Sciences University
Bathinda, India

Felix Uchenna Samuel
Faculty of Veterinary Medicine
National Animal Production Research Institute
Ahmadu Bello University
Zaria, Nigeria, and
Department of Food and Animal Science
Alabama A&M University
Normal, USA

Tulasiraman Sarath
Department of Veterinary Gynaecology and Obstetrics
Veterinary College and Research Institute
Tamil Nadu Veterinary and Animal Sciences University
Salem, India

Pardeep Sharma
Department of Veterinary Medicine
Dr G.C. Negi College of Veterinary and Animal Sciences
Palampur, India

Idris Sherif
Faculty of Veterinary Medicine
Ahmadu Bello University
Zaria, Nigeria

Abhiyuday P. Singh
Department of Veterinary Gynaecology & Obstetrics
College of Veterinary Science and Animal Husbandry
Jabalpur, India

Brejesh Singh
Department of Veterinary Medicine
College of Veterinary Science and Animal Husbandry
Jabalpur, India

Rashmi Singh
Post Graduate Institute of Veterinary
Education & Research
Jaipur, India

Satyavrat V. Singh
Department of Veterinary Medicine
College of Veterinary Science and Animal Husbandry
Acharya Narendra Deva University of
Agriculture and Technology
Ayodhya, Uttar Pradesh, India

Bhoomika Sirsant
Department of Veterinary Public Health and
Epidemiology, Bihar Veterinary College
Bihar Animal Sciences University
Patna, India

Sirigireddy Sivajothi
College of Veterinary Science, Sri Venkateswara Veterinary University
Proddatur, Andhra Pradesh, India

Simson Soren
Department of Veterinary Physiology
Lakhimpur College of Veterinary Science
Assam Agricultural University
North Lakhimpur, India

Benito Soto-Blanco
Department of Veterinary Clinics and Surgery
Veterinary School
Universidade Federal de Minas Gerais
Belo Horizonte, Brazil

Abhinav N. Suthar
Department of Medicine
College of Veterinary Science and Animal Husbandry
Kamdhenu University
Sardarkrushinagar, Gujarat, India

Ankaj Thakur
Department of Livestock Production Management
Dr G.C. Negi College of Veterinary and Animal Sciences
Palampur, India

Annadurai Thangamani
Department of Veterinary Gynaecology and Obstetrics
Veterinary College and Research Institute
Tamil Nadu Veterinary and Animal Sciences University
Salem, India

Amita Tiwari
Department of Veterinary Medicine
College of Veterinary Science and Animal Husbandry
Jabalpur, India

Mahendra P.S. Tomar
Department of Veterinary Anatomy
NTR College of Veterinary Science
Gannavaram, India

Shivangi Udainiya
Veterinary Polytechnic College
Nanaji Deshmukh Veterinary Science University
Bhopal, India, and

Department of Veterinary Medicine
College of Veterinary Science and Animal Husbandry
Jabalpur, India

Hridya Susan Varughese
Department of Veterinary Microbiology
Veterinary College, Karnataka Veterinary Animal and Fisheries Sciences University
Hebbal, India

Abhinov Verma
Department of Veterinary Anatomy, DUVASU
Mathura, India

Prerna Yadav
Post Graduate Institute of Veterinary Education and Research
Jaipur, India

Somu Yogeshpriya
Department of Veterinary Medicine
Veterinary College and Research Institute
Chennai, India

Preface

This book provides an essential resource for students, academicians, and practitioners and will be beneficial for audiences in the farm and industry sectors, and milk producers' union. The book provides practical, updated information about the normal reproduction, reproductive diseases, and management of goats. It covers the current thoughts and scientific modules for the betterment of understanding of the readers. The book illustrates the reproductive anatomy and physiology of both males and females in a systematic way.

The book is divided into three parts: normal reproduction, reproductive disorders, and reproductive management of goats. The main topics covered include breeding characteristics, pregnancy detection, diagnosis, treatment, and management of infertility, obstetrics, abortion, and care and management of kids. The book emphasizes current knowledge about the physiological and biochemical mechanisms in the regulation of reproduction. It will serve as a reference book for students, veterinary nurses, researchers, academicians, scientists, and professional workers engaged in small ruminant production, applicable to anyone who has a keen interest in the biology of normal reproduction, and reproductive diseases, and management of goats. Artificial insemination and advanced reproductive biotechnology are also described and discussed. Featuring contributions from experts in various fields, each section covers clinically relevant aspects of the reproductive anatomy and physiology of both males and females.

The main important topics include the evaluation of the normal physiological function of reproductive organs, breeding soundness, pregnancy diagnosis, diagnosis and treatment of infertility, abortion, obstetrics, surgery of the reproductive tract, care of kids, and the latest reproductive technology, illustrated throughout with figures and tables.

Tanmoy Rana
Department of Veterinary Clinical Complex, West Bengal
University of Animal & Fishery Sciences, Kolkata, India

Acknowledgment

I wish to thank all the authors of the first edition for their hard work, and sharing their expertise and knowledge to make the book fruitfully. I also express my gratitude to our Honourable Vice Chancellor, West Bengal University of Animal & Fishery Sciences, Kolkata, India, for giving me the opportunity to edit the book. I also convey my sincere gratitude and wholehearted thanks to all veterinarians, farm managers, and academicians for their expert opinions and thoughts to make the book a success. I would like to express my sincere regards to Dr Rituparna Bose, Commissioning Editor, Bhavya Boopathi, Managing Editor, and other members of Wiley Publishers who actively helped me during the editing of the book. I would also like to thank my family members for giving me great support and time to finalize the book.

Tanmoy Rana
Kolkata, India

Section 1

Goat Reproductive Health

1

Anatomy of the Reproductive System in the Buck and Doe

Abhinov Verma[1], *Mahendra P.S. Tomar*[2], *and Vikas Sachan*[3]

[1] *Department of Veterinary Anatomy, DUVASU, Mathura, India*
[2] *Department of Veterinary Anatomy, NTR College of Veterinary Science, Gannavaram, India*
[3] *Department of Veterinary Gynaecology, DUVASU, Mathura, India*

1.1 Introduction

Reproduction is crucial for the survival of species. It is the method used by living things to reproduce (Frandson et al. 2003). Since being domesticated, the goat has become seasonally polyestrous, meaning that it reproduces naturally at specific periods of the year. The photoperiod, rasse, and nutrition are the key determinants of this trait's variation (Delgadillo et al. 2012). Several areas of goat production are influenced by reproduction, so managing reproduction requires an understanding of this process. For survival of the species, the production of meat, milk, skin, and fiber, as well as the replenishment of breeding stock, a high rate of reproductive efficiency is crucial (Abebe 2008).

Male and female individuals in each species have specific anatomical and functional features (Nickel et al. 1973). Therefore, for easier understanding, this chapter is divided into two sections: the male reproductive system and female reproductive system in goats.

1.2 Male Reproductive System

The major function of this system is the production of spermatozoa and male sex hormone (Frandson et al. 2003). The male reproductive system consists of the following structures (Figures 1.1 and 1.2).

1) Scrotum
2) Testes
3) Epididymis
4) Ductus deferens
5) Accessory sex glands
6) Penis
7) Urethra

1.2.1 Scrotum

The testicles and nearby spermatic cord segments are located in the scrotum, which is a sac or pouch (Figure 1.1). It can take on a variety of shapes depending on the health of its subcutaneous muscular tissue. When exposed to cold, the latter constricts, causing the scrotum to rise and become thicker and wrinkled; when relaxed by heat, weariness, or debility, however, it becomes smooth and pendulous with a superior neck constriction (Frandson et al. 2003). It consists of layers which correspond with those of the abdominal wall, considered from without inward: skin, dartos, scrotal fascia, parietal layer of the tunica vaginalis (Getty 1975; Farooqui 2004; Pathak et al. 2014).

Elements of Reproduction and Reproductive Diseases of Goats, First Edition. Edited by Tanmoy Rana.

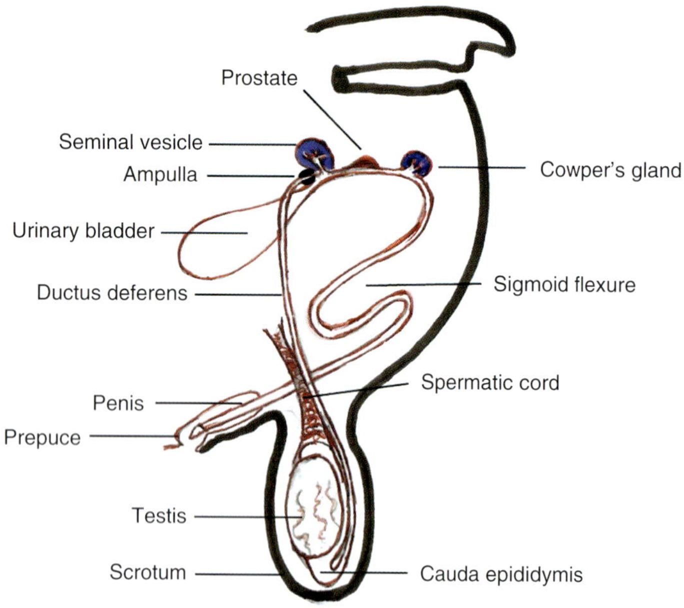

Figure 1.1 Diagrammatic presentation of the male reproductive system.

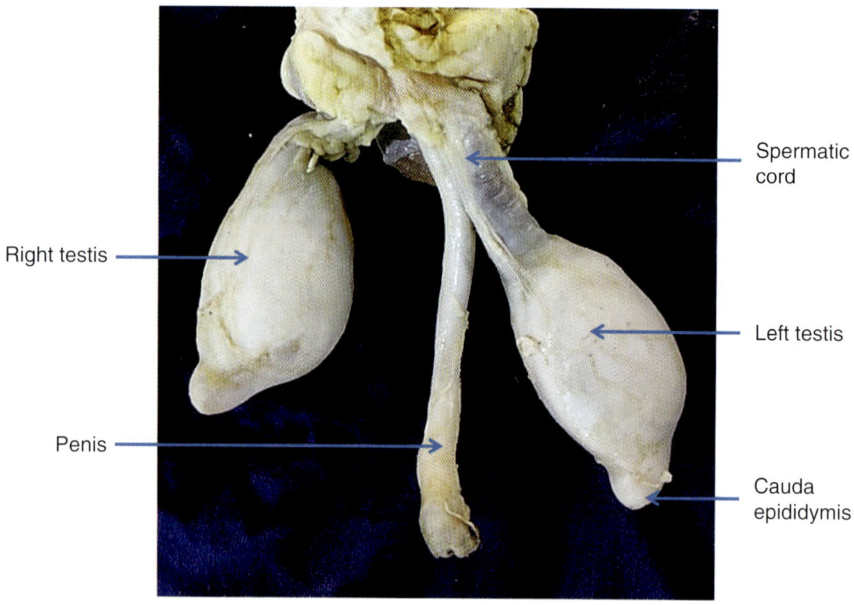

Figure 1.2 Photograph showing the organs of the male reproductive system.

The spermatic cord begins at the abdominal inguinal ring, where its constituent parts come together, extends obliquely downward through the inguinal canal, passes over the side of the penis and ends at the attached border of the testicle (Figure 1.2). It consists of the following structures.

1) Spermatic artery.
2) Spermatic vein.
3) Lymphatics.
4) Sympathetic nerves.
5) Ductus deferens.
6) Internal cremaster muscles.
7) Visceral layer of tunica vaginalis.

1.2.2 Testes

The testis is the seat of production of male germ cells. The testes are located in the inguinal region of the body and are enclosed in the scrotum (Frandson et al. 2003; Pathak 2006). They descend into the scrotum from the abdominal cavity during fetal development. Descent of the testes from the genital ridge in the fetus to an extracorporeal location after birth is a mandatory development process to ensure normal spermatogenesis in the mature testis (Farooqui 2004).

Each testis weighs about 130–160g with an elongated oval form and the long axis nearly vertical (Figure 1.1). It comprises two surfaces, two borders and two extremities. Both the surfaces, i.e. the medial and lateral surfaces, are convex and smooth. The cranial border is free and the caudal border is attached to the epididymis. The dorsal and ventral extremities are termed the head and tail, respectively. A testicle of an average sized adult buck is 6–7, 4–5, and 4–5cm in length, width, and thickness (in middle), respectively (Solaiman 2010). The testes are frequently of unequal size, with the left typically being larger, and their sizes fluctuate greatly. Testicular growth is extremely rapid from birth to puberty and then does not change significantly (Pathak et al. 2014). The testes of goats are broader in proportion to their length.

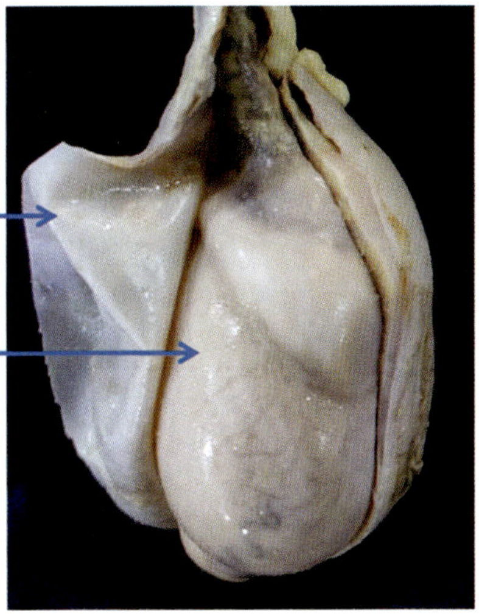

Figure 1.3 Photograph showing the testis and tunica vaginalis.

The tunica vaginalis, which is the visceral layer of the serous envelope surrounding the spermatic cord and testicle, covers the majority of the testicle's surface (Figure 1.3). This is reflected from the attached border of the gland, leaving an exposed area where the spermatic cord's vessels and nerves enter the testicle. The tunica albuginea, a robust capsule made of dense white fibrous tissue and unstriped muscle fibers, lies beneath the tunica vaginalis.

The spermatic artery supplies blood to the testicle. The artery is quite convoluted close to the testicle and descends in the anterior portion of the spermatic cord. It splits into many branches that enter the gland on the trabeculae and septa (septula testes) and ascend and descend on the testicular surfaces (Figure 1.4). The pampiniform plexus is a network formed by the testicular veins as they exit the testis and encircle the spermatic cord's artery. The lymphatic vessels often follow the veins' path before entering the lumbar lymph glands. The spermatic plexus, to which the vessels are primarily dispersed, is formed by the renal and posterior mesenteric plexuses, which supply the nerves.

The exocrine function of the testes is spermatogenesis under the influence of follicle-stimulating hormone (FSH) and testosterone, whereas their endocrine function is the synthesis and release of testosterone by Leydig cells under the effect

Figure 1.4 Photograph (sagittal section) showing the septula testis.

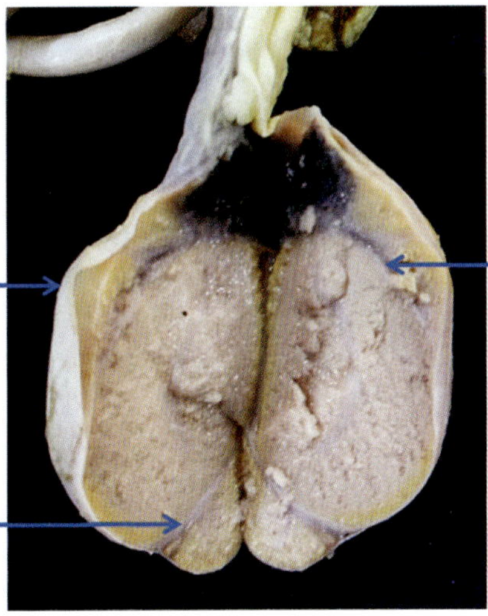

of luteinizing hormone (LH)/interstitial cell-stimulating hormone (ICSH). Castration is removal of the testicles in order to reduce buck aggression (König and Liebich 2020).

The blood supply to the testes is via the internal spermatic artery and innervation occurs via the renal and mesenteric plexuses.

1.2.3 Epididymis

The epididymis serves as the chief ductal system, besides providing nutrition for growth and maturation. The epididymis is attached to the caudal border of the testicle and somewhat overlaps the lateral surface. Its dorsal enlarged end is termed the head (caput epididymis), its ventral, slightly enlarged end is the tail (cauda epididymis), and the intermediate part is the body (corpus epididymis). The head is closely connected with the testicle by the efferent ducts, in continuation of the rete testis. The efferent ducts together form the ductus epididymis which runs inside the body of the epididymis. The ductus epididymis is very flexible and almost 60 m in length in the adult buck. The tail is continued by the ductus deferens/vas deferens which is attached to the posterior extremity of the testicle by the ligamentum epididymis.

1.2.4 Ductus Deferens

The ductus deferens extends from the tail of the epididymis to the pelvic urethra. It ascends in the inguinal canal, enclosed within the spermatic cord. At the vaginal ring, it separates from the other constituents of the spermatic cord, and turns backward and inward into the pelvic cavity to reach the pelvic urethra just caudal to the neck of the bladder. The two ducts lie very close together and empty on the roof of the urethra as enlarged ampullae.

1.2.5 Accessory Sex Glands or Annex Glands

Accessory sex glands are conspicuous outgrowths of the genital tract and can be regarded as part of the male reproductive system as they play an integral role in the fertility process. In the buck, they include the vesicular gland, prostate gland and bulbourethral or Cowper's gland.

The vesicular glands are paired sac-like lobulated glands, located on each side of the posterior dorsal surface of the neck of the urinary bladder. The excretory duct dips behind the prostate and opens in a mucous membrane pouch on the side of the colliculus seminalis, either alongside or concurrently with the ductus deferens. Each gland is 3–4 cm in length. In the buck, the disseminate part of the prostate gland surrounds the wall of the pelvic urethra. The prostatic ducts open in the pelvic urethra behind the colliculus seminalis. Each gland is covered by urethral muscles which are thin dorsally and ventrally, and thick laterally. At the ischial arch, on either side of the pelvic urethra, are the spherical bulbourethral glands which are covered by the urethral muscle. Their excretory ducts open directly into the urethral recess.

1.2.6 Penis

The penis, the organ of copulation, is made of fibroerectile tissue. Its length in bucks is roughly 0.4 m (Solaiman 2010). It extends from the ischial arch to the umbilical region of the abdominal wall (Figure 1.1). It is made up of the root, body, and glans. Two crura, which converge and merge beneath the ischial arch, connect the root of the penis to the lateral portions of the arch. The bulk of the organ, the body, starts at the point where the crura converge. Two sturdy flat bands, the suspensory ligaments of the penis, which converge with the tendon of origin of the gracilis muscles, bind it to the symphysis ischii at its beginning. The expanded free end of the penis is known as the glans penis.

Just behind the scrotum, it forms an S-shaped sigmoid flexure (Figure 1.1). The corpus cavernosum penis and the corpus cavernosum urethrae are the two main erectile structures that make up the penis. With the exception of its free extremity, the corpus cavernosum penis makes up the majority of the penile mass. The urethra is surrounded by a tube called the corpus cavernosum urethrae, which is connected with the glans penis at its anterior end. The prepuce is a very short tubular sheet covering the cranial free portion of the penis in the nonerectile state. The prepuce (foreskin) is the skin sheath that encloses and protects the free part of the penis when it is not erect. It is an analogue of the female labia majora.

1.2.7 Urethra

The urethra consists of two parts: the pelvic urethra and penile urethra. The urethral muscle encircles the pelvic urethra, which is located on the floor of the pelvic cavity. The penile urethra is inserted into the body of the penis and passes between the two penis crura. The corpus cavernosum penis' ventral surface has grooves where the urethra is located. The name "process urethrae" refers to the penile urethra's terminal part, which extends 1.5 inches beyond the glans penis. Uncastrated bucks have longer and larger urethras and various penile segments than do castrated bucks (Islam et al. 2021).

1.3 Female Reproductive System

The reproductive system of the doe comprises the following structures (Figures 1.5 and 1.6).

1) Ovaries.
2) Uterine or fallopian tubes or oviducts.
3) Uterus.
4) Vagina.
5) Vulva.
6) Mammary glands.

1.3.1 Ovaries

The ovaries are ovoid or almond-shaped structures located within the pelvic cavity suspended from the roof of the cavity by the mesovarium. They may show many other morphological shapes, e.g., heart shaped, long and narrow, many-sided and almost horseshoe shaped (Lyngset 1968). In most does, the right ovary is slightly larger than the left and measures approximately 14.4–17.7 mm in length and 10.0–13.5 mm in width while the left ovary measures 14.1–17.1 mm in length and 8.0–13.3 mm in width (Gupta et al. 2011; Bijna et al. 2016; Uddin et al. 2021). However, sometimes the trend may be reversed with a larger left ovary (Doğan et al. 2020). The size of the ovary depends on the physiological status of the animal; for example, during the estrous cycle, the development of antral follicles results in an increase in size whereas regression returns it to the previous size. Similarly, the ovaries become larger during pregnancy and show a gradual increase with advancement of gestational age (Jaji et al. 2012).

Each ovary is composed of two surfaces, two borders, and two extremities. The surfaces are medial and lateral and are smooth and rounded in prepubertal animals and irregular in cycling animals. The borders are the attached and free borders. The attached or mesovarial border is convex where the ovary is enclosed in a part of the broad ligament (mesovarium) through which the vessels and nerves reach the gland. The anterior extremity (tubal) is rounded and is related to the

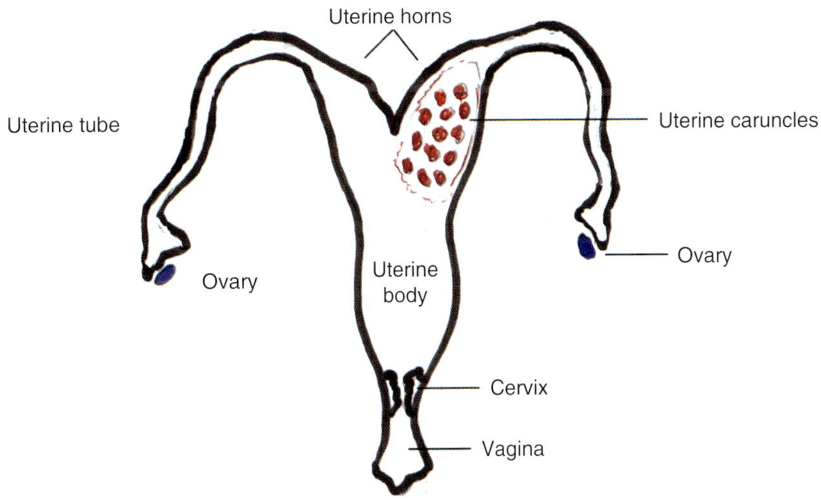

Figure 1.5 Diagrammatic presentation of the female reproductive system.

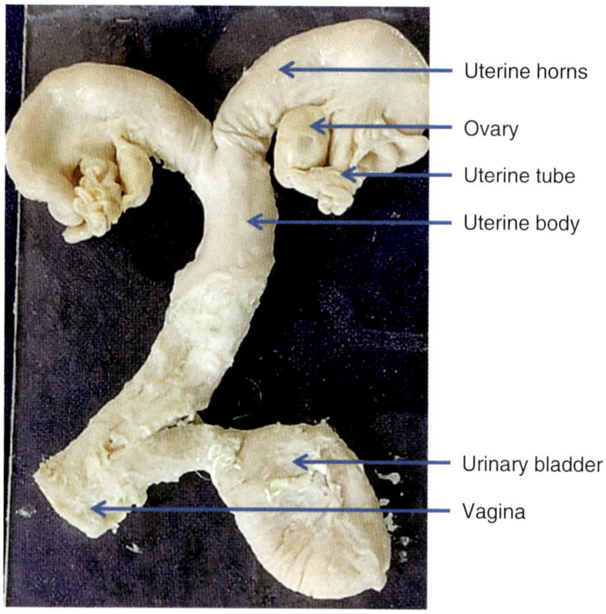

Figure 1.6 Photograph showing the organs of the female reproductive system.

fimbriated end of the oviduct. The posterior extremity (uterine) is also round, and connected with the uterine horn by the ovarian ligament. They are usually present adjacent to the lumbar wall of the abdomen. The ovarian ligament is a band of smooth muscle enclosed between the layers of the broad ligament. The ovarian stroma is a network of connective tissue. In young subjects, in the meshes of the stroma there are numerous follicles (folliculi oophori), containing oocytes in various stages of development (König and Liebich 2020; Uddin et al. 2021).

Depending on the stage of development, the oocyte is surrounded by one or many layers of follicle cells, i.e., primordial and primary follicles (single layer) and secondary and mature follicles (multilayered), forming the stratum granulosum, and by a condensation of the stroma termed the theca folliculi. A few follicles get recruited (depending on the breed) and show further development to become mature. The antrum of the mature follicle is filled by a fluid, the liquor folliculi. At one point, a collection of granulosa cells encloses the oocyte (cumulus oophorus–oocyte complex), connecting it with the follicle wall. Such follicles (folliculi oophori vesiculosi) enlarge to a diameter of 1 cm or more as they mature, becoming visible to the naked eye. The fully developed follicles are superficially situated and project slightly from the surface of the ovary. In cycling goats, these follicles rupture to release the oocyte (ovulation) and result in the formation of corpus/corpora luteum/lutea (CL). The CLs initially develop and in absence of fertilization, regress to become the corpus/corpora albicans (a fibrous scar). Therefore, in old animals, the ovaries commonly consist largely of fibrous tissue. The other follicles/oocytes which were not recruited regress and are phagocytized later (Eurell and Frappier 2006).

1.3.1.1 Vessels and Nerves

The ovarian arteries are paired and originate from the abdominal aorta. They are relatively large and flexible and reach the attached border of the ovary by passing between the layers of the mesovarium. The veins are large and numerous. They form a plexus similar to that of the spermatic cord. The lymph vessels pass to the lumbar glands. The nerves are derived from the sympathetic system through the renal and aortic plexuses. They accompany the arterial branches.

1.3.2 Uterine Tubes/Fallopian Tubes/Oviducts

The paired uterine tubes act as excretory ducts of the ovaries, as they convey the oocyte from the ovary to the uterus. They are not in direct continuity with the ovary but rather partly in continuity with, and partly attached to, it. Each flexible uterine tube ranges between 10.0 and 16.0 cm in length and approximately 0.2 cm in diameter and extends from the uterine extremity of the ovaries to the uterine horn. The right tube is slightly longer than the left in most does (Talukder et al. 2015). The ovarian end of the tube is funnel shaped and fimbriated, and then it widens considerably to form the ampulla tubae. Each is enclosed in a peritoneal fold, derived from the lateral layer of the broad ligament (the mesosalpinx). The uterine extremity of the tube communicates with the cavity of the uterine horn by a minute orifice, the ostium uterinum tubae. The ovarian extremity is expanded and somewhat funnel shaped, and is therefore termed the infundibulum tubae uterinae. The ovarian extremity of the tube appears normally to be applied to the ovary, so that the extruded oocytes pass into it and are conveyed to the uterus (Gupta et al. 2011; Doğan et al. 2019; Uddin et al. 2021).

1.3.2.1 Vessels and Nerves

The arterial supply to the oviduct is from branches of the uteroovarian artery. The veins are satellites of the arteries. The lymph vessels pass with the ovarian vessels to the lumbar glands. The nerves have a similar origin to those of the ovary.

1.3.3 Uterus

The uterus is a hollow musculomembranous tubular organ, which is continuous with the uterine tubes anteriorly and opens into the vagina posteriorly. Overall, the uterus in does is bicornuate (Kumar et al. 2020). It is situated chiefly in the posterior aspect of the abdominal cavity but extends a short distance into the pelvic cavity (in nonpregnant animals). It is suspended in the sublumbar region and the lateral walls of the pelvic cavity by the broad ligaments (two folds of peritoneum).

It consists of two horns (cornua uteri), the body (corpus uteri), and the neck (cervix uteri). The uterine horns are long, coiled, and entirely situated in the abdomen. They appear to vary considerably in position; commonly they are pressed up against the sublumbar muscles by the intestine (cecum, left parts of large colon, small colon, and small intestine). They are cylindrical when moderately distended and are approximately 4–5 inches long and 1–1.5 inches in diameter (nonpregnant animal) but reach up to 15–18 inches in length and 4–5 inches in diameter or even more during pregnancy and are highly variable depending upon the size and number of fetuses (Doğan et al. 2020). Morphometrically, the horn which has fetuses inside is larger than the other. The anterior extremity of each horn receives the isthmus of the uterine tube. Posteriorly, they increase slightly in caliber, converge and continue with the body. The dorsal border is slightly concave and is attached to the sublumbar region by the broad ligament while its ventral border (margo liber) is convex and free.

The body of the uterus is situated partly in the abdominal, partly in the pelvic cavity. It is cylindrical but considerably flattened dorsoventrally, so that in cross-section it is elliptical (Kumar et al. 2020). Its average length is 1–3 inches and its diameter is 1–2 inches in the nonpregnant animal while it reaches 9–10 inches in length and 10–12 inches in diameter during pregnancy (Doğan et al. 2020). Dorsally, it is related to the rectum and other parts of the intestine while it rests on the urinary bladder ventrally. The portion where the uterine horns originate from the body is called the fundus (fundus uteri) which is the wide anterior part. The neck of the uterus is the constricted posterior part which joins the vagina and possesses two openings (os/osteum uteri) – the internal and external os. It is about 1.5–2 inches long and 0.5–1.5 inches wide. It increases in dimension to reach 3–4 inches in length and 4–5 inches in diameter at parturition (Jaji et al. 2012; Doğan et al. 2020). The openings are closed by mucous plugs during the nonestrous (resting) period.

1.3.3.1 Attachments

Two large peritoneal folds, the broad ligaments of the uterus, hold the body and horns to the abdominal and pelvic walls. They extend to the dorsal border of the cornua and the lateral edges of the uterine body on either side from the sublumbar area and the lateral pelvic walls. They contain connective tissue, a significant quantity of smooth muscle fibers that are continuous with those of the uterus, the arteries and nerves of the uterus and ovaries, as well as connective tissue. The round ligament of the uterus, which projects from the lateral layer of each and folds into the parietal peritoneum above the abdominal inguinal ring, has its anterior extremity above the cornu's extremity and resembles a long, round appendix. It is a replica of the gubernaculum testis and contains muscles, blood vessels, and nerves. Due to its continuity with the vagina, the anterior section of the neck is in a more permanent position than the rest of the organ.

The contraction of the uterine wall and the folds of the mucous lining in the nonpregnant state completely obliterate the uterine cavity. It connects to the uterine tube at the end of each cornu by a minute opening on a small papilla. The cervical canal (cavity of cervix) is often sealed off by mucous folds and plugs. It has two orifices: one that opens into the body (orificium internum uteri) and one that opens into the vagina (orificium externum uteri).

1.3.3.2 Vessels and Nerves

The major arterial supply is from the uterine branch of the uteroovarian artery, which passes in the broad ligaments. It also gets a branch from the internal pudic artery. The veins form pampiniform plexuses and are satellite to the arteries. The lymph vessels are numerous and travel to the internal iliac and lumbar glands. The nerves are derived from the sympathetic through the uterine and pelvic plexuses.

1.3.4 Vagina

The vagina is the horizontally oriented musculomembranous tubular connection between the neck of the uterus (external os) and the vulva or vestibule and is located in the pelvic cavity. It is about 2.5–3.0 inches in length and, when slightly distended, about 1.5–2.0 inches in diameter (Uddin et al. 2021). It is connected laterally to the pelvic wall, ventrally to the urine bladder, and dorsally to the rectum. The peritoneal rectogenital pouch often reaches between the rectum and vagina for a short distance. As a result, the majority of the vagina is retroperitoneal and is encircled by a venous plexus, a quantity of loose connective tissue, and a varied amount of fat. The lumen of the cavity is a transverse slit under normal circumstances because of the apposition of the walls, which is more obvious when the rectum is full (Getty 1975). The intravaginal portion of the uterus neck occupies a considerable portion of the anterior end of the vagina, reducing the cavity to an annular recess known as the fornix vaginae. The transverse fold that covers the external urethral orifice serves as the only line of demarcation between the posterior section and the vulva in very young animals; this fold is extended on either side to produce the hymen, which narrows the entry to the vagina (König and Liebich 2020).

1.3.4.1 Vessels and Nerves

The arterial supply to the vagina is derived from the branches of the internal pudic arteries. The rich venous plexus drains into the internal pudic veins. The lymphatics join the internal iliac lymph glands. The innervation is basically sympathetic nerves derived from the pelvic plexus and supported by numerous ganglia located in the adventitia (König and Liebich 2020).

1.3.5 Vulva

The final section of the female genital system is known as the vulva. It opens externally at the vulvar cleft (rima vulvae) below the anus and is continuous with the vagina in the front. The vulva and vagina are not physically separated from one another. It measures 1–1.5 inches in length and approximately 1.5 inches in width. It is guarded by paired vertically oriented and rounded vulvar lips (labia vulvae) joining together at dorsal (at an acute angle) and ventral (rounded) commissures behind and below the ischial arch. It is related dorsally to the rectum and anus, ventrally to the pelvic floor, and laterally to the sacrosciatic ligament, the semimembranosus muscle and the internal pudic artery. When the labia are drawn apart, a rounded body is seen occupying a cavity in the ventral commissure which is called the glans clitoridis, the homologue of the glans penis, and the cavity in which it lies is the fossa clitoridis. The roof of the fossa is formed by a thin fold which overlies the glans clitoridis and is attached centrally to it (Gupta et al. 2011).

The external urethral orifice is covered by a fold of mucous membrane, the free edge of which is directed backward. The clitoris is the homologue of the penis and consists of similar parts (except the urethra and its muscle). The corpus clitoridis is attached to the ischial arch by two crura and its glans is in the form of a rounded and enlarged free end located in the fossa clitoridis in the ventral commissure of the vulva (Gupta et al. 2011). It is covered by a thin layer of pigmented skin that is continuous with and resembles the skin that lines the fossa; together, these two components make up the prepuce of the clitoris. The clitoris possesses erectile tissue similar to the corpus cavernosum penis. The ischiocavernosus is a weak muscle and is a homologue of the same muscle in the male. The bulbus vestibuli and the clitoris veins are connected by an intermediary plexus on either side.

1.3.6 Urethra

The female urethra is a small musculomembranous tube connecting the urinary bladder and the vagina. It lies centrally on the pelvic floor and is related dorsally to the vagina where it opens in the floor of the vaginal vestibule through a urethral orifice. The lumen is wider than the male urethra. The lumen has many mucosal folds based on the muscular wall. The urethral muscle (M. compressor urethrae) embraces the urethra and is continuous with the constrictor vestibuli. It is covered by a fibroelastic membrane (Getty 1975).

1.3.7 Mammary Glands

The mammary glands are anatomically related to the integumentary system but functionally they are closely associated with the reproductive system, therefore they are usually described with them. The mammary glands are modified cutaneous glands present in the udder which is located in the inguinal region. They are externally divided in two halves by a median intermammary groove where each half is composed of a mammary body and a teat. The mammary body is conical and its base is slightly concave and slopes cranioventrally in adaptation to the ventral abdominal wall. The lateral surface is convex and covered by a movable skin and fine hairs, while the medial surface is flattened.

Each half is internally made up of a single mammary unit, which contains the cavity system, duct system, and mammary glandular parenchyma. The lobulated lactiferous tissue aggregate at the base of each half makes up the mammary glandular parenchyma. The lactiferous ducts open irregularly into the corresponding sinus. The ducts are divided by slightly elevated folds on the interior layer of the duct system; these folds either extend for a brief distance or rise to the level of the lactiferous sinus. An annular fold partially divides the glandular and papillary portions of the lactiferous sinuses. The lactiferous sinus' glandular portion is a large, irregular pouch that receives the lactiferous duct openings (Adam et al. 2017).

The teat is funnel shaped with a wide base and narrow apex, and is directed cranioventrally and slightly laterally. The teat sinus is a funnel-shaped cavity, while the teat canal is a small narrow passage running for about 1.5–2.0 inches. The canal is lined by fine longitudinal ridges and opens externally via a teat orifice (Adam et al. 2017).

1.3.7.1 Vessels and Nerves

The arteries are derived from the external pudic artery, which enters the gland at the posterior part of its base. The veins form a plexus on either side of the base of the gland, which is chiefly drained by the external pudic vein. The lymph vessels are numerous and pass to the superficial inguinal and lumbar lymph glands. The nerves are derived from the inguinal nerves and the posterior mesenteric plexus of the sympathetic system.

Acknowledgment

The authors acknowledge Dr D.V.V.N. Durga Prasad (Assistant Professor, School of Veterinary and Animal Sciences, Centurion University of Technology and Management, Odisha, India) for all illustrations.

References

Abebe, G. (2008). Ethiopia sheep and goat productivity improvement program (ESGPIP). In: *Reproduction in Sheep and Goats* (ed. A. Yami and R.C. Merkel), 60–78. Langston, OK: Langston University.

Adam, Z.E.A.S., Ragab, G.A.N., Awaad, A.S. et al. (2017). Gross anatomy and ultrasonography of the udder in goat. *Journal of Morphological Science* 34 (3): 137–142.

Bijna, M., Karthiayini, K., and Lucy, K.M. (2016). Morphometry and histology of ovaries in Malabari goats. *International Journal of Science and Research* 7 (1): 291–293.

Delgadillo, J.A., Duarte, G., Flores, J.A. et al. (2012). Control of the sexual activity of goats without exogenous hormones: use of photoperiod, male effect and nutrition. *Tropical and Subtropical Agroecosystem* 15 (1): 15–27.

Doğan, G.K., Kuru, M., Bakır, B., and Sarı, E.K. (2019). Anatomical and histological analysis of the salpinx and ovary in Anatolian wild goat (*Capra aegagrus aegagrus*). *Folia Morphologica* 78 (4): 827–832.

Doğan, G.K., Kuru, M., Bakır, B., and Sarı, E.K. (2020). Anatomical and histological structure of cervix uteri, corpus uteri and cornu uteri of the Anatolian wild goat. *Turkish Journal of Veterinary Research* 4 (2): 63–68.

Eurell, J.A. and Frappier, B.L. (2006). *Dellmann's Textbook of Veterinary Histology*, 6e, 256–262. Ames, IA: Blackwell Publishing.

Farooqui, M. M. (2004). Morphological, histological and histochemical studies on male genital system of goat (*Capra hircus*). PhD thesis. DUVASU, Mathura.

Frandson, R.D., Wilke, W.L., and Fails, A.D. (2003). *Anatomy and Physiology of Farm Animals*, 6e. Philadelphia, PA: Lippincott Williams & Wilkins.

Getty, R. (1975). *Sisson and Grossman's: The Anatomy of the Domestic Animals*. New York: Saunders.

Gupta, M.D., Akter, M.M., Gupta, A.D., and Das, A. (2011). Biometry of female genital organs of black Bengal goat. *International Journal of Natural Sciences* 1 (1): 12–16.

Islam, R., Ahmed, S.S.U., Miazi, O.F. et al. (2021). Gross anatomy of urethra and penis in uncastrated and castrated buck of black Bengal goat. *International Journal of Morphology* 39 (1): 138–142.

Jaji, A.Z., Buduwara, R.A., Akanmu, A.I. et al. (2012). Pregnancy related biometric changes in the ovaries and uterus of the Sahelian goat. *Sokoto Journal of Veterinary Sciences* 10 (1): 18–21.

König, H.E. and Liebich, H.G. (2020). *Veterinary Anatomy of Domestic Animals*, 7e, 433–470. Stuttgart: Georg Thieme Verlag.

Kumar, M., Ray, S., Singh, K.N. et al. (2020). Gross anatomical studies on the ovary and uterus of black Bengal goat. *Journal of Entomology and Zoology Studies* SP-8 (2): 28–30.

Lyngset, O. (1968). Studies on reproduction in the goat: the normal genital organs of the non-pregnant goat. *Acta Veterinaria Scandinavica* 9: 208–222.

Nickel, R., Schummer, A., and Seiferle, E. (1973). *The Viscera of Domestic Mammals*. Hamburg: Verlag Paul Parey.

Pathak, A. (2006). Correlative anatomy of testis and accessory sex glands of gaddi goat (*Capra hircus*). PhD thesis. DUVASU, Mathura.

Pathak, A., Katiyar, R.S., Sharma, D.N., and Farooqui, M.M. (2014). Postnatal developmental anatomy of testes and epididymis of Gaddi goats. *International Journal of Morphology* 32 (4): 1391–1398.

Solaiman, S.G. (2010). *Goat Science and Production*. Ames, IA: Wiley Blackwell.

Talukder, A.K., Rahman, M.A., Islam, M.T., and Rahman, A.N.M.A. (2015). Biometry of genitalia, incidence of gynecological disorders and pregnancy loss in black Bengal goat: an abattoir study. *Journal of Embryo Transfer* 30 (1): 51–57.

Uddin, A.B.M.J., Akter, T., Siddiqui, M.S.I. et al. (2021). Biometry and histomorphometry of female reproductive system of black Bengal goats of Bangladesh. *Bangladesh Journal of Veterinary Medicine* 19 (1): 21–30.

2

Puberty and Sexual Maturity in the Buck and Doe

Ashok Baindha, Mohan Lal, Vipin Chandra, and Rashmi Singh

Post Graduate Institute of Veterinary Education and Research, Jaipur, India

2.1 Puberty

Puberty is generally defined as the point of sexual development at which the animal becomes capable of reproduction (first ovulation in the female and first spermatozoa in the ejaculate of the male), but often animals are not fully sexually mature at this stage. In both male and female goats, puberty may be reached without having achieved adequate physical growth to support reproduction. In the doe, this may be expressed as first ovulation not coinciding with first estrus, while in the male ejaculate quality and quantity are insufficient to achieve extensive breeding success. In immature bucks, the penis has adhesions that prevent it from being fully extended. At puberty, these adhesions dissolve and the penis can be fully extended.

2.2 Seasonal Breeding

Sexual development in the goat, as in other mammals, is a process of gradual maturation, a result of the interaction between the brain and gonads, initiated during embryonic development. Sexual development is influenced by both genetic and environmental factors (Amoah and Bryant 1984). The onset of puberty in goats typically occurs at 6–8 months of age in does and 4–6 months in bucks, dependent on nutrition, location, breed, and season of birth. Goats show a seasonal pattern in reproductive activity related to the annual variations of photoperiod. The onset and length of their breeding period throughout the year are dependent on different environmental and physiological factors (latitude and climate, food availability, breed, and breeding system).

Nutrition is among the most significant factors influencing reproductive development and the onset of puberty. Inadequate nutrition delays the occurrence of the first estrus. Increasing the level of nutrition generally advances the onset of puberty, but overfeeding before puberty will decrease subsequent fertility and impair mammary gland development. "Flushing," or "focused feeding," is a strategy in which a nutritional boost is supplied in a short period to enhance reproductive efficiency in ruminants without affecting body condition. This practice leads to a positive energy balance, which increases leptin and insulin concentrations, enhances glucose uptake, and is associated with increased folliculogenesis and ovulation rate. Dietary supplementation with beta-carotene, a vitamin A and retinoid precursor, at 50 mg/goat/day has reportedly produced this effect in does. Another strategy involves supplementing the diet of does with up to 0.45 kg/head/day of a 10–12% crude protein grain for ~2 weeks before and after breeding.

Along with nutrition, geographical location also has a significant effect on the achievement of puberty in goats. Geographical location, particularly the degree of latitude, has a significant impact on the timing and length of the breeding season. At locations close to the equator, tropical breeds of goats often are seasonal breeders and breed throughout the year. In temperate regions, the natural breeding season is mostly restricted to the fall and winter to allow for kidding in the spring and summer, when nutritional resources are adequate. In these regions, spring-born animals will undergo puberty at a younger age simply because physiological maturity coincides with periods of decreased day length (Amoah and Bryant 1984). Under tropical and subtropical conditions, where temperature and photoperiod are less variable, an

Elements of Reproduction and Reproductive Diseases of Goats, First Edition. Edited by Tanmoy Rana.

extended breeding period can be seen in certain breeds if appropriate resources are available to allow for year-round kidding.

The environmental cue most dominantly affecting seasonal breeding in small ruminants is the annual change in day length (short-day breeders). As the day length decreases in late summer and fall, does initiate estrus activity and males become more sexually active. However, following extended exposure to decreasing day length, animals become accustomed to the short day length and will again stop cycling.

The fact that their sexual activity is seasonal affects the distribution of their production over the year and this is a problem in both dairy and meat production systems which attempt to have constant production year round.

Goats are spontaneously ovulating, seasonally polyestrous animals with peak breeding activity occurring in the fall when the day length is shortening. As day length decreases, melatonin secretion from the pineal gland increases which activates pulsatile gonadotropin hormone-releasing hormone (GnRH) release from the hypothalamus. Hypothalamic GnRH secretion stimulates the release of luteinizing hormone (LH) and follicle-stimulating hormone (FSH) from the anterior pituitary and promotes the growth of follicles, stimulating the onset of the hypothalamic-pituitary-gonadal axis in short-day breeders.

Differences exist in the onset and length of the breeding season among various breeds of goats, and even between individual animals within a breed. In some breeds, such as pygmy goats, puberty may be reached as early as three months of age, but breeding should be delayed until the animal has reached at least 60% of its mature body weight to achieve higher conception rates and safer parturition. Larger goat breeds (e.g., Nubian, LaMancha, Boer, Saanen) can be safely bred when ~70 lb (32 kg). Angora kids should weigh a minimum of 27 kg and are frequently not bred until they are 1.5–2.5 years old. Season of birth also has a significant impact on the timing of puberty in both doelings and bucklings, with sensitivity to changes in day length already being in effect during the prenatal stages of development. Puberty in spring-born kids has to be achieved in the same year's fall breeding season or will be delayed until the following year's breeding season.

Other stressors such as transportation or illness may cause a temporary stoppage of estrus activity. In seasonal breeding does, the breeding season is framed by transitional periods during which gonadotropin levels are increasing but not to levels that will trigger estrus and ovulation. On average, the goat's estrus cycle is of 21 days, and the high frequency of the short estrual cycle is characteristic and tends to occur at the beginning of the reproductive season and in young animals. The average duration of standing estrus is 36 hours but can range from 24 to 48 hours depending on age, breed, season, and presence of a male.

Often the onset of estrus activity can be hastened through appropriate management techniques (i.e., introduction of males) during this transitional period. In the male, seasonal breeding is associated with changes in testis size and libido and the development of a distinct buck odor.

Reproductive failure is the most costly problem facing goat producers, whether they are producing meat or milk. Meat goat producers whose herds exhibit poor reproductive success earn less and have higher costs of production per kid produced than those whose herds reproduce successfully. Dairy producers with longer dry periods have higher feed costs because of increased periods of feeding without production in return.

The reproductive system of the goat is complex, but having a basic understanding of it will help farmers to better manage the reproductive success of their animals.

2.3 Puberty in Bucks

The most important animal in the herd is the buck. He provides half of the genetics of the herd, and using a sound, high-quality buck can make significant improvements to the herd.

Bucks reach puberty earlier than females and must either be separated from them by the age of four months or be castrated to prevent unwanted breeding. Buck kids can be used as herd sires at 8–10 months, but should not be used as heavily as mature bucks. A veterinarian should conduct a breeding soundness exam to test bucks for fertility and soundness before the breeding season. Also when selecting a buck, a veterinarian should perform a breeding soundness exam. A general physical exam can check the buck for structural soundness and abnormalities in the sex glands and organs. The scrotal circumference (at the widest point) should be measured since this correlates with fertility and semen production. As a general rule, dairy bucks should measure 25–28 cm at 100 pounds, meat bucks should measure 26–29 cm at 100 pounds, and larger bucks should measure at least 34–36 cm. A semen sample should be taken and evaluated. A normal concentration is two billion sperm per cubic centimeter of semen, in which 70% should be motile. The sperms' morphology should be evaluated to determine whether they are mature and if there are abnormalities. At least 80% of the sperm should be normal. Finally, the buck's libido should be monitored. A sound buck is of no use if he will not service does.

A full-grown, healthy buck should easily service up to 50 does. As a rule, bucks should not be bred to their daughters as inbreeding tends to expose genetic problems and lead to weaker stock. When bringing a new buck into the herd, producers should spend time and effort to locate a superior buck, one that has the traits the producer has identified as being important. A buck that has production records (has been on a test or has relatives that have been on a production test) is the surest bet. At the very least, producers should observe both the herd and the parents of the buck.

In any mating system, certain production practices help with record keeping to maintain selection decisions. One such practice is using visual markers to identify bred does. Animals can be fitted with a harness containing a crayon that will mark the females in heat when mounted. This procedure helps identify efficient females in the herd. Some goat producers use artificial insemination (AI) for breeding. This requires excellent heat detection skills and is more labor-intensive than natural service, but allows the economical use of outstanding sires.

Breeding goats can involve different strategies. Each of these strategies will have different consequences for the herd, and wise producers will pick a strategy that fits their philosophies and goals. No single strategy fits all situations, but each strategy is a wise choice for certain goals and production systems.

2.4 Puberty in Does

Female goats (does) reach puberty at 6–8 months of age, depending on their breed and nutrition. Does should be at 60–75% of their adult weight at breeding to prevent difficulty in kidding. Does will have higher lifetime production and be more profitable if they are bred to the kid as yearlings. Does should kid every year thereafter until at least the age of seven or eight, if they remain healthy.

Most goats are seasonal breeders, reacting to shorter days as a cue for breeding. Breeding season may be manipulated through the use of lights and hormone therapy. The presence of a buck (an uncastrated male goat) stimulates the reproductive cycle (estrus) and the behaviors of the does indicate they are in the fertile part of their cycle (in heat). The doe's estrous cycle normally occurs from August or September until January, with October to December being the peak time for breeding. The estrous cycle is normally 18–22 days long. Does in estrus are at the proper stage for breeding; at this time, they will be receptive to the buck. Estrus lasts for 12–36 hours. Signs of heat include tail wagging, swollen vulva, mounting behavior, decrease in milk yield if lactating, and a general increase in activity and bleating.

Kids are born about 150 days after breeding. Plan breeding so that the kids are born during the height of forage production in the spring, making efficient use of the pasture. Keeping accurate breeding records allows producers to know when kids are due and help them prepare for their arrival.

Another decision to consider in a breeding season is to match the breeding season to a potential market outcome to take advantage of higher market prices or traditional cycles.

2.5 Estrous Cycle

The estrous cycle consists of all morphological and physiological changes in the ovaries and genital tract leading to estrus expression (phase of receptivity toward males) and ovulation and the preparation of the genital tract for copulation, fertilization, and embryo implantation (Fatet et al. 2011). During the course of the breeding season, females can undergo several estrous cycles successively and the number of successive cycles is dependent on the length of the breeding season and the breed of goat. The length of the estrous cycle is defined by the interval between two successive expressions of estrus or two successive ovulations. The estrous cycle in goats is 21 days, on average, but can vary with different breeds or environmental conditions.

A relatively high frequency of short cycles is characteristic of goats and tends to occur in young does and earlier in the breeding season. Longer cycles may be observed later in the season when does are transitioning into anestrus.

The mean duration of standing estrus has been reported to be 36 hours, although it can range from 24 to 48 hours depending on age, breed, season, and presence of a male. Estrus detection is based on behavioral signs, bleating, flagging of the tail, reddened vulva, vaginal discharge (which causes the tail hairs to stick together), and occasional "riding" by other does. These behaviors are more pronounced in the presence of an intact male.

2.5.1 Physiology and Endocrinology of the Estrous Cycle of the Goat

During the estrous cycle, the ovaries undergo several morphological (follicular recruitment and growth), biochemical (follicle maturation), and physiological (endocrine regulations) changes leading to ovulation. These cyclical changes in the gonads are referred to as the ovarian cycle.

Follicular growth evolves in a wave-like manner throughout the cycle (Figure 2.1). A follicular wave is characterized by the sequence of three gonadotropin-dependent events in follicular growth: recruitment, selection, and dominance. Studies using repeated ultrasonography suggest that there are between two and six waves of follicle development during estrous cycles in goats, with three or four waves being the most prevalent. The last wave provides the ovulatory follicle. When double ovulations occur, they are usually of follicles derived from the same wave but in a few cases, they derive from two consecutive follicle waves.

The ovarian cycle is classically divided into two phases: the follicular phase and the luteal phase (Figure 2.1). The follicular phase corresponds to the wave of follicular development that will provide the ovulatory follicle and involves the maturation of follicles that are dependent on the gonadotropins until ovulation. During the follicular phase, FSH secreted by the anterior pituitary stimulates follicular growth. A cohort of antral follicles, which are gonadotropin dependent and with a diameter of 2–3 mm, is recruited and the follicles enter their terminal phase of growth. Only two or three of these follicles reach a size of 4 mm in diameter and are selected to enter the dominance phase. Under the influence of LH, the follicles reach the preovulatory stage (6–9 mm) while the subordinate follicles degenerate (follicular atresia). The increase in the peripheral concentrations of estradiol 17-beta causes a positive feedback effect on the hypophysis–gonadotropin axis, due to the follicular growth inducing the goat's estrus behavior (Fatet et al. 2011). The consequent increase in GnRH secretion induces an increase in the preovulatory LH peak, which will induce ovulation between 20 and 26 hours later, and finally, the luteinization of follicular cells will occur.

The beginning of the follicular phase, before the estrual behavior is observed, is known as proestrus. The estrus phase includes the events of the sexual behavior of the goat until ovulation. Consequently, a response to estrus and ovulation will mainly depend on the time of pregnancy and nutrition as providing the goat with short-energy supplementation can increase the rate of ovulation. The luteal phase begins when the corpus luteum is formed after follicle luteinization (duration 16 days). The luteal phase starts from the time of ovulation. About five days after the onset of estrus, cells of the

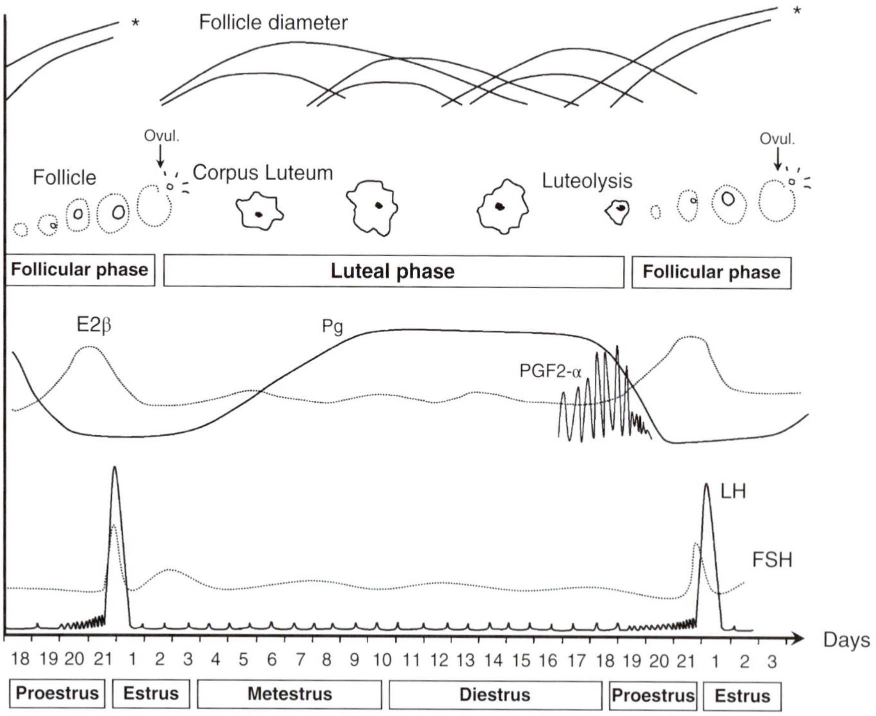

Figure 2.1 Schematic representation of the different physiological events occurring during the estrous cycle in goats: pattern of follicle development, ovarian cycle, and endocrine regulations.

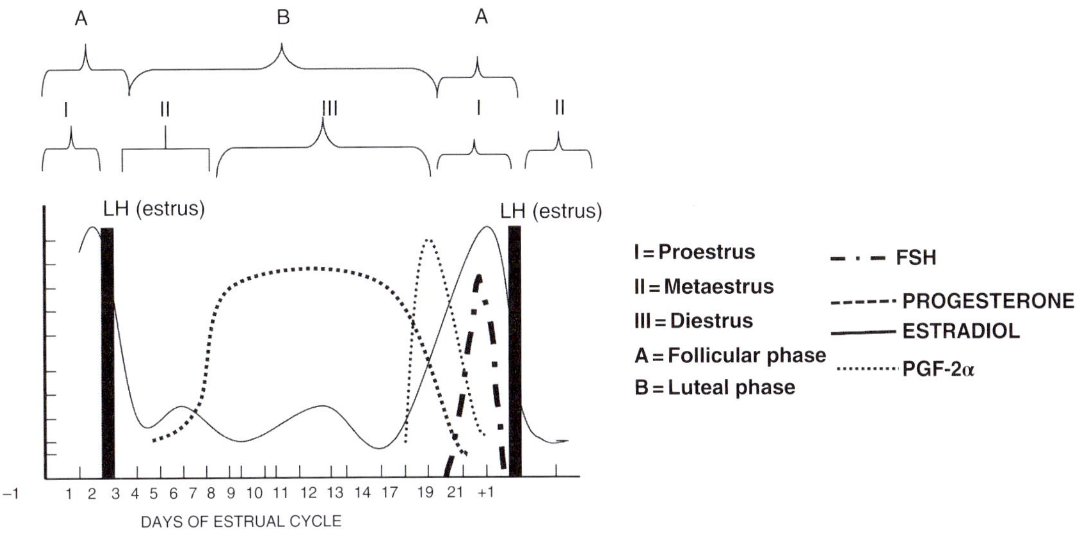

Figure 2.2 Schematic representation of the estrous cycle of the goat.

ovulating follicle turn into luteal cells and form the corpus luteum (CL). They secrete progesterone, causing its concentrations to increase and remain at a high level (>1 ng/ml) for 16 days. During this phase, LH is released in pulsatile fashion and its frequency is negatively correlated with progesterone. Now, progesterone has a negative feedback effect on LH. Luteolysis begins around days 16–17 of the estrus cycle, releasing uterine prostaglandins, influenced by oxytocin. With the above, the concentration of progesterone decreases, causing a strong increase in the frequency of pulses of LH and its amplitude, which causes ovulation.

During this luteal phase, gonadotropin-dependent follicular growth continues in a wave-like manner but progesterone inhibits ovulation. At the end of the luteal phase, 16–18 days after oestrus, prostaglandin F2-alpha secreted by the nongravid uterus induces CL regression – called luteolysis – and the decrease of progesterone secretion (Fatet et al. 2011). The decrease of plasma concentrations of progesterone gradually removes the inhibition of gonadotropic hormone secretion and a new follicular phase then commences.

The luteal phase is also called the postestrous period, which can be divided into metaestrus (Figure 2.2), when peripheral concentrations of progesterone begin to rise, and diestrus when peripheral concentrations of progesterone are high up to the start of luteolysis.

2.5.2 Folliculogenesis

In mammals, germ cells originate from the extraembryonic endoderm and migrate by amoeboid movement into the coelomic cavity, to reach the urogenital mesodermal crest. Subsequently, the germ cell is transformed into the oogonium, which should populate the gonad by mitotic processes. At the end of mitosis, the oogonium enters the meiotic cycle until prophase I, where it acquires the primary oocyte state. Therefore, folliculogenesis begins when the primordial follicle is formed, due to the union of the primary oocyte and granulosa cells. In primordial follicles, the primary oocytes leave their state of latency spontaneously and continue to other phases of growth, during which the differentiation and proliferation of the oocyte coexist with the surrounding cells and by the effect of the growth factors synthesized in the ovarian microenvironment; all these events are independent of the gonadotropins.

Different types of follicles are present during folliculogenesis.

- *Primordial follicle*: this follicle begins the process of follicular growth and maturation, to guarantee increasingly mature units that can lead the ovary toward ovulation or atresia.
- *Primary follicle*: characterized by a significant change occurring when the flattened cells surrounding the oocyte increase in size into a more cuboidal form, grow in diameter and consolidate as a structure with oocytes having a diameter >22.12 mm and a layer of 25–40 cuboidal cells called granulosa cells. It also increases the volume of the oocyte and the formation of the zona pellucida.

- *Secondary follicle*: the transition to this stage depends on FSH stimulus. At this stage, granulosa cells develop the ability to synthesize growth factors and steroids.
- *Tertiary and ovulatory follicle*: maturation of secondary follicles under the influence of gonadotropins leads to the formation of tertiary follicles and the ovulatory follicle.

2.5.3 Cyclical Changes in the Cytology and Secretions of the Genital Tract

During the estrous cycle, changes occur in the genital tract to facilitate sperm transport and fertilization and then to prepare for embryo implantation. Vaginal, cervical, and uterine mucosa congest and become edematous at the time of estrus due to high estrogen levels. In addition, uterine, cervical, and vaginal glands secrete important quantities of aqueous mucus, which is clear at the beginning of estrus, becoming more viscous and compact as the period of estrus continues.

The cervical mucus plays a central role in cervical function by controlling and directing sperm migration. Estrogens stimulate the secretion of sialomucin by mucus cells located at the bottom of the large cervical folds within the cervix. Sulfomucins are also secreted in smaller quantities by mucus cells on the upper parts of the cervical folds. At estrus, the cervical mucus becomes more watery and penetrable to sperm, allowing their migration through the cervix. Cervical secretion is inhibited by the postovulation rise in peripheral progesterone. Different studies have recorded cytological changes in the genital tract of the female goat during the estrous cycle. The relationships between vaginal exfoliated cells and ovarian steroids secretion cycle have been well established in goats. This pattern of exfoliation of vaginal cells could be used to determine the estrous cycle status. In this respect, superficial cells appear to be associated with the proestrus, estrus, and early metaestrus. Intermediate and parabasal cells are observed in larger quantities during the progesterone-dominated luteal phase. Exfoliated cells in the vaginal lumen are the result of rising peripheral estrogen which causes the vaginal wall to thicken. As the outermost layer moves further from the vascular supply, the cells keratinize and detach from the wall.

The distribution of mast cells also varies depending on physiological changes during the estrous cycle in the goat reproductive tract and ovarian tissues. The numbers of mast cells in the ovary, uterus, uterine cervix, and uterine tubes are highest on proestrus and lowest on metaestrus. Mastocytes are derived from hematopoietic precursors and represent critical effector cells in allergic diseases. It is assumed that these cells might operate as sentinel cells to help mediate the uterine host defense systems and might have a role in the uterus pertaining to embryo implantation.

2.5.4 Estrous Behavior

Estrous behavior includes two phases: proceptivity and receptivity (Figure 2.3). Proceptivity consists in seeking out and stimulating the male partner. Receptivity consists of the expression of the immobilization reflex in response to male nudges, inducing serial mounting and copulation. At the beginning of estrus, proceptivity always precedes receptivity, then both behavior components are expressed simultaneously. The duration of estrous behavior is about 36 hours but varies from 24 to 48 hours

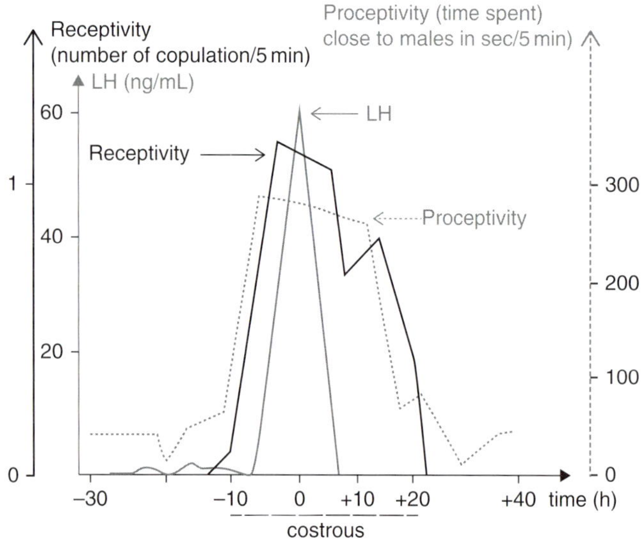

Figure 2.3 Evolution of sexual behavior during the estrous cycle.

depending on age, individuals and breeds, season, and the presence of a male. Angora goats and Mossi goats are known to have short estrus lasting only 22 and 20 hours. Creole goats exhibit 27 hours of estrous behavior and French Alpine goats are reported to experience 31 hours of estrus. In Boer goats, the mean duration of the estrous period is about 37 hours and it is about 58 hours in Matou goats in central China.

The interval from the beginning of estrus to the LH surge varies with breeds and individuals: 14.5 hours in the Alpine goat, 14–22 hours in the Mossi goat in Burkina Faso, and as short as eight hours in the Boer goat. The exact timing of ovulation relative to the onset of estrus is variable, ranging from nine to 37 hours, and is reported generally as occurring toward the end of standing estrus.

The continuous presence of a male and service during the estrous period may reduce the duration of estrus although it did not affect ovulation times or ovulation rates.

2.5.5 External Symptoms of the Estrus

The external symptoms of estrus that can be mentioned as important are moving the tail, increased vocalizations, decreased appetite, mounting behaviors, increased urine excretion, inflammation of the vulva, and discharge of vaginal mucus.

2.6 Pregnancy

After successful mating (natural or AI) and conception, does attain pregnancy. The gestation period in a goat is five months (150 days) and is affected by nutrition and stress factors. Pregnancy diagnosis is not of immediate concern in extensive goat operations that utilize extended natural mating, but the early determination of pregnancy can be a useful management tool with more intensive production conditions or when AI and embryo transfer are employed. Pregnancy diagnosis will identify the females that require repeat breeding or insemination and/or will allow the separation of pregnant and open females for different management. When fetal numbers can be determined as part of the pregnancy diagnosis, different feeding regimes can be applied to single and multiple litter-bearing females.

To be most useful to the producer, pregnant animals need to be identified as early as possible in gestation and provide an estimate of fetal numbers. Techniques have either focused on the detection of physical changes resulting from pregnancy (fluid accumulation and presence of a detectable fetus) through palpation and ultrasound. Techniques have also been concerned with identifying maternal and fetal physiological signals (progesterone or uterine proteins) associated with pregnancy. The most promising technique currently available for pregnancy diagnosis is real-time ultrasound scanning. Real-time ultrasound through the skin allows reliable pregnancy diagnosis as early as 35 days into gestation. Techniques using pregnancy-specific protein B are now available for use in small ruminants. Does can be tested for pregnancy at 30 days or later using a simple blood test.

2.7 Measures to Increase Reproductive Performance in Goats

Other than nutrition, breed, season, and location, several other important measures will affect breeding indirectly, such as trimming feet, grouping of animals, deworming, using the "buck effect" to synchronize does, and vaccination.

- *Trimming feet*: feet and legs should be examined closely for sores, overgrown hooves, and sources of strange smells that could be associated with infections or foot rot. Start trimming the feet of animals several weeks before the breeding season to make sure that they will be in top shape during that period of increased activity. The buck in particular will cover a lot of territory. A lame buck will cover does only sporadically, or might give up altogether. Similarly, limping does may not let bucks breed them.
- *Grouping of animals*: goats are very social animals and should be grouped together several weeks before the breeding season so that the pecking order of the animals may be established. Forming groups just before the breeding season will disrupt the pecking order. The fighting that will ensue to establish a new pecking order within the newly formed groups will be a source of stress and will influence reproductive performance. Young does should have reached approximately 70–75% of their estimated mature body weight to be bred successfully without adversely affecting their mature size.

- *Deworming*: deworming breeding does and buck(s) before the start of the breeding season is an important management tool. If flushing is planned, it is advisable to deworm before flushing. Wormy does will not increase their body condition during the flushing period and therefore flushing may not increase the ovulation rate. In addition, wormy does will not breed well, or may not breed at all, or may conceive and abort later.
- *The "buck effect"*: segregating does from bucks is crucial in the development of sound breeding programs that should be paralleled with feed resources and market demands. The best way to separate does from bucks is to develop a secure buck pasture. The buck pasture should be far enough from the breeding doe herd, otherwise bucks will attempt to go through fences to breed does in estrus. In goats, estrus can be induced with the strategic exposure of anestrus does to intact males. This response is dependent on the depth of seasonal anestrus and associated with first ovulation in 2–3 days after the introduction of the buck. The first ovulation is usually silent and of low fertility. The second ovulation five days later is accompanied by a fertile estrus. The response to the male effect is influenced by the sexual aggressiveness of the buck, the intensity of the stimulation, and the body condition of the does. Immediate contact results in a greater response than fence-line contact or intermittent contact. The pheromones responsible for inducing estrus are present in buck hair but not in urine, and are not associated with buck odor during the breeding season.
- *Vaccination*: although some producers have had no problems so far without implementing a vaccination program, it is recommended that goats be vaccinated against overeating disease (enterotoxemia) and tetanus. For twice-a-year vaccination, breeding does should be vaccinated before the start of the breeding season and 4–6 weeks before kidding. If vaccinated once a year, it is preferable to vaccinate breeding does before kidding because some immunity will be passed on to the newborns. The choice of vaccines is as follows.
  - *Clostridium perfringens* types C and D + tetanus toxoid in one vaccine, against overeating disease and tetanus. This vaccine is labeled for goats.
  - Multivalent clostridial vaccine (8-way vaccine): one example of a multiway clostridial vaccine, labeled for sheep, is Covexin® 8. Covexin8 is more reactive and may cause a higher incidence of adverse reactions at the injection site. It may be used in herds that have had problems with blackleg and malignant edema (gas gangrene). Although blackleg and malignant edema are common and costly infections in sheep and cattle, they are uncommon in goats.

References

Amoah, E.A. and Bryant, M.J. (1984). Effect of pattern of lighting and time of birth on occurrence of puberty in female goat kids. *Animal Production* 38 (1): 83–89.

Fatet, A., Pellicer-Rubio, M.-T., and Leboeuf, B. (2011). Reproductive cycle of goats. *Animal Reproduction Science* 124: 211–219.

Further Reading

Browning, R. and Leite-Browning, M.L. (2008). Reproductive, growth and fitness traits among Boer, Kiko, and Spanish meat goats semi-intensively managed in the southeastern US. In: *Proceedings of the Ninth International Conference on Goats, Queretaro, Mexico*. Little Rock, AR: International Goat Association.

Chemineau, P., Berthelot, X., Daveau, A. et al. (1993). Can melatonin be used in out-of-season reproduction in domestic mammals? *Contraception, Fertilité, Sexualité* 21 (10): 733–738.

Chemineau, P., Guillaume, D., Migaud, M. et al. (2008). Seasonality of reproduction in mammals: intimate regulatory mechanisms and practical implications. *Reproduction in Domestic Animals* 43 (Suppl. 2): 40–47.

Foster, D.L. (1994). Puberty in sheep. In: *The Physiology of Reproduction* (ed. E. Knobil and J.D. Neill), 411–451. Baltimore, MD: Lippincott Williams & Wilkins.

Freitas, V.J.F., Lopes-Junior, E.S., Rondina, D. et al. (2004). Puberty in Anglo-Nubian and Saanen female kids raised in the semi-arid of north-eastern Brazil. *Small Ruminant Research* 53: 167–172.

Gonzalez-Stagnaro, C. (1983). Comportamiento reproductivo de las razas locales de rumiantes en el Tropico Americano. In: *Reproduction des Ruminants en Zone Tropicale* (ed. P. Chemineau, D. Gauthier, and J. Thimonier), 1–80. Paris: Institut National de la Recherche Agronomique.

Gourdine, J.L., Bidanel, J.P., Noblet, J., and Renaudeau, D. (2006). Effects of season and breed on the feeding behavior of multiparous lactating sows in a tropical humid climate. *Journal of Animal Science* 84: 469–480.

Hafez, E.S.E. and Hafex, B. (2000). *Reproduction in Farm Animals*, 7e. Hoboken, NJ: Blackwell.

Hawken, P.A., Beard, A.P., Esmaili, T. et al. (2007). The introduction of rams induces an increase in pulsatile LH secretion in cyclic ewes during the breeding season. *Theriogenology* 68 (1): 56–66.

Knights, M. and Garcia, G.W. (1997). The status and characteristics of the goat (Capra hircus) and its potential role as a significant milk producer in the tropics: a review. *Small Ruminant Research* 26: 203–215.

Leboeuf, B., Delgadillo, J.A., Manfredi, E. et al. (2008). Management of goat reproduction and insemination for genetic improvement in France. *Reproduction in Domestic Animals* 43 (Suppl. 2): 379–385.

Luginbuhl, J. M. (2015). Preparing meat goats for the breeding season. NC State Extension Publications. https://content.ces.ncsu.edu/preparing-meat-goats-for-the-breeding-season (accessed 3 December 2023).

Martin, G.B., Rodger, J., and Blache, D. (2004). Nutritional and environmental effects on reproduction in small ruminants. *Reproduction, Fertility, and Development* 16 (4): 491–501.

Morrow, D.A. (1986). *Current Therapy in Theriogenology*. Toronto: W. B. Saunders.

Raposo, R.S., Silva, L.D.M., Lobo, R.N.B. et al. (1999). Perfil citológico vaginal de cabras cíclicas da raça Saanen. *Ciência Animal* 9 (2): 75–79.

Seyedmehdi, M. (2003). Georgia Small Ruminant Research and Extension Center, Fort Valley State University. American Dairy Goat Association National Convention.

Shelton, M. (1978). Reproduction and breeding of goats. *Journal of Dairy Science* 61 (7): 994–1010.

Stewart, J. L. (2021). Puberty and estrus in goats. www.msdvetmanual.com/management-and-nutrition/management-of-reproduction-goats/puberty-and-estrus-in-goats (accessed 4 November 2022).

Walkden-Brown, S.W. and Bocquier, F. (2000). Nutritional regulation of reproduction in goats. In: *Proceedings of the Seventh International Conference on Goats, Tours, France*. Little Rock, AR: International Goat Association.

3

Reproductive Biology of the Buck and Doe

Ashok Baindha, Mohan Lal, Rashmi Singh, and Vipin Chandra

Post Graduate Institute of Veterinary Education and Research, Jaipur, India

3.1 Introduction

Goats have been considered among the earliest domesticated animals and are the lifeline of 70–90% of the farmers living in rural areas of India. Their adaptability to the harsh environment (better resistance to heat stress and drought, better utilization and digestibility of pastures) allows local populations to improve animal production in a variety of climatic conditions ranging from extremes of tropical rainforests to dry deserts. Goats are widely found in tropical areas and are used primarily for meat production, but also in some regions for milk, fiber, and hide production. In temperate regions, they are bred mainly for dairy production, but also for meat and fiber. They are more tolerant of hot climates and give more production per unit investment. These benefits make goats the "poor man's cow" because of their immense contribution to the rural economy.

3.2 Reproduction in Goats

Reproduction is considered a primary trait of economic importance in animal production systems. Within this context, there is a need to adequately manage the reproduction of bucks and does to increase reproductive efficiency and herd production. Through reproductive management, goat herds may improve production levels. To understand and manipulate the reproductive processes of goats, it is important to be aware of their reproductive systems and functions.

In most areas of the world, goats are mated once yearly in the fall, during their natural mating season, for spring kidding. Animals bred at this time are more likely to get pregnant and have multiple kids. A longer breeding season allows for flexibility in breeding and matching kidding dates to times when the climate is more favorable and forage is available for the lactating doe. In addition, dates of ethnic/alternative markets should also be considered in the decision about when to breed females. How long the males are kept in with females for mating determines how long kidding will last, but a 40–45-day breeding season will guarantee that each doe has had at least two opportunities to come into heat. The male-to-female ratio in this breeding system is approximately one male per 30–40 females, but in synchronized breeding, this ratio should be one male with 20 or fewer females.

Likewise, under range conditions, bucks are often maintained with the doe herd throughout the year for continuous breeding. In such a system, proper health management is difficult and only limited supervision can be provided during kidding. Care is also required to routinely remove offspring from the herd to avoid mother/son and father/daughter matings. Although buck exposure is continuous, kidding under continuous mating will eventually follow seasonal breeding patterns, depending on the location of the farm and the breed of goat used.

However, globally, in intensive milk production systems, the use of basic reproductive techniques has been applied more extensively; for example, the estrus synchronization technique, artificial insemination (AI), is being used more commonly by goat producers. Artificial insemination makes it possible to obtain or transfer genetic material domestically and internationally. Many goat producers, both meat and dairy, utilize AI to produce animals that are more desired by markets and consumers as well as animals that will do well at local, state, and national livestock shows.

Elements of Reproduction and Reproductive Diseases of Goats, First Edition. Edited by Tanmoy Rana.

3.3 Male Reproductive Tract

The male reproductive tract can be divided into several segments (Table 3.1). The buck's reproductive anatomy is shown in Figure 3.1. Bucks possess a structure called a filiform appendage which is an extension of the urethra beyond the end of the penis. The urethra is the duct which carries urine or sperm out of the buck's body. The penis is the organ of copulation which allows the buck to deposit semen into the vagina of the doe. It is covered by the prepuce, a fold of skin that protects the penis (Fernandez n.d.).

The accessory sex glands, including the ampullae, seminal vesicles, prostate and bulbourethral glands, secrete fluids into the urethra during ejaculation. These fluids contain sugars to nourish the sperm, buffers to prevent rapid changes in pH, and other chemicals that serve to protect and propel the sperm out of the urethra and into the vagina. The ampullae are found at the terminus of the vas deferens which is the duct that leads from the testis to the urethra. When the veterinarian performs a vasectomy, the vas deferens is the duct he cuts to make a "teaser buck" infertile.

The vas deferens is connected to the tail of the epididymis, a large, winding tubule that can be felt on the side of the testis. Sperm cells that have been produced in the testis undergo a series of maturational steps as they pass from the head of the epididymis and through its body to the tail of the epididymis where they are stored. The testis (plural *testes*) is the site where sperm are manufactured and male steroids, especially testosterone, are produced. The scrotum is the pouch of skin that houses and protects the testes. The scrotum helps regulate the temperature of the testes by raising them closer to the body or lowering them away from the body. Sperm production cannot occur in the buck at or above normal internal body

Table 3.1 Reproductive organs and functions of male goats.

Organ	Major functions
Prepuce	Encloses free end of the penis for penetration
Penis	Copulation organ
Urethra	Transports spermatozoa and urine, and forms semen
Vas deferens	Transports spermatozoa
Epididymis	Concentration, nutrition, storage, maturation, and transport of spermatozoa
Spermatic cord	Supports and regulates the temperature of the testicles
Scrotum	Supports, protects, and regulates the temperature of the testicles
Testis or testicles	Produce spermatozoa and testosterone
Accessory glands	Production of seminal fluids to provide energy, buffer, and nourishment to the spermatozoa

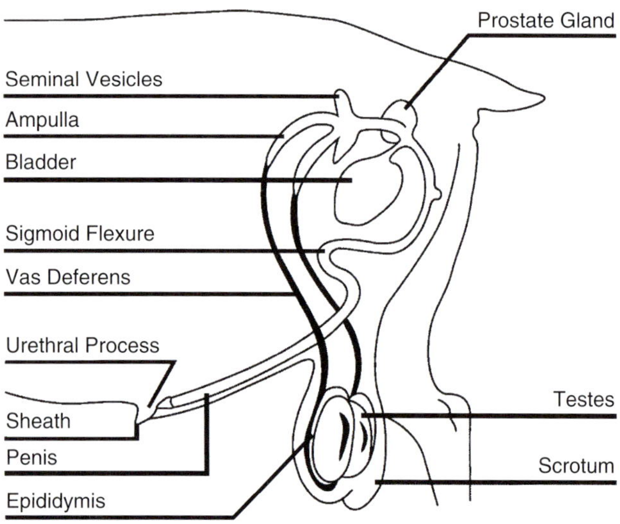

Figure 3.1 Anatomy of the buck's reproductive tract.

temperature. This is of special concern to goat producers who live in hotter climates if the external temperature rises above 103 °F for extended periods and the goats cannot cool themselves.

3.3.1 Prepuce

The prepuce is the sheath or foreskin that protects the penis.

3.3.2 Penis

This organ is responsible for male copulation and deposits semen in the female tract. The corpus spongiosum and corpus cavernosum are expandable tissues that enlarge and fill with blood when arousal occurs. In this excitatory state, the penis is erect, facilitating copulation and the ejaculation of semen in the female genital tract. In the buck, erection is achieved through extension of the sigmoid flexure that allows an increase of up to 12 inches and by filling the cavernous tissues with blood. In the nonerect state, the penis is contained in the sheath.

3.3.3 Urethra

The urethra is a duct common to the urinary and reproductive tracts. A distal portion of the urethra is connected to the urinary bladder. The distal portion is inserted in the penis and serves in discharging urine and semen.

3.3.4 Vas Deferens

The vas deferens, or ductus deferens, are a pair of ducts tied to the tail or cauda of the epididymis. They pass along the spermatic cord to the pelvic cavity where they merge with the urethra. The vas deferens transports spermatozoa from the epididymis to the urethra. It connects the epididymis to the ampulla and accessory sex glands. These glands are located in the pelvic region and provide the spermatozoa with the fluids that make up the ejaculate.

3.3.5 Spermatic Cord

The spermatic cord is composed of muscles and fiber tissues and a portion of the vas deferens. The cord connects the testicles to veins and arteries that irrigate the testicles in conjunction with the scrotum to position the testicles outside the body, and to help regulate the temperature of the testicles.

3.3.6 Epididymis

This is the first external duct of the testicles and is divided into three parts: the head, body, and tail. The epididymis transports, matures, nourishes, and stores spermatozoa produced in the testes. It is the site where the spermatozoa acquire motility.

3.3.7 Scrotum

The scrotum is the sac-like pouch formed by the skin that is responsible for protecting the testicles and the epididymis which is located in the inguinal region between the legs. The scrotum also aids in thermoregulation of the testicles.

3.3.8 Testes

The testes or testicles are oval shaped and paired. They are the main reproductive organs of a buck. The testicles are housed in the scrotum.

They are symmetrical in shape and size, elastic to firm in consistency and mobile in the scrotal sac. The primary sex organs are the testes, which produce the male gametes (spermatozoa) and sex hormones (i.e., testosterone). Sperm production (spermatogenesis) takes place inside the germinal epithelium, whereas Leydig cells in the interstitial tissue are responsible for hormone production. The testes are located in the scrotum, which aids in temperature regulation and maintains the testes at 3–5 °C below body temperature for optimal function. Spermatozoa produced by the testis enter the epididymis, also located in the scrotum, which serves as the site of sperm maturation (sperm acquire motility and fertilizing capacity) and storage before ejaculation.

Just like in the ovaries, events in the testis are controlled by the gonadotropins LH and FSH. In contrast to the female, where all eggs that will ever develop are present at birth, spermatozoa are produced by continuous division throughout the reproductive life of the male. In the final step of spermatogenesis, cells develop the characteristics of the functional spermatozoa (head, midpiece, and tail). Spermatozoa are then released from the germinal epithelium and pass to the epididymis, where fluid is removed and the sperm suspension is concentrated. Here sperm are stored in a dormant state before ejaculation or are voided in the urine in sexually inactive males. There is considerable variation in ejaculate volume and sperm concentration, dependent on season, age, and sexual activity. A buck of 8–14 months of age should have 25 cm of scrotal circumference. A normal range for volume and concentration is 0.5–1.5 ml and 1.5–5.0 billion sperm/ml.

3.3.9 Accessory Glands

The accessory glands are located next to the urethra and consist of the vesicular, prostate, and bulbourethral glands. The accessory glands are responsible for producing seminal fluid that nourishes, serves as a buffer, and provides other substances needed for the motility and fertility of spermatozoa. The spermatic fluid and spermatozoa combined form the semen. Accessory gland fluids empty into the urethra.

3.3.10 Thermoregulation

The temperature inside a testicle is 2 °C below body temperature. In cold weather, the testicles rise near the abdominal cavity; in hot weather, muscular relaxation permits the testes to hang down from the body. This relaxed state maintains the optimum temperature for spermatogenesis to proceed and the spermatozoa to survive. Structures responsible for thermoregulation include the cremaster and dartus muscles and the pampiniform plexus. A buck's low fertility rate may be attributed to environmental conditions and the incapacity to regulate the optimum testicular temperature.

3.4 Female Reproductive System

The basic structures of the doe's reproductive system are shown in Figure 3.2. The vulva is the exterior segment of the reproductive tract (Table 3.2). When the doe is in estrus, or in "heat," the vulva will often appear swollen and reddened (Fernandez n.d.).

3.4.1 Clitoris

The clitoris is located in the lower portion of the vulva. It is the excitatory organ of a doe's reproductive tract.

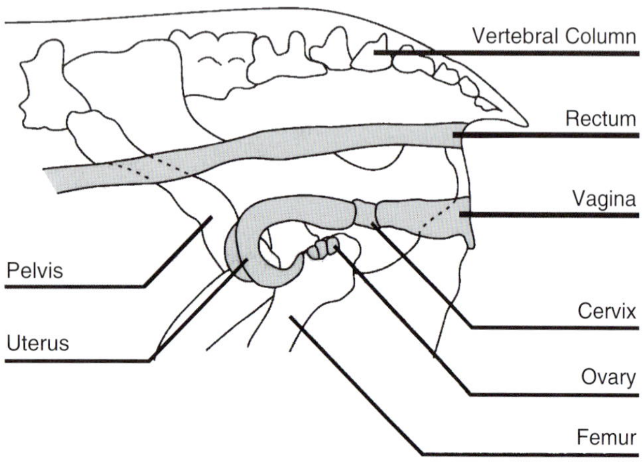

Figure 3.2 Anatomy of the doe's reproductive tract.

Table 3.2 Reproductive organs and functions of female goats.

Organ	Functions
Clitoris	Excitatory organ
Vulva	External genital structure
Vagina	Copulation and birth canal; site of sperm deposit during natural mating
Cervix	Transports spermatozoa Protects the uterus against foreign microorganisms
Uterus	Site for spermatozoa capacitation Embryo and fetus retention and nourishment
Oviducts	Transport spermatozoa and ova, further site of spermatozoa capacitation Site of fertilization of the ova
Ovaries	Produce the ova Produce estrogens (Graafian follicles) Produce progesterone (corpus luteum)

3.4.2 Vulva

The vulva is the external genitalia, consisting of the vestibule and the labia. The vestibule, generally 3 cm in length, is common to the urinary and genital tract. The vestibule joins the vagina with the urethral orifice (Leite-Browning 2009).

The labia consist of the labia majora and minora, the outer and inner folds of skin outside the vagina. The labia majora are homologous to the scrotum in males, and are the visible external portion of the female tract.

3.4.3 Vagina

The vagina is a large and tubular elastic structure 9–15 cm in length, located between the cervix and the vulva. It is the copulation organ of the female and is located directly in front of the vulva where the buck will deposit semen during mating, and it expands during the birth of the fetus. The vagina is part of the birth canal and also serves as a barrier to bacteria and foreign objects.

3.4.4 Cervix

The cervix is a fibrocartilaginous structure composed of three or four cartilage rings. It connects the uterus with the vagina. The cervix has an anterior and a posterior opening or os. The cervix is usually closed but it opens during heat under the influence of estrogen to facilitate the penetration of the sperm cells. The cervix is also opened during parturition for passage of the fetus. During pregnancy, the cervix enlarges like the uterus. The inner layer of the cervix has secretory cells that produce thick mucus, or "plug," that accumulates during pregnancy to protect the uterine environment against pathogens or infectious agents and foreign bodies.

The cervix secretes mucus to create a physical barrier that traps bacteria and flushes them out of the reproductive tract. However, during estrus, sperm must be allowed to pass through the cervix for conception to occur. When the doe is in estrus, the consistency of the cervical mucus changes, becoming more fluid so the sperm can pass through. This can sometimes be seen during estrus when the vulva appears to be wet or the area around the vulva appears to be dirtier or muddier than usual because the mucus flows out of the doe's vagina and vulva.

3.4.5 Uterus

The uterus is a smooth, muscular organ that stretches during pregnancy along with the growth of a fetus or fetuses. The uterus protects and provides nourishment to the embryo and fetus during pregnancy. A doe's uterus is bicornuate, which means that it has two long cornus or horns that connect the uterine body to the oviducts. Does have a small uterus, generally 3 cm in length and 2 cm wide.

The uterus is also the site where the sperm cells reach maturation or capacitation, and where the embryo migrates and develops throughout the pregnancy until parturition.

The uterus has three important layers. An inner glandular layer, i.e., the endometrium or internal layer of the uterus, is formed by glands that secrete endometrial milk that nourishes the embryo. The endometrial glands also secrete prostaglandin F2-alpha or PGF2-alpha, a hormone responsible for luteolysis or degradation of the corpus luteum (CL) at the end of the estrous cycle or days before parturition. A middle muscular layer pushes the fetuses out of the uterus during birth and an outer encapsulating layer provides support and attachment to the body of the doe. The uterus is separated from the vagina by a cartilaginous structure named the cervix (see above).

3.4.6 Oviducts

Oviducts are tiny, convoluted tubes located on each side of the uterus that connect the ovary to the uterine horns. They catch the ova as they are released from the ovaries and direct them into the rest of the reproductive tract. The oviducts are divided into three distinct segments that transport the ova and spermatozoids in opposite directions. Once the ova are released from the ovary during ovulation, they are captured in the oviduct. The oviduct is the site where the ova are fertilized, in a segment known as the ampulla. The oviduct is also the site where further capacitation of the spermatozoa occurs.

3.4.7 Ovaries

The ovaries are almond shaped, paired, and located on each side of the pelvic cavity. They produce the ova or female gametes and sex steroid hormones such as estrogen and progesterone. Estrogens are responsible for the development of the secondary sex characteristics of does and the physical and behavioral changes that does display during heat. Progesterone is responsible for changes in the uterine environment for embryo implantation, as well as for maintaining pregnancy and promoting mammary gland growth and development.

3.4.8 Supporting Structures

The female reproductive tract is located in the pelvic cavity and is supported by the broad ligament. This ligament supports the ovaries, oviducts, and uterus. Blood vessels and nerves pass through the broad ligament to supply blood to the female tract.

3.5 Seasonal Sexual Activity

Goats are usually "seasonally polyestrous," which means that they have estrus cycles during late summer, fall, and winter. The estrous cycle length of goats is 20–21 days, with a range of 17–24 days. Does are in heat (estrus) for approximately 30 hours, and ovulate 33 hours after the onset of estrus. Most goat breeds are prolific, and mature females shed more than one egg when ovulating.

Reproduction in goats is commonly described as seasonal with differences in seasonality between breeds and locations. The onset and length of the breeding season in goats are dependent on several factors: latitude and climate, breed, physiological stage, presence of a male, and breeding system but mainly photoperiod.

The main environmental factor affecting seasonal breeding in small ruminants is the annual change in day length. Photoperiodic control of reproductive patterns is mediated through circadian rhythmic secretions of melatonin by the pineal gland during darkness, which influences the gonadotropin-releasing hormone pulse generation and the hypothalamic–pituitary–gonadal feedback loop.

Animals bred in tropical and equatorial regions subjected to less change in photoperiod and temperature will display a longer breeding season than those bred in temperate and polar regions which exhibit more distinct seasonal effects.

3.5.1 At High Latitudes

Sexual activity in female goats can be assessed by their spontaneous ovulatory activity and demonstration of sexual behavior. Two distinct periods are observed throughout the year in temperate latitudes: a period of deep anestrus, when neither estrous behavior nor ovulations are noted, and the breeding period, with both estrous behavior and cyclic ovarian activity observed.

During the transition periods, anovulatory estrus or silent ovulations (ovulation not accompanied by estrous behavior) can also be seen. Seasonal breeding is observed in most breeds of goats originating from high latitudes (>35°) and in some local breeds from subtropical latitudes (25–35°). In temperate regions, the breeding period is the fall and winter. With increasing latitude, the breeding season tends to be restricted to the autumn months and most kids are born in spring. Exposure to males can extend the period of ovulatory activity both before and after the period of spontaneous ovulations.

3.5.2 At Lower Latitudes

In equatorial, tropical, and subtropical regions, changes in day length are less pronounced. Seasonality in reproduction is therefore less marked and most local goats in the tropics can breed all year round and have a relatively short postpartum anestrus. However, environmental factors (forage availability and temperature changes) have a strong influence which often does not allow these potentials to be fully expressed.

3.6 Estrous Cycle

The events of the estrous cycle are largely controlled by the hormonal interactions of the ovaries with the secretory glands (pituitary, hypophysis) located at the base of the brain. In addition to internal stimuli, this system is also responsive to external stimulation such as changes in day length and the presence and absence of males. Follicles in the ovaries, containing primary oocytes (eggs), develop in successive waves until some will rupture and release a secondary oocyte during ovulation. The released egg passes through the oviduct to join with spermatozoa, whereas the ruptured follicle transforms into a corpus luteum. The development of the follicle is under the control of gonadotropins (follicle-stimulating hormone-FSH, and luteinizing hormone-LH) released by the pituitary gland. The gonadotropins, via a hormonal feedback loop, also control the release of estrogens by the ovary, which control the estrous behavior displayed by the doe (flagging, mounting, etc.). Following ovulation, the luteinized follicle (corpus luteum) secrets progesterone, which prepares the uterus for a possible pregnancy, and suppresses the secretion of gonadotropins to halt further follicular development. Failure to establish pregnancy will result in the release of prostaglandin from the non-pregnant uterus, which will regress the corpus luteum and allow a new cycle to proceed.

Goats are spontaneously ovulating, polyestrous animals, bred in a wide range of production systems. Estrous cycle is a cascade of hormonal events which changes the female reproductive system morphology to prepare the animal for pregnancy. During the estrous cycle, ovaries undergo several morphological, biochemical, and physiological changes leading to ovulation.

3.6.1 Follicular Dynamics

A large pool of resting primordial follicles is laid down during fetal development in sheep and goats, with the first follicles being formed at about 70 days of gestation. It takes about six months for a follicle to develop from the resting stage to the preovulatory stage and approximately 34–43 days from initial antrum formation to the preovulatory phase. This pool is nonrenewable and during the lifetime of the animal, follicles develop into primary, secondary, and tertiary stages before ovulating. In domestic ruminants, the number of follicles ovulated during a female's reproductive life is minimal compared to the number of follicles she is born with, which suggests degeneration or atresia as the main fate of the follicle, not the ovulation. This seems to follow a selection process to ensure ovulation of only those follicles with oocytes that optimize the fertilization odds.

The dynamics of follicle wave development in goats have received less attention than in cattle or sheep. Follicular development can be divided into two phases: the gonadotropin-independent (FSH and LH) phase, where the follicle grows from primordial to the antral follicle, and another phase, which is FSH and LH dependent, where the follicle will reach preovulatory status, which in the presence of an adequate frequency and amplitude of LH pulses will ovulate. Follicle development during estrous cycles in goats follows a wave-like pattern and there are between two and six waves of follicle development during estrous cycles, with three or four waves being the most prevalent. On any day of the estrous cycle, there are 5–10 follicles which are ≥3 mm in diameter in the ovaries and follicles ovulate at between 6 and 9 mm in diameter. Due to the large variation in the number of waves, the onset of each wave and interwave interval is highly variable. The number of follicles that start growing in each wave is not well established, but about four follicles with a diameter >3 mm begin their growth in response to the transient peak of FSH. In goats, the diameter of the dominant follicle in anovulatory waves ranges from 6 to 6.7 mm, while the ovulatory follicle can reach up to 8.2 mm in diameter. However, the diameter of the nonovulatory dominant follicle and the ovulatory follicle is similar.

3.6.2 Follicular Dominance

A higher propensity of goats ovulating >1 follicle raises curiosity about the dominance of follicles in a wave. The existence of follicular dominance in small ruminants remained controversial for a long time. However, studies now suggest that dominance is also operative in the goat, especially during wave 1 and the ovulatory wave. The total number of small follicles decreased in correlation with the development of the largest follicle of wave 1 and this follicular pattern is one of the characteristics described for the phenomenon of dominance in cattle. Furthermore, in goats with monoovulatory cycles, the diameter of the two largest follicles differs significantly three days before ovulation.

Nevertheless, follicular dominance in goats is less absolute than in monoovulatory species such as cattle, but the evidence suggests the presence of similar relationships with two potential ovulatory follicles developing rather than one. The concept of codominance was introduced to explain that the two largest follicles can be observed in each wave.

3.7 Pregnancy

Does typically release more than one ovum during or shortly after estrus. What causes twinning is not completely clear but good nutrition, age of the doe, and breed are factors that are thought to contribute to twinning. There is a genetic component to twinning, and does that do not produce twins should be culled from the herd.

The ova are fertilized by sperm cells and begin dividing as they continue down the oviduct to the uterus. The developing embryos implant in the uterus by the 18th day after mating. This is the period during which the vast majority of failed pregnancies occur. Miscommunication between the doe and embryos causes the doe to terminate the pregnancy and return to estrus, giving the appearance that conception never occurred.

Pregnancy is established once fertilization of the ovum by the spermatozoon occurs. Fertilization occurs in the oviduct and requires the proper timing of insemination and ovulation, as spermatozoa remain viable for only 12 hours in the female reproductive tract, and the life span of the ovulated egg is limited to 12–24 hours. A healthy sperm will penetrate the zona pellucida surrounding the egg using enzymes contained in the cap of the sperm head. Fusion of the sperm cell with the egg will prevent the penetration of other spermatozoa. Fertilized eggs move from the oviduct toward the uterus and initiate cell division within 24 hours. The developing embryo will continue to divide and remain free floating until it attaches to the uterine wall 15–20 days after fertilization.

The uterus requires priming with progesterone for attachment of the embryo and membrane development to occur. In goats, in contrast to sheep, the corpus luteum is the primary source of progesterone throughout gestation. The developing fetus is contained in the placenta, a membrane that facilitates the exchange between maternal and fetal circulation. While the placenta experiences the most rapid growth between 90 and 110 days, fetal growth increases exponentially during the last trimester of pregnancy. Gestation length in the goat is approximately 150 days but is affected by breed and sex of kids, and tends to increase with age and decrease with litter size.

Pregnancy in goats tends to be a quiet period but does entering the last third of pregnancy face high nutritional demands because of rapid fetal growth. This is a critical time to manage does' nutrition because their nutritional needs nearly double. However, they are often unable to consume large quantities of feed because there is not enough space in their abdomens for both developing fetuses and more feed. For this reason, the quality of the feed must be higher. Unfortunately, the increased nutritional demand usually occurs during winter when the cost of feeding is higher.

The udder is also preparing for milk production. Udder growth and fluid production in the udder begin about 7–10 weeks before birth. Proper nutrition and good healthcare during pregnancy will result in heavier kids at birth and improved milk production. Heavier kids survive better than lightweight kids at birth, and better milk production will help the kids to grow rapidly.

Late pregnancy is an excellent time to prepare for the upcoming kidding season. One of the most overlooked preparations is contacting the veterinarian. Spring tends to be a busy period for vets, and taking the time now to establish plans with the vet for the kidding season will pay dividends when the kids start to arrive. Check the kidding kit and replace items that are damaged, contaminated, expired, or used up. Check to see if there is any frozen colostrum in the freezer and be prepared to collect fresh colostrum for freezing if needed. Clean out the kidding shed, check heating lamps, and put down fresh bedding.

3.8 Kidding

Kidding will begin about 150 days after mating. Signs of parturition can be observed with changes in does as their due dates approach. The ligaments connecting the hip bones will become more pliant and stretch. This will create hollowing of the hips. The udder will begin to swell and fill with fluid. The color of the fluid will change from honey-colored to milky, and it may drip from the teats as birth becomes imminent. The vulva may swell and show a mucus discharge. The doe may become restless, kick or butt her sides, and stop eating.

Parturition is initiated by regression of the corpus luteum approximately 24 hours before delivery, associated with an increase in estrogen. In preparation for parturition, the ligaments in the pelvic region relax, uterine contractions stimulated by oxytocin are initiated, and placental membranes rupture. Kids are usually born within 2–3 hours of initiation of labor. The rise in estrogen concentration at parturition is also involved in initiating maternal behavior and acceptance of the newborn. Maternal behavior is also fostered through stimulation of the cervical region as the kids pass through the birth canal.

Kidding or parturition begins with dilation of the cervix and contractions of the uterus. The doe's water will usually break during this period, which can last for several hours. The next phase of parturition is fetal expulsion. The kids enter the birth canal and are quickly pushed through. If the doe has not managed to expel the kids within an hour after hooves become visible, she will need assistance or the help of a veterinarian. Finally, the fetal membranes, or afterbirth, will be expelled. This can require several hours as well. The entire process from start to finish can take up to 12 hours. In most cases, does will not require assistance and kidding will happen naturally.

3.9 Lactation

Whether raising goats for dairy or meat, milk production by does is critically important to a herd's productivity. The udder begins secreting colostrum when the kids are born, but converts to milk production within a few days after birth. Colostrum is critically important to newborn kids, and it is important to ensure that kids suckle and receive colostrum within the first 24 hours after birth, preferably the first 2–4 hours. Colostrum is high in immunoglobulins or antibodies. It provides kids with a temporary immune system that will protect them against disease until their immune system is capable of making antibodies. Vaccinating does 30 days before kidding will boost the production of antibodies in the colostrum and better protect kids against diseases. Milk production increases until about the fifth week after kidding, then declines until about week 8. Milk production will usually decline gradually from week 8 until weaning.

3.10 Female with Newborn Kids

Due to temperature fluctuations, most goats are seasonal breeders, with more active breeding happening during seasons with shorter day lengths and little to no breeding during long day lengths. In females, reproduction is controlled by the estrous cycle. This represents the time from one standing heat (estrus) to the next. This cycle is usually 21 days, with the actual time for standing heat being 1–3 days. This cycle continues throughout the life of the female and is interrupted only by season, pregnancy, and lactation (milking).

3.11 Control of Sexual Activity and Optimization of Fertility Results

Techniques used to control reproduction in goats allow greater distribution of milk and meat production throughout the year, thus meeting the supply needs of industries and consumers. In dairy systems, milk supply is lagging behind the growing market demand for goat milk products due to the seasonality of production (Fatet *et al.* 2011). Producers aim at a consistent supply of goat milk all year round. In meat production systems, productivity relies on the number of offspring born and weaned and the frequency at which they are produced.

The main reproductive concerns are an optimum litter size (with a high survival to weaning) and the ability to breed does at a given period to fit a specific market demand. Therefore, controlling reproduction of goats is necessary to group kidding over a limited period of time and also to facilitate nutrition adjustments in relation to the physiological stage and lactation needs of batches of animals. Production out of the natural breeding season can be achieved by inducing ovulation via hormonal treatments, manipulation of the photoperiod or by the male effect. Nutritional strategies can also modulate the estrous cycle and affect reproductive performance.

Controlling goat reproduction offers three main advantages.

- The choice of a kidding period at a precise season of the year (determined by forage availability or by marketing of products).
- The synchronization of kiddings over a limited period of time (labor optimization, reduction in kid mortality, constitution of homogeneous feed lots of mothers and kids).
- The management of genetic resources (genetic selection, storage of genetic material).

Sustainable management in ruminant production systems clearly requires the development of sustainable methods to control reproduction. One of the major challenges with the hormonal control of estrus is to reduce the effects of repeated use of equine chorionic gonadotropin (eCG), specifically the production of anti-eCG antibodies which reduce the fertility of artificially inseminated females. The use of exogenous hormones (currently used by the majority of dairy goat breeders employing AI) is also causing growing consumer concern. eCG is an animal product extracted from pregnant mare serum and it may contain unknown pathogens. Progestogens are produced chemically and are free of pathogens but they give rise to residues in animal products or effluents that act as endocrine disrupters when concentrated in certain environments. These might therefore represent a risk for human health. Consequently, European regulations, which already restrict their use in livestock breeding, might become more restrictive in the future.

Clearly, natural, hormone-free methods such as the male effect, photoperiodic treatments without melatonin, nutritional strategies, other innovative ways of controlling sexual activity and the adaptation of parent stock to breeding constraints are promising research topics. Progress in fundamental research on the control of folliculogenesis and ovulation, on the mechanisms that govern social interactions and on the cellular and molecular mechanisms involved in the seasonality of reproduction is essential. This will produce new knowledge leading to the design of improved methods for manipulating reproduction in goats and will optimize productivity while reducing risks for the environment and human health. The development of hormone-free methods that allow artificial insemination will also contribute to faster genetic progress in the future.

3.12 Estrus and Male Mating Behavior

Does in estrus exhibit a number of characteristic behaviors. They may become quite vocal; they have been reported to bleat very loudly or moan. Does will wag their tails frequently, stop eating or at least reduce their feed intake and attempt to find a buck. They may attempt to mount other does and will stand to be mounted by does that attempt to ride them. Does may not exhibit all the behaviors listed, and under adverse conditions, such as extreme heat or at the beginning of the breeding season, may not exhibit any signs at all. The vulva may become swollen and reddened and may appear moist, dirty or muddy because of vaginal discharge. In the presence of a buck, the doe in estrus will stand to be mounted. Does that are not in estrus will attempt to escape mounting attempts by the buck or other does. Standing estrus in does usually lasts for 24 hours, and ovulation occurs during the latter portion of estrus or soon afterward.

Bucks will sniff and lick the vulva of does in an attempt to determine their breeding status. The buck will often raise his head and curl his lip in a behavior called the Flehmen (pronounced FLAYmen) response (Figure 3.3). Bucks will often test

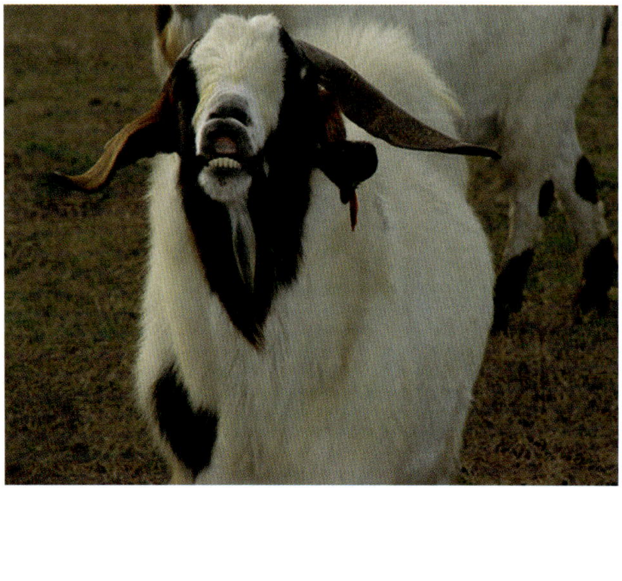

Figure 3.3 Buck exhibiting the curled lip and wrinkled nose typical of the Flehmen response.

a doe's receptivity by kicking at her side with his foreleg and licking or biting across her back and shoulders. The buck will attempt to mount the doe, and if she stands, copulation will occur very quickly. Copulation in goats usually lasts less than two minutes, but they will often mate several times while the doe is in estrus. Bucks must be carefully monitored during the breeding season, especially young bucks, because they spend so much of their time mating that they fail to eat. Bucks can lose up to 25 pounds over the course of the breeding season.

References

Fatet, A., Pellicer-Rubioa, M.-T., and Leboeuf, B. (2011). Reproductive cycle of goats. *Animal Reproduction Science* 124: 211–219.

Fernandez, D. (n.d.). Introduction to goat reproduction. Animal Science Cooperative Extension Program, University of Arkansas at Pine Bluff. www.uapb.edu/sites/www/Uploads/SAFHS/FSA-9607.pdf (accessed 4 November 2023).

Leite-Browning, M.L. (2009). Biology of reproduction of goats. Alabama Cooperative Extension System. Alabama A&M and Auburn Universities. https://silo.tips/download/biology-of-reproduction-of-goats# (accessed 4 November 2023).

Further Reading

Dávila, F.S. and Muñoz, G.P. (2020). Reproduction in small ruminants (goats). In: *Animal Reproduction in Veterinary Medicine* (ed. F. Aral, R. Payan-Carreira, and M. Quaresma). IntechOpen https://doi.org/10.5772/intechopen.93481 (accessed 4 November 2023).

Dávila, F.S., González, A.S.B., and Barragán, B.B. (2017). Reproduction in goats. In: *Goat Science*. Intechopen http://dx.doi.org/10.5772/intechopen.70003.

Sharma, A. and Sood, P. (2019). Follicular dynamics in goats. *Haryana Veterinarian* 58: 1–7.

4

Selection Criteria for the Buck and Doe

Ashok Baindha[1], *Mohan Lal*[1], *and Nirmal Singh Rajawat*[2]

[1] *Post Graduate Institute of Veterinary Education and Research, Jaipur, India*
[2] *College of Veterinary and Animal Sciences, Rajasthan University of Veterinary and Animal Sciences, Bikaner, India*

4.1 Introduction

Goat farming is one of the traditional occupations of livestock owners in India. Like poultry farming, goat farming is very profitable and employs a large number of people and helps to decrease the unemployment problem in the country. Goats are rightly called the "poor man's cow" since it can provide good returns that can serve as an investment source.

It is important to understand the criteria used to select and replace breed does and bucks in order to improve the productivity of goat herds. Among all the species of farm animals, goats (*Capra hircus*) have the widest ecological range and have been poor people's most reliable livelihood resource since their domestication during the Neolithic revolution about 10 millennia ago. Traditionally, the goat has served as a source of livelihood and financial security to large sections of society, mainly comprising resource-poor people. In the present scenario of changing agro-climatic conditions, this small ruminant farm animal has tremendous potential to be the "future animal" for rural and urban prosperity.

There were 148.88 million goats in India as per the 2019 census, showing an increase of 10.1% over the previous census. Rajasthan state had the highest goat population across India, at about 20.4 million in 2019.

First, Table 4.1 lists some commonly used terms for male and female domestic goats (*Capra hircus*) at different stages of reproductive development.

Anyone involved in goat production should have the skills to evaluate the physical characteristics of individual bucks for their potential as breeding stock. Producers should be able to visually evaluate goat structure and muscling.

For a buck to be sound on his feet and legs, he must be structurally correct. Correct structure enables the buck to move properly and proper movement allows bucks to comfortably mount does during breeding.

To be able to evaluate or select structurally correct bucks, producers must first have an understanding of the parts of a goat (Figure 4.1) as well as each part's correct structure. Remember, selection should begin with a look at performance records followed by visual evaluation. The visual appraisal can be a good indicator of frame size, muscling, body structure, feet and leg structure, and breed character.

The correct skeletal structure is essential for any animal to move to feed and water. This structure can be observed in shoulder angle, pastern angle, levelness of the hips, and top line from neck to rump. The angle of the shoulder should be approximately 45°, while the pastern angle should be approximately 50–55° or slightly more. Skeletal angles in the shoulders, hips, and legs are all important for ease of movement. When angles are within appropriate ranges, the animal is generally level across its top line and able to move freely.

When making visual selection decisions for correct structure, it is important to know all the external parts of a goat. Each part has an ideal characteristic for breeding bucks.

Elements of Reproduction and Reproductive Diseases of Goats, First Edition. Edited by Tanmoy Rana.

Table 4.1 Commonly used terms for male and female goats.

Term	Definition
Doeling	A doeling is a female goat less than a year old.
Doe or nanny	A doe is a mature female goat.
Buckling	A buckling is a young male less than a year old.
Buck or billy	A buck is an adult male goat.
Yearling	A yearling is a female or male goat that is a year old.
Wether	A wether is a castrated male goat.

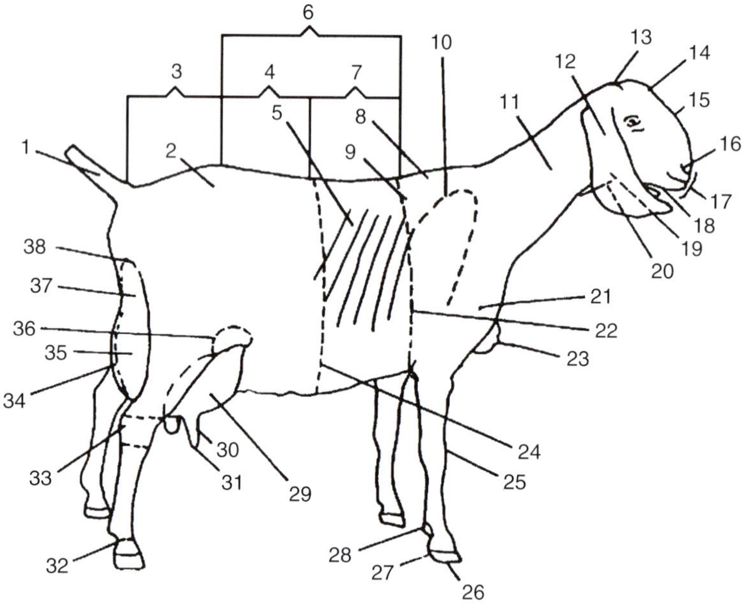

Figure 4.1 Body parts of the goat. 1 Tail. 2 Hip. 3 Rump. 4 Loin. 5 Rib. 6 Back. 7 Chine. 8 Withers. 9 Crop. 10 Shoulder blade. 11 Neck. 12 Ear. 13 Poll. 14 Forehead. 15 Bridge of nose. 16 Nostril. 17 Muzzle. 18 Jaw. 19 Throat. 20 Dewlap. 21 Point of shoulder. 22 Heart girth. 23 Brisket. 24 Barrel. 25 Knee. 26 Sole. 27 Heel. 28 Dewclaw. 29 Fore udder. 30 Teat. 31 Orifice. 32 Pastern. 33 Hock. 34 Medial suspensory ligament. 35 Rear udder. 36 Stifle joint. 37 Rear udder attachment. 38 Escutcheon.

4.2 Why Selection is Important

Proper selection is the first and the most important step in goat rearing. Records are the basis of selection and hence proper identification of animals and record keeping are essential (Figure 4.2). It is important to understand the criteria used to select and replace breeding does and bucks in order to improve the productivity of goat farm.

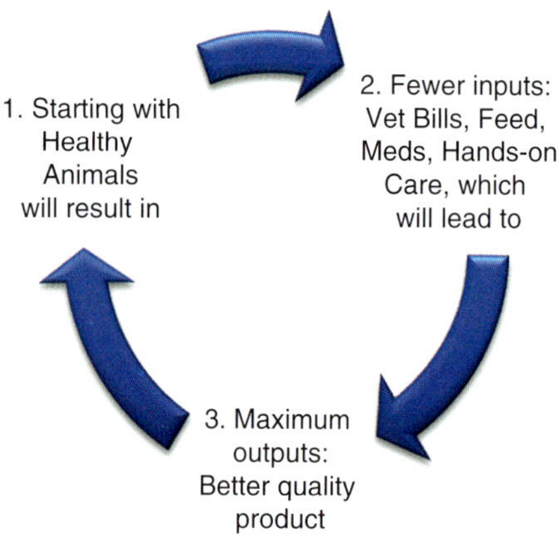

Figure 4.2 The importance of selection.

4.3 Setting a Breeding Objective

The first step in improving the genetics of a herd through selection and breeding is setting a breeding objective. A breeding objective describes the goats that you would like to breed that are appropriate for your production system and market. Setting a breeding objective will help you determine which breed, or crosses of breeds, you are going to produce, identify your genetic priorities and plan the selection methods that will allow you to achieve these.

To set your breeding objective you must identify the key characteristics, or traits, that:

- deliver meat and/or fiber products suited to your target market
- contribute the most to your profitability
- are heritable and have genetic variation across the herd
- can continue to be improved within the limitations of your environment and production system.

Typical traits that goat producers are aiming for in their selection and breeding program include:

- growth rate
- conformation such as feet, udder, and jaw
- frame size
- carcase and meat characteristics
- fertility and fecundity
- ease of kidding
- mothering ability
- temperament
- fiber characteristics
- milk production
- physical characteristics such as skin color.

It is important to remember that the more traits you include in your breeding objective, the slower the rate of progress will be for each trait. Therefore, it is important to identify those traits that are most important in your business. A breeding objective should be measurable and include a timeframe within which the improvements will be made. A common mistake producers make when setting a breeding objective is to have no measure of success; for example: big, white goats with red heads that produce heavy carcases and have multiple births.

4.4 Breeding and Selection Tools

When selecting bucks or does to purchase or retain, there are three main tools available to you to aid in your decision.

- Selection using visual appraisal.
- Selection using raw data.
- Selection using performance data.

A breeder should seek to use all three tools in combination depending on the traits that make up the breeding objective. This approach will be far more likely to lead to success in meeting the breeding objective than using one tool in isolation.

4.4.1 Selection Using Visual Appraisal

Visual selection is quick, efficient, and cost-effective for a large number of traits. It can occur at various times throughout a goat's life and should be an ongoing process. Visual selection is an important tool that needs to be utilized, particularly for traits that raw data or estimated breeding values (EBVs) are not available for. Examples include confirmation traits, temperament, and physical traits such as skin color.

While visual selection can be used for traits that can be measured, such as growth rates, it is important to remember that what a goat looks like is not necessarily what they will pass on through their genes to their progeny. This is due to the phenotype of the goat (what they look like) being a combination of the genes of the goat with the environment within which it has been bred and raised.

$$\text{Phenotype (P)} = \text{Genes (G)} + \text{Environment (E)}$$

Environmental factors that play a significant role in the phenotype of the goat will include their birth type (single or twin), age of their dam (maiden or mature doe), the season in which the goat was born and whether they have been supplementary fed.

4.4.1.1 Selection Criteria for Bucks

The characteristics of the buck are more crucial than those of does because a goat herd will be produced from many does, but many of those will be bred by a single buck. Therefore, it is critical to ensure that the buck has the kind of strong, desirable conformation that is being developed in the entire goat herd. The buck is considered as half of the herd as he is the sire of all the kids whereas the does are the dams of only a few kids each. So selection of the buck is far more important than any other step in breeding.

A replacement herd sire or buckling can be selected from the contemporary group at weaning (3–4 months of age) based on weaning weight. Subsequently, a postweaning growth evaluation can be made by 6–8 months of age. At eight months of age, a buckling can serve a small number of females in a herd. At two years of age, bucks are considered adults capable of serving a large number of does in heat. In general, a good herd sire should be selected based on structural and breeding soundness.

Salient points that should be keep in mind while selecting a breeding buck are as follows.

- The breed characteristics should be checked before choosing the buck for mating. A breeder must know the breed characteristic and it is advisable to choose purebred bucks for mating. Crossbreeding can be undertaken to improve the non-descript livestock.
- The buck should be big and well-developed with a broad back, good length and depth of the body, good ribcage, and muscular hind- and forequarters with good conformation as demonstrated in Figure 4.3.
- The health of the breeding animal is of prime importance. The breeding male should not show any symptoms of disease. Animals with bad breath should not be selected as they may have a tooth problem which may later affect their libido.
- A buck of 1–2 years of age should be selected for breeding. The age of the breeding male can be determined by examining the teeth (Figure 4.4). A central pair of permanent incisors signifies that the animal's age is one year. If there are two pairs of incisors, the animal's age is two years.
- Check the body weight of the breeding male. A buck of more than 30 kg should be selected for mating. In any case, the animal should not be less than 25 kg.
- The chest girth of the buck should be optimum. The chest should not be narrow. During mating, the chest rests on the female which provides the male with a stable posture during mating.

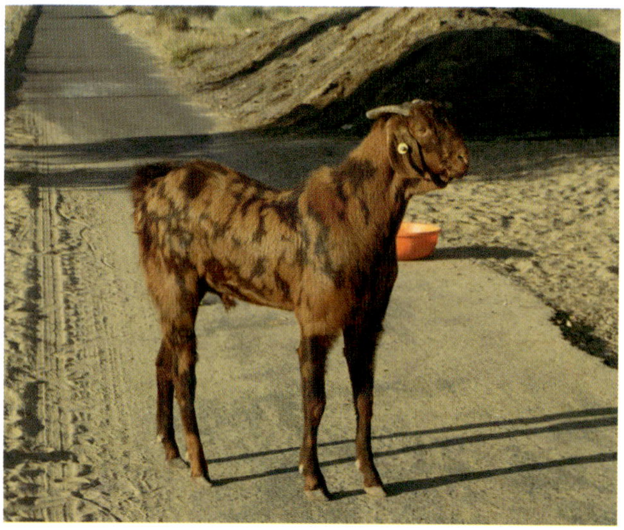

Figure 4.3 A healthy buck.

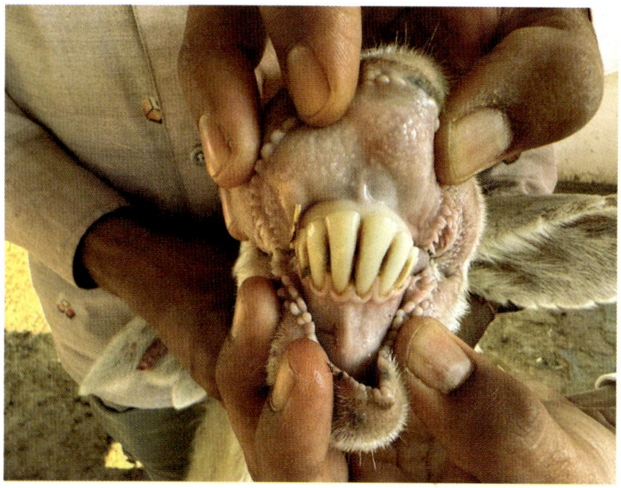

Figure 4.4 Dentition of the goat.

- The legs should be long but ensure that the body is not narrow. Long legs help in mounting and better gripping of females. Further, the legs should be set under the body and not out at the sides.
- The hooves of the animal should be checked for any pathological change. Bucks with perfectly placed hooves with intact hoof walls should be selected for mating. The toes should face forward and should not be split.
- The gait of the buck should be observed along with the response to stimuli. Always select active and alert males for mating. Limb deformities, laminitis, arthritis, etc. lead to loss of libido and animals do not mate readily.
- Both testes should be present with no pathological changes. A cryptorchid buck with single testes can also mate but always select an animal with both testes descended in the scrotum. Awell-placed epididymis on the ventral aspect of the testes with no pathological changes confirms normal physiology of reproduction.
- The testicles should have a firm consistency, elasticity on palpation, good mobility in the scrotal sac, and be oval shaped. Adult bucks should have a scrotal circumference of 25 cm on average (Figure 4.5).

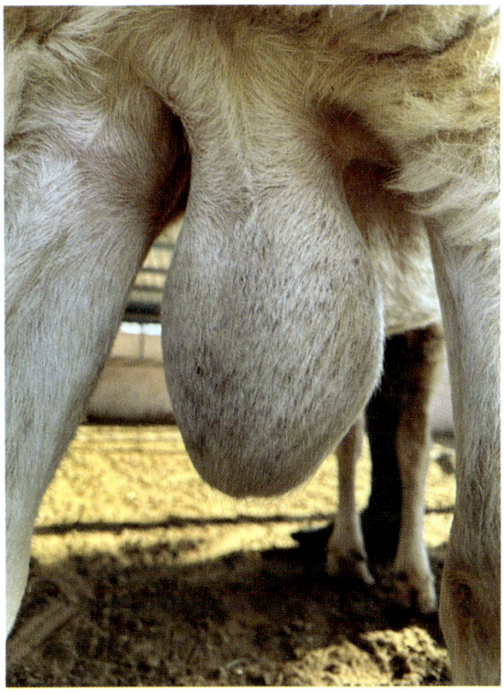

Figure 4.5 The scrotum and its measurement.

Sound hind legs are vital to the mating ability of bucks because during mating, most of the buck's weight is supported by the hind legs. A buck with hind leg defects may suffer pain while moving or mounting, which may interfere with his desire to mate. In an aging buck with faulty conformation, defects become more apparent and may tend to decrease his ability to breed larger groups of does.

The buck's legs should be free of excessive swelling at any of the joints, and joint flexures should be smooth and free of locking in any position. A goat with straight hind legs, or post legs, is predisposed to swollen hocks and arthritis in the hind leg joints. A goat with post leg or sickle hocks also may have more difficulty moving earlier in life, leaving it lame or unable to move freely throughout a pasture or, in the case of bucks, to breed does.

Other visual characteristics to consider when evaluating bucks relate to how filled out the animal appears. Bucks selected for breeding should exhibit volume and capacity. The indicators of volume are as follows.

- Width of the chest floor, which is the lower chest between the two front legs.
- Depth of body, which is the depth from the top of the animal's back to the bottom of their belly.
- The roundness of the ribcage.
- Uniformity of body depth refers to the animal being the same depth at the top of the shoulders to the fore flank compared to the top of the hips to the rear flank.

Goats with more volume are generally easier fleshing. That is, they produce external fat easily and are usually lower maintenance than goats that lack volume. Bucks should be selected with volume in mind to transmit these traits to their offspring.

The muscling of an animal is also important to the meat animal industry. Heavily muscled animals tend to produce more meat and less fat than animals with less muscle. Consumers prefer goats with larger loin chops and less fat. Indications of muscling can be seen over the animal's top and in the loin area, length of the hip, width between the rear legs, and hindquarters.

Leg structure, volume, and muscle all play a role in the correct structure of goats. Structure helps determine how well an animal will function. It can also affect the longevity of an animal. So, it is important to consider structure when selecting bucks to maintain a healthy and viable operation.

There are several undesirable feet and leg characteristics that animals can exhibit. To evaluate animals, we should be aware of these issues.

- *Pigeon-toed*: an animal is pigeon-toed or toed-in if when viewed from the front, the toes turn toward each other rather than pointing straight forward.

- *Bow-legged*: an animal is bow-legged if when viewed from the front, the knees curve out away from each other or if viewed from the rear, the hocks curve out away from each other.
- *Splay-footed or toed-out*: an animal is splay-footed or toed-out if when viewed from the front, the toes turn out away from each other rather than pointing straight forward.
- *Knock-kneed*: an animal is knock-kneed if when viewed from the front, the knees lean toward each other and are not in a straight line with the legs.
- *Cow-hocked*: an animal is cow-hocked if when viewing the hind legs from the rear, the hocks, which are the hind leg joints, are turned inward or are placed too close together. This causes the toes to turn outward.
- *Sickle-hocked*: an animal is sickle-hocked if when viewing the rear legs from the side, the hock has too much angle or set. A line dropped perpendicular from the pin bones to the ground should lie parallel to the cannon bone. A sickle-hocked animal has hocks that angle too much, which causes its feet to stand too far underneath its body. Often these animals will droop excessively from hocks to pins.
- *Post-legged*: an animal is post-legged if the hock has too little angle or set. The animal is too straight through the joint, which results in a very stiff, restricted movement due to the lack of flexibility. More goats become unsound because of being post-legged than sickle-hocked.
- *Buck-kneed*: an animal is buck-kneed, or "over at the knees," if the full extension of its knee cannot occur. When observed from the side, the legs appear slightly bent. This is usually seen in goats that are too straight in the shoulder.
- *Calf-kneed*: the opposite of buck-kneed. This means that the animal stands "back at the knees," when viewed from the side.
- *Weak pasterns*: pasterns, which are the leg bones between the hoof and fetlock, can be determined by visually looking at their angle. Weak pasterns have more than the normal slope to them which can indicate a structural fault. As mentioned previously, the correct pastern angle should be approximately 50–55° or slightly more.

4.4.1.2 Selection Criteria for Does

The nucleus of a production herd is a good doe (Figure 4.6). The maintenance of mature does in the breeding stock should be based on higher reproductive performance. Does are expected to wean kids annually. A doe should also exhibit good structure. Does which are to be selected as dams should be local animals with the following characteristics.

- Good body development is necessary for high milk production.
- The doe should be well developed and healthy looking, with her feet placed squarely on the ground rather than on her pasterns. She should stand squarely on her feet.

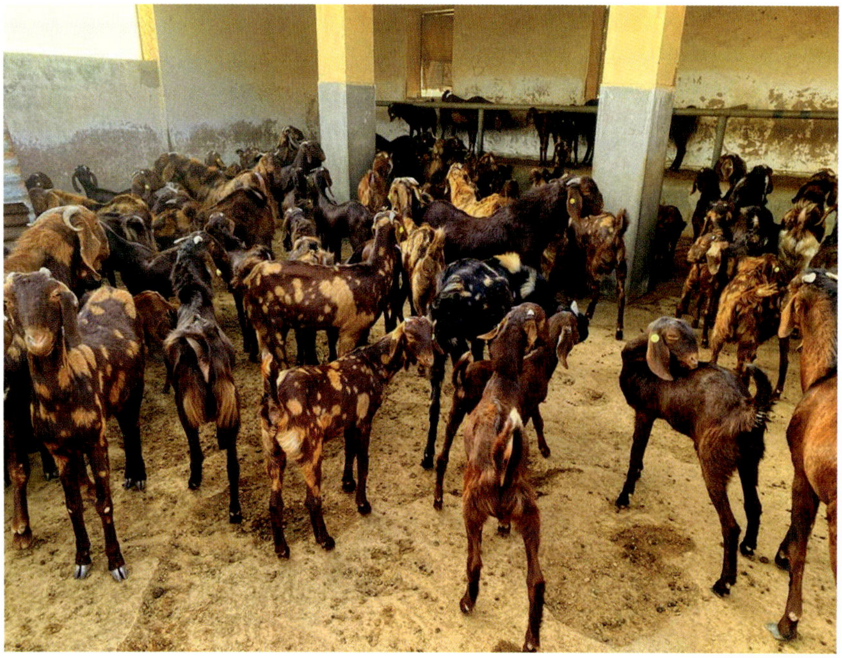

Figure 4.6 A goat flock.

- The animal should be free from any disease condition. The eyes of healthy animals are bright and alert. The skin should be loose, supple, and free from dryness.
- The jaw should be long and powerful and conditions like an overshot jaw, undershot jaw, or broken mouth should not be selected for breeding.
- She should have a regular reproductive cycle, early kidding ability with first kidding at around 16–18 months, good mothering nature, and high productivity with persistence in milking.
- An udder's milk capacity cannot be determined by its size. A good milk goat's udder should be smooth and supple rather than meaty. The udder of a recently milked goat should be compressed.
- For milk-type goats, the body should be wedge-shaped and sharp. The back should be strong, straight, and muscular and the ribs should be deep and wide apart. A wide ribcage and broad back indicate better feed intake capacity. A broad rump region indicates more space for carrying the fetus. Wide space between the thighs provides room for development of the udder.
- A large, spherical, well-attached udder should be between the thighs. The udder should have a broad base, elastic skin, and a prominent milk vein with thick teats slightly pointing forward (Figure 4.7).

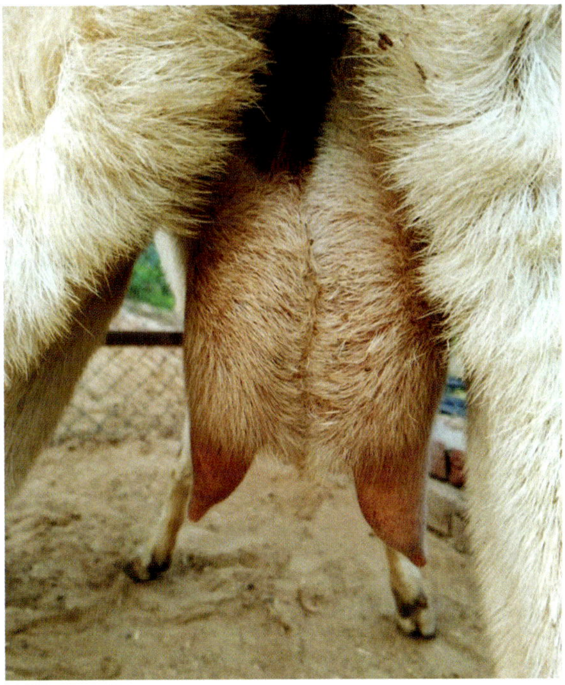

Figure 4.7 Udder of a doe.

- A good milker may have poor flesh, while a bad milker may have good flesh.
- They should have a truly feminine appearance and exhibit docile behavior.
- For meat type selection, does with a rectangular conformation and blocky appearance are preferable. They should have good muscle conformation and proper fat reserve. Selection of animals born as twins or triplets may increase the kidding percentage in the herd.

Other valuable traits include the following.

- A doe must be capable of breeding with no more than two services (rate to effect a pregnancy) required to conceive in a breeding season. She must be able to carry a pregnancy to term.
- She must be prolific with a history of kidding multiple births and have raised the kids up to weaning unassisted. Bear in mind that the reproductive merit of a doe cannot only be measured by the number of kids she has kidded, but by the number of heavy kids she has weaned.
- Does must have good milk production as indicated by the weaning weight of the kids.

4.4.1.3 Selection of Replacement Doelings

Replacing doelings in a breeding program is a multi-step process based on breed, season of birth, and management practices. The first screening begins at weaning when the doelings are 3–4 months of age. It is based on weight and development. Doelings are selected from their contemporary group in a herd and kept for further evaluation. At 6–8 months of age, the doelings should be reevaluated based on growth and development within their group. Only doelings that have achieved good growth and are structurally sound should be kept as replacement stock. Further selections are made at the yearling stage when the female is ready to breed. At this stage, the choice is based on cyclicity and pregnancy. Young does that do not show estrous cycles or do not become pregnant are cull candidates. The final selection is made after young does have weaned their first kids.

Replacement prospects are determined according to whether the does adequately raise their kids. This practice is only valid when doelings are under the same management practice.

Other traits to consider when selecting replacement doelings include the following.

- Females must be feminine, which includes good structural conformation including good feet and legs.
- The vulva must not be infantile. A small vulva with a tuff of hair is a sign of intersexuality.

- The length of the upper jaw should be equal to the lower teeth touching the superior dental pad. Mouth malformation will provoke bad bites and will prevent the animal from eating efficiently. This trait can also be transmitted to offspring.
- Watch for a higher average daily weight gain during development in comparison to their contemporary group.

4.4.2 Selection Using Raw Data

For traits that can be measured, such as weight, the use of raw data can improve the accuracy of selection and breeding decisions in comparison to visual selection for these traits. While the eye can be deceived and using actual raw data will remove any uncertainty or bias that visual selection can result in, it should be remembered that the raw data is a combination of the goat's gene and the environment in which it has been bred and raised. Therefore, as with visual selection, using raw data in isolation will not necessarily result in the best genes being retained or purchased. In many cases, however, raw data and visual selection may be the only tools available to base your selection decisions on. If this is the case, the following rules should be followed in order to minimize the environment effect that different goats may experience. They relate to both selecting bucks and does to be retained from your own herd and purchasing bucks and does from an outside herd.

- Goats that are to be selected from should have all run in the one group. If the numbers of goats are too large to run in one group, it is important to select from within the groups separately as paddock differences may need to be taken into account when selecting.
- Goats should be managed so they are given a good commercial opportunity to express their genetic potential. A group of well-grown goats will exhibit greater variation and facilitate better selection decisions compared to a group that has been held back through either health problems or lack of nutrition.
- Depending on the goats being selected, factors such as birth type (single or twin), age of the dam (maiden or mature doe), spread of kidding date and number of kids raised all have a significant impact on what you see and the raw data that might be presented. The younger the goat, the greater the impact these factors can have. Colored ear tags can assist in identifying these factors without having to have detailed records to look up for every goat.

4.4.3 Selection Using Performance Data

One of the best ways to compare individual goats is by using data. Producers collect these data starting when kids are born and add information throughout a goat's life.

When selecting bucks based on data, there are two options: EBVs and individual performance within a herd. EBVs are the preferred selection parameter because these numbers focus on genetic estimates for performance across a breed. EBVs are measurements of heritable traits such as the number of kids born, weaning and postweaning weights, and carcase traits. While an individual's performance within a herd is still useful information, the performance of that individual will be influenced by management and environmental factors in addition to genetics.

EBVs allow breeders to make more accurate selection and breeding decisions on a range of commercially important traits. EBVs take into account the known environmental influences that can affect a goat's visual or measured performance such as birth type (single, twin), age of dam and whether the goats have been run together or separately. Information from relatives and the heritability of each trait are also used to determine an EBV.

In addition, records allow producers to make informed decisions for both selecting replacement animals and culling poorly performing animals. This is especially important for identifying animals within the herd that do not produce offspring that meet minimum production standards. Producers can also utilize records on progeny to make culling decisions once does and bucks produce offspring. Performance data collected on individual goats can be interpreted at the farm level.

Common performance data include the following items.

- *Birth weight*: most kids should weigh between 5 lb and 8lb at birth, depending on the mature size of their parents. Larger kids may cause kidding difficulties, while smaller kids may require producer assistance for the first few days after birth. This adds to the labor requirements at kidding and can increase the likelihood of death losses.
- *Birth date*: to best manage groups of does and kids, does in the herd should give birth as close to the same date as possible. A good goal is for all kids within the herd to be born within two heat cycles, or 42 days. Kids born outside this 42-day window often weigh less than the average at weaning. Producers should consider culling does that do not kid within this timeframe.

- *Birth type and rearing type*: birth type refers to kids born as a single, twin, or triplet. To be profitable, many operations need their does to produce twins and does should rear those kids as twins. Yearling does are the exception, as most will produce a single kid. Selecting bucks, as well as does, born as twins can help to boost the genetic likelihood of twinning but nutrition also plays a large part in twinning rates.
- *Weaning weight*: many kids produced by livestock farmers are sold at weaning, so heavier weaning weights can increase the profitability of an operation. A good goal is to have meat goat kids weigh 35–50 lb or more by 90 days of age. However, this is not a realistic goal for all breeds. Kids born as singles normally weigh more at weaning than kids born as twins or triplets. Other factors, such as the sex of the kid and age at weaning, also influence the weaning weight. Keep in mind that a pair of twins will probably weigh more at weaning than a single kid. Thus, the weight of the pair, even if its individuals each weigh less than the single-born kids, determine the income produced by the doe.

4.4.3.1 Adjusting Weaning Weights

As alluded to earlier, animal performance is based on both genetics and the environment. Producers can adjust weaning weights in order to compare individual kids born on the same farm, since these animals have theoretically all been exposed to the same environmental conditions.

Weaning weights can be adjusted for:

- age at weaning
- birth type (single, twin, triplet)
- rearing type (single, twin, triplet)
- sex of the kid
- age of the dam or mother.

To adjust for the age at weaning:

1) determine an age to adjust to; weaning weights are typically adjusted to 90 days of age but could also be adjusted to other ages such as 60 or 120 days
2) subtract the birth weight from the weaning weight; this is the weight gained
3) divide by the age of the kid (in days) when it was weighed; this is the average daily gain
4) multiply the average daily gain by the weaning age you are adjusting to (usually 90 days)
5) add the birth weight.

$$\text{Estimated 90-day weight} = ((\text{[weaning weight} - \text{birth weight]}/\text{age at weaning}) \times 90) + \text{birth weight}$$

The estimated 90-day weight can then be adjusted for more factors. Table 4.2 lists adjustment factors to account for the age of the doe, sex of the kid, birth type, and rearing type.

An example of adjusting a weaning weight is given below.

A twin doe kid was born on January 2nd, weaned on April 4th, and raised as a twin. The dam is two years old.

- Birth weight = 7 lb
- Weaning weight = 45 lb
- Actual age at weaning = 91 days
- Weaning age to adjust to = 90 days

1) Adjust the weaning weight for 90 days. Use the following formula:

$$\text{Estimated 90-day weight} = \left[\left\{\left(\text{weaning weight} - \text{birth weight}\right)/\text{age at weaning}\right\} \times 90\right] + \text{birth weight}\left[\left\{\left(45-7\right)/91\right\} \times 90\right] + 7 = 44.58\,\text{lb.}$$

2) Now adjust the weaning weight for doe age, sex of the kid, and type of birth and rearing, by multiplying by the adjustment factors found in the table:
   1.09 = adjustment factor for a two-year-old doe
   1.11 = adjustment factor for a doe kid
   1.18 = adjustment factor for a twin raised as a twin

$$44.58\,\text{lb} \times 1.09 \times 1.11 \times 1.18 = 63.65\,\text{lb.}$$

Table 4.2 Kid preweaning and weaning weight adjustment factors.

Item to be adjusted	Class	Adjustment factor
Doe age in years	1	1.10
Doe age in years	2	1.09
Doe age in years	3+	1.00
Sex	Buck	1.00
Sex	Wether	1.08
Sex	Doe	1.11
Type of birth and rearing[a]	1/1	1.00
Type of birth and rearing[a]	1/2	1.14
Type of birth and rearing[a]	2/1	1.04
Type of birth and rearing[a]	2/2	1.18
Type of birth and rearing[a]	3/1	1.08
Type of birth and rearing[a]	3/2	1.23
Type of birth and rearing[a]	3/3	1.27

[a] Type of birth and rearing:
1/1 = single raised as a single.
1/2 = single raised as a twin.
2/1 = twin raised as a single.
2/2 = twin raised as a twin.
3/1 = triplet raised as a single.
3/2 = triplet raised as a twin.
3/3 = triplet raised as a triplet.

Therefore, the adjusted 90-day weight of this doe kid is 63.65 lb. This calculation allows producers to better compare kids and make more informed selection decisions.

Further Reading

Browning, R., Jr., Payton, T., Donnelly, B. et al. (2006). Evaluation of three meat goat breeds for doe fitness and reproductive performance in the southeastern United States. *Proceedings of 8th World Congress on Genetics Applied to Livestock Production, Belo Horizonte, Brazil* (13–18 August 2006). Peru: Instituto Prociencia.

Browning, R. and Leite-Browning, M. L. (2008). Reproductive, growth, and fitness traits among Boer, Kiko, and Spanish meat goats semi-intensively managed in the southeastern US. *Proceedings of 9th International Conference on Goats in Queretaro*, Mexico (31 August-5 September 2008). Little Rock, AR: International Goat Association.

Hafez, E.S.E. and Hafex, B. (2000). *Reproduction in Farm Animals*, 7e. Hoboken, NJ: Blackwell.

Meat and Livestock Australia (2006). Module 5: goat selection and breeding. www.mla.com.au/globalassets/mla-corporate/generic/extension-training-and-tools/gig_module-5_web.pdf (accessed 13 October 2023).

Notter, D. (2008). *The 2007 Boer Goat National Genetic Evaluation. Boer Goat Improvement Network Notebook, No. 4*. Centennial, CO: National Sheep Improvement Program.

Sastry, N.S.R. and Thomas, C.K. (2015). *Livestock Production Management*. Chennai, India: Kalyani Publishers.

Singh, R.R. and Islam, M.M. (2013). *Farm Animal Management. Principles and Practices*. New Delhi: New India Publishing Agency.

TNAU Agritech Portal (2009). Breeding management of sheep and goat. Expert system for sheep and goat. www.agritech.tnau.ac.in (accessed 13 October 2023).

5

Impact of Nutrition on Reproduction in Goats

Sanjay Kumar[1], *Kaushalendra Kumar*[1], *Rajni Kumari*[2], *Amitava Roy*[3], *and Tanmoy Rana*[4]

[1] *Department of Animal Nutrition, Bihar Veterinary College, Patna, India*
[2] *ICAR-RCER, Patna, India*
[3] *Department of Livestock Farm Complex, West Bengal University of Animal & Fishery Sciences, Kolkata, India*
[4] *Department of Veterinary Clinical Complex, West Bengal University of Animal & Fishery Sciences, Kolkata, India*

5.1 Introduction

Goat rearing is one of the important agricultural enterprises in rural parts of India and has proved very useful to humans throughout the ages, largely because of goats' adaptability to varying environmental conditions under which the breeds and strain types have evolved and in which they are maintained. They have tremendous ability to survive, and often thrive on sparse vegetation unsuitable for feeding of other livestock. Goats can be profitably raised with low investment under most forms of nomadic grazing and also intensive farming systems. The vast majority of this poorer section of the rural population depends on goat rearing for income and meat and milk for home consumption. Goat rearing requires low cost input and hence is suited to landless laborers, marginal farmers, and industrial workers (Birthal and Joshi 2006).

The livestock sector alone contributes nearly 25.6% of the total value of output in the agriculture, fishing, and forestry sector. The overall contribution of the livestock sector to total GDP was nearly 4.11% at current prices during 2012–2013. The goat population declined by 3.82% since the previous census and the total number of goats in the country was 135.17 million numbers in 2012. In the 19th Livestock Census (2012), the contribution of goats to the total livestock population was 26.40% in comparison with the 18th Livestock Census in which it was 26.53%. The goat population decreased by 3.18% in rural areas and 15.66% in urban areas of the country.

The goat is a versatile animal. It is known as the "poor man's cow" in India and as the "wet nurse" of infants in Europe. Goats can be kept with little expense and provide a dependable source of income to 40% of the rural population below the poverty line in India and to many who do not possess any land (Kumar 2007). The nutrition of goats is the most important factor affecting performance and expense, being about 70% of production costs. Poor nutrition results in low rates of production, often defined by growth, reproduction, and immune system. In many animal production systems, approximately two-thirds of improvements in livestock productivity can be attributed to improved nutrition. In economic terms, feed cost accounts for about 70% of the total cost of livestock production (Merkel et al. 1997). It is estimated that up to a fivefold increase in tropical livestock productivity can be attained if there is optimal feed resource utilization.

5.1.1 Nutritional Constraints

Nutritional constraints for improvement of goat production consist of insufficient feed supply, less efficient utilization of available feed resources, and reduced feed value of the available resources. Very poor-quality crop residues and browsing and grazing in natural pastures are the main sources of feed in most areas. Due to seasonal rainfall distributions, there are noticeable seasonal differences in the quality and quantity of feed supply. There is severe shortfall of feed supply during the dry season and the feeds available during this period are of very poor quality (low in protein with high-fiber diet), which results in low voluntary intake and digestibility by animals. Seasonal shortage of forage on small and medium farms is considered to be a main limitation for goat production due to small farm area and overstocking of livestock

Elements of Reproduction and Reproductive Diseases of Goats, First Edition. Edited by Tanmoy Rana.

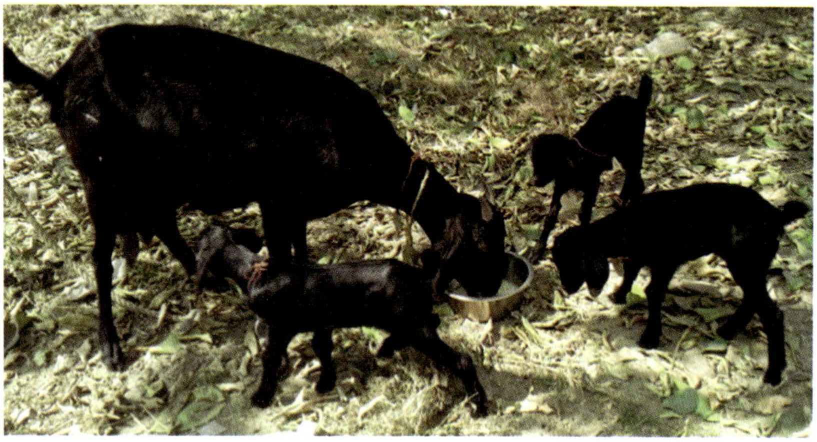

Figure 5.1 Feeding of poor-quality feed.

(Oteino et al. 1992; Onim et al. 1992). In a participatory rural appraisal, during the rainy season, low dry matter (DM) intake from grazed forages and uncertain availability with high cost of oil seed cakes were recognized to be the main nutritional constraints for dairy goat production in Tanzania (Ingratubun et al. 2000). During the critical period, the problem is exacerbated due to deficiency of substitute feeds.

Poor nutritional strategies result in low productive and reproductive performance and reduce the growth rate in young goats. Malnourished animals are more prone to diseases and parasitic infestation and in severe cases animals lose body condition and could ultimately die. In mixed farming areas, natural grazing may may occur but browsing is decreasing due to encroachment of the human population side by side with increasing demand for land for cultivation (Oteino et al. 1992; Said and Tolera 1991). Residual crop and stubble grazing are the main sources of feed in these situations (Figure 5.1).

During the dry season, straw and stover residues are stored and fed to animals when both the quantity and quality of available fodder from natural pastures declines significantly. However, efficient utilization of crop residues as animal feed is also limited by their seasonal supply and poor nutritive value (low nutrient content, poor digestibility, and low voluntary intake by animals).

Deficiencies of energy and protein are the major nutritional factors limiting productivity of goats in the region. Sufficient ruminal microbial population is crucial to digest and extract the nutrients contained in fibrous feedstuffs. During the dry season, when the protein content of fodder is generally below 6–7%, ruminal microbial growth and digestion are inadequate. This directly hampers protein and energy absorption by the animal. Furthermore, conditions related to an inadequate nitrogen supply for ruminal microbes, such as low microbial protein synthesis and intestinal amino acid absorption, can limit forage intake, further impairing animal performance (i.e., growth, live body weight, and reproduction). During the dry season, supply of extra protein may increase the microbial growth and fiber digestion rate often with increased forage intake, thus improving nutrient absorption for better animal productivity.

Certainly before other supplementation considerations, it is most practical and economical to first correct nitrogen deficiencies for ruminal microbes to increase supplies of energy-yielding substrates and amino acids available for use by the host animal. Nevertheless, in addition to amino acid absorption in the small intestine by microbial action, some proteins are not degraded in the rumen and reach the intestine intact. Furthermore, feedstuffs vary considerably in the proportion of protein not degraded by ruminal microbes, often termed "bypass" protein. It is important to note that both energy and amino acids are required for protein synthesis by growing animals. Thus, high dietary levels of bypass protein may require more energy absorption by correcting the ruminal nitrogen deficiency.

5.1.2 Nutritional Impact on Reproduction of Buck and Doe

Insufficient intake of energy, protein, vitamins, and micro- and/or macrominerals has been associated with suboptimal reproductive performance. Of these nutritional effects on reproduction, energy balance is probably the single most important nutritional factor related to poor reproductive function in animals. Metabolic available energy in buck and doe is used in the following physiological states in order of importance: (i) basal metabolism, (ii) activity, (iii) growth, (iv) energy reserves, (v) pregnancy, (vi) lactation, (vii) additional energy reserves, (viii) estrous cycles and initiation of pregnancy, and (ix) excess energy reserves.

Based on this list of metabolic priorities for energy, reproductive function is compromised because available energy is directed toward meeting minimum energy reserves and milk production. Restricting energy intake during late gestation increases the length of postpartum anestrus and reduces subsequent pregnancy rates. The impact of insufficient energy intake during late gestation cannot be overcome by increasing energy intake post partum. To produce more milk and high-quality meat, goats should be provided leguminous fodders and concentrate mixture in their diet. A balanced leguminous ration with a minimum level of 6% total protein and adequate energy, minerals such as calcium, phosphorus, etc., and vitamins need to be provided to ensure optimum production. Insufficient nutrition leads to delayed reproduction in both buck and doe which includes protein deficiency, energy deficiency, and mineral supplementation.

5.2 Goat Feeding

Proper feeding of goats is as important as feeding of any other farm animals. Lack of attention in feeding may lead to poor performance. The ultimate performance of a goat depends on it being fed during growth, pregnancy, lactation, and dry periods (Devendra 1986). Therefore, a scientific feeding program must be followed.

- Goats are very efficient ruminants which obtain about 80% of their nutrient requirements through grazing and browsing.
- They require higher DM (3–4% of live weight) compared to large animals.
- A higher level of protein is also required by goats for meat production.
- They like tree leaves and bushes and also dry green feeds.
- They have a higher metabolic rate than cattle and therefore, their maintenance need is comparatively higher.
- They require little concentrate mixture if enough forage is available.
- On an average, a milch goat requires 3.5–5.0 kg of fodder per day, of which 1 kg should be dry fodder like dry arhar leaves or pea or gram bhusa or legume hay.
- Due to their smaller stomach capacity, feed may be offered to them 3–4 times a day.
- Immediately after birth, kids must receive colostrum and thereafter kids up to two months must be fed milk at 1/10 of their body weight.
- Kids from two to four months of age should receive creep feed at 450 g daily along with green grass, water, etc.
- Four-month-old dry pregnant goats should be given concentrate mixture at 450 g with 14–16% crude protein and green grass *ad libitum*.
- The milking doe should be provided concentrate mixture at 350 g for each liter of milk.
- During the breeding season, the buck should be given concentrate mixture at 400 g daily with green pasture.
- Water should be provided *ad libitum*.

5.2.1 Nutrient Requirements for Goats (Percent or per kg Feed) (NRC Recommendations)

5.2.1.1 Growing/Finishing Kids

Table 5.1 Small breeds (slaughter weight 20–25 kg).

Body weight (kg)	DM (kg)	DCP (%)	TDN (%)	Ca (%)	P (%)	Carotene (mg)
5.0	0.20	12	70	0.23	0.21	1.0
10	0.45	10	65	0.23	0.21	1.0
15	0.60	7	65	0.21	0.20	1.0
20	0.80	6	60	0.20	0.19	1.0
25	1.00	5.5	60	0.20	0.19	1.0

Ca, calcium; DCP, dicalcium phosphate; DM, dry matter; P, phosphorus; TDN, total digestible nutrients.

Table 5.2 Large breeds (slaughter weight 30–35 kg).

Body weightt (kg)	DM (kg)	DCP (%)	TDN (%)	Ca (%)	P (%)	Carotene (mg)
10	0.40	12	70	0.23	0.21	1.0
15	0.68	10	65	0.21	0.20	1.0
20	0.88	7	65	0.20	0.19	1.0
25	1.10	6	60	0.20	0.19	1.0
30	1.20	5.5	60	0.19	0.18	1.0
35	1.40	5.0	55	0.19	0.18	1.0

Ca, calcium; DCP, dicalcium phosphate; DM, dry matter; P, phosphorus; TDN, total digestible nutrients.

Table 5.3 Doe: nonlactating pregnant (first 15 weeks of gestation).

Body weight (kg)	DM (kg)	DCP (%)	TDN (%)	Ca (%)	P (%)	Carotene (mg)
25	0.75	4.5	50	0.30	0.23	1.5
30	0.90	4.5	50	0.27	0.21	1.5
40	1.00	4.5	50	0.27	0.21	1.5
50	1.25	4.5	50	0.24	0.19	1.5
60	1.50	4.5	50	0.22	0.17	1.5

Ca, calcium; DCP, dicalcium phosphate; DM, dry matter; P, phosphorus; TDN, total digestible nutrients.

Table 5.4 Doe: nonlactating pregnant (last sixweeks of gestation).

Body weight (kg)	DM (kg)	DCP (%)	TDN (%)	Ca (%)	P (%)	Carotene (mg)
25	1.07	5.0	55	0.27	0.21	3.3
30	1.20	5.0	55	0.24	0.20	3.3
40	1.60	5.0	55	0.23	0.17	3.3
50	1.75	4.5	53	0.22	0.16	3.5
60	2.10	4.5	53	0.22	0.16	3.7

Ca, calcium; DCP, dicalcium phosphate; DM, dry matter; P, phosphorus; TDN, total digestible nutrients.

Table 5.5 Doe: lactating (first half of lactation period).

Body weight (kg)	DM (kg)	DCP (%)	TDN (%)	Ca (%)	P (%)	Carotene (mg)
25	1.0	5.0	65	0.30	0.22	2.7
30	1.20	6.0	62	0.29	0.21	2.8
40	1.60	5.0	60	0.28	0.20	3.0
50	2.00	5.0	60	0.27	0.20	3.1
60	2.40	4.5	60	0.27	0.20	3.3

Ca, calcium; DCP, dicalcium phosphate; DM, dry matter; P, phosphorus; TDN, total digestible nutrients.

Table 5.6 Doe: lactating (latter half of lactation period).

Body weight (kg)	DM (kg)	DCP (%)	TDN (%)	Ca (%)	P (%)	Carotene (mg)
25	1.00	5.5	60	0.30	0.22	2.7
30	1.20	5.5	60	0.28	0.20	2.9
40	1.60	5.0	55	0.27	0.19	3.1
50	1.75	4.5	55	0.25	0.18	3.3
60	2.10	4.5	55	0.24	0.17	3.3

Ca, calcium; DCP, dicalcium phosphate; DM, dry matter; P, phosphorus; TDN, total digestible nutrients.

Table 5.7 Bucks (breeding adult and yearling).

Body weight (kg)	DM (kg)	DCP (%)	TDN (%)	Ca (%)	P (%)	Carotene (mg)
30	1.20	6.0	65	0.20	0.18	1.5
40	1.50	5.0	64	0.20	0.18	1.5
50	1.70	5.0	60	0.18	0.16	1.5
60	2.00	4.5	50	0.14	0.15	1.8
70	2.10	4.0	50	0.16	0.14	2.0
80	2.40	4.0	50	0.15	0.13	2.2

Ca, calcium; DCP, dicalcium phosphate; DM, dry matter; P, phosphorus; TDN, total digestible nutrients.

Table 5.8 Cheap concentrate mixture (percentage).

Ingredients	Mix 1	Mix 2	Mix 3	Mix 4	Mix 5
Maize (crushed)	30	20	25	–	30
Wheat bran	20	20	25	25	20
Barley	–	10	5	20	10
Oats	10	10	10	25	–
Gram (crushed)	10	10	15	10	20
Groundnut cake	20	20	10	10	10
Gram/Arharchuni	6	6	6	6	6
Molasses	2	2	2	2	2
Common salt	0.5	0.5	0.5	0.5	0.5
Mineral mixture	1.5	1.5	1.5	1.5	1.5
Vitamin additives	0.5	0.5	0.5	0.5	0.5

Table 5.9 Mineral mixture for goats.

Bone meal, sterilized	42%
Ground limestone chalk	30%
Common salt	20%
Sulfur	5%
Ferrous sulfate	3%
Rate of mixing in concentrate mixture	2%

Table 5.10 Daily nutrient requirements of goats (maintenance, growth, and early gestation).

Body weight (kg)	Daily gain (g)	Dry matter intake kg/d	Dry matter intake % Live weight	Energy ME (Mcal)	Energy TDN (kg)	Protein Total (g)	Protein Digestible (g)	Ca (g)	P (g)
5	0	0.19	3.8	0.35	0.10	15	10	0.5	0.4
	25	0.22	4.4	0.52	0.14	22	15	0.8	0.6
	50	0.21	4.2	0.69	0.19	29	20	1.1	0.9
10	0	0.32	3.2	0.58	0.16	25	17	0.9	0.7
	25	0.36	3.6	0.75	0.21	32	22	1.2	0.9
	50	0.37	3.7	0.92	0.25	39	26	1.5	1.2
	75	0.35	3.5	1.09	0.30	46	31	1.9	1.5
15	0	0.44	2.9	0.79	0.22	33	23	1.2	0.9
	25	0.45	3.0	0.86	0.24	36	25	1.5	1.1
	50	0.50	3.3	1.13	0.31	48	33	1.9	1.4
	75	0.50	3.3	1.30	0.36	55	37	2.2	1.7
20	0	0.54	2.7	0.98	0.27	41	28	1.5	1.1
	50	0.60	3.0	1.32	0.36	56	38	2.1	1.6
	100	0.62	3.1	1.66	0.46	70	48	2.8	2.1
30	0	0.74	2.5	1.33	0.37	56	38	2.1	1.5
	50	0.80	2.7	1.67	0.46	71	48	2.7	2.0
	100	0.48	2.8	2.01	0.56	89	58	3.4	2.5
40	0	0.95	2.4	1.82	0.50	77	53	2.8	2.1
	50	0.98	2.4	2.0	0.55	85	58	3.1	2.4
	100	1.04	2.5	2.34	0.65	99	67	3.8	2.9
50	0	1.08	2.2	1.94	0.54	82	56	3.0	2.3
	50	1.15	2.3	2.28	0.63	96	66	3.6	2.8
	100	1.20	2.4	2.62	0.72	111	75	4.3	3.3
	150	1.24	2.5	2.96	0.82	125	85	5.0	3.8
	Daily requirement of goats (last 8 weeks of gestation and last 8 weeks of lactation)								
20	100	0.72	3.6	2.17	0.60	92	90	3.0	2.1
30	100	0.98	3.3	2.71	0.75	115	100	4.0	2.8
40	120	1.21	3.0	3.05	0.84	129	115	4.0	2.8
50	120	1.43	2.9	3.61	1.00	153	120	5.0	3.5
	First 10 weeks of lactation								
20	0.20	1.13	5.6	2.74	0.76	116	88	4.0	2.8
30	0.20	1.53	5.1	3.29	0.91	139	105	5.0	3.5
40	0.20	1.90	4.8	3.79	1.05	160	121	5.0	3.5
50	0.20	2.25	4.5	4.16	1.15	176	133	6.0	4.2

Dry matter intake calculated as 76.3 g/kg (0.75).

- Twenty percent was added to the ME requirement for first kidding goats (20–25 kg weight) and 10% for second kidding goats (40 kg weight) to compensate for body growth.
- Includes ME requirement for 1 kg 4% fat correction of milk.

Ca, calcium; FCM, fat correction of milk; P, phosphorus; TDN, total digestible nutrients.
Source: Kearl (1982).

5.2.1.2 Nutrition for Newborn Kids

It is crucial that kids nurse their mothers (does) in the first eight hours of their life to consume colostrum at a minimum rate of 10–20% of their body weight, preferably within 2–3 hours after birth. Colostrum contains vitamins and antibodies that will protect kids from many diseases including enterotoxemia and tetanus. Kids born as twins and triplets may need supplementation of colostrum gathered from other high-producing does and even cows. Extra colostrum from high-producing does with dead kids can be stored in the freezer. It is not recommended to thaw frozen colostrum in a microwave or on high heat as this could possibly denature the nutrients. Thawing at room temperature is preferred. Replacement kids should stay with their milking mothers for as long as possible. Early weaning of replacement kids can leave them undernourished and will have a detrimental effect on their production potential (Gipson et al. 2005).

5.2.1.3 Creep Feeding

The size of adult goat varies, ranging from 25 to 50 kg according to breed. Therefore, a wide variation in the birth weight of kids is recorded. Depending upon breed and nutritional status of the pregnant doe, the birth weight of kid ranges from 1 to 5 kg. Thus, to spare goat milk for human consumption and to achieve a faster gain in kids, it is required to provide them a balanced starter feed, known as creep ration, up to 10 weeks of age.

After feeding colostrum and milk to kids for 6–7 days, they should be separated from their dams and kept away on starter ration. They should be allowed restricted suckling 2–3 times a day. Free-choice legume hay, minerals, and drinking water should be made available along with the starter ration. Starter/creep rations should supply about 12–18% dicalcium phosphate and 70–78% total digestible nutrients (TDN) to the kids.

5.2.1.4 Feeding of Dry Goats

Dry goats should be fed enough to rebuild their lost body reserves. Good leguminous fodder can meet their maintenance and other needs. If good fodder is not available then the goat should be fed with 400 g concentrate mixture twice a day, in the morning and evening.

5.2.1.5 Feeding of Growing Kids

After weaning of growing kids, a complete ration providing 9–10% DCP and 60–65% TDN with 20–25% DM from good-quality roughage will meet their requirements. Fodders containing less protein and energy should be balanced with the concentrate mixture (Figure 5.2).

Table 5.11 Starter/creep rations.

Ingredients	Example 1	Example 2	Example 3	Example 4	Example 5
Maize	60	40	20	15	–
Barley/oat	–	23	45	40	40
Groundnut cake	20	20	20	20	22
Fish meal	10	10	10	10	10
Molasses	–	–	–	10	20
Wheat bran	7	7	2	3	5
Mineral mixture	2	2	2	2	2
Common salt	1	1	1	1	1
DCP	**18**	**17**	**17**	**17**	**17**
TDN	**78**	**77**	**75**	**71**	**70**

Notes: 1. Add 150 g TM-5/Aurofac®. 2. Add 25 g Vitablend®/Rovimix®. 3. Linseed cake, sesame cake, kusum cake or mustard cake may be used to replace groundnut cake. 4. Jower, bajra, and ragi may be used to substitute 1/3 cereal grains. 5. Rice bran and small millets may be used to replace wheat bran on a weight basis.
DCP, dicalcium phosphate; TDN, total digestible nutrients.

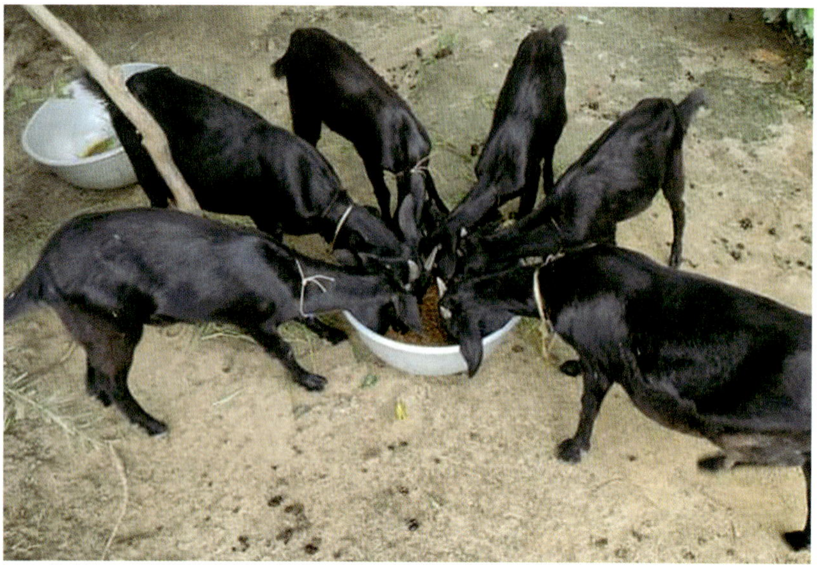

Figure 5.2 Feeding of growing goats.

5.2.1.6 Feeding of Pregnant Goats

The pregnant goat should be fed nutritious food in order to bear the burden of pregnancy and rebuild lost body reserves. For these purposes, the pregnant dry goat should be fed leguminous fodder *ad libitum* and concentrate at a level of 0.5–0.7 kg/day.

5.2.1.7 Feeding of Lactating Goats

When formulating the ration for lactating goats, many factors should be taken into consideration including body weight of goat, milk yield, fat % in milk, stage of lactation, weather conditions, availability of forages, and cost of feed ingredients. In general, 1 kg concentrate mixture over the maintenance will be sufficient for every 3 kg of milk production (Figure 5.3).

The amount of concentrate should be given twice a day in the morning and evening. If green fodder is not available, the goat should be fed good-quality leguminous hay. A few examples of concentrate mixtures for lactating goats are given in Table 5.12.

5.2.1.8 Feeding of Breeding Bucks

Breeding bucks should be fed at a rate of 3.0–3.5% of live weight and the ration should provide 4–6% DCP and 50–60% TDN with sufficient minerals and vitamins to maintain normal health and fertility (Figure 5.4).

Good pasture alone will maintain the buck in good health. If pasture is not available, feed good-quality hay and concentrate up to 0.7 kg/day.

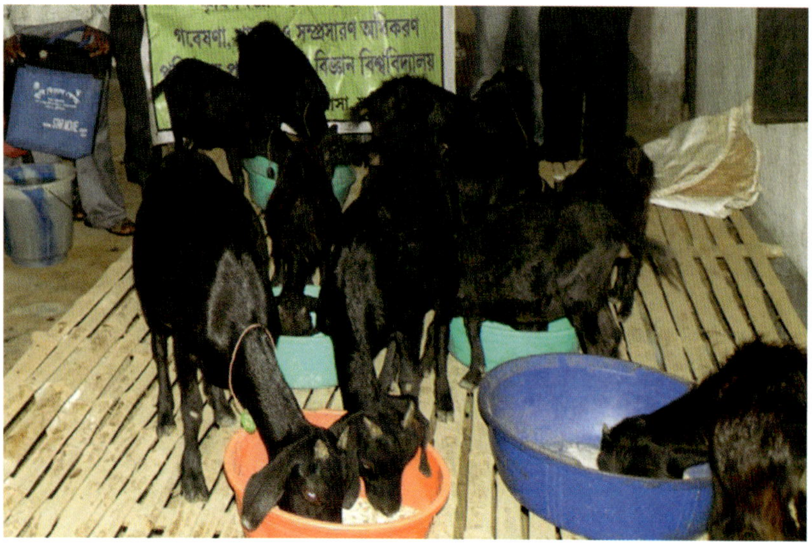

Figure 5.3 Feeding of lactating goats.

Table 5.12 Concentrate mixtures for lactating goats.

Example	Ingredient	Percent in feed
Type I	Gram	15.0
	Maize	37.0
	Groundnut cake	25.0
	Wheat bran	20.0
	Mineral mixture	2.5
	Common salt	0.5
Total		**100**
Type II	Maize	37.0
	Oat	37.0
	Wheat bran	16.0
	Soyabean meal	9.0
	Common salt	1.0
Total		**100**

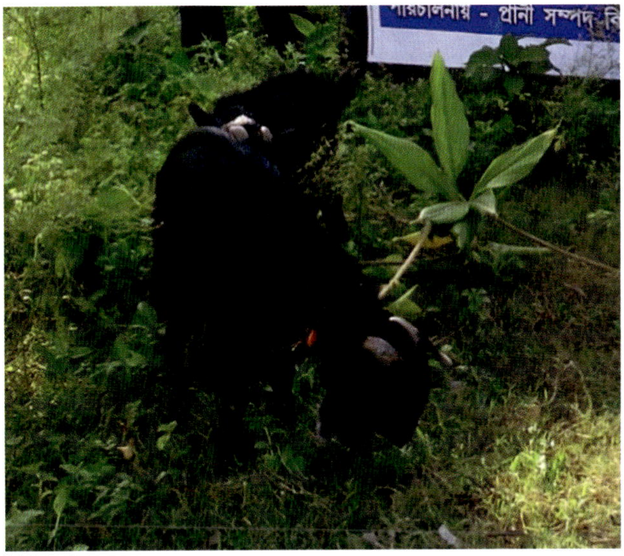

Figure 5.4 Grazing of bucks.

Table 5.13 Nutrient requirements of goats for general feeding practice.

Nutrients	Requirement
Dry matter	• For meat type goat 3–4% • For lactating goat 5–7%
Protein	
I. For maintenance	45–65 g DCP/100 kg live weight
II. For growth	70 g DCP/l milk
Energy	
I. For maintenance	725.8 g SE/100 kg body wt/d
II. For growth	3.0 g SE/g live weight gain
III. For milk production	300 g SE/kg milk
Water	450–700 ml/d for a goat weighing 18–20 kg
DM intake	Total water intake ratio 1 : 4
Minerals	
I. Calcium	147 mg/kg live weight
II. Phosphorus	72 mg/kg live weight

DCP, dicalcium phosphate; DM, dry matter; SE, starch equivalent.

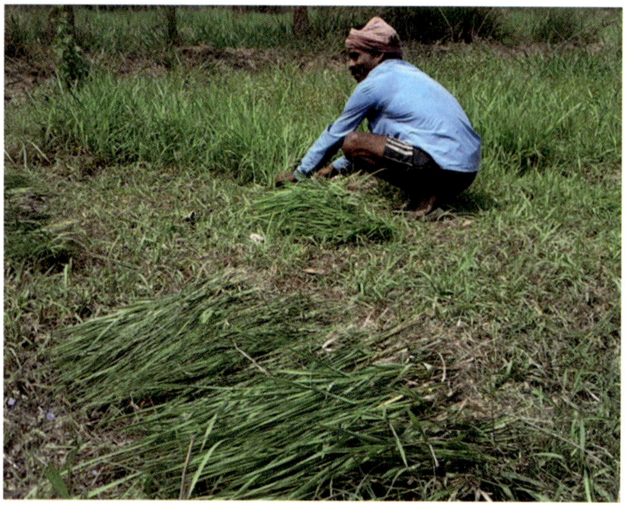

Figure 5.5 Pasture for feeding of goats.

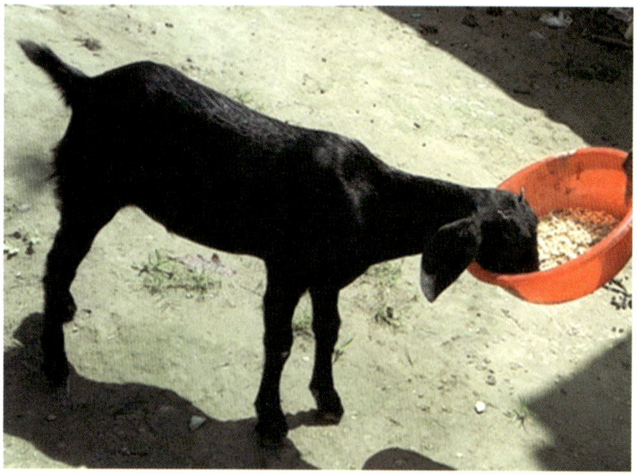

Figure 5.6 Feeding of concentrates.

5.2.2 Essential Nutrients

5.2.2.1 Carbohydrates

Sugars, starches (found in grains), and fiber (cellulose) are carbohydrates that are converted into volatile fatty acids (energy) by rumen flora (beneficial bacteria). The normal goat diet (browse, forbs, and grasses) is high in cellulose and requires digestion by rumen flora to be converted into energy. Fresh pastures and young plants may have highly digestible fiber and provide high energy compared to older plants. Higher energy levels come from lower fiber feeds. Energy is represented as total digestible nutrients (% TDN) in feed analysis reports. It is important to supply half of the goat ration in the form of hay or pasture to avoid high energy-related problems. Maintain at least 12% crude fiber in the diet (Figure 5.5).

Energy requirements for different physiological stages such as maintenance, pregnancy, lactation, and growth vary. The maintenance requirement for energy remains the same for most goats except dairy kids which require 21% higher energy than the average. It is important to feed high-energy rations at the time of breeding, late gestation, and lactation. Lactating does have the highest energy demand.

5.2.2.2 Proteins

Proteins are digested and broken down into amino acids and are eventually absorbed in the small intestine. Those amino acids are building blocks for body proteins (muscles). The rumen plays a major role in breaking down consumed protein into protein through bacterial fermentation. Feeds like forages, hays, pellets (alfalfa), barley, peas (screenings, whole, split), corn, oats, distilled grains, and meals (soybean, canola, cottonseed meals) are common sources of protein for goat rationing (Figure 5.6).

Protein requirements are higher during growth (kids), milk synthesis (lactation), and mohair growth. Producers may need to supplement protein during the year, especially in late fall or winter. It is very important for a commercial goat operation to determine cost-effective rationing as proteins can be an expensive feed ingredient. Good-quality hay does not need much protein supplement for goats. If the hay has about 12–13% protein content then provide ½ lb of protein source in the form of corn, barley, peas, or oats (with 20% protein in total). If the hay is of average quality, add 1 lb of protein as supplement.

5.2.2.3 Minerals and Vitamins

Goats need certain minerals and vitamins for their maintenance as well as proper functioning of their physiological systems. Feeding of fat-soluble vitamins (A, D, E, K) is necessary due to the goat's inability to make these vitamins. Rumen flora can make vitamin B in sufficient quantities for goat metabolism. Vitamin C is essential for the immune system to work efficiently.

Minerals can be classified as macro- and microminerals. Calcium, phosphorus, magnesium, sodium, potassium, sulfur, and chlorides are a few of the macrominerals needed in a goat's diet. Microminerals usually supplemented in goat rations are iron, copper, cobalt, manganese, zinc, iodine, selenium, molybdenum, and others. Feed tags report microminerals as parts per million (ppm) and macrominerals on a percentage basis.

Feeding of calcium and phosphorus (2:1 ratio) is recommended for better structural and bone strength, while other minerals are necessary for other bodily systems. Minerals should be added to the feed, keeping in mind the quality of forages as some forages can be high in some minerals and low in others. Free-choice supply of loose minerals and salts always works well. If the supplied minerals include enough salts then the producer should be careful in providing separate free-choice salt.

It is important to feed enough copper (10–80 ppm) to goats as they have a tendency to be copper deficient. High levels of molybdenum in a goat's diet can easily offset the copper levels in the body. Goats are not sensitive to copper, whereas in sheep even 20 ppm of copper can be very toxic. Selenium (0.1–3 ppm) is another mineral required for goats. Most of the soils in Manitoba are deficient in selenium, and forages from those soils may need selenium supplementation.

5.2.2.4 Fats

Fats can also be a source of energy for goats, which they can obtain while browsing. Excess energy produced by carbohydrates is stored in the form of fat, especially around internal organs. The stored fat in the body is used during high-energy periods, especially lactation. Supplying fats may not be a cost-effective idea for goat production.

5.2.3 Rotational Grazing

Rotational grazing by goats is best accomplished by dividing (fencing) the farm or ranch into a number of smaller pastures and thereafter controlling goat movement to/from these smaller units across time. Stocking density refers to the number of goats per pasture and is usually expressed as number of mature goats/acre. Stocking densities may be adjusted to reflect herd characteristics (age, size, lactation status, etc.) but in any case, for a given pasture size, the greater the stocking density, the shorter the grazing duration required to defoliate the forage down to the proper stubble height (which varies by major types of plants being grazed).

For extensively managed rotation schemes (usually larger acreages, more arid environments, with many species of browse plants), the stocking rate can vary widely; one mature goat/2–5 acres is typical. The duration of grazing for each pasture is primarily dependent on the grazing density chosen; 6–12-week periods are commonly used. The frequency (timing) of grazing pastures can be adjusted to "rest" them for various intervals so as to allow sufficient time for proper recovery of the forage plants. For intensively managed rotation schemes (usually found on relatively small operations in humid areas), stocking rates may average 2–3 mature goats/acre/grazing season. Grazing durations of 5–7 days may be used in conjunction with stocking rates ranging from 10 to 50 goats/acre. Note that grazing frequencies should be chosen to promote the necessary regeneration of plant root reserves.

5.3 Nutritional Health Problems

5.3.1 Pregnancy Toxemia (Ketosis or Twins Disease)

Does with a body condition score of 4 carrying twins or triplets need high-energy diets during their last trimester to cover the needs of the fetuses. Malnutrition during the last weeks of pregnancy leads to the breakdown of body fat reserves that secrete ketones. Due to lack of energy, the glucose concentration in the brain decreases and nervous signs appear. At this stage, the doe seldom survives. Autolysis of dead fetuses produces toxins causing whole-body toxemia of the doe and

Table 5.14 Acceptable quantities of macro- and microminerals in a goat's diet.

Macrominerals (%)		Microminerals (ppm)	
Calcium (Ca)	0.3–0.8	Iron (Fe)	50–1000
Phosphorus (P)	0.25–0.4	Copper (Cu)	10–80
Sodium (Na)	0.2	Cobalt (Co)	0.1–10
Potassium (K)	0.8–2.0	Zinc (Zn)	40–500
Chloride (Cl)	0.2	Manganese (Mn)	0.1–3
Sulfur (S)	0.2–0.32	Selenium (Se)	0.1–3
Magnesium (Mg)	0.18–0.4	Molybdenum (Mo)	0.1–3
		Iodine (I)	0.5–50

eventually death. Treatment is usually unsuccessful. Intravenous injection of 5% dextrose can be helpful in the early stages. However, proper feeding of does during pregnancy can prevent pregnancy toxemia.

5.3.2 Urinary Calculi

Excessive feeding of grain to males, particularly castrated males, can block the urinary tracts with calcium phosphate calculi. The calcium:phosphate ratio in a goat's diet should be 1:1 or 2:1.

5.3.3 Acidosis, Enterotoxemia, and Founder

A sudden increase or excessive feeding of grains can also cause problems for the doe. The lactic acid content of the rumen can increase to toxic levels (acidosis) due to feeding of starches that exceed need. Acidosis can cause vasoconstriction of blood vessels around the hooves (founder). High levels of starches in the diet also speed up bacterial growth in the intestines (enterotoxemia). The rapid bacterial growth means more endotoxin production and death occurs quickly. This usually happens with rapidly growing kids. Vaccination can prevent this disease.

5.3.4 Polioencephalomalacia

This is another disease caused by high levels of grain feeding accompanied by stress. Thiamine deficiency is the main cause of this problem.

5.4 Conclusion

Feeding goats is a science and an art which should be scientifically formulated to gain optimum feed utilization. Feed should be used carefully to avoid wastage and ensure that different types of feeds are used in the context of a balanced feeding system. The proper feeding management of goats with locally available feed resources will improve the production efficiency and profitability of farmers.

References

Birthal, P.S. and Joshi, P.K. (2006). *High Value Agriculture for Accelerated and Equitable Growth: Policy Brief. No. 24*. New Delhi: National Centre for Agricultural Economics and Policy Research.

Devendra, C. (1986). Feeding systems and nutrition of goats and sheep in the tropics. *Proceedings of the Workshop on the Improvement of Small Ruminants in Eastern and Southern Africa*, Nairobi, Kenya.

Gipson, T.A., Merkel, R.C., Hart, S. et al. (2005). *Meat Goat Production Handbook*. Langston, OK: American Institute for Goat Research.

Ingratubun, G.F., Owen, E., Massawe, N.F. et al. (2000). Effect of upgrading small east African goats on feed resource utilization in the Uluguru mountains in Tanzania; a farmers' perspective. *Livestock Research for Rural Development* 12 (3).

Kearl, L.C. (1982). Nutrient requirements of ruminants in developing countries. https://digitalcommons.usu.edu/etd/4183/ (accessed 2 October 2022).

Kumar, S. (2007). Commercial goat farming in India: an emerging agri-business opportunity. *Agricultural Economics Research Review* 20: 503–520.

Livestock Census (2012). *19th Livestock Census – 2012. All India Report*. New Delhi: Department of Animal Husbandry, Dairying and Fisheries.

Merkel, R.C. and Subandriyo Small Ruminant Collaborative Research Support Program (1997). *Sheep and Goat Production Handbook for Southeast Asia*. Davis, CA: Small Ruminant Collaborative Research Support Program, University of California, Davis.

Onim, J.F.M., Fitzhugh, H.A., and Getz, W.R. (1992). Developing and using forages. In: *On-farm Research and Technology for Dual-purpose Goats* (ed. P.P. Semenye and T. Hutchcroft). Kenya: Small Ruminant Collaborative Research Support Program and Kenya Agricultural Research Institute.

Oteino, K., Onim, J.F.M., and Semenye, P.P. (1992). Feed production and utilization by dual purpose goats in smallholder production systems of Western Kenya. In: *The Complementarity of Feed Resources for Animal Production in Africa. Proceedings of the Joint Feed Resources Networks Workshop, Gaborone, Botswana, 4-8 March 1991* (ed. J.E.S. Stares, A.N. Said, and J.A. Kategile). Addis Ababa, Ethiopia: African Feeds Research Network. ILCA (International Livestock Centre for Africa).

Said, A.N. and Tolera, A. (1991). Wheat straw utilization in Ethiopia. In: *Wheat Research in Ethiopia: A Historical Perspective* (ed. H. Gebre-Mariam, D.G. Tanner, and M. Hullaka), 353–378. Addis Ababa: IAR/CIMMYT.

6

Effect of Parasitic Infection on Reproductive Health

Bhupamani Das[1], *Abhinav N. Suthar*[2], *Ankit S. Prajapati*[2], *and Ramesh M. Patel*[3]

[1] Department of Clinics, College of Veterinary Science and Animal Husbandry, Kamdhenu University, Sardarkrushinagar, Gujarat, India
[2] Department of Medicine, College of Veterinary Science and Animal Health, Kamdhenu University, Sardarkrushinagar, Gujarat, India
[3] Department of Clinics, College of Veterinary Science and Animal Health, Kamdhenu University, Sardarkrushinagar, Gujarat, India

6.1 Introduction

Among all species of farm animals, goats have the widest ecological range and have been poor people's most reliable livelihood resource since their domestication during the Neolithic revolution about 10 million years ago. The domestic goat (*Capra aegagrus hircus*) is a widely distributed small ruminant species that is kept mainly for meat, milk, hides, and hair. Unlike cattle and sheep, goats are primarily browsing animals and have an extremely varied plant diet that has allowed them to adapt to many diverse conditions. In goats, reproductive efficiency includes the ability of the doe to ovulate, be mated, conceive with semen from a fertile goat, carry fetuses to term and, finally, produce a live-born kid which will be weaned at the appropriate time at an optimal bodyweight. The term implies efficient conception through active gametes, uninterrupted pregnancy, normal delivery of the newborn, unimpaired lactation of the doe, and survival and optimal growth of the kid.

In goat flocks, increased reproductive efficiency is the cornerstone for profitability so the naturally occurring anestrus period can impede reproductive efficiency. Hence, maintenance of high reproductive performance should be a priority for all involved (Amiridis and Fthenakis 2012).

Although goats are important sources of food and other products, they have not received adequate attention as far as parasitic diseases are concerned. This is due to the underdeveloped environments in which goats are normally raised. Parasitic infections are widespread in goats (Papadopoulos and Fthenakis 2012) and their adverse effects on health, production, and welfare have been repeatedly documented (Taylor et al. 2007). Gastrointestinal parasitic infections are currently among the major challenges in goat health management due to the widespread anthelmintic resistance in many parts of the world (Papadopoulos et al. 2012; Torres-Acosta et al. 2012) which increases potential adverse effects on the health and welfare of animals (Figure 6.1). Helminths and protozoan parasites are common among pregnant animals and produce more severe infections. However, severity depends on various factors, including parasitic load, interpregnancy intervals, nutritional status, poor hygiene and lack of safe drinking water, climate, immunity status, and the presence of coexisting infection. Examples of how reproductive status can influence parasitic infections are as follows: an increase in fecal parasitic output during the periparturient period, the heavier trichostrongylid infections of animals compared to kids from single parities.

This chapter reviews and discusses the interactions between parasitic disease and reproductive efficiency in goats. It is noteworthy that many arthropods can transmit various infective agents, which may negatively affect reproductive health (Figure 6.2).

Elements of Reproduction and Reproductive Diseases of Goats, First Edition. Edited by Tanmoy Rana.

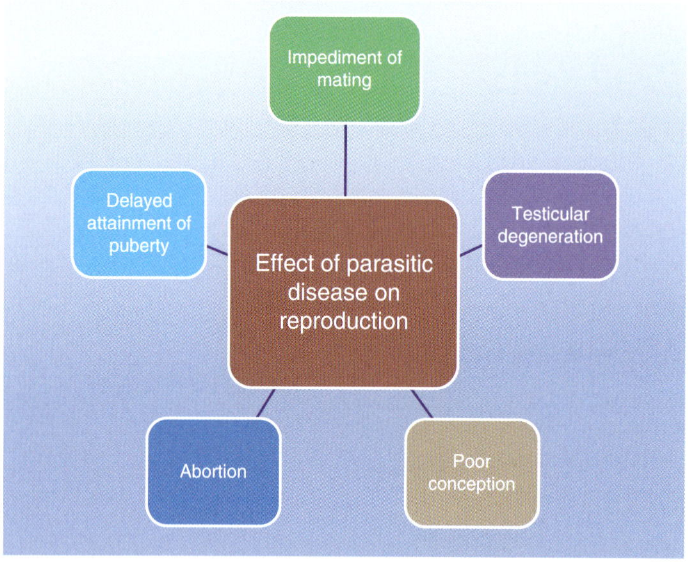

Figure 6.1 Effect of parasitic disease on reproduction in goats.

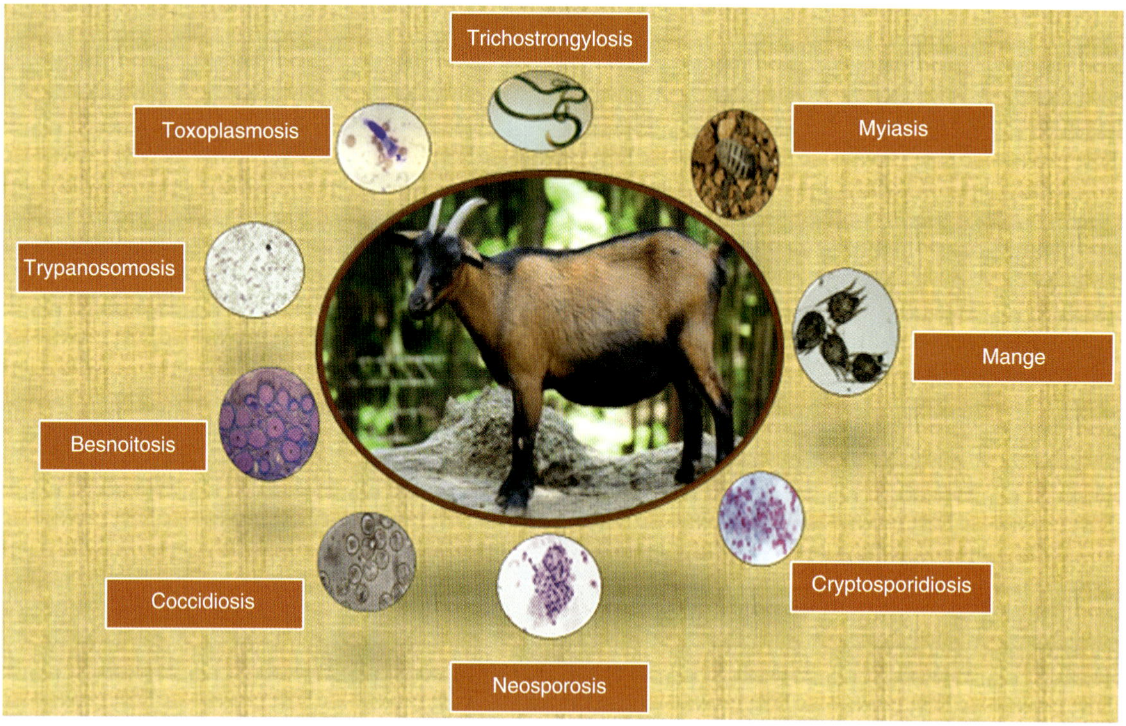

Figure 6.2 Parasitic causes of reproductive failure in goats.

6.2 Parasitic Diseases and Reproductive Health

6.2.1 Gastrointestinal Helminths

Many species of nematode and cestode cause gastritis and enteritis in sheep and goats. The most important of these are *Haemonchus contortus*, *Teladorgia* (*Ostertagia circumcincta*), *Trichostrongylus axei*, intestinal species of *Trichostrongylus*, *Nematodirus* spp., *Bunostomum trigonocephalum*, *Oesophagostomum columbianum*, *Cooperia curticei*, *Strongyloides papillosus*, *Trichuris ovis*, and *Chabertia ovina*.

The principal stomach worm of sheep and goats, *Haemonchus contortus*, causes hyperacute, acute, and chronic infection. The hyperacute disease is characterized by death within one week of heavy infection without significant signs. The acute disease is characterized by severe anemia (Figure 6.3) accompanied by generalized edema, while the chronic stage is accompanied by progressive weight loss. The condition can be fatal when the animal is pregnant or during lactation.

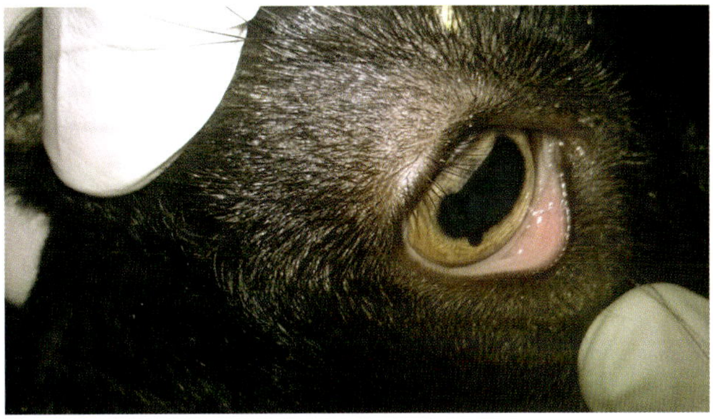

Figure 6.3 Pale mucous membrane in a hemonchosis affected goat. *Source:* Courtesy of Bhupamani Das.

The lesions, pathogenesis, and signs of *O. circumcincta* and *T. axei* infections are characterized by depressed appetite, impaired gastric digestion and reduced use of metabolizable energy and protein. *Ostertagia* is the principal genus involved in the periparturient rise in fecal egg count in small ruminants. Heavy infections may cause diarrhea and depressed milk production. The same type of inhibited development can also be seen with hemonchosis. Adult *B. trigonocephalum* and larvae of *Gaigeria pachysalis*, the hookworm, produce severe anemia by their voracious blood-sucking activity.

The strongyle nematode *Trichostrongylus axei*, also known as the hairworm, is a parasitic roundworm belonging to the family Strongylidae that affects cattle, sheep, goat, and other ruminants. The developing larvae burrow superficially in the crypts of the mucosa and develop to egg-laying adults in 18–21 days. The parasite is responsible for causing delayed attainment of puberty in goats because of the severe clinical presentation, including persistent diarrhea (Figure 6.4) and weight loss. Villous atrophy results in impaired digestion and malabsorption – protein-losing enteropathy.

Nematodirus infection is characterized by sudden onset, loss of bloom, and profuse diarrhea. Heavy infection results passing of large number of eggs through feces. The nodular worm *O. columbianum* also causes heavy diarrhea with excess mucus as well as streaks of blood. As diarrhea progresses, the animal becomes more emaciated and weak. In *Chabertia* infection, severe damage to the mucosa of colon results, along with congestion, ulceration, and small hemorrhages. Likewise, *Strongyloides* spp. penetrate skin and aid penetration of other pathogens, causing foot root. Heavy infection with whipworm is not common but may be seen in very young animals.

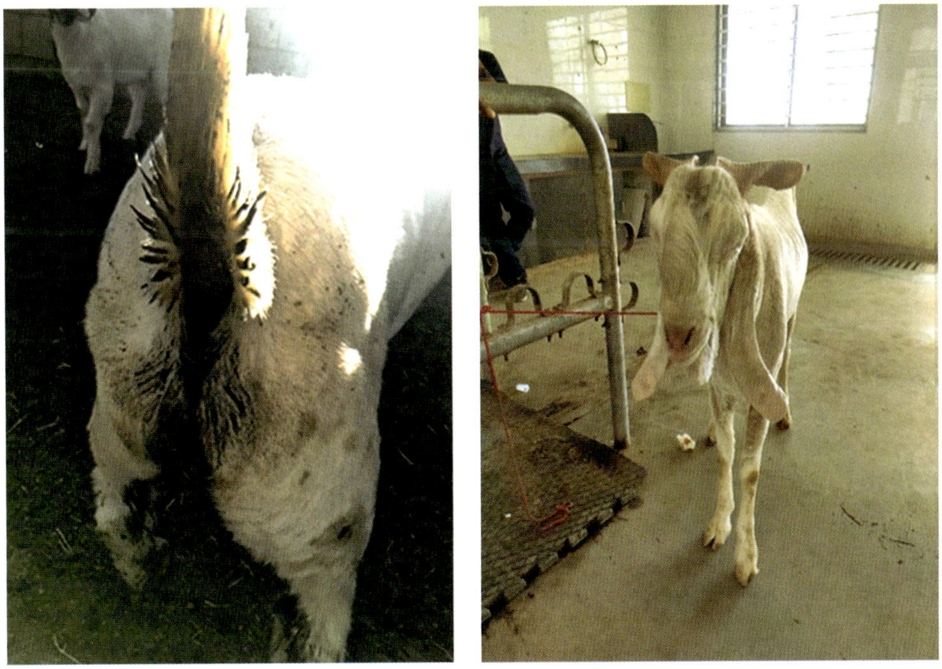

Figure 6.4 Weak and emaciated goat due to diarrhea caused by parasitic nematodes. *Source:* Courtesy of Bhupamani Das.

The pathogenicity of *Moniezia expansa* in small ruminants has long been debated. They are relatively nonpathogenic but heavy infection may cause emaciation and diarrhea.

6.2.1.1 Periparturient Rise During the Prepartum Period

The relaxation of acquired immunity to parasites around kidding and its consequences have been well documented (Armour 1980; Gibbs 1986; Barger 1993). This is manifested with a rise in fecal parasitic output and had initially, for nematode infections, been associated with increased prolactin concentration. Fleming (1993, 1996) investigated the potential role of prolactin and prostaglandin F2 and found that total egg production by *Haemonchus contortus* in infected animals increased after administration of prolactin, but not after administration of prostaglandin F2 to those animals.

Prolactin is a peptide hormone, responsible for initiating and sustaining lactation in animals (Castro et al. 2011). It acts in a cytokine-like manner and is an important regulator of the immune system (Rovensky et al. 1991). Blood concentration of prolactin in pregnant animals starts to increase from the 115th to 135th day of gestation (Banchero et al. 2006). Beasley et al. (2010a,b) reported that in small ruminants experimentally infected with *Trichostrongylus colubriformis*, the rise in fecal egg counts at the end of pregnancy was preceded by a decrease in the immunological competence of the animals, shown by a reduced number of eosinophils and decreased total antibody and IgG-1 titers. The changes coincided with increased prolactin concentration at the end of pregnancy but, nevertheless, the authors considered that they were unrelated to hormonal effects; this confirmed a similar earlier hypothesis by Coop et al. (1977). As significant differences have been reported in blood concentrations of prolactin according to season (Gomez and Lopez 1991), the periparturient rise in fecal parasitic output should have differed in accordance with the time of year. It is possible that a combination of immunological, parasitic, and nutritional factors may determine the whole process.

Parasites can also play a role in increasing metabolic pressure in pregnant animals. The increased parasitic output in the prepartum period has significant consequences for the epidemiology of reproductive diseases.

6.2.1.2 Number of Ovulations and Conception

The period immediately before and around conception is quite vulnerable and during that time, adverse developmental origin of the fetus might occur because of the reduced availability of nutrients to the dam (Fleming et al. 2012). The significance of increased energy available to female animals preconception has been well recognized (Clark 1934; Walkden-Brown et al. 1999; Dobson et al. 2012). Increased energy is provided by giving additional quantities of food, called flushing, which needs a good body condition score of 3–3.5 (Lovatt 2010). This results in a greater number of kids born per female.

Due to long-term energy drainage as proposed by Coop and Kyriazakis (1999) and reduced nutrient availability, parasites can result in delayed estrus development and reduced cycling rate. Ovulation rate also decreases as body condition deteriorates due to chronic conditions caused by the parasite (Dobson et al. 2012). It thus becomes evident that parasitism by the above helminths affects reproductive efficiency in goats.

6.2.1.3 Late Attainment of Puberty

Puberty is the endpoint of a series of events affecting the development of the hypothalamo-pituitary-gonadal axis leading to reproductive competence. From a practical point of view, puberty for females is the age at which the animal can support pregnancy to term. It is a complex mechanism involving primarily the reactivation of the gonadotropin-releasing hormone (GnRH) secretory system, affected by various factors (Senger 2003; Ebling 2005). Management of mating performance of goats requires increased energy availability. Parasitic infections can have an effect on puberty through interaction with energy intake, causing a delay in attaining puberty. Similar results are seen in other animals showing delay in puberty in infected animals compared to noninfected animals (Díaz-Torga et al. 2001).

6.2.1.4 Metabolic Problems

In small ruminants, pregnancy is a metabolically demanding period. During the first 100 days of pregnancy, there is slow fetal growth (Blanchart and Sauvant 1974). During the second month of pregnancy when fetal attachment has been established and placental growth is completed, the fetus can acquire 15–20% of its birth weight; finally, in the last month of pregnancy, an ovine fetus can develop rapidly, to 75–80% birth weight (Fthenakis et al. 2012). Hence, the energy requirement of pregnant does increases as the end of pregnancy approaches. But this situation can be aggravated in cases of heavy parasitic infections, as parasites increase the energy requirements of their host (Coop et al. 1977; Dakkak 1990) as well as protein synthesis by the host, and consequently protein requirements, due to tissue invasion and damage (Solomons 1993).

Helminth parasites such as *Fasciola hepatica* and *Dirocoelium dentriticum* in pregnant small ruminants have led to increased hydroxybutyrate concentration in blood, indicating a potential association between parasitic infections and pregnancy toxemia (Papadopoulos et al. 2013).

6.2.2 Ectoparasites

Ectoparasite infestation is a major veterinary problem affecting livestock in many parts of the world (Hourrigan 1979). Although these infections have been known since very ancient times, they remain an unresolved problem for animal production. They are responsible for severe economic losses to the livestock industry through abortion, reduced milk production, losses in weight and fertility, and poor hide quality in developing and developed countries (Otranto and Stevens 2002; Oryan et al. 2008).

6.2.3 Myiasis

Myiasis is the infestation of living vertebrate animals and humans by the larvae of certain fly species (Diptera), which feed on the host's living or dead tissues and body fluid. Myiasis in goats and sheep is a major animal welfare issue, causing pain and suffering if left untreated, and can result in serious tissue injury, productivity losses, reproduction losses, and death. The oestrid flies that cause myiasis in goats are *Wohlfahrtia magnifica*, *Przhevalskiana silenus*, *Oestrus ovis*, *Lucilia sericata*, and *Chrysomya albiceps* (Otranto and Puccini 2000; Sotiraki and Hall 2012).

The single obligate parasite causing traumatic myiasis of goats and sheep in Europe is the sarcophagid, *Wohlfahrtia magnifica*, Wohlfahrt's wound myiasis fly. All calliphorids and sarcophagids can infest sheep and goats and there is no known predisposition of certain genetic types for different hosts. Other flies include goat warble flies (*Przhevalskiana silenus*) and sheep nasal bot flies (*Oestrus ovis*). *P. sinensis* has been reported mainly from goats (Oryan et al. 2009). In contrast, infection rates and larval burdens with *O. ovis* are generally greater in sheep than goats.

Traumatic and wound myiasis caused by calliphorid and sarcophagid flies is also of great concern for the small ruminant rearer. Due to their continuous attack, especially to the perineal area, these fly larvae can cause severe injury which subsequently leads to impediment to mating. Sotiraki and Hall (2012) reported cases of infestation of the genital region of a goat in northern Morocco with larvae of *Lucilia sericata* and *Chrysomia albiceps* (Figure 6.4). Moreover, traumatic myiasis of the male genitalia of a goat in southern Greece was due to infestation by larvae of *W. magnifica* which clearly indicates the effect of these flies on reproduction.

6.2.3.1 Inability to Mate

Genital myiasis caused by various dipteran insects can lead to vulvar edema and subcutaneous fistulae around the vulva in small ruminants and to partial exteriorizing of the penis and markedly thickened prepuce with subcutaneous fistulae along the tissue (Fragkou et al. 2013). These lesions can impede mating. Development of myiasis lesions takes place during the summer months (Wall 2012). It is also suggested that ectoparasitic infections with intense pruritus could lead to decreased mating activity in animals as they would be busy scratching rather than being sexually active.

6.2.4 Mange

Mange caused by *Chorioptes bovis* infests sheep and goats worldwide. Distribution of lesions is the same as in cattle, with papules and crust on the feet and legs. However, *C. bovis* can cause exudative dermatitis on the lower leg and scrotal lesions. Scrotal mange affects semen quality as constant dermatitis increases the temperature of the scrotal area. Affected animals have decreased reproduction, meat gain, and milk yield. In goats, *Sarcoptes scabei* var. *caprae* is responsible for a generalized skin condition characterized by marked hyperkeratosis. The continuous presence of itching and lesions at the base of tail, perineum, and udder causes generalized disequilibrium and lesions reappear after treatment, which makes the animal unfit for breeding.

Psoroptes cuniculi causes ear mange in goat but also can spread to the head, neck, and body. Infestation of *P. cuniculi* in goats can be common, with 80–90% of a herd infested. Disease can range from subclinical to scaling, crusting, inflammation, alopecia, ear scratching, head shaking and rubbing of ears and head to alleviate irritation. *Demodex caprae* is also relatively common in goats. Nonpruritic papules and nodules develop, especially over the face, neck, shoulder, and sides or udder. The disease is most commonly seen in kids, pregnant does, and dairy goats (Reichard and Thomas 2015).

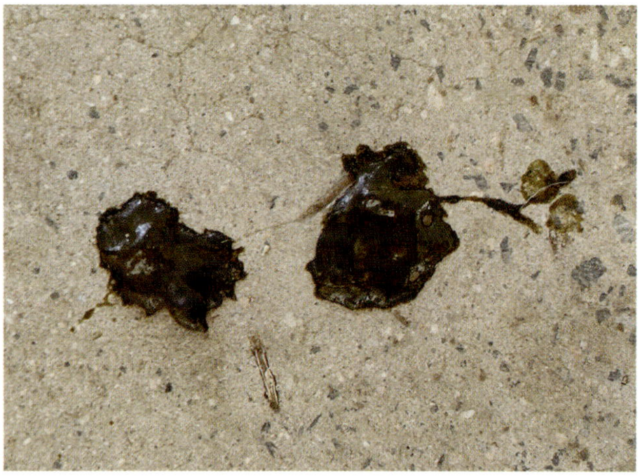

Figure 6.5 Diarrhea due to gastrointestinal helminths in a goat. *Source:* Courtesy of Bhupamani Das.

Ridler et al. (2012) proposed that ectoparasitic diseases can affect the scrotal circumference of small ruminants which has been associated with their reproductive performance (Gouletsou and Fthenakis 2010). Sarasa et al. (2011) reported that sarcoptic mange can cause reduction of testicular mass in Pyrenean ibex (*Capra pyrenaica*). This finding may have implications for goats, in which sarcoptic mange is a significant health problem (Figure 6.5).

6.2.5 Protozoan Disease

6.2.5.1 Besnoitiosis

Caprine besnoitiosis is an economically important parasitic disease caused by a coccidian protozoa belonging to the genus *Besnoitia*. While goats serve as the intermediate hosts of this parasite, the definitive host of *Besnoitia* has not been identified. The route of transmission of this coccidian to the goat is also not clearly understood.

The effect of besnoitiosis on the male goat reproductive system in Iran was studied by Oryan et al. (2008). They found that 18.9% (20/106) of male goats of different ages were infected with *Besnoitia* cysts, with mild to moderate mineralization in the testicles. Elsheikha et al. (2003) suggested that ingestion of infected tissues containing cysts through cannibalism and/or ingesting food or water contaminated with oocysts are the main routes of transmission of *Besnoitia* to intermediate hosts. However, experimental transmission of the bradyzoites of *Besnoitia* species infective to goats to the probable definitive host has not been successful, and the natural form of the definitive host has not been previously reported (Ng'ang'a and Kasigazi 1994). Njenga et al. (1999b) experimentally inoculated *Besnoitia* cysts from naturally chronic infected goats to healthy susceptible ones through subcutaneous inoculation, nasal instillation, intraconjunctival, and oral routes.

Deposition of the parasite in the dermis and deep epidermis of the scrotum initiates exudation and inflammatory cell infiltration from the surrounding capillaries to the infected area. Scrotal dermatitis, fibrosis, thickening, corrugation, and hair loss are the consequences of this long-standing damage (Dubey et al. 2004, 2005). In some cases, adhesion of the tunics of the surrounding tissues, i.e., scrotum, testicle, and epididymis, affects testicular blood circulation, movement, and ventilation which affects spermatogenesis. In addition, degenerating *Besnoitia* cysts that are localized in the testicular or epididymal parenchyma or the seminiferous tubules of the testis and ducts of the epididymis cause further damage and result in orchitis or epididymitis (Oryan and Sadeghi 1997).

Localization of *Besnoitia* cysts in the endothelial layer of small blood vessels and cyst emboli in blood circulation partially or completely occludes these vessels which reduces the blood supply to the affected tissues, leading to further degeneration and necrosis of the parenchymal cells (Cortes et al. 2005). Consequently, spermatogenesis is retarded or completely stopped (Njenga et al. 1999a).

The high morbidity of this disease in goat herds and its significant adverse economic impact on production make it highly significant. Infertility, weight loss, prolonged periods of convalescence, decreasing skin quality, and extensive carcase trimming are the adverse consequences of this parasitic disease in the goat industry. In general, there is little published evidence to corroborate an adverse association between parasitism and testicular function, although available results point in that direction. Possibly, changes in testicular function may lead to reduced production of testosterone, which is a determinant of an animal's sexual behavior and social ranking within a flock (Sekoni et al. 1992; Parkinson 1996).

6.2.6 Trypanosomosis

Reproductive disorders are a common occurrence in human and animal trypanosomosis and include irregular estrus, abortion, and neonatal death and infertility. The duration of the disorders varies considerably depending on the animal species and breed and the species and strain of trypanosomes. Despite the vast amount of research on trypanosomosis in domestic stock and the enormous volume of literature on many aspects of the disease, there is little data on the effect in small ruminants.

Natural infections with *Trypanosoma congolense*, *T. vivax*, *T. brucei*, and *T. evansi* have been described in goats. In goats, the disease produces acute, subacute, chronic, and subclinical forms, and *T. vivax*, *T. congolense*, and *T. evansi* are the most invasive trypanosomes for goats. In goats, due to low parasitemia, the species may also serve as a reservoir of trypanosome infection for other species, including humans in the case of *T. brucei rhodesiense*. *Trypanosoma congolense* (Osaer et al. 1999) infections can adversely affect onset of puberty and age at first lambing by depressing weight gain in affected animals. Sangare et al. (2010) reported azoospermia in *T. congolense* infection. The resulting infertility may have been due to one or a combination of the inadequate gonadotropin priming of follicles (Mcneilley et al. 1981), prevention of the LH surge required for ovulation (Reeves et al. 1971), and low glucose due to poor condition (Muller and Saaraofv 1972). More studies indicate that stress cortisol-hypothalamic opioid peptide and failure of LH surge may reduce fertility (Nanda et al. 1990).

6.2.7 Toxoplasmosis

Toxoplasmosis is an important zoonotic protozoal infection worldwide. All homeothermic animal species may be infected. Infection is generally asymptomatic and chronic in immunocompetent individuals. The main problem in goats affected by this organism is abortions. The organism is a protozoan called *Toxoplasma gondii*. Toxoplasma is a one-celled parasite. It is more of a problem in small ruminants and is a major cause of abortion (Figure 6.6), mummification, stillbirth, and weak kids. The cat is the carrier of the organism. Other susceptible animal species are Australian marsupials, New World monkeys, and meerkats. Goats become infected by eating grass, hay or grain contaminated by cat feces. The organism reaches the reproductive tract via the blood after invasion of the small intestine (Munday and Mason 1979).

Lopes et al. (2009) identified that *T. gondii*-infected animals produce smaller volumes of ejaculate than healthy animals, whilst parasitic agents may be transmitted through semen (De Moraes et al. 2010a,b). Fetopathies and abortions are a significant problem in pregnant does (Buxton and Rodger 2007). Does often become infected through consumption of oocyst-contaminated feed, given to the animals as an energy supplement (Buxton and Rodger 2007). If infection takes place before the 61st–80th day of gestation, embryonic death occurs, followed by absorption or expulsion of small embryos, rarely being noticed. If infection takes place later, up to the 110th–115th day of gestation, then abortion takes place. Finally, if infection takes place after that, congenitally infected lambs are born. In embryos, the organism causes coagulative necrosis in the placental cotyledons, as well as microglial foci, representing an immune response (Buxton and Rodger 2007).

Toxoplasmosis has been well studied around the world, with many scientific references describing all aspects of the disease (Buxton and Rodger 2007; Dubey 2009). If the goat is pregnant at the time of initial infection, *Toxoplasma* commonly invades the placenta and fetus approximately two weeks after initial infection of the doe. Fetuses infected in the first half of pregnancy are more likely to die than fetuses infected in the second half. Previously infected goats are usually resistant to abortion when challenged again by the organism. Symptoms are aborted fetuses, typically in the first half of pregnancy.

Toxoplasmosis is diagnosed by biological, serological or histological methods, or some combination of these. Clinical signs are nonspecific and are not sufficiently characteristic for a definitive diagnosis. Antemortem diagnosis may be accomplished by indirect hemagglutination assay or indirect fluorescent antibody assay (Dubey 2010). For animals other than humans, treatment of toxoplasmosis is seldom warranted.

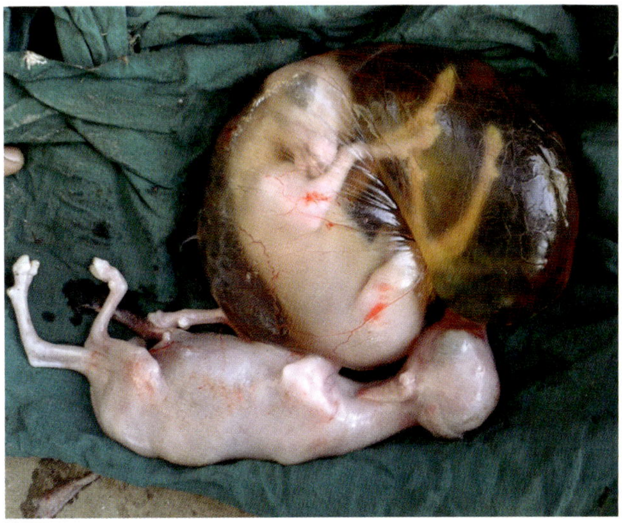

Figure 6.6 Abortion in a goat. *Source:* Courtesy of Prakash M. Chauhan.

6.2.8 Neosporosis

Neospora caninum is currently considered the main cause of abortion and neonatal death in cattle although it is emerging as one of the important reproductive problems in small ruminants. Many facets of the disease are unclear (Dubey and Schares 2011). In the initial literature, the infection was not always associated with abortion (Otter et al. 1997; Chanton-Greutmann et al. 2002), despite evidence showing the abortifacient role of the organism in experimental infections (Buxton et al. 1998, 2001). Progressively, however, reports from various parts of the world have associated the parasite with abortion in small ruminants (Masala et al. 2007; Howe et al. 2012; Moreno et al. 2012), although frequency and the clinical significance of the problem require further evaluation (Dubey and Schares 2011).

The organism establishes itself in the maternal caruncular septum, before crossing to the fetal placental villi. A direct fetopathic effect of the organism has been described to be the cause of abortion (Innes 2007; Gibney et al. 2008). For many years, the etiological diagnosis of abortion caused by *N. caninum* and *T. gondii* was unclear on histopathology due to similarity between the two organisms. However, advanced molecular techniques now enable detection of the parasite DNA and genetic characterization.

There is no approved treatment for neosporosis in small ruminants. Toltazuril and ponazuril are effective *in vitro*, but their efficacy in clinical neosporosis has not been reported. The prognosis is negatively associated with the severity of presenting clinical signs and with delayed treatment.

6.2.9 Cryptosporidiosis

Goat cryptosporidiosis is a parasitic disease with clinical signs showing in the 4–10-day-old kid. The disease is mainly caused by *Cryptosporidium parvum*. It causes high morbidity and mortality, the symptoms of which include lack of appetite and weight loss, yellow diarrhea with bad odor, abdominal pain, and weakness. The rapid loss of nutrients and fluid during diarrhea results in severe dehydration, ultimately leading to death (Pavlovic et al. 2010). Hence, it can be said that cryptosporidiosis is an indirect cause of reproductive failure due to high mortality in kids.

The source of cryptosporidial infection is oocysts that are fully sporulated and infective when excreted in feces. Large numbers are excreted during the patent period, resulting in heavy environmental contamination. Case fatality rates in cryptosporidiosis are generally low unless the condition is complicated by other factors (e.g., concurrent infections, energy deficits from inadequate intake of colostrum and milk, chilling from adverse weather conditions). A periparturient rise in the excretion of oocysts occurs in animals.

Oocysts are resistant to most disinfectants and can survive for several months in cool and moist conditions. Oocyst infectivity can be destroyed by ammonia, formalin, freeze-drying, and exposure to temperatures <32 °F (0 °C) or >149 °F (65 °C). Ammonium hydroxide, hydrogen peroxide, chlorine dioxide, 10% formol saline, and 5% ammonia are effective in destroying oocyst infectivity. Infectivity in calf feces is reduced after 1–4 days of drying.

Concurrent infections with other enteric pathogens, especially rotavirus and coronavirus, are common, and epidemiological studies suggest that diarrhea is more severe in mixed infections. Immunocompromised animals are more susceptible to clinical disease than immunocompetent animals, but the relationship between disease and failure of passive transfer of colostral immunoglobulins is not clear. Age-related resistance, unrelated to prior exposure, is seen in lambs but not calves. Infection results in production of parasite-specific antibodies, but both cell-mediated and humoral antibody are important in protection, as well as local antibody in the gut of neonates.

Diagnosis of this disease is based on detection of oocysts by examination of fecal smears with Ziehl–Neelsen stains, fecal flotation technique, and ELISA. Sheather's flotation sedimentation staining is the most sensitive (83%) and specific (99%) with relatively low cost per test. Currently, there are no currently licensed drugs available for *C. parvum* infection in food animals. However, paromomycin sulfate proved successful in preventing natural disease in a controlled field trial in goat kids.

6.2.10 Coccidiosis

Coccidiosis in goats is a complex, multifactorial problem. The disease depends on the various stresses to which the individual is subjected, the environment, the extent of contamination, and exposure to infection. It is a common cause of diarrhea in goat kid more than four weeks old. The disease occurs worldwide.

Seventeen species have been identified, including *E. alijevi*, *E. aspheronica*, *E. arloingi*, *E. caprina*, *E. caprovina*, *E. christenseni*, *E. gilruthi*, *E. hircee*, *E. jolchijevi*, and *E. ninakohlyakimovae*. Often several species infect the goat kid at the same time. Coccidia go through a complex lifecycle in the intestinal cells of goats. In the process, they produce large numbers of oocysts in the feces and rapid growth in intestinal cells while invading them. This may cause diarrhea and other signs of the disease. The disease starts shortly after weaning because of the stress of being suddenly separated from the dam. The scarring and damage to the intestinal lining following treatment may result in permanently unthrifty and stunted growth and these factors indirectly affect reproductive health by delaying attainment of puberty.

Goats develop some (not total) immunity to coccidiosis, with a need to achieve a balance between sufficient oocyst exposures to allow immunity without causing clinical disease. Wild goats rarely suffer from coccidiosis because they are browsers and feed over large areas. The nomadic existence of farmed goats in some countries means kids are exposed to small numbers of oocysts mainly produced by the adults. This allows a protective immunity to be built up and to be maintained without illness. However, when on a farm, especially when used for indoor goat milk production, young goats with high coccidial exposure may develop clinical signs.

In most countries, few or no treatments are licensed for goats, although products licensed for cattle and sheep are often available. Water and feed intake is usually decreased in unwell kids, so it is best to treat by drenching rather than rely on including any medicine in the drinking water or feed. It may be necessary to use electrolyte and nutritional solutions to feed unwell kids.

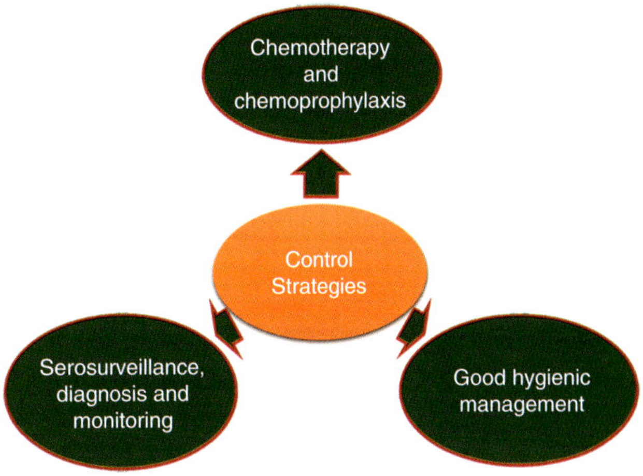

Figure 6.7 Strategies for control of parasitic diseases in goats.

6.3 Conclusion

Many factors are involved in male and female infertility of small ruminants, especially goats. Infectious parasitic diseases are one of the most important causes of infertility in both sexes. Protozoan parasitic infections may be an important risk factor for infertility, although the importance of these parasites is not clearly understood, especially in developing countries like India. Therefore, further investigations should be performed to study the relationship between parasitic infections and reproductive failure in goats. Moreover, via diagnostic techniques, surveillance, and regular monitoring of parasitic disease, the disease burden can be determined and good hygiene and chemotherapeutic agents can also be employed for better management of parasitic disease in goats (Figure 6.7).

References

Amiridis, G.S. and Fthenakis, G. (2012). Reproductive health management of sheep and goats. *Animal Reproductive Science* 130: 125.

Armour, J. (1980). Epidemiology of helminth disease in farm animals. *Veterinary Parasitology* 6: 7–46.

Banchero, G.E., Perez Clariget, R., Bencini, R. et al. (2006). Endocrine and metabolic factors involved in the effect of nutrition on the production of colostrum in female sheep. *Reproduction Nutrition Development* 46: 447–460.

Barger, I.A. (1993). Influence of sex and reproductive status on susceptibility of ruminants to nematode parasitism. *International Journal of Parasitology* 23: 463–469.

Beasley, A.M., Kahn, L.P., and Windon, R.G. (2010a). The periparturient relaxation of immunity in Merino ewes infected with *Trichostrongylus colubriformis*: endocrine and body compositional responses. *Veterinary Parasitology* 168: 51–59.

Beasley, A.M., Kahn, L.P., and Windon, R.G. (2010b). The periparturient relaxation of immunity in Merino ewes infected with Trichostrongylus colubriformis: parasitological and immunological responses. *Veterinary Parasitology* 168: 60–67.

Blanchart, D. and Sauvant, D. (1974). Consequences of pregnancy on the evolution of lactation. *Conference 'Information Day on the Feeding of the Dairy Goat'*, Paris, France (13 June), 76–87.

Buxton, D. and Rodger, S.M. (2007). Toxoplasmosis and neosporosis. In: *Diseases of Sheep*, 4e (ed. I.D. Aitken), 112–119. Oxford: Blackwell.

Buxton, D., Maley, S.W., Wright, S. et al. (1998). The pathogenesis of experimental neosporosis in pregnant sheep. *Journal of Comparative Pathology* 118: 267–279.

Buxton, D., Wright, S., Maley, S.W. et al. (2001). Immunity to experimental neosporosis in pregnant sheep. *Parasite Immunology* 23: 85–91.

Castro, N., Capote, J., Bruckmaier, R.M., and Arguello, A. (2011). Management effects on colostrogenesis in small ruminants: a review. *Journal of Applied Animal Science* 39: 85–93.

Chanton-Greutmann, H., Thoma, R., Corboz, L. et al. (2002). Abortion in small ruminants in Switzerland: investigations during two lambing seasons (1996–1998) with special regard to chlamydial abortions. *Schweizer Archiv für Tierheilkunde* 144: 483–492.

Clark, R.T. (1934). Studies of reproduction in sheep. 1. The ovulation rate of the ewe as affected by the plane of nutrition. *Anatomical Record* 60: 125–134.

Coop, R.L. and Kyriazakis, I. (1999). Nutrition–parasite interaction. *Veterinary Parasitology* 84: 187–204.

Coop, R.L., Sykes, A.R., and Angus, K.W. (1977). The effect of a daily intake of *Ostertagia circumcincta* larvae on body weight, food intake and concentration of serum constituents in sheep. *Research in Veterinary Science* 23: 76–83.

Cortes, H., Leitao, A., Vidal, R. et al. (2005). Besnoitiosis in bulls in Portugal. *Veterinary Record* 27: 262–264.

Dakkak, A. (1990). Gastrointestinal strongylosis and malabsorption of nutrients. *Annales de Parasitologie Humaine et Comparée* 65 (Suppl. 1): 73–76.

De Moraes, E.P., Batista, A.M., Faria, E.B. et al. (2010a). Experimental infection by Toxoplasma gondii using contaminated semen containing different doses of tachyzoites in sheep. *Veterinary Parasitology* 170: 318–322.

De Moraes, E.P., Freitas, A.C., Gomes-Filho, M.A. et al. (2010b). Characterization of reproductive disorders in ewes given an intrauterine dose of Toxoplasma gondii tachyzoites during the intrauterine insemination. *Animal Reproduction Science* 122: 36–41.

Díaz-Torga, G.S., Mejia, M.E., González-Iglesias, A. et al. (2001). Metabolic cues for puberty onset in free grazing Holstein heifers naturally infected with nematodes. *Theriogenology* 56: 111–122.

Dobson, H., Fergani, C., Routly, J.E., and Smith, R.F. (2012). Effects of stress on reproduction in ewes. *Animal Reproduction Science* 130: 135–140.

Dubey, J.P. (2009). Toxoplasmosis in sheep – the last 20 years. *Veterinary Parasitology* 163: 1–14.

Dubey, J.P. (2010). *Toxoplasmosis of Animals and Humans*, 2e. Boca Raton: CRC Press.

Dubey, J.P. and Schares, G. (2011). Neosporosis in animals – the last five years. *Veterinary Parasitology* 180: 90–108.

Dubey, J.P., Sreekumar, C., Rosenthal, B.M. et al. (2004). Redescription of Besnoitia tarandi (Protozoa: Apicomplexa) from the reindeer (*Rangifer tarandus*). *International Journal of Parasitology* 34: 1273–1287.

Dubey, J.P., Sreekumar, C., Donovan, T. et al. (2005). Redescription of *Besnoitia besnoitti* (Protozoa: Apicomplexa) from the donkey (Equus asinus). *International Journal of Parasitology* 35: 569–572.

Ebling, J.F.P. (2005). The neuroendocrine timing of puberty. *Reproduction* 129: 675–683.

Elsheikha, H.M., Mansfield, L.S., Fitzgerald, S.D., and Saeed, M.A. (2003). Prevalence and tissue distribution of *Besnoitia darlingi* cysts in the Virginia opossum (Didelphis Virginian) in Michigan. *Veterinary Parasitology* 115: 321–327.

Fleming, M.W. (1993). Acute or chronic administration of prolactin alters ovine infections of Haemonchus contortus. *Veterinary Parasitology* 50: 109–115.

Fleming, M.W. (1996). Effects of exogenous reproductive hormones on Haemonchus contortus populations in lambs. *Journal of Helminthology Society of Washington* 64: 269–274.

Fleming, T.P., Velazquez, M.A., Eckert, J.J. et al. (2012). Nutrition of females during the peri-conception period and effects on foetal programming and health of offspring. *Animal Reproduction Science* 130: 193–197.

Fragkou, I.A., Papadopoulos, E., Stavrakaki, S. et al. (2013). Observations in ovine myiosis in Greece, with special reference to clinical findings and treatment of genital myiosis. *Small Ruminant Research* 110: 104–107.

Fthenakis, G.C., Arsenos, G., Brozos, C. et al. (2012). Health management of ewes during pregnancy. *Animal Reproduction Science* 130: 198–212.

Gibbs, H.C. (1986). Hypobiosis and the periparturient rise in sheep. *Veterinary Clinics of North America: Food Animal Practice* 2: 345–353.

Gibney, E.H., Kipar, A., Rosbottom, A. et al. (2008). The extent of parasite-associated necrosis in the placenta and foetal tissues of cattle following *Neospora caninum* infection in early and late gestation correlates with foetal death. *International Journal of Parasitology* 38: 579–588.

Gomez, B.A. and Lopez, S.A. (1991). Effect of season on plasma concentrations of prolactin and cortisol in pregnant, non-pregnant and lactating ewes. *Animal Reproduction Science* 26: 251–268.

Gouletsou, P.G. and Fthenakis, G.C. (2010). Clinical evaluation of reproductive ability of rams. *Small Ruminant Research* 92: 51180–51183.

Hourrigan, J.W. (1979). Spread and detection of psoroptic scabies of cattle in United States. *Journal of the American Veterinary Association* 175: 1278–1280.

Howe, L., Collett, M.G., Pattison, R.S. et al. (2012). Potential involvement of Neospora caninum in naturally occurring ovine abortions in New Zealand. *Veterinary Parasitology* 185: 64–71.

Innes, E.A. (2007). The host–parasite relationship in pregnant cattle infected with Neospora caninum. *Parasitology* 134: 1903–1910.

Lopes, W.D., da Costa, A.J., Santana, L.F. et al. (2009). Aspects of toxoplasma infection on the reproductive system of experimentally infected rams (Ovis aries). *Journal of Parasitology Research* 2009: 602803.

Lovatt, F. (2010). Clinical examination of sheep. *Small Ruminant Research* 92: 72–77.

Masala, G., Porcu, R., Daga, C. et al. (2007). Detection of pathogens in ovine and caprine abortion samples from Sardinia, Italy, by PCR. *Journal of Veterinary Diagnostic Investigation* 19: 96–98.

Mcneilley, A.S., Moraq-Hunrrr, B., and Fraser, H.M. (1981). Inadequate corpus luteum function after the induction of ovulation in anoestrus ewe by LH-RH agonist. *Journal of Reproduction and Fertility* 63: 137–144.

Moreno, B., Collantes-Fernández, E., Villa, A. et al. (2012). Occurrence of Neospora caninum and Toxoplasma gondii infections in ovine and caprine abortions. *Veterinary Parasitology* 187: 312–318.

Muller, H.E. and Saaraofv, M. (1972). The pathogenic role of Trichomonas foetus neuraminidase. *Zentral-blatt fur Hygiene* 222: 275–279.

Munday, B.L. and Mason, R.W. (1979). Toxoplasmosis as a cause of perinatal death in goats. *Australian Veterinary Journal* 55 (10): 485–487.

Nanda, A.S., Ward, W.R., and Donson, H. (1990). Naloxone antagonizes the morphine suppression of the oestradiol-induced surge of luteinising hormone in dairy cows. *Animal Production Science* 22: 289–296.

Ng'ang'a, C.J. and Kasigazi, S. (1994). Caprine besnoitiosis: studies on the experimental intermediate hosts and the role of the domestic cat in transmission. *Veterinary Parasitology* 52: 207–210.

Njenga, M.J., Munyua, S.J., Mutiga, E.R. et al. (1999a). Semen characteristics of goats with subacute, acute and chronic besnoitiosis. *Journal of the South African Veterinary Association* 70: 18–20.

Njenga, M.J., Kang'ethe, E.K.M., Bwangamoi, O. et al. (1999b). Experimental transmission of *Besnoitia caprae* in goats. *Journal of the South African Veterinary Association* 70: 151–163.

Oryan, A. and Sadeghi, M.J. (1997). An epizootic of Besnoitiosis in goats in Fars Province of Iran. *Veterinary Research Communication* 21: 559–570.

Oryan, A., Kafi, M., and Morgan-Azghadi, N. (2008). Besnoitiosis of the reproductive tract of male goats. *Comparative Clinical Pathology* 17: 185–191.

Oryan, A., Razavi, S.M., and Bahrami, S. (2009). Occurrence and biology of goat warblefly infestation by *Przhevalskiana silenus* (Diptera, Oesterae) in Iran. *Veterinary Parasitology* 166: 178–181.

Osaer, S., Goossens, B., Kora, S., and Jeffcoate, I. (1999). Effects of *Trypanosoma congolense* infection and diet on puberty, age at first lambing and haematology changes in Djallonké ewe lambs. *Veterinary Parasitology* 80: 215–230.

Otranto, D. and Puccini, V. (2000). Further evidence on the internal life cycle of *Przhevalskiana silenus* (Diptera, Oestera). *Veterinary Parasitology* 88: 321–328.

Otranto, D. and Stevens, J.R. (2002). Molecular approaches to the study of myasis causing larvae. *International Journal of Parasitology* 32: 1345–1360.

Otter, A., Wilson, B.W., Scholes, S.F. et al. (1997). Results of a survey to determine whether Neospora is a significant cause of ovine abortion in England and Wales. *Veterinary Record* 140: 175–177.

Papadopoulos, E. and Fthenakis, G.C. (2012). Update on parasitic diseases of sheep. *Veterinary Parasitology* 189 (1): 1–136.

Papadopoulos, E., Gallidis, E., and Ptochos, S. (2012). Anthelmintic resistance in sheep in Europe: a selected review. *Veterinary Parasitology* 189: 85–88.

Papadopoulos, E., Mavrogianni, V.S., Mitsoura, A. et al. (2013). Potential association between trematode infections and development of pregnancy toxaemia in sheep. *Helminthologia* 50: 161–166.

Parkinson, T.J. (1996). Normal reproduction in male animals. In: *Veterinary Reproduction & Obstetrics*, 7e (ed. G.H. Arthur, D.E. Noakes, H. Pearson, and T.J. Parkinson), 551–571. London: Saunders.

Pavlovic, I., Ivanovic, S., Jujovic, M., and Tomic, Z. (2010). Goat cryptosporidiosis and its importance at goat production pathology. *Biotechnology in Animal Husbandry* 26 (3–4): 187–192.

Reeves, J.J., Apdmura, A., and Scallt, A.V. (1971). Pituitary responsiveness to purified luteinizing hormone-releasing hormone (LH-RH) at various stages of the oestrous cycle in sheep. *Journal of Animal Science* 32: 124–126.

Reichard, M.V. and Thomas, J.E. (2015). *Mange in Sheep and Goats. MSD Veterinary Manual.* Rahway, NJ: Merck & Co., Inc.

Ridler, A.L., Smith, S.L., and West, D.M. (2012). Ram and buck management. *Animal Reproduction Science* 130: 180–183.

Rovensky, J., Vigas, M., Marek, J. et al. (1991). Evidence for immunomodulatory properties of prolactin in selected in vitro and in vivo situations. *International Journal of Immunopharmacology* 13: 267–272.

Sangare, M., Bengaly, Z., Marichatou, H. et al. (2010). Influence of an experimental *Trypanosoma congolense* infection on the reproductive function of Djallonke and Sahelian rams in subhumid zone. *Biotechnology, Agronomy, Society and Environment* 14: 409–416.

Sarasa, M., Serrano, E., Soriguer, R.C. et al. (2011). Negative effect of the arthropod parasite, Sarcoptes scabiei, on testes mass in Iberian ibex, Capra pyrenaica. *Veterinary Parasitology* 175: 306–312.

Sekoni, V.O., Sanusi, A., Abatan, M.O.I. et al. (1992). Loss of libido and terminal sterility in a Friesian bull naturally infected with *Besnoitia besnoiti* in Northern Nigeria, a case report. *Theriogenology* 37: 533–549.

Senger, P.L. (2003). Puberty. In: *Pathways to Pregnancy and Parturition* (ed. P.L. Senger), 128–143. Redmond, OR: Current Conceptions Inc.

Solomons, N.W. (1993). Pathways to the impairment of human nutritional status by gastrointestinal pathogens. *Parasitology* 107: S19–S35.

Sotiraki, S. and Hall, M.J. (2012). A review of comparative aspects of myiasis in goats and sheep in Europe. *Small Ruminant Research* 103 (1): 75–83.

Taylor, M.A., Coop, R.L., and Wall, R.L. (2007). *Veterinary Parasitology*, 3e, 874. Oxford: Blackwell.

Torres-Acosta, J.F.J., Mendoza-de-Gives, P., Aguilar-Caballero, A.J., and CuéllarOrdaz, J.A. (2012). Anthelmintic resistance in sheep farms: update of the situation in the American continent. *Veterinary Parasitology* 189: 89–96.

Walkden-Brown, S.W., Martin, G.B., and Restall, B.J. (1999). Role of male-female interaction in regulating reproduction in sheep and goats. *Journal of Reproduction and Fertility* 54: 243–257.

Wall, R. (2012). Ovine cutaneous myiasis: effects on production and control. *Veterinary Parasitology* 189: 44–51.

7

Seasonal Perspectives on Reproduction of the Buck and Doe

Felix Uchenna Samuel[1,2], *Khumran Mada*[3], *Peter Ibrahim Rekwot*[3], *and Aliyu Abdullahi Mohammed*[4]

[1] *National Animal Production Research Institute, Faculty of Veterinary Medicine, Ahmadu Bello University, Zaria, Nigeria*
[2] *Department of Food and Animal Science, Alabama A&M University, Normal, USA*
[3] *Faculty of Veterinary Medicine, Ahmadu Bello University, Zaria, Nigeria*
[4] *Department of Animal Sciences, Usman Danfodio University, Sokoto, Nigeria*

7.1 Introduction

Mammals have evolved diverse physiological strategies to synchronize their reproductive seasons with specific periods of the year, ensuring the birth of offspring during times of ample food availability and favorable temperature conditions. As a result, species influenced by seasonal environmental changes exhibit distinct periods that either facilitate or hinder reproduction, influencing gametogenesis and the display of reproductive behaviors (Burtschell et al. 2023).

The crucial factor governing this physiological phenomenon is the annual photoperiod cycle. However, certain modulating factors also come into play, including environmental temperature, the nutritional state of the animals, social interactions, date of birth, and the lactation period. These factors can exert an influence on the overall reproductive pattern of mammals, further shaping their ability to adapt and thrive in their respective environments (Rosa and Bryant 2003; Goel and Kharche 2009).

The photic stimulus captured by the retina determines, through the retina-hypothalamus axis, whether or not the biosynthetic pathway of the hormone melatonin is activated (Aubry and Williams 2022). Among the various functions of this neurotransmitter, an important aspect is regulation of gonadotropin-releasing hormone (GnRH), which induces release of follicle-stimulating (FSH) and luteinizing (LH) hormones. The neurons that synthesize and release GnRH are found in the hypothalamus, but recent studies show the participation of other molecules, such as kisspeptins, in the regulation of the hypothalamic-pituitary-gonadal (HPG) axis (Saleh and Holtz 2022).

Gametogenesis and the synthesis of sex hormones, which play a crucial role in the development of phenotypic characteristics and secondary sexual manifestations, are activated by FSH and LH (Ramya et al. 2023).

Certain species, including small ruminants, buffaloes, and horses, are classified as seasonally polyestric, and their reproductive processes are sensitive to changes in photoperiod. The synthesis and release of sex hormones are regulated by the adenohypophysis in response to variations in luminosity throughout the year. In contrast, continuous polyestric species, such as cattle, are not influenced by luminosity, and the production and secretion of gonadotropins occur steadily, following the period of the estrous cycle (Inskeep 2011).

Species that exhibit an increase in reproductive activity in response to a decrease in photoperiod and a rise in melatonin concentration in the bloodstream are categorized as short-day species. Examples include goats and certain breeds of sheep and buffalo. On the other hand, species like horses, whose reproductive activities are stimulated by an increase in light intensity and a consequent decrease in melatonin concentration, are referred to as long-day species (Contreras-Correa et al. 2023).

These distinct reproductive strategies reflect the remarkable adaptability of different species to their environments and the intricate interplay between photoperiod, melatonin, and sex hormones in regulating their reproductive cycles.

In goats, seasonal patterns in sexual behavior and reproduction are common and influenced by several factors such as breed, location, and climate. The timing and duration of the breeding season are particularly affected by latitude, physiological stage, presence of males, breeding system, and, most notably, photoperiod. The regulation of reproductive patterns through

Elements of Reproduction and Reproductive Diseases of Goats, First Edition. Edited by Tanmoy Rana.

photoperiod is mediated by melatonin secretions from the pineal gland during periods of darkness. Melatonin influences the generation of GnRH pulses and the feedback loop involving the hypothalamus, pituitary gland, and gonads (Veliz-Deras et al. 2023).

At higher latitudes, female goats experience two distinct periods throughout the year: a deep anestrus phase characterized by the absence of estrous behavior and ovulation, and a breeding period during which both estrous behavior and cyclic ovarian activity are observed. In temperate regions, the breeding season typically occurs in fall and winter. However, the specific timing of the breeding season varies between regions; for example, in France, it spans from September to March whereas in Australia, it occurs from April to August, centered around the winter solstice. As latitude increases, the breeding season tends to be limited to autumn, resulting in most kids being born in spring (Cann et al. 2023).

In lower latitudes, such as equatorial, tropical, and subtropical regions, day length changes are less pronounced, leading to less marked seasonality in reproduction. Many local goat breeds in these areas have the ability to breed throughout the year, with shorter postpartum anestrus periods. Nevertheless, environmental factors, particularly forage availability and temperature changes, significantly influence this seasonality. Inadequate nutrition can lead to prolonged anestrous and anovulatory periods, reduced fertility and prolificacy, and increased spring mortality rates. The timing of mating and kidding in these regions often depends on climatic and management factors, with some areas experiencing estrus induction due to monsoon rains, causing kidding to be delayed until after the monsoon season. Despite year-round kidding potential in tropical goats, a peak period still occurs in spring, and fewer kidding events are observed in autumn. These variations highlight the remarkable adaptability of goats to diverse environmental conditions and the intricate interplay of photoperiod and other factors that govern their reproductive cycles (Cann et al. 2023).

7.2 Influence of Photoperiod on Reproductive Seasonality

The reproductive seasonality in goats and sheep is greatly influenced by photoperiod, which refers to the duration of light in a given location and is directly related to the latitude and season of the year. Animals living in regions with wide variations in photoperiod throughout the year often exhibit seasonality in their physiological, behavioral, and morphological functions (Figure 7.1) (Mandal et al. 2022).

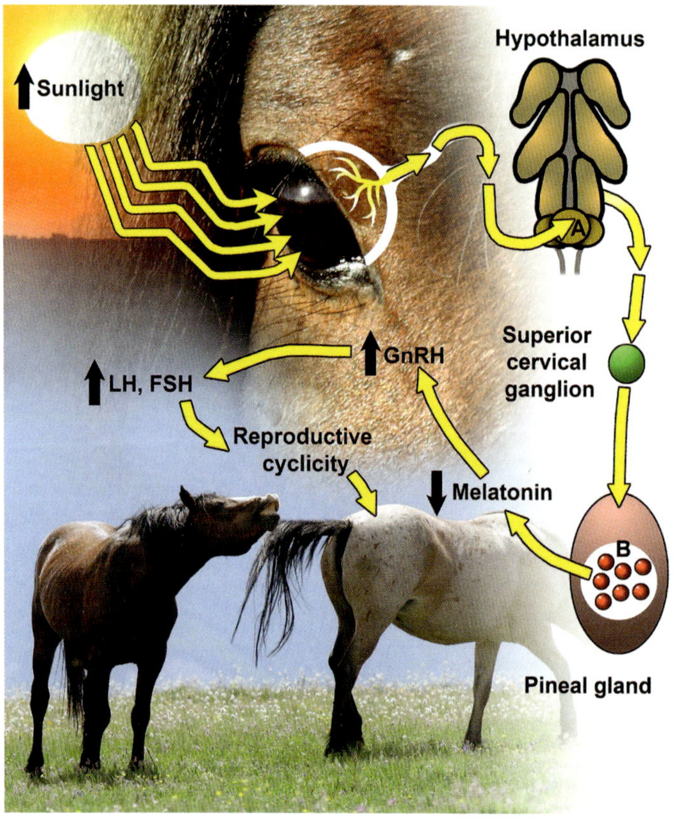

Figure 7.1 Photoperiod and reproduction. *Source:* Adapted from Ransom et al. (2013).

The annual photoperiodic variation is directly proportional to the latitude and altitude of the region, and its amplitude directly affects the reproduction of seasonal animals. Depending on the species and its gestation period, animals experience phases of activity and reproductive quiescence alternately throughout the year. As animals get closer to the Equator, the breeding season becomes smaller and less defined (Goldman and Nelson 2020).

Apart from photoperiod, other environmental conditions can also influence the seasonality of reproduction in animals, such as food availability and climate. In regions with lower latitudes, these factors may have smaller variations throughout the year. The annual cycle of rain directly affects the availability of food for offspring and lactating mothers, while environmental temperature is related to the survival and adaptation of newborns (Abecia et al. 2012). However, among the environmental variables, the length of daily luminosity is the most prominent synchronizing agent used by the animal organism since it remains constant between years (Goldman and Nelson 2020).

Horses are considered "long-day" breeders, and their reproductive activity is stimulated by an increase in daylight, food availability, and temperature during the days, particularly in spring (Nagy et al. 2000). On the other hand, goats and some sheep and buffalo breeds are commonly classified as "short-day" breeders because their sexual activity is triggered by the decrease in daily luminosity during late summer and early autumn, leading to reproductive anestrus in late winter (Abecia et al. 2012). These species are classified as seasonal or seasonally polyestrous since they have consecutive estrous cycles only during the female reproductive season. In contrast, tropical and subtropical breeds are considered nonseasonal or continuous polyestrous and rely on variables like food availability and quality as the main drivers for their breeding season. As latitude increases, the dependence on photoperiod becomes greater, and the period of reproductive activity becomes more restricted (Arroyo et al. 2007).

During the breeding season in goats and sheep, there are changes in sexual behavior, increased synthesis of FSH and LH, and successive estrous cycles. In females, regular intervals of estrous behavior and ovulation (17–21 days) are observed if pregnancy does not occur (Rosa and Bryant 2003). The transition from the anestrus phase to the reproductive season is gradual, with small cycles occurring as the first corpus luteum (CL) forms, typically about 5–6 days after its formation. Some discrepancies may occur at the beginning and end of the sexual season when some ovulations are not accompanied by estrous behavior (Souza-Fabjan et al. 2023).

Even during the anestrus phase, follicle growth and regression occur, as well as production of pituitary hormones LH and FSH. However, while there are no observable differences in plasma FSH concentrations between reproductive seasons, the concentration of progesterone (P4) remains nearly undetectable during the anestrus phase. Similarly, the frequency of LH release is lower during the anestrus season compared to the breeding season (Runcan and da Silva 2022).

In males, seasonal variations in breeding behavior and physiology are less pronounced than in females, but changes in hormonal activity, spermatogenesis, and testicular weight can be observed. For example, an increase in testicular weight and sperm production was observed in males of the Ile-de-France breed between the anestrus season and breeding season. Rams typically show sexual activity stimulated by photoperiod about 1–1.5 months earlier than ewes (Delgadillo et al. 2023). This differential sensitivity to photoperiod is significant, as ewes can ovulate within a few days after hormonal stimulation, while rams require about 45 days to establish complete spermatogenesis (Rosa and Bryant 2003).

7.3 Circadian Rhythm and Reproduction in Mammals

The circadian rhythm is an internal biological rhythm that persists close to 24 hours even under constant ambient conditions such as constant light, darkness, and temperature. This internal rhythm is inherent and genetically determined, meaning it exists independently of the external environment in which organisms are located (Kennaway 2005). However, the biological rhythmicity in organisms is also influenced by external environmental cues, as the circadian rhythm can be synchronized with the rhythmicity of the external environment (Sousa et al. 2008).

In mammals, the suprachiasmatic nucleus (SCN), located in the anterior hypothalamus near the optic chiasm and divided by the third ventricle, acts as the central pacemaker responsible for generating the circadian rhythm (Makrygianni and Chrousos 2023). The SCN plays a crucial role in regulating various biological and psychological processes in the organism, including digestion, wakefulness and sleep, cell renewal, temperature control, locomotion, water intake, corticosterone release, and reproduction (Abecia et al. 2012).

In response to the light–dark cycle, the pineal gland receives signals from the nervous system to synthesize and release melatonin (Hasan et al. 2023). Melatonin serves as a photobiological transducer, preparing organisms physiologically or behaviorally for cyclic external environmental change. In species that exhibit seasonality, melatonin plays a crucial role in modulating the HPG axis, which regulates the reproductive physiology of these animals (Feng et al. 2023). Removing or denervating the pineal gland leads to loss of the ability to respond to seasonal functions, while responses to circadian rhythms continue (Feng et al. 2023).

Although the precise mechanisms of melatonin's action on mammalian reproduction are not fully understood, its influence on the secretion of gonadotropins (FSH and LH), gonad activity (gametogenesis and steroid synthesis), and sexual behavior is well established. Melatonin plays a critical role in coordinating reproductive processes in response to changing environmental conditions and serves as a vital link between the circadian rhythm and the seasonal regulation of reproduction in mammals (Clarke et al. 2009).

7.4 Other Factors That Influence Reproductive Seasonality

The breeding period of animals is not exclusively controlled by the length of daylight but is also affected by a range of environmental elements including temperature, food availability, and interactions with other members of their species (Rosa and Bryant 2003; Asmarasari et al. 2023).

Environmental temperature, encompassing both high and low temperatures, can influence the onset of reproductive behavior in certain animals. Research has shown that mares may undergo their initial ovulation shortly after experiencing specific combinations of maximum and minimum temperatures. Likewise, sheep exposed to lower temperatures during the summer may commence their reproductive activity earlier compared to those in areas with typical seasonal temperatures. Consequently, environmental temperature, along with photoperiod, acts as a trigger for the circadian rhythm governing reproduction (Nagy et al. 2000; Joseph et al. 2023).

In temperate regions, photoperiod predominantly influences the reproductive season, while other environmental factors may affect the timing and duration of the breeding season. However, in tropical regions, nutrition is a more significant factor and can lead to some seasonal acyclicity. Nutrition directly or indirectly affects various reproductive processes, such as puberty. The timing of reproduction in seasonal species is regulated through nutrition to ensure that offspring are born during periods when abundant food is available for both the young and their lactating mothers. It is not only the energy intake but also the quality of protein in the diet that plays a crucial role Furthermore, variations in precipitation and rainfall in specific regions can also impact the timing of birth for certain species (Thimonier et al. 1986).

Several factors, such as lactation and poor physical condition of the mother, can have negative effects on the return of ovarian cyclicity and the timing of the first ovulation after seasonal anestrus. Additionally, hierarchical relationships and interactions within the herd can influence reproductive factors in both males and females (Rosa and Bryant 2003).

In conclusion, the process of animal reproduction during the reproductive season is intricate and influenced by a combination of photoperiod and various environmental factors (Ibeagha-Awemu and Khatib 2023).

7.5 Melatonin

7.5.1 Synthesis

Melatonin, also known as N-acetyl-5-methoxytryptamine and often referred to as the "dark marker hormone," is primarily produced by the pineal gland when the body is not exposed to light signals (Sousa et al. 2008). It is intriguing that melatonin can also be rhythmically generated at different times of the day in various tissues, including the retina, gastrointestinal tract, immunocompetent cells, and ovaries (Pontes et al. 2006). Although these additional sources of melatonin primarily function as autocrine or paracrine hormones, the highest concentration of melatonin in the bloodstream is attributed to its synthesis by the pineal gland (Figure 7.2).

The SCN, located in the hypothalamus, plays a vital role in receiving rhythmic signals captured by retinal photoreceptors through neurotransmitters like glutamate and pituitary adenylate cyclase activating polypeptide (PACAP) These signals from the SCN are then transmitted to the paraventricular nucleus (PVN) within the hypothalamus, and further relayed through the thoracic part of the spinal cord back to the superior cervical ganglion (GCS). Lesions in the SCN can significantly lower the levels of melatonin circulating in the body (Haddad et al. 2023).

During the dark phase, norepinephrine (NA) is released by the sympathetic postganglionic fibers of the GCS. This norepinephrine interacts with alpha-1 and alpha-adrenergic receptors on the membranes of cells in the pineal gland, triggering the expression of genes involved in the biosynthesis of melatonin. Consequently, melatonin is released in higher

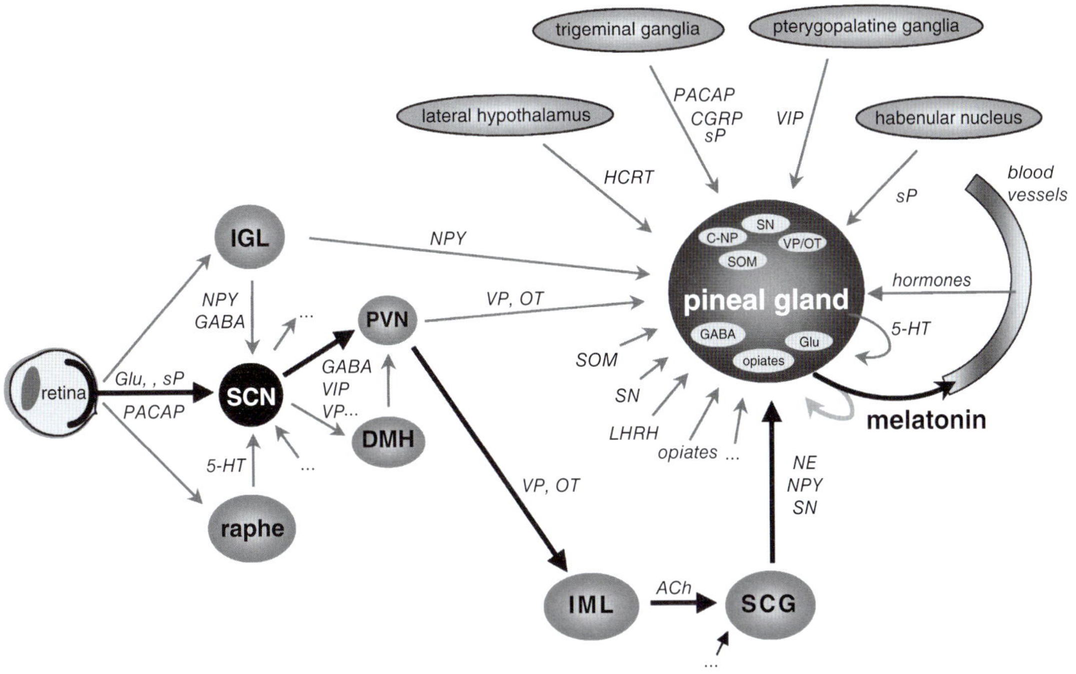

Figure 7.2 Synthesis of melatonin. *Source:* Adapted from Simonneaux and Ribelayga (2003).

quantities at the beginning of the dark phase, reaching levels approximately 100 times higher than during the day (Haddad et al. 2023).

The synthesis of melatonin commences with the essential amino acid tryptophan, which is taken from the bloodstream and undergoes a series of biochemical transformations. Initially, tryptophan is hydroxylated by tryptophan-5-hydroxylase (T-5-H) to form 5-hydroxytryptophan. Subsequently, 5-hydroxytryptophan is decarboxylated by 5-hydroxytryptophan decarboxylase (5-HDT) to produce 5-hydroxytryptamine (serotonin). Then, arylalkylamine-N-acetyltransferase (AANAT or NAT) acetylates serotonin to generate N-acetylserotonin, which is finally methylated by the enzyme cytosolic hydroxyindole-O-methyltransferase (HIOMT), now known as acetylserotonin O-methyltransferase (ASOMT), resulting in the production of melatonin (Figure 7.1) (Simonneaux and Ribelayga 2003; Reiter et al. 2009).

In summary, the synthesis and release of melatonin are intricately regulated by environmental light–dark cycles and play crucial roles in various physiological processes, including the regulation of circadian rhythms and the modulation of reproductive functions.

7.5.2 Regulation, Excretion, Transport, and Metabolism of Melatonin

The synthesis of serotonin from tryptophan occurs during both the day and night. However, during the daytime, the pineal gland shows higher serotonin levels compared to the night due to the significant conversion of serotonin into melatonin during nocturnal hours. Animals exposed to constant light have their nocturnal increase in melatonin inhibited or reduced (Horodincu and Solcan 2023).

NA acts on alpha-1 and alpha-adrenergic receptors on the pinealocytes' plasma membrane. Notably, NA triggers melatonin biosynthesis primarily through the stimulation of alpha-adrenergic receptors during the dark phase. This stimulation involves the Gs protein bound to GTP, leading to adenylate cyclase (AC) activation and up to 10-fold increase in cyclic AMP (cAMP) concentrations. The most substantial cAMP elevation occurs when alpha-1-adrenergic receptors are activated simultaneously. Activation of these receptors alone does not affect cAMP accumulation but significantly increases intracellular free calcium ion (Ca^{2+}) concentration and activates protein kinase C (PKC) (Tan et al. 2023).

In rodents, cAMP activates cAMP-dependent protein kinase, which binds to DNA, triggering transcriptional activity. This leads to a significant increase in AANAT mRNA expression. However, in the latter part of the night, a negative feedback mechanism reduces AANAT mRNA expression. cAMP activates elements that inhibit the transcription of the

AANAT gene, and posttranscriptional mechanisms involving proteolysis degrade the AANAT protein. This proteolysis allows for a faster adjustment in the amount of AANAT protein compared to transcriptional processes. In response to light exposure, melatonin synthesis rapidly decreases as the enzyme is degraded within 3.5 minutes (Tan et al. 2023).

The secretion of melatonin follows a cyclic pattern, resulting in low plasma melatonin concentrations during the day and high concentrations during the night. The rhythmicity of melatonin synthesis is mainly driven by the activity of the AANAT enzyme. The gene expression of this enzyme varies throughout the day, increasing significantly during the night, leading to a more than 100-fold nocturnal activity increase. In contrast, the HIOMT enzyme increases only by 50% during the night. Hence, the AANAT enzyme plays a critical role as a limiting factor or regulator of the rate of melatonin synthesis in the pineal gland. The activity of the HIOMT enzyme is also regulated to modulate melatonin secretion, but this regulation occurs on a longer timescale compared to AANAT, partly due to its high protein stability (half-life >24 hours) (Horodincu and Solcan 2023).

It is important to note that the nocturnal secretion profile of melatonin can vary between species. For instance, in sheep, melatonin concentrations reach a plateau shortly after the beginning of the night (within 10–30 minutes), remain elevated throughout the night, and decrease just before or close to the onset of daylight. Individual variability in melatonin secretion within the same species is related to the size of the pineal gland and the number of pinealocytes it contains, rather than the activity of its enzymes in the biosynthetic pathways (Gómez-Brunet et al. 2012).

Melatonin is not stored due to its lipophilic nature and is promptly released after synthesis in the pinealocytes. It can easily diffuse across cell membranes and cross the blood–brain barrier. Furthermore, a majority of circulating melatonin (60–80%) is bound to plasma proteins like albumin and alpha-1-acid glycoprotein. Melatonin has a short half-life (around 20 minutes in sheep) and is primarily metabolized by the liver enzyme melatonin 6-hydroxylase (Skene et al. 2001).

7.5.3 Site of Action of Melatonin in the Central Nervous System

Due to melatonin's wide-ranging effects on various physiological processes, identifying all the locations in the body where it operates can be challenging. Moreover, researchers have found high-affinity melatonin receptors in various bodily tissues (Gómez-Brunet et al. 2012). To investigate potential melatonin targets within the hypothalamic-gonadal axis (HHG), scientists have used 2-(125I)-iodomelatonin (125I-melatonin), a high-affinity agonist probe. This investigation has led to the identification of potential melatonin action sites within the HHG axis. However, the number and types of these identified structures vary significantly between species. Only two structures, the pars tuberalis (PT) of the pituitary and, to a lesser extent, the NSQ (nucleus suprachiasmaticus), show the presence of melatonin receptors in nearly all species (Malpaux 2006).

The significance of the PT lies in its role as the pathway for all blood vessels carrying hormones, such as GnRH, from the hypothalamus to the adenohypophysis. This anatomical location suggests the PT could play a crucial role in influencing hypothalamic-pituitary function and potentially impact the release of LH. However, studies in sheep have shown that directly releasing melatonin into the PT did not modify LH secretion. Instead, LH release was stimulated by microimplants of melatonin placed in the basal middle hypothalamus or the third ventricle of the brain (Malpaux et al. 1993, 1997). Therefore, it appears that the hypothalamus is a significant target for mediating melatonin's effects on the reproductive neuroendocrine axis while the pituitary's influence is indirect (Horodincu and Solcan 2023).

7.5.4 Melatonin Receptors

The utilization of the radioactive probe 125I-melatonin has allowed for the identification of the specific sites of action and receptors involved in melatonin's effects. These receptors were initially referred to as ML-1 and ML-2 based on their unique properties (Carrillo-Vico et al. 2003). The ML-1 receptor, now known as the MT1 receptor, is a high-affinity melatonin receptor classified as a G protein-coupled receptor (Gi and Gq), as demonstrated by research. Further studies have revealed different subtypes of this receptor class, with two subtypes, MT1 and MT2, found in mammals (Malpaux 2006). The MT1 receptors are more abundant in the hypothalamus, while MT2 receptors are predominantly found in the retina (Carrillo-Vico et al. 2003).

In contrast, the ML-2 receptor, initially known as ML-2 ligand with lower melatonin affinity, is now recognized as the MT3 melatonin receptor. This receptor is believed to play a crucial role in protecting cells against oxidative stress.

Both high-affinity receptors, MT1 and MT2, are associated with G proteins, PTX-sensitive (Gi) and PTX-insensitive (Gq), and they are involved in various cellular activation and blockade mechanisms that are not yet fully understood. Activation of MT1 and MT2 receptors leads to the inhibition of AC activity, resulting in reduced cAMP production and activation of protein kinase A (PKA), leading to a decrease in cellular response. On the other hand, the Gq protein and the beta subunit of the Gi protein can activate phospholipase C (PLC), which causes an increase in calcium and diacylglycerol (DAG), triggering intracellular responses, such as protein activation. Additionally, MT2 receptor activation may influence the concentration of guanosine monophosphate (cGMP) and increase PKC activity, possibly through stimulation of the PLC and DAG pathway (Singh et al. 2020).

The regulation of melatonin receptors is influenced by various factors, including the developmental stage of the animal, time of year, and the presence of melatonin itself. In sheep, it has been observed that only the MT1 receptor is expressed, suggesting that this particular subtype is primarily responsible for the seasonal effects of melatonin on reproduction in this species (Malpaux 2006).

7.5.5 GnRH and Gonadotropin Secretion Pattern in the Breeding Season and Anestrus

Fertility in mammals begins at puberty and is regulated through complex communication between the brain, pituitary gland, and gonads, involving both neural and hormonal pathways. The process starts with the hypothalamus releasing GnRH in a pulsatile manner through nerve endings in the middle eminence. This GnRH then travels to the pituitary gland via the hypophyseal portal system. Subsequently, the pituitary gland stimulates the synthesis and secretion of two important hormones, LH and FSH. These gonadotropins, in turn, play a critical role in stimulating the production of steroids and gametes in the gonads.

The pulsatile pattern of GnRH release from the brain is instrumental in determining the secretion pattern of LH in the pituitary. Sex steroids also contribute to enhancing control in gonadotrophs. During the breeding season, synthesis and secretion of GnRH peak in response to positive estrogen feedback, leading to the preovulatory levels of LH. The frequency of GnRH/LH pulses is essential in reproductive physiology as it regulates the entire follicular development in the ovarian cycle and influences various behavioral characteristics related to reproduction.

The transition from the "breeding season" to the "anestrus season" involves significant changes in the hormonal neurosecretion system. The pulsatile GnRH secretion is interrupted during anestrus, although gonadotropin secretion continues. Follicular waves persist in the ovaries without proper growth and regression due to the low frequency of GnRH and LH pulses. This leads to reduced estrogen concentrations, which prevent the induction of the LH preovulatory surge and ovulation.

During the breeding season, progesterone (P4) acts as the primary inhibitor of the pulsatile frequency of GnRH, allowing the preovulatory LH surge to occur. However, in the transition to anestrus, long photoperiods activate an inhibitory neural system, making estradiol the major negative feedback steroid that controls the pulsatile frequency of GnRH. When the last corpus luteum of the reproductive season regresses, the pulsatile frequency of GnRH and LH ceases, causing a lack of final growth in follicles from follicular waves and a subsequent absence of preovulatory estradiol, which would otherwise induce the LH surge and estrus behavior.

In autumn, with the decrease in photoperiod and an increase in melatonin synthesis, the activity of the inhibitory neural system diminishes. In the absence of progesterone, LH secretion increases, leading to elevated estradiol levels, which ultimately trigger the LH surge and initiate the first ovulation of the breeding season. The negative action of estradiol on LH secretion primarily occurs through a reduction in the pulsatile secretion of GnRH, rather than a greater decrease in the pituitary's response to GnRH.

The specific mechanisms by which changes in photoperiod induce different responses in the GnRH neurosecretory system, despite a similar pattern of estradiol secretion in various seasonal species, continue to be the subject of study. Research is ongoing to fully understand these intricate regulatory processes of reproductive cycles in mammals.

7.5.6 The Role of Melatonin in the Ovaries

Melatonin influences ovarian physiology both indirectly and directly. Indirectly, it affects the secretion of GnRH/FSH/LH, regulating steroidogenesis and gametogenesis. It also acts directly on ovarian cells, impacting follicular growth, atresia, steroidogenesis, cell maturation, ovulation, and embryonic development. Melatonin's presence in the follicular fluid at the time of ovulation acts as a potent antioxidant, protecting the oocyte from oxidative stress. Melatonin interacts with conventional membrane receptors (MT1 and MT2) and possibly nuclear receptors (RZR/ROR superfamily) to exert its effects. It influences steroid hormone production, including progesterone, and affects the follicular response to hormones like LH. Melatonin also has antiapoptotic actions, reducing the degradation of antral follicles. Additionally, it may play a role in final oocyte maturation and embryonic development, as supplementation in *in vitro* embryo production has shown improved outcomes in various animal species.

Overall, melatonin's interaction with gonadal steroids and its direct actions on the ovaries play vital roles in regulating seasonal reproduction and various reproductive processes in animals.

7.6 Control of Sexual Activity

The control of sexual activity in goats involves various hormonal and nonhormonal methods. Some of the main approaches include hormonal treatments, photoperiodic treatments, melatonin treatment, and the buck effect. Additionally, adapted nutrition can also influence the reproductive cycle.

7.6.1 Hormonal Treatment

Hormonal regimens using progestagens, eCG, and prostaglandins have been established for synchronizing estrus and ovulation during both the breeding and nonbreeding seasons. The treatment involves the use of a vaginal sponge impregnated with a progestagen, followed by injections of a PGF2-alpha analogue and eCG. This treatment is effective in achieving conception rates of about 60–65% during out-of-season artificial insemination (AI) with frozen-thawed semen.

7.6.2 Photoperiodic Treatment

Seasonality of reproduction in goats is strongly dependent on photoperiod. Manipulation of the photoperiod can be used to achieve out-of-season breeding. Animals are subjected to alternating long and short days, and melatonin implants can be used to provide short-day effects. Photoperiodic treatments can induce sexual activity in both males and females, but they may not be sufficient to synchronize ovulation for AI. They are often combined with hormonal treatments or the buck effect to achieve synchronization.

7.6.3 Melatonin Treatment

Melatonin, synthesized by the pineal gland, plays a crucial role in perceiving day length changes and controlling seasonal reproductive activity in animals. Melatonin treatment, typically administered through subcutaneous implants, can advance cyclical ovulatory activity in ewes and goats. It improves the timing of fertilization and the fecundity of females. Melatonin treatment can be used alone or in combination with other hormonal treatments or artificial photoperiodic treatment to stimulate sexual activity and sperm production in males.

7.6.4 Buck Effect

The "ram effect" is when noncycling (anestrous) ewes are stimulated to ovulate by the sudden introduction of a ram. Similarly, the male effect in goats involves the introduction of a buck or teaser buck to stimulate sexual activity in anovulatory females. This technique is particularly effective in breeds with moderate seasonality and may require pretreatment with photoperiod to optimize the response in highly seasonal breeds.

7.6.5 Adapted Nutrition

Nutrition plays a significant role in modulating various aspects of the reproductive cycle. Targeted nutrition can optimize ovulation rate, increase potential litter size, and advance puberty. Adequate nutrition during pregnancy can also influence embryo survival and the long-term performance of offspring. These approaches can be combined and tailored to specific breeds and environmental conditions to optimize reproductive performance in goats.

References

Abecia, J.A., Forcada, F., and González-Bulnes, A. (2012). Hormonal control of reproduction in small ruminants. *Animal Reproduction Science* 130 (3–4): 173–179.

Arroyo, L.J., Gallegos-Sánchez, J., Villa-Godoy, A. et al. (2007). Reproductive activity of Pelibuey and Suffolk ewes at 19 north latitude. *Animal Reproduction Science* 102 (1–2): 24–30.

Asmarasari, S.A., Azizah, N., Sutikno, S. et al. (2023). A review of dairy cattle heat stress mitigation in Indonesia. *Veterinary World* 16 (5): 1098–1108.

Aubry, L.M. and Williams, C.T. (2022). Vertebrate phenological plasticity: from molecular mechanisms to ecological and evolutionary implications. *Integrative and Comparative Biology* 62 (4): 958–971.

Burtschell, L., Dezeure, J., Huchard, E., and Godelle, B. (2023). Evolutionary determinants of reproductive seasonality: a theoretical approach. *Peer Community Journal* 3: article e56.

Cann, P., Le Danvic, C., Porte, C. et al. (2023). Variation of ewe olfactory secretome during a ram effect. *Frontiers in Veterinary Science* 9: 1033412.

Carrillo-Vico, A., Garcia-Perganeda, A., Naji, L. et al. (2003). Expression of membrane and nuclear melatonin receptor mRNA and protein in the mouse immune system. *Cellular and Molecular Life Sciences CMLS* 60: 2272–2278.

Clarke, I.J., Smith, J.T., Caraty, A. et al. (2009). Kisspeptin and seasonality in sheep. *Peptides* 30: 154–163.

Contreras-Correa, Z.E., Messman, R.D., Swanson, R.M., and Lemley, C.O. (2023). Melatonin in health and disease: a perspective for livestock production. *Biomolecules* 13 (3): 490.

Delgadillo, J.A., Espinoza-Flores, L.A., López-Magaña, D. et al. (2023). Maintenance of permanent sexual activity throughout the year in seasonal bucks using short photoperiodic cycles in open barns. In: *Encyclopedia of Reproduction*, 2e (ed. M. Skinner), 415–419. New York: Academic Press.

Feng, J., Yang, J., Jiang, Z. et al. (2023). Melatonin modulates the hypothalamic-pituitary neuroendocrine axis to regulate physiological color change in teleost fish. *International Journal of Biological Sciences* 19 (9): 2914.

Goel, A.K. and Kharche, S.D. (2009). Advances in reproductive techniques in goats – a review. *Indian Journal of Small Ruminants* 15 (1): 1–34.

Goldman, B.D. and Nelson, R.J. (2020). Melatonin and seasonality in mammals. In: *Melatonin*, 225–252. Boca Raton: CRC Press.

Gómez-Brunet, A., Santiago-Moreno, J., Malpaux, B. et al. (2012). Ovulatory activity and plasma prolactin concentrations in wild and domestic ewes exposed to artificial photoperiods between the winter and summer solstices. *Animal Reproduction Science* 132 (1–2): 36–43.

Haddad, M., Khazali, H., Janahmadi, M., and Ghanbarian, H. (2023). Inhibition of the retinal orexin receptors affects the hypothalamic-pituitary-gonadal axis through retinal pituitary adenylate cyclase activating polypeptide (PACAP) in male Wistar rats. *General and Comparative Endocrinology* 337: 114242.

Hasan, K.N., Das, J., and Acharyya, A. (2023). Melatonin as a biological "time keeper" and its potential application in fish reproduction: a review. *Biologia* 78: 1–14.

Horodincu, L. and Solcan, C. (2023). Influence of different light spectra on melatonin synthesis by the pineal gland and influence on the immune system in chickens. *Animals* 13 (13): 2095.

Ibeagha-Awemu, E.M. and Khatib, H. (2023). Epigenetics of livestock health, production, and breeding. In: *Handbook of Epigenetics* (ed. T. Tollefsbol), 569–610. New York: Academic Press.

Inskeep, E.K. (2011). Ruminant reproduction: recent findings and future challenges, a summary. *Reproduction in Domestic Ruminants VII* 1.

Joseph, J., Charalambous, R., Pahuja, H. et al. (2023). Impacts of climate change on animal welfare. CABI Reviews. www.cabidigitallibrary.org/doi/10.1079/cabireviews.2023.0020 (accessed 24 December 2023).

Kennaway, D.J. (2005). The role of circadian rhythmicity in reproduction. *Human Reproduction Update* 11 (1): 91–101.

Makrygianni, E.A. and Chrousos, G.P. (2023). Neural progenitor cells and the hypothalamus. *Cells* 12 (14): 1822.

Malpaux, B. (2006). Seasonal regulation of reproduction in mammals. In: *Knobil and Neill's Physiology of Reproduction*, 3e (ed. J.D. Neill), 2231–2281. Amsterdam: Elsevier.

Malpaux, B., Daveau, A., Maurice, F. et al. (1993). Short-day effects of melatonin on luteinizing hormone secretion in the ewe: evidence for central sites of action in the mediobasal hypothalamus. *Biology of Reproduction* 48 (4): 752–760.

Malpaux, B., Viguié, C., Skinner, D.C. et al. (1997). Control of the circannual rhythm of reproduction by melatonin in the ewe. *Brain Research Bulletin* 44 (4): 431–438.

Mandal, D.K., Kumar, M., and Tyagi, S. (2022). Effect of seasons and photoperiods on seminal attributes and sperm morphology in Holstein Friesian× Sahiwal crossbred dairy bulls. *International Journal of Biometeorology* 66 (11): 2223–2235.

Nagy, P., Guillaume, D., and Daels, P. (2000). Seasonality in mares. *Animal Reproduction Science* 60–61: 245–262.

Pontes, O., Li, C.F., Nunes, P.C. et al. (2006). The Arabidopsis chromatin-modifying nuclear siRNA pathway involves a nucleolar RNA processing center. *Cell* 126 (1): 79–92.

Ramya, S., Poornima, P., Jananisri, A. et al. (2023). Role of hormones and the potential impact of multiple stresses on infertility. *Stresses* 3 (2): 454–474.

Ransom, J.I., Hobbs, N.T., and Bruemmer, J. (2013). Contraception can lead to trophic asynchrony between birth pulse and resources. *PLoS One* 8: e54972.

Reiter, R.J., Tan, D.X., Manchester, L.C. et al. (2009). Melatonin and reproduction revisited. *Biology of Reproduction* 81 (3): 445–456.

Rosa, H.J.D. and Bryant, M.J. (2003). Seasonality of reproduction in sheep. *Small Ruminant Research* 48 (3): 155–171.

Runcan, E.E. and da Silva, M.A.C. (2022). Reproduction and the reproductive system. *Medicine and Surgery of Camelids* 3: 423–480.

Saleh, M. and Holtz, W. (2022). LH pattern and ovarian response in ovsynch-synchronized superovulated goats induced to ovulate with GnRH or hCG. *Theriogenology* 185: 61–69.

Shinomiya, A., Shimmura, T., Nishiwaki-Ohkawa, T., and Yoshimura, T. (2014). Regulation of seasonal reproduction by hypothalamic activation of thyroid hormone. *Frontiers in Endocrinology* 5: 12.

Simonneaux, V. and Ribelayga, C. (2003). Generation of the melatonin endocrine message in mammals: a review of the complex regulation of melatonin synthesis by norepinephrine, peptides, and other pineal transmitters. *Pharmacological Reviews* 55 (2): 325–395.

Singh, S., Rana, A., Kaur, S. et al. (2020). Pharmacology of melatonin and its receptors. *Frontiers in Pharmacology of Neurotransmitters* 293–324.

Skene, D.J., Papagiannidou, E., Hashemi, E. et al. (2001). Contribution of CYP1A2 in the hepatic metabolism of melatonin: studies with isolated microsomal preparations and liver slices. *Journal of Pineal Research* 31: 333–342.

Sousa, C.E.C., Cruz-Machado, S.S., and Tamura, E.K. (2008). Circadian rhythms and reproduction in mammals. *Bulletin of the Center for Reproductive Biology* 27 (1–2): 15–20.

Souza-Fabjan, J.M., Alves, B.R., Batista, R.I. et al. (2023). Reproductive biotechnologies applied to the female sheep and goat. In: *Sustainable Agriculture Reviews 59: Animal Biotechnology for Livestock Production 3* (ed. V. Yata, A. Mohanty, and E. Lichtfouse), 1–57. Cham: Springer Nature.

Tan, D.X., Reiter, R.J., Zimmerman, S., and Hardeland, R. (2023). Melatonin: both a messenger of darkness and a participant in the cellular actions of non-visible solar radiation of near infrared light. *Biology* 12 (1): 89.

Thimonier, J., Terqui, M., and Chemineau, P. (1986). Conduite de la Reproduction des Petits Ruminants dans les Differentes Parties du Monde. *Proceedings of the Atomic Energy Agency*, Vienna, Institut national de recherches agronomiques, Nouzilly, France, 135–147.

Veliz-Deras, F.G., Meza-Herrera, C.A., De Santiago-Miramontes, A. et al. (2023). An enhanced body condition improved sexual behavior, ovarian structure and function, and reproductive fitness in rangeland-crossbred dairy goats. *Agriculture* 13 (7): 1337.

8

The Buck Effect: A Management Tool for Improving Reproductive Efficiency in Goats

Mohammad M. Islam and Chirag P. Parmar

Pashupalan Sanshodhan Kendra, Kamdhenu University, Ramna Muvada, Gujarat, India

8.1 Introduction

Estrus synchronization is the process of manipulating the estrous cycle that results in standing estrus (heat) in most animals in a short time (Das et al. 2022). Estrus synchronization is a valuable management tool that has been successfully employed in enhancing reproductive efficiency. Estrus synchronization is vital in goats as the duration of both the estrous cycle and estrus is variable (Rahman et al. 2008) and they can exhibit silent estrus (Greyling and van der Nest 2000). One of the advantages of estrus synchronization is that many does are bred over a short period. As a result, management can be concentrated during short periods and does can be bred at a time that will be suitable for gaining the best marketing opportunities. Synchronization will also allow producers to schedule kidding to take advantage of feed supplies, labor, upward price trends and implementation of breeding technologies such as artificial insemination.

Although the merits of estrus synchronization are best realized in large animal breeding establishments, this technique can also be used to benefit the smallholder producer.

In the past, synchronization of estrus in goats has focused primarily on dairy goats to allow for optimal timing of milk production. However, recent interest in meat goat production has resulted in attempts to use dairy goat, sheep, and cattle synchronization regimens in meat goat management systems. Estrus synchronization through hormonal application is used nowadays to improve the reproductive efficiency of goats. Estrus synchronization in does, as in cows and ewes, is achieved either by reducing the length of the luteal phase of the estrous cycle with prostaglandin F_2-alpha (PGF_2-alpha) and/or its analogues, such as cloprostenol, or extending it artificially with exogenous progesterone or more potent progestogens (Karatzas et al. 1997). As an alternative to intramuscular administration, the vaginal administration route has many advantages, including direct delivery of the drug to the site of action, which results in reduced systemic side-effects (Major and McConville 2017) and no gastrointestinal absorption and hepatic first-pass metabolism of the drug (Roumen and Dieben 2006).

These hormonal applications have so far failed to be consistently effective and besides, some of these biologicals are not easily available or too expensive for farmers in developing countries like India. Therefore, harnessing the reproduction potential of livestock species in developing countries may require development of management strategies such as pheromones and biostimulation to effectively improve reproduction. Use of the "buck effect" can help to advance breeding season and provide a relatively good degree of synchrony (Tibary 2009). The buck effect can also be used in combination with progestogen to increase the degree of synchrony.

Induction of synchronous estrus behavior and ovulation in anovulatory females after introduction of a buck is called the "buck effect" (Ungerfeld et al. 2004). This response is widely used to advance and synchronize breeding in goats (Chemineau 1987; Walkden-Brown et al. 1993a,b,c; Veliz et al. 2002). Detailed studies of pheromones in goats, sheep, cattle, pigs, insects, and rodents have shown that male pheromones have a significant effect on reproductive activity in females (Wani et al. 2013). In addition, it has been reported that in sheep and goats, the male effect is more than a pheromone-triggered response, and is a multifaceted process involving sociosexual signals (Delgadillo et al. 2009).

Traditionally, goat keepers used this as a tool to manipulate goat reproduction without knowing much about the underlying physiology. However, it was studied by Chemineau (1987) and pheromonal, behavioral, tactile, and other cues were

Elements of Reproduction and Reproductive Diseases of Goats, First Edition. Edited by Tanmoy Rana.

reported to be involved in this phenomenon. The buck effect is now one of the well-established means of manipulating goat reproduction without using much criticized hormonal therapy in today's health-conscious and "organic"-oriented developed world, where meat-producing small ruminants, though concentrated mainly in the developing world, have and will continue to have a great marketing potential.

The expression of normal estrus behavior by does indicates their well-being and thereby their production capability. In contrast to the typical exploitation of production potential of the "animal machine," recent ethological integration with animal husbandry principles and practices is mainly directed toward bridging the age-old demand–supply gap. Estrus behavior is associated with sensible animal farming whereby the reproductive performances of females can be improved without much influence on their normal behavior, thus having regard to the various issues relating to animal welfare. This association is relatively recent and therefore requires special attention.

8.2 The Buck Effect

The induction of cyclic reproductive activity in females well before the initiation of spontaneous cycling by introduction of males is characteristically known as the "male effect" (Underwood et al. 1944). Social interactions between animals of the same species may lead to important changes in their reproductive status. Exposure of seasonally anovulatory goats and ewes to males can stimulate and synchronize their sexual activity (Chemineau 1987; Rosa and Bryant 2002).

This phenomenon of sexual biostimulation is known as the buck effect in goats and the ram effect in ewes, or "teasing," and has been extensively studied in goats and sheep (Shelton 1980; Ungerfeld et al. 2004). In these species, the response of females to the introduction of males involves a rapid increase of luteinizing hormone (LH) secretion that culminates in a preovulatory surge provoking ovulation (Chemineau et al. 1986). Sex pheromones produced by the ram or buck from sudoriferous glands act on receptors within the ewe or doe olfactory bulb, stimulating neurons in the ventromedial and arcuate nuclei in the hypothalamus, leading to an increase in kisspeptin secretion and the onset of estrus (Ergul Ekiz et al. 2013; Fabre-Nys et al. 2017).

In sheep, the first ovulation is not accompanied by behavioral estrus whereas in goats, a variable number of females show estrus behavior at the first induced ovulation 2–4 days after male introduction. Most goats have a short ovarian cycle of 5–7 days, followed by a second ovulation, which is associated with estrus behavior and a normal luteal phase (Chemineau 1987; Flores et al. 2000). The responses of females to teasing are variable and may depend on several internal and external factors operating in both sexes, such as variation of the females' responsiveness to the presence of males because of photoperiod, genetic factors, or the quality of the stimulus provided by the male. One of the major factors affecting the efficacy of response to the male effect depends on the strength of seasonality of female and male goats. In this respect, the response to the male effect varies within breeds through the seasonal anestrous period, and among breeds from different latitude origins (Walkden-Brown et al. 1999). When ewes and rams are in constant contact (sight or smell), the pheromones are much less effective at inducing estrus (Ghosh 2021).

The buck effect is a well-documented phenomenon in goats (Gelez and Fabre-Nys 2004) in which the primer pheromone produced in sexually mature males increases the LH pulse frequency and induces estrus in recipient females during the anestrous period (Chemineau 1987). The gonadotropin-releasing hormone (GnRH) pulse generator generates intermittent GnRH discharges into the portal vessels and thereby regulates the pulsatile LH secretion into the peripheral circulation (Karsch 1984). Therefore, the central target of the buck effect pheromone is thought to be the hypothalamic GnRH pulse generator. The introduction of sex pheromones from a novel male to anestrous ewes or does can also trigger an LH surge that induces ovulation in 46–50% of ewes and 10–16% of does without any other treatment (Davila et al. 2017).

The buck effect is a multisensory phenomenon involving olfactory, visual, tactile, and auditory cues. A high percentage of females respond to male stimulation when all cues are active (Chemineau 1987). In goats, olfactory cues from the male appear to be involved in mediating the buck effect (Over et al. 1990). In ewes, the male odor stimulates an increase in frequency of LH pulses, and induces ovulation in a high proportion of them. However, in other trials a lower proportion of ovulating goats were seen in the male odor group compared to those teasing with full male contact (Walkden-Brown et al. 1993b). However, in the dwarf Creole goat from the French West Indies in the Caribbean, peripherally induced anosmia does not prevent the response to the male effect, although the proportion of females showing estrus or ovulation decreases (50% in anosmic females vs 89% in control females) (Chemineau et al. 1986). Further evidence is provided by experiments in which seasonally anovulatory females have ovulated in response to ram fleece or buck hair rubbed directly on the muzzle or applied in a face mask (Knight et al. 1983; Claus et al. 1990).

Overall, these results indicate that olfactory cues are involved in the response of females to the male effect, but whole male–female behavioral interactions are likely to play some stimulatory role. Although at a lower percentage than with full buck contact, some does ovulate in response to male odor and vocalizations (19.5% vs 41.2%) (Shelton 1980).

8.2.1 Synchronization of Estrus by the Buck Effect

There is considerable scope for improving the reproductive management of goats by using the buck effect to initiate and synchronize reproductive activity in anovulatory does (Chemineau 1987). Amongst responsive does, a high proportion ovulates within three days of buck introduction, with variable exhibition of estrus and generally poor fertility. Typically, a second ovulation, accompanied by fertile estrus, occurs some 7–12 days later, after a short luteal phase of about five days with low release of luteal progesterone. The ovulation rate may be enhanced at this second ovulation (Chemineau 1987; Restall 1988). The proportion of goats responding to the buck stimulus depends on nutritional status, breed, buck aggressiveness, and parity of does (Walkden-Brown et al. 1999; Rosa and Bryant 2002).

After an isolation period, the stimulation of females by sexually active males previously photo-stimulated with artificial light induces and synchronizes ovulation in anovulatory goats (Luna-Orozco et al. 2012).

The buck effect is currently only used during seasonal or locational anestrus because the response is thought to be blocked in cyclic females by periods of elevated progesterone (Hawken et al. 2009). Buck exposure induces an increase in pulsatile LH in goats in the early and late luteal (LL) phases of the estrous cycle.

After introduction of a buck among the does, ovulation is detected around the third day of contact (Delgadillo et al. 2017; Pellicer-Rubio et al. 2019).

The high concentrations of progesterone in females in the midluteal phase appear to block the buck effect. However, ram introduction to cyclic ewes stimulates an increase in pulsatile LH secretion, independent of ewe genotype or stage of the estrous cycle (Hawken et al. 2007).

Exposure of a male and its effect on estrus and ovulation was extensively studied in Creole meat goats. The result reveals that 94% of noncyclic females ovulate 2.8 ± 0.2 days after introduction of the buck. In cyclic females, 99.3% of females come into estrus within 21 days after introduction of males, the highest frequency (25%) on the first day and lowest (<1%) on the fifth to sixth days (Chemineau 1983). This highest frequency of cyclic does coming into estrus on the first day of male introduction indicates that the male effect can also be used to stimulate synchronization of estrus.

As per Keskin (2003), using the buck effect for estrus synchronization is more economical than exogenous hormone administration and is recommended in extensive production, when animals are in an estrus cycle. The estrus can effectively be synchronized by the buck effect in cycling Shami (Damascus) goats. The time interval (mean ± SEM) between the introduction of bucks and the onset of estrus is 52.4 ± 4.69 hours with a range of 22–196 hours. Sharma et al. (2022) reported cent per cent estrus response with a duration of 70.33 ± 40.39 hours for estrus induction and 30.50 ± 0.56 hours of estrus duration.

Conception rate at the first buck-induced estrus, in the Creole goat, is lower than at the second induced estrus: 23% (56 estruses) vs 74% (70 estruses), respectively (Thimonier et al. 1983). This very low conception rate at first induced estrus is probably a consequence of the short ovarian cycle. The luteal failure probably does not allow the establishment of pregnancy (Chemineau 1983).

It is possible to advance the breeding season and to induce ovarian activity without the use of exogenous hormonal treatment (Avdi et al. 2004). Females which are in ovarian inactivity throughout spring all ovulate after buck introduction. During the transitional period, the male effect is as effective as synchronizing treatments involving Synchromate®-B (SMB) in inducing estrus in goats with reduced seasonal inhibition of reproduction (Mellado et al. 2000). Exposure to the buck after a period of isolation can be used to advance the breeding season and provides some degree of synchronization of estrus. Temporary kid removal (48 hours) after 28 days of lactation improves the response to the buck effect in lactating does. Introduction of the buck stimulates does and induces ovulation within 24–96 hours although only two-thirds of the does have an accompanying estrus. However, a great proportion of the induced ovulations by the buck effect is followed by a short luteal phase (short CL life span) and does return to estrus usually in two modes, i.e., 3–8 days and 7–12 days after introduction of the buck (Tibary 2009).

8.2.2 The Buck Effect as Tool for Improving Reproductive Efficiency in Goats

The buck effect is more efficient at inducing sexual activity in breeds of low seasonality, such as those from tropical and subtropical zones, than in breeds from middle and high latitudes (Chemineau 1987). The appearance of short luteal phases and delayed ovulation in goats treated with the male effect during seasonal anestrus depends on the stage of follicle development at the time of buck introduction (Gonzalez-Bulnes et al. 2006). A single injection of progesterone stimulates the emergence of a new follicular wave, able to grow and give adequate ovulation after induction of the buck effect (Chemineau 1987; Gonzalez-Bulnes et al. 2006). Most females treated with progesterone show estrus behavior and ovulation with luteal phases of normal length; moreover, the interval from male introduction to fertile estrus is reduced, allowing better synchronization of matings and births (Gonzalez-Bulnes et al. 2006).

Estrus can also be induced in anestrous does by a ram instead of a buck but the time taken by the ram is longer in comparison to the buck. Moreover, estrus synchronization is not achieved by ram teasing. Teasing with buck and ram induces heat respectively in 6/6 and 5/6 postpartum anestrous does which is significantly ($P < 0.05$) higher than in control does (2/6). When teased with aproned intact males, does show behavioral estrus, and subsequently ovulate within 2.6, 9.5, and 23 days of male introduction in buck-teased, ram-teased, and nonteased does, respectively. Estrus synchronization in does is 5/6 vs 1/6 within three days of introduction of buck and ram, respectively (Mondal 2005).

Early studies assumed that females must be preconditioned by a period of complete segregation (odor, sight, sound, and touch), from males in order to obtain a good ovulatory response (Chemineau 1987; Walkden-Brown et al. 1993c; Ungerfeld et al. 2004). Later results suggest that the previous isolation of seasonally anovulatory female goats from bucks is not critical to stimulate their reproductive activity by the male effect, if sexually active males are used, at least under subtropical conditions (Veliz et al. 2006).

The degree of contact between the two sexes may affect the response of the females to the male effect. Pearce and Oldham (1988) exposed ewes to various degrees of contact with rams (full physical contact, contact through an openwork fence, contact through an opaque fence, contact with rams' wool in face masks or complete isolation from males). Contact through an opaque fence is less effective than through an openwork fence, and the maximum effect is achieved in all cases when the ewes are allowed full physical contact with the males. In Angora goats, 41% of 85 does separated from bucks by a wire fence (weak stimulation) ovulated, compared with 69% (out of 66) when put in direct contact with the males (strong stimulation) (Shelton 1980). In both ewes and goats, a high response of females is obtained when both sexes are in full physical contact, showing that the degree of female response is influenced by the type of contact with males.

The continuous presence of the buck until ovulation is not necessary to maximize the response to the buck effect. Indeed, in local goats from subtropical Mexico exposed to bucks for 16 hours per day, the percentage of females that show estrus behavior (96%) is like that of control females which are in contact with a male for 24 hours (92%) (Rivaz-Munoz et al. 2007). Continuous presence of a male and service during the estrous period may reduce the duration of estrus although it did not affect ovulation times or ovulation rates in Nubian dairy goats (Romano and Fernandez Abella 1997).

However, when lambing occurs during the breeding season, the continuous presence of a ram with the ewes starting lambing advances the resumption of postpartum ovarian activity by approximately 30 days and causes a peak of estrus around day 40 after lambing. This practice can be advantageously integrated when designing more efficient management of reproduction in ewe flocks (Lassoued et al. 2004). The conception rate presented by Sharma et al. (2022) at induced estrus by a buck was 66.67% (4/6) and 83.33% (5/6) of three cycles overall. It was stated that the buck effect was efficient in synchronizing estrus and beneficial for improving conception rate in Surti does. Chaudhary et al. (2018) also stated that the buck effect was as effective as PGF2-alpha treatment for synchronization of estrus in Surti goats.

The parity of female goats does not influence their estrus and ovulatory responses to the buck effect. The interval between introduction of the buck and onset of estrus behavior do not differ significantly ($P > 0.05$) between multiparous (1.9 ± 0.1 days) and nulliparous (1.7 ± 0.2 days) females. The proportion of females displaying a short estrous cycle is greater ($P < 0.05$) in multiparous (13/21, 62%) than in nulliparous (5/19, 26%) females (Luna-orazco et al. 2008). However, the bucks are less responsive to maiden goats compared to mature goats, and fertility of nulliparous goats during the nonbreeding season is lower than multiparous goats after induced ovulation by the buck effect. In one study, all multiparous goats (20/20) displayed estrus behavior within the first 10 days of buck exposure, while 70% (14/20) of the nulliparous goats showed estrus ($P > 0.05$) (Veliz et al. 2009).

The immediate circulating LH response to the presence of the buck (as recorded number of pulses) is higher in dominant than in subordinate does, and this is associated with a higher number of dominant goats ovulating in response to the buck effect. The dominant does show significantly ($P < 0.05$) more LH pulses (2.0 ± 0.18 ng/ml vs 1.2 ± 0.25 ng/ml) and a higher mean plasma LH concentration (0.25 ± 0.03 ng/ml vs 0.14 ± 0.03 ng/ml) than the subordinate goats during the first six hours of exposure to the buck (Alvarez et al. 2009).

8.3 Synchronization of Estrus by Hormonal Protocol

Hormonal regimens based on progestogens, equine chorionic gonadotropin (eCG) and/or prostaglandins have been established for over four decades, allowing estrus and ovulation synchronization during both the breeding and non-breeding seasons. Synchronization of estrus is a technique by which most of the females in a population or herd can be brought into estrus at a predetermined time. It is a valuable management tool that has been successfully employed to enhance reproductive efficiency, particularly in ruminants (Kusina et al. 2000). In small ruminants, estrus synchronization is achieved either by reducing the length of the luteal phase of the estrus cycle with PGF_2-alpha or by extending the cycle artificially with exogenous progesterone or more potent progestogens (Kusina et al. 2000; Hafez and Hafez 2000).

The prostaglandins, especially PGF_2-alpha and its analogues, have been recognized as being luteolytic in domestic animals. Although they are ineffective when administered between the fourth and sixth days of the caprine estrus cycle (Ott 1982), this disadvantage could be overcome by giving two injections at an 11-day interval when all cycling goats should have a regressible CL. Medan et al. (2004) synchronized estrus with a single injection of 125 µg of a synthetic analogue of PGF_2-alpha after detection of CL by ultrasonography and reported 56.00 ± 2.70 hours interval for onset of estrus after the injection.

Several workers used a dose of 5–12.5 mg PGF_2-alpha (dinoprost tromethamine) for synchronization of estrus in does (Ahmed et al. 1998; Parmar et al. 2020). Akusu and Egbunike (1984) gave two intramuscular (IM) injections of PGF_2-alpha 11 days apart with two different doses of 5 and 10 mg/animal in two groups, each containing five does. All the animals of both groups showed synchronized estrus after 43.2 ± 10.73 and 59 ± 15.25 hours following the second injection with 5 and 10 mg PGF_2-alpha respectively. Parmar et al. (2020) reported an induction interval of 52.33 ± 1.15 hours estrus from the second PGF_2-alpha injection with cent per cent estrus response, 28.72 ± 0.54 hours duration of estrus and 44.44% conception rate at induced estrus, when does were injected with 12.5 mg dinoprost tromethamine at 11 days apart.

In Egypt, El-Amrawi et al. (1993) injected cycling Saanen goats twice with 8 mg PGF_2-alpha with an interval of 11 days between injections; 100% exhibit ed estrus within 48 hours after the second injection, with an 80% conception and kidding rate. Our indigenous goats (Black Bengal) show 100% synchronization of estrus with two injections of PGF_2-alpha at 11 days apart with a dose rate of 10 mg per injection after 113.3 ± 90.01 hours of the second injection with a conception rate of 83.3% (Pandey et al. 1985).

Effective synchronization of estrus with good conception rate in does can also be achieved by a double injection of PGF_2-alpha analogue, i.e., cloprostenol intramuscularly at 125 µg per injection at 13 days apart with 100% estrus response after 52.6 ± 4.8 hours following the second injection (Ahmed et al. 1998), at 10 days apart with 64% estrus response after 11–96 hours following the second injection (Kusina et al. 2000) and at 10 days interval with 83.3% estrus response after 20.4 ± 0.9 hours following the second injection (Perera et al. 1978).

Estrus synchronization in goats can be achieved by using a combination of two or more different hormonal treatments to achieve maximum pregnancy rates. Gupta et al. (2021) reported a 51.72% estrus response when GnRH injection was administered on day 0 and 9, and injection and PGF_2-alpha on day 7 (standard ovsynch protocol). However, in Mahabubnagar local goats, Kanduri et al. (2022) observed 80%, 52.37 ± 3.59 hours, 38.25 ± 1.76 hours and 80% estrus response, onset of estrus after PGF_2-alpha injection, duration of estrus and conception rate, respectively.

Estrus can be synchronized in goats by locally prepared progesterone sponges with good fertility rate. Kausar et al. (2009) prepared polyurethane sponges with medroxyprogesterone acetate (MAP: 60 mg) inserted intravaginally in a group of eight female postpartum goats (Beetal × Dwarf). By this treatment all the experimental goats exhibited estrus within 21–100 hours of removal of sponges on the 17th day. The average time from sponge withdrawal to the onset of estrus was 65.4 ± 24.0 hours. Several other workers also used intravaginal progesterone sponges with different doses for 14–16 days and achieved 50–80% estrus synchronization effect after 38–53 hours of sponge removal (Ahmed et al. 1998; Kusina et al. 2000; Greyling and Van Niekerk 1991). Dogan et al. (2016) assessed the four progestogen treatments for different duration on estrus synchronization and pregnancy rate in Anatolian black goats and stated that the reduction in the duration of progestogen treatment can be used without affecting reproductive efficiency. Kumar et al. (2018) reported a 75% pregnancy rate by only inserting vaginal sponge impregnated with progesterone for 12 days.

Pregnant mare serum gonadotropin (PMSG) is usually used in combination with progesterone or progestogen intravaginal sponges. PMSG can be injected intramuscularly before or after removal of the sponge in anestrous and cycling goats (Corteel 1975). A dose rate of 375–750 IU of PMSG is recommended to synchronize estrus. Any increase beyond this depresses rather than enhances the conception rate. However, a dose of 300 IU has been reported to synchronize estrus in goats (Bongso et al. 1982). A 40–60 mg progesterone-impregnated vaginal sponge for 14–16 days and 300–500 IU PMSG injection intramuscularly at or before two days of sponge removal gives good synchronization effect (75–100%) in does following 40–52 hours of sponge removal (Ahmed et al. 1998; Greyling and Van Niekerk 1991; Greyling and van der Nest 2000).

The ovarian response of goats to estrus synchronization varies with the type of intravaginal sponge, kind of progestogens, breed, nutritional status (Mani et al. 1992), stress, environment, and male effect (Romano 1993).

8.4 Behavior of Goats During Estrus

The mean number of estrus periods per doe per annum recorded for the Boer goat doe is 11.7 ± 4.4 (Greyling and Van Niekerk 1987) and in theAngora, it is 4.7 ± 2.5 (Marincowitz 1962). A high frequency (approximately 30%) of long estrous cycles (40–60 days) is observed in the Boer goat doe (Greyling and Van Niekerk 1987).

The mean estrous cycle length is a minimum of 18.32 days in the Chegu goat (Thakur and Singh 2002) followed by 18.56 ± 0.57 days in Beetal × Black Bengal goats (Singh et al. 2002), 19.27 ± 1.94 days in Black Bengal (Ahmed 1992) and 20.7 ± 0.7 days in mature Boer does (Greyling 2000) with a range of 15–24 days (Ahmed 1992). The incidence pattern of the estrus cycle in Beetal × Black Bengal goats is short (<10 days), medium (10–28 days), and long (>28 days) at 20.87%, 65.14%, and 13.99%, respectively (Singh et al. 2002).

Similarly, the mean estrus duration is recorded to be a minimum of 29.28 hours in the Chegu (Thakur and Singh 2002) followed by 35.52 ± 2.39 hours in tropical Indian goats (Goel et al. 1992) and 37.4 ± 8.6 hours in mature Boer goats (Greyling 2000). Estrus duration in the tropical Indian goat ranges between 12 and 60 hours (Goel et al. 1992). There is no significant difference recorded between multiparous, biparous, or primiparous Boer goats (38.2 vs 34.0 vs 38.6 hours, respectively) (Greyling 2000).

The mean estrus duration was similar to that of normally cycling goats in synchronized does using progesterone-impregnated intravaginal sponges alone or in combination with PMSG. Estrus durations of 29.8 ± 6.7 hours (Kausar et al. 2009), 31.5 ± 15.1 hours (Greyling and van der Nest 2000) and 40.7 ± 14.5 hours (Greyling and Van Niekerk 1991) have been recorded following synchronization of estrus using intravaginal progesterone-impregnated sponges at 60 mg/sponge for 14–16 days with or without 300–500 IU PMSG intramuscularly on the day of sponge removal.

In comparison to progesterone sponges, PGF_2-alpha shows a shorter duration of estrus following synchronization of estrus. The mean estrus durations using PGF_2-alpha (dinoprost tromethamine) are 18 hours (Pandey et al. 1985) and 21.75 ± 1.03 hours (Ishwar and Pandey 1992). As per Akusu and Egbunike (1984), estrus duration is 39 ± 15.76 and 22.4 ± 8.6 hours following the second injection of PGF_2-alpha at 11 days apart with dose rates of 5 mg and 10 mg, respectively.

The estrus duration was significantly ($P < 0.05$) low in does which were treated with the buck effect (21.90 ± 0.87 hours) versus untreated does (47.00 ± 1.00 hours) (Mondal et al. 2009).

Estrous behavior includes two phases: proceptivity and receptivity. Proceptivity consists of seeking out and stimulating the male partner. Receptivity consists of expression of the immobilization reflex in response to male nudges, inducing serial mounting and copulation. At the beginning of estrus, proceptivity always precede receptivity; then both behavior components are expressed simultaneously. The duration of estrous behavior is about 36 hours but varies from 24 to 48 hours depending on age, individuals and breeds, season, and presence of a male (Ghosh 2021).

In the absence of a buck, it is difficult to detect estrus does (Hafez and Hafez 2000; Noakes 2001). Does at estrus become more active and attentive. Behavioral symptoms included restlessness, nonspecific bleating, wagging of tail, frequent micturition, and tendency to cluster around the buck, turn their head back when approached by the male allowing him to tease while swollen external genitalia, estral discharge or moist appearance of the external genitalia were recorded as physical signs of estrus. Restlessness was observed in 94.25% estrus, whereas nonspecific bleating, wagging of tail, frequent micturition, and tendency to cluster around the buck were noticed in 91.95%, 94.83%, 31.60%, and 62.07% estrus, respectively. The swollen external genitalia were found to be the most common physical symptom (95.40%) (Ghosh and Das 2002).

As per studies carried out by Mondal (2005) in indigenous goats of the Rohilkhand region, the most common sign of behavioral estrus is a swollen vulva (93.8%) in does. Rubbing neck and body with the male (37.5%) (Figure 8.1), putting the nose under the male's flank (31.3%), and tail fanning (59.83%) are other important estrus behavioral signs.

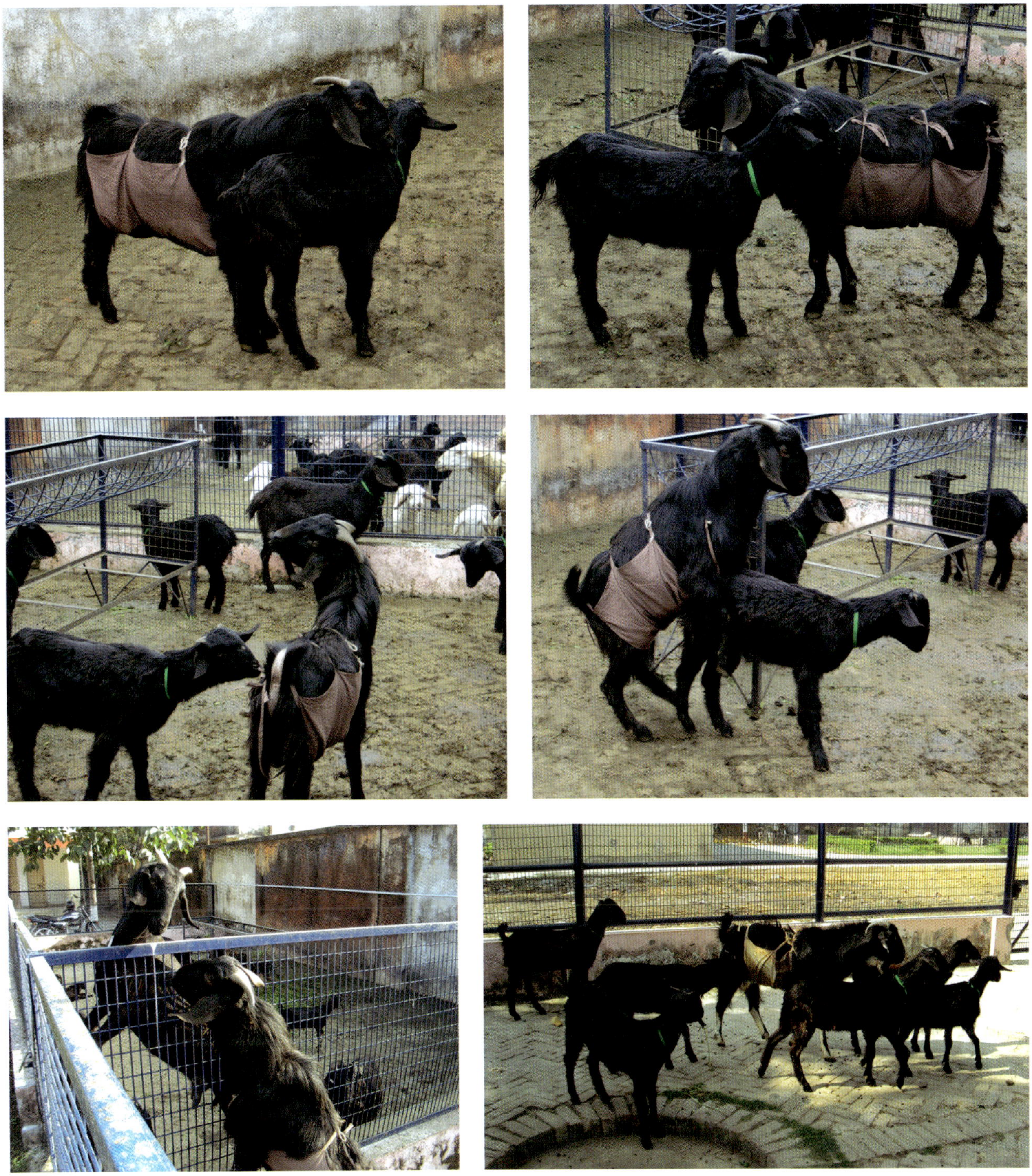

Figure 8.1 Estrus-related behaviors in goats.

8.5 Hormones Related to Estrus and Their Changes in Goats

Estradiol-17-beta and progesterone are ovarian hormones that have several practical applications in the management of reproduction in animals. They are involved in estrus manifestations, the ovulatory process, cyclic regression of the corpus luteum, establishment of pregnancy, and parturition.

8.5.1 Estradiol-17-beta

Estradiol-17-beta is the primary biologically active estrogen secreted from theca and granulosa cells of the growing ovarian follicles. It induces the behavioral symptoms of estrus and exerts both positive and negative feedback controls on LH and follicle-stimulating hormone (FSH) release from the pituitary (Hafez and Hafez 2000). The concentration of this gonadal steroid varies with the stages of reproduction.

Prior to estrus, the circulatory levels of estradiol-17-beta start rising from day 19 (22.3 ± 4.2 pg/ml) of the previous cycle (Leyva-Ocariz et al. 1995) and attain their peak at or around the day of estrus. Recorded levels of estradiol-17-beta by Yede et al. (2021) at estrus were 34.11 ± 1.04 and 32.92 ± 1.31 pg/ml in does treated with different hormonal treatments and 35.69 ± 2.10 pg/ml in Surti does having no treatment, respectively. Similar concentration (35.20 ± 16.3 pg/ml) was also reported by Cetin et al. (2021) in hairy goats at the Small Ruminants Research Center, Van Yüzüncü Yıl University, Van, Turkey, during the estrus phase. Levels of 28 ± 6 and 24 ± 5 pg/ml were also observed in crossbred (Alpine-Nubian) and native goats in Venezuela, respectively (Leyva-Ocariz et al. 1995) during estrus.

The blood level of estradiol-17-beta on the day of estrus in Indian native goats such as Surti (15.54 ± 1.0 pg/ml) and Marwari (15.39 ± 1.59 pg/ml) is much less in comparison to exotic goats (Pathak et al. 1992). As per Khanum et al. (2008), this level is also less in dwarf goats (*Capra hircus*) of Pakistan, with 7.7 ± 1.7 pg/ml at estrus, and drops down to lower levels within 3–4 days post estrus, while the peak value of estradiol-17-beta (14.0 ± 1.2 pg/ml) is observed on the 18th day of the cycle, i.e., 1–2 days prior to estrus. However, the value of estradiol-17-beta at estrus may be as high as 152.6 ± 31.6 pg/ml (Akusu et al. 2004); 46.1 ± 5.9, 41.6 ± 5.2, and 93.1 ± 39.5 pg/ml in does suckled for 60 days, does suckled for 120 days, and nonlactating does respectively (Gaafar et al. 2005) and 1.16 ng/ml (Bauernfeind and Holtz 1991).

The blood level of estradiol-17-beta starts decreasing gradually as the luteal phase advances, i.e., up to day 13 of the cycle, and then starts increasing, reflecting the new follicular phase reaching a peak on day 20 of the cycle (Pathak et al. 1992; Yede et al. 2021). The value during the luteal phase is, however, varied among the studies. The lowest recorded value is 4–6 pg/ml (Pathak et al. 1992) followed by 10–20 pg/ml (Bono et al. 1983; Yede et al. 2021); 12.5–15 pg/ml (Leyva-Ocariz et al. 1995); 45.7 ± 3.1, 30.8 ± 1.4, and 61.04 ± 6.5 pg/ml in does suckled for 60 days, does suckled for 120 days, and nonlactating does respectively (Gaafar et al. 2005) and 0.9 ng/ml (Bauernfeind and Holtz 1991).

The estradiol-17-beta remains at lower concentrations for 30–50 days of gestation, then gradually increases and reaches 270 ± 13.0 pg/ml a few days before parturition (Khanum et al. 2008). Yede et al. (2021) observed a 12–16 pg/ml concentration in Surti does at day 30 post breeding. In Indian goats, the overall average concentration of serum estradiol-17-beta is 142.43 ± 22.51 and 158.30 ± 24.90 pg/ml for Surti and Marwari goats, respectively, for the entire pregnancy period while the values (259.3 ± 11.41 and 260.8 ± 12.36 pg/ml respectively) increased much higher a day prior to parturition (Patel et al. 1992).

There are seasonal differences in secretion of the ovarian steroid hormones following induced estrus using intravaginal progesterone sponges (40 mg FGA) for 12 days and 500 IU PMSG IM injection at sponge withdrawal. In autumn, the concentration of estradiol-17-beta at estrus (15.3 ± 5.0 versus 12.2 ± 3.8 pg/ml; $P < 0.01$) is significantly higher than in spring (Blaszczyk et al. 2004).

Exposure of cyclic does to males increases LH pulse frequency in the early luteal (EL) and LL groups ($P < 0.01$) but not in the midluteal (ML) group ($P > 0.1$). Male exposure also increases basal and mean concentrations of LH in the LL group ($P < 0.05$). There is no significant effect of male exposure on basal concentrations of LH in the EL or ML groups ($P < 0.1$). There is no change in mean concentrations of LH in the ML group and the apparent increase in this variable in the EL group is not significant ($P < 0.1$). LH pulse frequency increases due to positive feedback caused by estradiol-17-beta. The physiological implications of increased pulsatile LH secretion during the early and late luteal phase of female goats are currently unknown (Hawken et al. 2009). As per Chemineau et al. (1986), contact with males induces a rapid and dramatic increase in the frequency and amplitude of plasma LH pulses. Before introduction of the males, there were 0.3 pulses per three hours in five Saanen goats, with a mean amplitude of 0.5 ng/ml. After buck introduction this increased to 2.2 pulses per three hours with a mean amplitude of 1.2 ng/ml.

8.5.2 Progesterone

Progesterone is a principal steroid hormone secreted mainly by the CL. The adrenal cortex and placenta also secrete some progesterone during certain specific physiological stages like pregnancy. The circulatory concentration of progesterone directly reflects the function of the CL indicating the stage of cycle. Progesterone in blood plasma is a reliable and convenient means of monitoring ovarian activity in livestock, including goats (Thibier et al. 1981).

The level of progesterone in blood changes throughout the estrous cycle. At or around estrus, the peripheral concentration of progesterone fluctuates at basal levels of 0.1–0.8 ng/ml. The level begins to rise from day 3 of the cycle, reaching a peak (3–10 ng/ml) between days 9 and 14 and remains elevated till days 16–17 of the cycle (Thorburn and Schneider 1972; Thibier et al. 1981; Wani 1989; Bauernfeind and Holtz 1991; Pathak et al. 1992; Leyva-Ocariz et al. 1995; Nandy et al. 2001; Zarkawi and Al-Masri 2002; Gaafar et al. 2005; Khanum et al. 2008). With the start of luteolysis on days 16–17, the progesterone level declines rapidly to the basal value (below 1 ng/ml) and remains at this level until the next estrus and ovulation (Pathak et al. 1992).

A progesterone level below 1 ng/ml at the time of estrus is consistent in the literature (Yede et al. 2021; Saribay et al. 2020; El-Tarabany et al. 2019). However, the initial increase as well as peak values appearing in relation to days of luteal phase of cycle are reportedly variable among different studies. This variation is attributed to the difference in climate, breed, management, assay methodology, and antisera used (Leyva-Ocariz et al. 1995). The lowest mean plasma progesterone levels during pregnancy are 4.5–5.5 ng/ml (Thorburn and Schneider 1972) followed by 5.41 ± 1.91 and 4.31 ± 1.51 ng/ml for Surti and Marwari goats respectively (Patel et al. 1992); 4.3–11 ng/ml (Khanum et al. 2008); 8.56 ± 0.39 ng/ml (Hirata and Mori 1995); 13.84 ± 3.77 ng/ml (Zarkawi and Al-Masri 2002); 4.6 ± 2.8 and 24.5 ± 3.1 ng/ml at two and 12 weeks of pregnancy respectively (Gaafar et al. 2005).

Progesterone secretion during the luteal phase is positively related to social dominance in goats. This may explain the difference in conception time between dominant and subordinate does, where dominant females conceive earlier. As per a study conducted by Alvarez et al. (2010), during days 11–17 following prostaglandin synchronization, the plasma progesterone levels are higher in high-ranking ($P < 0.05$), compared to low-ranking does. Progesterone levels are 96.2 ± 5.8, 79.5 ± 5.3, and 81.3 ± 5.3 ng/ml for high-, medium-, and low-ranking does respectively.

There are seasonal differences in the secretion of ovarian steroid hormones following induced estrus using intravaginal progesterone sponges (40 mg FGA) for 12 days and 500 IU PMSG i/m injection at sponge withdrawal. In autumn, the concentration of progesterone at estrus (0.42 ± 0.11 vs 0.27 ± 0.08 ng/ml; $P < 0.01$) is significantly higher than in spring (Blaszczyk et al. 2004).

After male introduction, the concentration of progesterone decreases over 12 hours of sampling in females in the LL group. There is no change in progesterone concentrations in females in the EL or ML groups (Hawken et al. 2009). As per Chemineau (1983), a high proportion of females is in estrus within six days of male exposure and it is proposed that this divergence in the distribution of estrus is driven by the presence of males. Interestingly, these females have significantly lower concentrations of progesterone (2.95 ± 0.53 ng/ml vs 5.06 ± 0.68 ng/ml) than females that come into estrus after this date.

8.6 Conclusion

The buck effect is mostly used for inducing estrus in goats which are noncyclic for a long period of time but recent research has proved that it can also be used for synchronization of estrus in goats for achieving uniform kidding. Hence, the buck effect could be used as a management tool for improving reproductive efficiency in goats.

References

Ahmed, J. (1992). Reproductive patterns of Black Bengal goats (*Capra hircus*). Recent Advances in Goat Production. *Proceedings of the V International Conference on Goats*, 2–8 March 1992, International Goat Association, New Delhi, India.

Ahmed, M.M.M., Makawi, S.E., and Jubara, A.S. (1998). Synchronisation of oestrus in Nubian goats. *Small Ruminant Research* 30: 113–120.

Akusu, M.O. and Egbunike, G.N. (1984). Fertility of the West-African Dwarf goat in its native environment following $PGF_2\alpha$ induced oestrous. *Veterinary Quarterly* 6 (3): 173–176.

Akusu, M.O., Nduka, E., and Soyebo, B.A. (2004). Peripheral plasma levels of progesterone and oestradiol-17β of west african dwarf goats during the oestrus cycle. https://cgspace.cgiar.org/items/c2d93951-7659-441b-8ff5-b4400e70da94 (accessed 12 November 2022).

Alvarez, L., Ramos, A.L., and Zarco, L. (2009). The ovulatory and LH response to the male effect in dominant and sub-ordinate goats. *Small Ruminant Research* 83: 29–33.

Alvarez, L., Arvizu, R.R., Luna, J.A., and Zarco, L.A. (2010). Social ranking and plasma progesterone levels in goats. *Small Ruminant Research* 90: 161–164.

Avdi, M., Leboeuf, B., and Terqui, M. (2004). Advanced breeding and "buck effect" in indigenous Greek goats. *Livestock Production Science* 87: 251–257.

Bauernfeind, M. and Holtz, W. (1991). Progesterone and estrogen levels in serum of cycling goats measured by enzyme immunoassay. *Small Ruminant Research* 6: 95–102.

Blaszczyk, B., Udala, J., and Gaczarzewicz, D. (2004). Changes in oestradiol, progesterone, melatonin, prolactin, and thyroxin concentrations in blood plasma of goats following induced oestrus in and outside the natural breeding season. *Small Ruminant Research* 51: 209–219.

Bongso, T.A., Fatimah, I., and Dass, S. (1982). Synchronization of oestrous of goats treated with progestagen-impregnated intravaginal sponges and PMSG, and reproductive performance following natural mating or A.I. with frozen semen. *Journal of Animal Reproduction Science* 5: 111–116.

Bono, G., Cairoli, F., Tamanini, C., and Abrate, L. (1983). Progesterone, estrogen. LH, FSH and PRL concentration in plasma during the estrous cycle in goat. *Reproduction, Nutrition, Development* 23: 217–222.

Çetin, N., Eşki, F., Mis, L. et al. (2021). Dynamics of oxidants, antioxidants and hormones during different phases of pregnancy in hairy goats. *Kafkas Universitesi Veteriner Fakultesi Dergisi* 27 (1): 117–121.

Chaudhary, M.M., Khasatiya, C.T., Patel, S.B. et al. (2018). Serum endocrine profile in relation to estrus synchronization in Surti does. *Indian Journal of Veterinary Sciences and Biotechnology* 13 (3): 44–48.

Chemineau, P. (1983). Effect of oestrus and ovulation of exposing Creole goats to the male at three times of the year. *Journal of Reproduction and Fertility* 67: 65–72.

Chemineau, P. (1987). Possibilities for using bucks to stimulate ovarian and oestrous cycles in anovulatory goats – a review. *Livestock Production Science* 17: 135–147.

Chemineau, P., Levy, F., and Thimonier, J. (1986). Effects of anosmia on LH secretion, ovulation and oestrous behaviour induced by males in the anovular Creole goats. *Animal Reproduction Science* 10: 125–132.

Claus, R., Over, R., and Dehnhard, M. (1990). Effect of male odour on LH secretion and the induction of ovulation in seasonally anoestrus goats. *Animal Reproduction Science* 22: 27–38.

Corteel, J.M. (1975). The use of progestagens to control the oestrous cycle of the dairy goat. *Annales de Biologie Animale Biochimie Biophysique* 15: 353–363.

Das, D.N., Paul, D., and Mondal, S. (2022). Biotechnological tools to enhance sustainable livestock production. In: *Emerging Issues in Climate Smart Livestock Production* (ed. S. Mondal and R. Singh), 317–337. Philadelphia: Elsevier.

Davila, F.S., Bosque-Gonzalez, A.S.d.B., and Barragan, H.B. (2017). Reproduction in goats. In: *Goat Science* (ed. S. Kukovics), 87–105. Herceghalom, Hungary: Intech Open.

Delgadillo, J.A., Gelez, H., Ungerfeld, R. et al. (2009). The 'male effect' in sheep and goats – revisiting the dogmas. *Behavioural Brain Research* 200: 304–314.

Delgadillo, J.A., Chemineau, P., and Keller, M. (2017). Using socio-sexual stimulations for sustainable goat production under subtropical latitudes. In: *Sustainable Goat Production in Adverse Environments*, vol. I (ed. J. Simoes and C. Gutiérrez), 89–99. Cham: Springer.

Dogan, I., Nur, Z., and Dogan, S. (2016). Different progestagen treatment duration on estrous synchronization during the natural breeding season in non-lactating Anatolian black goats. *Animal Reproduction* 13 (4): 806–810.

El-Amrawi, G.A., Hussein, F.M., and El-Bawab, I.E. (1993). Fertility of Saanen goats following induction of oestrus using $PGF_{2}\alpha$. *Assiut Veterinary Medical Journal* 29: 241–248.

El-Tarabany, M.S., El-Tarabany, A.A., and Atta, M.A. (2019). Effect of season on hormonal profile and some biochemical parameters at different stages of estrous cycles in Baladi goats. *Biological Rhythm Research* 50 (2): 1–10.

Ergul Ekiz, E., Ekiz, B., and Kocak, O. (2013). Effects of ram presence during synchronization period and previous experience on certain estrus parameters and sexual behaviors in Kivircik ewes. *Turkish Journal of Veterinary and Animal Sciences* 37: 189–193.

Fabre-Nys, C., Cognie, J., Dufourny, L. et al. (2017). The two populations of kisspeptin neurons are involved in the ram-induced LH pulsatile secretion and LH surge in anestrous ewes. *Endocrinology* 158: 3914–3928.

Flores, J.A., Véliz, F.G., Pérez-Villanueva, J.A. et al. (2000). Male reproductive condition is the limiting factor of efficiency in the male effect during seasonal anestrus in female goats. *Biology of Reproduction* 62: 1409–1414.

Gaafar, K.M., Gabr, M.K., and Teleb, D.F. (2005). The hormonal profile during the oestrus cycle and gestation in Damascus goats. *Small Ruminant Research* 57: 85–93.

Gelez, H. and Fabre-Nys, C. (2004). The "male effect" in sheep and goats: a review of the respective roles of the two olfactory systems. *Hormones and Behavior* 46: 257–271.

Ghosh, S. (2021). Reproduction in goats: a review. *International Journal of Recent Advances in Multidisciplinary Research* 8 (5): 6797–6802.

Ghosh, S.K. and Das, A. (2002). Studies on behavioural and physical symptoms of estrus in Black Bengal goat. In: *XVIII Annual Convention and National Symposium on Reproductive Technologies for Augmentation of Fertility in Livestock*, 128. Izatnagar, India: Indian Veterinary Research Institute.

Goel, A.K., Tyagi, S., and Agarwal, K.P. (1992). Ovulation characteristics of synchronized non-descript goats in tropical zone of India. Recent Advances in Goat Production. *Proceedings of the V International Conference on Goats*, 2–8 March 1992, International Goat Association, New Delhi, India.

Gonzalez-Bulnes, A., Carrizosa, J.A., Urrutia, B., and Lopez-Sebastian, A. (2006). Oestrus behaviour and development of preovulatory follicles in goats induced to ovulate using the male effect with and without progesterone priming. *Reproduction, Fertility, and Development* 18: 745–750.

Greyling, J.P.C. (2000). Reproduction traits in the Boer goat doe. *Small Ruminant Research* 36: 171–177.

Greyling, J.P.C. and van der Nest, M. (2000). Synchronization of oestrus in goats: dose effect of progestagen. *Small Ruminant Research* 36: 201–207.

Greyling, J.P.C. and Van Niekerk, C.H. (1987). Occurrence of oestrus in the Boer goat doe. *South African Journal of Animal Science* 17: 147–149.

Greyling, J.P.C. and Van Niekerk, C.H. (1991). Different synchronization techniques in Boer goat does outside the normal breeding season. *Small Ruminant Research* 5: 233–243.

Gupta, P.S.P., Tej, J.N., Johnson, P. et al. (2021). Efficiency of different synchronization protocols on oestrous response and rhythmic changes in 17β oestradiol and progesterone hormone concentration in Salem Black goats. *Biological Rhythm Research* 52 (1): 11–21.

Hafez, E.S.E. and Hafez, B. (2000). Sheep and goats. In: *Reproduction in Farm Animals*, 7e. Baltimore: Lippincott, Williams & Wilkins.

Hawken, P.A.R., Beard, A.P., Esmaili, T. et al. (2007). The introduction of rams induces an increase in pulsatile LH secretion in cyclic ewes during the breeding season. *Theriogenology* 68: 55–66.

Hawken, P.A.R., Esmaili, T., Jorre de st Jorre, T., and Martin, G.B. (2009). Do cyclic female goats respond to males with an increase in LH secretion during the breeding season? *Animal Reproduction Science* 112: 384–389.

Hirata, S. and Mori, Y. (1995). Monitoring reproductive status by fecal progesterone analysis in ruminants. *Journal of Veterinary Medical Science* 575: 845–850.

Ishwar, A.K. and Pandey, J.N. (1992). Oestrus synchronization and fertility in black Benegal goats following administration of progesterone and gonadotrophins. *Research in Veterinary Science* 52 (2): 141–146.

Kanduri, A.K.R., Reddy, K.C.S., Ramana, V.K. et al. (2022). Effect of different estrus synchronization protocols on reproductive performance in Mahabubnagar local goats. *Pharma Innovation Journal* SP-11(3): 1448–1452.

Karatzas, G., Karagiannidis, A., Varsakeli, S., and Brikas, P. (1997). Fertility of fresh and frozen-thawed goat semen during the nonbreeding season. *Theriogenology* 48: 1049–1059.

Karsch, F.J. (1984). The hypothalamus and anterior pituitary gland. In: *Reproduction in Mammals: 3 Hormonal Control of Reproduction*, 2e (ed. C.R. Austin and R.V. Short), 1–20. Cambridge: Cambridge University Press.

Kausar, R., Khanum, S.A., Hussain, M., and Shah, M.S. (2009). Estrus synchronisation with medroxyprogestrone acetate impregnated sponges in goats (*Capra hircus*). *Pakistan Veterinary Journal* 29 (1): 16–18.

Keskin, M. (2003). Influence of buck effect and exogenous hormone treatments on oestrus synchronization and litter size in Shami (Damascus) goats. *Turkish Journal of Veterinary and Animal Sciences* 27: 453–457.

Khanum, S.A., Hussain, M., and Kausar, R. (2008). Progesterone and estradiol profiles during estrous cycle and gestation in dwarf goats (*Capra hircus*). *Pakistan Veterinary Journal* 28 (1): 1–4.

Knight, T.W., Tervit, H.R., and Lynch, P.R. (1983). Effect of boar pheromones, rams wool, and presence of buck on ovarian activity in anovular ewes early in the breeding season. *Animal Reproduction Science* 6: 129–134.

Kumar, E.S.A., Reddy, K.R., Reddy, A.G. et al. (2018). Efficacy of estrus synchronization protocols on reproductive performance in goats. *Pharma Innovation Journal* 7 (3): 3–6.

Kusina, N.T., Tarwirei, F., Hamudikuwanda, H. et al. (2000). A comparison of the effects of progesterone sponges and ear implants, $PGF_2\alpha$, and their combination on efficiency of oestrus synchronization and fertility of Mashona goat does. *Theriogenology* 53: 1567–1580.

Lassoued, N., Naouali, M., Khaldi, G., and Rekik, M. (2004). Influence of the permanent presence of rams on the resumption of sexual activity in postpartum barbarine ewes. *Small Ruminant Research* 54: 25–31.

Leyva-Ocariz, H., Munro, C., and Stabenfeldt, G.H. (1995). Serum LH, FSH, estradiol-17β and progesterone profiles of native and crossbred goats in a tropical semiarid zone of Venezuela during estrous cycle. *Animal Reproduction Science* 39: 49–58.

Luna-orazco, J.R., Fernandez, I.G., Gelez, H., and Delgadillo, J.A. (2008). Parity of female goats does not influence their oestrus and ovulatory responses to the male effect. *Animal Reproduction Science* 106: 352–360.

Luna-Orozco, J.R., Guillen-Muñoz, J.M., De Santiago-Miramontes, M.A. et al. (2012). Influence of sexually inactive bucks subjected to long photoperiod or testosterone on the induction of estrus in anovulatory goats. *Tropical Animal Health and Production* 44: 71–75.

Major, I. and McConville, C. (2017). Vaginal drug delivery for the localised treatment of cervical cancer. *Drug Delivery and Translational Research* 7: 817–828.

Mani, A.U., McKelvey, W.A.C., and Watson, E.D. (1992). The effect of low level of feeding on response to synchronization of oestrus, ovulation, and embryo loss in goats. *Theriogenology* 38: 1013–1022.

Marincowitz, G. (1962). The sexual activity of Angora doe on mixed Karooveld. *South African Journal of Agricultural Science* 2 (5): 211–217.

Medan, M., Watanbe, G., Gamal, A.B.S.Y. et al. (2004). Early pregnancy diagnosis by means of ultrasonography as a method of improving reproductive efficiency in goats. *Journal of Reproduction and Development* 50 (4): 391–397.

Mellado, M., Olivas, R., and Ruiz, F. (2000). Effect of buck stimulus on mature and pre-pubertal norgestomet-treated goats. *Small Ruminant Research* 36: 269–274.

Mondal, S.K. (2005). Studies on 'male effect' and reproductive behaviour in sheep and goats under mixed flock system. PhD thesis. IVRI, Izatnagar, India.

Mondal, S.K., Joshi, H.C., Majumdar, A.C. et al. (2009). Reproductive responses of anoestrous indigenous doe to male introduction during postpartum. *Indian Journal of Animal Sciences* 79 (6): 554–560.

Nandy, D.K., Kumar, P., and Singh, K. (2001). Reproductive behaviour of goat in different seasons. *International Journal of Animal Sciences* 16 (1): 167–170.

Noakes, D.E. (2001). Endogenous and exogenous control of ovarian cyclicity. In: *Arthur's Veterinary Reproduction and Obstetrics* (ed. D.E. Noakes, T.J. Parkinson, and C.W. Gary), 3–53. London: W.B. Saunders.

Ott, R.S. (1982). Breeding techniques for dairy goats. *International Goat and Sheep Research* 1: 1–15.

Over, R., Cohen-Tannoudji, M., Claus, R., and Signoret, J.P. (1990). Effect of pheromones from male goats on LH-secretion in anoestrus ewes. *Physiology & Behavior* 48: 665–668.

Pandey, J.N., Ishwar, A.K., and Singh, R.A. (1985). Oestrous synchronization in goats using prostaglandin (Lutalyse). *Indian Journal of Animal Sciences* 55 (7): 551–552.

Parmar, C.P., Dhami, A.J., Patel, J.A., and Belsare, V.P. (2020). Efficiency of different estrus synchronization protocols in Surti goats. *Indian Journal of Veterinary Science and Biotechnology* 15 (3): 21–23.

Patel, A.V., Pathak, M.M., Mehta, V.M., and Janakiraman, K. (1992). Circulating hormone levels in pregnant goats. Recent Advances in Goat Production. *Proceedings of the V International Conference on Goats*, New Delhi, India.

Pathak, M.M., Patel, A.V., Jaiswal, R.S. et al. (1992). Circulating hormone levels in cyclic goats. Recent Advances in Goat Production. *Proceedings of the V International Conference on Goats*, 2–8 March 1992, International Goat Association, New Delhi, India.

Pearce, G.P. and Oldham, D.M. (1988). Importance of non-olfactory ram stimuli in mediating ram induced ovulation in the ewe. *Journal of Reproduction and Fertility* 84: 333–339.

Pellicer-Rubio, M.T., Boissard, K., Grizelj, J. et al. (2019). Vers une maitrise de la reproduction sans hormones chez les petits ruminants [Reproduction mastering without hormones in small ruminants]. *INRA Productions Animales* 32 (1): 51–66.

Perera, B.M.A.O., Bongso, T.A., and Abeynaike, P. (1978). Oestrus synchronisation in goats using cloprostenol. *Veterinary Record* 102: 314.

Rahman, A.N.M.A., Abdullah, R.B., and Wan-Khadidjah, W.E. (2008). Synchronization and superovulation in goats: a review. *Journal of Biological Sciences* 8: 1129–1137.

Restall, B.J. (1988). The artificial insemination of Australian goats stimulated by the buck effect. *Proceedings of the Australian Society of Animal Production* 17: 302–305.

Rivaz-Munoz, R., Fitz-Rodriguez, G., Poidron, P. et al. (2007). Stimulation of estrous behaviour in grazing female goats by continuous or discontinuous exposure to males. *Journal of Animal Science* 85: 1257–1263.

Romano, J.E. (1993). Effect of service on oestrus duration in dairy goats. *Theriogenology* 40: 77–84.

Romano, J.E. and Fernandez Abella, D. (1997). Effect of service on duration of oestrus and ovulation in dairy goats. *Animal Reproduction Science* 47: 107–112.

Rosa, H.J.D. and Bryant, M.J. (2002). The "ram effect" as a way of modifying the reproductive activity in the ewe – a review. *Small Ruminant Research* 45: 1–16.

Roumen, F.J. and Dieben, T.O. (2006). Comparison of uterine concentrations of ethinyl estradiol and etonogestrel after use of a contraceptive vaginal ring and an oral contraceptive. *Fertility and Sterility* 85: 57–62.

Saribay, M.K., Naseer, Z., Dogruer, G. et al. (2020). Variations in serum metabolites in response to season, cyclicity, and pregnancy in estrus synchronized Damascus goats. *Tropical Animal Health and Production* 52: 1519–1525.

Sharma, H.C., Khasatiya, C.T., Chaudhari, N.F., and Tyagi, K.K. (2022). Efficacy of various estrus synchronization protocols on reproductive performance in Surti does. *Haryana Veterinarian* 61 (SI): 53–55.

Shelton, M. (1980). Goats: influence of various exteroceptive factors on initiation of oestrus and ovulation. *International Goat and Sheep Research* 1: 156–162.

Singh, D.K., Singh, L.B., and Das, P. (2002). Effect of parity and season on incidence and duration of oestrous cycle in Beetal Halfbreds with Black Bengal goats. In: *XVIII Annual Convention and National Symposium on Reproductive Technologies for Augmentation of Fertility in Livestock*, 114. Izatnagar, India: Indian Veterinary Research Institute.

Thakur, Y.P. and Singh, M. (2002). Reproductive parameters of chegu goats in their breeding tract. In: *XVIII Annual Convention and National Symposium on Reproductive Technologies for Augmentation of Fertility in Livestock*, 138. Izatnagar, India: Indian Veterinary Research Institute.

Thibier, M., Pothelet, D., Jeanguyot, N., and deMontigny, G. (1981). Estrous behaviour, progesterone in peripheral plasma and milk of dairy goats and onset of breeding season. *Journal of Dairy Science* 64 (3): 513–519.

Thimonier, J., Chemineau, P., and Gauthier, D. (1983). Augmenter la fertilite des ruminants en zone tropicale: une realité. *Reproduction des Ruminants En Zone Tropicale, Pointe-a-pitre*. Guadelope, FWI.

Thorburn, G.D. and Schneider, W. (1972). The progesterone concentration in the plasma of the goat during the oestrus cycle and pregnancy. *Journal of Endocrinology* 52: 23–36.

Tibary, A. (2009). Estrus synchronization and AI: method for successful and timely pregnancy. *81st Western Veterinary Conference, 15–19 February, 2009, V552*, Washington State University, USA.

Underwood, E.J., Shier, F.L., and Davenport, N. (1944). Studies in sheep husbandry in W.A.V. The breeding season of Merino, crossbred and British ewes in the agricultural districts. *Journal of Agriculture of Western Australia* 2: 135–143.

Ungerfeld, R., Forsberg, M., and Rubianes, E. (2004). Overview of the response of anoestrous ewes to the male effect. *Reproduction, Fertility, and Development* 16: 479–490.

Veliz, F.G., Moreno, S., Duarte, G. et al. (2002). Male effect in seasonally anovulatory lactating goats depends on the presence of sexually active bucks, but not estrous females. *Animal Reproduction Science* 72: 197–207.

Veliz, F.G., Poindron, P., Malpaux, B., and Delgadillo, J.A. (2006). Maintaining contact with bucks does not induce refractoriness to the male effect in seasonally anestrous female goats. *Animal Reproduction Science* 92: 300–309.

Veliz, F.G., Meza-Herrera, C.A., De Santiago-Miramontes, M.A. et al. (2009). Effect of parity and progesterone priming on induction of reproductive function in Saanen goats by buck exposure. *Livestock Science* 125: 261–265.

Walkden-Brown, S.W., Restall, B.J., and Henniawati (1993a). The male effect in the Australian Cashmere goat. 1. Ovarian and behavioural response of seasonally anovulatory does following the introduction of bucks. *Animal Reproduction Science* 32: 41–53.

Walkden-Brown, S.W., Restall, B.J., and Henniawati (1993b). The male effect in the Australian Cashmere goat. 2. Role of olfactory cues from the male. *Animal Reproduction Science* 32: 55–67.

Walkden-Brown, S.W., Restall, B.J., and Henniawati (1993c). The male effect in the Australian Cashmere goat. 3. Enhancement with buck nutrition and use of oestrous females. *Animal Reproduction Science* 32: 69–84.

Walkden-Brown, S.W., Martin, G.B., and Restall, B.J. (1999). Role of male-female interaction in regulating reproduction in sheep and goats. *Journal of Reproduction and Fertility* 52 (Suppl): 243–257.

Wani, G.M. (1989). Plasma progesterone concentration during oestrous cycle in goat. *Indian Journal of Animal Reproduction* 10 (1): 44–46.

Wani, A.A., Dhindsa, S.S., Shafi, T.A. et al. (2013). The role of pheromones in animal reproduction – a review. *Progressive Research* 8 (1): 14–18.

Yede, A.B., Khasatiya, C.T., Singh, V.K., and Kumar, D. (2021). Rhythmic changes in serum progesterone and estradiol-17β in surti goats under different synchronization protocols. *Indian Journal of Animal Research* 55: 1–6.

Zarkawi, M. and Al-Masri, M.R. (2002). Use of radioimmunoassay to measure progesterone levels during different reproductive stages in female Damascus goats. *Tropical Animal Health and Production* 34: 535–539.

9

Estrus Synchronization and Mating Systems in Goats

Ravi Ranjan[1], *Rajesh Kumar*[2], *Chetana Gangwar*[1], *and Pramod Kumar*[3]

[1] *Animal Physiology and Reproduction Division, ICAR-Central Institute for Research on Goat, Mathura, India*
[2] *Department of Veterinary Gynaecology and Obstetrics, College of Veterinary Science and Animal Husbandry, Acharya Narendra Deva University of Agriculture and Technology, Ayodhya, India*
[3] *Department of Veterinary Physiology and Biochemistry, College of Veterinary Science and Animal Husbandry, Acharya Narendra Deva University of Agriculture and Technology, Ayodhya, India*

9.1 Introduction

Synchronization of estrus is a technique by which a significant number of females in a flock are brought into estrus at a predetermined time (De Ziegler et al. 2007). The development of estrus synchronization techniques is directed at more intensive production and facilitating genetic improvement. The aims of these reproductive technologies are to speed up the genetic improvement of small ruminants and reduce the generation intervals. Estrus synchronization plays a major role in fixed time breeding, artificial insemination (AI), laparoscopic ovum pick-up (LOPU) for oocyte or embryo collection and embryo transfer (ET). This technique was developed in the early 1960s and since then a number of synchronizing methods have been introduced (Habeeb and Kutzler 2021).

Approaches to synchronizing estrus in livestock focus on manipulation of either the luteal or the follicular phase of the estrous cycle. In the doe, the window of opportunity is generally greater during the luteal phase, which is of longer duration and more responsive to manipulation. Different approaches have been concerned with either extending the luteal phase by supplying exogenous progesterone or shortening this phase through regression of the corpus luteum.

There are several ways to control the estrous cycle such as light manipulation, the male effect and hormone treatments with progesterone, prostaglandins (PG), equine chorionic gonadotropin (eCG), and gonadotropin-releasing hormone (GnRH).

9.2 Estrous Cycle

Knowledge of the estrous cycle is an important aspect of synchronization. It makes it possible to understand the various mechanisms which govern various protocols used during synchronization. Estrous cycle characteristics are summarized in Table 9.1.

9.2.1 Principles of Estrous Synchronization

The principal physiological basis for estrus synchronization is the fact that luteal progesterone exerts a negative feedback effect on the hypothalamus and subsequent suppression of LH release from the anterior pituitary gland and thus inhibits the maturation of Graafian follicles in the cyclic animal. Indeed, control of the time of ovulation occurs by maintaining a progesterone block on the hypothalamus by exogenous progesterone supplementation even after natural luteolysis or

Elements of Reproduction and Reproductive Diseases of Goats, First Edition. Edited by Tanmoy Rana.

Table 9.1 Species variation in estrous cycle characteristics.

Animal	Type of estrous cycle	Length of estrous cycle (days)	Duration of estrus	Time of ovulation	Time of insemination
Goat	Seasonal polyestrus in fall	18–21 Average: 19.5	1–4 days Average: 39 hours	21–36 hours after start of estrus	18 hours after the onset of the heat

removing the progesterone block by pharmacological luteolysis. Therefore, the two main methods of controlling the time of estrus are:

- holding the animal in an artificial luteal phase with exogenously administered progesterone until endogenous regression of the corpus luteum has occurred in all animals as the CL has an inherent life span
- induction of premature but predictable regression of the cyclic corpus luteum with prostaglandin F_2-alpha which in turn removes the negative feedback effect of progesterone and thus restarts synchronized follicular activity.

9.2.2 Progestagen-based Synchronization of Estrus

Administration of natural progesterone or its synthetic analogues, namely medroxyprogesterone acetate (MPA), methylacetoxyprogesterone (MAP), fluorogestone acetate (FGA), and norgestomet, might be an effective method of estrus synchronization in does. Various routes (intravaginal, intramuscular and subcutaneous) and doses of progesterone or progestagens have been tested with varying success (Hashemi et al. 2006; Abu et al. 2008; Knights and Singh-Knights 2016; Sun et al. 2019; Salim et al. 2020). In fact, progesterone and synthetic progestagens suppress estrus and ovulation. Moreover, progesterone has little effect on the life span of the corpus luteum unless treatment begins within four days after estrus. As stage of cycle is seldom known, classically progesterone administration for 18 days was advised (long-term progesterone therapy), a period after which all animals undergoes natural luteolysis. Since prolonged progesterone therapy results in lower fertility rates (Rubianes and Menchaca 2003; Fonseca et al. 2005), currently short-term progesterone therapy has been advocated as fertility is improved and infection minimized.

9.2.2.1 Orally Active Progestagens as Feed Supplement

Early studies on synchronization of estrus centered around the use of orally active progestagens like MPA, melengestrol acetate (MGA), and chloramidinone acetate (CAP). These compounds are usually fed for 18 days in a concentration of 0.25 mg/kg body weight. Estrus occurs within three days after withdrawal of progesterone feeding. Extensive data from studies conducted over a five-year period with MGA showed acceptable response in grouping heat periods, but a conception rate that was only 70% of that obtained in controls. The main disadvantage with oral treatment appears to be the inability to control the precise daily dose absorbed by each animal.

9.2.2.2 Intravaginal Sponges

The progesterone-impregnated intravaginal sponge has been the most common choice across the globe for estrus synchronization in small ruminants (Kirdli et al. 2002) during breeding and nonbreeding seasons. FGA and MPA are commercially available but fluorogestone acetate is the most commonly used synthetic progestagen in vaginal sponges (Whitley and Jackson 2004). Intravaginal sponges are usually inserted over a period of 9–12 days and used in conjunction with pregnant mare serum gonadotropin (PMSG) or follicle-stimulating hormone (FSH), particularly for out-of-season breeding, injected at the time of sponge removal or 48 hours before (Wildeus 2000). Furthermore, Sen and Onder (2016) used intravaginal sponges (30 mg fluorogestone acetate) for 11 days with or without 500 IU PMSG in Saanen goats and concluded that synchronization of estrus shortened the kidding period but use of PMSG may cause high kid mortality.

Intravaginal sponges have high retention rates (>90%) and females usually exhibit estrus within 24–48 hours after sponge withdrawal. The physical presence of the devices and the impact of the hormones may induce purulent vaginitis (Martins et al. 2009; Penna et al. 2013) but do not interfere with fertility. Furthermore, Endo et al. (2020) suggested that a mixture of mucoadhesive polymer and silicone fluid has the potential for sustained release of progesterone for estrus synchronization.

9.2.2.3 Intravaginal Coil/Controlled Internal Drug Release Device

The first report of the use of controlled internal drug release devices (CIDRs) for synchronizing estrous in ewes was made by Welch et al. (1984). A CIDR is a T-shaped intravaginal device made up of progesterone-impregnated medical silicone elastomers molded over a nylon core (Wheaton et al. 1992, 1993) and was developed as an alternative to intravaginal progestogen sponges. This product has been used in New Zealand and Australia with success for the past several years. Many types of CIDR are available and those intended for use in cattle, sheep, and goats were designated as CIDR-B, CIDR-S, and CIDR-G respectively. Some workers suggested that use of CIDRs did not require a milk or meat withdrawal period because CIDR-subjected goats have lower or similar milk progesterone concentrations than those found in goats who were in diestrus or pregnant (Rowe et al. 2010).

Unlike progesterone-based pessaries and sponges, CIDR devices did not impede vaginal secretions and are less foul smelling, have better retention rate, induce tight synchrony and consist of natural progesterone (Knights and Singh-Knights 2016). Long-term (more than 10 days) use of CIDR results in low progesterone concentration at the time of insert removal, ovulation of persistent or aged follicles, and reduced fertility (Johnson et al. 1996; Vinoles et al. 2001). To overcome the problem, short-term CIDR application along with PGF2-alpha at removal has been suggested (Beck et al. 1993).

Many studies reported effect time, i.e., long (13–16 days) or short duration (5–9 days) of CIDR insertion (Oliveira et al. 2001; Motlomelo et al. 2002; Romano 2004; Nogueira et al. 2011; Inya and Sumretprasong 2013), with the majority of protocols including PGF2-alpha and eCG treatment at or prior to insert removal. Moreover, Motlomelo et al. (2002) opined that MAP, FGA, and CIDR are equally effective in synchronization of estrus in Boer goats, when progestin withdrawal is followed by 300 IU PMSG intramuscularly. Vilarino et al. (2011) reused CIDR-Gs associated with short-term protocols which yielded an acceptable pregnancy rate (60%) in goats but it was significantly lower than with use of a new device.

9.2.2.4 Injectable Progesterones

Intravaginal pessaries are not always available and promising results have been obtained using injectable progesterone (Bongso et al. 1982; Niswender et al. 2000; Al-Merestani et al. 2003; Chao et al. 2008; Chemineau et al. 1999; Suresh et al. 2021) so this might be a good choice for synchronizing estrus in does. Furthermore, Khatun et al. (2022) reported that intramuscular injection of synthetic progesterone (12.5 or 15 mg) for 14 days might be used for estrus synchronization in Black Bengal goats. Similarly, Alvarado-Espino et al. (2019) proposed a pessary-free ultra-short protocol for estrus synchronization in acyclic multiparous and nulliparous Alpine goats which is composed of 20 mg injectable progesterone followed by 100 IU hCG 24 hours later. Moreover, estrus was tightly synchronized after hCG injection and resulted in an acceptable pregnancy rate following fixed-time artificial insemination (FTAI).

9.2.2.5 Subcutaneous Implants

This method involves the use of a subcutaneous polymer implant impregnated with highly potent progesterone SC21009 (norgestomet) which is inserted in the ear for nine days, the start of the treatment being preceded by an injected dose of progestagen estrogen (2.5 mg estradiol valerate and 1.5 mg norgestomet in goats). Removal of the implant is followed by satisfactory estrus response and normal fertility.

- Shorter progestagen treatments result in higher fertility than long-term treatments, but adequate control of CL through use of PGF2-alpha is required.
- The use of GnRH 30 hours after progesterone withdrawal synchronized onset of ovulation in does.
- The injection of 400–500 IU eCG (PMSG) at the time of progestagen removal increases the estrus response and degree of synchronization.

9.2.3 Prostaglandin (PGF2-alpha)-based Synchronization of Estrus

Control of the estrous cycle using PGs is based on the fact that PGF2-alpha causes luteolysis of the susceptible CL (McCracken et al. 1970). As prostaglandins are quickly metabolized in the lungs, PGs do not build up in tissues (Piper et al. 1970) so they are good substitutes for progestagens because of public health and animal welfare concerns (Martin et al. 2004). Indeed, natural PGF2-alpha (dinoprost tromethamine and carboprost) produces normal luteolysis through slow degeneration (Abecia et al. 2011) and synthetic analogues of PGF2-alpha (cloprostenol sodium) typically have a more potent and prolonged effect (Gordon 1997; Omontese et al. 2012). When the goat CL is receptive on day 3 of the estrus cycle, prostaglandins should be given (Gonzalez-Bulnes and Veiga-Lopez 2008).

Prostaglandins are usually administered through intramuscular or subcutaneous routes but the intravulval submucosal route has been tried with varying success. Factors affecting estrus response to the prostaglandin are dose (Greyling and van Niekerk 1987) and route of administration, the interval between PG doses (Lassal et al. 2004), age of CL (Rubianes and Menchaca 2003), the season, and the use of other hormones as co-treatment (Omontese et al. 2014). In order to improve estrus response rates, PG protocols have been modified using gonadotropins such as FSH, eCG, and GnRH. Moreover, Matsumoto et al. (2021) reported that intravaginal insertion of estradiol benzoate capsules with sustained drug delivery base is applicable for synchronization of estrus.

One advantage of prostaglandin use is lack of tissue residue as it is rapidly and completely metabolized in the lung on intramuscular administration (Evans et al. 2004) but a few workers have reported variability in ovulation timing due to compromised follicular function (Hawken et al. 2007). Furthermore, the drugs do not create problems of antibody production (Baril et al. 1996), follicular cyst (Santiago Moreno et al. 1999) or vaginitis (Penna et al. 2013), as occurs with use of other hormones.

Usually, two PGF2-alpha injections must be given at intervals of 9–11 days. By doing this, practically all the animals would be in the middle of their luteal phase, which would improve their response to the second treatment (Amiridis and Cseh 2012). Two doses of cloprostenol sodium at 11-day interval result in a higher estrus response (92.8% vs 75%) compared to single shot in Red Sokoto goats(Omontese et al. 2013). Furthermore, Maia et al. (2017) studied the effect of two doses of 37.5 µg d-cloprostenol injected at 7-, 10-, and 11.5-day intervals and observed that 7- and 11.5-day intervals promoted high estrus synchrony following the second dose; moreover, overall estrus induction response did not differ significantly among different groups. Wondem et al. (2022) compared the efficacy of three estrus synchronization protocols (P4+eCG+PGF2-alpha; single-shot PG, and double-shot PG) for estrus synchronization in Abergella goats during the breeding season and concluded that double-shot PG could be a more effective method of synchronization of estrus in fixed-time AI. Different agents used for synchronization of estrus are summarized in Table 9.2.

Table 9.2 Timeline of different agents used for synchronization of estrus in goats.

Name of agent	Ingredients	Dose	Route of administration	References
Veramix® (Pharmacia & Upjohn, Canada)	Medroxyprogesterone acetate	60 mg for 18 days in goats	Intravaginal sponge	Goel and Agrawal (1991)
Choronogest® (Intervet, France)	Fluorogestone acetate	45 mg for 9–12 days in sheep	Intravaginal sponge	Freitas et al. (1996)
Synchromate®-B (Sanifi Animal Health, USA)	Norgestomet	3 mg for 9 days	Subcutaneous implant	Rowe and East (1996)
CIDR (Inter Ag, New Zealand)	Progesterone	330 mg	Intravaginal sponge	Waldron et al. (1999)
Natural progesterone (SDF Fine Chemicals, India)	Progesterone	350 mg for 12–14 days in sheep	Intravaginal sponge	Das et al. (2000)
Crestar® ear implant (Intervet, Holland)	Norgestomet	3 mg ear implant + IM injection of 1.5 mg noregestomet +2.5 mg estradiol valerate	Subcutaneous implant	Kharche et al. (2002)
Lutalyse (Upjohn Co., USA)	Dinoprost tromethamine	7.5 mg single injection, IM	IM	Kharche et al. (2002)
Lutalyse (Upjohn Co., USA)	Dinoprost tromethamine	Double injection at 11 days apart, 7.5 mg × 2, IM	IM	Goel and Agrawal (2003)
Clostenol (Sarabhai Zydus Animal Health Ltd, India)	Cloprostenol	1 ml	IM	Kharche et al. (2008)

9.3 The Male Effect

Estrus can be induced with the strategic exposure of anestrous does and ewes to intact males or androgen-treated castrates. This response is dependent on the depth of seasonal anestrus and associated with a first ovulation in 2–3 days. This effect is mediated through changes in pulsatile GnRH release from the hypothalamus, selectively increasing tonic LH. The first ovulation is usually silent and of low fertility, with premature regression of the first CL. The second ovulation five days later is accompanied by a fertile estrus with a luteal phase of normal length. The response to the male effect is influenced by such factors as the serving capacity and sexual aggressiveness of the buck and ram, and the intensity of the stimulation, with immediate contact resulting in a greater response than fenceline contact or intermittent contact and body condition.

9.4 Applications of Synchronization of Estrus

- To reduce the age of puberty during prepubertal period of goats.
- To reduce the time required for detection of estrus.
- To allow breeding of goats at a fixed time without estrus detection.
- To facilitate the use of AI in a breeding program designed to accelerate genetic improvement.
- To synchronize and determine parturition dates so that parturitions take place when facilities and staff are available.
- To increase reproductive rate by induction of ovarian activity in anestrous females, particularly seasonal breeders.
- To provide a useful management aid for scheduling the use of animals and facilities.
- To implement assisted reproductive technologies in reproduction such as embryo transfer, cloning and transgenesis, etc.

9.5 Female Mating Systems

Reproductive performance of a goat flock is assessed by breeding efficiency, kidding percentage, and kidding rate. Generally, it ranges between 80–90%, 90–150%, and 1.0–1.80 in Indian goat breeds. Breeding tools such as selection are adopted on goat farms to enhance reproductive efficiency. Does and female kids play a crucial role in improving reproduction in goats.

Mating systems in goats include natural and artificial mating using AI techniques.

9.5.1 Selection of Superior Males

Choice of future bucks should include pure-bred males as individuals and progeny of pure-bred parents, large in size (sire and doe) as per breed standards, and doe (mother) with good milk yield record. Height and body length of selected individuals should be very good. They should bear genetic potential for good feed conversion efficiency. Body weight of candidate males at different production stages should be very good (30–35% higher than average); as an example, the body weight of a Barbari male should be about 2, 9, 17, 23, and 29 kg at birth, 3, 6, 9, and 12 months of age under semiintensive feeding systems. Testes should be well developed and descended and equal in size. A buck should have good libido and be able to fertilize females. A good buck should be able to transmit its characteristics to its progeny and should not be a carrier of any genetic disease.

The best method of buck selection is construction of a selection index on the basis of the nine-month body weight of that particular male and 90 days milk yield of its dam. Those who attain the top rank along with the above described characteristics should be selected, tested (semen quality and libido) and then used for breeding.

For good conception, a buck should be utilized after attaining proper physical and physiological maturity. In large goat breeds such as Jamunapari, Jakhrana, Beetal and Sirohi, the proper age of breeding is after 18 months, in medium breeds such as Osmanabadi, Sangamneri, Marwari, Barbari, Gaddi, and Malabari it is 16 months and in small breeds such as Black Bengal 12 months. A buck should be used twice in a week and 2–3 females should be covered in a day. One male is sufficient to cover 30 females but one should always keep one standby buck.

A semiintensive feeding system is ideal to boost a buck's performance and selection. Breeding males should be fed 400–500 g dry fodder, 500–1000 g green fodder, and 200–300 g concentrate per day as a maintenance ration. However, during the breeding season in summer (April–June) and autumn (September–November), a buck should be provided 200, 250, and 300 g additional concentrate for small, medium, and large breeds respectively. In order to avoid inbreeding, a particular buck should be used for one year for small flocks and 1.5 years for medium to large flocks. However, in large flocks a breeding chart could be prepared through which unrelated males and females can be used for breeding. Farmers with small flocks often rotate (exchange) their buck after one year of use in their flocks. However, such bucks should be vaccinated against all infectious diseases and screened for brucellosis as per schedule.

Those bucks whose progeny (daughters) have high milk yields (in case of milch breed), deliver multiple births or have good growth rates should be identified for semen collection and extensive utilization through AI with frozen semen.

9.5.2 Breeding Management

9.5.2.1 Decide Breeding Period

Even though Indian goats are bred throughout the year, most goat breeds have two peaks of breeding, one in May–July and another in September–November; more than 80% of does come into heat and are bred during these months. Rather than breeding does throughout year, it is worthwhile to identify the breeding seasons and breed the does during these restricted periods for efficient management of kidding and kids. Initially, the frequency of goats coming into heat during different months should be recorded and the decision of breeding period based on this.

9.5.2.2 Allotment of Does to Each Buck

The allotment of does to each buck should be done prior to the breeding season by preparing a breeding chart. This is essential for avoiding inbreeding and achieving the maximum number of progeny per buck.

9.5.2.3 Flushing of Does Before Breeding Season

The method of flushing does is to withdraw concentrate feed for a week with good exercise through the increasing grazing period, irrespective of grazing available. The does are then fed additional concentrate at 100 g each and 100 g of sprouted matki (*Phaseolus aconitifollus*) and moth bean (kulhathi) (*Vigna aconitifolia*) for three weeks. This should be done one month before the onset of the breeding season.

9.5.2.4 Isolation of Does Showing No Signs of Heat

Does showing no signs of heat should be kept in a separate pen in order to undertake reproductive healthcare.

Besides any specific treatment, provide 100 g of sprouted matki/grains for a period of 15 days in addition to usual concentrate mixture and also provide Cocu-Tabs as per recommendation. Does may be mated when 10–15 months old so that they kid at the age of 15–20 months. As a rule, a goat should not be mated until it is one year old. The average gestation period is 150 ± 3 days. It is better to breed a female once a year but some goats can be bred twice in 18 months. Goats are at their maximum breeding efficiency from four to seven years.

9.5.3 Breeding Policy and Road Map for Goat Improvement and Conservation

- Selective breeding and grading up are two breeding approaches recommended for goat improvement after thorough review of past goat improvement and development programs. Under this policy registration large numbers of flocks should be involved as essential components of the program. Selective breeding may be implemented through nucleus schemes.
- Improvement of goats in a flock (which are increasing in number and decreasing in size) requires a regular supply of potential semen. Therefore, the technologies of frozen semen and AI need perfection in caprines and simultaneously capacity building of veterinary officers and goat keepers.
- The nondescript goat population is extensive and needs immediate attention. Upgrading of nondescript goats by improver stock suitable for that particular breed may be utilized for this purpose. AI with a good potential buck has tremendous potential for improvement. Programs will be long term so input support (services) to farmers and data recording on production, reproduction, and pedigree are equally important.
- Improvement in the genetic potential of goats needs a regular supply of superior bucks and semen through establishment of nucleus farms, kids' nursery farms, and buck mother farms. To ensure continuous improvement, such nucleus farms should have sound selection and breeding programs and management of goats.

- Formation of goat breeder's cooperatives/societies/SHGs. Such groups should be financially and technically supported. The process of credit to allow goat keepers to adopt technologies and expand their flocks should be simplified.
- Establishment of more multiplier flocks of each breed and proper recording of data for open nucleus breeding system-based genetic improvement.

9.5.4 Artificial Insemination

It is said that centuries ago Bedouin horse breeders stole the semen of famous stallions by inserting a sponge into the vagina of a mare before service and then successfully transferring the sponge to their own mares.

The first documented use of AI in domestic animals was done by the Italian physiologist L. Spallanzani in 1780. A new landmark in the field of AI was established in 1949, when Polge et al. (1949) discovered a practical method for the long-term preservation of semen of certain species by deep freezing to temperatures of −79 °C, by means of dry ice (CO_2). AI is the deliberate introduction of semen into a female reproductive tract for the purpose of achieving a pregnancy through fertilization by means other than mating/natural service. In India, AI in goats is relatively less developed compared to cattle and buffalo, the main reason being lack of emphasis on the economic importance of goats.

The human population is predicted to reach 1.7 billion and the goat population will be 216 million by 2050 (ICAR-CIRG, Vision 2050). Therefore to meet requirements for milk, meat, and associated byproducts of the ever increasing human population, it is imperative to increase goat productivity. This could be possible by increasing highly productive descript (33%) goat population and reducing nondescript (67%) and less productive goats by promoting scientific goat farming. There are 71 million breedable does and 17 million breeding bucks available in India as per the 12th Livestock Census Report. One buck by natural mating can cover a maximum of 50 does in a year, but using stored frozen semen, 3000 does can be covered in a year. Therefore, to cover 71 million breedable does, we need 1.5–2 million bucks in a natural system, compared to only 50 000 bucks needed for frozen semen AI technology.

Artificial insemination is the first generation of reproductive biotechnology by which we can replace nondescript and less productive goats with a productive goat population. AI and semen cryopreservation represent a pivotal tool for long-term *ex situ in vitro* conservation, in order to exchange valuable germplasm of livestock and endangered species. Encouraged by the experimental work on AI in goats, several AI centers and veterinary clinics in different parts of the country have started by maintaining 2–4 stud goats. Mixed AI centers would reduce the cost of these operations. However, few centers are operating exclusively for goats (Table 9.3).

9.5.4.1 Methods of AI

- Intravaginal
- Intracervical
- Intrauterine

Intravaginal and intracervical AI are used by most workers. The other methods are used for research purposes.

For intracervical AI, the estrous goat is lifted for clear visualization of the genitalia (Figure 9.1). A lubricated glass vaginal speculum is inserted through the vagina for visualization of the cervical opening under sunlight. Then a fresh or frozen thawed semen straw is inserted through the speculum and through the cervical opening and semen is deposited there and waits for 2–3 minutes. Clitoral massage should be done for better fertility. AI should be done twice at a 12-hour interval. If a goat comes into estrus in the morning, then AI should be done in the evening of the same day and morning of the next day.

Table 9.3 How AI will be helpful.

Total goats in the country	148.88 million	
Breedable does	85 million	
Breedable bucks	15 million	
	Natural mating	**AI with frozen semen**
Number of goats covered by one buck in a year	50	2000
Bucks required to cover breedable goats	**2 million**	**50 000**

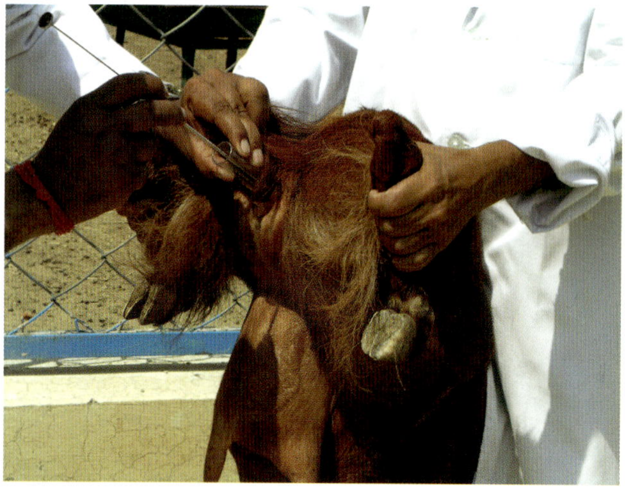

Figure 9.1 Artificial insemination.

- Nonspermicidal, sterile lubricant
- Semen thaw unit
- Insemination reports
- Fresh cooled or frozen semen
- Vaginal swabs
- Liquid nitrogen storage tank

Goats have a complex cervical anatomy, with 3–6 cartilaginous cervical folds horizontally aligned. It is very difficult to pass an AI gun throughout the cervix. The conception rate is highly correlated with depth of penetration so the above technique is more suited to goats and easy to perform. The total time taken is 2–3 minutes. The pregnancy rate is 20–55% (FAO 2012).

9.5.4.2 AI Equipment and Supplies

- Carrying case
- Kit warmer
- AI gun
- AI gun sheaths
- AI light
- Vaginal speculum
- Straw tweezers
- Straw cutter

9.5.4.3 Factors Affecting AI

The success of any AI program is largely dependent on three primary factors.

- The use of live/viable fresh cooled or frozen semen.
- The appropriate timing of insemination in relation to estrus and ovulation.
- The proper deposition of semen in the doe.

Other factors affecting AI include the following.

- The breed.
- Age of buck and doe.
- Condition of buck and doe.
- Nutrition.
- Season of insemination.
- The use of fresh, cooled, chilled, frozen semen.
- The technique involved.
- Time of insemination.
- The extender used.
- Dose of inseminated semen.
- The method (vaginal, cervical, cervicouterinal, laparoscopic) used.

9.5.4.4 Fertility with Frozen Semen

Although laparoscopic AI involving deposition of frozen-thawed semen directly into the uterus generally results in 60–70% fertility (Salamon and Maxwell 1995), the conception rate of cryo-preserved semen following transcervical AI (TCAI) is still very low (16–40%; Kumar and Naqvi 2014). Premature capacitation as a consequence of freezing and thawing curtails the lifespan of spermatozoa which therefore have a shorter time to achieve fertilization compared to fresh sperm. Therefore, further research efforts are required to develop better freezing protocols and diluents that minimize the ultrastructural and biochemical alterations in spermatozoa resulting from the freezing/thawing process, particularly if intended for TCAI because spermatozoa have to survive longer to traverse through the cervical mucosa before reaching the site of fertilization.

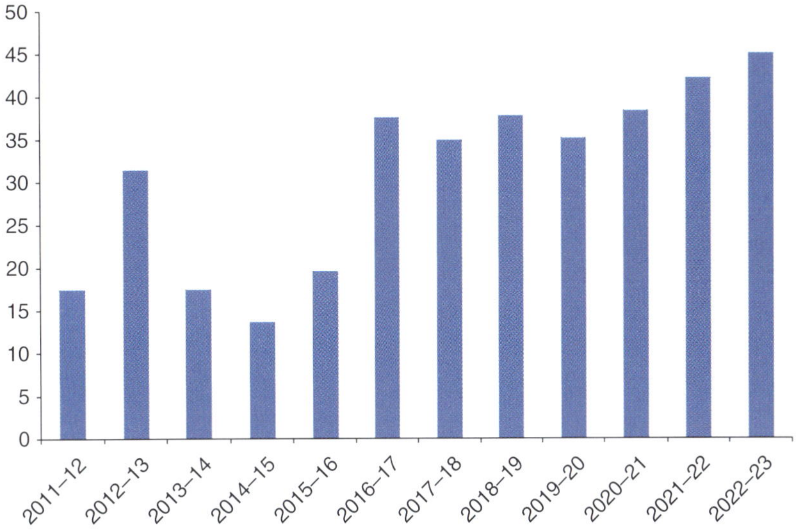

Figure 9.2 Kidding percentage through AI at ICAR-CIRG in different years.

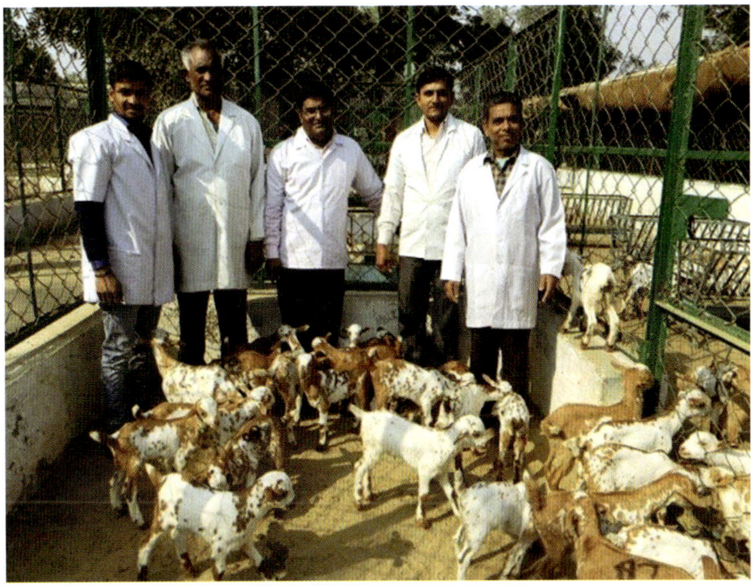

Figure 9.3 Kids born through AI.

The kidding rate was 37.57% during 2016–2017 at ICAR-CIRG, Mathura, UP, India in four breeds of goat – Jamunapari, Barbari, Jakhrana, and Sirohi – through frozen semen AI technology (Figures 9.2 and 9.3).

9.5.4.5 Applications

The pioneering work on techniques in goat carried out at the Indian Veterinary Research Institute, Izatnagar, and Veterinary College, Mathura, revealed around 50% conceptions after first insemination with washed spermatozoa diluted in EYC diluents. Though AI in goats has been attempted on an experimental basis at various organized farms and research institutions in India, serious and coordinated efforts are still lacking for taking up AI in goats on a large scale as has occurred in cattle and buffalo. Research work on the freezability of buck semen with the use of citrate-yolk milk and tris-citrate acid yolk diluents was carried at Veterinary College Anand, Guwahati, Tirupati, Ranchi, Bombay, Akola, NARI and Mathura including the Central Institute for Research on Goats (CIRG). Irrespective of glycerol percentage (3–9%) and equilibration time (0–6 hours), postthaw motility varied between 42% and 66%. There was a 71.43% pregnancy rate with a kidding rate of 1.27 by pellet semen. Conception rate was poor (35–45%) due to deposition of frozen semen over the opening of the cervix. Improvement in fertility (55–65%) was observed with a deep cervical insemination technique.

9.5.4.6 Laparoscopic Insemination

Laparoscopic insemination entails elaborate equipment and special skills. Laparoscopic AI (LAI) with frozen semen yields higher pregnancy rates and allows a reduction in the concentration of the seminal dose (200 vs 100 million spermatozoa/inseminated goats with the CAI and LAI techniques, respectively). Gibbons et al. (1997) obtained a 69% pregnancy rate by LAI with 100 million frozen spermatozoa/insemination dose under optimal conditions in an Angora herd. Similarly, other authors with different breeds (cashmere: Ritar et al. 1990; dairy goats: Baril et al. 1992) reported a 20% increase in pregnancy rates when applying LAI in relation to average values of CAI.

Pregnancy rates achieved with LAI are approximately 60–80% (Cseh et al. 2012), making use of this technique an attractive option for producers with large numbers of animals requiring insemination. Pregnancy rates of 56.67% were observed with frozen thawed semen through LAI by Anakkul et al. (2014). In concurrence with these findings, Ritar et al. (1990) reported 52.1% pregnancy rates in cashmere goats and Gibbons and Cueto (2011) reported 54% pregnancy rates in Angora goats with frozen semen through LAI.

9.5.4.7 Important Applications of AI

- The technique helps to introduce a new or desirable genotype into the livestock population at a faster rate.
- High-quality semen produced by superior sires can be used to breed large numbers of does.
- AI helps in genetic management.
- The maintenance of a large number of males, which would otherwise be required, is reduced.
- AI permits reproduction when suitable males are not available for natural mating.
- The technique provides accurate breeding records for good herd management.
- AI improves the efficiency of on-farm progeny testing schemes by a better elimination of the flock effect.
- Valuable sires which are incapable of mating due to age or injury may be utilized through electric ejaculation.
- AI prevents stray mating and also solves the problems of mating of dams of unequal size.
- The technique helps control disease transmission, since males used for insemination are under health control and do not circulate from one flock to another.
- The technique can be used as a means of sex control through separation of X- and Y-spermatozoa before use.
- Artificial insemination has been used experimentally to yield hybrids between species that do not voluntarily mate.

9.5.4.8 Limitations

- There is a possibility of dissemination of hereditary defects or uncontrolled diseases.
- Lack of awareness on the part of goat keepers of the economic advantages of using selected progeny-tested males.
- Conception rate with AI is lower than that of natural matings.
- Due to lack of cheap and practical techniques of estrus synchronization in tropical goats, the farmer has to spend a lot of time in heat detection and breeding operations.
- Lack of interest on the part of concerned agencies to encourage the concept of mixed AI centers (cow, buffalo, goat) which is quite feasible in the existing AI set-up in India.
- Illiteracy among farmers, religious taboos and sentiments also serve as limiting factors.
- There is a need for scientists to exchange experience, discussions, and mutual understanding of the problems of AI in goats.
- A sound program does not exist for training extension workers in AI of goats at the national and provincial level.

References

Abecia, J.A., Forcada, F., and Gonzalez-Bulnes, A. (2011). Pharmaceutical control of reproduction in sheep and goats. *Veterinary Clinics of North America: Food Animal Practice* 27: 67–79.

Abu, A.H., Iheukwumere, F.C., and Onyekwere, M.U. (2008). Effect of exogenous progesterone on oestrus response of West African Dwarf (WAD) goats. *African Journal of Biotechnology* 7 (1): 59–62.

Al-Merestani, M.R., Zarkawi, M., and Wardeh, M.F. (2003). Improving the reproductive efficiency, pregnancy diagnosis and monitoring the resumption of luteal activity in indigenous damascus goats. *Reproduction in Domestic Animals* 38 (1): 36–40.

Alvarado-Espino, A.S., Menchaca, A., Meza-Herrera, C.A. et al. (2019). Use of injectable progesterone and hCG for fixed-time artificial insemination during the non-breeding season in goats. *Theriogenology* 127: 21–25.

Amiridis, G. and Cseh, S. (2012). Assisted reproductive technologies in the reproductive management of small ruminants. *Animal Reproduction Science* 130: 152–161.

Anakkul, N., Suwimonteerabutr, J., Tharasanit, T. et al. (2014). Sperm distribution and fertilization after unilateral and bilateral laparoscopic artificial insemination with frozen-thawed goat semen. *Theriogenology* 82 (8): 1137–1144.

Baril, G., Remy, B., Vallet, J.C., and Beckers, J.F. (1992). Effect of repeated use of progestagen-PMSG treatment for estrus control in dairy goats out of breeding season. *Reproduction in Domestic Animals* 27 (3): 161–168.

Baril, G., Remy, B., Leboeuf, B. et al. (1996). Synchronization of estrus in goats: the relationship between eCG binding in plasma: time of occurrence of estrus and fertility following artificial insemination. *Theriogenology* 45: 1553–1559.

Beck, N.F.G., Davies, B., and Williams, S.P. (1993). Oestrous synchronization in ewes: the effect of combining a prostaglandin analogue with a 5-day progestagen treatment. *Animal Production* 56: 207–210.

Bongso, T.A., Fatimah, I., and Dass, S. (1982). Synchronisation of oestrus of goats treated with progestagen-impregnated intravaginal sponges and PMSG, and reproductive performance following natural mating or AI with frozen semen. *Animal Reproduction Science* 5 (2): 111–116.

Chao, L.M., Takayama, K., Nakanishi, Y. et al. (2008). Luteal lifespan and fertility after estrus synchronization in goats. *Journal of Veterinary Science* 9 (1): 95–101.

Chemineau, P., Baril, G., Leboeuf, B. et al. (1999). Implications of recent advances in reproductive physiology for reproductive management of goats. *Journal of Reproduction and Fertility. Supplement* 54: 129–142.

Cseh, S., Faigl, V., and Amiridis, G.S. (2012). Semen processing and artificial insemination in health management of small ruminants. *Animal Reproduction Science* 130 (3–4): 187–192.

Das, G.K., Naqvi, S.M.K., Gulyani, R. et al. (2000). Effect of two doses of progesterone on estrus response and fertility in acycling crossbred Bharat Merino ewes in a semi-arid tropical environment. *Small Ruminant Research* 37 (1–2): 159–163.

Endo, N., Rahayu, L.P., Yamamura, T. et al. (2020). Intravaginal administration of progesterone using a new technique for sustained release in goats. *Journal of Reproduction and Development* 66 (5): 489–492.

Evans, A.C.O., Duffy, P., Crosby, T.F. et al. (2004). Effect of ram exposure at the end of progestagen treatment on oestrus synchronisation and fertility during the breeding season in ewes. *Animal Reproduction Science* 84: 349–358.

FAO (2012). *Livestock Country Reviews (3). Pig Sector in Kenya*. Rome: Food and Agriculture Organization.

Fonseca, J.F., Torres, C.A.A., Costa, E.P. et al. (2005). Progesterone profile and reproductive performance of estrus-induced Alpine goats given hCG five days after breeding. *Animal Reproduction* 2 (1): 54–59.

Freitas, V.J., Baril, F.G., and Saumande, J. (1996). Induction and synchronization of estrus in goats: the relative efficiency of one versus two fluorogestone acetate impregenated vaginal sponges. *Theriogenology* 46: 1251–1256.

Gibbons, A. and Cueto, M. (2011). Cryopreservation and diffusion of goat genetic material in the Argentine Patagonia. *Revista Brasileira de Reprodução Animal* 35 (2): 108–112.

Gibbons, A., Willems, P., and Cueto, M. (1997). *Inseminación artificial con semen congelado por vía vaginal o laparoscopía en cabras de raza Angora*, vol. 2, 165–170. Estoril, Portugal: I Congreso Ibérico de Reproducción Animal.

Goel, A.K. and Agrawal, W.D. (1991). Induction and synchronization of oestrus in anoestrus (a cyclical recipient goats). *Indian Journal of Animal Reproduction* 12 (2): 187–189.

Goel, A.K. and Agrawal, K.P. (2003). Ovulation in Jakhrana goats native to tropical climates. *Small Ruminant Research* 50 (1–2): 209–212.

Gonzalez-Bulnes, A. and Veiga-Lopez, A. (2008). Ovarian follicular dynamics and dominance effect in sheep. *Societa Italiana di Fisiologia Veterinaria. VI Congress Nazionale*. Stointino (Sassari), Italy.

Gordon, I. (1997). *Controlled Reproduction in Farm Animals Series, Controlled Reproduction in Sheep and Goats*, vol. 2. New York: CABI.

Greyling, J.P.C. and van Niekerk, C.H. (1987). Occurrence of oestrus in the Boer goat doe. *South African Journal of Animal Science* 17: 147–149.

Habeeb, H.M.H. and Kutzler, M.A. (2021). Estrus synchronization in the sheep and goat. *Veterinary Clinics of North America. Food Animal Practice* 37 (1): 125–137.

Hashemi, M., Safdarian, M., and Kafi, M. (2006). Estrous response to synchronization of estrus using different progesterone treatments outside the natural breeding season in ewes. *Small Ruminant Research* 65 (3): 279–283.

Hawken, P.A.R., Beard, A.P., Esmaili, T. et al. (2007). The introduction of rams induces pulsatile LH secretion in cyclic ewes during the breeding season. *Theriogenology* 68: 56–66.

Inya, T. and Sumretprasong, J. (2013). Serum progesterone profiles in Saanen crossbred goats during a 5-day progestin-based estrous synchronization protocol. *Kasetsart Journal (Natural Science)* 47: 94–100.

Johnson, S.K., Dailey, R.A., Inskeep, E.K., and Lewis, P.E. (1996). Effect of peripheral concentrations of progesterone on follicular growth and fertility in ewes. *Domestic Animal Endocrinology* 13: 69–79.

Kharche, S.D., Goel, A.K., Jindal, S.K, and Sinha, N.K. (2002). Estrous response to different synchronizing agents in nondescript goats. *XVIII Annual Convention of ISSAR and National Symposium in Reproductive Technology for Augmentation of Fertility in Livestock* (14–16 November 2002). IVRI, Izatnagar, India.

Kharche, S.D., Goel, A.K., Jindal, S.K. et al. (2008). Effect of somatic cells co-culture on cleavage and development of in-vitro fertilized caprine embryos. *Indian Journal of Animal Sciences* 78 (7): 686.

Khatun, A., Hoque, S.A.M., Ali, M.Y., and Mamy, K. (2022). Estrus synchronization in Black Bengal goats using synthetic progesterone. *Journal of Agriculture, Food and Environment* 3 (1): 33–38.

Kirdli, R.T., Abdullah, A.Y.M., and Husein, Q. (2002). Protocols for estrus synchronization in awassi ewes under arid environmental conditions. *Asian-Australasian Journal of Animal Sciences* 15 (7): 957–962.

Knights, M. and Singh-Knights, D. (2016). Use of controlled internal drug releasing (CIDR) devices to control reproduction in goats: a review. *Animal Science Journal* 87 (9): 1084–1089.

Kumar, D. and Naqvi, S.M.K. (2014). Effect of time and depth of insemination on fertility of Bharat Merino sheep inseminated trans-cervical with frozen-thawed semen. *Journal of Animal Science and Technology* 56 (1): 1–6.

Lassal, A., Hernandez-Ceron, J., Rodrıguez-Maltos, R., and Gutierrez, C.G. (2004). The influence of the corpus luteum on ovarian follicular dynamics during estrous synchronization in goats. *Animal Reproduction Science* 84: 369–337.

Maia, A.L.R.S., Brandao, F.Z., Souza-Fabjan, J.M.G. et al. (2017). Reproductive parameters of dairy goats after receiving two doses of d-cloprostenol at different intervals. *Animal Reproduction Science* 181: 16–23.

Martin, G.B., Milton, J.T., Davidson, R.H. et al. (2004). Natural methods for increasing reproductive efficiency in small ruminants. *Animal Reproduction Science* 82: 231–245.

Martins, G., Figueira, L., Penna, B. et al. (2009). Prevalence and antimicrobial susceptibility of vaginal bacteria from ewes treated with progestin-impregnated intravaginal sponges. *Small Ruminant Research* 81 (2–3): 182–184.

Matsumoto, S., Tanaka, T., and Endo, N. (2021). Intravaginal administration of estradiol benzoate capsule for estrus synchronization in goats. *Journal of Reproduction and Development* 67 (2): 83–88.

McCracken, J.A., Glew, M.E., and Scramuzzi, R.J. (1970). Corpus luteum regression induced by prostaglandin F2α. *Journal of Clinical Endocrinology and Metabolism* 30: 544–546.

Motlomelo, K.C., Greyling, J.P.C., and Schwalbach, L.M.J. (2002). Synchronisation of oestrus in goats: the use of different progestagen treatments. *Small Ruminant Research* 45: 45–49.

Niswender, G.D., Juengel, J.L., Silva, P.J. et al. (2000). Mechanisms controlling the function and life span of the corpus luteum. *Physiological Reviews* 80 (1): 1–29.

Nogueira, D.A., Lopes, E.S. Jr., de Peixoto, R.M. et al. (2011). Using the same CIDR up to three times for estrus synchronization and artificial insemination in dairy goats. *Acta Scientiarum. Animal Sciences* 33: 321–325.

Oliveira, M.A.L., Guido, S.I., and Lima, P.F. (2001). Comparison of different protocols used to induce and synchronize estrus cycle of Saanen goats. *Small Ruminant Research* 40: 149–153.

Omontese, B.O., Rekwot, P.I., Makun, H.J. et al. (2012). Induction of estrus in Sahel goats using fluorogestone acetate (FGA) sponges and equine chorionic gonadotrophin (eCG). *Sokoto Journal of Veterinary Sciences* 10 (2): 21–25.

Omontese, B.O., Rekwot, P.I., Makun, H.J. et al. (2013). Oestrus induction using fluorogestone acetate sponges and equine chorionic gonadotrophin in red Sokoto goats. *South African Journal of Animal Science* 43 (1): 68–73.

Omontese, B., Rekwot, P., Rwuaan, J., and Nwannenna, A. (2014). Comparison of short-term vs. longterm progestin treatments for synchronisation of oestrus in Red Sokoto does during the rainy season. *Basic & Clinical Pharmacology & Toxicology* 115 (1): 370.

Penna, B., Libonati, H., Director, A. et al. (2013). Progestin-impregnated intravaginal sponges for estrus induction and synchronization influences on goats vaginal flora and antimicrobial susceptibility. *Animal Reproduction Science* 142 (1–2): 71–74.

Piper, P.J., Vane, J.R., and Wyllie, J.H. (1970). Inactivation of prostaglandins by the lungs. *Nature* 225: 600–604.

Polge, C., Smith, A.U., and Parkes, A.S. (1949). Revival of spermatozoa after vitrification and dehydration at low temperatures. *Nature* 164 (4172): 666.

Ritar, A.J., Ball, P.D., and O'May, P.J. (1990). Artificial insemination of Cashmere goats: effects on fertility and fecundity of intravaginal treatment, method and time of insemination, semen freezing process, number of motile spermatozoa and age of females. *Reproduction, Fertility and Development* 2 (4): 377–384.

Romano, J.E. (2004). Synchronization of estrus using CIDR, FGA or MAP intravaginal pessaries during the breeding season in Nubian goats. *Small Ruminant Research* 55: 15–19.

Rowe, J.D. and East, N.B. (1996). Comparison of two sources of gonadotropin for estrus synchronization in does. *Theriogenology* 45 (8): 1569–1575.

Rowe, J.D., Tell, L.A., Carlson, J.L. et al. (2010). Progesterone milk residues in goats treated with CIDR-G inserts. *Journal of Veterinary Pharmacology and Therapeutics* 33: 605–609.

Rubianes, E. and Menchaca, A. (2003). The pattern and manipulation of ovarian follicular growth in goats. *Animal Reproduction Science* 78: 271–287.

Salamon, S. and Maxwell, W.M.C. (1995). Frozen storage of ram semen. II. Causes of low fertility after cervical insemination and methods of improvement. *Animal Reproduction Science* 38: 1–36.

Salim, M.A.E.W., Nikhaila, A.M.M.A., Adam, A.A.G., and Eissa, H.I.A. (2020). Effect of synchronization protocols on timing and duration of estrus in Nubian goats. *University of Khartoum Journal of Agricultural Sciences* 17 (2): 270–282.

Santiago Moreno, J., Acosta Rodríguez, M., González De Bulnes, A. et al. (1999). Evaluation of the small ruminant cystic ovarian disease using transrectal ultrasonography. *Archivos de Zootecnia* 48: 157–165.

Sen, U. and Onder, H. (2016). The effect of estrus synchronization programmes on parturition time and some reproductive characteristics of Saanen goats. *Journal of Applied Animal Research* 44 (1): 376–379.

Sun, S., Liu, S., Luo, J. et al. (2019). Effects of repeated exposure to an estrus synchronization protocol on reproductive parameters in dairy goats. *Canadian Journal of Animal Science* 99 (3): 489–496.

Suresh, S., Annayappa, S., Narasimhamurthy, M. et al. (2021). Relative efficacy of short term progestagen and PGF2α with PMSG or GnRH or both on estrus synchronization in Hassan breed of ewes. *Pharma Innovation Journal* 10 (5S): 790–793.

Vilarino, M., Rubianes, E., and Menchaca, A. (2011). Re-use of intravaginal progesterone devices associated with the short-term protocol for timed artificial insemination in goats. *Theriogenology* 75 (7): 1195–1200.

Vinoles, C., Forsberg, M., Banchero, G., and Rubianes, E. (2001). Effect of long-term and short-term progestagen treatment on follicular development and pregnancy rate in cyclic ewes. *Theriogenology* 55: 993–1004.

Waldron, D.F., Willingham, T.D., Thompson, P.V., and Bretzlaff, K.N. (1999). Effect of concomitant injection of prostaglandin and PMSG on pregnancy rate and prolificacy of artificially inseminated Spanish goats synchronized with controlled internal drug release devices. *Small Ruminant Research* 31 (2): 177–179.

Welch, R.A.S., Andrews, W.D., Barnes, D.R. et al. (1984). CIDR dispensers for oestrus and ovulation control in sheep. *Proceedings of the 10th International Congress on Animal Reproduction and Artificial Insemination*. University of Illinois.

Wheaton, J.E., Carlson, K.M., Windels, H.F., and Johnston, L.J. (1992). *Use of Controlled Internal Drug Release Dispensers (CIDR) for Controlled Breeding of Sheep*, 123–133. Ames, IA: Iowa State University Extension.

Wheaton, J.E., Carlson, K.M., Windels, H.F., and Johnson, L.J. (1993). CIDR: a new progesterone-releasing intravaginal device for induction of estrus and cycle control in sheep and goats. *Animal Reproduction Science* 33: 127–142.

Whitley, N.C. and Jackson, D.J. (2004). An update on estrus synchronization in goats: a minor species. *Journal of Animal Science* 82 (E-Suppl): E270–E276.

Wildeus, S. (2000). Current concepts in synchronization of estrus: sheep and goats. *Journal of Animal Science* 77: 1–14.

Wondem, B., Taye, M., Alemayhu, K. et al. (2022). The efficacy of estrus synchronization protocols and artificial insemination in the Albergella goats on-station and on-farm condition of Northern Ethiopia. *Journal of Applied Animal Research* 50 (1): 518–525.

de Ziegler, D., Fraisse, T., de Candolle, G. et al. (2007). Outlook: roles of FSH and LH during the follicular phase: insight into natural cycle IVF. *Reproductive Biomedicine Online* 15 (5): 507–513.

10

Preparation for the Breeding Season

Ashok Baindha, Vipin Chandra, Rashmi Singh, and Mohan Lal

Post Graduate Institute of Veterinary Education and Research, Jaipur, India

10.1 Purpose of Goat Breeding

Goats are reared for livelihood generation, employment generation (Singh 2021), and as a source of earning in the form of:

- dairy production and dairy goat sales
- meat production and meat goat sales
- raising goats for fiber
- renting goats for brush clearing
- agri-tourism
- goat care services
- goat farm online marketing and education.

A good breeding stock is the foundation of any profitable sheep and goat enterprise.
Desirable characteristics of male and female animals are as follows.
Male:

- faster growth rate
- sexual aggressiveness
- health, fertility, and vigor.

Female:

- reproduce regularly at specified times
- early lambing/kidding ability
- good mothering ability with good milk yield
- production of lambs/kids with good growth rate
- have a long productive life.

Factors to be considered in selecting a breed of animal include:

- market demand in the area
- type of operation and breeding program
- the cost and availability of good seed stock
- the quantity and quality of available seed stock
- climatic condition and topography.

Elements of Reproduction and Reproductive Diseases of Goats, First Edition. Edited by Tanmoy Rana.

10.2 Establishing a Reproducing/Breeding Flock

The old adage "the sire is half of the flock" is very relevant to sheep and goat husbandry. Future productivity of the flock depends on proper selection of the male. The rate of progress from selection of males alone will probably be about twice as great as or more than selection of females. It is also essential to select the right type of females. When selecting breeding males and females, consider the following guidelines.

- *Health*: select males and females that are vigorous with clear eyes and healthy skin. Animals that stand with their head down and the "tail enders" when they are driven are probably sick. They should be avoided for establishing a breeding flock.
- *Soundness*: males to be used for breeding should have sound reproductive organs. They should have two well-developed testicles that are approximately the same size, well descended into the scrotum.

10.3 Examination for Breeding Soundness in Goats

Does and bucks should be examined before the breeding season to optimize the likelihood of reproductive success (Harighi *et al.* 2022). Breeding soundness examinations in does are typically performed only after discovering tht the doe did not become pregnant during the breeding season (Stewart 2022). Bucks should be in moderate body condition (3–4 out of 5) because they can lose more than 10% of their body condition during the breeding season. Does should be in marginal body condition (2–3 out of 5) to maximize response to focused feeding programs and to minimize the risk of developing pregnancy toxemia in the last trimester.

Breeding animals should be in overall good health. Anemia due to heavy parasite infections and chronic debilitating diseases, such as pneumonia, can lead to loss of libido and/or infertility. Foot abnormalities, from overgrown hooves to severe laminitis, should be treated appropriately to ensure the ability of bucks to mount and does to be mounted. Bucks with caprine arthritis and encephalitis (CAE) virus infection may have painful, enlarged stifles and even if they are able to mount, are usually reluctant to ejaculate because of pain. Does infected with CAE may have mastitis and should be culled. A complete assessment of the reproductive organs and semen quality should be performed routinely on all bucks before the breeding season, whereas does may be assessed only if they do not conceive.

The external genitalia of doelings should be examined for abnormalities such as an enlarged clitoris, hypotrophic vulva, or increased urogenital distance that suggest intersex, a condition common in homozygous polled females, especially in Alpine, Saanen, and Toggenburg breeds. Intersex goats are sterile and should be culled. Examination of the external genitalia may also help to detect adhesions or rectovaginal fistulas in multiparous does that had a previous dystocia. These conditions may be surgically corrected in valuable does; however, does are more commonly culled because treatment may be unrewarding.

A speculum can be used to examine the walls of the vagina, vestibules, and cervix to search for lesions in does with fertility issues. Transabdominal and/or transrectal ultrasonography can be used to examine the uterus and ovaries for cysts, hydrometra (pseudo-pregnancy), or other abnormalities. Occasionally, a doeling may have a shortened vagina and no cervix, and segmental aplasia of various parts of the tract that warrant culling. In valuable breeding does, surgical laparoscopy or laparotomy may be performed to check for causes of infertility such as oviductal blockage, tumors, adhesions, or segmental aplasia that may not be visible on speculum examination or via ultrasonography.

Palpation of the penis and prepuce of bucks is performed to ensure there are no masses or lesions that may prevent protrusion, intromission, or ejaculation. The penis can be assessed during electroejaculation or via manual exteriorization. The buck may be placed on its rump or laid on its side with pressure applied to the sigmoid flexure by an assistant while the prepuce is stabilized for penis exteriorization. Shearing wounds (especially in Angoras), prior balanoposthitis, and old fly-strike wounds and scarring around the prepuce may make protrusion of the penis impossible, and animals should be culled if severely affected. Persistent penile frenulum may also prevent exteriorization in young bucks and should be surgically corrected before breeding. Prior amputation of the urethral process to prevent obstruction by a calculus is common and has no apparent deleterious effect on breeding ability.

Although cryptorchidism is rare, a thorough reproductive examination in young breeding bucks should include confirmation that both testicles have descended completely. The testicles should be evaluated for size (scrotal circumference), consistency, and symmetry. Testicular hypoplasia occurs in only ~2% of intact bucks and is mostly associated with intersex condition; however, it may also be a manifestation of chronic malnutrition. Scrotal circumference is positively correlated with semen production capacity and should be >25 cm in mature bucks (>14 months). Scrotal circumference can vary by season and decrease by as many as 3 cm outside the breeding season.

The testicles and epididymides should be symmetrical and slightly firm on palpation. Any asymmetry or changes in tone may indicate infection or injury and can adversely affect fertility. Orchitis and epididymitis are both rare, occurring in ~1% of breeding bucks, and affected bucks should be tested for *Brucella melitensis*, because bred does are at risk of stillbirths and abortions. Other causes of orchitis and epididymitis in bucks are of minimal concern for transmission; however, treatments are generally unrewarding. Caseous lymphadenitis, spermatic granuloma, and calcification of the testicles (which also may be due to *Corynebacterium pseudotuberculosis* infection) all reduce or eliminate the buck's fertility, and infected bucks should be culled. In extreme cases, ultrasound may be used to determine whether one or both testicles are affected and if hemicastration is an option to preserve breeding potential.

Buck semen can be collected via use of either an artificial vagina or an electroejaculator. The former yields a higher quality sample but it requires the presence of a doe in heat to perform. Electroejaculation is more convenient and thus used more commonly. Once semen is obtained, it should be maintained at 37 °C (98.6 °F) and evaluated as quickly as possible. Grossly, the semen should be cloudy, white, and free of urine, blood, pus, or dirt. Occasionally, semen will be an off-yellow color and may be normal, though semen this color should be examined more closely for urine contamination.

Semen should be evaluated microscopically for motility, morphology, and presence of WBCs. Gross motility can be measured by placing a drop of undiluted semen on a warmed slide and evaluating microscopically on low-magnification (typically 100×). A satisfactory sample should exhibit anywhere from general oscillation to vigorous swirling. Sporadic oscillation usually indicates poor semen viability, though it may also be due to low concentration. Individual and progressive motility should also be assessed at higher magnification (400×) by diluting the semen with prewarmed isotonic diluent (e.g., 0.9% saline) or extender. Sperm cells should be counted to determine the percentage of progressively motile sperm, with a minimum of 30% considered acceptable.

Sperm morphology should also be assessed microscopically at 1000× to assess percentage of normal cells versus those with head, midpiece, or tail defects. Morphological analyses can be performed with light microscopy by preparing a slide with eosin-nigrosin staining of sperm cells, or with a phase-contrast microscope, by preparing a wet-mount slide of formalin-killed sperm. Parameters for morphological assessment are extrapolated from those used in bulls, with a minimum of 70% normal being acceptable. Recently, sperm with distal droplets have been reclassified as normal sperm cells in bulls and may be considered normal in bucks too, because these defects do not appear to affect fertility in ruminants. Bucks with questionable sperm morphology may be deferred and rechecked in seven weeks, after a full spermatogenic cycle has passed. Notably, semen quality can be affected by photoperiod, so bucks evaluated outside the breeding season should always be deferred and rechecked in the fall.

10.4 Onset of Puberty

This process generally occurs when bucklings and doelings reach 60–70 lb or 30–50% of adult body weight. Depending on the breed, the onset of puberty occurs at 3–7 months of age. Puberty in both bucklings and doelings is controlled by sexual hormones: testosterone in the bucklings and estrogen in doelings. These hormones cause physiological and behavioral changes in both sexes leading up to puberty. Environmental factors such as nutrition and season affect the onset of puberty. Precocity is the term used to describe an animal that exhibits early puberty or achieves puberty at an earlier age compared to the breed average.

The ovaries are essentially inactive from birth until puberty. They become active as the hypothalamus and anterior pituitary gland begin to produce stimulatory hormones such as gonadotropin-releasing hormone (GnRH), follicle-stimulating hormone (FSH), and luteinizing hormone (LH). Photoperiod, an environmental factor, also greatly affects the onset of puberty of does. In does, puberty and estrus cyclicity in general depend on photoperiodic changes. The onset of puberty typically occurs during the short days of autumn. Spring-born animals are exposed to long days and achieve puberty during the short days of autumn in the same year. However, puberty in doelings can be manipulated through management techniques such as permanent exposure to the buck, enhanced nutrition, and breeding management practices. In bucks, puberty involves testicular growth and spermatogenesis (spermatozoa production); bucks do not appear to depend on photoperiodic changes and attain puberty during either the long or short days. The season of birth also does not appear to significantly affect the onset of puberty in bucks.

10.5 Breeding During Puberty

Once puberty is reached, it is best to breed a doeling when she reaches approximately 70% of her mature body weight, depending on the breed. A sexually mature and healthy doeling with adequate size can be bred, carry a pregnancy, and deliver a kid without affecting her growth potential. If a doe becomes pregnant before achieving 70% of her estimated mature body weight, growth and development may be suppressed. In addition, she could suffer abortion, increased interval postpartum, and encounter rebreeding problems.

10.6 Preparation of Males for Breeding

Care of males is just as important as care and management of females. Buck can donate good-quality semen under good management practices throughout the year. The male will have limited fertility during the hot summer months and they increase in both fertility and libido in October and November. It is important to provide proper care and environment for at least six weeks prior to breeding, as well as during breeding. Therefore, for the production of good-quality semen the males should be cared for as follows.

- The male should be fed with extra rations six weeks before the actual period of mating.
- Each male should be fed with about 200–500 g of extra concentrate per day depending up on its body weight.
- Each buck should be examined for health and semen viability before it is allowed to mate.
- Feet should be trimmed and inspected for foot rot and other disease.
- The buck should be dewormed with recommended dose of dewormer.
- The hair around the prepuce should be kept trimmed.
- The external reproductive organs, particularly the testes, must be well developed and free from obvious abnormalities and hardness.
- During the summer season, bucks should be kept in cool housing and during the cooler season in warm housing. Provide shade before breeding starts in hot weather; this is more advantageous for males than females.

10.7 Preparation of Females for Breeding

- *Age-wise distribution*: the does are most productive at 3–4 years of age, but all the animals in the flocks cannot be in this age group. It is customary to have all ages represented in the same flock. Young ewes or does that have not reached their mature size at the time of breeding often require extra care or feed. Likewise, older does are sometimes kept for a year even though their teeth may have begun to spread and these require extra care. For these reasons, these animals may be kept divided at breeding time. Animals which are 2–3 years old may be grouped together.
- *Health and soundness*: health and soundness are always essential for the success of any breeding operation. Unsound ewes and does with tooth malformations, excess wear on the teeth, broken mouth and bad gums, those with unsound udders or nonfunctional teats, and those animals that are not sound on their feet and legs should be removed before breeding begins. Freedom from diseases and parasites is also a necessity for does, to remain thrifty and capable of gaining weight. Drenching for internal parasites can be done before breeding begins.
- *Flushing*: this means providing extra rations about 15–30 days before the breeding season. This results in females achieving a good health condition before breeding. Flushing will provide the following benefits.
  - It will increase the incidence of estrus.
  - It will increase the conception rate in females.
  - It will decrease early embryonic mortality by strengthening the fetal membrane integrity.
  - It will increase the rate of ovulation and the chance of getting twins and triplets.

  Flushing is usually accomplished by providing each ewe with fresh pasture, good-quality hay and 250 g of concentrate mixture per day.
- *Estrus stimulation*: a helpful practice for stimulating and to some extent synchronizing breeding is the “buck entry technique” (buck effect), i.e., putting vasectomized males with females about 10 days to two weeks prior to the beginning of

breeding. The same effects can result from fenceline contact, which involves turning a ram or buck into an adjoining shed. As a result of this, a large portion of the ewes will ovulate and conceive during the early part of the breeding season.

- *Synchronizing estrus*: synchronization is a management tool that has received a lot of attention from researchers. Synchronization occurs naturally to some extent simply by weaning lambs/kids all at the same time, a traditional practice followed in commercial sheep operations. Use of hormone treatment for synchronizing estrus is common in research institutions but not to any great extent in commercial sheep businesses.
- *Male to female ratio for breeding*: one male can be used to breed 30–40 females but they have to be replaced once in a year and the new ram/buck has to be introduced from an outside flock, to avoid inbreeding. In farm conditions, where the males are selected from the farm animals, one male can be used to breed 20–30 females. To avoid inbreeding, the sire and dam of the males and females has to be verified and the males are allowed to breed females in such a way that they are not closely related to each other.
- *Puberty and time of first mating*: the time of first estrus accompanied by ovulation is known as puberty, but this does not denote complete sexual maturity. Females should not be mated until they are physically large enough to cope with both pregnancy and rearing of lambs. If mated too young, the female may remain stunted and any kid born will tend to have low birth weight and vigor with a lower chance for survival. As a guideline, females should be mated only when they reach 70% of the average adult body weight. Breeding of ewe lambs and kids is more common than in past years, but it is still a practice limited to flocks in which lambs/kids are well grown out.

The females (kids) that reach puberty and breeding during their first year (before cutting teeth) have a greater lifetime production than those not exposed. However, any system of management that involves breeding of ewe lambs/kids requires extra care and more feed. Regardless of whether bred as kids or not, doe kids have to be handled in separate groups during the breeding season.

In male animals, puberty occurs when sperm appears in the ejaculate. More visible signs include increased aggressiveness and sexual desire, a change in body conformation to look more masculine, rapid growth of testes and penis, and separation of the penis from the sheath so that extension of the penis is possible.

10.8 Estrous Cycle

Does will exhibit estrus or heat at regular intervals during the breeding season. Estrus is the fertile period and if the female does not conceive, it is repeated on average 19–21 days in does (range 17–24 days, though 8–10% of animals may have short cycles of 6–10 days; these intervals may be 1–2 days shorter in young animals).

10.8.1 Estrus

Estrus is the period of the cycle when the female displays sexual behavioral activity and it is the only time when she will accept the male. The estrus period lasts for about 34–38 hours in does. The number of ova shed has an influence on the length of the period. Does with multiple ovulations are probably in heat longer than those with only one ovum shed. Generally, ewes do not show visible signs of estrus if a ram is not present. The signs of estrus are more marked in the doe. The outward signs include the following.

- Reddening of the vulva.
- Tail wagging.
- Mounting other animals.
- Seeking males.
- Frequent bleating.
- Presents her back to the buck.
- Stands for mating.

Generally, young females don't show aggressive estrus behavior.

The males are attracted by smell, sight, and sound and exhibit the following behavior.

- Curling of the lip (Flehmen' reaction).
- Sniff the vulva.

- Push the doe with head (nuzzling).
- Paw the doe (nudging).
- Mount and mate.

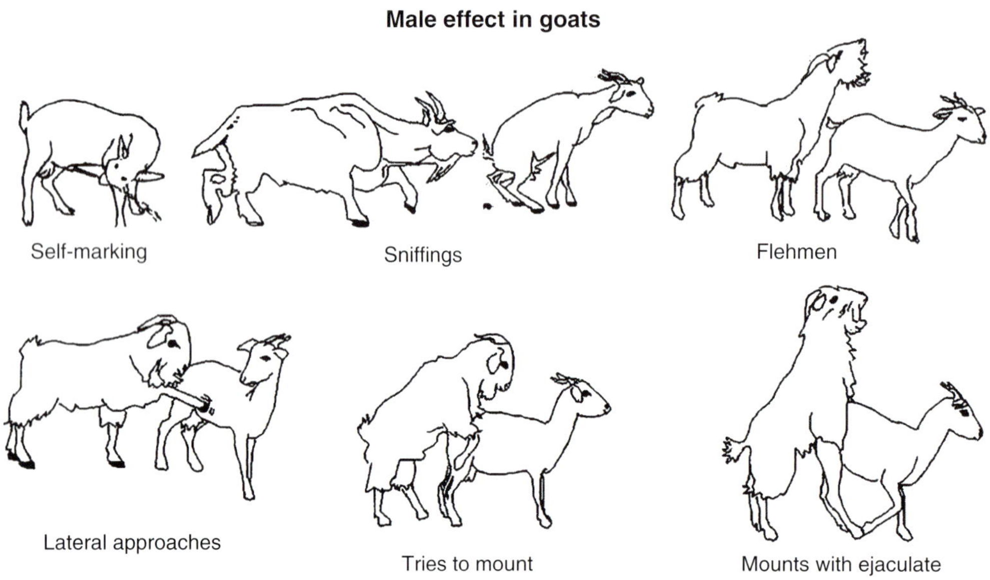

The male will mount and serve the female more than once if access is allowed. In general, the only sure sign of estrus is that the female will stand and allow the male to mount (standing reflex).

10.8.2 Identification of Goat in Heat

One of the problems in scientific manipulation of breeding programs is the detection of goats in heat. It is difficult to identify does in heat by physical signs. The techniques generally used are as follows.

- *Using an intact male*: in this method an intact buck or ram is let in to the flock. The buck will follow the doe in estrus. However, there is a chance that the buck or ram will mate with the doe if it is not controlled properly.
- *Use of intact male fitted with apron*: in this case an apron is tied on the abdomen of the male to cover the penis. The apron is made of a soft piece of cloth measuring 60 × 45 cm with strings on four sides to tie it properly. This prevents mating. The apron should be washed daily and checked for holes or tears to avoid unwanted mating. There are two distinct disadvantages to this method. First, there is a risk of fertile mating if the apron is not securely fastened and checked frequently. Second, inflammation, irritation, and infection of the penis and prepuce area can occur, resulting in inhibited sexual desire and mounting behavior. The bucks are apronised and allowed into the flock in the morning and evening for about 15–20 minutes.
- *Introduction of teaser bucks*: teaser bucks can help to detect females in heat, which are separated out for breeding with the desired ram. Once estrus is detected in a flock, the marked animals should be removed from the flock, so that the buck can detect any other female in estrus. If this is not done, the buck may only pay attention to the first female and ignore others that may be in heat. The teaser will sniff the vulva of a female in heat, nuzzling, nudging, and mounting her. The female in heat will stand and allow the male to mount. The teaser male is mainly used for detection of females in estrus, but also to stimulate estrus and ovulation. In some places, the males are introduced to the females which have been previously isolated from the males for several weeks, resulting in large numbers of females coming into heat at the same time. This is called the "male effect," "teaser effect" or "ram effect." This method of estrus synchronization is effective only at certain times of the year, usually just before the onset of the natural breeding season, when the majority of the females are not yet cycling. The animals generally will come to heat within five or six days after introduction of the buck/ram. Use of an intact male fitted with an apron is only suitable for small groups of animals teased for short periods.

10.8.3 Ovulation

Ovulation is the process in which the mature Graafian follicle ruptures and releases the ovum. In does, ovulation is spontaneous. The time of ovulation is related to the onset of estrus. It occurs 30–36 hours after the onset of estrus in does.

10.8.4 Time of Mating

Mating activity during the breeding period is higher in the morning and evening. The majority of does remain in heat for a period of 34–38 hours after the onset of estrus. Breeding of does at about 12–14 hours after the onset of heat gives a higher conception rate. Therefore the suggestion is that does detected to be in heat in the evening should be mated the next morning and those found in heat in the morning should be mated in the evening for better results. This time period allows the released egg and sperm to meet in the proper place in the reproductive tract.

10.9 Goat Nutrition During Breeding

Nutrition during the goat breeding season is critical. It has been determined that a lack of proper nutrition can actually decrease a doe's chances of becoming pregnant. A lack of selenium and vitamin E can also cause white muscle disease (nutritional muscular dystrophy) in new kids. Overall nutrition is important anyway, for both does in heat and bucks in rut, due to the extended, significant physical energy that goats burn up throughout the entire breeding season and process.

As usual, make sure your goats have plenty of quality forage, hay, and grain. Consider adding minerals and vitamins, from sources such as black oil sunflower seeds (BOSS). They are a great source of extra vitamin E, zinc, iron, and selenium, which can add butter fat to the goats' milk and make their coats shinier. You may want to limit these seeds for bucks, however, as there has been some evidence that they can cause urinary calculi in bucks.

Goats can often suffer from a deficiency of copper, selenium, and vitamin E which can lead to serious health problems. Sometimes this can occur when they are raised in pens and do not get enough natural "browse" to eat. So farmers need to give supplements like selenium and vitamin E and possibly a "copper bolus" for extra copper. This has to be inserted way down in the goat's throat, so the goat cannot spit it back out or chew it. Farmers may need to use a device called a bolus gun to make this process easier.

10.10 Breeding Systems

Selection simply means using some goats for reproduction and some for food. Selection ensures that the more desirable goats produce more offspring than the less desirable goats. Other concepts include the following breeding strategies.

- Inbreeding.
- Line breeding.
- Line crossing.
- Crossbreeding.

These strategies have slightly different definitions, but the important thing is that pairing of animals for reproduction can have varying outcomes, depending on the relationship of the animals mated. The comparisons of inbreeding/line breeding and crossbreeding traits and potential consequences are as follows.

10.10.1 Inbreeding

Inbreeding is mating between direct family members such as father–daughter, brother–sister, etc. which can lead to genetic problems, deformities, and deaths. Even so, some farms use inbreeding in an attempt to emphasize certain desirable genetic traits in their goats, or to avoid spending money on goats from outside their goat families. Regardless, it is not ideal and should generally be avoided.

10.10.2 Line Breeding

Line breeding is different from inbreeding just in degree. Both of these strategies involve mating related animals. Inbreeding can be arbitrarily set as the mating of first-degree relatives (offspring and parents, or siblings), although this is only one possible definition among many. Line breeding can then be considered as the mating of related animals, but of close relationship less than first degree. Line breeding (or inbreeding) results in uniformity of offspring, especially if adopted as a long-term strategy with appropriate selection. Since the parents are related, line-bred animals increase in genetic, appearance, and performance uniformity.

Line breeding and inbreeding are the usual strategies for the establishment of breeds. Predictability is the major attribute that breeders find useful; they want a specific type of goat producing a specific product. Problems are more common with inbreeding and include loss of general vigor and especially loss of reproductive performance. Obviously, selection can help offset these. As a result, many line-bred and inbred resources are indeed productive, vigorous, and reproductively sound.

10.10.3 Line Crossing

Line crossing is the crossing of different lines within a breed, and while it has some of the same consequences as crossbreeding, it does contain this within a single breed. As a result, the variability is not as great as a cross between breeds, so the boost from hybrid vigor is not as great. With line crossing, the benefits of crossbreeding can be achieved without loss of breed character and type. Consistency of production is still diminished, and each individual situation will indicate whether this is a good trade-off or not.

The phenomena associated with crossbreeding and line crossing will have differing consequences for different breeders, largely due to differences in the breeders' philosophies. That is, what do they want and how do they want to get there? These questions are essential for all goat breeders but are not frequently asked. In the absence of a guiding philosophy and set of goals, breeding programs fail to make the progress possible with such guidance.

Line crossing takes time and commitment, while crossbreeding can be a quick fix and is a tempting strategy for a variety of reasons. One outcome of crossbreeding is phenomenal initial results, especially if the parents are intelligently selected.

10.10.4 Crossbreeding

Crossbreeding is the philosophical and biological opposite to line breeding and involves the mating of animals of two different breeds. Crossbreeding is a fascinating phenomenon, partly because different things happen depending on which stage of crossbreeding is considered.

The first stage is the initial cross. When two different breeds are crossed, the initial result is very uniform, benefitting from the specific combination of the genetic array of the parental breeds. Since each parental breed is uniform, and each kid gets half from each breed, every kid is pretty much like the next. This first kid crop is reaping the benefits of homogeneous parental breeds. If these kids are in turn used for reproduction, variability then increases since these kids are half one thing, half another. Variability is not all bad, and if combined with selection, the excellent goats can be skimmed off the herd and used for advantages in shows and other situations. They may indeed have excellent type and performance. What they lack, though, is the ability to consistently pass along this excellence to the next generation.

Many of the advantages of crossbreeding, such as increased vigor and reproductive efficiency, are somewhat the disadvantages of line breeding. Conversely, the disadvantages of crossbreeding, such as lack of consistency and predictability, are the advantages of line breeding.

10.11 Mating Methods

Animals may be mated using a variety of methods, broadly categorized as follows.

- *Natural mating*: this involves the normal act of mating between a male and female animal.
  - Pasture mating or flock mating.
  - Pen mating.
  - Hand mating.

- *Artificial mating*:
  - Artificial insemination.
  - Embryo transfer technology.

10.11.1 Natural Mating

This can be practically implemented in the flock as a whole as follows.

- *Pasture mating or flock mating*: pasture mating is probably the most widely used system. A male is allowed in with a group of females for a longer period of time both day and night. Females are bred as they become ready for mating. This is a traditional Indian method of breeding. Farmers do not keep any record of mating. Pasture mating is less efficient for male animals. In such flocks, generally more than one male is kept. This method requires little time and effort on the part of the farmer.
- *Pen mating*: in this system, the does are divided into batches varying from 20 to 25. They are stalled in the shed every night with a painted buck selected for the particular group. A proper record of the covered goats is kept by using different colors, changing them after every 16 days. The bucks should be removed from the flock after two estrous cycles. The male is separated during the day time from the female. This system has its own demerits. A buck may develop attraction for one particular goat in heat and serve it a number of times while others remain unattended, resulting in empty does and low fertility rate. The buck sometimes exhausts itself overnight by serving more than a dozen times and the last served does may not receive an optimum number of spermatozoa and remain unconceived.
- *Hand mating*: in this system, a teaser buck detects the does in heat, which are marked and separated out for breeding with the desired buck. The females are allowed to mate one by one. In this system, a buck may not be allowed to mate more than three does a day. This method ensures the expected time of kidding and allows the farmer to know that the animal has actually being bred. Hand mating reduces the risk of injuries to animals and is beneficial when mating an older male with a younger female. It also improves the breeding efficiency of the male, resulting in an increased number of females that can be bred in a shorter period of time.

10.11.2 Artificial Mating

- *Artificial insemination*: this offers the best means of distributing germplasm from a nucleus breeding flock to many small flocks within each ecosystem. Fresh as well as frozen semen is used. The speculum method of insemination is used for does. Generally, artificial insemination leads to a lower reproductive rate than natural service and frozen semen gives an even lower pregnancy rate, around 40%. Cervical insemination is generally carried out to improve conception rates.
- *Embryo transfer technology*: this currently requires surgery in sheep so it may not become practical in production, but it offers great promise in enhancing genetic progress.

10.11.3 Buck Rag

A "buck rag" is created by taking a rag, rubbing it all over a buck, then keeping it in a jar and using it to help does come into heat. Just letting a doe smell the rag can sometimes trigger her to come into heat. If she comes into heat, place her with a buck to be bred. Some does may not show signs of heat unless a buck is present. Sometimes a doe needs to be taken to the buck on a lead (leash) and held so the buck can mount her. The pheromones emitted by a buck that cause a doe to go into heat do not come from his urine or his smell, they are in his hair.

10.12 Goat Gestation Period

To estimate the expected kidding date, start from the approximate date the doe may have been bred and add the usual "gestation" days (the length of time it takes a doe to deliver a kid from the time she first got pregnant). The average gestation period for a goat is 145–155 days. Miniature breeds average about 145 days. Other breeds average about 150 days.

10.13 Pregnancy Diagnosis

There are multiple ways to tell if your doe is pregnant. Some are more reliable than others. Some involve more effort and expense than others.

10.13.1 Natural Signs of Pregnancy

One way to know the goat is pregnant is to look for the typical signs, which include the following.

- Missed heat cycle.
- Puffy vulva.
- Goat appears wider than normal.
- Movement felt on goat's right side (movement on left side is the rumen).
- Udder starts developing (often about a month before kidding).

10.13.2 Ultrasound

An ultrasound is one of the most reliable tests for goat pregnancy. However, it tends to be more expensive since it is usually performed by a trained technician. The great thing about an ultrasound is that it can sometimes detect how many kids are going to be born. It is usually more accurate when there are one or two kids but with larger numbers of kids, it is harder to be exact.

10.14 Separating Male and Female Goats

The most common system is to keep bucks and does separated most of the time, and only put them together for intentional, controlled breeding. However, sometimes it may not be practical to keep bucks separated. In those cases, there are other ways to stop a buck from breeding.

10.14.1 Castration

One sure way to stop a buck from breeding is to castrate him. After that, he's referred to as a "wether" rather than a "buck." Typically, a male goat can be castrated when he's fairly young (a "buckling") using elastrator pliers which apply an elastrator band (a small latex rubber ring) around the goat's testicles. Banding is a fairly common procedure for castrating goats. Usually after about two weeks, the testicles simply shrivel up and fall off. Surprisingly, there is usually minimal pain for the goat (treatable at the start with some medication).

A buckling should probably not be castrated before 10 weeks of age or there may be an increased risk of urinary calculi (occurs when the urethra gets blocked and the urine cannot exit), which can be fatal. Conversely, one should not wait too long to castrate, or the testicles may be too big to fit into the open elastrator band. If the testicles are too large for that, a veterinarian will need do it surgically. Otherwise, if the testicles are not too big, a breeder will usually be able to castrate goats themselves after instruction by an experienced vet.

Surgical castration is considered the riskiest form of goat castration with a high risk of possible side-effects including infection.

10.14.2 Buck Apron (Goat Antimating Apron)

Another less permanent method to keep goats from breeding is to use an "antimating apron" or "buck apron." This is a weighted apron that hangs around the buck's waist, held in place by a girth strap, and gets in the way when he tries to breed a doe. Another benefit of antimating aprons is that they can help avoid urine scald because they block the buck from urinating on his own face or front legs. Constant urination on the goat's face and legs can irritate and burn the skin and even remove the hair in those areas due to the acid in the urine.

One downside of an antimating apron is that the apron can move around and sometimes the buck may be able to get around it and still breed.

References

Harighi, M.F., Wahid, H., Khumran, A.M., and Baiee, F. (2022). Breeding soundness examination (BSE): a decision-making tool that requires a particular guideline for male goats. *Tropical Animal Health Production* 54 (3): 174.

Singh, R. (2021). Importance of goat farming in India. www.pashudhanpraharee.com/importance-of-goat-farming-in-india (accessed 30 October 2022).

Stewart, J.L. (2022). Breeding soundness examination in goats. www.msdvetmanual.com/management-and-nutrition/management-of-reproduction-goats/breeding-soundness-examination-in-goats (accessed 30 October 2022).

11

Gestation and Parturition

Pramod Kumar[1], Rajesh Kumar[2], Satyavrat V. Singh[3], and Sarita Devi[4]

[1] Department of Veterinary Physiology and Biochemistry, College of Veterinary Science and Animal Husbandry, Acharya Narendra Deva University of Agriculture and Technology, Ayodhya, Uttar Pradesh, India
[2] Department of Veterinary Gynaecology and Obstetrics, College of Veterinary Science and Animal Husbandry, Acharya Narendra Deva University of Agriculture and Technology, Ayodhya, Uttar Pradesh, India
[3] Department of Veterinary Medicine, College of Veterinary Science and Animal Husbandry, Acharya Narendra Deva University of Agriculture and Technology, Ayodhya, Uttar Pradesh, India
[4] Department of Medicine, College of Veterinary Science and Animal Husbandry, Kamdhenu University, Sardarkrushinagar, Gujarat, India

11.1 Introduction

The majority of goats are raised under a smallholder farming system with compromised nutritional resources (Sibanda et al. 1999). Goats are cloven-hooved animals belonging to order Artiodactyla, suborder Ruminatia (ruminants or cud-chewing animals), subfamily Capra, which includes *Ovis aries* (sheep) and *Capra hircus* (goats). *Capra hircus* is the domestic goat which originated from western Asian goats. Goats are members of the Bovidae group of mammals which possess even number of toes, a compartmentalized fore-stomach, and horns. Being herbivorous by nature, goats utilize certain noncarbohydrate carbon substrates for the production of glucose as an energy source (gluconeogenesis, i.e., formation of new sugars). Goats should be maintained on a cycle at par with natural conditions.

11.2 Gestation

The term *gestation* is used to denote the period of intrauterine development of the embryo and fetus. The word originated from a Latin root word *gestare* literally meaning "carry or bear." Length of gestation is calculated as the interval from fertile mating to kidding or parturition. A pregnant goat is usually overlooked until the last one-half to one-third of the gestation period. On the other hand, the goat is one of the few ungulate species which frequently displays false pregnancy, also known as faux pregnancy (Underwood et al. 2015) or hydrometra. However, the literature regarding gestation and antenatal development of the goat is very scanty.

11.2.1 Endocrinology of Gestation

In domestic animals like ruminants, horses, and pigs with a uterine-dependent estrous cycle, modification of synthesis and release of PGF2-alpha is essential for the establishment of pregnancy. In order to abrogate a default PGF2-alpha synthetic program, different signals are involved in different mammalian species (Table 11.1). The e phenomenon is termed maternal recognition of pregnancy (MRP). Developing caprine conceptuses secrete a protein (trophoblastin) from the trophoectoderm between days 16 and 21 (Newton et al. 1996), which serves as an antiluteolytic signal in particular. The trophoblastins belong to a group of signaling proteins called interferon type I; thus, caprine blastocyst secreted trophoblastin, which is currently termed caprine interferon tau (cIFN-τ) (the lower-case Greek letter tau designate its trophoblastic origin), extends the life of the corpus luteum. Bazer (2013) reported that interferon tau is a novel pregnancy signaling protein and is very stable at low pH (2–3).

Elements of Reproduction and Reproductive Diseases of Goats, First Edition. Edited by Tanmoy Rana.

Table 11.1 Time of production and agents of maternal recognition of pregnancy (MRP) in mammals.

Species	Placental takeover of P4 production (days)	Agent of MRP	Day of production	References
Goat	—	cIFNτ	16 and 21	Newton et al. (1996)
Ewe	50	oIFNτ	9/10–21	Flint et al. (1994)
Cow	180–240	bIFNτ	12–38	Flint et al. (1994)
Sow	11–30	Oestradiol	11–30	Geisert et al. (1990)
Human	60–70	hCG	11	Ticconi et al. (2007)
Mare	70	Proteins/estrogen?	14–16: 15–30	Ziecik et al. (2011)
Dog and cat	—	None	—	Pineda and Dooley (2003)

oIFNτ, ovine interferon tau; bIFNτ, bovine interferon tau; hCG, human chorionic gonadotropin.

The plasma level of progesterone, which is produced almost entirely by the corpora lutea of the pregnant goat and not by the placenta, remains high until about four days prepartum (Chemineau et al. 1982). Surgical ablation of the ovary or pharmacological luteolysis at any stage of gestation results in termination of gestation in does. Furthermore, the caprine placenta produces a substantial amount of prostaglandin E2, which is believed to be luteotropic in nature in this species (Ford et al. 1995). Bovine and ovine placentas produce sufficient progesterone to maintain pregnancy beyond a certain period of gestation (beyond day 50 in sheep and day 250 in cattle). However, the caprine placenta cannot produce sufficient progesterone to sustain pregnancy (Senger 2005).

A battery of PAGs, including pregnancy-specific protein B, are produced by trophoblastic binucleate cells and are detectable in the peripheral circulation of the dam from 21 days after insemination and continuing throughout gestation (Humblot et al. 1990). Goats with two or more conceptuses tend to have higher concentrations of PAGs compared to goats carrying single fetuses. Compromised placental function results in declining PAG concentrations many days or weeks before abortion. Estrone sulfate produced from the fetus or placenta begins to rise in peripheral blood at 40–50 days of gestation, reaching a peak at parturition then declining to a nadir one day after parturition. Moreover, PAGs can be used for detection of pregnancy beyond day 40–50.

Placental lactogen, which is also produced by the placenta and thus can be used for pregnancy diagnosis and prediction of litter size, follows a similar pattern. Placental lactogen is first detectable at about 60 days of gestation and stimulates mammary gland development (Byatt et al. 1992; Takashi et al. 2013). Goats with false pregnancies/hydrometra will have a prolonged elevation in progesterone but will not show increases in PAGs, placental lactogen, or estrone sulfate. Thus, these hormones can be used for differential diagnosis of pregnancy.

The placenta of the goat is cotyledonary and syndesmochorial. The caruncles are concave. The fetal trophectoderm is composed of uninucleate and binucleate cells. The fetal binucleate cells migrate to and fuse with the uterine epithelium to form syncytial plaques (Wooding et al. 1993). This migration continues throughout pregnancy. As pregnancy advances, the placenta also commences to produce progesterone using the maternal cholesterol. In some species such as sow, goat, and camel, the CL is required throughout the period of gestation because the placenta cannot produce enough progesterone to sustain the pregnancy (Table 11.1).

The gestation period can be roughly divided in to three phases based on the size of the individual and the tissue and organs (Figure 11.1).

11.2.2 The Ovum or Blastula

This period lasts about 10–12 days in ruminants, extending from the time of conception/fertilization to development of the zygote and primitive fetal membrane in the uterus. The morula (16–32 cells) enters into the uterus at day 4–5 in ruminants. At about 6–10 days, the zona pellucida breaks. At about 12 days the blastocyst is about 1.5 mm in diameter. During this period defective ova die and are absorbed.

11.2.3 Embryo and Organogenesis

This period extends from 12–15 days to 45 days of gestation in ruminants. During this period, major tissues and organs are formed and by the end of this period the species of the embryo is readily recognizable. A circular or elongated gestation sac or embryonic vesicle of 4.1 mm to 1 cm diameter has been detected from day 17 to 21 of pregnancy by various researchers (Martínez et al. 1998; Medan et al. 2004; Singh et al. 2004; Padilla-Rivas et al. 2005; Suguna et al. 2008; Kumar et al. 2015). Moreover, the embryo proper can be detected using ultrasonography on day 26–35 of pregnancy (Martínez et al. 1998; Medan et al. 2004; Singh et al. 2004; Padilla-Rivas et al. 2005; Suguna et al. 2008; Martínez et al. 1998; Singh et al. 2004; Suguna et al. 2008), which can be used for differential diagnosis of pregnancy with hydrometra (Hesselink and Taverne 1994). Earliest detection of the developing heart occurred on day 19 of pregnancy and can be counted from day 28 onwards (Hesselink and Taverne 1994; Martínez et al. 1998; Medan et al. 2004; Padilla-Rivas et al. 2005; Suguna et al. 2008).

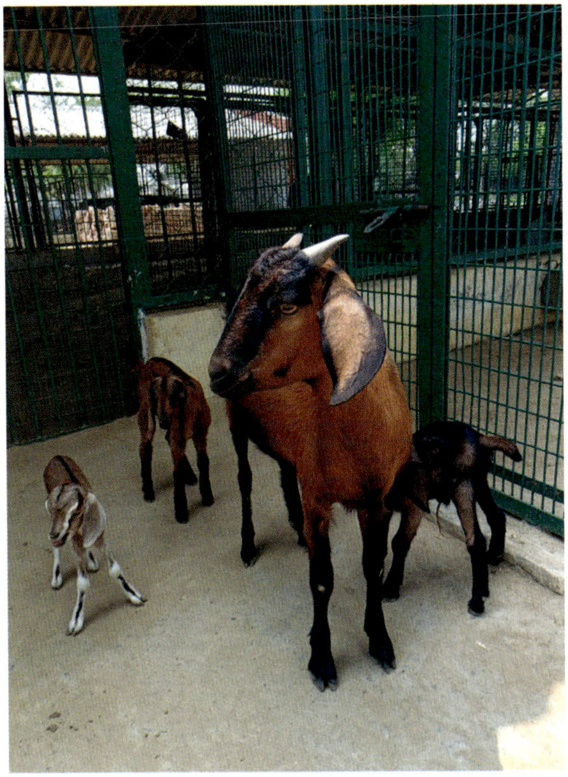

Figure 11.1 Nondescript goat with triple kids.

11.2.4 Fetus and Fetal Growth

This period extends from 45 days of gestation to kidding. During this period the caruncle and cotyledons develop and enlarge to support nutrition to the fetus. The fetus resides in a thermoneutral environment, i.e., thermally protected from variations of body temperature during changes in the dam's internal milieu (Faurie et al. 2001).

Fetal development is most rapid during the last month of pregnancy and the growth rate can be retarded, even halved, if the dam suddenly suffers severe undernutrition around day 120 of gestation (Mellor and Matheson 1979). In late gestation, there is preferential utilization of nutrients in favor of the fetus at the cost of the dam's body tissues (Osuagwuh and Aire 1990). Energy availability for fetal development is dependent upon the live weight of the dam and changes in live weight are suggestive of antenatal fetal development (Amoah et al. 1996). Undernutrition during late pregnancy results in weight loss in the dam (Dayeh et al. 1996; Sibanda et al. 1999; Al-Totanji and Lubbadeh 2000). Available evidence suggests that the last month of pregnancy is nutritionally the most critical period for pregnant goats (Rastogi et al. 2003). Changes in the weight of pregnant does can be used to assess fetal growth (Akingbade et al. 2001).

Although undernutrition in late gestation results in reduced kid birth weight and survival, overfeeding during late gestation should also be avoided as it can increase the occurrence of dystocia. In addition to adverse effects on fetus and dam, prolonged undernutrition during pregnancy also affects the offspring's future fertility (Anonymous 2013).

11.2.5 Factors Affecting Gestation Length

Gestation is defined as the total number of days between service and parturition (Mellado et al. 2000). The average gestation period for various goat breeds is 145–150 days (Table 11.2) and the duration is genetically determined, though lower heritability estimates for reproductive traits have been reported (Sahoo et al. 2023). Environmental, fetal, and maternal variables can alter it to some extent. Various factors affecting length of gestation are described below.

11.2.5.1 Sex of Fetus

Mellado et al. (2000) suggested that the gestation length of a goat bearing males (single or multiple), females (single or multiple) or mixed sexes does not differ significantly. However, some workers suggested that a male fetus may be carried for one or two days more than a female. Fetal sexing in goats is appropriate because it will lead to better planning during the marketing of fetuses while still *in utero* (Amer 2008). Utilizing ultrasonography can help with early fetal sexing in singleton pregnant does.

Table 11.2 Gestation length in different goat breeds.

Breed	Days	References
Alpine	151.4	Mellado et al. (2000)
Angora	150	Hafez and Hafez (2006)
Ardi	150	Ali et al. (2022)
Berari	149.98	Kale et al. (2021)
Black Bengal	144	Roy et al. (2007)
Crossbred	150.6	Mellado et al. (2000)
Jamunapari	150	Hafez and Hafez (2006)
Mehsana	148.97	Patel and Pandey (2013)
Nubian	151.0	Mellado et al. (2000)
Saanen	150	Hafez and Hafez (2006)
Toggenburg	151.7	Hafez and Hafez (2006)

11.2.5.2 Parity

Generally, first-kidding does have one or two kids, and in subsequent kiddings, triplets and quadruplets are not uncommon. Twins or triplets are usually more common than single kids. Quadruplets are not rare. Parity has a significant effect on length of gestation (Mellado et al. 2000). The first and second gestation are generally one to two days shorter than in multiparous goats. Prolonged gestation (152–160 days) in goats is beneficial because it results in heavier litters at birth and higher viability of neonatal kids (Mellado et al. 2000).

11.2.5.3 Season

Many studies have suggested that breeding season or kidding season has a significant effect on length of gestation (Gangwar and Yadar 1987; Ruvuna et al. 1988; Deshpande and Mehta 1992; Mellado et al. 2000). Moreover, births are much more likely to occur during daylight hours than at night and are most frequent around midday. If parturition occurs during the breeding season, the doe will resume ovarian activity and can conceive again.

11.2.5.4 Litter Size

There is no consensus among different researchers about the effect of litter size on gestation length. Earlier studies have shown that the number of kids born is not a significant factor affecting gestation length (Sinha and Sahni 1982; Gangwar and Yadar 1987), but later studies reported that litter size is a significant factor affecting gestation period (Singh and Singh 1983; Ruvuna et al. 1988; Deshpande and Mehta 1992). Many factors including age, parity, breed, season, live weight, and nutrition affect the rate of twinning in goats (Robertson et al. 2020). Some researchers suggest that quadruplets are born only three days earlier than single kids and the gestation period is shortened by 3–6 days in monotocous breeds.

Available evidence suggests that, unlike in cattle, longer gestation length in does increases the chances of kid survival, produces heavier kids at birth, and reduces neonatal death rate. Some scientists recommended that gestation up to 160 days should be considered normal in goats.

11.3 Parturition or Kidding

Kidding is a physiological process of parturition in which the pregnant uterus delivers the fetus and placenta. Parturition is a natural phenomenon that normally takes place unaided, but it is one of the most stressful events in life, for both newborn and dam (Padbury et al. 1988; Mainau and Manteca 2011).

Elevated fetal derived cortisol level is the initial signal for the cascade of endocrine events that initiate parturition (Nagel et al. 2019); the cortisol level reaches its zenith at or just after birth of the first kid (Hydbring et al. 1997, 1999). Liggins (1994) suggested that elevated fetal cortisol level is mandatory for preparation and maturation so that the fetus can survive *ex utero*. The most important fetal contribution to the initiation of parturition, at least in domestic bovids, is the secretion of glucocorticoids from the fetal adrenal gland (Liggins 1979; Nathanielsz 1978). Furthermore, both P_4 and cortisol (C) were higher in does bearing multiple fetus than does with singleton pregnancies (Probo et al. 2022).

Parturition is signaled by a series of events in pregnant does that alert the owner to impending kidding, like swollen udder and red swollen vulva. Relaxation of the pelvic ligaments, as a result of an increase in circulating estrogen levels in late gestation, is another signal (Underwood et al. 2015). At about the same time, the vulva enlarges and may become slightly longer. In most goats there is rapid enlargement and engorgement of the udder as well, but udder enlargement may not be an accurate indicator of impending parturition, because it may occur as early as the third or fourth month of gestation in goats kidding for the first time. Some does have early engorgement of the udder to the point that milking is required. Other does do not show udder enlargement until the point of, or just shortly after, parturition. Estrus synchronization shortens the length of the kidding period, concentrates parturition time during daylight hours and increases reproductive performance in Saanen goats.

11.3.1 Stages of Parturition or Labor

Parturition in goats is divided mainly into three stages: stage I, dilation of cervix; stage II, expulsion of fetus; and stage III, expulsion of fetal membranes.

11.3.1.1 Stage I Dilation of Cervix

The first stage is also referred as prelabor and usually goes unnoticed. This stage is characterized by the onset of myometrial contractions as progesterone levels drop and estrogen levels increase and stage may last from two to 12 hours. Maternal plasma concentrations of estrogen rise within 24 hours of parturition in normal goats (Rawlings and Ward 1977). Pluriparous does may show very little discomfort, and the first stage may last only a few hours. The doe is restless and most signs are reflective of abdominal discomfort.

Frequently the doe will lie down and rise, paw at the bedding, and maybe urinate or defecate. The endometrial mass causes pressure on the urinary tract, resulting in straining during urination (Eljarah et al. 2012). During this period, the cervix relaxes and releases the cervical seal that is seen at the vulva as thick, tenacious, yellowish-brown mucus. The contracting uterus pushes the placenta, fetus, and fetal fluids toward the cervix.

11.3.1.2 Stage II Expulsion of Fetus

The second stage of labor begins when the water bag is pushed out, the doe continues to squat and exhibits restless behavior, pawing the ground and biting her side, often making soft sounds with the concomitant abdominal press that is characteristic of active labor. Depending on the number of fetuses present, this stage will last from one to three hours, with most does delivering all fetuses within two hours. Does typically are in lateral recumbency during this stage, but some older, more experienced does may remain standing for delivery. After the placenta reaches the vagina, the chorioallantois ruptures, lubricating the vaginal canal, and the amnion, or water bag, is partially delivered through the vulvar opening. This also ruptures and the kid is delivered. In multiple births, the doe may rest between deliveries, or they may occur one after the other.

11.3.1.3 Stage III Expulsion of Afterbirth

The third stage of parturition is delivery of the placenta or placentae, depending upon number of kids and involution of the uterus. In the goat, the placenta is usually delivered within one hour of kidding and is considered retained if not expelled by 12 hours. In some multiple births, placental expulsion may be intermingled with delivery of kids. The mass and volume of the postpartum uterus decline drastically from delivery until about day 12 post partum. Involution is macroscopically complete by day 28 post partum.

Hypocalcemia in goats occurs around the time of parturition and is caused by decreasing levels of calcium to less than 10 mg/dl. Hypocalcemia in does causes both metabolic and oxidative stress during periparturient periods while also retarding uterine involution during postpartum periods (Bayoumi et al. 2021). The rapid decline in mass and volume of the uterus is ascribed to contraction of the myometrium together with vasoconstriction and loss of tissue fluids.

Lochia is normally discharged for up to three weeks. This is a nonodorous, reddish-brown discharge that represents the debris remaining in the uterine lumen from parturition as well as some of the residual tissue and fluid from uterine involution.

11.3.2 Endocrinology of Kidding

Fetal maturation triggers increasing cortisol synthesis that initiates the onset of parturition. Like sheep and cattle, the parturient mechanism in does is probably initiated by an elevated cortisol level (Hudson et al. 1976) because of an increased fetal adrenal responsiveness to adrenocorticotropin (Ford et al. 1998). One day before parturition, maternal cortisol concentrations in the goat tend to increase above those values that could be explained by diurnal variation (Olsson and Dahlborn 1989). The high cortisol values at parturition may partially be a result of the stress and pain that accompany this event and seem to be correlated with the increased need for glucocorticoids, to accelerate mammary growth and initiate lactation (Kitts 1985). Also, fetal corticosteroids increase during the last 13–11 days of gestation, and particularly sharply during the last three days (Currie and Thorburn 1977). After the prepartum fetal cortisol rise (Bassett and Thorburn 1969), placental synthesis should be redirected from progesterone toward estrogens, leading to an increase in the estrogen/progesterone ratio (Ford et al. 1998).

Cortisol and the C-19 steroids diffuse through the placenta and stimulate the placental aromatization enzyme system, 17-alpha hydroxylase/17,20-lyase which controls the conversion of progestrone to estrogen via androgen. This prepartum decline in progesterone concentration has been positively correlated with initiation of parturition (Ford et al. 1998; Laura et al. 2004; Probo et al. 2011). Furthermore, Probo et al. (2011) suggested that progesterone decline is only significant one day prepartum in pathological parturitions. The prepartum increase in estrogen concentration was gradual (Capezzuto et al. 2008) and reached a peak at the time of parturition followed by prompt and significant reduction (Probo et al. 2011). On the other hand, the progressive rise in estradiol-17-beta detected 3–4 days before parturition (Currie et al. 1988) stimulates the uterine production of PGF2-alpha (Ford et al. 1998), whose concentrations increase 24 hours before delivery (Umo et al. 1976).

The physiological role of PGF2-alpha in the initiation of luteal regression in the pregnant doe is still unclear, and the possibility that it could be the cause or the consequence of the progesterone fall is still a matter of debate (Ford et al. 1998); moreover, important differences in PGF2-alpha concentrations post partum exist between species (Perera et al. 1981; Kindahl et al. 1982; Lindell et al. 1982; Stewart et al. 1984), and might be related to the type of placentation (Fredriksson et al. 1984). Furthermore, estrogen begins to influence uterine muscle by stimulating the production of contractile protein and the formation of gap junctions; the former increases the contractile potential of the uterus, and the latter facilitate the contractile process through increased communication among smooth muscle cells.

Thus, important changes that set the stage for kidding start weeks before the actual process begins. In the end, the uterus is converted from a quiescent to a contractile organ, and importantly, the cervix relaxes and opens to allow the fetus to be delivered (Jainudeen and Hafez 2000). The cervical wall revealed a marked increase in the liberation of hydroxyproline from collagen and a change in the pattern of extractable glycosaminoglycans, as induction advanced (Fitzpatrick and Dobson 1979).

Prostaglandins initiate regression of the CL, resulting in progesterone withdrawal and allowing the myometrium to become more contractile. They exert a direct effect on the uterine musculature. This is brought about by its ability to decrease sacroplasmic binding of calcium ions, thus freeing them to interact in the contractile process. This initial increase in the contractility of uterine muscles is important for the start of the first stage of labor. Prostaglandins have an indirect effect on uterine contractility by making the uterine musculature more sensitive to oxytocin. The elevated prepartum concentration of prostaglandin F brings about luteolysis and a subsequent decline in progesterone concentration (Umo et al. 1976). The concentration of plasma T4 was also lowest on the day of kidding and increased during the postpartum period. Plasma insulin concentrations were low in the day of kidding (Khan and Ludri 2002a,b). The insulin concentration fell late in pregnancy, but there was a transient increase two days after parturition (Khan and Ludri 2002b).

However, Alila-Johansson et al. (2003) opined that circadian variation of cortisol secretion in goats is completely masked by external factors, and lighting conditions do not have immediate effects on daily secretion patterns. The seasonal variation in overall cortisol levels is most probably related to the changes in photoperiod. Cortisol is involved in relaxation of the cervix by dissolving the ground substance that binds fibroblasts and fibrocytes together and also stimulates the release of oxytocin from the posterior pituitary. Luteolysis occurrs in pregnant goats in mid and late gestation due to increased PGF2-alpha, with an associated release of prolactin and decrease in plasma progesterone (McMahon et al. 1979).

Relaxin has an important role in partition by relaxing the cervix and softening the tissues that surround the pelvic canal, which in turn allows the fetus to have maximal space for its passage through the pelvis. The relaxin and PGs cause

Table 11.3 Reproductive traits associated with gestation and parturition in some goat breeds.

Breed	Age at first kidding (m)	Kidding interval (m)	Kid mortility (%)	Litter size
Alpine	16.9	—	—	1.8
Barbari	15	8	5	1.6
Beetal	20	11	5	1.4
Jakharana	18	11	5	1.5
Jamunapari	20	11	5	1.3
Nubian	16.9	—	—	2.1
Saanen	16.9	—	—	1.8
Sirohi	16	10	5	1.2
Surti	18	9	5	1.5
Toggenburg	16.9	—	—	1.8

Source: Mellado et al. (2000), Castañeda-Bustos et al. (2014), and Singh et al. 2023.

softening of the cervix and the body of the uterus by increasing the proportion of collagen in the tissues; they dilate the cervix, relax the sacroiliac joints, and widen the birth canal.

Induced parturition in dairy goats can also be used as a strategic farm management tool (Pollock et al. 2021).

11.3.3 Factors Affecting Rate of Kidding

Various reproductive traits are depicted in Table 11.3. Kidding rate has a very low heritability range (0–0.15), and management practices have an influence on kidding rate (Sahare et al. 2009). Abortion and stillbirth rates vary based on the caliber of the producers, the management structure, and the production system, but if the rate is more than 5–8%, it should be investigated (Holler 2012). Higher fecundity rate has been reported in goats with higher parity compared to does with first parity (Mellado et al. 2006). A greater condition score or live weight, as well as better nutrition in the days before ovulation, can all lead to an increase in the twinning rate (De Santiago-Miramontes et al. 2009). Factors such as season, diet, age, and breed can affect the kidding rate (Robertson et al. 2020).

It has been demonstrated that lower nutrition levels during mating lower the likelihood of kidding (Urrutia-Morales et al. 2012) and extremely high rates of fetal loss have been associated with nutritional stress in late pregnancy (Urrutia-Morales et al. 2012). On the other hand, nutritional supplementation like methionine during gestation improves the birth weight of kids (Castillo-Gutierrez et al. 2022). Does in their first pregnancy have more fetal loss than adult goats (Mellado et al. 2004).

The most frequent reasons for neonatal death in goats include premature birth, dystocia, primary predator, infection, congenital anomalies, and the number of young (Nogueira et al. 2016; Robertson et al. 2020).

11.4 Problems of Caprine Gestation

11.4.1 Superfecundation

This is when a doe in a single estrus copulates with more than one male and ovulates each time. Heteropaternal superfecundation may be defined as the fertilization of two or more ova during the same estrus cycle as a result of more than one coital act from different males; this results in fetuses of the same age being born in the same litter but with different paternity (Berry et al. 2020).

11.4.2 Superfetation

This is the simultaneous occurrence of different stages of developing offspring in the same dam (Raghuwanshi et al. 2014).

11.4.3 Hydrometra

Accumulation of aseptic fluid *in utero* is termed hydrometra or psuedo-pregnancy (Underwood et al. 2015; Maia et al. 2018). Does may have characteristically distended abdomens or "deliver" large volumes of cloudy fluid at expected due dates, a phenomenon termed a "cloud burst." The incidence varies between 3.0% and 20.8% (Hesselink 1993). The etiopathophysiology is not clearly understood (Wittek et al. 1997). The condition is accompanied with persistence of the CL. The condition can be diagnosed with ultrasonography and treated with prostaglandins or oxytocin, which results in luteolysis and voiding of large amounts of fluid (Pieteres and Taverne 1986; Purohit and Mehta 2012).

11.5 Pharmacological Induction of Kidding

The benefits of induced kidding are predictable timing of parturition, tight synchrony between kiddings, and improved kid survival. It can be used for improved management of farm activities, efficient utilization of personnel resources, and optimum supervision of parturition events to avoid dystocia or to provide prompt assistance for difficult kidding and postnatal kid care.

The natural or synthetic prostaglandins or dexamethasone can be used for artificial initiation of parturition in goats (Bretzlaff et al. 1983; Thakur and Verma 1990; Romano et al. 2001; Youngquist and Threlfall 2006; Pollock et al. 2021).

References

Akingbade, A.A., Nsahlai, I.V. IV, Bonsi, M.L. et al. (2001). Reproductive performance of South African indigenous goats inoculated with DHP-degrading rumen bacteria and maintained on Leucaena leucocephala/grass mixture and natural pasture. *Small Ruminant Research* 39 (1): 73–85.

Ali, A., Derar, D.R., and Elshahed, M. (2022). Management factors affecting reproductive performance and causes of infertility of Ardi goats in Saudi Arabia. *Journal of the Saudi Society of Agricultural Sciences* 21 (2): 93–97.

Alila-Johansson, A., Eriksson, L., Soveri, T., and Laakso, M.L. (2003). Serum cortisol levels in goats exhibit seasonal but not daily rhythmicity. *Chronobiology International* 20 (1): 65–79.

Al-Totanji, W. and Lubbadeh, W. (2000). Effect of feeding different levels of energy and protein during the last two months of gestation on Shami goats performance in Jordan valley. *Dirstat Agricultural Sciences* 27: 165–175.

Amer, H.A. (2008). Determination of first pregnancy and foetal measurements in Egyptian Baladi goats (Capra hircus). *Veterinaria Italiana* 44 (2): 429–437.

Amoah, E.A., Gelaye, S., Guthrie, P., and Rexroad, C.E. Jr. (1996). Breeding season and aspects of reproduction of female goats. *Journal of Animal Science* 74 (4): 723–728.

Anonymous (2013). *Livestock Infertility and Its Management*. New Delhi, India: National Academy of Agricultural Sciences.

Bassett, J.M. and Thorburn, G.D. (1969). Foetal plasma corticosteroids and the initiation of parturition in sheep. *Journal of Endocrinology* 44 (2): 285–286.

Bayoumi, Y.H., Behairy, A., Abdallah, A.A., and Attia, N.E. (2021). Peri-parturient hypocalcemia in goats: clinical, hematobiochemical profiles and ultrasonographic measurements of postpartum uterine involution. *Veterinary World* 14 (3): 558–568.

Bazer, F.W. (2013). Pregnancy recognition signaling mechanisms in ruminants and pigs. *Journal of Animal Science and Biotechnology* 4 (1): 23.

Berry, D.P., Bohan, A., O'Brien, A.C. et al. (2020). Heteropaternal superfecundation frequently occurs in multiple-bearing mob-mated sheep. *Animal Genetics* 51 (4): 579–583.

Bretzlaff, K.N., Hill, A., and Ott, R.S. (1983). Induction of luteolysis in goats with prostaglandin F2 alpha. *American Journal of Veterinary Research* 44 (6): 1162–1164.

Byatt, J.C., Warren, W.C., Eppard, P.J. et al. (1992). Ruminant placental lactogens: structure and biology. *Journal of Animal Science* 70 (9): 2911–2923.

Capezzuto, A., Chelini, M.O., Felippe, E.C., and Oliveira, C.A. (2008). Correlation between serum and fecal concentrations of reproductive steroids throughout gestation in goats. *Animal Reproduction Science* 103 (1–2): 78–86.

Castañeda-Bustos, V.J., Montaldo, H.H., Torres-Hernández, G. et al. (2014). Estimation of genetic parameters for productive life, reproduction, and milk-production traits in US dairy goats. *Journal of Dairy Science* 97 (4): 2462–2473.

Castillo-Gutierrez, D., Hernández-Arteaga, L.E.S., Flores-Najera, M.J. et al. (2022). Methionine supplementation during pregnancy of goats improves kids' birth weight, body mass index, and postnatal growth pattern. *Biology* 11 (7): 1065.

Chemineau, P., Gauthier, D., Poirier, J.C., and Saumande, J. (1982). Plasma levels of LH, FSH, prolactin, oestradiol-17beta and progesterone during natural and induced oestrus in the dairy goat. *Theriogenology* 17 (3): 313–323.

Currie, W.B. and Thorburn, G.D. (1977). Parturition in goats: studies on the interactions between the foetus, placenta, prostaglandin F and progesterone before parturition, at term or at parturition induced prematurely by corticotrophin infusion of the foetus. *Journal of Endocrinology* 73 (2): 263–278.

Currie, W.B., Gorewit, R.C., and Michel, F.J. (1988). Endocrine changes, with special emphasis on oestradiol-17 beta, prolactin and oxytocin, before and during labour and delivery in goats. *Journal of Reproduction and Fertility* 82 (1): 299–308.

Dayeh, R.A.A., Tabba, M.J., and Harb, M.Y. (1996). Effect of different feeding levels on the productive and reproductive performance of Shami (Damascus) goats in the Jordan Valley. *Dirstat Agricultural Sciences* 23: 131–142.

De Santiago-Miramontes, M.A., Malpaux, B., and Delgadillo, J.A. (2009). Body condition is associated with a shorter breeding season and reduced ovulation rate in subtropical goats. *Animal Reproduction Science* 114 (1–3): 175–182.

Deshpande, S.B. and Mehta, V.M. (1992). Effect of nongenetic factors on gestation length, weight of placenta and placental expulsion time in Surti and Marwari goats. *Indian Journal of Animal Science* 62: 155–158.

Eljarah, A., Sod, G., Gill, M. et al. (2012). Bloody vaginal discharge in a goat with an endometrial stromal polyp. *Large Animal Review* 18: 317–319.

Faurie, A.S., Mitchell, D., and Laburn, H.P. (2001). Feto-maternal relationships in goats during heat and cold exposure. *Experimental Physiology* 86 (2): 199–204.

Fitzpatrick, R. and Dobson, H. (1979). The cervix of the sheep and goat during parturition. *Animal Reproduction Science* 2 (1–3): 209–224.

Flint, A.P.F., Guesdon, F.M.J., and Stewart, H.J. (1994). Regulation of trophoblast interferon gene expression. *Molecular and Cellular Endocrinology* 100 (1–2): 93–95.

Ford, M.M., Young, I.R., and Thorburn, G.D. (1995). Prostaglandins and the maintenance of pregnancy in goats. *Journal of Reproduction and Fertility Supplement* 49: 555–559.

Ford, M.M., Young, I.R., Caddy, D.J., and Thorburn, G.D. (1998). Fetal and maternal endocrine changes approaching parturition in the goat: lack of evidence for prostaglandins E2 and F2alpha as signals for luteolysis. *Biology of Reproduction* 58 (4): 1065–1070.

Fredriksson, G., Kindahl, H., and Edqvist, L.E. (1984). Periparturient release of prostaglandin F2 alpha in the goat. *Zentralblatt fur Veterinarmedizin Reihe A* 31 (5): 386–392.

Gangwar, S.D. and Yadar, M.C. (1987). Factors affecting gestation length in Indian goats. *Indian Journal of Dairy Science* 11: 365–366.

Geisert, R.D., Zavy, M.T., Moffatt, R.J. et al. (1990). Embryonic steroids and the establishment of pregnancy in pigs. *Journal of Reproduction and Fertility. Supplement* 40: 293–305.

Hafez, B. and Hafez, E.S.E. (2006). *Reproduction in Farm Animals*, 7e. Oxford: Blackwell.

Hesselink, J.W. (1993). Incidence of hydrometra in dairy goats. *Veterinary Record* 132 (5): 110–112.

Hesselink, J.W. and Taverne, M.A. (1994). Ultrasonography of the uterus of the goat. *Veterinary Quarterly* 16 (1): 41–45.

Holler, L.D. (2012). Ruminant abortion diagnostics. *Veterinary Clinics of North America. Food Animal Practice* 28 (3): 407–418.

Hudson, S., Mullford, M., Whittlestone, W.G., and Payne, E. (1976). Bovine plasma corticoids during parturition. *Journal of Dairy Science* 59 (4): 744–746.

Humblot, P., De Montigny, G., Jeanguyot, N. et al. (1990). Pregnancy-specific protein B and progesterone concentrations in French Alpine goats throughout gestation. *Journal of Reproduction and Fertility* 89 (1): 205–212.

Hydbring, E., MacDonald, E., and Olsson, K. (1997). Radiotelemetrically recorded blood pressure and heart rate changes in relation to plasma catecholamine levels during parturition in the conscious, unrestrained goat. *Acta Physiologica Scandinavica* 161: 295–302.

Hydbring, E., Madej, A., MacDonald, E. et al. (1999). Hormonal changes during parturition in heifers and goats are related to the phases and severity of labor. *Journal of Endocrinology* 160: 75–85.

Jainudeen, M.R. and Hafez, E.S.E. (2000). Gestation, prenatal physiology and parturition. In: *Reproduction in Farm Animals*, 7e (ed. B. Hafez and E.S.E. Hafez), 140–155. Oxford: Wiley-Blackwell.

Kale, V.B., Pawshe, C.H., Ingawale, M.V. et al. (2021). Reproductive traits in Berari goats of Vidharbha region of Maharashtra. *Indian Journal of Veterinary Science and Biotechnology* 17 (1): 82–84.

Khan, J.R. and Ludri, R.S. (2002a). Hormone profile of crossbred goats during the periparturient period. *Tropical Animal Health and Production* 34 (2): 151–162.

Khan, J.R. and Ludri, R.S. (2002b). Changes in blood glucose, plasma non-esterified fatty acids and insulin in pregnant and non-pregnant goats. *Tropical Animal Health and Production* 34 (1): 81–90.

Kindahl, H., Alonso, R., Cort, N., and Einarsson, S. (1982). Release of prostaglandin F2 alpha during parturition in the sow. *Zentralblatt fur Veterinarmedizin Reihe A* 29 (7): 504–510.

Kitts, D.D. (1985). Peripartal endocrine changes and the initiation of lactation in ewes of diverse breeds. *Growth* 49 (2): 176–189.

Kumar, K., Chandolia, R.K., Kumar, S. et al. (2015). Two-dimensional and three-dimensional ultrasonography for pregnancy diagnosis and antenatal fetal development in Beetal goats. *Veterinary World* 8 (7): 835–840.

Laura, A.S., Kumar, M.S., William, G., and Sandra, L.A. (2004). Predicting the onset of parturition in the goat by determining progesterone levels by enzyme immunoassay. *Small Ruminant Research* 52: 203–209.

Liggins, G.C. (1979). Initiation of parturition. *British Medical Bulletin* 35 (2): 145–150.

Liggins, G.C. (1994). The role of cortisol in preparing the fetus for birth. *Reproduction, Fertility, and Development* 6: 141–150.

Lindell, J.O., Kindahl, H., Jansson, L., and Edqvist, L.E. (1982). Post-partum release of prostaglandin F(2alpha) and uterine involution in the cow. *Theriogenology* 17 (3): 237–245.

Maia, A.L.R.S., Brandão, F.Z., Souza-Fabjan, J.M.G. et al. (2018). Hydrometra in dairy goats: ultrasonic variables and therapeutic protocols evaluated during the reproductive season. *Animal Reproduction Science* 197: 203–211.

Mainau, E. and Manteca, X. (2011). Pain and discomfort caused by parturition in cows and sows. *Applied Animal Behaviour Science* 135: 241–251.

Martínez, M.F., Bosch, P., and Bosch, R.A. (1998). Determination of early pregnancy and embryonic growth in goats by transrectal ultrasound scanning. *Theriogenology* 49 (8): 1555–1565.

McMahon, G.R., Shearman, R.P., Shutt, D.A., and Smith, I.D. (1979). Prostaglandin F2 alpha-induced prolactin release and luteolysis in the goat. *Australian Journal of Biological Sciences* 32 (1): 109–114.

Medan, M., Watanabe, G., Absy, G. et al. (2004). Early pregnancy diagnosis by means of ultrasonography as a method of improving reproductive efficiency in goats. *Journal of Reproduction and Development* 50 (4): 391–397.

Mellado, M., Amaro, J.L., García, J.E., and Lara, L.M. (2000). Factors affecting gestation length in goats and the effect of gestation period on kid survival. *Journal of Agricultural Science* 135 (1): 85–89.

Mellado, M., Valdez, R., Lara, L.M., and García, J.E. (2004). Risk factors involved in conception, abortion, and kidding rates of goats under extensive conditions. *Small Ruminant Research* 55 (1–3): 191–198.

Mellado, M., Valdéz, R., García, J.E. et al. (2006). Factors affecting the reproductive performance of goats under intensive conditions in a hot arid environment. *Small Ruminant Research* 63 (1–2): 110–118.

Mellor, D.J. and Matheson, I.C. (1979). Daily changes in the curved crown-rump length of individual sheep fetuses during the last 60 days of pregnancy and effects of different levels of maternal nutrition. *Quarterly Journal of Experimental Physiology and Cognate Medical Sciences* 64 (2): 119–131.

Nagel, C., Aurich, C., and Aurich, J. (2019). Stress effects on the regulation of parturition in different domestic animal species. *Animal Reproduction Science* 207: 153–161.

Nathanielsz, P.W. (1978). Endocrine mechanisms of parturition. *Annual Review of Physiology* 40: 411–445.

Newton, G.R., Ott, T.L., Woldesenbet, S. et al. (1996). Biochemical and immunological properties of related small ruminant trophoblast interferons. *Theriogenology* 46 (4): 703–716.

Nogueira, D.M., Gummow, B., Gardiner, C.P. et al. (2016). A survey of the meat goat industry in Queensland and New South Wales. 2. Herd management, reproductive performance and animal health. *Animal Production Science* 56: 1533–1544.

Olsson, K. and Dahlborn, K. (1989). Fluid balance during heat stress in lactating goats. *Quarterly Journal of Experimental Physiology (Cambridge, England)* 74 (5): 645–659.

Osuagwuh, A.I. and Aire, T.A. (1990). Intrauterine growth rates of the west African dwarf goat and some foetal organs in relation to strategic feed supplementation during pregnancy. *Zentralblatt fur Veterinarmedizin Reihe A* 37 (3): 198–204.

Padbury, J.F., Agata, Y., Polk, D.H. et al. (1988). Catecholamine and endorphin responses to delivery in term and preterm lambs. *Developmental Pharmacology and Therapeutics* 11 (1): 44–50.

Padilla-Rivas, G.R., Sohnrey, B., and Holtz, W. (2005). Early pregnancy detection by real-time ultrasonography in Boer goats. *Small Ruminant Research* 58: 87–92.

Patel, A.C. and Pandey, D.P. (2013). Growth, production and reproduction performance of Mehsana goat. *Journal of Livestock Sciences* 4: 17–21.

Perera, B.M., Abeygunawardena, H., Thamotharam, A. et al. (1981). Peripartal changes of estrone, progesterone and prostaglandin in the water buffalo. *Theriogenology* 15 (5): 463–467.

Pieteres, M.C. and Taverne, M.A. (1986). Hydrometra in goats: diagnosis with real-time ultrasound and treatment with prostaglandins or oxytocin. *Theriogenology* 26: 813–812.

Pineda, M.H. and Dooley, M.P. (2003). *McDonald's Veterinary Endocrinology and Reproduction*, 5e. Ames, IA: Iowa State Press.

Pollock, J.M., Miner, K., Buzzell, N. et al. (2021). Induction of parturition in a large number of pregnant dairy goats and its benefits as a management tool in a commercial scale goat operation. *Theriogenology* 172: 1–7.

Probo, M., Cairoli, F., Kindahl, H. et al. (2011). Peripartal hormonal changes in Alpine goats: a comparison between physiological and pathological parturition. *Reproduction in Domestic Animals* 46 (6): 1004–1010.

Probo, M., Cotticelli, A., Bucci, R. et al. (2022). Association between a single measurement of progesterone and cortisol blood concentrations at two to one week before parturition, and number of fetuses in the Teramana goat. *Meycyna Weterynaryina-Veterinary Medicine Science and Practice* 78 (2): 74–78.

Purohit, G.N. and Mehta, J.S. (2012). Hydrometra in goats (Capra hircus): clinical analysis of 26 cases. *Ruminant Science* 1 (2): 117–119.

Raghuwanshi, D.S., Patil, A.D., and Narwade, P.S. (2014). Superfoetation in osmanbadi does. *Intas Polivet* 15 (2): 223–224.

Rastogi, A., Dutta, N., and Kusumakar, S. (2003). Effect of strategic feed supplementation during gestation on intake, blood-biochemical profile and reproductive performance of goats. *Asian Australasian Journal of Animal Sciences* 16 (12): 1725–1731.

Rawlings, N. and Ward, W. (1977). Progesterone and the initiation of parturition in the goat. *Theriogenology* 7 (6): 317–329.

Robertson, S.M., Atkinson, T., Friend, M.A. et al. (2020). Reproductive performance in goats and causes of perinatal mortality: a review. *Animal Production Science* 60: 1669–1680.

Romano, J.E., Rodas, E., and Ferreira, A. (2001). Timing of prostaglandin F2a administration for induction of parturition in dairy goats. *Small Ruminant Research* 42: 199–202.

Roy, N., Ishwar, A.K., and Singh, S.K. (2007). Reproductive performance of black Bengal goats – a note. *Indian Journal of Small Ruminants* 13 (1): 84–85.

Ruvuna, F., Cartwright, T.C., Blackburn, H. et al. (1988). Gestation length, birth weight and growth rates of pure-bred indigenous goats and their crosses in Kenya. *Journal of Agricultural Science* 3: 363–368.

Sahare, M.G., Sawaimul, A.D., Ali, S.Z., and Kolte, B.R. (2009). Kidding percentage and twinning ability in Osmanabadi goat in Vidarbha climatic condition. *Veterinary World* 2 (2): 60–61.

Sahoo, S., Alex, R., Vohra, V. et al. (2023). Estimation of genetic parameters and genetic change of first parity reproductive traits in Alpine × Beetal goats. *Reproduction in Domestic Animals* 58: 1188–1198.

Senger, P.L. (2005). *Pathways to Pregnancy and Parturition*. Pullman, WA: Current Conceptions.

Sibanda, L.M., Ndlovu, L.R., and Bryant, M.J. (1999). Effects of a low plane of nutrition during pregnancy and lactation on the performance of Matebele does and their kids. *Small Ruminant Research* 32: 243–250.

Singh, D.K. and Singh, C.S.P. (1983). Effect of kid's genotype on gestation period, birth weight of placenta in black Bengal goats. *Indian Journal of Animal Science* 53: 678–680.

Singh, M.K., Singh, S.K., and Chauhan, M.S. (2023). Exploring potential of goat based dairy farming in India and way forward. *Indian Journal of Animal Sciences* 93 (3): 243–250.

Singh, N.S., Gawande, P.G., Mishra, O.P. et al. (2004). Accuracy of ultrasonography in early pregnancy diagnosis in doe. *Asian-Australasian Journal of Animal Sciences* 17 (6): 760–768.

Sinha, N.K. and Sahni, K.L. (1982). A note on the factors affecting gestation period of certain Indian breeds of goats. *Veterinary Research Journal* 5: 73–77.

Stewart, D.R., Kindahl, H., Stabenfeldt, G.H., and Hughes, J.P. (1984). Concentrations of 15-keto-13, 14-dihydro-prostaglandin F2 alpha in the mare during spontaneous and oxytocin induced foaling. *Equine Veterinary Journal* 16 (4): 270–274.

Suguna, K., Mehrotra, S., Agarwal, S.K. et al. (2008). Early pregnancy diagnosis and embryonic and fetal development using real time B mode ultrasound in goats. *Small Ruminant Research* 80 (1–3): 80–86.

Takashi, T., Hayashi, K., and Hosoe, M. (2013). Biology of the placental proteins in domestic ruminants: expression, proposed roles and practical applications. *Japan Agricultural Research Quarterly* 47 (1): 43–51.

Thakur, M.S. and Verma, S.K. (1990). Use of dexamethasone for induction of parturition in goats. *Archiv fur Experimentelle Veterinarmedizin* 44 (3): 459–463.

Ticconi, C., Zicari, A., Belmonte, A. et al. (2007). Pregnancy-promoting actions of HCG in human myometrium and fetal membranes. *Placenta* 28: S137–S143.

Umo, I., Fitzpatrick, R.J., and Ward, W.R. (1976). Parturition in the goat: plasma concentrations of prostaglandin F and steroid hormones and uterine activity during late pregnancy and parturition. *Journal of Endocrinology* 68 (3): 383–389.

Underwood, W.J., Blauwiekel, R., Delano, M.L. et al. (2015). Biology and diseases of ruminants (sheep, goats, and cattle). *Laboratory Animal Medicine* 623–694.

Urrutia-Morales, J., Meza-Herrera, C.A., Tello-Varela, L. et al. (2012). Effect of nutritional supplementation upon pregnancy rates of goats under semiarid rangelands and exposed to the male effect. *Tropical Animal Health and Production* 44 (7): 1473–1477.

Wittek, T., Richter, A., Erices, J., and Elze, K. (1997). Incidence, diagnosis, therapy and subsequent fertility in goats with hydrometra. *Tierärztliche Praxis* 25: 576–582.

Wooding, F.B., Hobbs, T., Morgan, G. et al. (1993). Cellular dynamics of growth in sheep and goat synepitheliochorial placentomes: an autoradiographic study. *Journal of Reproduction and Fertility* 98 (1): 275–283.

Youngquist, R.S. and Threlfall, W.R. (2006). *Current Therapy in Large Animal Theriogenology*, 2e. New York: Elsevier Health Sciences.

Ziecik, A.J., Waclawik, A., Kaczmarek, M.M. et al. (2011). Mechanisms for the establishment of pregnancy in the pig. *Reproduction in Domestic Animals* 46: 31–41.

12

Lactation

Manoj Kumar Kalita[1], Simson Soren[2], Jitumoni Das[1], and Prerona Patowary[3]

[1] Department of Animal Reproduction, Gynaecology and Obstetrics, Lakhimpur College of Veterinary Science, Assam Agricultural University, North Lakhimpur, India
[2] Department of Veterinary Physiology, Lakhimpur College of Veterinary Science, Assam Agricultural University, North Lakhimpur, India
[3] Department of Veterinary Clinical Medicine, Ethics and Jurisprudence, Assam Agricultural University – Goat Research Station, Burnihat, India

12.1 Introduction

Lactation, the intricate process of milk synthesis, secretion, and excretion, begins after calving or lambing and continues until the lactating female naturally or artificially dries off (Ventrella et al. 2019). The mammary gland comprises parenchyma and stroma, including the ductal system, with tissue distribution varying across lactation stages and yields. Mammary glands undergo enlargement during late gestation and the initial to middle lactation phases due to increased epithelial cell count and lumen area (Biswas et al. 2022). Post late lactation, a decline in the secretory structure results in reduced mammary gland volume.

Across various lactation stages (Figure 12.1), goats and sheep consistently exhibit similar mammary gland patterns. In recent years, small ruminants have gained prominence in the dairy sector, particularly in underdeveloped regions, with significant economic and societal impacts (Lerias et al. 2014). Goat farming has a pivotal economic role in countries within the Mediterranean and Middle Eastern regions, exemplified by well-organized goat farming in France, Italy, Spain, and Greece. India boasts a substantial goat population of 148.88 million, accounting for 27.80% of its total livestock count, driven by domestic goat milk consumption and global population growth (20th Livestock Census 2019).

The global interest in goat milk products, including cheese and yogurt, is another pivotal factor influencing the goat milk market. This surge is driven by rising disposable income and the prevalence of cow milk allergies and gastrointestinal conditions (Coni et al. 1999). Goat milk is increasingly sought after due to perceived advantages over conventional medical treatments, particularly in developed nations. Goats play a crucial role in providing dairy and meat products to rural populations, especially in developing countries, making them a suitable option for landless and marginal farmers due to their adaptability, stress tolerance, and low maintenance costs (Devendra 2013).

Goats are often referred to as "the poor man's cow" due to their affordability compared to cows, making them accessible to underprivileged segments of society (Alexandre and Mandonnet 2005). However, insufficient volume and seasonal demand have hindered goat milk industrialization. Despite a growing goat population and increased milk production, marketing efforts for goat milk remain inadequate. Goat milk's mineral and vitamin richness and creamy texture position it as a substitute for various dietary supplements, showing promise as an alternative to both cow and human milk (Pietrzak-Fiecko and Kamelska-Sadowska 2020).

Goat milk consumption, surpassing that of other milk types, prevails in many parts of the world due to choice or necessity. It serves as a crucial source of daily calcium, phosphate, and protein in underdeveloped countries. With enhanced protein and fat digestibility, alkalinity, buffering ability, and therapeutic nutritional benefits, goat milk stands apart from human or cow milk. It contains more medium-chain fatty acids (MCTs), catering to malabsorption patients and growing children's energy needs (Coni et al. 1999). The rising demand for healthy foods has fueled interest in dairy goats and goat milk products, particularly among infants and those with cow milk allergies (Zenebe et al. 2014). These unique attributes contribute to the long-term sustainability of the dairy goat sector, especially for individuals experiencing allergic responses

Elements of Reproduction and Reproductive Diseases of Goats, First Edition. Edited by Tanmoy Rana.

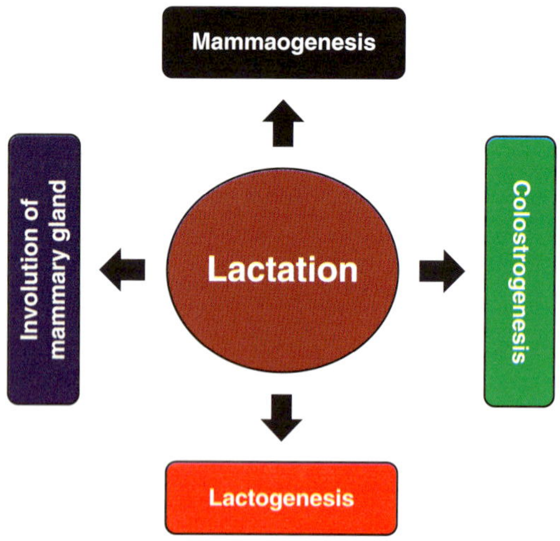

Figure 12.1 Stages of lactation.

to cow milk (Coni et al. 1999). Goat milk is often better tolerated due to the flavor of its curd and smaller fat globules.

Beyond its role as a nutrient source, goat milk harbors potent antioxidant, antibacterial, and antiallergic properties, making it a valuable nutraceutical. Recent research highlights the link between goat milk's structural and functional attributes and its potential in mitigating common milk-related health concerns.

This emphasis on neonatal sustenance through maternal lactation underscores the essential role of mothers in converting nutrients into highly nutritious milk. Neonates benefit from this synthetic and secretory process as their primary task during the early postnatal phase is nursing. Selective breeding has led to some animals overproducing milk, exceeding the needs of their young. The thriving multi-billion dollar dairy industry in the Western world relies on substantial milk yields, resulting in a diverse array of dairy products. This chapter delves into mammary gland development (mammogenesis), anatomical variations, and milk ejection from the gland.

12.2 Mammary Glands are Sophisticated Sweat Glands

Depending on the species, the mammary ridges can produce one or several mammary glands. For instance, animals like pigs, dogs, and cats have a sequence of individual glands that develop in consistent locations along the entire mammary ridges' course. Paired mammary glands, as seen in humans and elephants, emerge from the thoracic region of the mammary ridges. In animals like cows, mares, and goats, mammary glands develop at the inguinal area of the mammary ridge (Wallace 1953; Purup et al. 1993).

The main mammary bud forms from the denser epidermal epithelium that constructs the mammary ridges. During development, the primary mammary bud extends into the underlying dermis. Continued growth results in secondary mammary buds generating protrusions away from the parent bud (Wallace 1953; Johnsson 1984; Ellis et al. 1998). As embryonic development progresses, these secondary buds elongate and branch. These branched buds eventually begin canalizing, forming small ducts within each bud. Subsequently, each bud evolves into a duct with a lumen. By birth, the lactiferous ducts expand, leading to larger ducts that exit the mammary gland externally (Sejrsen et al. 1983; Johnsson et al. 1985).

12.2.1 Postnatal Growth

The postnatal growth of the mammary gland is regulated by endocrine factors. Full anatomical maturation and the capacity for milk synthesis and release occur in females after reaching puberty, undergoing pregnancy, and giving birth.

From birth until puberty, the growth of the mammary gland follows an isometric pattern, expanding at a similar rate to other tissues. Unlike the rest of the body, there is no observable increase in the size of the mammary glands during this period (Wallace 1953; Purup et al. 1993).

12.2.2 Between Puberty and Pregnancy

Upon the onset of puberty, the mammary gland undergoes accelerated growth compared to the rest of the body, a phenomenon termed allometric growth. Over successive estrous cycles, the mammary gland constructs a complex duct and alveolar structure, forming the cellular foundation for subsequent milk synthesis (Holcombe et al. 1988). Under the influence of estrogen, the ducts exhibit branching during the initial estrous or menstrual cycles, accompanied by an increase in diameter. The commencement of the luteal phase triggers the terminal segments of each branch to generate early alveoli, a process orchestrated by progesterone. These alveoli constitute the functional secretory components of the mammary gland (Figure 12.2).

The presence of prolactin and growth hormone (somatotropin) accelerates duct formation more effectively than estrogen alone and both these hormones surge during the onset of puberty. Although repeated and cyclic exposure to estrogen and progesterone stimulates limited mammogenesis, complete and rapid development necessitates subsequent endocrine input during the gestational phase (Buskirk et al. 1997; Swanson 1960). This input is crucial for the maturation of the mammary framework, established between puberty and pregnancy.

12.2.3 Mammary Development During Pregnancy

In the dam, complete alveolar development takes place during the final trimester of pregnancy. In this timeframe, terminal alveoli gradually aggregate into clusters referred to as lobules. An analogy would be a bunch of grapes where a lobule corresponds to a collection of grapes on a single stem (Figure 12.2).

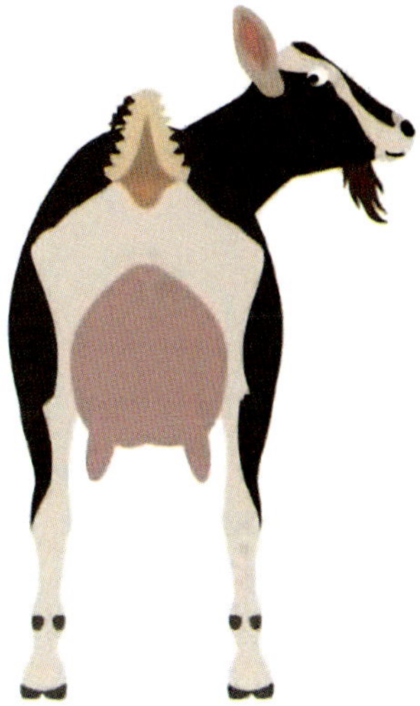

Figure 12.2 Anatomical position, number, and teat morphology of goat.

These lobulo-alveolar structures expand, constituting nearly 90% of the mammary gland's cellular mass by parturition in the last trimester of pregnancy (Stelwagen et al. 1993). The mammary epithelium's capacity for milk production hinges on pivotal hormones such as placental lactogen (PL), prolactin, and adrenal cortical hormones. The levels of all these hormones notably surge just prior to delivery. The initiation of the mammary gland's milk secretion capability is meticulously synchronized with the onset of parturition, ensuring immediate access to milk for the newborn (Akers and Cleale 1990; Knight et al. 1994).

12.3 Colostrogenesis

This intricate process can be described as the prepartum transfer of components, primarily immunoglobulins, from the maternal bloodstream into mammary secretions within a distinct and limited period. Notably, goat colostrum exhibits an IgG concentration about 2.8 times higher than that in blood serum.

The initiation of colostrogenesis is governed by estradiol and progesterone, whereas lactogenic hormones control its termination, given the hormonally regulated nature of the entire process. In cattle, prolactin diminishes the expression of the mammary IgG1 receptor during the onset of lactogenesis (Barrington et al. 1999). According to Brandon et al. (1971), the transfer of IgG from the maternal circulation to mammary secretion commences several weeks prior to parturition and halts abruptly just before parturition, implying that colostrogenesis precedes lactogenesis. Ciupercescu (1977) investigated the duration during which IgG is transferred from the bloodstream to colostrum.

Several factors influence the final composition of colostrum, encompassing species, breed, age, nutrition, litter size, length of dry period, and health status (Csapo et al. 1994; Awadeh et al. 1998; Maunsell et al. 1998). Despite not being fully comprehended, colostrogenesis generally occurs and stores colostrum in the mammary gland during late pregnancy, following the research of Linzell and Peaker (1971). The input of colostrum's secretion components into the mammary gland is regulated by several mechanisms (Patton and Jensen 1975) and influenced by both local and systemic factors (Castro et al. 2011).

12.3.1 Colostrum Composition

Colostrum, the initial secretion produced by the mammary gland around or just before parturition, constitutes a blend of bioactive substances (Hernandez-Castellano et al. 2014a). The composition of colostrum differs from mature milk in established lactation, marked by a higher concentration of immunoglobulin G (IgG) in colostrum, particularly IgG1, which stands as a notable distinction among ruminants (Micusan and Borduas 1977). Colostrum is a complex mixture encompassing components crucial for the nutrition of newborn ruminants, including fat, lactose, vitamins, and minerals (Ontsouka et al. 2003; Hernández-Castellano et al. 2014b).

Observations by Hadjipanayiotou (1995) spotlight the evolution of fat, protein, and lactose concentrations in the early postpartum period of small ruminants, particularly goats and ewes. Lactose displayed a similar pattern in both species, declining on the first day of lactation (3%) and later increasing. Yet, protein and fat amounts diverged between ewes and goats on the first day (19% vs 16% protein, 11% vs 8% fat, respectively). This discrepancy could be attributed to varying immunoglobulin levels, causing a substantial protein content drop on the second day of lactation.

While primarily serving a nutritional purpose, colostrum's protein composition actively contributes to defense against infections and postpartum environmental challenges. Additionally, colostrum contains ingredients such as vitamins, hormones, growth factors, cytokines, enzymes, and metabolites from alveolar epithelial cells and immunocompetent cells (Linzell and Peaker 1975; Lee et al. 1980; Blum and Hammon 2000; Vetter et al. 2013). Among these, immunoglobulins, especially IgG, have been extensively researched due to their pivotal role in protecting neonatal ruminants from infections (Moreno-Indias et al. 2012). The three most significant immunoglobulins in colostrum are IgG, IgM, and IgA.

Temporal changes in colostral IgG concentration postpartum were noted by Castro et al. (2006). Rudovsky et al. (2008) conducted a study on goat colostrums, revealing the concentrations of various Ig subclasses, including 49.1, 3.19, and 2.00 mg/ml of IgG, IgM, and IgA respectively, at parturition. These values account for 90.3%, 6.0%, and 3.7% of the total colostrum immunoglobulin content. Recent discoveries have identified the enzyme chitotriosidase (ChT) as a component in goat colostrum, released by activated macrophages.

12.3.2 The Importance of Colostrum in Newborn Ruminants

The postpartum behavior of both the mother and the newborn ruminant, along with the applied management practices, has an important influence on the animal's survival prospects (Nowak et al. 2000). Lamb mortality rates vary between 10% and 25%, and goat kid mortality ranges from 7% to 50%, contingent on the farm (Mellor and Stafford 2004). This situation compromises animal welfare and impacts the overall benefits for farmers as well. Research by Logan and Pearson (1978) revealed that the immune system of a newborn ruminant seems to possess limited capability for manufacturing its own immunoglobulins during the initial month of life.

As a result, the correlation between colostrum administration and the survival of newborn ruminants has been extensively studied (Argüello et al. 2004; Castro et al. 2005, 2009, 2011). Colostrum feeding plays a pivotal role in helping newborn ruminants regulate their body temperature. In fact, a study by Dwyer and Morgan (2006) found that more active newborn lambs with increased colostral nourishment exhibited improved thermoregulation, effectively managing their body temperatures compared to less active counterparts.

Observations by Dos-Santos et al. (1994) demonstrated that newborn goat kids experienced an elevation in rectal temperature following colostrum feeding. Beyond temperature regulation, colostrum's significance is underscored by its abundant magnesium content, a vital element for initiating peristalsis. Colostrum's role in enhancing meconium expulsion also prevents bacterial colonization of the intestinal mucosa, as confirmed by various researchers (García de Jalón et al. 1990; Barza et al. 1993).

12.4 Lactogenesis

As Cowie et al. (2011) state, the onset of milk secretion is referred to as lactogenesis. This physiological process, delineated by Linzell and Peaker (1975), can be divided into two distinct phases. The first stage commences when the gland is adequately developed during pregnancy, initiating the release of specific milk components like caseins and lactose in small amounts. The second stage, characterized by the commencement of abundant milk secretion in relation to parturition, marks the transition to heightened milk production.

12.4.1 Basic Composition of Goat Milk

The constitution of milk varies based on multiple factors, encompassing breed, environment, and breeding strategies applied across different countries. For young mammals, milk functions as the primary nutritional source after colostrum, preceding their capacity to digest alternative nourishment. Goat and sheep milks exhibit diminished immunoglobulin content compared to equivalent colostrum. While goat and sheep milks contain higher lactose quantities compared to colostrum, their fat and protein percentages are comparatively lower (Haenlein and Caccese 1984). In terms of core composition, goat milk closely resembles cow milk. On average, caprine milk comprises 12.2% total solids, with 3.8% fat, 3.5% protein, 4.1% lactose, and 0.8% ash (Jenness 1980; Favier and Dorsainvil 1987). Contrasted with cow milk, goat milk presents higher fat, protein, and ash contents while exhibiting lower lactose levels. Although goat milk's total casein content is slightly inferior to that of cow milk, it holds a greater presence of nonprotein nitrogen. Goat, cow, and human milk all have comparable totals of solids and caloric content (Pirisi et al. 2007; Park et al. 2007).

In a comparison between goat milk and sheep milk, the latter contains elevated fat and protein percentages (6.82% and 5.59% respectively) compared to goat milk (3.70% and 3.57% respectively). However, the lactose content remains comparable in both species' milk (4.88% in sheep milk and 4.92% in goat milk) (Alichanidis and Polychroniadou 1996).

12.4.1.1 Lipids

The fat percentage of goat milk exhibits breed-related variation, spanning from 2.45% to 7.76% (Haenlein and Caccese 1984). According to available reports, the average fat globule diameters for goat, cow, buffalo, and sheep milks are 3.49, 4.55, 5.92, and 3.30 μm, respectively (Haenlein and Caccese 1984; Jenness 1980). In goat milk, the smaller fat globules result in enhanced dispersion and a more uniform fat mixture, presenting a larger fat surface area that promotes improved lipase digestion.

In goat milk fat, approximately 97–99% consists of free lipids, predominantly triglycerides, with 1–3% accounting for bound lipids, primarily in the form of polar and neutral lipids (Chandan et al. 1992). Goat milk fat notably contains a significantly higher proportion of short- and medium-chain fatty acids (MCT) (C4:0–C14:0) in comparison to cow and human milks (Park 1994). This unique composition has been harnessed for the treatment of various patient conditions associated with fat malabsorption, signifying its therapeutic potential (Jensen et al. 1990).

12.4.1.2 Protein

Goat milk is composed of five key proteins: s2-casein (s2-CN), beta-casein (beta-CN), kappa-casein (kappa-CN), beta-lactoglobulin (beta-Lg), and beta-lactalbumin (beta-La) (Haenlein and Caccese 1984; Jenness 1980). While beta-casein is the predominant casein fraction in goat milk, s1-casein takes precedence in cow milk (Jenness 1980). In comparing goats and cows, noteworthy variations arise in the amino acid composition of goat milk's casein fractions. Aspartate, lysine, and tyrosine show greater abundance in alpha-caseins compared to beta-casein, whereas leucine, proline, and valine exhibit higher levels in the latter (Jenness 1980). In terms of casein micelles, those in goat milk are characterized by lower solvation, reduced heat stability, and a heightened susceptibility to beta-casein loss compared to bovine micelles (Juarez and Ramos 1986).

Across multiple species' milks, a common pattern emerges in terms of amino acid content. The amino acids glutamate (with glutamine, comprising 20%), proline (10%), and leucine (10%) predominate (Davis et al. 1994). Notably, goat and other nonprimate milks contain elevated levels of glutamate and proline, alongside diminished leucine quantities, in contrast to human milk's three most prevalent amino acids (Davis et al. 1994). Among sulfur-containing amino acids, primate milks demonstrate higher cystine levels and lower methionine levels when compared to goat and other nonprimate milks (Davis et al. 1994).

12.4.1.3 Carbohydrates

Lactose constitutes a major portion of goat milk, with a slightly lower content of 0.2–0.5% compared to cow milk (Chandan et al. 1992). This disaccharide, formed by combining glucose and a galactose molecule, is synthesized by the mammary gland. In contrast to goat milk, the milk of lower mammalian species contains higher fat content and reduced lactose levels. Although monosaccharides and oligosaccharides are present in goat milk, their specific concentrations relative to cow milk remain undisclosed (Chandan et al. 1992).

12.4.1.4 Minerals

Goat milk contains approximately 134 mg of calcium and 141 mg of phosphorus per 100 g. In comparison, human milk has only one-fourth to one-sixth of these mineral quantities. In terms of minerals, goat milk surpasses cow milk in calcium, phosphorus, potassium, magnesium, and chlorine content, while showing lower levels of sodium and sulfur. A close inverse correlation exists between lactose concentration and the molar sum of sodium and potassium in goat milk and other species' milks (Haenlein and Caccese 1984; Jenness 1980).

The presence of sodium does not exhibit significant connections with potassium, chlorine, or lactose. However, chloride shows a positive correlation with potassium and a negative correlation with lactose (Park and Chukwu 1989). Factors such as diet, breed, stage of lactation, and the individual animal influence trace mineral concentrations. On average, goat milk boasts a higher mineral content compared to cow milk. Conversely, goat milk's lower hydration level is accompanied by an inverse correlation between micelle mineralization and hydration (Remeuf and Lenoir 1986).

12.4.1.5 Vitamins

Goat milk exhibits a higher vitamin A content compared to cow milk. This distinction arises because goats convert all beta-carotene into vitamin A within the milk, rendering caprine milk whiter than its bovine counterpart. Goat milk serves as a suitable source of vitamin A, niacin, and an excess of thiamin, riboflavin, and pantothenate for human infants. However, if exclusively fed on goat milk, a human infant could receive an excess of protein, calcium, phosphorus, vitamin A, thiamin, riboflavin, niacin, and pantothenate in relation to the requirements set by the Food and Agriculture Organization and World Health Organization (FAO-WHO) (Jenness 1980).

Vitamin B levels in both goat and cow milks are influenced by rumen synthesis and exhibit a degree of dietary independence. However, goat milk falls short in terms of folic acid and vitamin B_{12} when compared to cow milk. The latter boasts five times the amount of folate and vitamin B_{12} found in goat milk, and as folate is essential for hemoglobin synthesis, this distinction is noteworthy (Jenness 1980; Park 1994). Pyridoxine (B_6), vitamins C and D, and other essential nutrients must be supplemented in both goat and cow milk to address these deficiencies, contrasting with cow milk's higher folate and vitamin B_{12} content (Haenlein and Caccese 1984; Jenness 1980).

12.4.2 Milk Contains Hormones and Growth Factors

Milk comprises a range of chemicals akin to those present in blood, leading to the natural presence of hormones and growth factors from the bloodstream of lactating females. Additionally, milk can contain exogenous substances such as alcohol, narcotics, antibiotics, and other compounds if consumed by the dam. In earlier times, before controlled nutrition for dairy calves, milk could taste like onions during spring due to cows grazing on wild onions in pastures. The chemicals responsible for the characteristic onion scent dissolve in lipids, facilitating their entry into milk (McFadden et al. 1990).

The presence of hormones in milk is linked to two transmission pathways. The alveolar epithelium possesses hormone receptors on its cells, enabling these hormones to permeate the alveolar cells. Subsequently, the hormone can be secreted into the milk. Prolactin, synthesized by the pituitary, is a primary example of a hormone released in this manner. Prolactin, originating in the anterior lobe of the pituitary gland, travels through the blood and mammary cells, and ultimately into the milk. Apart from prolactin, other hormones like gondadotropin hormone-releasing hormone (GnRH), growth hormone (somatotropin), and thyroid hormone (thyroxine), along with their releasing factors, have been identified in milk. Importantly, it should be noted that protein hormones undergo digestion into amino acids in the gastrointestinal tract, diminishing their biological effects and minimizing physiological impacts on neonates (or consumers) (Forsyth 1997).

12.4.3 Ovarian Steroids

Due to their lipid solubility, estrogens and progesterones can passively move from the bloodstream into the milk. Milk encompasses all steroid hormones (Malekinejad and Rezabakhsh 2015). The concentrations of estrogen and progesterone in milk exhibit a strong correlation with their levels in the blood, mirroring the cyclic hormone synthesis carried out by the ovaries. This phenomenon allows for the swift evaluation of a female's reproductive status by analyzing steroid levels in milk, particularly progesterone. The use of cowside ELISA technology enables the measurement of progesterone levels in milk.

Ongoing research and enhancements are recommended in the realm of progesterone testing methods utilizing "inline" assay technologies within the milking parlor (Bruinje and Ambrose 2019). Such an approach would involve integrating a small sensor into each milking machine, converting progesterone concentrations into electrical signals transmitted to a computer. The adoption of this technology could empower producers to monitor individual cows' daily and estrous cycle stages, pregnancy status, and certain ovarian pathologies (such as cystic ovarian disease). The introduction of such advanced technology has the potential to revolutionize dairy cow reproductive management practices.

12.4.4 Growth Factors in Milk May Provide New Insights to Neonate Health

It is widely recognized that colostrum contains notable concentrations of various growth factors. The initial milk produced postpartum is termed colostrum, and it carries antibodies that confer a passive immune system to the newborn. The accumulation of growth factors in colostrum is believed to have evolved to support the growth and development of neonates.

Among the growth factors found in colostrum are insulin-like growth factors 1 and 2 (IGF1 and 2), epidermal growth factor (EGF), and transforming growth factors (TGF) alpha and beta (Ginjala and Pakkanen 1998). Research has shed light on these growth factors within milk. Their presence holds potential significance due to their substantial physiological impact. First, the identification of these growth factors introduces a fresh avenue of exploration into the role of mammary secretions in infant development and well-being, extending beyond mere nutritional supply. Second, there must exist a molecular protective mechanism safeguarding these growth factors from being digested by the gastrointestinal tract (Macias and Hinck 2012). Gaining deeper insights into these realms could potentially unveil novel understandings of the growth and defense mechanisms of various proteins, as well as their impact on newborn health.

12.4.5 Immunity Transfer in Small Ruminants

12.4.5.1 Lactation Provides Immunoprotection and Nutrition for the Neonate

Immunoglobulins are present in lacteal secretions across all species and are found in both colostrum and regular milk (Bramhell 1970; Butler 1974; Hemmings 1976). The initial milk releases from the mammary gland, known as colostrum, are vital for neonatal survival due to the presence of immunoglobulins (antibodies) in the dam's milk. These immunoglobulins are consumed by the newborn and transported unchanged into the mucosal cells of the stomach, providing passive immunity. In species with an epitheliochorial placenta like ruminants (and other animals), maternal immunoglobulins cannot be transferred *in utero* because the placenta acts as a barrier. Therefore, consuming colostrum shortly after birth becomes crucial for providing the necessary immunological protection to the newborn. In contrast, immunoglobulins are transferred from mother to fetus through the placenta in humans and other animals with hemochorial placentation.

The predominant serum immunoglobulin passed from mother to fetus or through lacteal secretions to the newborn is IgG. Mammary gland local plasmacytes can produce IgA and IgM. The concentration and relative proportion of these immunoglobulin classes in a species' lacteal secretions reveal the primary mode of passive immunity transmission and the origin of immunoglobulins (humoral or local) (Bramhell 1970; Butler 1974; Hemmings 1976). As a result, the fetus is born with partial passive immunity. Even in monkeys, milk immunoglobulins play a critical role in newborn immunoprotection. Colostrum is provided for the initial 2–3 days of lactation, after which milk composition becomes largely stable.

Milk synthesis increases during breastfeeding and peaks shortly after parturition. The synthetic rate decreases after peak secretion, which usually occurs around weaning. It is important to note that the neonate's growth is closely linked to the dam's milk production. Instances of agalactia (inability to produce milk) or mastitis (mammary gland inflammation) can sometimes lead to failure to thrive in neonates (Davis 2017). It is noteworthy that in certain breeds of sheep and goats, the reproductive goal is to produce triplets and quadruplets. However, this objective contradicts the anatomical breastfeeding capacity limitations of the dam, as both species only have two teats. Consequently, the newborn's nutrition may be compromised due to insufficient milk supply to meet their requirements.

12.4.6 The Neuroendocrine System During Lactation and Mammary Gland Development

The neuroendocrine system's role in regulating the mammary gland's structure and function, spanning from development to milk release, has been well established. The neurological system primarily initiates the milk evacuation mechanism, while the endocrine system mainly synchronizes mammary development and function with the animal's reproductive stage. The hypothalamic–pituitary axis serves as the link between these two systems. The interplay of various substances such as prolactin, oxytocin, growth hormone, and others, alongside the coordination of hormone-releasing organs like the ovaries, placenta, mammary gland, etc., enables these closely interconnected organs to govern the entire process of milk production (Klein 2013).

12.4.7 Reproductive Hormones

The development of the mammary gland is regulated by a variety of hormones. Estrogens, progesterone, prolactin, PL, glucocorticoids, growth hormone, and insulin play a role in the mammogenesis of various species (Cowie et al. 2011). After administration of estrogen to prepubertal sheep over a brief period, the mammary epithelium's DNA synthesis capacity was enhanced (Ellis et al. 1998). Conversely, for goats during a similar prepubertal period, ovarian activity appears to be essential for mammary development (Dessauge et al. 2009). Ovariectomy negatively impacted prepubertal mammary development, epithelial cell proliferation, and gene expression in goats.

Placental lactogen bears structural resemblance to both prolactin and growth hormone, depending on the species (Tucker 2000). Pituitary removal has been linked to extensive mammary growth in ewes and goats (Forsyth 1986). The relationship between milk production and the number of offspring, along with the increase in plasma PL levels during gestation and before parturition in sheep, indicates that the placenta plays a role in mammogenesis (Forsyth 1986).

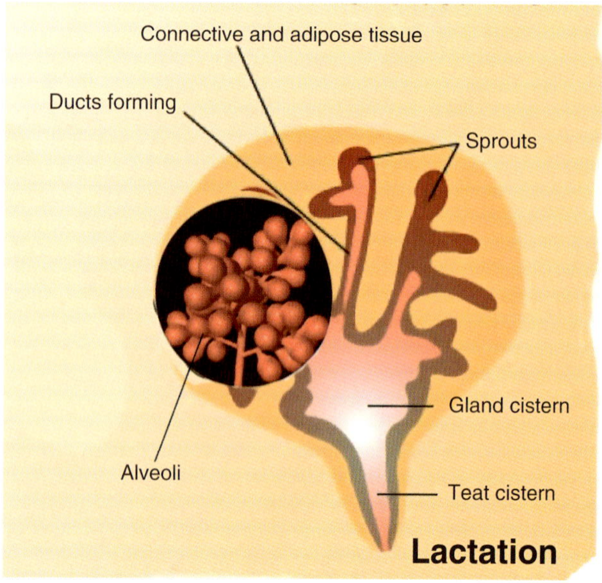

Figure 12.3 Cistern of doe.

Prolactin has been shown to function as a promoter of mammary epithelial cell differentiation in sheep and goats when prolactin is scarce (Forsyth 1986). Prolactin levels increase during the last trimester of pregnancy, coinciding with the start of lactogenesis stage I in healthy pregnancies (Hayden et al. 1979). Prolactin, produced in response to milking stimulation, is a significant mammogenic hormone and contributes to mammary tissue proliferation during lactation. According to Flint and Knight (1997), prolactin is as vital as growth hormone in maintaining goat milk supply.

Estrogen, progesterone, and endogenous prolactin are necessary for tubule-alveolar development completion (Schams et al. 1984). Oxytocin is traditionally associated with milk release from the mammary gland. In goats, most milk is stored in large cisterns, which can be emptied by suction on the teat (Figure 12.3). Some goats produce ample milk but have low plasma oxytocin levels after milking, suggesting reduced oxytocin dependence for milk removal (Marnet and McKusick 2001).

Metabolic hormones like growth hormone, thyroid hormone, glucocorticoids, and insulin are involved in milk secretion and may influence the mammary response to reproductive hormones, indirectly affecting milk synthesis and release (Neville et al. 2002). Growth hormone administration stimulated parenchymal growth in prepubertal and pubertal sheep lambs (Johnsson et al. 1986). Bovine somatotropin (bST), a growth hormone used in dairy herds, has been associated with maintaining cell numbers in lactating goat mammary glands (Knight et al. 1990). Exogenous growth hormone had minimal effect on goat mammary cell proliferation during early lactation (Sejrsen et al. 1999) but it was linked to increased secretory tissue in midlactation (Knight et al. 1990). The mammary hormones include growth hormone, leptin, prolactin, and parathyroid hormone-related peptide (PTHrP). The mammary gland is considered an endocrine organ that secretes hormones with potential local or systemic roles in mammary biology (Neville et al. 2002).

12.4.7.1 Nervous Systems

Milk ejection is a functional neuroendocrine process involving sensory neurons in the teat or nipple, the release of oxytocin from the neurohypophysis, and the contraction of myoepithelial cells lining alveoli and portions of ducts (Tsingotjidou and Papadopoulos 2008). This ejection phase rapidly moves milk from alveoli and smaller ducts into the mammary gland's larger ducts and cisterns. Myoepithelial cells, which surround each alveolus in a mesh-like pattern, are spindle-shaped contractile cells similar in structure to smooth muscle cells. "Milk letdown" is a common term for milk ejection. Efficient and timely milk evacuation is essential for both neonatal milk extraction and preventing pressure atrophy in milk harvesting. Milk secretion capacity generally increases with milk removal frequency and decreases pressure atrophy (Marnet and McKusick 2001).

The principal sensory stimulus for milk ejection is tactile stimulation of the teat. The sounds of the newborn, visual cues of the infant, or the presence of a milking facility can also trigger the release of oxytocin from the neurohypophysis (Laboussiere et al. 1978). Afferent nerve fibers synapse with oxytocin-producing neurons in the paraventricular and supraoptic nuclei, leading to oxytocin release. Once sufficient stimulation frequency is achieved, neurons in these nuclei start firing and release oxytocin from their terminals in the neurohypophysis. Oxytocin is subsequently released into the bloodstream and the dam's circulation (Linzell 1963). Figure 12.4 illustrates the physiology of milk ejection.

12.5 Involution of Mammary Gland

Dairy cows achieve their highest milk production when they are pregnant for approximately 70% of each lactation cycle. A nonlactating phase is necessary between lactations to ensure sufficient milk supply for the next cycle (Roche 2003). As the need for milk as the sole source of sustenance diminishes, newborns suckle less frequently, leading to an increase

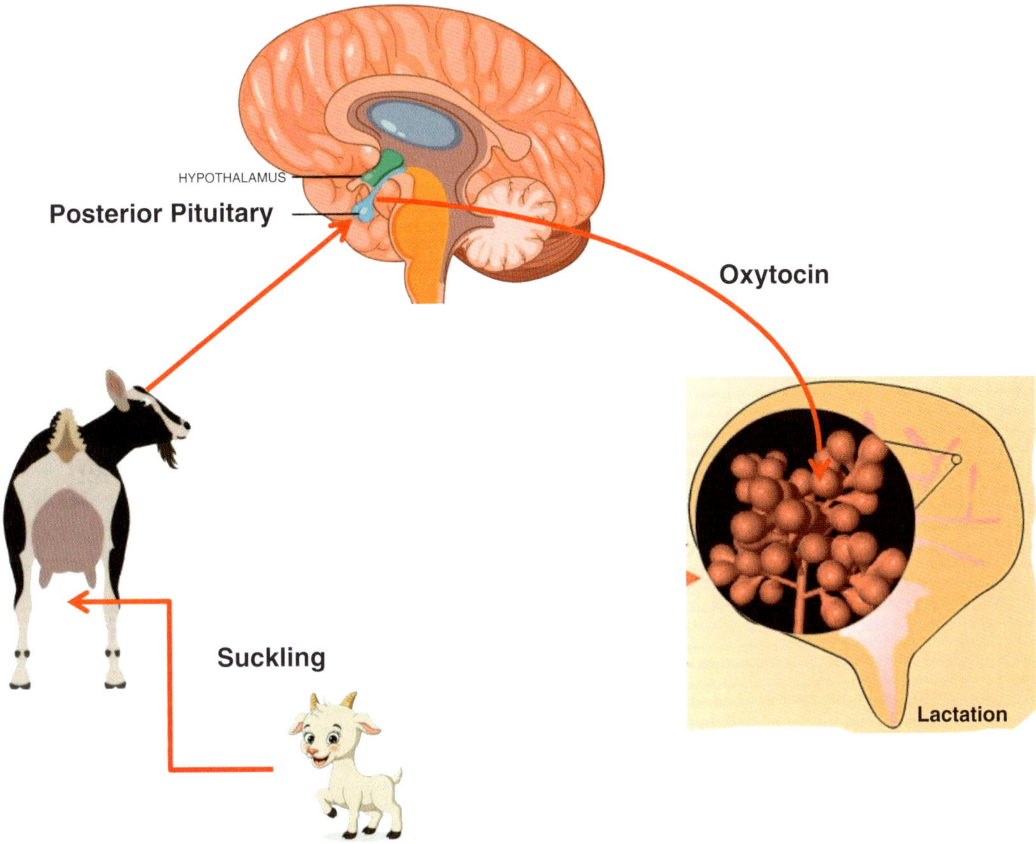

Figure 12.4 Physiology of milk ejection in goat.

in pressure within the mammary gland. This rise in pressure causes the secretory cells to become progressively less active, a phenomenon known as pressure atrophy. Rapidly escalating intramammary pressure, if not controlled, can halt milk synthesis within a few days, with the alveolar epithelium's milk-producing capacity diminishing to near-complete atrophy (Wiseman and Werb 2002).

To enhance milk production profitability, management strategies have been developed that emphasize the importance of a controlled involution phase between successive lactations (Zhao et al. 2019). Evaluating tissue morphological changes and specific cell types is crucial for assessing the extent of mammary involution following milk production cessation. The morphological shifts more accurately reflect changes in the secretory state of the mammary gland, particularly evident during the dry period in dairy cows (De Vries et al. 2011).

The resumption of secretory cell activity occurs only after another pregnancy. Prolactin, adrenal cortical hormones, and PL once again stimulate alveolar cells to produce milk for the subsequent lactation cycle during a subsequent pregnancy. During involution, immune cells such as lymphocytes and macrophages infiltrate mammary tissue. Mammary involution is a pivotal process, allowing the gland to recover and generate new secretory tissue for the upcoming lactation cycle (Akers 1985).

12.6 Lactation Curve

Lactation curves serve as valuable tools for management decisions and selection in the dairy industry. Predicting total milk supply can be accomplished using lactation curve data from a single test day (Wood 1974) or a series of test days early in lactation (Goodall and Sprevak 1985). Armed with this information, dairy farmers can better manage their herds during the early lactation phase based on individual production (Doyle 1983; Auernhammer et al. 1987).

The knowledge of genetic influences on the lactation curve empowers dairy producers to confidently select animals aligned with their specific production goals. Opting for persistent does offers several advantages, including stable year-round milk availability in seasonal milk-producing goats, which is economically significant. Reduced stress stemming from negative energy balance in early lactation can lead to fewer metabolic and reproductive issues. Maintaining a consistent diet and increasing roughage intake could lower doe feeding costs (Sölkner and Fuchs 1987).

A few studies have employed mathematical functions to model lactation curves. Among these, the multiphasic function provides valuable insights into scale (starting and peak yields) and shape (time of peak yield and persistency) of the lactation curve. Traits like breed, parity, kidding season, and production level influence these aspects and affect both the scale and shape of the curve. Breed also affects the scale and shape. Further exploration is needed regarding the use of the multiphasic function as a lactation curve model for dairy goats. Enhanced genetic and physiological studies are necessary to comprehensively understand the biological characteristics of lactation curve stages in dairy goats and determine their applicability in management and selection. Such understanding aids farmers in making informed selection and management choices by enabling them to compare each doe's milk output to a "standard" curve.

12.7 Heat Stress

Dairy goats experience heat stress (HS), which notably elevates rectal temperature and respiration rate, particularly in the initial days. This HS also exerts a detrimental influence on milk production and milk constituents. Animals subjected to HS are more vulnerable to diseases, implying potential compromise to their immune system. About half of the decline in milk yield can be attributed to reduced dry matter intake, even though the productive and physiological responses of dairy animals to HS are well documented (Rhoads et al. 2009). The other half of the milk yield losses could stem from augmented maintenance requirements, suppressed growth hormone secretion (Mitra et al. 1972), reduced udder blood flow (Lough et al. 1990), downregulation of milk protein genes, and upregulation of apoptosis genes in the mammary gland (Collier et al. 2006). The adverse impact of HS during high temperature-humidity index (THI) conditions extends beyond diminished milk supply to encompass a decline in milk quality, reproductive issues, escalated healthcare costs, compromised immune function, and even animal mortality, thereby diminishing dairy farm profits.

Despite extensive research on dairy cows, limited knowledge exists regarding the repercussions of HS in dairy goats. Due to their greater metabolism and enhanced water-conserving capabilities compared to cows, goats are believed to endure higher THI values better (Silanikove 2000). Studies on East African goats (Maloiy and Taylor 1971) and domestic Swedish goats (Olsson et al. 1995) have shown that their respiration rate increases from 30 to over 200 breaths/min as environmental temperatures climb from 20 to 40 °C. This suggests that respiration-driven water evaporation plays a significant role in heat dissipation in goats. Lactating Saanen goats subjected to moderate or severe HS for four days (THI = 81 or 89) experienced a 3% or 13% reduction in milk output, according to Sano et al. (1985). Brown et al. (1988) found that dairy goats exposed to moderate HS conditions for five weeks (34 °C and 25% humidity; THI = 79) exhibited decreased milk output in Alpine goats but not Nubian goats, highlighting breed-specific HS responses. Moreover, warmer and more humid conditions favor disease vector survival, heightening disease exposure risk in animals.

The link between HS and dairy animals' susceptibility to infectious and noninfectious diseases further complicates the scenario. HS has been observed to lead to instances of lameness in lactating dairy cows during summer (Cook et al. 2007). Summer also witnesses an upswing in intramammary infections in sheep and dairy cattle, resulting in substantial economic losses (Sevi and Caropresse 2012). Thompson et al. (2014) found that HS during the dry period had an adverse effect on the immune response of cows challenged with *Staphylococcus aureus* later in lactation; noncooled cows showed lower neutrophil counts and milk somatic cell counts (SCC) compared to cooled cows. Love (2015) reported that the increase in SCC in response to an lipopolysaccharide challenge in dairy goat milk took four hours, as opposed to the two hours observed in thermal neutral (TN) conditions, with SCC in TN conditions recovering more swiftly.

Interestingly, the late lactation milk output of HS-exposed goats was akin to that of goats raised under TN conditions, despite reported feed intake reduction. While the milk fat level in HS goats remained unchanged, the protein content decreased. Nitrogen retention in goats under TN conditions was similar to that in goats under HS, suggesting that the consumed nitrogen might have been utilized for metabolic processes beyond milk protein production.

12.8 Dry Period for Cell Proliferation

The intermission between lactation cycles is a vital consideration for goat farmers, especially when determining the optimal initiation of a new lactation cycle without jeopardizing the animal's well-being (Carnicella et al. 2008). Typically, a dry period of around 50 days is recommended to allow the mammary gland to recover and facilitate gland tissue renewal.

While this dry period is crucial for dairy cows, its necessity for goats appears less evident. Reasons such as the replenishment of bodily reserves, regeneration of mammary tissue, and optimizing benefits from endocrine events near parturition have been proposed to justify the dry period's requirement. In cows or glands subjected to continuous milking, milk production diminishes despite consistent mammary DNA and cell counts (Zahradeen et al. 2009). Endocrine hormones and nutritional status do not appear to contribute to the reduction in milk supply in continuously milked glands. Studies on continuous lactation suggest that reduced functioning of the mammary parenchyma is the primary factor responsible for low milk production. The influence of bST supplementation, which enhances lactation persistence and milk production, has not been adequately considered alongside current milk production levels. Continuous milking has been shown to decrease milk production in subsequent lactations (Capuco et al. 2001).

In goats, it seems that after delivery, there is a simultaneous occurrence of new cell proliferation and old cell involution, resulting in even higher milk yields in goats that either lack a dry period or have a shorter one. Research on Murciano-Granadinas goats revealed that the absence of a dry period led to reduced milk production (1.73 l/d), whereas goats with dry periods of 27 and 56 days produced 2.68 and 2.53 l/d of milk respectively. In this context, a shortened dry period did not affect milk yield and even facilitated quicker production initiation for the herd (Caja et al. 2006). Consequently, it is essential to determine the optimal dry period for each goat breed, considering its unique characteristics and the specific management requirements of goat farming.

12.9 Conclusion

Lactation in goats encompasses diverse facets, capturing the attention of goat farmers, dairy producers, and consumers alike. This intricate process involves the production and secretion of milk by mammary glands that undergo dynamic transformations during pregnancy, lactation, and involution.

Goat milk's unique composition sets it apart from other species, with varying levels of fat, protein, lactose, minerals, vitamins, and enzymes. Notably, goat milk boasts higher concentrations of short- and medium-chain fatty acids, potentially conferring human health benefits, along with lower levels of allergenic alpha-s1 casein. Colostrum, the initial milk postpartum, is a repository of immunoglobulins, primarily IgG, furnishing passive immunity to newborn ruminants. Its bioactive components, including growth factors, cytokines, and antimicrobial peptides, bolster neonatal gastrointestinal tract development and organ function.

Lactation curves chart milk production shifts over time, shaped by factors including breed, parity, nutrition, and environment, divided into peak, persistence, decline, and dry periods. HS emerges as a substantial challenge for dairy goats, impacting milk quantity and quality by disrupting feed intake, blood flow, and synthesis. A well-structured dry period, the interval between lactations, facilitates mammary gland rejuvenation, reproductive performance, and overall health. Further research into optimal dry periods and lactation curve stages is necessary, aiming to enhance production, management practices, and animal well-being for goat farmers.

References

20th Livestock Census. All India Report. Department of Animal Husbandry and Dairying, Government of India. (2019). https://dahd.nic.in/sites/default/filess/Key%20Results%2BAnnexure%2018.10.2019.pdf (accessed 28 January 2024).

Akers, R.M. (1985). Lactogenic hormones: binding sites, mammary growth, secretory cell differentiation, and milk biosynthesis in ruminants. *Journal of Dairy Science* 68 (2): 501–519.

Akers, R.M. and Cleale, R.M. (1990). Effect of somatotropin during the dry period on subsequent milk production and induced secretion of somatotropin, prolactin and insulin pre and postpartum. *Journal of Dairy Science* 73 (Suppl. 1): 154.

Alexandre, G. and Mandonnet, N. (2005). Goat meat production in harsh environments. *Small Ruminant Research* 60: 53–66.

Alichanidis, E. and Polychroniadou, A. (1996). Special features of dairy products from ewe and goat milk from the physicochemical and organoleptic point of view. Proceedings of the IDF/Greek National Committee of IDF/CIRVAL Seminar.

Argüello, A., Castro, N., Capote, J. et al. (2004). Effect of colostrum administration practices on serum IgG in goat kid. *Livestock Production Science* 90: 235–239.

Auernhammer, H.G., Wendl, G. and Harkow, S. (1987). Lactation curves for performance oriented ratio calculation of dairy cows. Proceedings of the III Symposium on Automation in Dairying, Wageningen, The Netherlands.

Awadeh, F.T., Abdelrahman, M.M., Kincaid, R.L., and Finley, J.W. (1998). Effect of selenium supplements on the distribution of selenium among serum proteins in cattle. *Journal of Dairy Science* 81: 1089–1094.

Barrington, G.M., Besser, T.E., Gay, C.C. et al. (1999). Regulation of the immunoglobulin G1 receptor: effect of prolactin on in vivo expression of the bovine mammary immunoglobulin G1 receptor. *Journal of Endocrinology* 163: 25–31.

Barza, H., Marinescu, M., and Blaga, L. (1993). Disorders of foals 0–10 days of age. Part I. *Revista Romana de Medicina Veterinaria* 3: 9–20.

Biswas, S.K., Banerjee, S., Baker, G.W. et al. (2022). The mammary gland: basic structure and molecular signaling during development. *International Journal of Molecular Sciences* 23 (7): 3883.

Blum, J.W. and Hammon, H. (2000). Colostrum effects on the gastrointestinal tract, and on nutritional, endocrine and metabolic parameters in neonatal calves. *Livestock Production Science* 66: 151–159.

Bramhell, F.W.R. (1970). The transmission of passive immunity from mother to young. In: *Frontiers of Biology*, vol. 18 (ed. A. Neuberger and E.L. Tatum), 201–210. Amsterdam: North Holland.

Brandon, M.R., Watson, D.L., and Lascelles, A.K. (1971). Mechanism of transfer of immunoglobulin into mammary secretion of cows. *Australian Journal of Experimental Biology and Medical Science* 49: 613–623.

Brown, D.L., Morrison, S.R., and Bradford, G.E. (1988). Effects of ambient temperature on milk production of Nubian and Alpine goats. *Journal of Dairy Science* 71: 2486–2490.

Bruinje, T. and Ambrose, D. (2019). Technical note: Validation of an automated in-line milk progesterone analysis system to diagnose pregnancy in dairy cattle. *Journal of Dairy Science* 1: 102.

Buskirk, D.D., Faulkner, D.B., Hurley, W.L. et al. (1997). Growth, reproductive performance, mammary development, and milk production of beef heifers as influenced by prepubertal dietary energy and administration of bovine somatotropin. *Journal of Animal Science* 74: 2649–2662.

Butler, J.E. (1974). Immunoglobulins of the mammary secretions. In: *Lactation: A Comprehensive Treatise*, vol. 111 (ed. B.L. Larson and V.R. Smith), 217–243. New York: Academic Press.

Caja, G., Salama, A.A.K., and Such, X. (2006). Omitting the dry-off period negatively affects colostrum and milk yield in dairy goats. *Journal of Dairy Science* 89: 4220–4228.

Capuco, A.V., Wood, D.L., Baldwin, R. et al. (2001). Mammary cell number, proliferation, and apoptosis during a bovine lactation: relation to milk production and effect of bST. *Journal of Dairy Science* 84: 2177–2187.

Carnicella, D., Dario, M., Ayres, M.C.C. et al. (2008). The effect of diet, parity, year and number of kids on milk yield and milk composition in Maltese goat. *Small Ruminant Research* 77: 71–74.

Castro, N., Capote, J., Álvares, S., and Argüello, A. (2005). Effects of lyophilized colostrum and different colostrum feeding regimens on passive transfer of immunoglobulin G in Majorera goat kids. *Journal of Dairy Science* 88: 3650–3654.

Castro, N., Capote, J., Martin, D., and Arguello, A. (2006). The influence of dietary conjugated linoleic acid on blood serum and colostrum immunoglobulin G concentration in female goats before and after parturition. *Journal of Animal Physiology and Animal Nutrition* 90: 429–431.

Castro, N., Capote, J., Morales-delanuez, A. et al. (2009). Effects of newborn characteristics and length of colostrum feeding period on passive immune transfer in goat kids. *Journal of Dairy Science* 92: 1616–1619.

Castro, N., Capote, J., Batista, M. et al. (2011). Management effects on colostrogenesis in small ruminants: a review. *Journal of Applied Animal Research* 39: 85–93.

Chandan, R.C., Attaie, R. and Shahani, K.M. (1992). Nutritional aspects of goat milk and its products. *Proceedings of the V International Conference on Goats II*, New Delhi, India.

Ciupercescu, D.D. (1977). Dynamics of serum immunoglobulin concentrations in sheep during pregnancy and lactation. *Research in Veterinary Science* 22: 23–27.

Collier, R.J., Stiening, C.M., Pollard, B.C. et al. (2006). Use of gene expression microarrays for evaluating environmental stress tolerance at the cellular level in cattle. *Journal of Animal Science* 84 (E. Suppl): E1–E13.

Coni, E., Bocca, B., and Caroli, S. (1999). Minor and trace element content of two typical Italian sheep dairy products. *Journal of Dairy Research* 66 (4): 589–598.

Cook, N.B., Mentink, R.L., Bennett, T.B., and Burgi, K. (2007). The effect of heat stress and lameness on time budgets of lactating dairy cows. *Journal of Dairy Science* 90: 1674–1682.

Cowie, A.T., Forsyth, I.A., and Hart, I.C. (2011). *Hormonal Control of Lactation*. London: Springer.

Csapo, J., Csapo-Kiss, Z., Martin, T.G. et al. (1994). Composition of colostrum from goats, ewes and cows producing twins. *International Dairy Journal* 4: 445–458.

Davis, S.R. (2017). Triennial lactation symposium/bolfa: mammary growth during pregnancy and lactation and its relationship with milk yield. *Journal of Animal Science* 95 (12): 5675–5688.

Davis, T.A., Nguyen, H.V., Garcia-Bravo, R. et al. (1994). Amino acid composition of human milk is not unique. *Journal of Nutrition* 124: 1126.

De Vries, L.D., Casey, T., Dover, H. et al. (2011). Effects of transforming growth factor-β on mammary remodeling during the dry period of dairy cows. *Journal of Dairy Science* 94 (12): 6036–6046.

Dessauge, F., Finot, I., Wiart, S. et al. (2009). Effects of ovariectomy in prepubertal goats. *Journal of Physiology and Pharmacology* 60: 127–133.

Devendra, C. (2013). Investments on pro-poor development projects on goats: ensuring success for improved livelihoods. *Asian-Australasian Journal of Animal Sciences* 26 (1): 1–18.

Dos-Santos, G.T., Bertolini, D.A., Prado, I.N. et al. (1994). Variabilidade em imunoglobulina G (IgG) no colostro de cabra de primeira ordena e absorção intestinal de IgC pelos cabritos récemnascidos. *Brazilian Archives of Biology and Technology* 37: 8.

Doyle, C.J. (1983). Evaluating feeding strategies for dairy cows: a modelling approach. *Animal Production* 36: 47–57.

Dwyer, C.M. and Morgan, C.A. (2006). Maintenance of body temperature in the neonatal lamb: effects of breed, birth weight, and litter size. *Journal of Animal Science* 84: 1093–1101.

Ellis, S., McFadden, T.B., and Akers, R.M. (1998). Prepubertal ovine mammary development is unaffected by ovariectomy. *Domestic Animal Endocrinology* 15: 217–225.

Favier, J.C. and Dorsainvil, E. (1987). Composition des fromages de chèvre. *Cahiers de Nutrition et de Dietetique XXII* 2: 117–123.

Flint, D.J. and Knight, C.H. (1997). Interactions of prolactin and growth hormone (GH) in the regulation of mammary gland function and epithelial cell survival. *Journal of Mammary Gland Biology and Neoplasia* 2: 41–48.

Forsyth, I.A. (1986). Variation among species in the endocrine control of mammary growth and function: the roles of prolactin, growth hormone, and placental lactogen. *Journal of Dairy Science* 69: 886–903.

Forsyth, I.A. (1997). Prolactin, growth hormone and placental lactogen: a historical perspective. *Journal of Mammary Gland Biology and Neoplasia* 2: 3–6.

García de Jalón, J.A., Delas-Heras, M., Ferrer, L.M., and Sancho, J.F. (1990). Sindrome de la boca mojada en corderos. In: *Medicina Veterinaria 7*. Barcelona, Spain: Pulso Ediciones.

Ginjala, V. and Pakkanen, R. (1998). Determination of transforming growth factor-beta 1 (TGF-beta 1) and insulin-like growth factor (IGF-1) in bovine colostrum samples. *Journal of Immunoassay* 19 (2–3): 195–207.

Goodall, E.A. and Sprevak, D. (1985). A Bayesian estimation of the lactation curve of a dairy cow. *Animal Production* 40: 189–193.

Hadjipanayiotou, M. (1995). Composition of ewe, goat and cow milk and of colostrum of ewes and goats. *Small Ruminant Research* 18: 255–262.

Haenlein, G.F.W. and Caccese, R. (1984). Goat milk versus cow milk. In: *Extension Goat Handbook*, vol. 1984 (ed. G.F.W. Haeinlein), 1–9. Washington, DC: USDA.

Hayden, T.J., Thomas, C.R., and Forsyth, I.A. (1979). Effect of number of young born (litter size) on milk yield of goats: role for placental lactogen. *Journal of Dairy Science* 62: 53–57.

Hemmings, W.A. (1976). Maternofoetal transmission of immunoglobulins. In: *Proceedings of the Symposium on Transmission of Immunoglobulins from Mother to Young*. London: Cambridge University Press.

Hernandez-Castellano, L.E., Almeida, A.M., Castro, N., and Argüello, A. (2014a). The colostrum proteome, ruminant nutrition and immunity: a review. *Current Protein and Peptide Science* 5: 64–74.

Hernández-Castellano, L.E., Almeida, A.M., Ventosa, M. et al. (2014b). The effect of colostrum intake on blood plasma proteome profile in newborn lambs: low abundance proteins. *BMC Veterinary Research* 10: 85.

Holcombe, D.W., Hallford, D.M., and Hoefler, W.C. (1988). Reproductive, hormonal and milk characteristics in ewe lambs treated with ovine growth hormone before breeding. *Theriogenology* 30: 517–528.

Jenness, R. (1980). Composition and characteristics of goat milk: review 1968–1979. *Journal of Animal Science* 63: 1605.

Jensen, R.G., Ferris, A.N., Lammi-Keefe, C.J., and Henderson, R.A. (1990). Lipids of bovine and human milks: a comparison. *Journal of Dairy Science* 73: 223.

Johnsson, I.D. (1984). Nutritional and hormonal influences on prepubertal mammogenesis in sheep and rats. PhD thesis, University of Reading.

Johnsson, I.D., Hart, I.C., Simmonds, A.D., and Morant, S.V. (1985). Pre-pubertal mammogenesis in the sheep. 2. The effects of level of nutrition on plasma concentrations of growth hormone, insulin and prolactin at various ages in female lambs and their relationship with mammary development. *Animal Production* 41: 333–340.

Johnsson, I.D., Hart, K., and Turvey, A. (1986). Pre-pubertal mammogenesis in sheep. The effects of restricted feeding or daily administration of bovine growth hormone and bromocriptine on mammary growth and morphology. *Animal Production* 42: 53–63.

Juarez, M. and Ramos, M. (1986). Physico-chemical characteristics of goat milk as distinct from those of cow milk. *International Dairy Bulletin* 202: 54.

Klein, B. (2013). *Cunningham's Text Book of Veterinary Physiology*, 5e. St Louis, MO: Elsevier.

Knight, C.H., Fowler, P.A., and Wilde, C.J. (1990). Galactopoietic and mammogenic effects of long term treatment with bovine growth hormone and thrice daily milking in goats. *Journal of Endocrinology* 127: 129–138.

Knight, C.H., Brown, J.R., and Sejrsen, K.A. (1994). Comparison of growth hormone-induced mammogenesis in pregnant and lactating goats. *Endocrinology and Metabolism* 1 (Suppl. B): 52.

Laboussiere, J., Combaud, J.F., and Petrequin, P. (1978). Influence respective de la fréquence quotidienne des evacuations mammaires et des stimulations du pis sur l'entretien de la secretion lactée chez la brebis. *Annales de Zootechnie* 27: 127–137.

Lee, C.S., Wooding, F.B., and Kemp, P. (1980). Identification, properties, and differential counts of cell populations using electron microscopy of dry cows secretions, colostrum and milk from normal cows. *Journal of Dairy Research* 47: 39–50.

Lerias, J.R., Hernandez-Castellano, L.E., Suarez-Trujillo, A. et al. (2014). The mammary gland in small ruminants: major morphological and functional events underlying milk production – a review. *Journal of Dairy Research* 81 (3): 304–318.

Linzell, J.L. (1963). Some effects of denervating and transplanting mammary glands. *Quarterly Journal of Experimental Physiology* 48: 34–60.

Linzell, J.L. and Peaker, M. (1971). The permeability of mammary ducts. *Journal of Physiology* 216: 701–716.

Linzell, J.L. and Peaker, M. (1975). The distribution and movements of carbon dioxide, carbonic acid and bicarbonate between blood and milk in the goat. *Journal of Physiology* 244: 771–782.

Logan, E.F. and Pearson, G.R. (1978). Distribution of immunoglobulins in intestine of neonatal calf. *Annales de Recherches Vétérinaires* 9: 319–326.

Lough, D.S., Beede, D.K., and Wilcox, C.J. (1990). Effects of feed intake and thermal stress on mammary blood flow and other physiological measurements in lactating dairy cows. *Journal of Dairy Science* 73: 325–332.

Love, S. (2015). Milk yield, milk composition, and milk metabolomics of dairy goats challenged with mammary LPS under heat stress conditions. MSc thesis, Autonomous University Barcelona.

Macias, H. and Hinck, L. (2012). Mammary gland development. *Wiley Interdisciplinary Reviews: Developmental Biology* 1 (4): 533–557.

Malekinejad, H. and Rezabakhsh, A. (2015). Hormones in dairy foods and their impact on public health – a narrative review article. *Iranian Journal of Public Health* 44 (6): 742–758.

Maloiy, M.O. and Taylor, C.R. (1971). Water requirements of African goats and haired-sheep. *Journal of Agricultural Sciences* 77: 203–208.

Marnet, P.G. and McKusick, B.C. (2001). Regulation of milk ejection and milk ability in small ruminants. *Livestock Production Science* 70: 125–133.

Maunsell, F.P., Morin, D.E., Constable, P.D. et al. (1998). Effects of mastitis on the volume and composition of colostrum produced by Holstein cows. *Journal of Dairy Science* 81: 1291–1299.

McFadden, T.B., Daniel, T.E., and Akers, R.M. (1990). Effects of plane of nutrition, growth hormone and unsaturated fat on mammary growth in prepubertal lambs. *Journal of Animal Science* 68: 3171–3179.

Mellor, D.J. and Stafford, K.J. (2004). Animal welfare implications of neonatal mortality and morbidity in farm animals. *Veterinary Journal* 168: 118–133.

Micusan, V.V. and Borduas, A.G. (1977). Biological properties of goat immunoglobulins G. *Journal of Immunology* 32: 373–381.

Mitra, R.G., Christison, G.I., and Johnson, H.D. (1972). Effect of prolonged thermal exposure on growth hormone (GH) secretion in cattle. *Journal of Animal Science* 34: 776–779.

Moreno-Indias, I., Sánchez-Macías, D., Castro, N. et al. (2012). Chemical composition and immune status of dairy goat colostrum fractions during the first 10 h after partum. *Small Ruminant Research* 103: 220–224.

Neville, M.C., McFadden, T.B., and Forsyth, I. (2002). Hormonal regulation of mammary differentiation and milk secretion. *Journal of Mammary Gland Biology and Neoplasia* 7: 49–66.

Nowak, R., Porter, R.H., Lévy, F. et al. (2000). Role of mother young interactions in the survival of offspring in domestic mammals. *Reviews of Reproduction* 5: 153–163.

Olsson, K., Josater-Hermelin, M., Hossaini-Hilali, J. et al. (1995). Heat stress causes excessive drinking in fed and food deprived pregnant goats. *Comparative Biochemistry and Physiology* 110: 309–317.

Ontsouka, C.E., Bruckmaier, R.M., and Blum, J.W. (2003). Fractionized milk composition during removal of colostrums and mature milk. *Journal of Dairy Science* 86: 2005–2011.

Park, Y.W. (1994). Hypo-allergenic and therapeutic significance of goat milk. *Small Ruminant Research* 14: 151.

Park, Y.W. and Chukwu, H.I. (1989). Trace mineral concentrations in goat milk from French-Alpine and Anglo-Nubian breeds during the first 5 months of lactation. *Journal of Food Composition and Analysis* 2: 161.

Park, Y.W., Juárez, M., Ramos, M., and Haenlein, G.F.W. (2007). Physico-chemical characteristics of goat and sheep milk. *Small Ruminant Research* 68 (1–2): 88–113.

Patton, S. and Jensen, R.G. (1975). Lipid metabolism and membrane functions of the mammary gland. *Progress in the Chemistry of Fats and Other Lipids* 14: 163–277.

Pietrzak-Fiecko, R. and Kamelska-Sadowska, A.M. (2020). The comparison of nutritional value of human milk with other mammals milk. *Nutrients* 12 (5): 1404.

Pirisi, A., Lauret, A., and Dubeuf, J.P. (2007). Basic and incentive payments for goat and sheep milk in relation to quality. *Small Ruminant Research* 68: 167–178.

Purup, S., Sejrsen, K., Foldager, J., and Akers, R.M. (1993). Effect of exogenous bovine growth hormone and ovariectomy on prepubertal mammary growth, serum hormones and acute in vitro proliferative response of mammary explants from Holstein heifers. *Journal of Endocrinology* 139: 19–26.

Remeuf, F. and Lenoir, J. (1986). Relationship between the physico-chemical characteristics of goat's milk and its rennetability. *International Dairy Bull* 202: 68.

Rhoads, M.L., Rhoads, R.P., Van Baale, M.J. et al. (2009). Effects of heat stress and plane of nutrition on lactating Holstein cows: I. Production, metabolism, and aspects of circulating somatotropin. *Journal of Dairy Science* 92: 1986–1997.

Roche, J.R. (2003). Effect of pregnancy on milk production and bodyweight from identical twin study. *Journal of Dairy Science* 86 (3): 777–783.

Rudovsky, A., Locher, L., Zeyner, A. et al. (2008). Measurement of immunoglobulin concentration in goat colostrum. *Small Ruminant Research* 74: 265–269.

Sano, H., Ambo, K., and Tsuda, T. (1985). Blood glucose kinetics in whole body and mammary gland of lactating goats exposed to heat stress. *Journal of Dairy Science* 68: 2557–2564.

Schams, D., Rüsse, I., Schallenberger, E. et al. (1984). The role of steroid hormones, prolactin and placental lactogen on mammary gland development in ewes and heifers. *Journal of Endocrinology* 102: 121–130.

Sejrsen, K., Huber, J.T., and Tucker, H.A. (1983). Influence of amount fed on hormone concentrations and their relationship to mammary growth in heifers. *Journal of Dairy Science* 66: 845–855.

Sejrsen, K., Purup, S., Vestergaard, M. et al. (1999). Growth hormone and mammary development. *Domestic Animal Endocrinology* 17: 117–129.

Sevi, A. and Caroprese, M. (2012). Impact of heat stress on milk production, immunity and udder health in sheep: a critical review. *Small Ruminant Research* 107: 1–7.

Silanikove, N. (2000). The physiological basis of adaptation in goats to harsh environments. *Small Ruminant Research* 35: 181–193.

Sölkner, J. and Fuchs, W. (1987). A comparison of different measures of persistency with special respect to variation of test-day milk yields. *Livestock Production Science* 16: 305–319.

Stelwagen, K., Grieve, D.G., Walton, J.S. et al. (1993). Effect of prepartum bovine somatotropin in primigravid ewes on mammogenesis milk production and hormone concentrations. *Journal of Dairy Science* 76: 992–1001.

Swanson, E.W. (1960). Effect of rapid growth with fattening of dairy heifers on their lactational ability. *Journal of Dairy Science* 43: 377–387.

Thompson, I.M.T., Tao, S., Monteiro, A.P.A. et al. (2014). Effect of cooling during the dry period on immune response after Streptococcus uberis intramammary infection challenge of dairy cows. *Journal of Dairy Science* 97: 7426–7436.

Tsingotjidou, A.S. and Papadopoulos, G.C. (2008). The milk-ejection reflex in the sheep: an anatomical study on the afferent pathway. *Anatomia Histologia and Embryologia* 37: 245–250.

Tucker, H.A. (2000). Hormone, mammary growth, and lactation: a 41-year perspective. *Journal of Dairy Science* 83: 874–884.

Ventrella, D., Forni, M., Bacci, M.L., and Annaert, P. (2019). Non-clinical models to determine drug passage into human breast milk. *Current Pharmaceutical Design* 25 (5): 534–548.

Vetter, A., Argüello, A., Baumrucker, C., and Bruckmaier, R.M. (2013). Short communication: fractional milking distribution of immunoglobulin G and other constituents in colostrum. *Journal of Dairy Science* 96: 5919–5922.

Wallace, C. (1953). Observations on mammary development in calves and lambs. *Journal of Agricultural Science* 43: 413–421.

Wiseman, B.S. and Werb, Z. (2002). Stromal effects on mammary gland development and breast cancer. *Science* 296 (5570): 1046–1049.

Wood, P.D.P. (1974). A note on the estimation of total lactation yield from production on a single day. *Animal Production* 19: 393–396.

Zahradeen, D., Butswat, I.S.R., and Mbap, S.T. (2009). A note on factors influencing milk yield of local goats under semi-intensive system in Sudan savannah ecological zone of Nigeria. *Parity* 1: 442.

Zenebe, T., Ahmed, N., Kabeta, T., and Kebede, G. (2014). Review on medicinal and nutritional values of goat milk. *Academic Journal of Nutrition* 3 (3): 30–39.

Zhao, X., Ponchon, B., Lanctot, S., and Lacasse, P. (2019). Invited review: accelerating mammary gland involution after drying-off in dairy cattle X. *Journal of Dairy Science* 102: 6701–6717.

13

Reproductive Techniques

Felix Uchenna Samuel[1,2] *and Peter Ibrahim Rekwot*[3]

[1] *Faculty of Veterinary Medicine, National Animal Production Research Institute/Ahmadu Bello University, Zaria, Nigeria*
[2] *Department of Food and Animal Science, Alabama A&M University, Normal, USA*
[3] *Faculty of Veterinary Medicine, Ahmadu Bello University, Zaria, Nigeria*

13.1 Introduction

Goats are multiparous or polytocus animals, which play significant economic role by providing meat, leather, and fiber. The global goat population is estimated to be 850 million and the majority are found in developing countries. However, the demand for goat and its products in developed nations is increasing, and in order to meet this demand, the maximization of reproduction is aimed at increasing the reproductive efficiency (conception, fecundity, kidding rate) of goats (Daramola et al. 2021). However, reproductive performance depends on the relationship between genetic and environmental factors. Significant environmental factors include nutrition, ambient temperature, stocking density, age groups, etc. Although goat breeds have an excellent ability to accommodate and adapt to fluctuations in environment, this often involves some degree of reproductive failure (Zarazaga et al. 2005; Simões et al. 2021).

Numerous factors affect a doe's ability to reproduce: length of the breeding season, cyclic activity, fertilization rate, growth, etc. Hence, reproductive efficiency in does is stated in terms of kidding rate, kidding interval, birthweight, or weaning weight, among others (Mustefa et al. 2019). The goat is an excellent candidate for applied reproductive technology because of its overall hardiness, high fecundity, good mothering capacity, and extended breeding season (Simões et al. 2021). Commonly employed techniques include artificial insemination (AI), synchronization, and superovulation or multiple ovulation and embryo transfer (MOET).

13.2 Reproductive System of the Doe

The ovaries (reproductive gland), tubular genital organs (uterus, uterine tubes, vagina, vestibule), and external genital organs (vulva, clitoris, urethra) make up the doe's reproductive system (Smith 2007).

13.2.1 Reproductive Gland: Ovaries

The function of the ovaries includes the production of eggs and secretion of different hormones, depending on the reproductive cycle. The ovaries are paired structures located within the pelvic cavity. Their surface is uneven and ovoid in shape due to the presence of the corpora lutea (sing. corpus luteum) and follicles. Each ovary consists of a superficial epithelium, an albuginea (a dense capsule), a cortical and a medullary zone. The cortex (cortical zone) contains the follicles. The medulla (medullary zone) is vascular. Both follicles and vessels are surrounded by the stroma, the connective tissue framework of the ovary. Each ovary has two ends: a tubal end that is near the uterine tube's infundibulum and a uterine end that is opposite the tubal end and is where the ovary's proper ligament attaches it to the uterus. The mesovarium, a peritoneal fold and the most cranial portion of the wide ligament, suspends each ovary from the roof of the abdominal cavity.

Elements of Reproduction and Reproductive Diseases of Goats, First Edition. Edited by Tanmoy Rana.

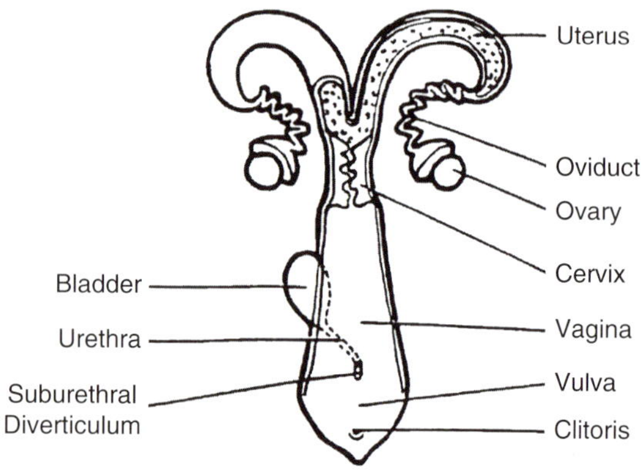

Figure 13.1 Reproductive system of a doe.

A suspensory ligament of the ovary can be identified at the free border of the mesovarium, and is attached to the diaphragm (Figure 13.1).

13.2.2 Tubular Genital Organs

The purpose of the tubular genital organs (uterine tubes, salpinges, sing. salpinx, or fallopian tubes) is to safeguard the spermatozoa while they "swim" toward the ovaries and to direct the ova (sing. ovum) toward the uterine horns once the eggs have been fertilized (Figure 13.1). Between the uterine horns and the ovaries are two extremely tiny, flexible, movable tubes that range in length from 10 to 16 cm called the salpinges. Each uterine tube has an abdominal aperture with an infundibulum, or funnel-shaped end, that is pointed in the direction of the ovary. It is followed by an isthmus, which opens into the corresponding uterine horn, and an ampulla, which is the wide portion and site for fertilization. The uterine horn gradually joins the salpinx in the doe.

A fringe of processes known as fimbriae, some of which are linked to the ovary, is present on the infundibulum. The second mesosalpinx segment of the wide ligament suspends each uterine tube. An area known as the ovarian bursa is bounded by the ovary, mesovarium, and mesosalpinx.

13.2.3 Uterus

The uterus is a unique organ with two symmetrical horns, one body, and the cervix at the neck. Its role is to protect and nourish the embryo or fetus until birth.

The uterine horns are coiled and range in length from 12 to 15 cm each. The intercornual ligament connects the horns before they come into contact with the uterus's body. The uterine velum keeps the horns apart inside the uterus. The mesometrium, which is a component of the wide ligament, is related to the mesometrium border on the horns, which also have free and convex borders.

The uterine body is only 2–3 cm long. It is held in place by the mesometrium, a fold of the peritoneum, and a portion of the broad ligament. Myometrium refers to the uterine musculature as a whole, whereas endometrium refers to the mucosal layer. Caruncles are tiny protrusions present on the endometrium of the uterine horns and body. In four rows, there are more than 100 caruncles. They have a pedunculated shape and a flat or slightly concave surface. The placenta surrounds the caruncles during gestation (pregnancy). Cotyledons are the parts of the placenta that connect the caruncles, and a placentome is the result of the union of the two. The cotyledons release villi, which settle inside the caruncles' spongy surface (Figure 13.1).

The cervix extends for 3–4 cm into the uterus body. The cervical canal is regular. External uterine ostium (orifice) refers to the communication with the vagina, whereas internal uterine ostium (orifice) refers to the communication with the uterus body (orifice). The vaginal fornix, a circular recess surrounding the latter's protrusion into the vagina, is present. There are three to four circular folds on the cervix's endometrium that interdigitate with one another (Figure 13.1).

13.2.4 Vagina

The cervix extends for 3–4 cm into the uterus body. It has three to four circular folds on the cervix's endometrium that interdigitate with one another. The cervical canal has the external uterine orifice which communicates with the vagina, and the internal uterine orifice which communicates with the uterus body. The vaginal fornix, a circular recess surrounding the latter's protrusion into the vagina, is present (Figure 13.1).

13.2.5 External Genital Organs

The perineum, which includes the vulva, is the region ventral to the anus. The pudendal fissure is defined by two labia (sing. labium) and two commissures (dorsal and ventral, the sites where the two labia meet). Labia are delicate, yet thick structures. The ventral commissure is directed downward, while the dorsal commissure is rounded (Figure 13.1b).

The ventral wall of the vestibule contains the clitoris, a primitive homologue of the penis. The mucosa of the vestibule contains two crura and the body of the clitoris. The only thing visible is the glans clitoridis. The clitoris is 2–2.5 cm in length (Figure 13.1).

The female urethra lies within the pelvic floor, covered by the floor of the vagina. It opens by the external urethral ostium on the floor of the vagina, between it and the vestibule. At this level, the suburethral diverticulum, a tiny pouch caudal to the aperture, is connected to the urethra's opening.

13.3 Reproductive Techniques in Goats

Animal production depends greatly on reproduction, and productivity is the secret to economic development. It is well known that one of the most significant reasons for financial losses in the animal industries is reproductive inefficiency. Despite the impressive progress made in reproductive physiology in recent years, infertility caused by a low conception rate and a high embryonic mortality rate continues to be significant (Verma et al. 2012). Modern reproductive biotechnologies and techniques can be used by agricultural research and its applications in order to satisfy future needs and maintain agricultural productivity (Holtz 2005). This drive has necessitated the development of various assisted reproductive techniques to obtain a large number of offspring from genetically superior animals or obtain offspring from infertile (or subfertile) animals, in addition to disease control (Widayati 2012; Mapletoft 2013). Reproductive techniques are intended for widespread use in breeding animal populations to decrease generational gaps and transmit genetic material.

Reproductive methods such as artificial insemination (AI), embryo transfer (ET), manipulation of *in vitro* fertilization (IVF), cloning, and transgenesis have been created over generations to help attain this goal as well as sperm separation techniques, including selection of spermatozoa for chromosomal sex (commonly named sex sorting) (Morrell and Rodriguez-Martinez 2011).

13.3.1 Significance of Reproductive Technologies in Animal Production

The economic benefits that could result from a rise in the number of genetically superior offspring, as well as the need to protect the genetic diversity of infertile or subfertile animals, have been the main forces behind the emergence and development of reproductive technologies. In other words, the development of reproductive technology offered the potential for a wider application of superior germplasm (Zuidema et al. 2021). However, increasing productivity has been met with challenges and also with diseases due to varying environmental conditions.

The introduction and widespread use of modern reproductive technologies have created a variety of new opportunities for research, treatment, and manipulation of the reproductive process both *in vitro* and *in vivo*, with the goal of enhancing reproductive efficiency in a variety of domestic livestocks (Alan et al. 2021). By combining superior genetics into their operations, estrus synchronization and AI can be employed to maximize the reproductive potential in many species of livestock. Many farmers benefit from estrus synchronization timed AI protocols since they cuts down on the time and labor needed for estrus identification and lessen the frequency of animal handling. Additional methods that can increase reproductive effectiveness and pregnancy rates include sexing sperm, synchronization, and fixed-time insemination, superovulation, ET, and *in vitro* embryo creation. If procedures and protocols are correctly followed, reproductive technology can also be utilized to control reproductive illnesses.

The main objectives of using reproductive biotechnologies in livestock are to increase production, reproductive efficiency, and rates of genetic improvement (Singla and Singh 2022).

13.3.2 Synchronization/Induction of Estrus

Estrus synchronization could change the randomness of estrus behavior through the application of exogenous sex hormones or use of pheromonal cues so that estrus occurs within a predetermined time. There are many reports of induction or synchronization of estrus in goats. The male effect, female effect, hormonal methods, administration of melatonin, etc. to induce periods of cyclicity in goats are well documented.

13.3.3 Male Effect (Buck Effect)

The buck effect describes how the presence of a buck induces synchronous estrus activity and ovulation in anovulatory females (Ungerfeld et al. 2004; Landaeta-Hernández et al. 2023). This reaction is widely used to speed up and coordinate goat breeding (Veliz et al. 2002). The buck effect is one of the well-known methods for limiting goat fertility without the controversial use of hormone therapy. Every species has a means of exchanging information, and many of them rely on chemoreceptor organs, which enable the perception of pheromones and act as intermediaries in intraspecies communication related to mating recognition.

The benefits of the male effect include cost savings, avoidance of an unfavorable immune response through the use of chorionic gonadotropin, and a decrease in hormonal residues in treated females, all of which are in accordance with ecological and sustainable production principles in the animal industry.

In the southern United States, managing goats for almost year-round breeding and kidding has mostly relied on the male effect. The majority of the female animals ovulate when a previously isolated (for at least 2–3 weeks) rutting buck is abruptly reintroduced to transitional does. The buck effect causes sensory stimulation as a result of their scent, behaviors, and vocalizations. Genetic selection of female animals born outside the traditional kidding season has resulted in some populations of goats that appear to be in transition during most of the months when they are not exhibiting spontaneous estrous cycles. These populations now use the buck effect more frequently as a result of this.

It is well known that does that are around bucks show greater behavioral signs of estrus. Early in the estrus cycle, sterile service by vasectomized bucks of artificially inseminated does shortens the duration of estrus and increases the likelihood of conception. The duration between the removal of pessaries or the second prostaglandin injection in synchronized does and the onset of estrus is also shortened by the continual presence of bucks at this time after the removal of progestins or after the second injection of prostaglandin (37.6 hours in exposed does versus 48.3 hours in control animals) (Juan et al. 2016).

13.3.4 Female Effect

When a group of synchronized does are kept in close proximity to or together with untreated does during the nonbreeding season, a large proportion of anovulatory does are induced to ovulate. This could make it more difficult to evaluate data from studies where participants were randomly assigned to receive various treatments within the same pens (Romano 2002).

13.3.5 Hormonal Methods for Synchronization of Estrus and Ovulation

The aim of any synchronization program is to group animals so they enter into the same physiological state as simultaneously as possible. In estrus synchronization, the goal is to bring all does on heat at the same time, allowing animals to be heat checked as a group, with individual does bred after they show estrus. This saves time, allowing one to take advantage of AI for breeding. In practice, most estrus synchronization techniques cause a group of does to enter estrus over the period of roughly 48 hours, necessitating morning and evening heat tests before, during, and after this desired time period.

When employing AI, does are bred 12 hours after they are first discovered in estrus according to the AM–PM rule, meaning that if a doe is identified in estrus in the morning, she will be bred that evening, and if in the evening, she will be bred the next morning. Producers have access to a variety of helpful techniques for estrus synchronization in goats during the breeding season. These include progesterone-based or prostaglandin-based protocols as well as combined methods utilizing both progesterone- and prostaglandin-based treatments (Baldassarre and Karatzas 2004).

13.3.5.1 Progesterone-based Synchronization

Treatments using either the synthetic progesterone derivatives, known as progestogens, or the natural hormone progesterone are used in progesterone-based synchronization. A regulated intravaginal drug-releasing device, for instance, contains natural progesterone (CIDR®, Pfizer Inc.) (Figure 13.2). Progestogens include substances such as melengestrol acetate (MGA), altrenogest, and norgestomet. These substances imitate the progesterone-secreting corpus luteum (CL), which is found on the ovary. A doe will not display estrus if she has a CL that is secreting progesterone. The CL also functions to maintain pregnancy, if the doe has been bred successfully.

Whether using the natural hormone or a progestogen, similar physiological responses occur within the animal. However, there are variations among the different progestogens in terms of dosages needed, effectiveness, and price The synchronization process consists of a single CIDR introduced gently into a doe's vagina with the device remaining in place for specified periods until removed. The CIDR causes increased serum levels of progesterone to be released which constitute a physiological block at the hypothalamic level, preventing the doe from coming into estrus until the device is removed. Upon removal of the CIDR, the doe comes into heat about 36–72 hours later and can be bred by AI. The vaginal *in situ* period of CIDRs varies, typically ranging from nine to 21 days. Any does not settled after AI at the first estrus following CIDR removal will remain synchronized for the second estrus three weeks later.

Figure 13.2 CIDR and its applicator.

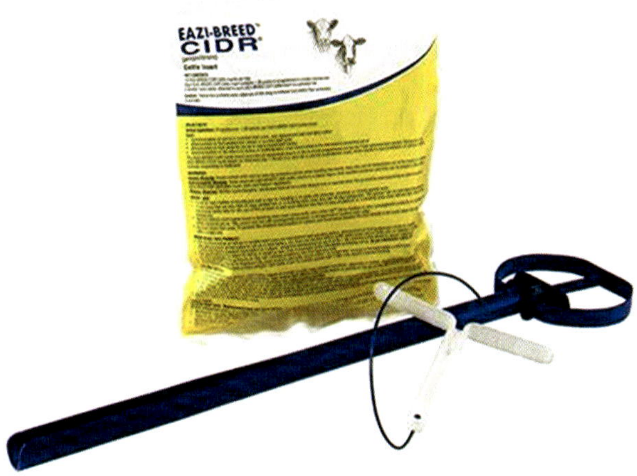

CIDRs can be purchased from commercial animal health and livestock suppliers and do not require a prescription. However, because they are only approved for use in sheep in the United States, their use in goats would be considered extra-label (Wondim et al. 2022).

13.3.5.2 Prostaglandin-based Synchronization

Prostaglandin F2-alpha (PGF) is a naturally occurring hormone that can be used to synchronize estrus. It is effective only if the CL is present on the ovaries. The CL is the ovarian structure responsible for the production of progesterone (Wondim et al. 2022). In a normal estrous cycle, secretion of PGF from the uterus destroys the CL and the doe comes into heat. PGF is sold as the product dinoprost (Lutalyse®, Pfizer, Inc.) (Figure 13.3). To obtain PGF, or any of its synthetic analogues, a prescription is required.

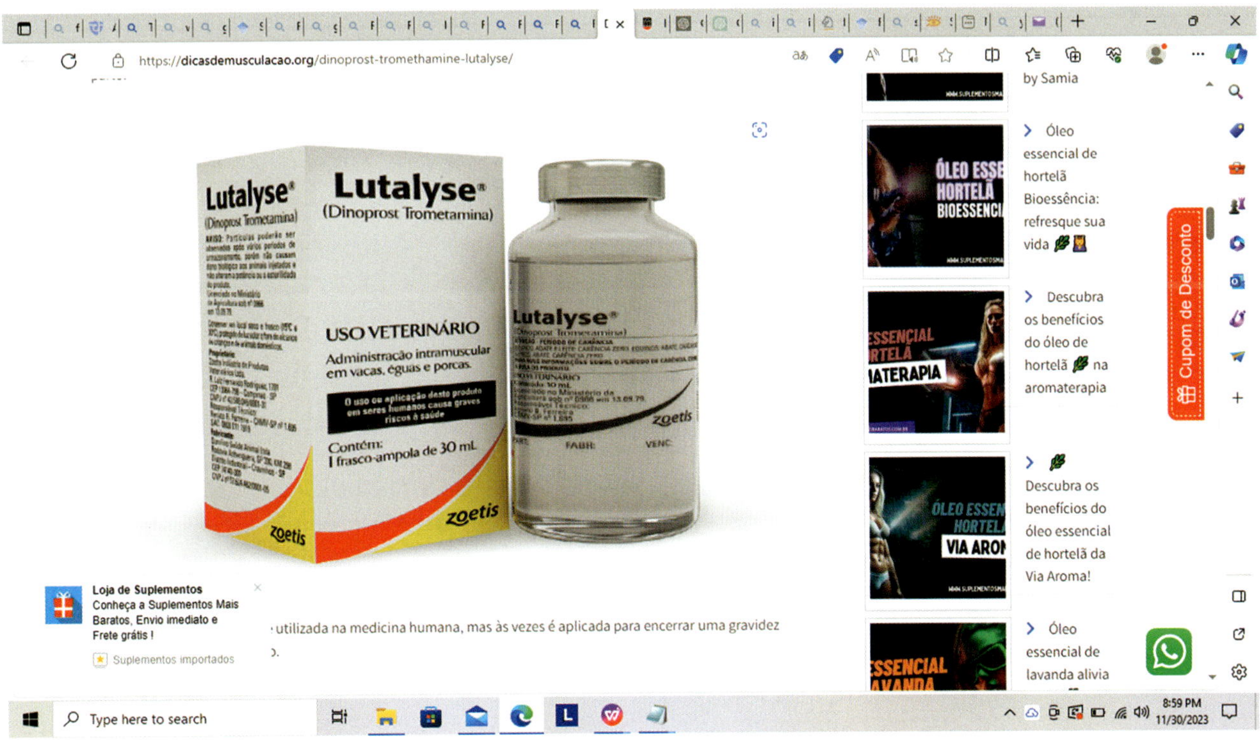

Figure 13.3 Lutalyse®: a dinoprost trimethamine preparation (PGF2-alpha).

Two treatments are normally administered during synchronization with PGF, the first on day 1 and the second on day 10. The dosage of Lutalyse per injection can range from 7.5 to 15 mg. The dosage of 15 mg has been found to produce consistent and reliable results (Bowdridge et al. 2013). However, lower doses can also be effective (Al Yacoub et al. 2011). Does will come into heat after either the first or second PGF injection and can be bred by AI at either time. Animals are often only heat monitored after the second PGF injection in order to better conserve labor. Within 36–96 hours of the second PGF injection, 80–90% of treated does will exhibit estrus When PGF is utilized, there is no loss of fertility at the synchronized estrus.

13.3.5.3 Combined CIDR and PGF Synchronization

A combination of CIDRs and PGF has been found to be effective for estrus synchronization in goats. This protocol can reduce infertility associated with longer term CIDR use, resulting in good synchronization and fertility at the estrus immediately post treatment. A relatively simple combined CIDR-PGF protocol involves a short, six-day CIDR treatment. A CIDR is inserted on day 1 in the morning and six days later is removed (morning or evening on day 6). An injection of PGF must be given at the time of either CIDR insertion or CIDR removal. If PGF is given at the time of CIDR removal, does will come into estrus 36–72 hours later and can be bred by AI based on estrus detection (Wondim et al. 2022).

It is vital to remember that estrus synchronization can also be used in conjunction with natural breeding, even though producers will see the highest genetic improvements when coupling estrus synchronization methods with AI. Producers can take advantage of grouping females for breeding and subsequent kidding periods by using estrus synchronization in this situation, which makes overall reproductive management of the doe herd more predictable (Rege et al. 2022). Based on research in cattle, there are few studies that have assessed buck-to-doe ratios when females have synchronized estrus. It is advised that only adult males be used for this task. A mature buck should be able to handle ratios of 1:15–20 synchronized females with good pregnancy rates (Crilly et al. 2022).

13.3.6 Ovulation Synchronization

Ovulation synchronization is a method that allows producers to synchronize ovulation rather than simply synchronizing estrus. The major advantage of ovulation synchronization is that it does not require heat detection prior to breeding. The method includes ovulation synchronization and breeding by AI at a fixed time during the treatment protocol. This is referred to as "timed AI." Ovulation synchronization further focuses labor requirements to the preselected day of breeding only because heat checking is not used and breeding dates can be precisely scheduled in advance of the breeding season. Pregnancy rates are comparable to those obtained for AI breed-by-estrus protocols (Bowdridge et al. 2013; Holtz et al. 2008; Sohnrey and Holtz 2005).

Ovulation synchronization-TAI protocols have been successfully developed for goats. These utilize several different hormones in sequence to control CL function, stimulate follicular development, and regulate ovulation. Progesterone-free protocols are also available and utilize treatment combinations of PGF and the ovulatory hormone, gonadotropin-releasing hormone (GnRH) or PG600 (Bowdridge et al. 2013; Holtz et al. 2008) (Figure 13.4). Using PG600 or equine chorionic gonadotropin (eCG) to stimulate the ovaries in goats may result in an increase in the number of offspring born. It is not advised to use this hormone on goats repeatedly, either within one breeding season or across breeding seasons. Similar to cattle, goats will produce antibodies against this hormone, usually following two eCG doses. As a result, females will become permanently resistant to the effects of this hormone (Roy et al. 1999; Rehman et al. 2021).

13.3.7 Melatonin

By secreting melatonin, the pineal gland regulates reproductive activity in species that breed seasonally, including sheep, goats, horses, and cats. However, it cannot be utilized to alter seasonal activity in the mare because doing so would require preventing the release of melatonin or neutralizing its effects in order to move the start date forward. It has been employed commercially to hasten the start of the breeding season in ewes and does, who are short-day breeders.

The hormone is injected subcutaneously near the base of the ear and comes in the form of an implant containing 18 mg of melatonin. It is important that bucks be separated from does so that they are out of sight, sound, and smell at least seven days before the insertion of the implant. They must remain separated for at least 30 days and not more than 40 days, when bucks should then be reintroduced. Peak mating activity occurs 25–35 days later. The breeding season can be successfully advanced by two to three months with good fertility (Tölü et al. 2022).

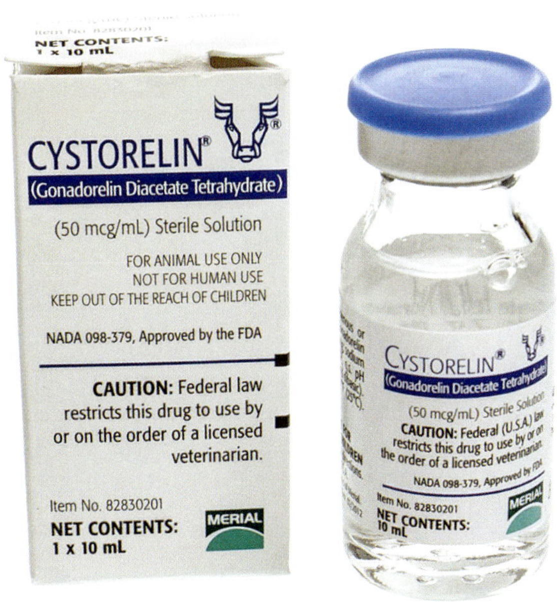

Figure 13.4 GnRH preparation (Cystorelin®).

13.3.8 Artificial Insemination

The process of artificial insemination involves semen collection, evaluation and processing and then the introduction of the semen into the reproductive system of a female on estrus. Laparoscopic insemination and transcervical insemination are the two primary methods of AI utilized in goats (Cseh et al. 2012). Comparing laparoscopic insemination to transcervical insemination, pregnancy rates are often greater. However, because it involves small surgical operations and the administration of anesthesia, laparoscopic insemination necessitates highly qualified inseminators, who are frequently veterinarians or people working under their supervision. In contrast, transcervical insemination methods do not involve anesthesia or surgical intervention and the producer can be trained to use them (Cseh et al. 2012).

13.3.8.1 Laparoscopic Insemination

A small surgical incision is made into the doe's abdominal cavity during laparoscopic insemination, and the semen dose is then directed into each uterine horn. Usually, qualified veterinarians and veterinary assistants who are proficient in the procedure carry it out. Briefly, for laparoscopic insemination, the doe is anesthetized and restrained in dorsal recumbency with her rear quarters elevated above her head. Abdominal incisions are made on either side of the midline and the abdominal cavity inflated with carbon dioxide to enhance visualization of the uterus and ovaries. Insemination is done by laparoscopic identification of the uterine horn and deposition of semen into the uterine lumen using a sterile insemination needle. This technique takes about 5–10 minutes. After deposition of the semen, the incisions are sutured and the doe is returned to a recovery pen where she will recover in about 10 minutes (Abecia et al. 2021).

Laparoscopic insemination has a pregnancy rate of between 60% and 80%, making it a desirable choice for farmers who have a lot of animals that need insemination. In contrast, farmers with fewer animals might find that this solution is not economical. Laparoscopic insemination might become a more appealing option, particularly for smaller producers, when ovulation synchronization and TAI procedures are used since specific insemination dates can be easily prepared (Cseh et al. 2012).

13.3.8.2 Transcervical Insemination

The cervical canal of a doe has four tightly closed, cartilaginous rings that act as structural support to the cervix and, along with cervical mucus, form a protective physical barrier against the entry of foreign particles. For optimum pregnancy rates using transcervical insemination, semen must be deposited intrauterine or into the uterine horns (Gutierrez et al. 2022).

During this insemination technique, all four cervical rings must be traversed in order for semen to be deposited into the uterus. It can be difficult to pass the insemination rod during transcervical artificial insemination due to the small size of the doe's reproductive tract and tightness of the cervical rings as well as their typical lack of alignment, especially for nulliparous or young primiparous does. The protocols outlined for nonsurgical embryo transfer in goats are similar to several of the transcervical insemination techniques that are already available (Cseh et al. 2012).

13.3.8.3 Standard AI Method (Tube Speculum)

The basic transcervical AI technique uses a regular French-style insemination gun and a tube-like speculum. The external cervical os, which serves as the entrance to the cervical channel, is visualized using a speculum with a detachable lamp that is put into the doe's vaginal vault. The 1/4 cc or 1/2 cc straws of frozen sperm must be suitably thawed before usage. A clean sheath is placed on top of the semen straw after it has been prepared and inserted into the insemination gun to safeguard it and prevent cross-contamination between does. Sheaths can have either conventional (rounded) or apex (pointed) ends, which can help to achieve deeper cervix penetration. The insemination gun is passed through the speculum and through the cervix to deposit the semen into the uterine body.

The main benefit of the conventional approach is that it is a straightforward, simple-to-learn procedure that works quite well with older, multiparous does. The main drawback of this method is that it is challenging to slide the insemination gun through a young doe's small cervix or through a cervix that is extremely convoluted. In many cases, use of the standard technique results in deposition of the semen in the cervix if all the cervical rings cannot be passed. Pregnancy rates due to the standard technique are low, typically in the range of 20–30% (Sohnrey and Holtz 2005).

13.3.8.4 Deep Cornual (Uterine) Insemination (Catheter-Within-Catheter) Method

A novel method for transcervical insemination of goats was developed by Sohnrey and Holtz (2005). In their method, semen is introduced deep into the uterine horn (cornua) by means of a catheter-within-catheter technique.

In order to gain entry to the uterine body and uterine horns, this method uses a soft pediatric urine catheter with a small diameter that has been hardened with an insemination gun stylet. The doe's hindquarters are elevated to make it easier to pass through the cervix, and a Pozzi tenaculum forceps is used to hold the cervix and line up the cervical rings. Once the catheter is in the uterine horn, the stylet is withdrawn and fresh or frozen-thawed semen is injected into the top part of the uterine horn using a tiny diameter insemination tube that is threaded through the urine catheter. The urinary catheter is then repositioned into the opposite uterine horn and the second half of the semen sample is deposited deep into that horn to complete the insemination. The entire procedure takes about 5–10 minutes by a skilled technician and does not involve any surgical entry or anesthesia of the doe (Sohnrey and Holtz 2005).

The pregnancy rates of deep cornual insemination are greater than those for laparoscopic insemination (Sohnrey and Holtz 2005). A further study by Holtz et al. (2008) found that ovulation synchronization with TAI of a single dose of frozen semen resulted in pregnancy rates of 58% and kidding rates of 53%. These pregnancy rates are equivalent to those for beef cattle using frozen semen for first-service insemination following TAI (Lamb et al. 2010).

13.3.8.5 NCSU Simplified Catheter-based Method

Work by North Carolina State University (NCSU) resulted in the development of a modified insemination technique (Farin and Knox, unpublished) based on the deep uterine technique reported by Sohnrey and Holtz (2005) and the nonsurgical embryo transfer technique. According to Sohnrey and Holtz (2005), this method depends on the use of the pediatric urinary catheter, insemination gun stylet, and Pozzi tenaculum forceps to pass through the cervix and reach the uterus. According to the NCSU procedure, the catheter tip is inserted into the uterine body and its location is checked using a digital palpator through the vaginal vault or a predefined measurement. Once the pediatric catheter is in place, the stylet is removed, a syringe barrel is attached to the distal end of the catheter, and the semen sample is injected into the uterine body through the catheter itself. The entire procedure takes about 5–8 minutes.

Pregnancy rates following estrus synchronization and AI or ovulation synchronization and TAI using the simplified catheter method for transcervical insemination are comparable to those reported for the deep cornual insemination (catheter-within-catheter) method (Holtz et al. 2008). Furthermore, pregnancy rates are greater for either of the catheter-based methods compared to the standard AI technique (Bowdridge et al. 2013; Holtz et al. 2008; Sohnrey and Holtz 2005).

13.3.9 Embryo Technologies

Embryo transfer is a reproductive technology that involves the exploitation of the genetic potentials of the dams. ET can also be used to quickly reintroduce new breeds or genetic lines into herds that already exist. Effective record keeping and extensive reproductive control are necessary for the successful implementation of ET within a goat herd. Additionally, a thorough evaluation of cost–benefit ratios must be taken into account (Alkan et al. 2021).

As major advances were being made in methods of semen collection, extension, and preservation in goats between the 1970s and 1990s, there was a parallel research effort focused on females that facilitated the commercialization of AI. Due to the fast development of such technologies in dairy cattle, corresponding similar research in dairy goats occurred at almost the same pace. For females, superovulation and ET are seen as methods for rapid multiplication for superior animals. Although recovery and transfer of embryos from females does not match the enormous potential genetic contribution of individual bucks, it does allow production of more kids per female, which is very beneficial to produce more offspring from high-producing does. *In vitro* production of embryos by combining ovum pick-up, IVF, and ET, enabled embryo manipulation techniques to develop. It is now possible to freeze embryos, store them for future use or transport them internationally, which can bypass certain disease situations, initiate production of kids from reproductively immature doelings, and evaluate embryos before transfer (Luo et al. 2019). Dairy goats of all breeds could ovulate 1–3 eggs per estrus cycle, but 10–20 available oocytes can be obtained from these goats after superovulation treatment with appropriate doses of follicle-stimulating hormones (FSHs). The principle of superovulation is to artificially add exogenous gonadotropin so that more follicles have the opportunity to continue development. Finally, these follicles will be able to complete the conversion from FSH dependent to LH dependent, and will establish the status of the dominant follicle.

Pregnant mare serum gonadotropin (PMSG) and FSH are widely used for superovulation in the goat industry. Primary methods for inducing follicle stimulation and oocyte production use PMSG or eCG; because of its long half-life, only a single injection of PMSG was required for inducing superovulation in goats and cows. Due to the 72-hour half-life of PMSG, goat ovaries are prone to display a large number of anovulatory follicles and early degeneration of the corpus luteum after PMSG injection, thus FSH was applied for superovulation of dairy goats. Superovulation with FSH was reported in 1958, and when ET programs changed to porcine FSH, injected twice daily over a period of four days, more consistent superovulatory results were achieved (Luo et al. 2019).

Embryo transfer involves the following procedures: (i) selection and preparation of donors, (ii) collection of embryos, (iii) handling, evaluation, and storage of embryos, (iv) selection and preparation of recipients, and (v) practical embryo transfer.

The basic steps in the ET process are illustrated in Figure 13.5. Donor females with superior genetic quality are superovulated with hormonal treatments that cause multiple ovulation. The donor doe is inseminated with semen from a genetically superior sire and the fertilized embryos undergo developmental changes within the uterus for approximately seven days. Thereafter, the embryos are recovered from the uterus of the donor female by uterine lavage (flushing). The recovered embryos are identified, assessed and 1–3 embryos are transferred into the uterus of a recipient female that is of lower genetic quality and whose reproductive cycle has been carefully synchronized to match the cycle of the donor female. In this technique, embryos are harvested and transferred from the uterus of the original donor into the uterus of a recipient doe at same gestational stage, and which can in turn complete the fetal development to term unaffected. This process can be repeated after 2–3 months, with the superovulation of the original donor female and breeding them again to produce more embryos for transfer.

Because protocols for freezing goat embryos are available, it is also feasible for recovered embryos to be frozen and held for transfer at a later date (Al Yacoub et al. 2011). While all transcervical (nonsurgical) procedures are used for ET in cattle, this is not the case in goats. Instead, laparotomy (abdominal surgery) or, more frequently, a combination of laparoscopy for embryo recovery and laparoscopy for embryo transfer into the recipient female are used (Amiridis and Cseh 2012). Embryo recovery by nonsurgical methods has been documented in goats (Melican and Gavin 2008). However, laparoscopic recovery is still used for the majority of donor flushes in goats. Producers who are considering an ET program for their herd must engage with a vet who is skilled in these procedures in order to have these operations done on the farm.

Effective donor and recipient management is a requirement for a successful ET program. The donor does are estrus synchronized, superovulated, and bred by AI to produce multiple numbers of embryos with desirable genetic potential. Multiple ovulation protocols for goats have been published and involve a combination of CIDR, PGF, or PGF-analogue injection, FSH treatment to induce follicular development, and GnRH treatment to induce ovulation (Menchaca et al. 2010; Rubianes and Menchaca 2003).

Using either laparoscopy or nonsurgical embryo recovery, between 0 and 18 embryos are produced per donor, with about 4–6 on average (Menchaca et al. 2010). It is crucial to remember that superovulation is an uncontrolled process. According to statistics from cattle, approximately 25% of donor cow flushes result in no embryos while the remaining 25% result in an excessive amount of embryos. The producer should therefore anticipate, on average, roughly 4–6 embryos to be created per donor every session when employing ET, and it is frequently advised that at least 3–4 donor females be set up for a particular ET session.

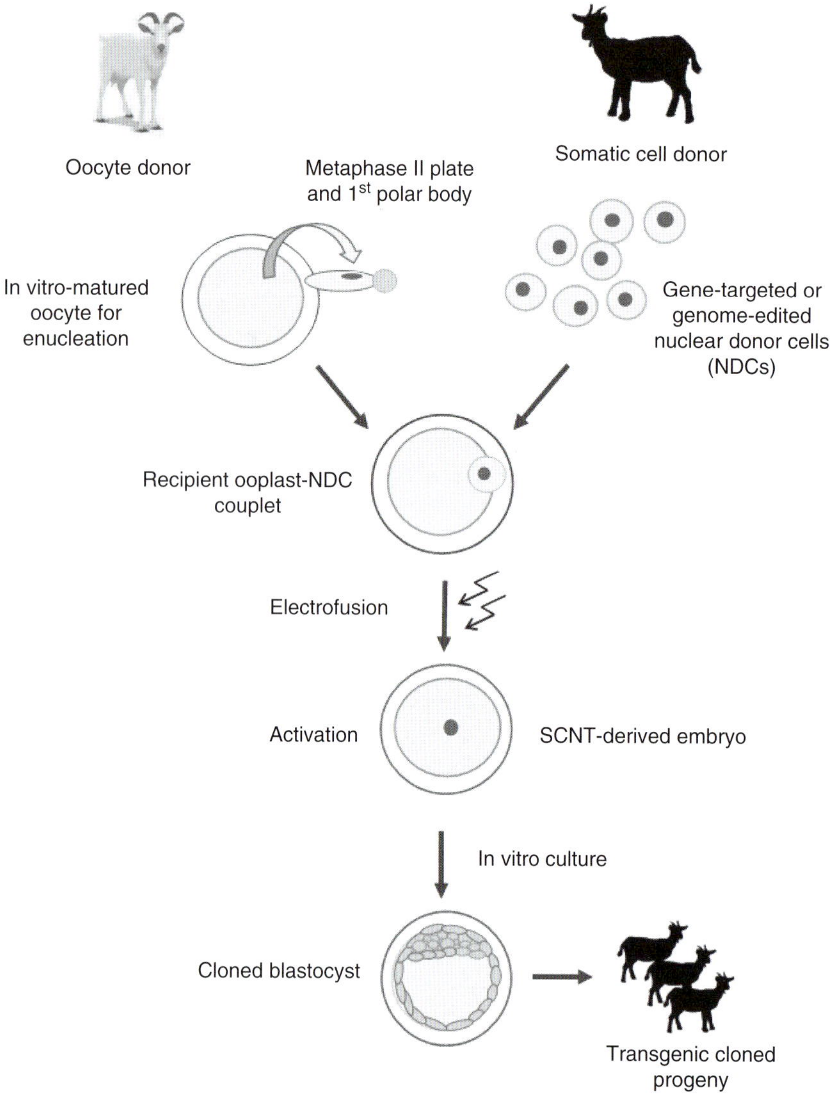

Figure 13.5 Somatic cell nuclear transfer in goats.

In conjunction with donor preparation, recipient females also need to be estrus synchronized so that they are at the same stage of the estrous cycle as the donor does. Heat detection is carried out on the recipient does to establish their estrus period but they must not bred. Recipient cycles can be synchronized by a variety of estrus or ovulation synchronization protocols. According to Shin et al. (2008), 1–3 embryos are transplanted into the recipient female's uterus through a laparoscopic procedure. For each donor doe planned for embryo recovery, a fair rule of thumb for predicting the number of recipient females required for an ET session is to have roughly 3–4 recipients synchronized. Embryos can be frozen and kept for future transfer if extras are created but no additional recipients are available. Additionally, if the producer is able to procure frozen embryos, the recipient does can be synchronized, estrus monitored, and 1–3 embryos can be transferred through laparoscopy into the recipient's uterus.

13.3.10 Cloning

One of the most rapidly developing reproductive biotechnology strategies in farm livestock is cloning by somatic cell nuclear transfer (SCNT). Cloning, often known as "asexual reproduction," is the process of creating a genetically identical individual from donor cells and duplicating genes. It entails the development of an animal or person whose genes come from just one other individual.

Cloning techniques include embryo splitting and nuclear transfer, which involves separating an embryo just as it is maturing after the egg has been fertilized by the sperm but before the embryo is transferred. It is optimally performed at the

6–8-cell stage, where it can be used as an expansion of IVF to increase the number of available embryos. Cloning can be used in conjunction with other assisted reproduction techniques to help conserve native livestock breeds, which have a proven track record of productivity and environmental adaptability and should not be lost from the global gene pool. Additionally, it makes it possible for commercial farmers to quickly achieve superior genotypes from nucleus breeding flocks and herds.

Cloning technology has the potential to spur the growth of the animal biotechnology sector in many nations and give environmentalists a new tool to help with the preservation of seriously endangered wildlife species. However, the inadequate remodeling and reprogramming of the transferred somatic cell nuclei in the cytoplasm of nuclear-transferred oocytes, which results in low pre- and postimplantation developmental potential and poor quality of SCNT-derived embryos, is caused by the abnormal adaptation of the transferred somatic cell nuclei to the biochemical conditions of the oocyte cytoplasmic microenvironment (Yang et al. 2018). The latter also contributes to the very high occurrence of anatomical, histological, and physiopathological abnormalities in cloned fetuses and offspring that are congenital deformities.

Only a few nuclear donor cell (NDC) types have been examined to determine if they can be used to create cloned embryos or fetuses in this livestock species. The ones that have undergone testing are from a variety of tissues taken from both adult animals of both sexes and ages as well as caprine fetuses. Mention should be made of the following NDCs: (i) fetal dermal fibroblasts (transgenic or nontransgenic) *in vitro* grown; (ii) juvenile and adult dermal fibroblasts; (iii) mural granulosa cells isolated from antral ovarian follicles; and (iv) cumulus oophorus cells (Skrzyszowska and Samiec 2021) (Figure 13.5).

13.3.11 Sex Determination of Embryo

The presence or lack of components typically found on the Y chromosome determines the embryo's sexual differentiation. Chromosome analysis of demi-embryos, immunological detection of embryonic H—Y antigen, use of Y-specific probes, fluorescence *in situ* hybridization, rapid sexing method for preimplantation using loop-mediated isothermal amplification (LAMP) reaction, and ultrasound examination of fetal structures are some of the techniques used commercially for the sexing of embryos (Shi et al. 2008). Predicting the sex of offspring increases the amount of males or females produced and aids in the selection of individuals with the best genetic make-up for the benefit of the following generation. Known sex of embryos produced for use in ET programs can more effectively help to manage producer resources. Semen sexing can be used in IVF and AI programs (Hussein and Karam 2022).

13.3.12 Sex Determination of Semen

Semen sexing is the process of separating spermatozoa into two subpopulations containing spermatozoa bearing X-chromosomes and Y-chromosomes. Sexing spermatozoa can be used for directed production of offspring of a desirable sex by modified flow cytometric cell sorting of fluorescent dye-loaded living spermatozoa. Goats have about 3–4% differences in DNA contents between their X- and Y-chromosome-bearing spermatozoa, this molecular weight difference being large enough to allow successful sorting. This technique involves the separation of X- and Y-bearing spermatozoa in small quantities based on the DNA content of the spermatozoa (Hussein and Karam 2022).

Through the use of sperm sexing technology (SST), livestock farmers will be able to predict the gender of their progeny before they are even conceived, increasing production, financial success, and genetic potential. There is a definite preference for one sex over the other in almost every area of commercial animal breeding. The sexed sperm can be used for artificial insemination (AI) or to create *in vivo* and *in vitro* embryos (Garner and Seidel 2008).

13.3.13 Transgenesis

A transgenic animal is one that has had a different gene purposefully put into its genome. Following gene transfer or as a result of molecular modifications of endogenous genomic DNA, transgenic animals have undergone genetic modification to contain a gene from a different species. Similar to how an organism's own genes are passed down to children, the new gene does the same (Seidel 2007).

There are various transgenesis techniques, including DNA microinjection, DNA transfer into gametes, and DNA electroporation. Transgenic farm animals can be employed for biomedical research as well as breeding. Transgenic individuals produced are equipped with disease resistance and improved quantitative and qualitative traits (Rajoriya et al. 2013).

13.3.14 *In vitro* Fertilization

The sperm and egg are fertilized *in vitro* under particular environmental and biochemical conditions. IVF involves the removal of unfertilized eggs (oocytes) from the donor ovaries. The oocytes develop in an incubator and are fertilized by sperm. Before being implanted into the recipient, the resultant zygotes undergo incubation and development in the laboratory (Niemann et al. 2005).

For IVF prior to fertilization, the buck ejaculate needs to be prepared. The most motile and viable spermatozoa from the whole fresh ejaculate or frozen-thawed sperm are selected. Techniques used for selection are swim-up and centrifugation in Percoll® or Ficoll® density gradient. The swim-up technique yielded more motile spermatozoa compared to Ficoll or Percoll density gradient centrifugation, but no differences were observed in terms of oocyte penetration and cleavage rate after IVF with fresh goat semen (Cowan and Becker 2010). For frozen-thawed goat semen, conventionally, motile spermatozoa are obtained by centrifugation on a discontinuous Percoll gradient.

Once the most viable and motile spermatozoa are selected, sperm capacitation is carried out in media supplemented with heat-inactivated estrus serum (20% with fresh semen, 2% with frozen-thawed semen). Capacitation of frozen-thawed sperm can also be achieved using 10% (v/v) estrus sheep serum in SOF medium and 0.5 g/ml of heparin for one hour (Cowan and Becker 2010). For fresh sperm capacitation, selected by swim-up, the supernatant is recovered and capacitated in mDM with 50 g/ml heparin for 45 minutes. After oocyte maturation and sperm capacitation, oocytes are transferred to microdrops of modified Tyrode's medium (TALP) (Cognié et al. 2003), supplemented with hypotaurine and glutathione. Different fertilization media have been used by different authors: BO (Kątska-Książkiewicz et al. 2004), SOF (Ongeri et al. 2001), and TALP-fert medium (Cognié et al. 2003).

References

Abecia, J.A., Cannas, A., Delgadillo, J.A. et al. (2021). Review: managing sheep and goats for sustainable high yield production. *Animal* 15 (1): 100293.

Al Yacoub, A.N., Gauly, M., Sohnrey, B., and Holtz, W. (2011). Fixed-time deep uterine insemination in PGF2alpha-synchronized goats. *Theriogenology* 76: 1730–1735.

Alan, D., Crowe, P., Lonergan, S., and Butler, T. (2021). Invited review: use of assisted reproduction techniques to accelerate genetic gain and increase value of beef production in dairy herds. *Journal of Dairy Science* 104 (12): 12189–12206.

Alkan, K.K., Alkan, H., Kaymaz, M., and Izgur, I.H. (2021). Multiple ovulation and embryo transfer during the breeding season in angora goats: a comparison of fresh and vitrified-thawed embryo transfer. *Veterinary Research Forum* 12 (2): 143–148.

Amiridis, G.S. and Cseh, S. (2012). Assisted reproductive technologies in the reproductive management of small ruminants. *Animal Reproduction Science* 130: 152–161.

Baldassarre, H. and Karatzas, C.N. (2004). Advanced assisted reproduction technologies (ART) in goats. *Animal Reproduction Science* 82–83: 255–266.

Bowdridge, E.C., Knox, W.B., Whisnant, C.S., and Farin, C.E. (2013). NCSynch: a novel, progestagen-free protocol for ovulation synchronization and timed artificial insemination in goats. *Small Ruminant Research* 110: 42–45.

Cognié, Y., Baril, G., Poulin, N., and Mermillod, P. (2003). Current status of embryo technologies in sheep and goat. *Theriogenology* 59 (1): 171–188.

Cowan, T. and Becker, G.S. (2010). Biotechnology in Animal Agriculture: Status and Current Issues. Congressional Research Service. https://nationalaglawcenter.org/wp-content/uploads/assets/crs/RL33334.pdf (accessed 2 January 2024).

Crilly, J.P., Wood, M., and Reilly, B. (2022). Such a tease! Production and uses of teaser rams, bucks, boars and bulls. *Clinical Practice* 44 (4): 228–238.

Cseh, S., Faigl, V., and Amiridis, G.S. (2012). Semen processing and artificial insemination in health management of small ruminants. *Animal Reproduction Science* 130: 187–192.

Daramola, J.O., Abioja, M.O., Iyasere, O.S. et al. (2021). The resilience of dwarf goats to environmental stress: a review. *Small Ruminant Research* 205: 106534.

Garner, D. and Seidel, J.G. (2008, 2008). History of commercializing sexed semen for cattle. *Theriogenology* 69 (7): 886–895.

Gutierrez, V.A., Sánchez-Dávila, F., Ledezma-Torres, R.A. et al. (2022). The use of oxytocin to cause cervical dilation for transcervical insemination in nulliparous goats: improving pregnancy and kidding rates. *Reproduction in Domestic Animals* 57 (8): 886–892.

Holtz, W. (2005). Recent developments in assisted reproduction in goats. *Small Ruminant Research* 60 (1–2): 95–110.
Holtz, W., Sohnrey, B., Gerland, M., and Driancourt, M.A. (2008). Ovsynch synchronization and fixed-time insemination in goats. *Theriogenology* 69: 785–792.
Hussein, S.A. and Karam, K.M. (2022). Early determination of fetal sex in goat: a comparison between real time PCR and ultrasonography. *IOP Conference Series: Earth and Environmental Science* 951: 012059.
Juan, E., Romano, A.A., Victor, O.F., and Amstalden, M. (2016). Continuous presence of male on estrus onset, estrus duration, and ovulation in estrus-synchronized Boer goats. *Theriogenology* 85 (7): 1323–1327.
Kątska-Książkiewicz, L., Ryńska, B., Gajda, B., and Smorąg, Z. (2004). Effect of donor stimulation, frozen semen and heparin treatment on the efficiency of in vitro embryo production in goats. *Theriogenology* 62 (3–4): 576–586.
Lamb, G.C., Dahlen, C.R., Larson, J.E. et al. (2010). Control of the estrous cycle to improve fertility for fixed-time artificial insemination in beef cattle: a review. *Journal of Animal Science* 88: 181–192.
Landaeta-Hernández, A.,.J., Rodolfo, U., and Peter, J.C. (2023). Biostimulation and pheromones in livestock: a review. *Animal Reproduction Science* 248 (2023): 107154.
Luo, J., Wang, W., and Sun, S. (2019). Research advances in reproduction for dairy goats. *Asian-Australasian Journal of Animal Sciences* 32 (8): 1284–1295.
Mapletoft, R. (2013). History and perspectives on bovine embryo transfer. *Animal Reproduction* 10 (3): 168–173.
Melican, D. and Gavin, W. (2008). Repeat superovulation, non-surgical embryo recovery, and surgical embryo transfer in transgenic dairy goats. *Theriogenology* 69: 197–203.
Menchaca, A., Vilarino, M., Crispo, M. et al. (2010). New approaches to superovulation and embryo transfer in small ruminants. *Reproduction, Fertility, and Development* 22: 113–118.
Morrell, J. and Rodriguez-Martinez, H. (2011). Practical applications of sperm selection techniques as a tool for improving reproductive efficiency. *Veterinary Medicine International* 1–9.
Mustefa, A., Banerjee, S., Gizaw, S. et al. (2019). Reproduction and survival analysis of Boer and their crosses with Central Highland goats in Ethiopia. *Livestock Research for Rural Development* 31: 166.
Niemann, H., Kues, W., and Carnwath, J. (2005). Transgenic farm animals: present and future. *Revue Scientifique et Technique* 24 (1): 285–298.
Ongeri, E.M., Bormann, C.L., Butler, R.E. et al. (2001). Development of goat embryos after in vitro fertilization and parthenogenetic activation by different methods. *Theriogenology* 55 (9): 1933–1945.
Rajoriya, R., Rajoriya, S., and Kumar, N. (2013). Transgenic animals: prospects for improving livestock productivity. *Journal of Bio Innovation* 2 (5): 240–259.
Rege, J.E.O., Ochieng, J.W., and Sones, K. (2022). The state of applications and impacts of biotechnology in the livestock sector. In: *Agricultural Biotechnology in Sub-Saharan Africa* (ed. J.E.O. Rege and K. Sones). Cham: Springer.
Rehman, A., Ahmad, E., Sattar, A. et al. (2021). Long term effects of immunization against inhibin on fresh and post-thawed semen quality and sperm kinematics during low and peak breeding seasons in Beetal bucks. *Small Ruminant Research* 201: 106442.
Romano, J.E. (2002). Does in proestrus-estrus hasten estrus onset in does estrous synchronized during breeding season. *Applied Animal Behaviour Science* 77 (4): 329–334.
Roy, F., Combes, B., Vaiman, D. et al. (1999). Humoral immune response to equine chorionic gonadotropin in ewes: association with major histocompatibility complex and interference with subsequent fertility. *Biology of Reproduction* 61: 209–218.
Rubianes, E. and Menchaca, A. (2003). The pattern and manipulation of ovarian follicular growth in goats. *Animal Reproduction Science* 78: 271–287.
Seidel, J.G. (2007). Overview of sexing sperm. *Theriogenology* 68 (3): 443–446.
Shi, L., Yue, W., Ren, Y. et al. (2008). Sex determination in goat by amplification of the HMG box using duplex PCR. *Animal Reproduction Science* 105 (3–4): 398–403.
Shin, S.T., Jang, S.K., Yang, H.S. et al. (2008). Laparoscopy vs laparotomy for embryo transfer to produce transgenic goats (Capra hircus). *Journal of Veterinary Science* 9: 103–107.
Simões, J., Abecia, J.A., Cannas, A. et al. (2021). Review: managing sheep and goats for sustainable high yield production. *Animal* 15 (1): 100293.
Singla, S.K. and Singh, B. (2022). Multiple ovulation and embryo transfer in livestock production. In: *Frontier Technologies in Bovine Reproduction* (ed. A. Kumaresan and A.K. Srivastava). Singapore: Springer.
Skrzyszowska, M. and Samiec, M. (2021). Generation of monogenetic cattle by different techniques of embryonic cell and somatic cell cloning – their application to biotechnological, agricultural, nutritional, biomedical and transgenic research. A review. *Annals of Animal Science* 21: 1–15.

Smith, M.C. (2007). Clinical reproductive physiology and endocrinology of does. In: *Current Therapy in Large AnimalTheriogenology*, 2e (ed. R.S. Youngquist and W.R. Threlfall), 535–537. Philadelphia: WB Saunders.

Sohnrey, B. and Holtz, W. (2005). Technical note: transcervical deep cornual insemination of goats. *Journal of Animal Science* 83: 1543–1548.

Tölü, C., Yazgan, N., Işıl, H. et al. (2022). Effects of melatonin implants on reproductive performance of dairy sheep and dairy goats. *Reproduction in Domestic Animals* 57 (6): 665–672.

Ungerfeld, R., Forsberg, M., and Rubianes, E. (2004). Overview of the response of anoestrous ewes to the male effect. *Reproduction, Fertility and Development* 16: 479–490.

Veliz, F.G., Moreno, S., Duarte, G. et al. (2002). Male effect in seasonally anovulatory lactating goats depends on the presence of sexually active bucks, but not estrous females. *Animal Reproduction Science* 72: 197–207.

Verma, O.P., Kumar, R., Kumar, A., and Chand, S. (2012). Assisted reproductive techniques in farm animals – from artificial insemination to nanobiotechnology. *Veterinary World* 5 (5): 301–310.

Widayati, D.T. (2012). Embryo transfer as an assisted reproductive technology in farm animals. *World Academy of Science, Engineering and Technology* 6: 10–21.

Wondim, B., Taye, M., Alemayehu, K. et al. (2022). The efficiency of estrus synchronization protocols and artificial insemination in the Abergelle goat on-station and on-farm conditions of northern Ethiopia. *Journal of Applied Animal Research* 50 (1): 518–525.

Yang, M., Perisse, I., Fan, Z. et al. (2018). Increased pregnancy losses following serial somatic cell nuclear transfer in goats. *Reproduction, Fertility, and Development* 30: 1443–1453.

Zarazaga, L.A., Guzmán, J.L., Domínguez, C. et al. (2005). Effect of plane of nutrition on seasonality of reproduction in Spanish Payoya goats. *Animal Reproduction Science* 87 (3–4): 253–267.

Zuidema, D., Kerns, K., and Sutovsky, P. (2021). An exploration of current and perspective semen analysis and sperm selection for livestock artificial insemination. *Animals* 11 (12): 3563.

14

Reproductive Failure in Does

Felix Uchenna Samuel[1,2], *Pauline Chiezey Ngozi*[1], *Adeniyi Njideka*[3], *Kolawole Jonathan Bamidele*[4], *and Hycinth Ndabatsado Kolo*[5]

[1] *National Animal Production Research Institute/Faculty of Veterinary Medicine, Ahmadu Bello University, Zaria, Nigeria*
[2] *Department of Food and Animal Science, Alabama A&M University, Normal, USA*
[3] *Department of Biological Sciences, Alabama A&M University, Normal, USA*
[4] *Faculty of Veterinary Medicine, Ahmadu Bello University, Zaria, Nigeria*
[5] *Department of Animal Health and Production, Federal University of Technology, Minna, Nigeria*

14.1 Introduction

Domestication has led to the transformation of the reproductive processes of farm animals from a free-grazing, seasonal mating system to an intensive production, year-round mating system. As a result, the reproductive efficiency of farm animals has declined due to environmental factors and the demands of economic production. These factors may result in partial or complete reproductive failure. Sterility is a permanent factor preventing procreation, and infertility or temporary sterility is the inability to produce viable young within a stipulated time characteristic for each species. Reproductive problems caused by nutritional deficiencies and infectious diseases and other environmental stresses are discussed in this chapter.

14.2 Ovarian Dysfunction

The ovary performs two main functions: the production of ova and secretion of ovarian hormones. These functions are intimately related and directed toward successful reproduction. In this section, the discussion will focus on abnormalities of estrus, ovary, and the uterus.

14.2.1 Anestrus

Anestrus denotes a state of complete sexual inactivity with no manifestations of estrus (Figure 14.1). It is not a disease but a sign of a variety of conditions. Although anestrus is observed during certain physiological states, e.g,. before puberty, during pregnancy, and lactation, and in seasonal breeders, it is most often a sign of temporary or permanent depression of ovarian activity (true anestrus) caused by seasonal changes in the physical environment, nutritional deficiencies, lactation stress, and aging (Figure 14.2). Certain pathological conditions of the ovaries or the uterus also suppress estrus.

14.2.2 Ovarian Abnormalities

Ovarian abnormalities that cause anestrus are of two types.

Ovarian hypoplasia (failure of the ovaries to develop): affected animals have underdeveloped reproductive tracts and never exhibit estrus. Ovarian hypoplasia tends to be associated with white coat color, being inherited as an autosomal recessive. Some mares with small inactive ovaries have an abnormal sex chromosome complement (e.g., XO) as well as low plasma estrogen and high LH levels. Freemartins, which are heifers born twinned with bulls, have poorly developed ovaries and fail to show estrus.

Elements of Reproduction and Reproductive Diseases of Goats, First Edition. Edited by Tanmoy Rana.

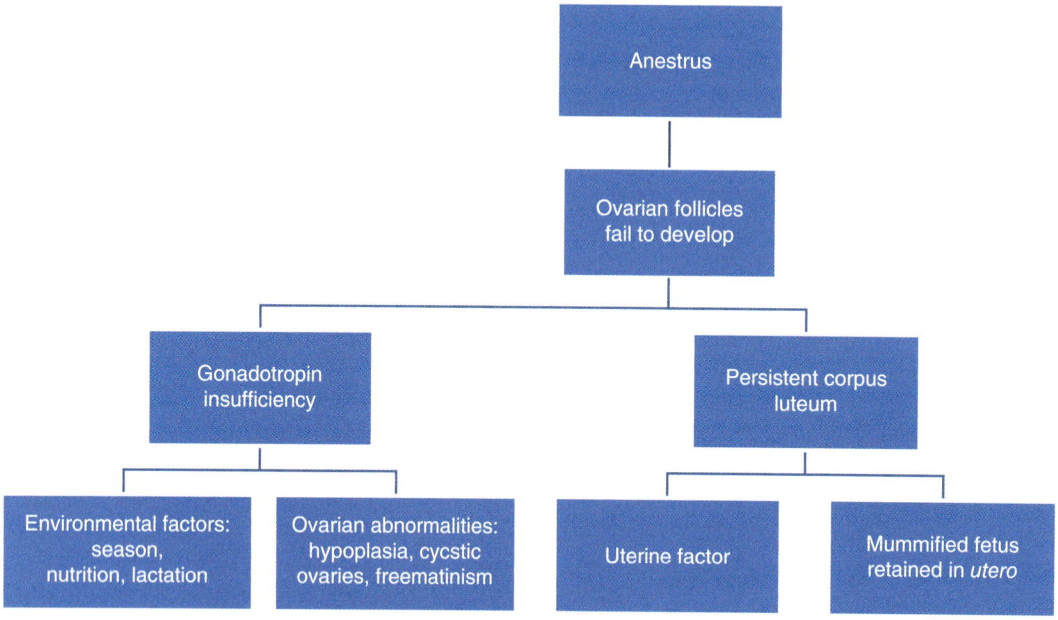

Figure 14.1 Anestrus during the natural breeding season. Persistence of the CL may be attributed to a failure of PGF2-alpha release.

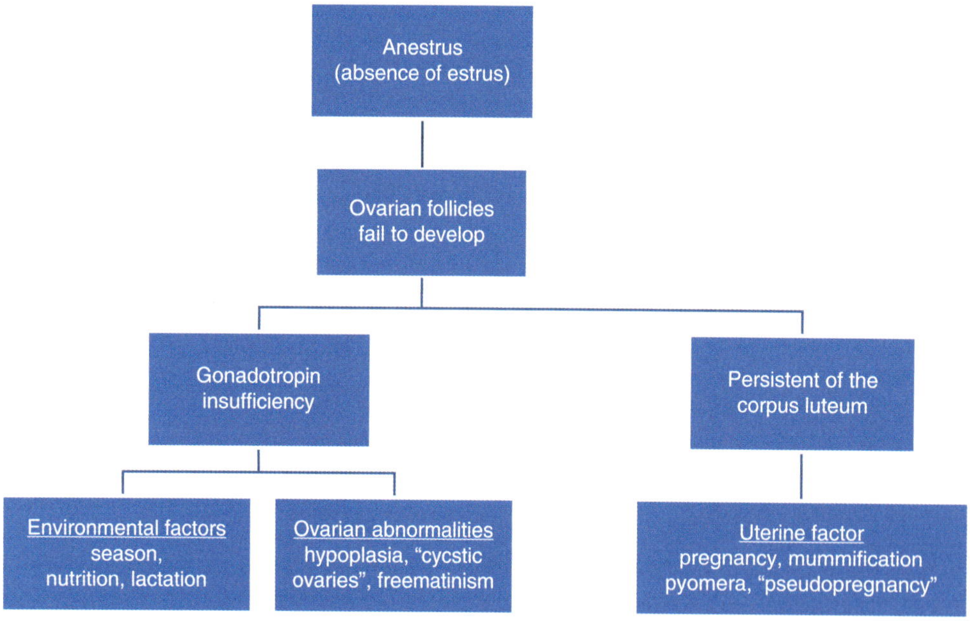

Figure 14.2 Possible causes leading to a failure of follicle development in the ovary and anestrus in farm animals. Note that pregnancy is an important cause for an absence of estrus.

Persistence of the CL associated with uterine pathology: conditions include pyometra, mucometra, fetal mummification, or maceration in cattle, goats, sheep, and pigs and pseudo-pregnancy in the mare, sow, and doe. Functional corpora lutea and a uterus containing either endometrial gland secretions or remnants of embryonic or fetal tissue characterize pseudo-pregnancy in the pig. Injections of estrogens (embryonic luteotropin) toward the end of the luteal phase of the estrous cycle also induce pseudo-pregnancy in the sow. Pseudo-pregnancy (hydrometra) in the doe is the accumulation of uterine fluid associated with persistence of the CL. The abdomen of the doe enlarges as in pregnancy, but udder development and kidding fail to occur. The term cloudburst is used when spontaneous discharge of a cloudy uterine fluid occurs around the expected time of parturition. Progesterone levels are elevated, making it difficult to differentiate this state from pregnancy; it can easily be diagnosed by real-time ultrasonography by the lack of placentomes in the fluid-filled uterus. The factors causing pseudo-pregnancy in the goat have not been established, but prolactin plays an important luteotropic role.

Both PGF2-alpha and repeated oxytocin treatments result in a decline in progesterone levels, estrous behavior, and the discharge of intrauterine fluid.

Prolonged diestrus results from spontaneous prolongation of the life of the cyclic CL beyond the normal 14–15 days. It is a major cause of anestrus during the natural breeding season. Persistence of the CL may be attributed to a failure of PGF2-alpha release.

14.2.3 Ovulatory Failure

Ovulatory failure may be due to failure of the follicle to ovulate during a normal cycle or to cystic ovaries.

Anovulatory estrus is more common in swine and horses than in cattle, goats, and sheep. The animal shows normal behavioral estrus and the ovarian follicle reaches preovulatory size but does not rupture. Anovulatory follicles become partly luteinized and then regress during the estrous cycle, as does a normal CL.

Cystic ovarian disease or "cystic ovaries" is common in dairy cattle and swine but has also been reported in goats. It is rarely encountered in beef cattle or other species. The disease is a common endocrine abnormality particularly among high milk-producing animals. Most ovarian cysts probably develop prior to the first ovulation post partum since more ovarian cysts are detected in cows examined at 30 days post partum than after breeding or after abnormal estrous behavior. Although some affected animals may exhibit intense mounting behavior (nymphomania), the majority fail to exhibit estrus (anestrus). One or both ovaries contain one or more large cysts exceeding 2.5 cm diameter. These are either follicular or luteal cysts. Follicular cysts undergo cyclic changes, i.e., they alternately grow and regress but fail to ovulate. Luteal cysts contain a thin rim of luteal tissue, also fail to ovulate, but persist for a prolonged period.

In the past, the differentiation of cyst type was based on rectal palpation, which was highly subjective. However, with the advent of transrectal ultrasonography, the accuracy of differentiation has been markedly improved. The available evidence indicates that luteal cysts may be caused by a failure in the LH release mechanism. This failure is not due to a deficiency or release of GnRH but more to an insensitivity of the hypothalamic–pituitary axis to elevated levels of estradiol.

The development of cystic ovaries has been related to high milk production, seasonal changes, hereditary predisposition, and pituitary dysfunction (Figure 14.3).

The cause and effect relationship between milk production and cystic ovarian disease is not clear, but high milk yield may be a response to hormonal changes in animals with ovarian cysts rather than the cause of the disease.

Development of cystic ovaries has been related to postpartum uterine infections. Endotoxins produced by microorganisms in the uterus may trigger PGF2-alpha release, which in turn stimulates the secretion of cortisol. The elevated cortisol levels suppress the preovulatory release of LH and lead to the development of cysts.

A relationship exists between cystic ovarian disease and heredity as the incidence has steadily declined in several herds after culling bulls whose daughters had cystic ovarian disease.

Cystic ovaries are also frequently encountered in dairy cows, does and sows fed higher levels of nutrients, and during the winter.

Several methods are available for the treatment of cystic ovarian disease.

- Manual rupture of the cyst by rectal palpation in cattle and laparoscopy in small ruminants.
- hCG and GnRH are equally effective for the treatment of follicular cysts, but GnRH, being of lower molecular weight, is less likely to stimulate antibody formation.
- Prostaglandin Fza or its analogues are effective for treatment of luteal cysts.
- Progesterone injections or progesterone intravaginal devices may also restore ovarian cycles in cows with ovarian cysts.

Cystic ovaries in swine are an important cause of reproductive failure and a major reason for culling, particularly older sows. Large multiple luteinized follicles are more common than small

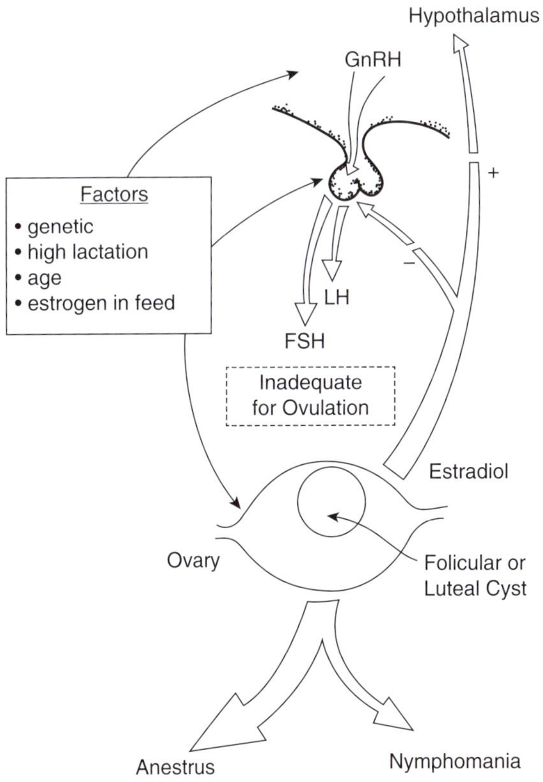

Figure 14.3 Hormonal patterns, types of ovarian cysts, and behavioral manifestation.

multiple cysts, and they contain progesterone. Estrous cycles that are irregular with prolonged periods between cycles may be mistaken for pregnancy. Signs of estrus are pronounced but nymphomania does not occur.

14.3 Disorders of Fertilization

Disorders of fertilization include failure of fertilization and atypical fertilization.

14.3.1 Fertilization Failure

Fertilization failure may result from death of the egg before sperm entry, structural and functional abnormality in the egg or sperm, physical barriers in the female genital tract preventing gamete transport to the site of fertilization, or ovulatory failure (Figure 14.4).

14.3.1.1 Abnormal Eggs

Several types of morphological and functional abnormalities have been observed in unfertilized eggs, including giant egg, oval-shaped egg, lentil-shaped egg, and ruptured zona pellucida. Failure to undergo fertilization and normal embryonic development may be due to inherent abnormalities of the egg or to environmental factors. For example, fertilization is lower in animals exposed to elevated ambient temperature prior to breeding. In sheep and goats, some conception failures at the beginning of the breeding season are associated with a high incidence of abnormal ova.

14.3.1.2 Abnormal Sperm

The physiological significance of abnormal sperm in relation to fertilization failure has been documented. Certain forms of male infertility are related to structural defects of the DNA protein complex. Sperm aging and injury may cause:

- alterations in the acrosomal cap, which may prevent defective spermatozoa from fertilizing the egg. In bulls, rams, and boars, a good correlation exists between fertility and acrosomal integrity
- leakage of vital intracellular constituents such as cyclic AMP or the formation of lipid peroxides from sperm plasmalogen when sperm are stored under anaerobic conditions
- a gradual decrease in the fertilizing capacity of aging spermatozoa in the female genital tract.

14.3.1.3 Structural Barriers to Fertilization

Congenital or acquired defects of the female genital tract interfere with transport of the sperm and/or the ovum to the site of fertilization.

Congenital defects are the result of arrested development of the different segments of the müllerian ducts (oviduct, uterus, and cervix) or an incomplete fusion of these ducts caudally. A classic congenital anomaly associated with the gene for white coat color is "white heifer disease" in cattle, in which the prenatal development of the müllerian ducts is arrested and the vaginal canal is obstructed by an abnormally developed hymen. It can be differentiated from the freemartin syndrome by the presence of normal ovaries, vulva, and labia.

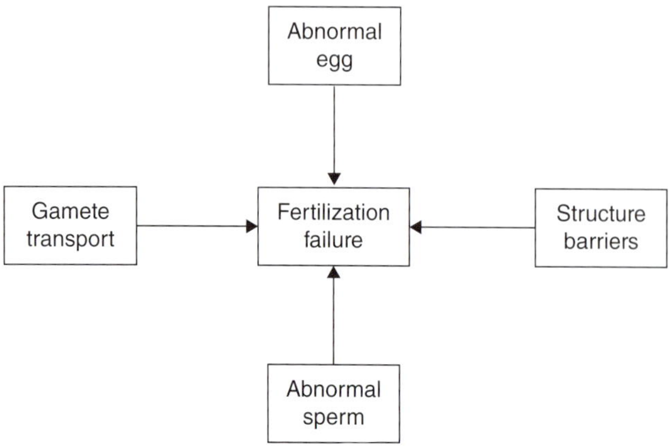

Figure 14.4 Causes of fertilization failure.

Common anatomical abnormalities include adhesions of the infundibulum to the ovary or uterine horns; this interferes with the pick-up of the egg or causes a mechanical obstruction of one part of the reproductive duct system. Bilateral or unilateral missing segments of the reproductive tract also cause anatomical sterility.

14.3.1.4 Phytoestrogens

Reproductive failure occurs more in sheep than in cattle grazing on plants that contain compounds with estrogenic activity, e.g., subterranean clover (*Trifolium subterraneum*) and red clover (*Trifolium pratense*). The estrogenic activity is due to plant isoflavones and related substances with hydroxyl groups. Cows, does, and ewes fed estrogenic forage may suffer impaired ovarian function, often accompanied by reduced conception rates and increased embryonic loss. In cows, clinical signs resemble those associated with cystic ovaries. The infertility is temporary, normally resolving within one month after cessation of the estrogenic feed. Ewes grazed on pastures containing estrogenic plants around the time of mating shed fewer ova and have a reduced chance of conception. Fertility is improved within three weeks after the animals are moved into nonestrogenic pastures.

The pathological changes in temporary infertility are due to the action of estrogens on the hypophyseal ovarian axis and on sperm transport. Small ruminants grazed for several seasons on estrogenic pastures mate and ovulate, but fertilization rate is depressed due to failure of sperm transport caused by severe changes occurring in the cervix.

14.3.2 Atypical Fertilization

Atypical fertilization may occur spontaneously as a result of aging of the gametes described below.

Aging of the egg is gradual, during which various functions are successively lost. An early effect of egg aging is that the resulting embryo is not viable and is resorbed before birth. Further aging leads to abnormalities in fertilization, particularly involving the pronuclei. The biophysical and biochemical reactions associated with sperm entry into the egg become slower, a condition leading to increased polyspermy (entry of more than one sperm).

Polyspermy occurs in several species of laboratory and farm animals. In swine, a delay in copulation or injection of progesterone given 24–36 hours before ovulation leads to some eggs having more than two pronuclei. It is not clear whether these potential triploid embryos are caused by failure to extrude the second polar body or to polyspermy, which may result from failure of the block to polyspermy during ovum aging. The incidence of polyspermy increases when mating or insemination is delayed, resulting in triploid embryos that do not survive.

14.4 Pregnancy Wastage

Pregnancy wastage is responsible for most gestation failures in farm animals. Pregnancy wastage can be divided into embryonic and fetal mortality (Figure 14.5). A small percentage of the wastage is involved in the normal reproductive process and may be regarded as unavoidable.

Termination of pregnancy may occur at various stages.

- Before maternal recognition of pregnancy, in which case length of the cycle is not affected (early embryonic mortality).
- After maternal recognition of pregnancy, associated with a delay in the length of the cycle (late embryonic mortality).
- During the fetal stage (fetal mortality).

Figure 14.5 Pregnancy wastage in farm animals.

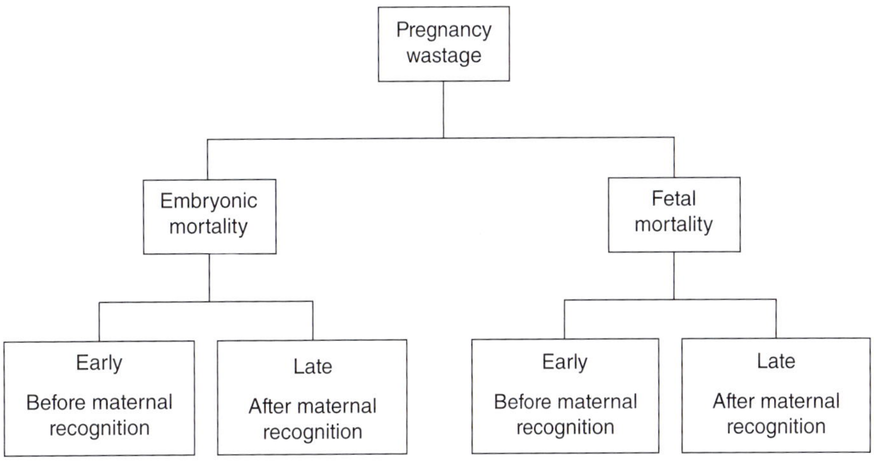

14.4.1 Embryonic Mortality

Embryonic mortality denotes the death of fertilized ova and embryos up to the end of implantation. About 25–40% of embryos are normally lost in farm species. It is also noted in large litters of swine and during multiple pregnancies in cattle and sheep. Mortality is more common during the early than the late gestation period. Early embryonic mortality should be regarded as a normal process of eliminating unfit genotypes in each generation, particularly in large litters of swine and multiple pregnancies in cattle and sheep.

In the past, it was believed that the bovine conceptus was resorbed but transrectal ultrasound examination has demonstrated that the conceptus and its breakdown products apparently are eliminated by expulsion through the cervix, which either goes unnoticed or appears as a vulval discharge of clear mucus.

Embryonic mortality after natural breeding or artificial insemination (AI) accounts for the majority of reproductive failures in domestic animals, with a mortality rate of up to 40% of all fertilized eggs. In cattle, most embryonic deaths occur between days 8 and 16 during hatching of the blastocyst and implantation without affecting cycle lengths. Since most embryos die between days 9 and 15, infertile ewes may experience normal as well as prolonged cycles.

Several methods are used to demonstrate embryonic mortality. In cattle embryonic mortality can be estimated as follows.

- Calculating the fertilization rate and number of fertilized eggs that fail to continue following slaughter at different intervals after mating. The return to estrus interval following mating is less accurate because an extended cycle length may be due to reasons other than embryonic mortality. Early embryonic deaths before regression of the CL are indistinguishable from failure of fertilization in that both cow and ewe return to estrus at the normal time. Death of one embryo in twin ovulating ewes may be undetected, as pregnancy will continue.
- Examining embryos collected by *in vivo* flushing of the reproductive tract at different days after breeding.
- Determining progesterone levels in blood or milk.
- Assessment of embryonic heart beat beyond 20 days by real-time ultrasonography.
- Counting the number of ovulations by laparoscopy for the loss of single embryos in sheep.

Several studies have demonstrated that embryonic mortality in swine is 20–30%, and that more than two-thirds of the reproductive wastage in the pig occurs between 8 and 18 days of gestation. The number of embryos that survive and the stage of pregnancy determine the effects of embryonic mortality on the estrous cycle of swine. For example, if all embryos are lost by day 4 of gestation, the sow returns to estrus after a normal cycle length, but if 1–4 embryos survive beyond day 4, the pregnancy would still terminate but the next estrous period is delayed by six days. For pregnancy to continue beyond day 10, at least four embryos must be present in both uterine horns, whereas for it to continue beyond 12 days, as few as one embryo is sufficient. Normal and subfertile mares have high fertilization rates, but subfertile mares have a higher embryonic loss rate before day 14 post ovulation.

14.4.1.1 Causes

Embryonic mortality can be due to maternal factors, embryonic factors, or embryo–maternal interactions (Table 14.1). Maternal failure tends to affect an entire litter, resulting in complete loss of pregnancy. In contrast, embryonic failure affects embryos individually, often leaving others in the litter unharmed. In other cases the maternal environment may be insufficient, allowing the support of only a few strong embryos. Embryonic loss is influenced by several factors (Figure 14.6).

14.4.1.1.1 Endocrine Factors

Accelerated or delayed transport of the egg, as a result of estrogen– progesterone imbalance, leads to preimplantation death. An abnormally undersized conceptus might not be able to counteract the uterine luteolytic effect, with consequent regression of the CL and termination of pregnancy. In swine, as stated previously, at least four living blastocysts are needed by day 10 of pregnancy to counteract the uterine luteolytic effects.

A critical period of embryonic survival is the late blastocyst stage. Normally, the developing CL secretes progesterone, which acts on the female tract in close synchrony with the development of the embryos. The cause and effect relationship between luteolysis and embryonic deaths is controversial. Apparently, embryonic mortality in cattle is not caused by a progesterone deficiency during the luteal phase of the cycle; luteal regression follows rather than precedes embryonic mortality. However, a diminished response to circulating luteotropic hormones may contribute to embryo mortality in subfertile cows.

Table 14.1 Causes of embryonic mortality.

	PERIOD OF MAXIMAL MORTALITY		
Species	**Days of gestation**	**Stage of development**	**Possible causes**
Cattle	8–16	Hatching of blastocysts and initiation of elongation and commencement of implantation	Progesterone deficiency; inbreeding; multiple pregnancy; blood group homozygosity; J antigen in sera; parity; timing of inseminations; chromosomal aberrations
Sheep	9–15	Transition from yolk sac to allantoic placentation	Inbreeding; increasing maternal age; hemoglobin types; overfeeding; multiple pregnancy; high environmental temperatures
Swine	8–16	Spacing of embryos; transuterine migration; maternal recognition of pregnancy	Inbreeding; chromosomal aberrations; overcrowding; overfeeding; increasing maternal age; high environmental temperature; transferrins
Horses	30–36	Corpus luteum of pregnancy regresses and accessory corpora lutea are formed; change from a yolk sac to an allantochorion placentation	Lactation; twinning; nutrition; chromosomal aberrations

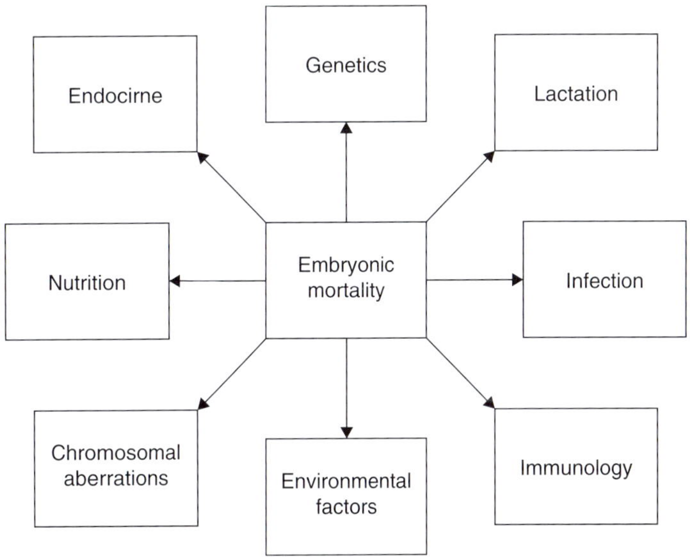

Figure 14.6 Causes of embryonic mortality.

14.4.1.1.2 Lactation

Embryonic mortality occurs during lactation in cattle, sheep, and horses and is characterized by prolonged estrous cycles after breeding. Mating of mares at foal heat leads to early embryonic mortality, which has been attributed to reduced effectiveness of uterine defense mechanisms, stress of lactation, and incomplete regeneration of the endometrium. Sows bred after weaning at seven days of lactation suffer high embryonic losses between days 9 and 20 of pregnancy.

14.4.1.1.3 Nutrition of the Dam

Caloric intake and specific nutritional deficiencies affect ovulation rate and fertilization rate, as well as causing embryonic death. Also extremes in the level of feeding are detrimental to embryo survival, as are extremes in the supply of specific dietary nutrients.

In dairy cows, high intakes of rumen-degradable protein may lead to embryonic mortality. This effect may be mediated through a reduction in the pH of the uterine environment during the luteal phase of the cycle in which the embryo must grow.

In swine, high caloric intake or continuous unlimited feeding increases ovulation rate, thereby increasing the incidence of embryonic mortality before implantation. However, following implantation, unlimited feeding decreases fetal death.

In sheep, full feeding before breeding also increases ovulation rate as well as embryonic mortality. Poor body condition of ewes at mating increases the incidence of embryonic mortality, whereas moderate feed restriction from day 20–100 of pregnancy is less likely to reduce lambing percentages. Undernutrition affects twin ovulators more than single ovulators because both embryos are lost in the former, while a single embryo survives in the latter. Thus, more twin than single ovulating ewes are barren.

In the mare, the critical period for embryonic resorption is between 25 and 31 days after ovulation. No resorption occurs if mares are maintained on an adequate plane of nutrition until 35 days after service.

14.4.1.1.4 Age of Dam

A higher incidence of embryonic mortality is observed in gilts and in sows after the fifth gestation. In the ewe, the incidence of late embryonic loss is higher in ewe lambs and ewes over six years than it is in mature ewes, which is due to factors associated with the embryo rather than the uterine environment.

14.4.1.1.5 Overcrowding In Utero

Because the degree of placental development is primarily influenced by the availability of space and vascular supply within the uterus, increasing the number of implantations decreases the vascular supply to each site and restricts placental development. This results in a high embryonic and fetal mortality rate and probably explains the higher incidence of embryonic mortality in cattle and sheep following twin rather than single ovulation. It should be noted, however, that uterine capacity does not limit the ability of the cow and ewe to carry twins, provided they are located in separate uterine horns. In cattle, embryo transfer experiments have shown a higher embryonic mortality rate in recipients which received two embryos in a single uterine horn. This loss may be due to overcrowding and intrauterine competition for nutrients.

In cattle and sheep with multiple ovulations, the number of embryos surviving is reduced to a fairly constant number (2–3 embryos per female) within the first three or four weeks of pregnancy, which implies that embryonic loss increases as the number of eggs shed increases. Mortality does not seem to be due to a deficiency of progesterone. In prolific breeds of sheep, late embryonic deaths occur in ewes with more than five ovulations.

Transuterine migration of embryos is of importance for equal distribution of embryos in the two horns of the uterus in polytocous species such as swine. In its absence, there is a high incidence of embryonic mortality in swine.

14.4.1.1.6 Thermal Stress

Embryonic mortality increases in a number of species following exposure of the mother to elevated ambient temperatures, especially in tropical areas. The effects of thermal stress on the early embryo are not apparent until the later stages of its development. Fertilized eggs of sheep and cattle, when subjected to high temperatures either *in vitro* or in *vivo,* are damaged but continue to develop, only to die during the critical stages of implantation. Reduced fertility of summer heat-stressed dairy cows may result from decreased viability and developmental capacity of 6–8-day-old embryos and may account for the well-documented seasonal reduction in the efficiency of AI during summer.

Heat stress between days 8 and 17 of pregnancy may also alter the uterine environment as well as growth and secretory activity of the conceptus. Apparently heat stress antagonizes the inhibitory effects of the embryo on the uterine secretion of PGFza.

14.4.1.1.7 Semen

A portion of all embryonic mortality is attributable to the male and the mating system. Genetic factors that are transmitted by the male to the embryo may be inherited, may arise from testicular tissue, or may occur in spermatozoa after they are released from the testis. Infertile matings by highly fertile bulls are primarily due to embryonic mortality, while those of bulls with low fertility are due to fertilization failure and embryonic deaths. In swine, semen stored for three days before insemination produced zygotes much more susceptible to early embryonic death, presumably owing to the reduced DNA content in aged spermatozoa.

14.4.1.1.8 Incompatibility

The inherited genotype of the male may include a variety of genetic factors that lead to incompatibility and early embryonic loss. There may be incompatibility between spermatozoa and mother, between spermatozoa and egg, or between zygote and mother. Immunological incompatibilities may block fertilization (prezygotic selection), or cause embryonic, fetal, or neonatal mortality. In cattle, homozygosity for certain blood groups and certain substances related to transferrin (beta-globulin) and J antigen in sera are associated with increased embryonic loss as well as decreased fertilization rate.

14.4.2 Fetal Mortality

14.4.2.1 Abortion

Abortion is the termination of pregnancy with the expulsion of a fetus of recognizable size before it is viable, which is arbitrarily defined as 260 days for cattle, 290 days for horses, and 110 days for swine. Fetal mortality is not an essential prelude to abortion. Abortions may be spontaneous or induced, infectious or noninfectious.

14.4.2.1.1 Noninfectious Abortions

Noninfectious abortions are more prevalent in cattle, particularly dairy cattle, than in sheep or horses. Noninfectious causes of spontaneous abortion may be due to genetic, chromosomal, hormonal, or nutritional factors (Table 14.2). Spontaneous abortion may also occur in animals bred immediately after puberty or immediately after parturition. Mares seem to be endocrinologically susceptible to abortion between the fifth and 10th months of pregnancy. Chromosomal abnormalities are known to cause embryonic losses in farm animals but their importance in abortion in farm animals is unknown.

Abortions are occasionally induced with high doses of estrogens, PGF l or glucocorticoids, particularly in young females bred at an early age and in meat-producing animals. Twin pregnancy is the most common cause of abortion in mares; over two-thirds of twin pregnancies terminate in abortions. The inability of a mare to successfully carry twin fetuses to term may be related to placental insufficiency arising from competition between the placentae. This may lead to the death of one fetus and eventually to the abortion of both fetuses.

In the past, habitual abortions at 3–4.5 months of gestation in Angora goats were attributed to a hereditary defect of the anterior pituitary gland. These abortions are associated with two different syndromes. The first of these syndromes is

Table 14.2 Noninfectious causes of pregnancy wastage in farm animals.

Causes	Cow	Mare	Sow	Ewe or Doe
Chemicals, drugs, and poisonous plants	Nitrates, chlorinated naphthalenes, arsenic, perennial broomweeds, pine needles	None	Dicoumarin, aflatoxin, wood preservatives (creosote, pentachlorophenols)	Lead, nitrate, locoweeds, lupines, sweet clover, onion grass, veratrum
Hormonal	High doses of estrogens, glucocorticoids, PGF2-alpha	High doses of estrogens or cortisone (?)	High doses of estrogens or PGF2-alpha	High doses of estrogens, cortisol or ACTH, PGF2-alpha, progesterone deficiency
Nutritional	Starvation, malnutrition, deficiencies of vitamin A or iodine	Reduced energy intake	Deficiencies of vitamin A, iron, and calcium	Lack of TDN or energy, deficiencies of vitamin A, copper, iodine, and selenium
Genetic or chromosomal	Embryonic mortality, fetal anomalies	Fetal anomalies	Embryonic mortality, congenital or genetic lethal defects	Lethal genetic defects
Physical	Douching or insemination of pregnant uterus, stress (transport, lever, surgery)	Manual dilation of cervix, natural service during pregnancy; rectal palpation of the very young blastodermic vesicle	Stress (transportation, fighting, injury), heat stress	Severe physical stress
Miscellaneous	Twinning, allergies, anaphylaxis	Twinning	Poor management	Twinning (?)

ACTH, adrenocorticotrophic hormone; PGF2-alpha, prostaglandin F2-alpha; TDN, total digestible nutrients.

related to nutritional stress. The hypoglycemia that occurs in the doe and fetus activates the fetal hypothalamic–pituitary axis and alters placental endocrine function. PGFl-alpha released by the placenta causes regression of the CL of pregnancy and expulsion of one or more recently dead fetuses. Improving the nutritional status of the does may reduce these losses. The other syndrome, resulting from hyperactivity of the maternal adrenal cortex, leads to an excessive accumulation of fetal fluids over a prolonged period. The aborted fetus shows varying degrees of decomposition.

14.4.2.1.2 Infectious Abortions

Infectious abortions account for a major percentage of the pregnancy wastage in farm animals. The major diseases, organisms, mode of transmission, and clinical findings are summarized in Table 14.3.

Cattle *Neospora caninum* is a recently recognized protozoan parasite, which was previously misidentified as *Toxoplama gondii*. It is a major cause of bovine abortion in many countries. *N. caninum* was found in fetal tissues of 34 of 688 cases of bovine abortion. The aborted fetuses ranged in gestational age from three to eight months.

Neospora sp. has the ability to be transmitted from dam to offspring for several generations. This mode of transmission would explain the maintenance of infection in a population of cattle despite the lack of a definitive host for the parasite. Congenitally acquired *N. caninum* infection can cause a substantial number of abortions during the initial pregnancy of heifers, with abortion risk attributable to *N. caninum* decreasing in subsequent pregnancies, possibly because of selective culling. Subsequent abortions can be expected in congenitally infected cows that have aborted previously.

Epizootic bovine abortion (EBA, foothill abortion) is a well-defined clinical condition that occurred in the 1950s, principally in the foothills and mountain areas surrounding the central valleys of California. It is characterized by abortions occurring in the last third of pregnancy, most commonly in beef cattle. The abortion rate may exceed 80% when large numbers of animals are exposed for the first time. The highest incidence is in heifers but older animals moved into endemic areas for the first time may subsequently abort. Usually a cow aborts only once, makes a complete recovery, and fertility is normal in subsequent gestations.

The cause is suspected to be a virus (*Chlamydia psittaci*). Feeding the tick *Ornithodoros coriaceus* on susceptible cattle during the second trimester of gestation can experimentally produce the disease. No vaccine is available because the causative agent has not been identified. Adjusting the calving season so that the middle trimester of pregnancy

Table 14.3 Summary of diseases causing pregnancy wastage in sheep and goats.

Disease	Transmission	Clinical findings
PROTOZOAL		
Toxoplasmosis (*Toxoplasma gondii*)	Ingestion	Late abortion; stillbirth
BACTERIAL		
Brucellosis (*Brucella ovis, Brucella melitensis*)	Spread from ram to ram through ewes Infected genital discharges	Late abortion, stillbirths, epididymitis Abortion; goats are highly suspectible
Vibriosis (*Campylobacter fetus* or *jejuni*)	Ingestion	Abortion in last trimester; stillbirths, metritis
Salmonellosis (*Salmonella dublin, S. typhimurium*)	Ingestion	Late abortion, neonatal mortality
Listeriosis (*Listeria monocytogenes*)	Ingestion (?)	Abortion after three months; retained fetal membranes and metritis
VIRAL		
Enzootic abortion of ewes (*Chlamydia psittaci*)	Ingestion	Late abortion; stillbirths, weak lambs
Rift Valley fever	Insects	Abortion

Source: Adapted from: Laing JA, Brinley-Morgan WJ, Sagner WC. Fertility and Infertility in Veterinary Practice, 4th edn. London: Baillière Tindall, 1988; Radostits OM, Blood DC, Gay GC. Veterinary Medicine, 8th edn. London: WB Saunders, 1994; Arthur GH, Noakes DE, Pearson H, Parkinson TM. Veterinary Reproduction and Obstetrics, 7th edn. London: WB Saunders, 1996.

does not coincide with the tick season has reduced the incidence of abortion. Animals that have experienced the disease will not abort again, and these should be maintained in the herd. There is no evidence that this disease spreads from cow to cow.

In a 10-year survey of 8995 bovine abortions and stillbirths in South Dakota, viruses were associated with 948 (10.58%) and bacteria with 1299 (14.490/0). Bovine herpesvirus 1 (IBR) was detected in 485 (5.41%), and bovine viral diarrhea virus (BVDV) in 407 (4.54%). The five bacteria most commonly associated with bovine abortion or stillbirth were *Actinomyces pyogenes*, 378 (4.22%); *Bacillus* spp., 321 (3.58%); *Listeria* spp., 121 (1.35%); *Escherichia coli*, 98 (1.09%); and *Leptospira interrogans*, 79 (0.88%).

Sheep and Goats Enzootic abortion of ewes (EAE) occurs in many parts of the world and has been diagnosed in the western United States. The rate of abortion in a newly infected flock may be as high as 30%. In flocks experiencing a reinfection, the rate is less than 5%. Ewes abort during the last month of pregnancy. Abortions continue until normal lambing time, and some fetuses are expelled alive at term but are diseased.

The causative agent of EAE is a member of the *Chlamydia* group. This disease must be differentiated from vibriosis. Diagnosis of EAE depends on finding the elementary bodies of the infectious agent in smears from the cotyledon or placental exudate. The disease produce immunity. A single infection produces lifetime immunity and the disease can be prevented by vaccination.

In a 10-year survey of 1784 of ovine abortions and stillbirths in South Dakota, infectious agents were found in 39%, noninfectious agents in 5%, and 56% of cases were undiagnosed. Together, *Toxoplasma gondii*, *Campylobacter* sp., and *C. psittaci* caused about 25% of all abortions and stillbirths.

Horses The equine herpesvirus I infection is primarily a disease of the upper respiratory tract. The horse first experiences exposure to this virus as a foal in the fall near weaning time. This epizootic disease in foals produces a massive exposure of mares that are in midpregnancy. Abortion usually occurs after the eighth month of pregnancy, with most abortions occurring between January and April because of seasonal breeding.

By far the most frequent cause of epizootics of abortion in mares is the equine herpesvirus I. This infection should be suspected until otherwise eliminated. Abortion from this infection rarely occurs in successive years, and in the absence of other control methods, it may not occur in a single band of mares for several years. Immunization is the best method of prevention.

In a survey of 3514 aborted fetuses, stillborn foals, or foals that died less than 24 hours after birth, and of 13 placentas from mares in Kentucky, fetoplacental infection caused by bacteria (628), equine herpesvirus (143), or fungi (61) was the most common diagnosis. A diagnosis was not established in 16% of the cases seen (585). Leptospirosis (78) was an important cause of bacterial abortion in mares, and infection by a nocardioform actinomycete (45) was an important cause of chronic placentitis.

14.4.2.1.3 Fetal Mummification

Fetal mummification is characterized by mortality of the fetus but it is not aborted. Instead, resorption of placental fluids, dehydration of the fetus and its membranes lead to a uterus which is tightly wrapped around the fetus. It is more common in cattle and swine than in sheep and horses.

Cattle The syndrome occurs mainly from the fifth to seventh months of gestation in all breeds of cattle. Affected cows conceive normally in the subsequent breeding period. Occasionally, bovine mummified fetuses are aborted spontaneously, but in most cases they are carried many months beyond the gestation period because the CL persists. It is suspected only when gestation is prolonged. In cases of incomplete abortion, bacteria enter through a partially dilated cervix to autolyze fetal soft tissues, leaving fetal bones floating within the uterine lumen. This condition is referred to as fetal maceration, which is a septic process unlike mummification. A high incidence of fetal mummification in the Jersey and Guernsey breeds tends to support a hereditary influence.

Sheep Twin-bearing ewes may abort a mummified fetus during late gestation and maintain the other lamb to full term, or they may deliver a mummified fetus attached to the placenta of a viable offspring.

14.5 Perinatal and Neonatal Mortality

14.5.1 Perinatal Mortality

Perinatal mortality refers to death of the offspring shortly before, during, or within the first 48–72 hours of life at normal term. Perinatal mortality, which includes stillbirths (born dead), accounts for most of the losses between birth and weaning. The extent of perinatal losses ranges from 5% to 15% in cattle and horses, up to 20–30% in sheep and pigs.

Most losses occur within 72 hours of birth. Asphyxia, starvation, chilling, and congenital malformations are major contributing factors. Species differences exist in the relative importance of these stresses. For example, trauma during prolonged or assisted birth occurs more frequently in cattle than in pigs, whereas asphyxiation may be more likely to occur in the pig as a result of premature rupture of the umbilical cord. The use of drugs to induce parturition might adversely affect neonatal survival. For example, induction of parturition in the sow with PGFza before day 111 of gestation and in the cow with corticosteroids before day 265 of gestation may result in a higher incidence of perinatal mortality.

Stillborn piglets resemble live littermates, but their lungs do not float in water. One to two piglets in approximately one-third of all litters are dead at birth with advancing parity, in extremes of litter size, and in litters in which the gestation period is less than 110 days. Two types of stillbirth occur in swine. In the first type, which is usually due to infectious causes, fetuses die prepartum whereas in the second type, which is due to noninfectious causes, piglets die during parturition. The presence of meconium on the skin, in the mouth, and in the trachea of the piglet differentiates the latter from the former.

A high incidence of piglet death is observed with uterine inertia, with prolongation of farrowing time or of the interval between births of piglets, in litters that contain less than four or more than nine piglets, and among piglets in the last third of the litter. These intrapartum deaths may be due to the low tolerance of piglets to anoxia and are usually associated with rupture of the umbilical cord prior to delivery. Since piglets suffer irreversible brain damage within five minutes after umbilical rupture or impeded umbilical flow, delivery must be completed rapidly.

In sheep, most losses between implantation and weaning occur during the perinatal period, as a result of starvation of the neonate, dystocia among lambs born to maiden ewes, ewes on poor pasture, or ewes with "clover disease."

14.5.2 Neonatal Mortality

Neonatal mortality (death of the neonate during the first few weeks of life) is related to heredity, environmental factors, nutrition, and infection. Several nutritional deficiencies may contribute to neonatal mortality.

Respiratory distress syndrome (RDS) is characterized by a failure of the fetal lungs to produce surfactant necessary to maintain the stability of the terminal air spaces of the lung after birth. RDS occurs in premature human infants and is invariably fatal. It has been reported in foals, calves, and piglets. RDS in calves, as in the human infant, is caused by a deficiency of a surfactant (phospholipid), and its diagnosis is based on levels in the amniotic fluid of two phospholipids – lecithin and sphingomyelin.

Neonatal mortality may also result from prolonged labor, poor maternal nutrition, weakness of the mother or the young, bacterial infection of the young through the umbilical cord, poor maternal behavior, or delayed onset of lactation. Exposure of the newborn pig to low environmental temperature leads to hypothermia, hypoglycemia, and death. Heat prostation and some deaths occur in newborn lambs exposed to high environmental temperature. Another source of danger to the neonate is the presence of mammalian or avian predators.

15

Postpartum Care of the Doe

Felix Uchenna Samuel[1,2], Ama Adadzewa Eshun[2], Bashir Maryam Darma[3], Mada A. Khumran[4], Allam Lushaikyaa[4], Hycinth Ndabatsado Kolo[5], and Mojetoluwa S. Afolabi[2]

[1] Faculty of Veterinary Medicine, National Animal Production Research Institute/Ahmadu Bello University, Zaria, Nigeria
[2] Department of Food and Animal Science, Alabama A&M University, Normal, USA
[3] Veterinary Teaching Hospital, Faculty of Veterinary Medicine, Bayero University, Kano, Nigeria
[4] Faculty of Veterinary Medicine, Ahmadu Bello University, Zaria, Nigeria
[5] Department of Animal Health and Production, Federal University of Technology, Minna, Nigeria

15.1 Introduction

Careful examination of the ewe or doe for the presence of additional fetuses should be performed by either ballottement of the abdomen or transabdominal ultrasonography. Vital signs and muscle tone also should be assessed as a means of detecting hypocalcemia. After parturition, the placenta is passed rather quickly but is not considered retained until 6–12 hours post partum (Kharche and Kouamo 2015). Dairy does should be milked soon after parturition. In meat and fiber production herds, the doe's or ewe's udder should be palpated for evidence of mastitis and to determine the quality and quantity of colostrum or milk production. Colostrum or milk should be expressed from each teat to ensure patency and detect any abnormal secretions (Sharun and Erdoğan 2019). Postpartal females should be monitored closely for appropriate infant–maternal bonding and to ensure that the lamb or kid is nursing appropriately. Observation is facilitated by placing the doe or ewe with her litter in a small pen for several days before being moved back into the main herd. Does and ewes also should be monitored closely for signs of hypocalcemia or ketosis (Mongini and Van Saun 2023). Maximizing dry matter intake by fresh does and ewes will help prevent metabolic disease and ensure maximum production.

Postpartum or puerperal care involves all the care and attention given to the doe after parturition with the aim of maintaining its reproductive efficiency (Peleki et al. 2023). The normal uterus of a goat is shown in Figure 15.1.

15.2 The Puerperium

The puerperium is that period after the completion of parturition, including the third stage of labor, when the genital system is returning to its normal nonpregnant state. In polyestrous species, it is important that there should be a normal puerperium since it is the practice under most systems of husbandry to breed from individuals of these species fairly soon after they have given birth. Thus any extension of the puerperium may have a detrimental effect on the reproductive performance of the individual animal.

The genital system does not completely return to the original pregravid state since, particularly after the first gestation, certain changes are not completely reversible (Costello et al. 2023). There are four main areas of activity.

- The tubular genital tract, especially the uterus, shrinks and atrophies due to tissue loss, thus reversing the hypertrophy that occurs in response to the stimulus of pregnancy. Myometrial contractions, which continue for several days after parturition, aid this process and help in the voiding of fluids and tissue debris; this is normally referred to as involution.

Elements of Reproduction and Reproductive Diseases of Goats, First Edition. Edited by Tanmoy Rana.

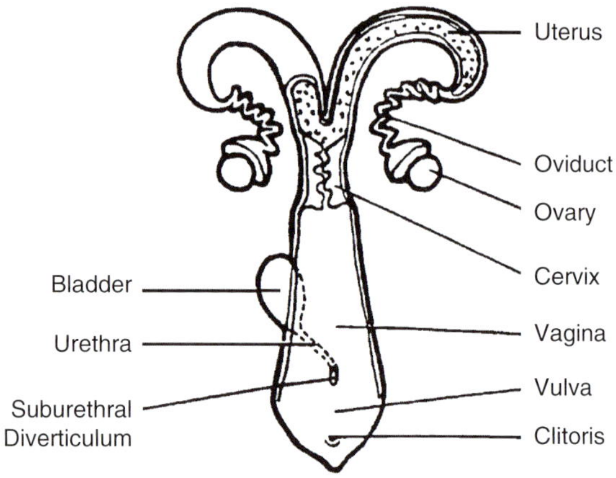

Figure 15.1 The uterus of a doe. *Source*: www.thegoatchick.com/kidding.html

- The structure of the endometrium and deeper layers of the uterine wall is restored.
- There is a resumption of ovarian function in polyestrous species and a return to cyclical activity.
- Bacterial contamination of the uterine lumen is eliminated.

15.2.1 Involution

There is rapid shrinkage and contraction of the uterus, particularly during days 3–10 post partum, as determined by measurements of uterine weight and length, diameter of uterine body and previously gravid horn (Badawi et al. 2014). According to these measurements, involution is complete by 20–25 days. Using sequential radiography and radiopaque markers, uterine involution has been shown to be complete by about 28 days in suckling ewes, although an unexplained increase in uterine dimensions has been reported at 42 days. Involution in the ewe is also due to collagen breakdown, since although tissue collagen concentrations remain fairly constant with advancing pregnancy, there is a 7–8-fold increase in uterine mass; the reduction in size can only be a reversal of this process (Noakes 2009).

The cervix constricts rapidly post partum; within 10–12 hours of a normal calving it becomes almost impossible to insert a hand through it into the uterus, and by 96 hours it will admit just two fingers. The cervix also undergoes atrophy and shrinkage due to the elimination of fluid and the reduction in collagen and smooth muscle. Marion and Gier (1968) found that the mean external diameter was 15 cm at two days post partum, 9–11 cm at 10 days, 7–8 cm at 30 days, and 5–6 cm at 60 days (Kelly 2022).

A useful guide that involution is occurring normally is to compare the diameter of the previously gravid horn with that of the cervix, since at about 25 days post partum the latter starts to exceed the former.

Prostaglandins may have a role in controlling uterine involution, although the postpartum rise in the metabolite of PGF2-alpha may be a reflection of the involution process rather than the cause (Noakes 2009). Eley et al. (1981) demonstrated a positive correlation between prostaglandin metabolite (PGFM) concentrations in the peripheral circulation and the diameter of the uterine horn. Using exogenous PGF2-alpha twice daily for 10 days starting from three days post partum, uterine involution was accelerated by 6–13 days; however, the number of animals was small and the frequency and duration of the treatment regimen were very atypical of the normal situation (Kelly 2022).

Since the increase in the uterine mass during pregnancy is due to a combination of increases in both collagen and smooth muscle, then involution must be associated with a reduction of these tissues. This has been shown very clearly in the study of Kaidi et al. (1991) in relation to collagen degradation, but in relation to the loss of smooth muscle the results were equivocal (Tian and Noakes 1991). The studies of the latter authors also showed that exogenous hormones such as estrogens, PGF2-alpha, and long-acting oxytocin analogues do not influence the rate of involution (Kelly 2022).

15.2.2 Restoration of the Endometrium

Endometrial restoration begins with a noticeable loss of fluid and tissue debris. This is sometimes referred to as the "second cleansing" or "secundus." The presence of such a discharge in cows is normal, although sometimes individuals will mistake it for an abnormal discharge due to uterine infection and request treatment (Noakes et al. 2018).

As in the cow, there are profound changes in the structure of the caruncles with degeneration of the surface, necrosis, sloughing, and subsequent regeneration of the superficial layers of the endometrium. There is evidence, determined by the slaughter of animals three days before the expected date of lambing, of prepartum hyaline degenerative changes. This occurs in the connective tissue at the base of, and adjacent to, the endometrial crypts and also involves both directly and indirectly the walls of the arteries and veins, thus reducing their lumens; the fetal villi are unaffected (Noakes et al. 2018). After dehiscence and separation of the placenta, there is further hyaline degeneration of caruncular tissue, which results in constriction of the blood vessels at the base of the maternal crypts. There is necrosis of the surface layer of the caruncle so that at about four days post partum, the most superficial layers are undergoing autolysis and liquefaction, which are responsible for the dark reddish brown or black coloration of the lochial discharge at this time. By 16 days post partum, necrosis of the whole superficial part of the caruncle has occurred with, in most cases, separation of the brown necrotic plaque so that it is lying free in the uterine lumen. The caruncles now have a clean, glistening surface, and the process of regeneration is completed by the reepithelialization of the caruncles by about 28 days (Noakes et al. 2018).

The quantity of lochia voided is variable. Initially it arises from blood, fetal fluids, and placental debris but as the puerperium proceeds, the liquefied, sloughed caruncular tissue contributes to it. The lochial discharge is usually yellowish-brown or reddish-brown; the volume voided varies greatly from individual to individual. Pluripara can void up to a total of 2000 ml, although it is more usually about 1000 ml. In primipara, it is rarely more than 500 ml and in some animals it is occasionally nil, owing to the complete absorption of the lochia. The greatest flow of lochia occurs during the first 2–3 days; by eight days it is reduced, and by 14–18 days post partum it has virtually disappeared. At about nine days it is frequently bloodstained, while before it ceases it becomes lighter in color and almost "lymph-like." Normal lochial discharge does not have an unpleasant odor.

The lochia is derived from the remains of fetal fluids, blood from the ruptured umbilical vessels and shreds of fetal membranes, but mainly from the sloughed surfaces of the uterine caruncles (Dadarwal et al. 2017). The slough occurs following degenerative changes and necrosis of the superficial layers, first described by Rasbech (1950). After the shedding of the allantochorion, the caruncle is about 70 mm long, 35 mm wide, and 25 mm thick. The endometrial crypts frequently contain remnants of the chorionic villi which were detached from the rest of the allantochorion at the time of placental separation. Within the first 48 hours post partum, there is evidence of early necrotic changes in the septal mass of the caruncle; the caruncular blood vessels become rapidly constricted and are nearly occluded. At five days the necrosis has proceeded rapidly, so that the stratum compactum is now covered by a leukocyte-laden necrotic layer. Some of this necrotic material starts to slough and contributes to the lochia. Small blood vessels, mainly arterioles, then protrude from the surface of the caruncle, from which there is oozing of blood, causing a red coloration of the lochia.

By 10 days, most of the necrotic caruncular tissue has sloughed and undergone some degree of liquefaction and by 15 days post partum sloughing is complete, leaving only stubs of blood vessels protruding from the exposed stratum compactum. This eventually becomes smooth by 19 days, owing to the disappearance of the vessels (Noakes et al. 2018).

Regeneration of the epithelium of the endometrium occurs immediately after parturition in those areas which were not seriously damaged and is complete in the intercaruncular areas by eight days. Complete reepithelialization of the caruncle, which is largely derived from centripetal growth of cells from the surrounding uterine glands, is complete from 25 days onwards, although the stage at which complete healing occurs is variable.

While these changes are taking place, the caruncles are becoming smaller so that at 40–60 days they consist of small protrusions 4–8 mm in diameter and 4–6 mm high. They also differ from those of nullipara because they are larger and have melanin pigmentation and a more vascular base (Kelleher et al. 2019).

15.2.3 Return of Cyclical Activity (Ovarian Rebound)

Although in temperate climates does normally become anestrus after kidding, there are numerous reports of ovarian activity occurring within a few days to two weeks post partum. Follicular growth is common but ovulation is unusual and when it does occur, it is usually associated with a silent heat. Failure of follicular maturation and ovulation is probably due to inadequate release of luteinizing hormone (LH) as a result of a deficiency in gonadotropin-releasing hormone (GnRH) synthesis and secretion (Kárpáti et al. 2023). As a result, basal LH levels and the pulse frequency of episodic LH secretion are inadequate to stimulate normal ovarian function. It is possible that the time of the year when the does kid has a profound effect, with those that kid early and within the normal breeding season being more likely to have normal ovarian rebound (Di Segni et al. 2022). The structure of the ovary is shown in Figure 15.2.

Anovulatory follicular waves occur periodically during pregnancy, with the emergence of follicles of up to a maximum of 6 mm in diameter. However, because of the prolonged period of inhibition during pregnancy, due to the continuous negative feedback effect of progesterone secreted by the corpus luteum and placenta, the pituitary is refractory post partum, as demonstrated by a lack of response to the administration of GnRH (Di Segni et al. 2022).

This eventually recovers with time. As a result of the absence or low output of gonadotropins, the ovary is relatively quiescent and the doe is in the anestrous phase. However, during this postpartum phase the ovaries frequently contain numerous large anovulatory follicles which quickly become atretic; these are sometimes incorrectly diagnosed as cysts (Kárpáti et al. 2023).

In the immediate postpartum period, both estradiol and progesterone are low. The anterior pituitary is capable of releasing FSH during the first few days post partum so that with the sporadic release of endogenous GnRH there is a gradual and sustained rise in plasma FSH (Kasoha et al. 2022).

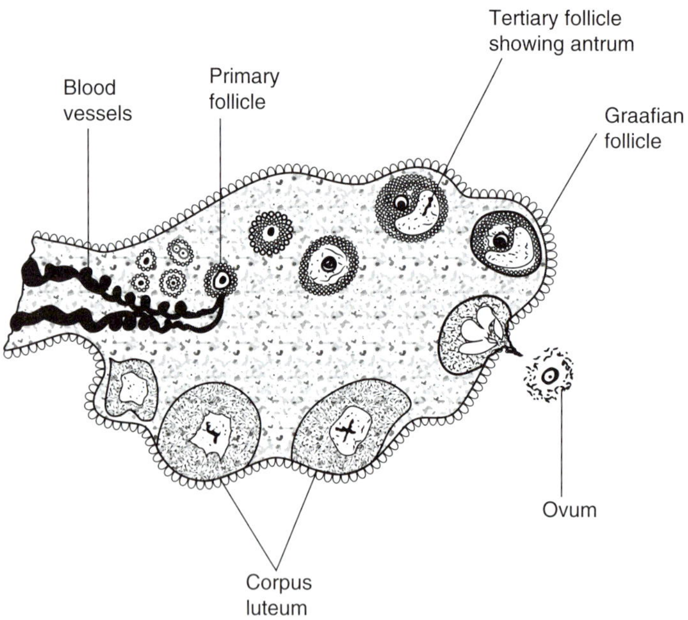

Figure 15.2 Structure of the ovary. *Source:* www.sarthaks.com/357263/draw-labelled-diagram-sectional-view-human-ovaryshowing-various-stages-follicles-growing#google_vignette Dr Vet.

15.2.4 Elimination of Bacterial Contamination

Although it would have been expected that similar events to those previously described for the cow and mare would occur, the author was unable to isolate bacteria from uterine swabs obtained from 10 ewes, 1–14 days post partum, at surgical hysterotomy. More recently, using sequential transcervical swabbing of 13 ewes during the first week post partum, bacteria were isolated from four ewes; thus in the other nine ewes the uterus was sterile (Goericke-Pesch and Packeiser 2022).

At calving, and immediately post partum, the vulva is relaxed and the cervix is dilated, thus allowing bacteria to gain entry into the vagina and thereafter the uterus. A wide range of bacteria may be isolated from the uterine lumen; Elliott et al. (1968) identified 33 different species, those most frequently isolated being Arcanobacterium (*Actinomyces [Corynebacterium] pyogenes*), *Escherichia coli*, streptococci, and staphylococci. In all studies there is a decrease with time in the percentage of uteri from which bacteria are isolated. The main mechanism involved in the elimination of the bacteria is phagocytosis by migrating leukocytes; however, persistence of uterine contractions, sloughing of caruncular tissue, and uterine secretions all assist in the physical expulsion of the bacteria. Early return to cyclical activity is probably important since the estrogen-dominated uterus is more resistant to infection. However, there is evidence that in some cases early return to estrus may be disadvantageous in that if the bacteria are not eliminated at the first estrus then the cow enters the first luteal phase where progesterone is the dominant hormone (Kelly 2022).

15.3 Factors Influencing the Puerperium

15.3.1 Uterine Involution

Many of the methods used to measure the rate of involution have been largely subjective and thus inaccurate; however, with the advent of transrectal ultrasound imaging, accurate measurements of uterine and cervical dimensions are now possible (Pascottini et al. 2023). Influential factors include the following.

- *Age*: most observers have found that involution is more rapid in primipara than pluripara.
- *Season of year*: if there is any influence, involution is probably most rapid in spring and summer.
- *Suckling vs milking*: results are contradictory; it may be a breed influence on the effect of time to return of cyclical ovarian activity.
- *Climate*: there is evidence that heat stress can accelerate and inhibit the speed of involution.

- *Periparturient abnormalities*: dystocia, retained placenta, hypocalcemia, ketosis, twin calves, and metritis delay involution. Periparturient problems cause an overall delay in the completion of this process of 5–8 days (Buch et al. 1955; Tennant and Peddicord 1968).
- *Delayed return to cyclical ovarian activity*: this inhibits involution.

15.3.2 Restoration of the Endometrium

There is little relevant documented evidence but retained fetal membranes and metritis inhibit healing, while ovarian rebound to cyclical activity may have an influence.

15.3.3 Return of Cyclical Activity (Ovarian Rebound)

Relevant factors include the following (Pascottini et al. 2023).

- *Periparturient abnormalities*: a number of authors have shown that a whole range of periparturient problems delay ovarian rebound.
- *Milk yield*: there is much contradictory evidence on the influence of current milk yield; some authors have demonstrated an effect of the lactation preceding calving. It is frequently difficult to differentiate the influence of nutrition and milk yield.

  Nutrition: in both beef suckler and dairy cows, inadequate feeding, especially of energy, during the dry period and after calving inhibits ovarian rebound. This will usually be shown as poor body condition score. Ovulation of the dominant follicle will occur after 3.2 ± 0.2, or 10.6 ± 1.2, follicular waves in beef cows in good and poor body condition score, respectively (Crowe 2000). The effect of nutrition on ovarian function is likely to be mediated by insulin and IGFs.
- *Breed*: while it has been known for some time that there is a longer delay in beef compared with dairy cows, there is evidence of a breed effect within the two groups, especially in the former.
- *Parity*: most observers have recorded a delay in primipara compared with pluripara – up to the fourth lactation. Conflicting opinions have probably arisen because of the problems of separating the influences of nutritional status, milk yield, and weight loss.
- *Season of the year*: there is good evidence that photoperiod has an effect. This has been shown by experimentally subjecting heifers to continuous darkness, which inhibited the return of cyclical activity. Suckler cows that calved between February and April were acyclic significantly longer than those that calved between August and December. By stimulating the effects of short day length using exogenous melatonin, it has been possible to delay the return to estrus and ovulation in postpartum beef cows.
- *Climate*: cows in tropical climates show a delay compared with those in temperate zones.
- *Suckling intensity and milking frequency*: the greater the frequency of milking and the intensity of suckling (number of calves), as well as calf presence, the longer the period of acyclicity. This can be reversed in beef suckler cows by restricting the access of the calf to suckle from 30 days post partum.

15.3.4 Elimination of Bacterial Contamination

The consequence of bacterial contamination is the development of metritis and endometritis.

- *Magnitude of bacterial contamination*: a massive bacterial flora may overwhelm natural defense mechanisms.
- *Nature of bacterial flora*: many obligate Gram-negative anaerobes, such as *Fusobacterium necrophorum* and *Bacteroides* spp., exhibit synergy with Gram-positive aerobic contaminants.
- *Delayed uterine involution.*
- *Retained placenta.*
- *Calving trauma to the uterus.*
- *Return of cyclical ovarian activity*: there is contradictory evidence since, with an early return to estrus, there is an early estrogen peak which should assist in the elimination of the bacteria. However, if the level of contamination is such that a significant bacterial flora persists after the first estrus, the subsequent luteal phase may allow the bacteria to proliferate (Richardson 2022).

References

Badawi, M.E., Makawi, S.E.A., Abdelghafar, R.M., and Ibrahim, M.T. (2014). Assessment of postpartum uterine involution and progesterone profile in Nubian goats (Capra hircus). *Journal of Advanced Veterinary and Animal Research* 1 (2): 36–41.

Buch, N.C., Tyler, W.J., and Casida, L.E. (1955). Postpartum estrus and involution of the uterus in an experimental herd of Holstein-Friesian cows. *Journal of Dairy Science* 38 (1): 73–79.

Costello, E.K., DiGiulio, D.B., Robaczewska, A. et al. (2023). Abrupt perturbation and delayed recovery of the vaginal ecosystem following childbirth. *Nature Communications* 14 (1): 4141.

Crowe, M. A. (2008). Resumption of ovarian cyclicity in post-partum beef and dairy cows. *Reproduction in domestic animals*, 43, 20–28.

Dadarwal, D., Palmer, C., and Griebel, P. (2017). Mucosal immunity of the postpartum bovine genital tract. *Theriogenology* 104: 62–71.

Di Segni, N., Busnelli, A., Secchi, M. et al. (2022). Luteinizing hormone supplementation in women with hypogonadotropic hypogonadism seeking fertility care: insights from a narrative review. *Frontiers in Endocrinology* 13: 907249.

Eley, D.S., Thatcher, W.W., Head, H.H. et al. (1981). Periparturient and postpartum endocrine changes of conceptus and maternal units in Jersey cows bred for milk yield. *Journal of Dairy Science* 64 (2): 312–320.

Elliott, D.S., Legates, J.E., and Ulberg, L.C. (1968). Changes in the reproductive processes of mice selected for large and small body size. *Reproduction* 17 (1): 9–18.

Goericke-Pesch, S. and Packeiser, E.M. (2022). Reproductive management in catteries: optimising health and wellbeing through veterinarian-breeder collaboration. *Journal of Feline Medicine and Surgery* 24 (9): 881–904.

Kaidi, R., Brown, P.J., David, J.S. et al. (1991). Uterine collagen during involution in cattle. *Matrix* 11 (2): 101–107.

Kárpáti, E., Fürlinger, D., Pleskó, A.M. et al. (2023). Various approaches to influence melatonin level in sheep reproduction. *Veterinarski Glasnik* 77: 1–7.

Kasoha, M., Takacs, Z., Dumé, J. et al. (2022). Postpartum assessment of the correlation between serum hormone levels of estradiol, progesterone, prolactin and ß-HCG and blood pressure measurements in pre-eclampsia patients. *Diagnostics* 12 (7): 1700.

Kelleher, A.M., DeMayo, F.J., and Spencer, T.E. (2019). Uterine glands: developmental biology and functional roles in pregnancy. *Endocrine Reviews* 40 (5): 1424–1445.

Kelly, E. (2022). Reproductive tract disease and estrus detection inaccuracy in Irish seasonal calving pasture-based dairy cows. Doctoral thesis. University College Dublin, School of Veterinary Medicine.

Kharche, S.D. and Kouamo, J. (2015). An overview of pregnancy diagnosis in small ruminants. *Indian Journal of Animal Sciences* 85 (4): 331–342.

Marion, G.B. and Gier, H.T. (1968). Factors affecting bovine ovarian activity after parturition. *Journal of Animal Science* 27 (6): 1621–1626.

Mongini, A. and Van Saun, R.J. (2023). Pregnancy toxemia in sheep and goats. *Veterinary Clinics: Food Animal Practice* 39 (2): 275–291.

Noakes, D. (2009). The puerperium. In: *Veterinary Reproduction and Obstetrics*, 9e (ed. D. Noakes, T. Parkinson, and G. England), 194–205. Philadelphia, PA: WB Saunders.

Noakes, D.E., Parkinson, T.J., and England, G.C. ed. (2018). *Arthur's Veterinary Reproduction and Obstetrics*. St Louis, MO: Elsevier Health Sciences.

Pascottini, O.B., Aurich, C., England, G., and Grahofer, A. (2023). General and comparative aspects of endometritis in domestic species: a review. *Reproduction in Domestic Animals* 58: 49–71.

Peleki, C., Kiosis, E., Polizopoulou, Z.S. et al. (2023). Effect of sugar beet pulp and anionic salts on metabolic status and mineral homeostasis during the peri-parturient period of dairy sheep. *Animals* 13 (2): 213.

Rasbech, N.O. (1950). The normal involution of the uterus in the cow. *Nordisk Veterinaermedicin* 2: 655–687.

Richardson, K. J. (2022). Increasing reproductive efficiency and progeny performance through improved embryonic and genetic selection in cattle. Doctoral dissertation, West Texas A & M University.

Sharun, K. and Erdoğan, G. (2019). A review: obstetrical emergencies in small ruminants. *Alexandria Journal for Veterinary Sciences* 62 (1): 1–16.

Tennant, B. and Peddicord, R.G. (1968). The influence of delayed uterine involution and endometritis on bovine fertility. *Cornell Vet* 58: 185–192.

Tian, W. and Noakes, D.E. (1991). Effects of four hormone treatments after calving on uterine and cervical involution and ovarian activity in cows. *Veterinary Record* 128 (24): 566–569.

Section 2

Disorders of the Male Reproductive System

16

Diseases of the Glans Penis and Prepuce

Felix Uchenna Samuel[1,2], *Ogunkunle Nathaniel*[2], *Adeniyi Njideka*[2], *Idris Sherif*[3], *Hycinth Ndabatsado Kolo*[4], *and Aliyu Abdullahi Mohammed*[5]

[1] *Faculty of Veterinary Medicine, National Animal Production Research Institute, Ahmadu Bello University, Zaria, Nigeria*
[2] *Department of Food and Animal Science, Alabama A&M University, Normal, USA*
[3] *Faculty of Veterinary Medicine, Ahmadu Bello University, Zaria, Nigeria*
[4] *Department of Animal Health and Production, Federal University of Technology, Minna, Nigeria*
[5] *Department of Animal Sciences, Usman Danfodio University, Sokoto, Nigeria*

16.1 Introduction

The glans penis in goats is the terminal part of the male reproductive organ and is located at the distal end of the penis. It is cone shaped and may vary in size and shape among different goat breeds and individual animals. It displays significant diversity among different species, adapting to their distinct reproductive strategies and ecological environments. Just like numerous other mammals, goats have developed distinct attributes in their reproductive system to match their ecological and reproductive requirements. The glans is covered by a specialized fold of skin called the prepuce, which protects it when not in use during copulation. The glans penis consists of erectile tissue, including the corpus cavernosum and corpus spongiosum, which allow it to engorge with blood and become erect during sexual arousal. The presence of the glans penis is essential for successful copulation and the deposition of semen into the female's reproductive tract (Spencer 2019; Lossi 2022).

16.2 Comparative Anatomy of the Glans Penis

The glans penis is a complex structure located at the tip of the penis in mammals. It displays considerable variation in shape and size across different species (Spencer 2019). For instance, primates typically have a prominent glans with distinctive features like ridges and grooves, while rodents may have a more hidden structure. In certain animals like dogs, the glans can be bulbous in shape, which aids in efficient copulation.

Birds have a unique reproductive system, and not all species have a penis. However, for those avian species that possess a penis, like ducks and ostriches, the glans plays a crucial role in the reproductive process. It usually takes on a phallus-like form, which is temporary and inflatable during copulation.

In reptiles and amphibians, if a glans penis is present, it is often simple and lacks specialized features. The shape and size of the glans in these species may vary depending on their mating behaviors and reproductive strategies.

Overall, the diversity of the glans penis across different animals reflects their adaptation to specific reproductive needs and behaviors.

Elements of Reproduction and Reproductive Diseases of Goats, First Edition. Edited by Tanmoy Rana.

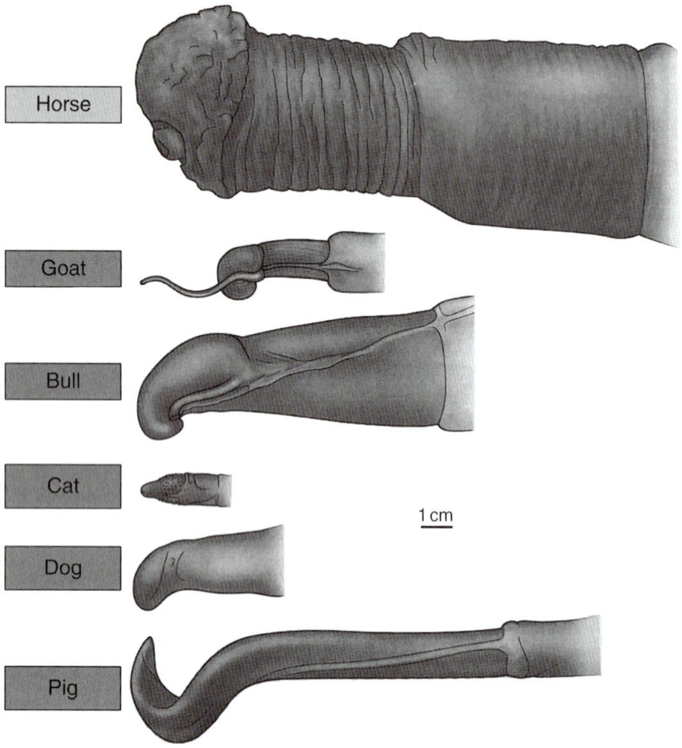

Source: Google Quizlet Inc., 2023.

16.3 Anatomy of the Glans Penis in Goats

The various anatomical features of the glans penis of a goat are summarized below (Islam et al. 2021).

16.3.1 Erectile Tissue

As in many mammals, the glans penis of goats contains erectile tissue responsible for engorgement and rigidity during copulation. The two main types of erectile tissue in the glans are the corpus cavernosum and the corpus spongiosum. When sexually aroused, these tissues fill with blood, causing the glans to enlarge and become erect, which is essential for successful penetration during mating.

16.3.2 Urethral Process

One unique feature of the goat's glans penis is the presence of a prominent structure called the urethral process. This elongated, thread-like projection emerges from the urethral opening of the glans. During copulation, the urethral process plays a crucial role in guiding semen into the female's reproductive tract with precision.

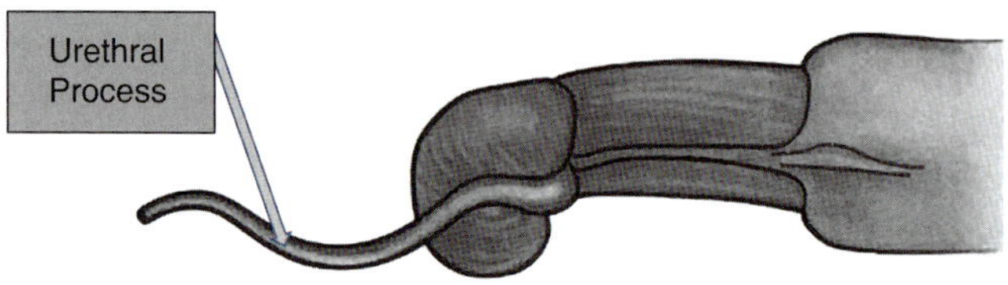

Source: Google Quizlet Inc., 2023.

16.3.3 Sensory Innervation

The glans penis of goats, like in many mammals, is highly sensitive and richly innervated with sensory nerve endings. These specialized nerve endings are responsible for tactile perception during copulation, contributing to sexual arousal and triggering the release of hormones necessary for successful mating.

16.3.4 Penetration Mechanism

During copulation, male goats exhibit a characteristic mating behavior known as "flagging" or "Flehmen response." This involves the male lifting its head, curling back its upper lip, and extending its neck to expose the glans penis while adopting a stiff-legged posture. This action facilitates the introduction of the glans into the female's reproductive tract for insemination.

16.3.5 Role of Glans Penis in Reproduction

The glans penis in goats plays a crucial role in the reproductive process. During mating, the male uses the erect glans penis and the urethral process to achieve successful penetration of the female's vagina. Once inside, the male ejaculates semen into the doe's reproductive tract, initiating the fertilization process and increasing the chances of conception (Bazer 2020).

16.3.6 Seasonal Breeding Behavior

In some goat species, breeding behavior is regulated by photoperiod and is linked to hormonal changes, including fluctuations in testosterone levels, which impact the development and function of the glans penis (Ponce-Covarrubias et al. 2023).

16.3.7 Prepuce

The prepuce is a fold of skin that surrounds and protects the glans penis when it is not in use during copulation. It serves as a sheath that covers the glans and retracts to expose the glans during mating or urination.

The prepuce has a well-developed muscle called the retractor preputii muscle, which contracts to retract the skin and expose the glans penis during sexual arousal or urination. This muscle is under hormonal control and is responsible for the "flagging" behavior observed in male goats during mating.

16.4 Physiology of the Glans Penis and Prepuce in Goats

16.4.1 Erection and Copulation

16.4.1.1 Sexual Arousal and Nitric Oxide Release

Sexual arousal in male goats is triggered by various sensory stimuli, including visual, olfactory, and auditory cues from receptive females. When exposed to these stimuli, sensory nerve endings in the glans penis are stimulated, initiating a neural response that leads to the release of nitric oxide (NO).

Nitric oxide is a potent vasodilator, meaning it relaxes the smooth muscles in the walls of the arteries supplying blood to the erectile tissue of the penis. This relaxation causes the arteries to dilate, allowing increased blood flow into two sponge-like erectile structures within the penis, known as the corpus cavernosum and corpus spongiosum (El-Shalofy et al. 2023).

16.4.1.2 Erection: Engorgement of the Glans Penis

As a result of the increased blood flow, the corpus cavernosum and corpus spongiosum become engorged with blood, causing the glans penis to become erect and firm. This erection is a vital physiological response required for successful mating and penetration.

The erection in male goats, as in many other mammals, is a reflexive response to sexual stimulation. Once the sensory nerve endings in the glans penis are stimulated and nitric oxide is released, the process of erection is initiated. It is an involuntary response that ensures the male is physically prepared for mating (Qi et al. 2023).

16.4.1.3 Role of the Retractor Preputii Muscle in Mating Behavior

When a male goat is sexually aroused and ready to mate, the retractor preputii muscle comes into play. This muscle is responsible for retracting the prepuce, which is the fold of skin covering the glans penis when not erect. This muscle contraction pulls back the prepuce, exposing the erect glans penis and making it accessible for mating.

The retractor preputii muscle's action is an integral part of the mating behavior in male goats. It facilitates successful copulation by revealing the erect penis, allowing for proper positioning and penetration during the mating process.

16.4.1.4 Mating Behavior and Ejaculation

With the glans penis exposed and erect, the male goat engages in mating behavior. This behavior involves various courtship displays, vocalizations, and physical interactions with the receptive female, all aimed at maximizing the chances of successful copulation. Upon successful penetration, ejaculation occurs. During ejaculation, semen containing sperm is expelled from the male's reproductive tract into the female's reproductive tract, facilitating fertilization if conditions are favorable (El-Shalofy et al. 2023).

16.4.2 Scent Marking and Territorial Behavior

The prepuce plays a crucial role in social interactions and reproductive behaviors. This specialized organ houses scent glands that secrete pheromones, chemical signals that carry vital information to other goats. By rubbing their prepuce on surfaces or other goats, males can establish dominance, attract females, and communicate their reproductive readiness. The following reference delves into the significance of the prepuce in male goat behavior, focusing on scent marking and territoriality (Bala and Babbar 2023).

16.4.2.1 Pheromonal Property of the Prepuce

The prepuce is a retractable fold of skin covering the glans penis in male goats. This sheath-like structure is present in various other mammals as well. Within the prepuce are specialized scent glands responsible for secreting pheromones, which are potent chemical substances that play a crucial role in communication within the goat community. The scent glands within the prepuce release pheromones that vary depending on the goat's age, health, and reproductive status. These chemical signals are perceived through the vomeronasal organ (Jacobson's organ) located in the roof of the goat's mouth. This unique organ is dedicated to detecting and processing pheromones, allowing goats to receive and interpret the information conveyed through these chemical signals (Bala and Babbar 2023).

16.4.2.2 Scent Marking: Establishing Dominance and Territory

Scent marking is an essential social behavior in goats. When a male goat rubs its prepuce on surfaces or other goats, it deposits pheromones, thereby marking its territory. The scent left behind serves as a territorial boundary, indicating ownership of a particular area and deterring intruders. Through scent marking, dominant males establish and maintain their status within the group hierarchy, ensuring their access to valuable resources such as food, water, and mating opportunities (Villagrán et al. 2023).

16.4.2.3 Attracting Females and Reproductive Signaling

In the breeding season, the prepuce's role becomes particularly vital for male goats. The pheromones secreted by the scent glands within the prepuce serve as powerful sexual attractants. Female goats (does) are highly sensitive to these chemical cues and can detect them from considerable distances. By rubbing their prepuce on surfaces and other goats, males disseminate their unique scent, indicating their reproductive readiness to potential mates. During this time, males compete fiercely for the attention of females. The dominant males, having established their territory through scent marking, have an advantage in attracting females. The quality and quantity of pheromones can also convey information about a male's genetic fitness and overall health, making them more attractive to potential mates.

16.4.2.4 Communication of Reproductive Readiness

Male goats utilize their prepuce as a means of communicating their reproductive readiness to females. This is particularly crucial in species with seasonal breeding patterns, where successful reproduction must be synchronized with optimal environmental conditions and resource availability. Through pheromone secretion via the prepuce, male goats can synchronize their reproductive cycles with those of the receptive females, enhancing the chances of successful mating and increasing the overall reproductive efficiency of the population. This reproductive synchronization is vital for maintaining genetic diversity and population stability.

16.5 Diseases of the Glans Penis and Prepuce in Goats

The glans penis and prepuce in goats, like any other anatomical structure, can be susceptible to various diseases and conditions that may affect their reproductive health and overall well-being. Below we describe some common diseases that can occur in the glans penis of goats.

16.5.1 Balanoposthitis

Balanoposthitis is a common medical condition in male animals, including goats, characterized by inflammation of the glans penis and the prepuce (sheath) surrounding it. It can arise due to various factors, such as bacterial, viral, or fungal infections, as well as irritants accumulating in the preputial cavity. The following reference explores the causes, symptoms, and potential management strategies for balanoposthitis in male goats (Lillo et al. 2023).

16.5.1.1 Causes of Balanoposthitis

- *Infections*: bacterial, viral, and fungal agents can all trigger balanoposthitis in male goats. Common bacterial causes include *Staphylococcus* spp., *Streptococcus* spp., and *Escherichia coli*. Viral infections may be caused by herpesviruses, while fungal infections can be attributed to *Candida* spp. or other fungi.
- *Irritants*: accumulation of urine or fecal matter in the preputial cavity can act as irritants and cause inflammation. These irritants provide a conducive environment for bacterial growth, exacerbating the condition.
- *Trauma*: injuries to the genital region can also lead to balanoposthitis. Scrapes, cuts, or abrasions can provide entry points for infectious agents, leading to inflammation.

16.5.1.2 Symptoms of Balanoposthitis

Balanoposthitis manifests with several noticeable symptoms.

- *Redness*: the glans penis and prepuce appear reddened due to inflammation.
- *Swelling*: the affected area may become swollen, leading to discomfort and pain.
- *Discharge*: a discharge may be present at the preputial orifice, which can be pus-like, bloody, or watery, depending on the causative agent.
- *Odor*: in cases of infection, a foul odor may emanate from the preputial cavity.
- *Discomfort and pain*: male goats may exhibit signs of discomfort, such as frequent attempts to lick or bite the affected area.

16.5.1.3 Diagnosing Balanoposthitis

To diagnose balanoposthitis in male goats, a veterinarian will conduct a thorough physical examination, considering the presenting symptoms. They may collect samples of the discharge for laboratory analysis to identify the causative agent accurately. Bacterial culture, viral polymerase chain reaction (PCR), or fungal staining can aid in determining the responsible pathogen.

16.5.1.4 Management and Treatment

The treatment of balanoposthitis in male goats depends on the underlying cause.

- *Infections*: antibiotics, antivirals, or antifungal medications are prescribed based on the specific pathogen detected. The treatment may need to be administered topically or systemically, depending on the severity of the infection.
- *Irritants*: proper hygiene practices are crucial to prevent irritants from accumulating in the preputial cavity. Regular cleaning and washing of the genital region can help reduce the risk of balanoposthitis.
- *Supportive care*: pain relief medications may be administered to alleviate discomfort and pain. Additionally, keeping the affected goat in a clean and stress-free environment can aid in the recovery process.
- *Prevention*: implementing good management practices, such as maintaining clean bedding and hygienic living conditions, can reduce the risk of balanoposthitis. Regular health checks and timely treatment of any injuries can also contribute to prevention.

16.5.2 Phimosis

Phimosis is a significant medical condition that can affect male goats, leading to the narrowing of the opening of the prepuce. This constriction makes it challenging or even impossible for the glans penis to be extruded during mating or urination. The following reference explores the causes, symptoms, and implications of phimosis in goats (Hopkins 2006).

16.5.2.1 Causes of Phimosis

- *Congenital*: phimosis can be present at birth as a congenital condition. Some goats may have a naturally narrow preputial opening due to genetic factors.
- *Scarring and inflammation*: trauma, injuries, or infections in the genital area can lead to scarring and inflammation, causing the preputial opening to narrow over time.
- *Infections*: inflammatory conditions or infections involving the prepuce can cause swelling and constriction of the opening, leading to phimosis.
- *Inadequate cleaning and hygiene*: poor hygiene practices may result in the accumulation of debris, smegma, and dirt around the preputial orifice, contributing to the development of phimosis.

16.5.2.2 Symptoms of Phimosis

- *Difficulty in mating*: male goats with phimosis may find it challenging or impossible to extrude the glans penis during mating, leading to fertility issues.
- *Urinary obstruction*: phimosis can obstruct the urinary flow, causing difficulty or pain during urination. In severe cases, this obstruction may lead to urinary retention, a potentially life-threatening condition.
- *Discomfort*: goats suffering from phimosis may exhibit signs of discomfort, such as frequent attempts to urinate or vocalizations indicating pain.
- *Swelling and inflammation*: the preputial area may appear swollen and inflamed due to the restricted opening.

16.5.2.3 Implications of Phimosis

- *Breeding difficulties*: phimosis can significantly impact a male goat's reproductive capacity. Inability to mate successfully can lead to reduced breeding efficiency and lower pregnancy rates in the herd.
- *Urinary complications*: the narrowing of the preputial opening can lead to urinary obstruction, causing discomfort, pain, and potential kidney damage if not promptly addressed.
- *Reproductive health*: phimosis may also lead to the accumulation of smegma and debris within the preputial cavity, increasing the risk of infections and reproductive health issues.

16.5.2.4 Management and Treatment

The management of phimosis in goats depends on the underlying cause and severity of the condition.

- *Medical treatment*: mild cases of phimosis may respond to medical treatment, including antiinflammatory medications and antibiotics to address any underlying infections.
- *Cleaning and hygiene*: ensuring proper hygiene and regular cleaning of the preputial area can help prevent or manage phimosis caused by debris and dirt accumulation.
- *Surgical intervention*: in severe cases of phimosis or when conservative treatments are ineffective, surgical correction may be necessary. The surgical procedure involves widening the preputial opening to allow for normal extrusion of the glans penis.
- *Preventive measures*: proper management practices, including maintaining a clean and hygienic environment, regular health checks, and timely treatment of injuries, can help prevent the development of phimosis.

16.5.3 Paraphimosis

Paraphimosis is a concerning medical condition that can affect male goats, wherein the retracted glans penis becomes stuck outside the prepuce and cannot be retracted back into the sheath. This condition is painful and can lead to severe consequences, such as swelling, impaired blood flow, and tissue damage if not promptly addressed (Stewart and Shipley 2021).

16.5.3.1 Causes of Paraphimosis

Paraphimosis in goats can result from various factors.

- *Inadequate cleaning*: poor hygiene and inadequate cleaning of the preputial region may lead to the accumulation of smegma and debris, causing the glans penis to become trapped outside the prepuce.
- *Sexual activity*: intense or prolonged sexual activity, especially during mating, can cause the glans penis to become engorged and fail to retract into the preputial sheath.
- *Trauma*: injuries or trauma to the genital area can cause the glans penis to become trapped outside the prepuce.
- *Inflammation and infections*: inflammatory conditions or infections involving the prepuce may lead to swelling and constriction of the preputial orifice, resulting in paraphimosis.

16.5.3.2 Symptoms of Paraphimosis

Paraphimosis in goats is characterized by the following symptoms.

- *Inability to retract glans penis*: the glans penis remains stuck outside the prepuce and cannot be retracted back into the sheath.
- *Swelling*: the preputial area may become swollen due to the engorgement of the glans penis and impaired blood flow.
- *Pain and discomfort*: goats suffering from paraphimosis may exhibit signs of distress, such as vocalizations, restlessness, or attempts to lick or bite the affected area.
- *Tissue damage*: prolonged paraphimosis can lead to tissue damage, as the glans penis becomes deprived of oxygen and nutrients, potentially resulting in necrosis.

16.5.3.3 Management and Treatment

Paraphimosis in goats requires prompt and appropriate management to prevent complications and promote recovery. The following steps may be taken.

- *Manual reduction*: in mild cases, manual reduction of the glans penis into the preputial sheath may be attempted by a veterinarian. This should be done gently and with caution to avoid causing further damage.
- *Lubrication*: applying a lubricant around the preputial orifice can aid in facilitating the retraction of the glans penis.
- *Warm compress*: applying a warm compress to the affected area may help reduce swelling and discomfort.
- *Sedation and anesthesia*: in more severe cases, sedation or general anesthesia may be necessary to relax the goat and facilitate the reduction of the glans penis.
- *Surgical intervention*: if manual reduction is unsuccessful or if tissue damage has occurred, surgical intervention may be required to address the condition and prevent complications.

16.5.3.4 Preventive Measures

To prevent paraphimosis in goats, proper hygiene and regular cleaning of the preputial region are crucial. Additionally, monitoring breeding activity and ensuring adequate rest and recovery periods for male goats can help minimize the risk of paraphimosis associated with sexual activity.

16.5.4 Urethral Obstruction

Urethral obstruction in goats is a critical condition that can result from various factors, with stones or calculi blocking the urethra being one of the potential causes. This blockage hinders the normal flow of urine, leading to difficulty urinating and subsequent complications involving the glans penis and surrounding structures. The following reference explores the causes, symptoms, and potential complications of urethral obstruction in goats (Stewart and Shipley 2021).

16.5.4.1 Causes of Urethral Obstruction

Urethral obstruction in goats can be caused by several factors.

- *Urinary stones or calculi*: the presence of mineral deposits, known as stones or calculi, in the urinary tract can obstruct the urethra, preventing the passage of urine.
- *Dehydration*: inadequate water intake can lead to concentrated urine, increasing the risk of stone formation and potential obstruction.

- *Diet*: certain diets high in minerals, such as calcium, phosphorus, and magnesium, can contribute to the formation of urinary stones and increase the likelihood of urethral obstruction.
- *Bladder or urethral tumors*: tumors in the bladder or urethra can cause physical blockage, leading to obstruction.
- *Inflammation or infections*: inflammatory conditions or infections in the urinary tract can cause swelling and narrowing of the urethra, leading to obstruction.

16.5.4.2 Symptoms of Urethral Obstruction

Urethral obstruction in goats can present with the following symptoms.

- *Straining to urinate*: affected goats may repeatedly attempt to urinate without producing much urine.
- *Vocalizations and signs of discomfort*: goats in distress may vocalize, display signs of agitation, and appear restless due to the pain and discomfort associated with obstruction.
- *Abdominal distension*: as urine accumulates in the bladder, the abdomen may become visibly distended.
- *Lack of urination*: complete obstruction can lead to the complete inability to pass urine, resulting in a life-threatening condition known as urinary retention.

16.5.4.3 Complications of Urethral Obstruction

If left untreated, urethral obstruction can lead to severe complications.

- *Hydronephrosis*: backflow of urine into the kidneys can cause swelling and damage to these vital organs, leading to a condition called hydronephrosis.
- *Urethral rupture*: the accumulation of urine and increased pressure within the urinary tract can lead to the rupture of the urethra, a potentially life-threatening situation.
- *Bladder rupture*: in severe cases, the bladder can rupture due to excessive urine retention, resulting in peritonitis, a serious and potentially fatal inflammation of the abdominal cavity.
- *Tissue necrosis*: prolonged obstruction can lead to tissue damage and necrosis in the urethra, bladder, and surrounding structures.

16.5.4.4 Management and Treatment

Urethral obstruction in goats is a veterinary emergency that requires immediate intervention. Treatment options include the following.

- *Catheterization*: passing a urinary catheter into the urethra can help relieve the obstruction and facilitate the drainage of urine.
- *Surgery*: in cases of severe obstruction or when catheterization is not possible, surgical intervention may be necessary to remove the stones or calculi causing the blockage.
- *Fluid therapy*: rehydration and fluid therapy are crucial to correct dehydration and reduce the risk of stone formation.
- *Pain management*: administration of pain medication can alleviate discomfort and distress in affected goats.
- *Dietary changes*: adjusting the goat's diet to reduce mineral intake and promote urinary health may help prevent recurrence.

16.5.5 Pizzle Rot

Pizzle rot is a significant health concern that primarily affects male goats, particularly those raised for meat production. This condition is caused by a bacterial infection and is often associated with unsanitary conditions and the excessive accumulation of urine and feces on the fleece surrounding the glans penis. Pizzle rot can lead to inflammation, ulceration, and the production of foul-smelling discharge. The following references explores the causes, symptoms, and potential management strategies for pizzle rot in goats (Stewart and Shipley 2021).

16.5.5.1 Causes of Pizzle Rot

Pizzle rot is primarily caused by bacterial infections, most commonly associated with the bacterium *Corynebacterium renale*. This pathogen thrives in moist and unsanitary conditions, making male goats raised for meat production particularly susceptible to the condition.

The following factors contribute to the development of pizzle rot.

- *Urine and fecal accumulation*: in unclean or overcrowded housing conditions, male goats may be exposed to excessive urine and feces on their fleece surrounding the glans penis. This creates an ideal environment for bacterial growth and infection.
- *High-protein diet*: diets rich in protein can lead to an increase in urinary ammonia concentration, further promoting the development of pizzle rot.
- *Wet and dirty bedding*: the use of wet or dirty bedding in goat pens can exacerbate the condition by prolonging contact with harmful bacteria.

16.5.5.2 Symptoms of Pizzle Rot

Pizzle rot presents with various noticeable symptoms.

- *Inflammation*: the glans penis and surrounding fleece become inflamed due to the bacterial infection.
- *Ulceration*: pizzle rot can cause the development of painful ulcers on the affected area.
- *Foul-smelling discharge*: infected goats may exhibit a noticeable, foul-smelling discharge from the glans penis.
- *Agitation and pain*: male goats suffering from pizzle rot may display signs of discomfort, such as restlessness, vocalizations, or attempts to lick or bite the affected area.

16.5.5.3 Management and Treatment

The management and treatment of pizzle rot in goats involve addressing both the infection and its underlying causes.

- *Hygiene and sanitation*: ensuring clean and sanitary living conditions is crucial to preventing pizzle rot. Regularly cleaning goat pens, providing dry and clean bedding, and maintaining proper ventilation can help reduce the risk of bacterial growth.
- *Trimming fleece*: regularly trimming the fleece surrounding the glans penis can minimize the accumulation of urine and feces, reducing the risk of infection.
- *Antibiotic treatment*: veterinary intervention is essential to administer appropriate antibiotics to treat the bacterial infection. Systemic or topical antibiotics may be prescribed, depending on the severity of the condition.
- *Dietary adjustment*: modifying the goat's diet to reduce protein levels can help decrease urinary ammonia concentration and reduce the risk of pizzle rot development.
- *Pain management*: administration of pain medication can help alleviate discomfort and pain associated with pizzle rot.

16.5.5.4 Preventive Measures

Implementing preventive measures is crucial in managing pizzle rot and promoting overall goat health.

- *Regular health checks*: regular veterinary check-ups can help identify and address early signs of pizzle rot.
- *Cleanliness and hygiene*: maintaining clean and hygienic living conditions is vital in preventing the development of pizzle rot.
- *Proper diet*: providing a well-balanced diet with appropriate protein levels can reduce the risk of urinary ammonia concentration and subsequent bacterial growth.

16.5.6 Contagious Ecthyma (Orf)

Contagious ecthyma, commonly known as orf or sore mouth, is a viral disease that affects goats and other small ruminants. This infectious condition can manifest in various parts of the goat's body, including the mouth, lips, and sometimes even the glans penis. The disease leads to the formation of painful, contagious sores, which can have significant impacts on feeding, mating, and overall health in affected goats. The following reference explores the symptoms, impact, and management of contagious ecthyma in goats (Stewart and Shipley 2021).

16.5.6.1 Symptoms of Contagious Ecthyma

Contagious ecthyma is characterized by the following symptoms.

- *Formation of lesions*: painful and contagious sores, often with a thick, scab-like crust, appear on the mouth, lips, and other parts of the body, including the glans penis in some cases.

- *Reduced feeding*: the presence of painful mouth sores can lead to difficulty in eating and reduced appetite, potentially leading to weight loss.
- *Reluctance to mate*: male goats with lesions on the glans penis may experience discomfort during mating, leading to reduced breeding activity.
- *Contagious nature*: contagious ecthyma can easily spread from one goat to another through direct contact or exposure to contaminated surfaces.

16.5.6.2 Impact on Feeding and Nutrition

The presence of painful sores in the mouth can significantly affect a goat's ability to eat and feed properly. Goats with oral lesions may experience difficulty in grasping and chewing food, leading to reduced food intake and, subsequently, weight loss. Proper nutrition is vital for the health and productivity of goats, and compromised feeding due to contagious ecthyma can result in decreased growth rates and lower milk production in lactating does.

16.5.6.3 Impact on Mating Behavior

In male goats, the formation of painful lesions on the glans penis can lead to reluctance to mate. The discomfort and pain experienced during breeding may result in reduced libido and mating activity, affecting the goat's reproductive efficiency and the overall breeding performance of the herd.

16.5.6.4 Management and Treatment

Managing contagious ecthyma in goats involves several measures.

- *Isolation*: isolate affected goats from the rest of the herd to prevent further spread of the virus.
- *Topical treatment*: the sores can be treated topically with antiseptic solutions to promote healing and prevent secondary bacterial infections.
- *Pain management*: administering pain relief medications can alleviate discomfort and improve feeding and mating behaviors.
- *Nutritional support*: providing palatable and easily consumable feed can encourage goats with oral lesions to eat and maintain proper nutrition.
- *Hygiene practices*: practicing good hygiene is essential to prevent the spread of the virus. Regularly clean and disinfect surfaces and equipment that may come into contact with infected animals.
- *Vaccination*: vaccination against contagious ecthyma is available in some regions and can be effective in preventing the disease or reducing its severity.

16.5.6.5 Preventive Measures

Implementing preventive measures is crucial to minimize the risk of contagious ecthyma.

- *Quarantine*: new animals introduced to the herd should be quarantined and monitored for signs of the disease before being integrated into the main herd.
- *Hygiene*: regularly clean and disinfect areas where goats congregate, especially during periods of outbreaks.
- *Monitoring*: regularly monitor the health of the herd and promptly isolate and treat any suspected cases of contagious ecthyma.

16.5.7 Vesicular Stomatitis

Vesicular stomatitis is a viral disease that can affect various livestock species, including goats. This infectious condition causes the formation of vesicles and ulcers in the oral and genital areas of goats, including the glans penis. The presence of vesicles and ulcers on the glans penis can lead to discomfort during mating and potentially reduce fertility. The following reference explores the impact of vesicular stomatitis on the oral and genital health of goats, with a specific focus on its effects on the glans penis and reproductive capabilities (Stewart and Shipley 2021).

16.5.7.1 Vesicular Stomatitis in Goats

Vesicular stomatitis is caused by the vesicular stomatitis virus (VSV), which belongs to the family Rhabdoviridae. The virus primarily affects the oral mucosa, leading to the formation of fluid-filled vesicles and subsequent ulceration. In some cases, vesicles and ulcers may also develop in the genital area, including the glans penis of male goats.

16.5.7.2 Impact on the Glans Penis

In male goats, vesicular stomatitis can lead to the development of vesicles and ulcers on the glans penis. These lesions can cause discomfort and pain, particularly during mating activities. The presence of painful ulcers on the glans penis may result in reluctance to mate, reduced breeding activity, and suboptimal reproductive performance in infected bucks.

16.5.7.3 Discomfort During Mating

The discomfort caused by the vesicles and ulcers on the glans penis can lead to a decrease in libido and mating behavior in male goats. The pain and irritation during mating may result in reduced breeding efficiency and lower pregnancy rates, leading to potential economic losses for goat producers.

16.5.7.4 Impact on Fertility

Vesicular stomatitis can indirectly impact fertility in goats due to reduced mating activity caused by the discomfort and pain associated with the lesions on the glans penis. Bucks may be less inclined to actively engage in mating, leading to lower rates of successful mating and subsequent pregnancies in the herd.

16.5.7.5 Management and Treatment

There is no specific treatment for vesicular stomatitis, and management focuses on supportive care and prevention of disease spread.

- *Isolation*: infected goats should be isolated from the rest of the herd to prevent further spread of the virus.
- *Hydration and nutrition*: providing proper hydration and nutrition to affected goats can support their immune response and overall health.
- *Pain management*: administering pain relief medications can help alleviate discomfort and encourage normal feeding and breeding behaviors.
- *Hygiene practices*: practicing strict biosecurity measures, such as regularly cleaning and disinfecting facilities and equipment, can help prevent the spread of the virus.

16.5.7.6 Preventive Measures

Preventing vesicular stomatitis is essential to maintain goat health and productivity.

- *Quarantine*: new animals introduced to the herd should be quarantined and monitored for signs of vesicular stomatitis before being integrated into the main herd.
- *Vector control*: controlling insect vectors, such as flies and mosquitoes, can help reduce the risk of virus transmission.
- *Surveillance*: regularly monitor the health of the herd and promptly report any suspected cases of vesicular stomatitis to veterinary authorities.

16.5.8 Tumors and Growths

Tumors and growths in goats, such as papillomas or squamous cell carcinomas, can occur on or near the glans penis. These growths can have significant implications for the reproductive health and mating behavior of male goats. Depending on their nature and severity, surgical intervention may be necessary to manage these conditions. The following reference explores the impact of tumors and growths on the glans penis of goats, their effects on mating behavior, and the potential need for surgical treatment (Stewart and Shipley 2021).

16.5.8.1 Types of Tumors and Growths

Several types of tumors and growths can develop on or around the glans penis in goats.

- *Papillomas*: papillomas are benign, wart-like growths caused by certain types of viruses. While they are generally noncancerous, papillomas can interfere with mating and cause discomfort.
- *Squamous cell carcinomas*: squamous cell carcinomas are malignant tumors that arise from the squamous cells lining the glans penis. These growths can be aggressive and may lead to significant complications if left untreated.
- *Fibromas*: fibromas are benign tumors composed of fibrous tissue and can develop on the glans penis or surrounding areas.

16.5.8.2 Impact on Mating Behavior

Tumors and growths on the glans penis can interfere with normal mating behavior in male goats. Depending on the location, size, and nature of the growths, affected goats may experience discomfort or pain during mating attempts. This discomfort can result in reduced libido and mating activity, leading to decreased breeding efficiency and lower reproductive performance in infected bucks.

16.5.8.3 Need for Surgical Intervention

The need for surgical intervention depends on the type and extent of the tumors or growths.

- *Papillomas*: in most cases, papillomas do not require surgical treatment and may resolve spontaneously over time. However, if the growths are causing significant interference with mating or if they are particularly large and persistent, surgical removal may be considered.
- *Squamous cell carcinomas*: squamous cell carcinomas are aggressive malignant tumors and generally require surgical intervention for proper diagnosis and treatment. Early detection and surgical removal are crucial to prevent further spread and potential complications.
- *Fibromas*: benign fibromas may or may not require surgical removal, depending on their size and location. While some fibromas may resolve on their own, others may need surgical excision if they cause discomfort or hinder normal mating behavior.

16.5.8.4 Management and Treatment

Management and treatment of tumors and growths on the glans penis involve the following.

- *Veterinary evaluation*: early diagnosis and proper evaluation by a veterinarian are essential to determine the nature of the growth and the most appropriate course of action.
- *Surgical intervention*: if surgical removal is deemed necessary, a veterinarian can perform the procedure under appropriate anesthesia and aseptic conditions.
- *Pain management*: administering pain relief medications post surgery can help alleviate discomfort and promote recovery.
- *Follow-up care*: regular follow-up examinations by a veterinarian are crucial to monitor the healing process and detect any potential recurrence or complications.

16.6 Trauma and Injuries

Injuries to the glans penis in goats can occur due to various reasons, including accidents, aggressive mating behaviors, or improper handling during breeding. These injuries may vary in severity, ranging from minor abrasions to more severe wounds that require veterinary attention. Timely and appropriate management is essential to prevent infections and promote healing in affected goats. The following reference discusses the causes, severity, and management of glans penis injuries in goats (Stewart and Shipley 2021).

16.6.1 Causes of Glans Penis Injuries

Several factors can lead to glans penis injuries in goats.

- *Accidents*: goats can sustain injuries to their genital area due to accidents, such as getting caught in fencing or equipment.
- *Aggressive mating behaviors*: during mating, male goats may display aggressive behaviors, including forceful thrusting or mounting, which can lead to injuries.
- *Improper handling during breeding*: improper handling of goats during breeding or artificial insemination procedures can result in unintended injuries to the glans penis.

16.6.2 Severity of Injuries

Glans penis injuries can vary in severity.

- *Minor abrasions*: minor injuries may involve superficial abrasions or small cuts on the glans penis, causing mild discomfort.

- *Lacerations*: more severe injuries may lead to lacerations or deeper wounds that can cause pain and bleeding.
- *Puncture wounds*: in some cases, puncture wounds can occur if the glans penis is pierced by sharp objects or during aggressive mating.
- *Fractures*: in rare cases of extreme force, the glans penis may suffer fractures, which can be extremely painful and require immediate veterinary attention.

16.6.3 Symptoms of Glans Penis Injuries

- *Pain and discomfort*: goats with glans penis injuries may exhibit signs of pain and discomfort, such as vocalizations, restlessness, or reluctance to mate.
- *Bleeding*: depending on the severity of the injury, bleeding may be visible around the glans penis.
- *Swelling*: the injured area may become swollen due to inflammation.
- *Abnormal mating behavior*: injuries can result in altered mating behavior, including decreased libido or avoidance of mating.

16.6.4 Management and Treatment

The management of glans penis injuries in goats involves the following.

- *Veterinary examination*: a thorough examination by a veterinarian is essential to assess the severity of the injury and determine the appropriate course of action.
- *Wound cleaning*: cleaning the wound and keeping it free from debris and dirt is crucial to prevent infection.
- *Antibiotics*: in cases of open wounds, administering antibiotics may be necessary to prevent or treat infections.
- *Pain management*: providing pain relief medications can alleviate discomfort and encourage normal behaviors.
- *Restricting mating*: depending on the severity of the injury, it may be necessary to temporarily restrict the goat from mating until the wound heals.
- *Proper husbandry*: ensuring proper husbandry practices and handling during breeding can help reduce the risk of injuries.

16.6.5 Preventive Measures

Implementing preventive measures can minimize the risk of glans penis injuries.

- *Safe environment*: providing a safe and well-maintained environment for goats can reduce the likelihood of accidents and injuries.
- *Monitoring mating behavior*: regularly monitoring mating behavior can help identify and address any aggressive behaviors that may lead to injuries.
- *Proper handling*: properly handling goats during breeding or artificial insemination procedures can minimize the risk of injuries.

16.7 Conclusion

Diseases affecting the glans penis and prepuce in goats can have significant implications for their reproductive health and overall well-being. Balanoposthitis, phimosis, paraphimosis, urethral obstruction, pizzle rot, contagious ecthyma, and vesicular stomatitis are some of the conditions that can affect the genital region of male goats. Timely diagnosis, proper management, and preventive measures are crucial in maintaining the health and productivity of goats in a herd. Veterinary intervention, good hygiene practices, and providing a clean and stress-free environment are essential components of effective disease prevention and control strategies for goat owners and managers.

References

Anderson, D.E. (2008). Surgery of the prepuce and penis. *Veterinary Clinics of North America: Food Animal Practice* 24 (2): 245–251.

Bala, B. and Babbar, B. K. (2023). Sex pheromones of preputial gland: their chemical identification and role in social & reproductive behaviour of house rat, *Rattus rattus*. https://assets.researchsquare.com/files/rs-2745121/v1/908912e1-cd62-42ac-80fb-8afd662abf3a.pdf?c=1680798571 (accessed 3 April 2023).

Bazer, F.W. (2020). Reproductive physiology of sheep (Ovis aries) and goats (Capra aegagrus hircus). *Animal Agriculture* 2020: 199–209.

El-Shalofy, A.S., Samir, H., and El-Sherbiny, H.R. (2023). Intramuscular administration of l-arginine boosts testicular hemodynamics, plasma concentrations of testosterone and nitric oxide in heat-stressed rams. *Theriogenology* 197: 127–132.

Hopkins, F.M. (2006). Diseases of the reproductive system of the bull. In: *Current Therapy in Large Animal Theriogenology*, 2e (ed. R.S. Youngquist and W.R. Threlfall), 310–322. St Louis, MO: Elsevier Health Sciences.

Islam, R., Uddin Ahmed, S.S., Golam Kibria, A.S.M. et al. (2021). Gross anatomy of urethra and penis in uncastrated and castrated buck of black Bengal goat. *International Journal of Morphology* 39 (1): 138–142.

Lillo, E., Pellegrini, F., Rizzo, A. et al. (2023). In vitro activity of ozone/oxygen gaseous mixture against a caprine herpesvirus type 1 strain isolated from a goat with vaginitis. *Animals* 13 (12): 1920.

Lossi, L. (2022). Anatomical features for an adequate choice of the experimental animal model in biomedicine: III. Ferret, goat, sheep, and horse. *Annals of Anatomy* 144: 151978.

Maxie, M.G. (2007). *Jubb, Kennedy and Palmer's Pathology of Domestic Animals*, 5e, vol. 3, 566–620. St Louis, MO: Elsevier Health Science.

Metzler, J.A., Price, E.O., Kitchell, R.L., and Bondurant, R.H. (1988). Sexual behavior of male dairy goats: effects of deafferentation of the genitalia. *Physiology & Behavior* 43 (2): 207–212.

Ponce-Covarrubias, J.L., García y González, E.C., Pineda-Burgos, B.C. et al. (2023). Annual sexual behavior in Boer bucks located in the Guerrero tropics in Mexico. *Ruminants* 3 (2): 149–157.

Qi, L., Iskols, M., Handler, A., and Ginty, D.D. (2023). Krause corpuscles of the genitalia are vibrotactile sensors required for normal sexual behavior. *bioRxiv*, preprint. https://doi.org/10.1101/2023.06.14.545006.

Scully, C.M. (2021). Management of urologic conditions in small ruminants. *Veterinary Clinics of North America: Food Animal Practice* 37 (1): 93–104.

Smith, M.C. and Sherman, D.M. (2009). *Goat Medicine*. Hoboken, NJ: Wiley.

Spencer, E. (2019). Animal anatomy and physiology. In: *Mosby's Comprehensive Review for Veterinary Technicians* (ed. M. Tighe and M. Brown), 1–23. St Louis, MO: Elsevier.

Stewart, J.L. and Shipley, C.F. (2021). Management of reproductive diseases in male small ruminants. *Veterinary Clinics of North America: Food Animal Practice* 37 (1): 105–123.

Villagrán, M., Ceva, M., Machiñena, A. et al. (2023). The environment matters: season and female contact affect the behavior of captive Addax nasomaculatus male antelope. *Acta Ethologica* 26 (2): 109–117.

17

Diseases of the Urethra

Felix Uchenna Samuel[1,2], *Ogunkunle Nathaniel*[2], *Kolawole Jonathan Bamidele*[3], *Idris Sherif*[3], *and Hycinth Ndabatsado Kolo*[4]

[1] *Faculty of Veterinary Medicine, National Animal Production Research Institute, Ahmadu Bello University, Zaria, Nigeria*
[2] *Department of Food and Animal Science, Alabama A&M University, Normal, USA*
[3] *Faculty of Veterinary Medicine, Ahmadu Bello University, Zaria, Nigeria*
[4] *Department of Animal Health and Production, Federal University of Technology, Minna, Nigeria*

17.1 Introduction

The goat's urethra is a specialized tube made up of smooth muscle and lined with mucous membrane. Its length, diameter, and structure may vary slightly among individual goats, but it generally follows a similar pattern. The urethra begins at the neck of the bladder, where it connects to the ureters, the tubes responsible for transporting urine from the kidneys to the bladder. From the bladder neck, the urethra extends downward through the pelvic region and the floor of the pelvis, passing through the urethral sphincter muscles. These sphincter muscles provide control over the release of urine, allowing goats to voluntarily retain urine until an appropriate time for urination. As the urethra continues its course, it passes through the external urethral orifice, which is the opening through which urine is expelled from the body during urination. In males, the urethra also serves as a conduit for the expulsion of semen during ejaculation (Hafez and Hafez 2013) (Figure 17.1).

17.2 General Function of the Goat's Urethra

The primary function of the urethra in goats is to eliminate urine from the body. Urine is a waste product produced by the kidneys during the filtration of blood. It contains water, electrolytes, and other waste substances that need to be removed from the body to maintain proper bodily functions and homeostasis. During urination, the muscular walls of the bladder contract, forcing urine into the urethra. The urethral sphincters, located at the junction between the bladder and urethra, act as valves to control the flow of urine. When these sphincters relax, urine is expelled from the urethra and exits the body through the urethral orifice.

17.3 Anatomy and Function of the Male Urethra

The urethra in goats, as in other mammals, is a muscular tube that extends from the urinary bladder to the external opening called the urethral orifice. In males, the urethra is responsible for the elimination of both urine and semen during ejaculation (Runcan and da Silva 2022).

The male urethra is a tubular structure that runs through the penis, connecting the urinary bladder to the external environment. It consists of three main segments: the prostatic urethra, the membranous urethra, and the spongy (penile) urethra. Each segment is surrounded by specific tissues and serves distinct functions (Ramírez-González and Sansone 2022).

Elements of Reproduction and Reproductive Diseases of Goats, First Edition. Edited by Tanmoy Rana.

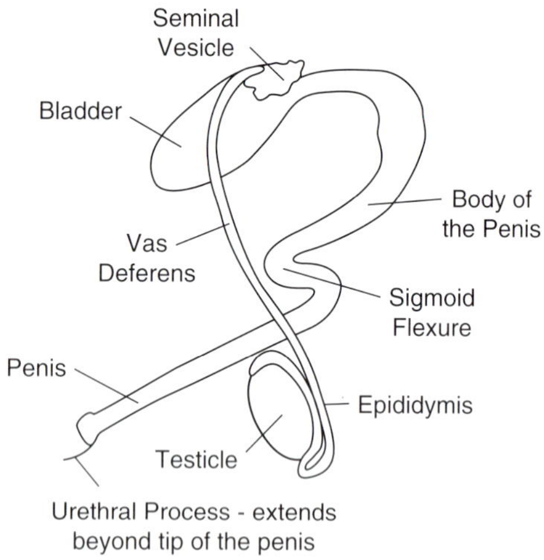

Figure 17.1 Anatomical representation of a buck's reproductive system. *Source:* www.infovets.com/books/smrm/B/B710.htm.

17.3.1 Prostatic Urethra

The prostatic urethra is the initial portion of the male urethra and extends through the prostate gland. This segment is approximately 3–4 cm in length and is lined with transitional epithelium. During ejaculation, the prostate gland contributes essential components to semen, including enzymes and nutrients that support sperm viability (Brenner 2022).

17.3.2 Membranous Urethra

The membranous urethra follows the prostatic urethra and measures around 1 cm in length. It passes through the pelvic floor muscles and is lined with stratified or pseudo-stratified columnar epithelium. This segment plays a crucial role in controlling the release of urine and semen by its position between the urinary and reproductive systems (Ramírez-González and Sansone 2022).

17.3.3 Spongy (Penile) Urethra

The longest segment of the male urethra is the spongy urethra, which extends through the length of the penis. It measures approximately 15 cm and runs within the corpus spongiosum, a sponge-like erectile tissue. The spongy urethra is lined with stratified columnar and pseudo-stratified columnar epithelium. During ejaculation, semen travels through this segment and exits the body through the external urethral orifice located at the tip of the penis (Ramírez-González and Sansone 2022).

17.3.4 Dual Role in Urine and Semen Elimination

17.3.4.1 Urinary Function

The primary function of the male urethra is the elimination of urine, a waste product produced by the kidneys. When the urinary bladder is full, it contracts and urine flows into the prostatic urethra. The presence of urine in the prostatic and membranous urethra signals the brain to initiate the micturition reflex. The external urethral sphincter, a ring-like muscle surrounding the urethra, relaxes and the detrusor muscle contracts, expelling urine from the body. This process is known as urination or voiding (Mitchell et al. 2022).

17.3.4.2 Reproductive Function

Apart from its urinary function, the male urethra also plays a critical role in reproduction. During sexual arousal, the penis becomes erect due to increased blood flow to the erectile tissues. This is a result of signals from the autonomic nervous system in response to sexual stimuli. When sexual stimulation reaches a threshold, the nervous system triggers ejaculation. During ejaculation, the smooth muscles in the walls of the epididymis, vas deferens, and seminal vesicles contract, pushing semen into the prostatic urethra. At the same time, the bladder neck sphincter closes to prevent retrograde ejaculation (semen entering the bladder). The semen then travels through the membranous and spongy urethra before being expelled through the penis.

17.3.4.3 Mechanisms of Separation During Ejaculation

One might wonder how the male urethra successfully separates urine and semen during ejaculation, preventing the simultaneous expulsion of both fluids. The key to this separation lies in the coordination of various physiological processes (Garaffa et al. 2010).

17.3.4.3.1 Closure of the Bladder Neck

During sexual arousal, the sympathetic nervous system stimulates the closure of the bladder neck sphincter. This prevents the backward flow of semen into the bladder during ejaculation.

17.3.4.3.2 Rhythmic Contractions

Ejaculation involves rhythmic contractions of various reproductive structures, including the epididymis, vas deferens, seminal vesicles, and prostate gland. These contractions propel semen forward through the male urethra and out of the body.

17.3.4.3.3 Inhibition of Urinary Reflex

The spinal cord plays a crucial role in coordinating the reflexes involved in ejaculation and urination. During ejaculation, inhibitory signals prevent the activation of the micturition reflex, effectively suppressing the urge to urinate.

17.4 Anatomy and Function of the Female Urethra

17.4.1 Anatomy

In female goats, the urethra is relatively short compared to other animals, but it serves its purpose efficiently. The urethra starts at the neck of the bladder and extends to the external urethral orifice located just below the vaginal opening. The female goat's urethra is encased in surrounding tissues and muscles, ensuring its proper functioning and preventing leakage of urine. The urethral sphincters, which are circular muscles around the urethra's opening, play a crucial role in controlling the flow of urine. These muscles remain contracted to maintain continence, and relaxation allows the release of urine during the micturition process (Radostits et al. 2010).

17.4.2 Function: Urine Elimination

The primary function of the urethra in female goats is to facilitate the elimination of urine from the body. Urination, also known as micturition, is a vital excretory process that helps maintain fluid balance and rid the body of waste products. As the kidneys filter blood to remove excess water, waste products, and toxins, the resulting liquid waste, or urine, is stored in the bladder until it needs to be expelled. When the bladder fills with urine, it stimulates stretch receptors that signal the nervous system to initiate the micturition reflex. This reflex triggers a series of coordinated muscular contractions. The detrusor muscle in the bladder wall contracts, while the urethral sphincters relax. The combination of these actions allows urine to flow from the bladder, through the urethra, and out of the body through the external urethral orifice.

In female goats, the urethra is shorter and opens into the vulva, separate from the reproductive tract. The opening is situated beneath the clitoral area (Radostits et al. 2010).

17.5 Diseases of the Urethra

Goats, like any other animals, can face certain health issues related to the urethra. Some of the common problems include the following (Radostits et al. 2010).

17.5.1 Urethral Prolapse

Urethral prolapse in goats is an uncommon but serious condition that requires prompt attention and appropriate management. Here we explore the factors contributing to urethral prolapse, clinical signs, and treatment options.

17.5.1.1 Factors Contributing to Urethral Prolapse

- *Hormonal imbalances*: hormonal changes, particularly an imbalance of estrogen, have been associated with the development of urethral prolapse. Estrogen is responsible for maintaining the integrity of the tissues in the urogenital area, and an imbalance can weaken the tissues, leading to prolapse.
- *Trauma*: physical trauma to the genital area can also be a factor in causing urethral prolapse. This trauma may occur during mating, parturition (giving birth), or other accidents or injuries involving the urogenital region.

17.5.1.2 Clinical Signs of Urethral Prolapse

- *Visible mass in the genital area*: one of the most obvious signs of urethral prolapse is protrusion of the urethral tissue through the external opening. This visible mass can be red or pink in color and may be mistaken for a prolapsed uterus in female goats.
- *Difficulty in urination*: goats with urethral prolapse may experience difficulty or pain while urinating. They may strain to pass urine due to the obstruction caused by the prolapsed tissue.

17.5.1.3 Treatment Options for Urethral Prolapse

Surgical treatment is usually required to address urethral prolapse effectively. The specific procedure may vary depending on the severity of the prolapse and the individual goat's condition. Here are some common surgical options.

- *Urethral repositioning*: in less severe cases, the veterinarian may attempt to reposition the prolapsed tissue back into its normal position and suture the area to prevent further prolapse.
- *Urethral amputation*: in more severe cases or instances of tissue necrosis, partial or complete amputation of the prolapsed tissue may be necessary.

In some cases, hormonal therapy may be prescribed to help balance hormone levels and reduce the risk of further prolapse.

17.5.2 Contagious Ecthyma (Orf)

Contagious ecthyma, also known as orf or sore mouth, is a viral disease that primarily affects the skin of goats and other ruminants. However, in some cases, it can lead to secondary complications in the urethra and urinary system. Here we explore the transmission, clinical signs, diagnostic methods, potential impact, preventive measures, and treatment options for contagious ecthyma of the urethra in goats.

17.5.2.1 Transmission

Contagious ecthyma is caused by the orf virus, which belongs to the Parapoxvirus genus. The virus can be transmitted through direct contact with infected animals or indirectly through contaminated objects or the environment. Goat kids are particularly susceptible to contracting the virus, and the infection is more common in younger animals with developing immune systems. Additionally, areas with poor hygiene and overcrowded conditions can facilitate spread of the virus.

17.5.2.2 Clinical Signs

The primary clinical signs of contagious ecthyma involve lesions on the skin, particularly around the lips, mouth, and teats. However, in some cases, the virus can also affect the urethra and urinary system. When the urethra is involved, clinical signs may include the following.

- *Difficulty in urination*: the presence of lesions or swelling in the urethra can lead to obstruction, making it difficult for the goat to pass urine normally.
- *Painful urination*: the irritation and inflammation caused by the virus in the urethra can result in pain and discomfort during urination.
- *Inflammation and edema*: the urethra may become swollen and inflamed due to the viral infection, leading to edema (fluid accumulation) in the affected area.
- *Secondary urinary tract infections (UTIs)*: the compromised urethral tissue can create an entry point for bacteria, leading to secondary UTIs.

17.5.2.3 Diagnostic Methods

Diagnosing contagious ecthyma involves a thorough clinical examination and considering the presence of skin lesions, particularly around the lips, mouth, and teats. For cases involving the urethra, additional examination of the genital and urinary areas is necessary to identify any swelling, lesions, or obstruction. Veterinary professionals may also take samples from the lesions and conduct laboratory tests, such as polymerase chain reaction (PCR) assays, to confirm the presence of the orf virus.

17.5.2.4 Potential Impact on the Urethra and Urinary System

Contagious ecthyma affecting the urethra can result in significant discomfort and pain for the goat. The obstruction of the urethra can lead to urinary retention, causing the bladder to become distended and potentially leading to secondary complications like UTIs. If not promptly and appropriately treated, these secondary infections can spread to the kidneys and other parts of the urinary system, posing serious health risks to the goat.

17.5.2.5 Preventive Measures

Preventing contagious ecthyma involves implementing good biosecurity practices. Preventive measures include the following.

- *Isolation*: isolate infected animals from healthy ones to prevent the spread of the virus.
- *Hygiene*: maintain proper hygiene by regularly cleaning and disinfecting equipment, facilities, and hands to reduce the risk of transmission.
- *Vaccination*: in some regions, vaccines are available to protect against contagious ecthyma. Consult with a veterinarian to determine the appropriate vaccination strategy for your goat herd.
- *Avoid overcrowding*: reduce overcrowding in living spaces to minimize the chances of virus transmission.

17.5.2.6 Treatment Options

Treatment for contagious ecthyma focuses on supportive care and managing secondary complications, especially if the urethra is affected. Veterinary interventions may include the following.

- *Pain management*: providing pain relief to alleviate discomfort during urination.
- *Antibiotics*: administering antibiotics to treat secondary UTIs.
- *Urethral catheterization*: in severe cases of urethral obstruction, a veterinarian may need to catheterize the goat to relieve urinary retention.
- *Topical treatments*: applying topical ointments or creams to soothe and promote healing of the lesions in the urethral area.
- *Symptomatic care*: ensuring the goat receives adequate nutrition, hydration, and rest to support its immune system during recovery.

17.5.3 Urinary Tract Infections (UTIs)

UTIs are a prevalent health concern in various animals, including goats. These infections occur when bacteria or other pathogens enter and multiply in the urinary system, leading to inflammation and discomfort. While both male and female goats can be affected, UTIs are more common in females due to their shorter urethra, which facilitates easier bacterial ascent to the bladder.

17.5.3.1 Causes of UTIs in Goats

UTIs in goats are often caused by bacterial infections. The most common pathogens involved include *Escherichia coli*, *Staphylococcus* spp., *Streptococcus* spp., and *Proteus* spp., among others. These bacteria can enter the urinary system through various means.

- *Ascending infection*: in female goats, the shorter urethra makes it easier for bacteria to travel up from the external environment, enter the urinary tract, and reach the bladder. This is a common route of infection for females.
- *Hematogenous spread*: bacteria may enter the bloodstream from other infected areas in the body and reach the kidneys, causing an ascending UTI.
- *Contaminated water or feed*: poor hygiene practices, contaminated water sources, or feed can introduce bacteria to the goat's system, increasing the risk of UTIs.
- *Catheterization or medical procedures*: in some cases, medical procedures involving catheters or improper sterilization can introduce bacteria into the urinary tract.

17.5.3.2 Symptoms of UTIs in Goats

Identifying UTIs in goats is crucial for early intervention and effective treatment. Some common symptoms of UTIs in goats include the following.

- *Frequent urination*: infected goats may exhibit more frequent attempts to urinate.
- *Painful urination*: goats with UTIs may strain or show signs of discomfort while urinating.
- *Blood in urine*: hematuria, or blood in the urine, can be indicative of a UTI.
- *Foul-smelling urine*: the presence of strong or abnormal odors in the urine might suggest an infection.
- *Decreased appetite*: goats may experience a loss of appetite due to the discomfort caused by the UTI.
- *Lethargy and reduced activity*: infections can lead to general malaise and reduced activity levels.

17.5.4 Urolithiasis

Urolithiasis, a common condition in goats, is characterized by the formation of urinary calculi or stones within the urinary tract. These stones can obstruct the urethra, leading to significant difficulties in urination, intense pain, and potential damage to the urinary organs. Urolithiasis poses a considerable health risk to goats, making it essential for goat keepers to be aware of its causes, symptoms, and preventive measures. This section explores the nature of urolithiasis in goats and the potential impact it can have on their urinary system (Bamal et al. 2023).

17.5.4.1 Formation of Urinary Calculi

Urolithiasis in goats results from the accumulation of minerals and other substances in the urinary tract, leading to the formation of calculi or stones. The most common type of urinary calculi in goats is composed of magnesium ammonium phosphate (struvite) or calcium carbonate. The formation of these stones is influenced by various factors, including diet, hydration, and individual goat factors.

Diet plays a crucial role in the development of urolithiasis. Goats that consume diets high in phosphates and calcium, combined with low water intake, are at increased risk. Concentrate-rich diets, such as those heavy in grains, can be problematic as they may lack adequate roughage, leading to insufficient fiber intake. The insufficient fiber can result in reduced rumination, decreased saliva production, and altered mineral balance in the urine, promoting stone formation.

17.5.4.2 Implications and Symptoms

When urinary calculi form and grow in size, they can eventually obstruct the urethra, which is particularly problematic in male goats due to their longer and narrower urethra. The obstruction prevents the normal passage of urine, leading to symptoms such as the following.

- *Straining to urinate*: goats with urolithiasis will attempt to urinate frequently but struggle to pass urine.
- *Abdominal distension*: the abdomen may become visibly swollen and tense due to the accumulation of urine.
- *Pain and discomfort*: affected goats may exhibit signs of discomfort, restlessness, and vocalization due to the pain caused by the urinary obstruction.
- *Kicking or biting at the flank*: goats may display this behavior as a response to the pain and discomfort.
- *Decreased appetite*: pain and discomfort can lead to a reduced desire to eat.
- *Lethargy*: affected goats may become lethargic and inactive.

17.5.4.3 Potential Damage and Complications

If left untreated, urinary obstruction caused by urolithiasis can lead to severe complications.

- *Rupture of the bladder*: the build-up of urine can lead to excessive pressure on the bladder, potentially causing it to rupture.
- *Urethral rupture*: the pressure from the obstructed urine can also cause the urethra to rupture, leading to a life-threatening situation.
- *Kidney damage*: chronic obstruction and back-up of urine can cause damage to the kidneys.

17.5.4.4 Preventive Measures

Preventing urolithiasis in goats involves implementing appropriate management practices.

- *Providing ample water*: ensuring goats have constant access to clean, fresh water encourages higher water intake, reducing the risk of stone formation.
- *Balanced diet*: feeding goats a balanced diet with appropriate levels of calcium, phosphorus, and roughage helps maintain a healthy urinary system.
- *Ammonium chloride supplementation*: in some cases, adding ammonium chloride to the diet can help prevent urinary calculi formation.
- *Regular exercise*: encouraging physical activity and movement can promote urinary health.

17.5.5 Urethral Obstructions

Urethral obstructions in male goats are serious medical emergencies that can lead to life-threatening consequences if not promptly addressed. These obstructions occur when the urethra becomes blocked, preventing the normal flow of urine. Several factors, such as urinary stones or a build-up of debris, can lead to this condition. Understanding the causes, symptoms, and urgency of urethral obstructions is crucial for goat keepers to recognize the signs early and seek immediate veterinary attention. This section sheds light on the severity of urethral obstructions in male goats and the importance of swift medical intervention (Smith et al. 2023).

17.5.5.1 Causes of Urethral Obstructions

Urethral obstructions in male goats are often attributed to the presence of urinary calculi, commonly known as urinary stones. These stones can form in the urinary tract due to mineral imbalances or dietary factors. The most common types of urinary stones in goats include struvite (magnesium ammonium phosphate) and calcium carbonate stones. As the stones grow in size, they can obstruct the narrow male urethra, making it difficult or impossible for the goat to urinate normally.

Another factor contributing to urethral obstructions is the build-up of debris, such as mucus, crystals, or sloughed tissue, which can accumulate in the urethra and obstruct the urine flow.

17.5.5.2 Symptoms of Urethral Obstructions

Urethral obstructions in male goats can manifest through various distressing symptoms.

- *Straining to urinate*: the goat may repeatedly attempt to urinate with little to no urine being passed.
- *Vocalization and discomfort*: due to the pain caused by the obstruction, goats may vocalize, appear restless, and exhibit signs of discomfort.
- *Abdominal distension*: the abdomen may become visibly enlarged and tense as urine accumulates.
- *Kicking at the flank*: goats may kick or bite at their flanks as a response to the pain.
- *Depression and lethargy*: the goat may appear lethargic and inactive due to the discomfort and distress.
- *Reduced appetite*: pain and discomfort can lead to a loss of appetite.

17.5.5.3 Importance of Immediate Veterinary Attention

Urethral obstructions in male goats are considered medical emergencies that require immediate veterinary attention. Without intervention, the condition can have severe consequences, including the following.

- *Rupture of the bladder*: the accumulation of urine can create excessive pressure on the bladder, potentially leading to bladder rupture.
- *Urethral rupture*: the pressure from the obstructed urine can cause the urethra to rupture, resulting in a life-threatening situation.
- *Kidney damage*: the back-up of urine can lead to kidney damage and impairment.
- *Septicemia*: in cases of prolonged obstruction, bacteria may enter the bloodstream, causing septicemia, a severe and potentially fatal infection.

17.5.5.4 Treatment and Management

When a male goat exhibits symptoms of urethral obstruction, immediate veterinary intervention is essential. The veterinarian may attempt to relieve the obstruction by catheterization or surgical means, depending on the severity and location of the blockage. Intravenous fluids and pain management are often necessary to stabilize the goat's condition.

17.5.5.5 Prevention

Preventing urethral obstructions involves adopting good husbandry practices and maintaining the overall health of the goat. Measures to minimize the risk include the following.

- *Providing adequate water*: ensuring goats have access to clean, fresh water encourages adequate hydration, reducing the likelihood of stone formation.
- *Balanced diet*: offering a balanced diet with appropriate levels of calcium, phosphorus, and roughage helps prevent mineral imbalances that can lead to stone formation.
- *Regular exercise*: promoting regular physical activity can support a healthy urinary system.

17.5.6 Urethritis

Urethritis is inflammation of the urethra, the tube that carries urine from the bladder to the external environment. In goats, urethritis can occur due to various factors, including infections, irritants, or injuries. Understanding the causes, symptoms, and management of urethritis in goats is crucial for maintaining their urinary health and overall well-being. This section explores the nature of urethritis in goats and highlights the importance of appropriate care and treatment (Wuillemin et al. 2023).

17.5.6.1 Causes of Urethritis in Goats

- *Infections*: bacterial, viral, or fungal infections can cause urethritis in goats. Pathogens can enter the urethra through contaminated water, unhygienic living conditions, or via sexual transmission.
- *Irritants*: exposure to irritants, such as harsh chemicals, can lead to inflammation of the urethra in goats. This can occur if goats come into contact with irritating substances in their environment or through improper use of medications.
- *Injuries*: trauma or injury to the urethra can cause inflammation. Such injuries may result from accidents, rough mating behavior, or improper handling during medical procedures.

17.5.6.2 Symptoms of Urethritis

The symptoms of urethritis in goats may vary depending on the underlying cause and severity of inflammation. The following are some common signs.

- *Frequent urination*: goats with urethritis may show increased attempts to urinate.
- *Painful Urination*: straining and vocalization during urination can indicate discomfort.
- *Blood in urine*: hematuria, or the presence of blood in the urine, may be observed.
- *Foul-smelling urine*: urethritis can lead to abnormal odors in the urine.
- *Swelling or redness*: inflammation of the urethra may cause visible swelling or redness around the genital area.

17.5.6.3 Management and Treatment

The management of urethritis in goats involves identifying and addressing the underlying cause. If an infection is suspected, a veterinarian may perform tests, such as urine analysis or bacterial cultures, to determine the pathogen responsible and prescribe appropriate antibiotics or antifungal medications.

To manage urethritis due to irritants or injuries, goats should be removed from the source of irritation or provided with a clean and comfortable living environment. Supportive care, including pain management and proper wound care, may also be necessary to aid healing.

17.5.6.4 Preventive Measures

Preventing urethritis in goats involves maintaining good hygiene practices and minimizing exposure to potential irritants and pathogens. Preventive measures include the following.

- *Clean water and living conditions*: providing clean and uncontaminated water and maintaining a hygienic living environment can reduce the risk of infections and irritations.
- *Proper medication use*: ensuring correct administration and dosage of medications can prevent adverse reactions and irritations.
- *Safe handling and management*: handling goats gently and carefully during medical procedures and mating can reduce the risk of urethral injuries.

17.6 General Management and Prevention

Proper management and care can help prevent some urethral issues in goats. Ensuring a balanced diet with adequate water intake can reduce the risk of urolithiasis. Providing a clean and hygienic living environment can also help prevent UTIs.

Regular health check-ups and prompt veterinary attention at the first sign of any urinary problem are crucial for maintaining the well-being of goats and addressing any urethral issues in a timely manner.

17.7 Conclusion

Diseases of the urethra can pose significant challenges to goat health and productivity. Understanding the symptoms, causes, diagnostic methods, and treatment options for these conditions is essential for goat farmers and veterinarians alike. By implementing preventive measures and early intervention, goat herds can be safeguarded against urethral diseases, leading to improved well-being, productivity, and economic viability of goat farming operations. Continued research and awareness are necessary to address these health issues and ensure the longevity and prosperity of goat herds globally.

References

Bamal, P.S., Kumar, V., John, J.K. et al. (2023). High urinary trace element concentrations: a possible indicator of urolithiasis in goats? *Journal of Trace Elements and Minerals* 4: 100060.

Brenner, E. (2022). Functional anatomy of the upper and lower urinary tract. In: *Handbook of Neurourology: Theory and Practice* (ed. L. Liao and H. Madersbacher), 1–34. Singapore: Springer Nature.

Garaffa, G., Minhas, S., and Ralph, D.J. (2010). Male sexual function. In: *The Scientific Basis of Urology* (ed. A. Mundy, J. Fitzpatrick, D. Neal, and N. George), 300–315. Boca Raton, FL: CRC Press.

Hafez, E.S.E. and Hafez, B. (ed.) (2013). *Reproduction in Farm Animals*. Hoboken, NJ: Wiley.

Mitchell, A., Strafford, M., and Tavares, S. (2022). The renal system and associated disorders. *British Journal of Nursing* 31 (19): 989–996.

Radostits, O.M., Blood, D.C., and Gay, C.C. (2010). *Veterinary Medicine. A Textbook of the Diseases of Cattle, Sheep, Pigs, Goats and Horses*, 8e. Oxford: Baillière Tindall.

Ramírez-González, J.A. and Sansone, A. (2022). Male reproductive system. In: *Fertility, Pregnancy, and Wellness* (ed. D. Vaamonde, A. Hackney, and J. Garcia-Manso), 23–36. St Louis, MO: Elsevier.

Runcan, E.E. and da Silva, M.A.C. (2022). Reproduction and the reproductive system. *Medicine and Surgery of Camelids* 3: 423–480.

Smith, J.S., Hespel, A.M., Garcia, J.D. et al. (2023). Delayed urethral obstruction after migration of a ballistic pellet in an Alpine wether. *Case Reports in Veterinary Medicine* 2023: 3531856.

Wuillemin, F., Vachon, C., Dunn, M., and Desrochers, A. (2023). Management of obstructive urethroliths, urethral pseudodiverticulum, and stricture by diverticulectomy, urethroplasty, and urethral stenting placement in a male goat. *Canadian Veterinary Journal* 64 (8): 733–741.

18

Diseases of the Inguinal Lymph Nodes

Felix Uchenna Samuel[1,2], *Mojetoluwa S. Afolabi*[2], *Kolawole Jonathan Bamidele*[3], *and Hycinth Ndabatsado Kolo*[4]

[1] *Faculty of Veterinary Medicine, National Animal Production Research Institute, Ahmadu Bello University, Zaria, Nigeria*
[2] *Department of Food and Animal Science, Alabama A&M University, Normal, USA*
[3] *Faculty of Veterinary Medicine, Ahmadu Bello University, Zaria, Nigeria*
[4] *Department of Animal Health and Production, Federal University of Technology, Minna, Nigeria*

18.1 Introduction

The lymphatic system is a complex network of vessels, nodes, and organs that play a vital role in maintaining fluid balance, filtering harmful substances, and facilitating immune responses within the body. In animals, including goats, the lymphatic system is integral to overall health and disease resistance. One crucial component of this system is the inguinal lymph nodes, which are located in the groin area of goats (Valdes and Valdes 2022).

18.2 Lymphatic System Overview

The lymphatic system is a parallel circulatory system that works alongside the blood circulation. It consists of lymphatic vessels, lymph nodes, lymphoid organs (such as the spleen and thymus), and lymphatic fluid (lymph). Lymphatic vessels carry lymph throughout the body, and lymph nodes act as filtering stations, where immune cells are stationed to detect and fight off infections, as well as abnormal cells, toxins, and debris (Albertin et al. 2023).

Lymphatic vessels originate as small capillaries that collect interstitial fluid (fluid that surrounds cells) and transport it toward larger vessels. The lymphatic system plays a vital role in maintaining fluid balance by returning excess interstitial fluid to the bloodstream, preventing tissue swelling (Figure 18.1).

18.3 Role of Inguinal Lymph Nodes

Inguinal lymph nodes are a specific group of lymph nodes located in the inguinal region of goats, which is the area where the hindlimbs meet the body. These nodes are strategically positioned to filter lymph from the lower abdomen, genitalia, and hindlimbs. Their primary role is to monitor lymph for potential pathogens, toxins, or foreign particles and initiate immune responses when necessary. The inguinal lymph nodes contain various immune cells, including lymphocytes (such as B cells and T cells) and macrophages. These cells collaborate to identify and neutralize invading microorganisms or abnormal cells. When an infection occurs in the lower body, the immune cells within the inguinal lymph nodes mount an immune response. This response involves the production of antibodies, the release of cytokines, and the recruitment of additional immune cells to the site of infection.

The inguinal lymph nodes serve as important indicators of the overall health status of goats. Changes in size, consistency, or tenderness of these nodes can be early signs of an underlying health issue, such as infection or inflammation. Monitoring the condition of the inguinal lymph nodes is crucial for timely disease detection and management (Lampejo et al. 2023).

Elements of Reproduction and Reproductive Diseases of Goats, First Edition. Edited by Tanmoy Rana.

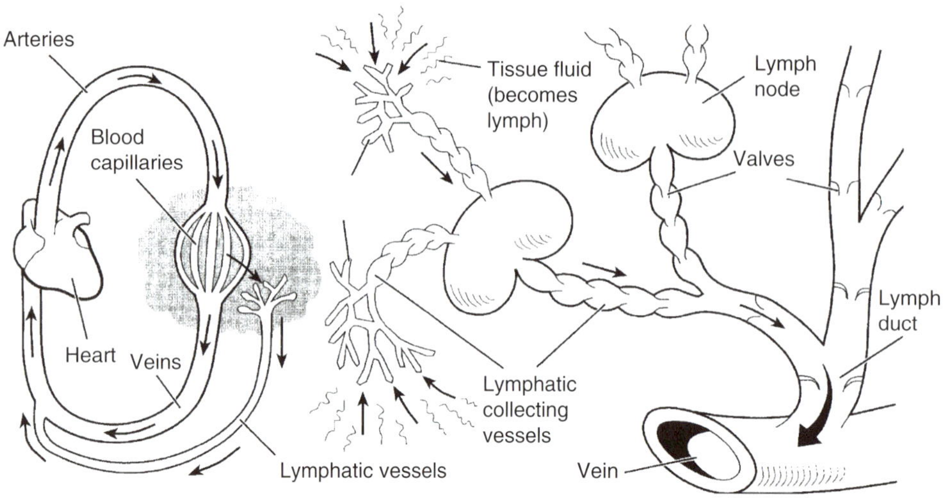

Figure 18.1 Lymphatic system.

18.4 Location and Structure

Inguinal lymph nodes are strategically located in the inguinal region of goats, which is situated in the groin area where the hindlimbs meet the body. These nodes are part of a larger network of lymph nodes distributed throughout the body. The inguinal lymph nodes can be palpated as small, bean-shaped structures beneath the skin in this region.

The structure of inguinal lymph nodes consists of various components that contribute to their function. Each node is encapsulated by a connective tissue capsule that houses a network of lymphatic vessels. These vessels allow lymph to flow into and out of the node. Within the node, there are different regions, including the cortex and the medulla. The cortex contains clusters of immune cells, such as lymphocytes, while the medulla contains specialized cells called medullary cords and sinuses (Albertin et al. 2023).

18.5 Immune Function

The inguinal lymph nodes are integral to the immune system's ability to detect and respond to infections and other challenges. Their immune function is multifaceted and includes the following key roles (Ozdowski and Gupta 2023).

- *Filtration and surveillance*: lymph from the surrounding areas, including the lower abdomen, genitalia, and hindlimbs, is collected and transported to the inguinal lymph nodes. Here, the lymph undergoes thorough filtration, as immune cells within the node scan for any foreign particles, pathogens, or abnormal cells. If any potential threats are identified, the immune response is initiated.
- *Immune response initiation*: the inguinal lymph nodes serve as sites where immune cells, particularly lymphocytes, interact with antigens. Antigens are molecules that can trigger an immune response. When immune cells encounter antigens from pathogens (such as bacteria, viruses, or parasites), they become activated. This activation leads to the production of antibodies and the recruitment of additional immune cells to combat the infection.
- *Antibody production*: B lymphocytes, a type of white blood cell, play a significant role in the production of antibodies. These antibodies are specific to the antigens encountered and help neutralize pathogens by binding to them. Antibodies can also mark pathogens for destruction by other immune cells.
- *Immune cell proliferation*: the inguinal lymph nodes provide an environment conducive to the proliferation and maturation of immune cells. This amplification of immune cells allows for a more robust response to infections.
- *Memory cell generation*: after an initial encounter with an antigen, memory B and T cells are generated within the lymph nodes. These memory cells "remember" the antigen and facilitate a faster and stronger immune response upon subsequent exposure. This is the basis of immunological memory.

18.6 Common Infectious Diseases Affecting Inguinal Lymph Nodes in Goats

18.6.1 Caprine Paratuberculosis (Johne Disease)

18.6.1.1 Etiology

Caprine paratuberculosis, commonly known as Johne disease, is a chronic infectious disease caused by the bacterium *Mycobacterium avium* subspecies paratuberculosis (MAP). This bacterium primarily affects the gastrointestinal tract and is known for its prolonged incubation period, during which infected goats can shed the bacteria into the environment without showing clinical signs (Stefanova et al. 2023).

18.6.1.2 Clinical Presentation

Johne disease progresses slowly and is characterized by several stages. In the early stages, infected goats may not display any clinical signs. As the disease advances, symptoms may include chronic weight loss, reduced appetite, diarrhea, and a rough, unkempt coat. The disease often leads to emaciation despite adequate feed intake. Infected goats may have swollen, firm, and palpable inguinal lymph nodes due to the chronic inflammation caused by the bacteria.

18.6.1.3 Diagnostic Methods

Accurate diagnosis of Johne disease is essential for effective management and prevention. Various diagnostic methods are available.

- *Fecal culture*: this method involves isolating the bacterium from fecal samples. It is a specific but time-consuming technique.
- *PCR (polymerase chain reaction)*: PCR amplifies DNA sequences specific to MAP, allowing for its detection in fecal samples. It is a rapid and sensitive method.
- *Serological tests*: blood tests can detect antibodies against MAP. However, serological tests might not be reliable during the early stages of infection.
- *Necropsy and histopathology*: postmortem examination and histological analysis of tissues, particularly the intestines and lymph nodes, can provide definitive diagnosis.

18.6.1.4 Treatment and Control

Currently, there is no cure for Johne disease and infected goats remain carriers for life. Management strategies focus on disease control and prevention.

- *Culling*: infected goats should be culled to prevent further spread of the disease within the herd.
- *Biosecurity*: implement strict biosecurity measures to prevent the introduction of MAP into the herd. Avoid purchasing animals from known infected herds.
- *Sanitation*: proper cleaning and disinfection of facilities, equipment, and feed/water sources can help reduce the risk of transmission.
- *Vaccination*: vaccines have been developed to reduce the prevalence of Johne disease. These vaccines aim to reduce clinical signs and shedding of the bacteria.
- *Herd testing*: regular testing of the herd using a combination of diagnostic methods can help identify and manage infected animals.
- *Calf management*: separating calves from infected mothers at birth and feeding them heat-treated colostrum and milk can reduce the risk of transmission.
- *Pasture management*: avoiding overgrazing and maintaining clean pastures can help minimize exposure to contaminated environments.

18.6.2 Caseous Lymphadenitis

18.6.2.1 Causative Agent

Caseous lymphadenitis (CLA) is a contagious bacterial infection in goats caused by *Corynebacterium pseudotuberculosis*. This bacterium primarily affects lymph nodes, causing abscesses filled with a thick, cheese-like material. CLA is highly contagious and can spread within a herd through direct contact with infected animals or contaminated environments (El Damaty et al. 2023).

18.6.2.2 Clinical Signs

The clinical signs of CLA can vary depending on the stage of the disease. Infected goats may initially exhibit no noticeable symptoms. As the disease progresses, the following clinical signs may become apparent.

- *Lymph node enlargement*: the inguinal lymph nodes are commonly affected, leading to swelling and palpable lumps in the groin area.
- *Abscess formation*: abscesses can develop in the affected lymph nodes. These abscesses are filled with a thick, caseous (cheese-like) material.
- *Fever*: infected goats may show signs of fever and general malaise.
- *Reduced appetite and weight loss*: the presence of abscesses and systemic infection can lead to decreased feed intake and subsequent weight loss.
- *Lameness*: CLA abscesses in the inguinal region can cause discomfort and lameness.

18.6.2.3 Diagnosis and Management

Early diagnosis and prompt management of CLA are crucial to prevent its spread and mitigate its impact on the herd. Diagnostic methods and management strategies include the following

18.6.2.3.1 Diagnosis

Physical examination: palpation of the inguinal region for swollen lymph nodes and abscesses is an initial step in diagnosing CLA.

- *Ultrasound*: ultrasound can be used to visualize the internal structures of the lymph nodes and confirm the presence of abscesses.
- *Aspiration and culture*: aspirating fluid from suspected abscesses and culturing the bacterium can provide a definitive diagnosis.

18.6.2.3.2 Management

Isolation: infected goats should be isolated to prevent the spread of the disease to other animals.

- *Abscess drainage*: abscesses can be drained by a veterinarian to reduce discomfort and promote healing.
- *Antibiotic treatment*: early treatment with antibiotics can help reduce abscess size and prevent the spread of infection.
- *Culling*: in severe cases or recurrent infections, culling affected goats may be necessary to prevent further spread.
- *Vaccination*: vaccines against CLA are available in some regions and can help reduce the prevalence of the disease within a herd.
- *Biosecurity measures*: strict biosecurity practices, including quarantine and monitoring of new animals, can prevent the introduction of CLA into the herd.
- *Hygiene and sanitation*: regular cleaning and disinfection of facilities and equipment can reduce the risk of bacterial contamination.

18.6.3 Brucellosis

18.6.3.1 Pathogen and Transmission

Brucellosis is a bacterial disease caused by various species of the genus *Brucella*, with *B. melitensis* being the most common species affecting goats. This zoonotic disease can also infect other animals, including cattle, pigs, and dogs, as well as humans. Transmission of brucellosis in goats occurs through contact with infected animals, consumption of contaminated feed and water, or exposure to contaminated materials. Infected goats can shed the bacteria in their milk, urine, and reproductive fluids, posing a risk to other animals and humans (Burns et al. 2023).

18.6.3.2 Symptoms in Goats

Brucellosis can lead to various symptoms in infected goats, although some individuals may show no signs. Clinical manifestations of brucellosis include the following.

- *Abortion*: one of the hallmark signs of brucellosis in goats is late-term abortion or stillbirths, often without apparent signs of illness in the doe.
- *Infertility*: infected bucks may experience reduced fertility, resulting in fewer pregnancies in the herd.

- *Retained placenta*: infected does may have difficulty expelling the placenta after giving birth.
- *Lameness*: in some cases, brucellosis can lead to joint inflammation, causing lameness.
- *Swollen joints*: enlarged joints, especially the knee joints, can be a symptom of brucellosis.
- *Generalized weakness*: goats may appear weak and lethargic, and have a decreased appetite.

18.6.3.3 Diagnosis and Control

Diagnosing and controlling brucellosis are essential to prevent its spread within goat herds and to other susceptible animals.

18.6.3.3.1 Diagnosis

- *Serological testing*: blood tests can detect antibodies against *Brucella* species. Positive serological results may indicate exposure to the pathogen, but further testing is needed for confirmation.
- *Culturing*: isolating the bacteria from clinical samples, such as blood, milk, or tissues, can confirm the presence of the pathogen.

18.6.3.3.2 Control

- *Culling*: infected animals should be culled to prevent further transmission.
- *Quarantine and testing*: new animals introduced to the herd should be quarantined and tested for brucellosis before integration.
- *Vaccination*: while vaccines are available for brucellosis, their use varies depending on the region and the specific *Brucella* species present.
- *Biosecurity measures*: strict biosecurity practices, including isolation of new animals, proper sanitation, and control of movement, can help prevent the introduction of brucellosis.
- *Testing and monitoring*: regular testing and monitoring of the herd are essential to detect and manage infections early.
- *Education*: educate herd owners and workers about the importance of proper hygiene, disease prevention, and zoonotic risks associated with brucellosis.

18.6.4 *Corynebacterium pseudotuberculosis* Infection

18.6.4.1 Clinical Features

Corynebacterium pseudotuberculosis is the causative agent of several infections in goats, including CLA, as discussed earlier. This bacterium can also cause other infections, such as ulcerative lymphangitis and external abscesses. The clinical features of these infections can include the following.

- *External abscesses*: infected goats may develop abscesses on the skin, often in the neck, chest, or shoulder regions. These abscesses are filled with thick, caseous material and can rupture, leading to the spread of infection.
- *Ulcerative lymphangitis*: this condition involves inflammation and ulceration of the lymphatic vessels, often resulting in swollen and painful limbs. Infected goats may exhibit lameness and reluctance to move (Nicoleti et al. 2023).

18.6.4.2 Diagnostic Approaches

Diagnosing *Corynebacterium pseudotuberculosis* infections involves a combination of clinical evaluation, physical examination, and laboratory tests.

- *Clinical signs*: external abscesses, swelling, and lameness are key indicators of these infections.
- *Aspiration and culture*: aspirating fluid from abscesses and culturing the bacteria can confirm the presence of *C. pseudotuberculosis*.

18.6.4.3 Treatment Options

Treatment of *C. pseudotuberculosis* infections often involves a combination of medical and surgical interventions.

- *Abscess drainage*: ruptured or mature abscesses should be drained by a veterinarian to promote healing and prevent further spread.

- *Antibiotic therapy*: antibiotics, such as penicillin or oxytetracycline, may be prescribed to treat active infections. However, treatment success can vary.

Supportive care: affected goats may require pain management, wound care, and supportive treatment to aid in recovery.

18.6.5 *Mycoplasma* Infections

18.6.5.1 Clinical Features

Mycoplasma species can cause various respiratory infections in goats, leading to pneumonia and other respiratory issues. Clinical features may include (Shi et al. 2023) the following.

- *Coughing and sneezing*: infected goats may exhibit coughing and sneezing due to respiratory irritation.
- *Nasal discharge*: clear or purulent nasal discharge may be present, indicating respiratory inflammation.
- *Labored breathing*: respiratory distress, rapid breathing, and increased effort to inhale and exhale can occur.

18.6.5.2 Diagnostic Approaches

Diagnosis of *Mycoplasma* infections involves a combination of clinical signs, physical examination, and laboratory tests.

- *Clinical evaluation*: respiratory symptoms and history of exposure help identify potential *Mycoplasma* infections.
- *Nasal swabs*: swabs from nasal discharge can be used for bacterial culture and identification.

18.6.5.3 Treatment Options

Managing *Mycoplasma* infections typically involves supportive care and antibiotic treatment.

- *Antibiotics*: veterinary-prescribed antibiotics, such as tetracyclines or macrolides, may be used to treat *Mycoplasma* infections. Treatment success may vary based on the specific *Mycoplasma* species and the extent of the infection.
- *Supportive care*: providing a clean and comfortable environment, ensuring proper nutrition and hydration, and minimizing stress can aid in recovery.

18.6.6 Pizzle Rot

Pizzle rot, also known as urinary calculi or urolithiasis, is a condition where mineral deposits accumulate in the urinary tract, potentially leading to blockages and infections. This can indirectly affect the inguinal lymph nodes due to the spread of infection. Symptoms include straining to urinate, restlessness, and painful swelling around the groin. Dietary adjustments, access to clean water, and veterinary care can help prevent and manage pizzle rot.

18.6.7 Caprine Arthritis Encephalitis (CAE)

Caprine arthritis encephalitis (CAE) is a viral disease that affects goats, causing chronic arthritis and other health issues. While it primarily impacts joints and mammary glands, the inguinal lymph nodes can also be affected. Bucks with CAE might display lameness, joint swelling, and decreased mobility. Preventive measures include screening, separation of infected animals, and avoiding the consumption of raw colostrum.

18.7 Noninfectious Causes of Inguinal Lymph Node Enlargement

In addition to infectious diseases, there are several noninfectious factors that can lead to enlargement of the inguinal lymph nodes in goats. These factors range from physical trauma to immune responses to neoplastic conditions (Besson et al. 2023).

18.7.1 Injury and Trauma

Inguinal lymph node enlargement can occur as a result of physical injury or trauma in the lower abdominal or hindlimb regions. Injuries such as kicks, punctures, or blunt force trauma can cause inflammation and swelling in the surrounding tissues, including the lymph nodes. The lymph nodes respond to the inflammation by increasing in size as part of the immune response. While injury-related lymph node enlargement is often temporary, it is essential to monitor the affected goat for any signs of infection that might develop as a secondary complication.

18.7.2 Allergic Reactions

Allergic reactions to various substances, such as certain feeds, medications, or environmental allergens, can trigger immune responses that lead to inguinal lymph node enlargement. Hypersensitivity reactions can cause inflammation in the lymph nodes as the immune system responds to the perceived threat. Allergic reactions are usually accompanied by other clinical signs, such as skin rashes, itching, and respiratory symptoms. Identifying and eliminating the allergen can help resolve the allergic reaction and reduce lymph node enlargement.

18.7.3 Neoplastic Conditions

Neoplastic conditions, including tumors or cancerous growths, can lead to enlargement of the inguinal lymph nodes. Lymph nodes play a role in filtering and detecting abnormal cells, and when cancerous cells or tumors develop nearby, the lymph nodes can become involved in the immune response against these abnormal cells. This can result in enlargement of the lymph nodes. Neoplastic conditions can be benign or malignant, and a thorough veterinary evaluation, including diagnostic imaging and biopsy, is necessary to determine the nature of the growth and its impact on the lymph nodes and overall health of the goat.

18.8 Diagnosis of Inguinal Lymph Node Diseases

Accurate diagnosis of diseases affecting inguinal lymph nodes in goats is essential for effective treatment and management. A combination of clinical examination, laboratory tests, and imaging techniques is often used to identify the underlying cause of lymph node enlargement and associated symptoms.

18.8.1 Clinical Examination

A thorough clinical examination is the first step in diagnosing inguinal lymph node diseases. This involves observing the goat's overall health, assessing vital signs, and conducting a physical examination. During the examination, the veterinarian will palpate the inguinal region to assess the size, consistency, tenderness, and mobility of the lymph nodes. Clinical signs such as fever, weight loss, and lameness will also be evaluated. The information gathered from the clinical examination helps guide further diagnostic steps.

18.8.2 Laboratory Tests

- *Culture*: fluid or tissue samples from enlarged lymph nodes can be collected and cultured to identify the presence of bacteria or other pathogens. Bacterial cultures can help diagnose infections such as CLA caused by *Corynebacterium pseudotuberculosis*.
- *PCR*: PCR is a molecular technique that amplifies DNA sequences specific to certain pathogens. It can be used to detect the genetic material of bacteria, viruses, or other microorganisms present in lymph node samples. PCR is particularly useful for detecting infectious agents with a low load, such as *Mycoplasma* species.
- *Serology*: blood samples can be tested for the presence of antibodies against specific pathogens. Serological tests can provide information about past or ongoing infections and immune responses. However, serology might not always be suitable for early-stage or acute infections.

18.8.3 Imaging Techniques

- *Ultrasound*: ultrasound imaging can provide real-time visualization of the lymph nodes and surrounding tissues. It allows veterinarians to assess the size, shape, internal structure, and blood flow patterns within the lymph nodes. Ultrasound is particularly valuable for detecting abscesses, fluid accumulation, or other abnormalities within the nodes.

- *Radiography (X-rays)*: X-rays can be used to assess the internal structures of the lymph nodes and surrounding tissues. While less detailed than ultrasound for soft tissue visualization, radiography can help identify calcifications, foreign bodies, or other structural abnormalities.

18.8.4 Combining Diagnostic Approaches

Effective diagnosis often involves a combination of these diagnostic approaches. For example, a veterinarian may perform a clinical examination, collect tissue samples for culture and PCR analysis, and use imaging techniques to obtain a comprehensive assessment of the lymph nodes and surrounding tissues. The choice of diagnostic tests depends on the suspected underlying cause and the clinical presentation of the goat.

18.8.5 Summary

In conclusion, a thorough and systematic approach to diagnosing diseases affecting inguinal lymph nodes in goats involves clinical examination, laboratory tests, and imaging techniques. Accurate diagnosis is crucial for determining the appropriate treatment and management strategies to ensure the health and well-being of the affected animals and the overall herd.

18.9 Treatment Strategies

18.9.1 Antibiotic Therapy

Antibiotics are commonly used to treat bacterial infections that affect the inguinal lymph nodes. The choice of antibiotic depends on the specific pathogen causing the infection. Antibiotic therapy aims to eliminate or reduce the bacterial load, control inflammation, and promote healing. It is essential to administer antibiotics as prescribed by a veterinarian, and treatment duration should be followed carefully to prevent the development of antibiotic resistance.

18.9.2 Surgical Interventions

Surgical interventions may be necessary for certain cases, such as abscesses that require drainage. A veterinarian can perform incision and drainage of abscesses to remove accumulated pus and debris. Surgical removal of enlarged lymph nodes (lymphadenectomy) might be considered for cases involving neoplastic growths or severe infections. Proper wound care and postoperative management are crucial to ensure successful healing.

18.9.3 Supportive Care

Supportive care is important for goats with inguinal lymph node diseases to aid in their recovery. This can include providing a clean and comfortable environment, ensuring proper nutrition and hydration, and minimizing stress. Pain management, wound care, and maintaining overall well-being contribute to the goat's recovery and immune response.

18.10 Prevention and Control Measures

18.10.1 Vaccination

Vaccination plays a vital role in preventing certain diseases that can affect the inguinal lymph nodes. Vaccines are available for diseases like CLA and can help reduce the prevalence and severity of infections. Consult with a veterinarian to develop a vaccination schedule tailored to the specific diseases prevalent in the region and the herd's risk factors.

18.10.2 Biosecurity Measures

Implementing biosecurity measures is essential to prevent the introduction and spread of infectious agents that can affect the inguinal lymph nodes. Biosecurity practices may include quarantining new animals before introducing them to the herd, restricting access to the farm, and implementing hygiene protocols to minimize the risk of disease transmission.

18.10.3 Proper Management Practices

Proper management practices contribute to maintaining overall herd health and preventing diseases. This includes providing a balanced and nutritious diet, clean and adequate housing, and regular health monitoring. Proper sanitation, waste management, and ensuring optimal environmental conditions help reduce stress and the risk of disease outbreaks.

18.11 Conclusion

The diseases that affect the inguinal lymph nodes of bucks can have significant implications for their overall health, reproductive capacity, and disease resistance. Timely diagnosis, appropriate treatment, and stringent biosecurity measures are key to mitigating the impact of these diseases. Goat keepers and veterinarians play a crucial role in maintaining the health of bucks and ensuring the well-being of their herds.

References

Albertin, G., Astolfi, L., Fede, C. et al. (2023). Detection of lymphatic vessels in the superficial fascia of the abdomen. *Life* 13 (3): 836.

Besson, S., Boucher, E., Laurin, D. et al. (2023). Stimulation of the immune system by a tumor antigen-bearing adenovirus-inspired VLP allows control of melanoma growth. *Molecular Therapy – Methods & Clinical Development* 28: 76–89.

Burns, R.J., Siengsanun-Lamont, J., and Blacksell, S.D. (2023). A review of coxiellosis (Q fever) and brucellosis in goats and humans: implications for disease control in smallholder farming systems in Southeast Asia. *One Health* 16: 100568.

El Damaty, H.M., El-Demerdash, A.S., Abd El-Aziz, N.K. et al. (2023). Molecular characterization and antimicrobial susceptibilities of corynebacterium pseudotuberculosis isolated from caseous lymphadenitis of smallholder sheep and goats. *Animals* 13 (14): 2337.

Lampejo, A.O., Ghavimi, S.A.A., Hägerling, R. et al. (2023). Lymphatic/blood vessel plasticity: motivation for a future research area based on present and past observations. *American Journal of Physiology Heart and Circulatory Physiology* 324 (1): H109–H121.

Nicoleti, J.L., Braga, E.S., Stanisic, D. et al. (2023). A serum NMR metabolomic analysis of the Corynebacterium pseudotuberculosis infection in goats. *Applied Microbiology and Biotechnology* 107: 4593–4603.

Ozdowski, L. and Gupta, V. (2023). Physiology, lymphatic system. StatPearls Publishing. www.ncbi.nlm.nih.gov/books/NBK557833/ (accessed 22 December 2023).

Shi, H., Hui, R., Zhou, M. et al. (2023). Abortion outbreak in pregnant goats and cows with coinfection of 'Candidatus Mycoplasma haemobos' and HoBi-like pestivirus. *Veterinary Microbiology* 279: 109690.

Stefanova, E.P., Quesada-Canales, Ó., Paz-Sánchez, Y. et al. (2023). Morphological assessment of concomitant lesions detected in goat herds naturally infected with paratuberculosis (Johne's disease). *Animals* 13 (10): 1693.

Valdes, J.J. and Valdes, E.R. (2022). Biological agents: threat and response. In: *Handbook of Security Science* (ed. A. Masys), 739–769. Cham: Springer International Publishing.

19

Diseases of the Prostate

Felix Uchenna Samuel[1,2], Ogunkunle Nathaniel[1,2], Kolawole Jonathan Bamidele[3], Idris Sherif[3], Hycinth Ndabatsado Kolo[4], Bashir Maryam Darma[5], and Mada A. Khumran[3]

[1] Faculty of Veterinary Medicine, National Animal Production Research Institute, Ahmadu Bello University, Zaria, Nigeria
[2] Department of Food and Animal Science, Alabama A&M University, Normal, USA
[3] Faculty of Veterinary Medicine, Ahmadu Bello University, Zaria, Nigeria
[4] Department of Animal Health and Production, Federal University of Technology, Minna, Nigeria
[5] Veterinary Teaching Hospital, Faculty of Veterinary Medicine, Bayero University, Kano, Nigeria

19.1 Introduction

The prostate gland is an accessory sex organ that contributes secretions into the seminal fluid, which aids in sperm delivery and fertilization capacity. Two basic types of cells make up the prostate gland: epithelial cells, which produce exocrine secretions, and stromal cells, which provide structure to the gland and help expel secretions into the urethra. The prostate gland in bucks, as in many other mammals, is an essential part of the reproductive system. It is a small, walnut-sized organ located just below the bladder and surrounds the urethra, the tube responsible for transporting urine and semen out of the body. The prostate's main function is to produce and secrete various fluids that help support sperm function and promote successful reproduction (Bazer 2020) Figure 19.1.

19.2 Cell Biology

The prostate gland comprises two main types of cells: parenchymal epithelial cells and stromal cells. The parenchymal epithelial cells are responsible for forming the acini and ducts within the gland, and they play a crucial role in secreting prostatic fluid. On the other hand, the stromal cells surround the acini and ducts, providing essential support and structure to the gland (Gauntner and Prins 2018).

19.2.1 Epithelial Cells

The prostate gland's acini and ducts, also known as the parenchyma, are created by three different types of epithelial cells, each with distinct characteristics and functions: basal cells, luminal cells, and neuroendocrine cells. Among these, prostate epithelial cell stem cells are found within the basal cell layer. Surrounding the glandular epithelium, there is a fibromuscular stroma, which aids in the expulsion of prostatic secretions into the urethra during ejaculation (Di Donato et al. 2023).

19.2.1.1 Luminal Epithelial Cells

The prostate gland's exocrine product is generated by secretory luminal cells, which form the inner lining of the glandular acini. These cells are cuboidal or pseudo-columnar in shape and are positioned atop a layer of basal cells resting on the basement membrane. Their primary function is to secrete various proteins and substances into the lumen of the glands at the apex of the cell (Lew et al. 2023).

Elements of Reproduction and Reproductive Diseases of Goats, First Edition. Edited by Tanmoy Rana.

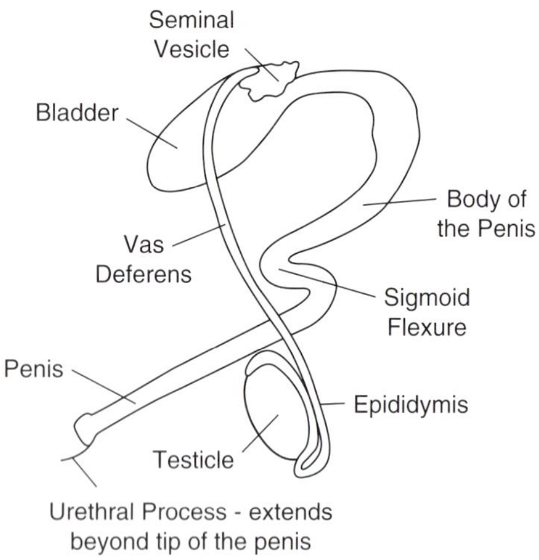

Figure 19.1 Anatomical representation of a buck's reproductive system. *Source:* www.nhptv.org/natureworks/whitetaileddeer.htm.

These luminal epithelial cells are crucial for producing and releasing prostatic fluid, a vital component of semen. They are situated on the innermost layer of the prostate gland's tubular structures, specifically the prostatic acini or ducts. The prostatic acini are responsible for both synthesizing and storing prostatic fluid. The luminal epithelial cells line the central space (lumen) of these acini, where prostatic fluid accumulates before being released during ejaculation (Di Donato et al. 2023).

19.2.1.1.1 Features of Luminal Epithelial Cells

Luminal epithelial cells possess specific characteristics that make them well suited for their functions in the prostate gland (Di Donato et al. 2023).

- *Columnar shape*: these cells are typically tall and columnar in shape, with elongated nuclei and more abundant cytoplasm compared to basal epithelial cells.
- *Secretory machinery*: luminal epithelial cells are specialized for secretion. They contain numerous organelles, such as Golgi apparatus and secretory vesicles, which are involved in the synthesis and packaging of prostatic fluid components.
- *Apical microvilli*: the apical (top) surface of luminal epithelial cells may have microvilli, which are tiny finger-like projections that increase the cell's surface area for more efficient secretion and absorption.

19.2.1.1.2 Functions of Luminal Epithelial Cells

The luminal epithelial cells of the prostate gland play crucial roles in the production and secretion of prostatic fluid, which serves various functions essential for reproduction (Pitzen and Dehm 2023).

- *Prostatic fluid production*: the main function of luminal epithelial cells is to produce and secrete prostatic fluid. This fluid constitutes a significant portion of semen and contains various substances, including enzymes, citric acid, calcium ions, and prostate-specific antigen (PSA).
- *Contribution to semen*: prostatic fluid contributes to semen's composition which, along with sperm from the testes and seminal fluid from other accessory glands, forms the ejaculate released during copulation. Prostatic fluid provides the necessary nutrients and protection for sperm, enhancing their motility and increasing their chances of successfully fertilizing the female's eggs.
- *Regulation of seminal liquification*: after ejaculation, the prostatic fluid plays a role in the liquification of semen, which initially coagulates to form a gel-like plug in the female reproductive tract. This liquification process allows sperm to disperse more freely, improving their movement within the female reproductive tract.
- *Neutralization of urethral pH*: prostatic fluid contains alkaline substances that help neutralize the acidic environment in the male urethra. This neutralization is important to protect sperm from the potentially harmful acidic conditions and maintain their viability until ejaculation.

19.2.1.2 Basal Epithelial Cells

Basal cells in the prostate gland are nonsecretory epithelial cells that have a flat to cuboidal shape. They can be distinguished from luminal cells based on their expression of specific proteins, including CK5, CK14, and the transcription factor p63. Notably, basal cells do not express PSA or prostatic acid phosphatase (PAP). Additionally, most basal cells do not have androgen receptors (ARs) directly, but may still respond to circulating androgens through paracrine signaling with AR-expressing luminal cells or stromal cells.

In addition to extracellular paracrine signaling, basal and luminal epithelial cells can communicate directly through gap junction proteins, enabling cytoplasmic signaling between these two cell types. This suggests that the unique functions of each cell type are co-regulated by the other. Moreover, junction-like structures are observed between cells in the basal layer, leading some researchers to propose the existence of a blood–prostate barrier similar to the one found in the testis. This barrier might explain why systemically administered antibiotics have poor perfusion into the prostate (Beshiri et al. 2023).

19.2.1.2.1 *Functions of Basal Epithelial Cells*

While the specific functions of basal epithelial cells are still being investigated, they are believed to serve several important roles in the prostate gland (Beshiri et al. 2023).

- *Stem cell maintenance*: basal epithelial cells are thought to act as stem cells or progenitor cells, responsible for generating and replenishing other cell types within the prostate gland. They have the ability to divide and differentiate into different cell lineages, contributing to the continuous renewal of the prostate tissue.
- *Cellular support*: basal epithelial cells provide support to the glandular cells that produce and secrete prostatic fluid. They help maintain the structural organization of the gland and ensure that the secretory cells are properly arranged for efficient secretion.
- *Hormonal regulation*: these cells may also be involved in responding to hormonal signals that regulate prostate function. Hormones like testosterone and other androgens play a significant role in prostate development and function, and basal epithelial cells may participate in these hormonal responses.
- *Immune function*: basal epithelial cells might play a role in the immune defense of the prostate gland. They could be involved in detecting and responding to pathogens or foreign substances, helping to protect the gland from infections and inflammation.

19.2.1.3 Epithelial Stem Cells

Prostate stem cells play a crucial role in replenishing the prostate epithelium throughout an individual's life. These stem cells reside within a specialized environment known as the stem cell niche, which is situated within the basal epithelial layer. While in this niche, the stem cells typically remain in a state of relative inactivity (quiescence) until they receive signals from the niche that stimulate their significant potential for proliferation. Our understanding of prostate stem cells has largely been derived from studies in rodent models.

The study of prostate stem cell biology is particularly significant due to the observation that cancer cells share many characteristics with stem cells. Cancer cells possess the ability to divide almost indefinitely, resist apoptosis (programmed cell death), migrate within tissues, and even spread to other tissues, in addition to acquiring altered metabolic states, among other traits.

Prostate stem cells exhibit three fundamental properties: (i) they have a slow growth rate or relative quiescence, (ii) they have a high capacity for replication, and (iii) they can regenerate a prostate-like gland. During development of the prostate gland, the stem cells undergo relatively high levels of proliferation to generate sufficient progeny for the formation of the gland. However, in the adult gland, the stem cells exist in a state of relative quiescence, which is regulated by both intrinsic growth control mechanisms within the stem cells themselves and external cues from the surrounding niche.

Several signaling pathways control the growth and self-renewal decisions of prostate stem cells. These pathways can originate from the stem cells themselves (autonomous) or from other cells within the niche, including progenitor cells and stromal cells (extrinsic). Some of these pathways include bone morphogenic peptide/transforming growth factor-beta (BMP/TGF-beta), wingless-integrated (Wnt)/beta-catenin, fibroblast growth factor (FGF), Notch, Hedgehog, and Ephrin pathways (Beshiri et al. 2023). These signaling pathways play critical roles in maintaining the balance between quiescence and proliferation in prostate stem cells, thereby ensuring the proper functioning of the prostate gland and influencing its potential for cancer development.

19.3 Prostatic Secretions

19.3.1 The Prostate Gland Contributes Secretions to the Seminal Plasma

The sex accessory tissues, such as the prostate, seminal vesicles, bulbourethral glands, and glands of Littre, have a primary function in producing seminal plasma, which is the nongamete portion of semen. Seminal plasma serves as a nutrient-rich, buffered transport medium for sperm during ejaculation and their subsequent journey into the female genital tract. While certain components in seminal plasma can enhance the fertilizing capacity of sperm, they are not essential for mature spermatozoa to successfully fertilize an egg.

Seminal plasma has a slightly alkaline pH, ranging from 7.2 to 7.8, which helps neutralize the acidic environment of the vagina, creating a more favorable environment for sperm survival. Prostaglandins present in seminal plasma play a role in stimulating the smooth muscle contractions along the female genital tract, aiding in the propulsion of sperm toward the egg.

Several other substances found in seminal plasma contribute to its properties. Zinc and immunoglobulin A (IgA) are two important components with bacteriostatic properties, helping to protect against bacterial infections. Additionally, a range of prostatic proteins is present in seminal plasma, which helps prevent the autoagglutination (clumping) of sperm.

In total, the secretions from the prostate gland account for approximately 25% of the ejaculate volume, which typically ranges from about 1 to 6 ml in human males (Ješeta et al. 2023). The combined contributions of all the sex accessory tissues ensure the successful delivery and survival of sperm within the female reproductive tract, supporting the process of fertilization.

19.3.2 Role of Prostatic Secretions in Coagulation/Liquefaction

Semen coagulates and forms a gelatinous mass soon after ejaculation due to clotting factors produced by the seminal vesicles. Although analogous to blood coagulation, the seminal coagulation process has a unique biochemistry that does not involve prothrombin, fibrinogen, or hematologic clotting factors. Furthermore, the seminal coagulation process is not inhibited by heparin or sodium citrate. Prostate-derived proteolytic enzymes, including seminin, plasminogen activators, and PSA, liquefy the coagulated semen after 15–60 minutes. This liquefaction frees the sperm to advance up the female reproductive tract. Defective or absent secretion of these liquefying factors from the prostate is one cause of reduced male fertility (Ješeta et al. 2023).

19.3.3 Regulation of Prostatic Secretion

The production of seminal plasma, including the prostatic component, is under hormonal control and driven by circulating androgens, which are always present in normal males. In the prostate, circulating testosterone is taken up by prostate cells, converted to dihydrotestosterone (DHT) which binds to luminal cell AR, dimerizes, and translocates to the nucleus. Nuclear AR binds response elements on androgen-regulated genes, initiating gene transcription with subsequent translation of secretory proteins or enzymes whose products are secreted into seminal fluid. Prostatic secretions are also under neural control (Ventura et al. 2002). Both the epithelial and stromal compartments in the prostate are innervated by the autonomic nervous system.

19.3.4 Components of Prostatic Fluid

19.3.4.1 Zinc

The prostate gland contains the highest concentration of zinc of any organ in the human body, as reported by Bertrand and Vladesco in 1921. This elevated zinc level in the seminal plasma, which is about 140 mg/ml, is nearly 100 times higher than the concentration of zinc in the blood serum, according to Eliasson's research in 1977. The exact physiological role of such high zinc concentrations in the prostate and seminal plasma remains unclear. While the prostate contains numerous zinc-containing metalloenzymes, the observed zinc concentration far surpasses what would be theoretically required for these enzymes to function.

Within the seminal plasma, zinc plays several roles. It acts to stabilize the chromatin within the sperm head, aiding in sperm function and viability. Additionally, zinc binds to semenogelin I and II in the seminal plasma, contributing to the regulation of liquefaction, a process involved in sperm release and movement (Heathcote and Washington 1973; Fair et al. 1976; Jonsson et al. 2005).

Furthermore, zinc serves as an antibacterial agent in both seminal plasma and nonejaculatory prostatic secretions. *In vitro* studies have demonstrated its activity against various Gram-positive and Gram-negative bacteria, as evidenced by research by Radhi et al. (2023). This antibacterial function may play a crucial role in protecting sperm and reproductive health.

Despite these known functions of zinc in the prostate and seminal plasma, the full extent of its physiological significance in these contexts is yet to be fully understood. Ongoing research continues to shed light on the intricate roles of zinc and its implications for male reproductive health.

19.3.4.2 Citric Acid

Citrate, a potent binder of metal ions, is one of the major anions present in human seminal plasma. In ejaculate, the average concentration of citrate is 376 mg/dl, which is 500–1000 times higher than its concentration in blood plasma. The molar concentration of citrate (20 mM) is comparable to the combined concentration of divalent metals in the semen, which includes calcium (7 mM), magnesium (4.5 mM), and zinc (2.1 mM). The primary source of citrate in seminal plasma is the prostate, while seminal vesicle secretions contribute to a much lower concentration of citrate, approximately 100-fold less. The elevated levels of citrate have been associated with a decreased ability of prostatic mitochondria to oxidize citrate, leading to an imbalance between citrate production and oxidation. Researchers measured citrate and isocitrate levels and found that the prostate has a ratio of 33:1, whereas other tissues demonstrated ratios of 10:1. This finding suggests that reduced aconitase activity may be responsible for the unusually high citrate levels in prostatic secretions (Yun et al. 2023).

19.3.4.3 Sodium, Potassium, Calcium, Magnesium, and Chloride

Although seminal plasma contains calcium and magnesium in higher concentrations than other body fluids, the relative contribution of the prostate to these levels has not been established. It is known, however, that the concentration of sodium, potassium, calcium, magnesium, and chloride within prostatic fluid varies between individuals and states of wellness or disease. This is in part a passive response to varied levels of citrate secretion in prostatic fluid during states of disease (Rodríguez-Díaz et al. 2023).

19.3.4.4 Spermine

Polyamines are small, positively charged organic molecules that have two or more primary amino groups. These molecules are found in all eukaryotic cells, where they have pleiotropic effects on a variety of physiological processes including cell proliferation. Spermine, so named as a polyamine that was first discovered in semen, is present in seminal plasma at concentrations of 50–350 mg/dl and imparts a unique odor to semen. The prostate gland has the highest concentration of spermine in the human body and is the primary source of this polyamine in seminal plasma. The enzyme ornithine decarboxylase (ODC) is the rate-limiting enzyme in the synthesis of polyamines and spermine. The expression of ODC is increased in benign prostatic hyperplasia (BPH) tissue, which suggests a possible role for polyamines in the pathogenesis of this disease. At physiological pH, spermine has four positive charges that bind strongly to acidic or negatively charged molecules such as phosphate ions, nucleic acids, or phospholipids.

Spermine is generated via a series of enzymatic reactions that use other polyamines as substrates, proceeding from ornithine to putrescine to spermidine to spermine. Spermine is oxidized enzymatically by diamine oxidase, which is found in the seminal plasma. The aldehyde products from this reaction are very reactive and toxic to both sperm and bacteria. This is one reason why prolonged exposure of sperm to seminal plasma will reduce its fertilizing capacity (Prylutskyi et al. 2023).

19.3.4.5 Prostaglandins

In 1934, von Euler coined the term *prostaglandins* to describe the active components in seminal plasma on the assumption that they were produced by the prostate. Over 20 years later, Eliasson determined that the majority of prostaglandins originate from the seminal vesicles, with the prostate gland's contribution being minimal (Eliasson 1959). Nevertheless, the name stands to this day.

Prostaglandins are expressed throughout the body but in humans, the highest concentrations by far are found in the seminal vesicles. The seminal plasma contains 15 different prostaglandins at a concentration of 100–300 mg/ml. Prostaglandins are 20-carbon hydroxyl fatty acids containing a cyclopentane ring and two side chains. They are classified into four major groups (A, B, E, and F) based on the structure of the cyclopentane ring and given a number based on the structure of the side chain (e.g., PGE3). The E group of prostaglandins predominates in the male reproductive tract, while the F group predominates in the female.

Prostaglandins have a variety of potent proposed physiological effects in the male and are involved in erection, ejaculation, sperm motility, and testicular and penile contractions. Additionally, seminal fluid prostaglandins deposited in the vagina affect cervical mucus, vaginal secretions, and uterine contractions (Hoxha et al. 2023).

19.3.4.6 Cholesterol and Lipids

The human prostate contributes to the lipid fraction of seminal plasma, which contains 185 mg/dl of total lipids, 103 mg/dl of cholesterol, and 83 mg/dl of phospholipids. The phospholipids have been further characterized as 44% sphingomyelin, 12.3% ethanolamine plasmalogen, and 11.2% phosphatidylserine. This ratio of cholesterol to phospholipid helps stabilize the sperm against temperature and environmental shock (Goyal and Saxena 2023b).

19.3.4.7 Immunoglobulins

Immunoglobulins are found in the seminal plasma at levels lower than in blood. Specifically, IgG is measured from 7 to 22 mg/dl and IgA from 0 to 6 mg/dl. IgM has also been detected in the seminal plasma at very low levels (Gahankari and Golhar 1993). Given the lower levels of immunoglobulins, it is theorized that these may simply be exudates, but IgA has been localized more so to the bulbourethral glands and suggests an immunological component to the bulbourethral gland function. IgG and IgA are likely secreted from the prostate (Carvalho et al. 2023).

19.3.4.8 Acid Phosphatase

Acid phosphatase activity is more than 200 times more abundant in the prostate than any other tissue. PAP is a glycoprotein dimer with seminal plasma levels of 0.3–1 g/l. The substrate for PAP in the seminal plasma may be phosphorylcholine phosphate, which is rapidly hydrolyzed by the enzyme. However, the physiological significance of the high levels of PAP and their function are not well understood. Serum acid phosphatase concentration was once widely measured as a biomarker for metastatic prostate cancer but this has been replaced by the more sensitive and specific assay for PSA (Ngo et al. 2023).

19.3.4.9 Prostate Specific Antigen

Prostate specific antigen is a 33 kD glycoprotein that acts as a serine protease and is produced almost exclusively in prostate epithelial cells, PSA is involved in lysing the ejaculatory clot with semenogelin as its substrate. The PSA gene (hKLK3) is a member of the kallikrein family which are all located on chromosome 19. Expression of PSA is dependent upon androgens.

Clinically, PSA is used as an important serum marker for prostate cancer and prostate disease since its presence in the circulation indicates a breakdown in the epithelial/basement membrane barrier. Unfortunately, while PSA is organ specific, it is not cancer specific and is found in the serum of patients with BPH as well as prostatitis. PSA is found in seminal plasma in concentrations from 0.5 to 5 mg/ml whereas PSA in serum of men 50–80 years of age without prostate disease is 1000-fold less at 1.0–4.0 ng/ml. The serum level of PSA in men with prostate cancer is generally elevated (>4.0 ng/ml), but not until its level is >10 ng/ml does this measurement suggest specificity for prostate cancer.

As prostate cancer cells remain A -dependent, even in the absence of androgens, circulating levels of PSA in patients with metastatic disease can reach into the hundreds and monitoring levels over time can be a useful indicator of progression and relapse after treatment failure (Unuma et al. 2023).

19.4 Diseases of the Prostrate

Diseases of the prostate in goats can affect their reproductive health and overall well-being. While goats are generally hardy and resistant to many diseases, they are not immune to prostate-related issues. Here are some common diseases of the prostate that can affect goats (Zachary and McGavin 2012).

19.4.1 Prostatitis

Prostatitis is inflammation of the prostate gland, and it can occur in goats due to various reasons, including bacterial infections. Infections may ascend from the urinary tract or be introduced through the bloodstream. Symptoms of prostatitis in goats include difficulty urinating, frequent urination, blood in the urine, and discomfort in the hindquarters.

19.4.2 Benign Prostatic Hyperplasia (BPH)

Benign prostatic hyperplasia is a noncancerous enlargement of the prostate gland, commonly seen in aging goats. As goats get older, hormonal changes can lead to the growth of prostate tissue, causing the gland to enlarge. BPH can lead to urinary obstruction and difficulty in passing urine, leading to discomfort and distress for the goat.

19.4.3 Prostatic Abscesses

Prostatic abscesses can develop as a result of bacterial infections in the prostate gland. These abscesses are pus-filled pockets that can cause severe pain, difficulty urinating, and systemic signs of illness such as fever and lethargy.

19.4.4 Prostate Cancer

Prostate cancer is a relatively rare condition in goats but can occur. Tumors may develop in the prostate gland, leading to various urinary and reproductive issues. Unfortunately, prostate cancer in goats often has a poor prognosis.

19.4.5 Prostate Calculi

Prostate calculi are mineral deposits that can form within the prostate gland or urinary tract. They can obstruct the urethra, making it difficult for the goat to urinate and leading to potential urinary blockages and related complications.

19.4.6 Prostatic Cysts

Prostatic cysts are fluid-filled sacs that can develop within the prostate gland. They may cause discomfort, pain, and issues with urination, especially if they grow large enough to compress surrounding structures.

19.5 Conclusion

The prostate gland is a crucial organ in the reproductive health of male goats, responsible for semen production and fertility. Various diseases can afflict the prostate gland, such as prostatitis, BPH, prostate abscess, and even prostate cancer. Early detection and proper treatment are essential to ensure the overall well-being and productivity of male goats. Goat farmers must be vigilant, implement preventive measures, and collaborate with veterinarians to maintain the health of their herds and secure the future of their goat farming endeavors.

References

Bazer, F.W. (2020). Reproductive physiology of sheep (Ovis aries) and goats (Capra aegagrus hircus). *Animal Agriculture* 2020: 199–209.

Beshiri, M., Agarwal, S., Yin, J.J., and Kelly, K. (2023). Prostate organoids: emerging experimental tools for translational research. *Journal of Clinical Investigation* 133 (10): e169616.

Carvalho, M., Gomes, R.M., Rocha, S.M. et al. (2023). Development of a novel electrochemical biosensor based on plastic antibodies for detection of STEAP1 biomarker in cancer. *Bioelectrochemistry* 152: 108461.

Di Donato, M., Giovannelli, P., Migliaccio, A., and Castoria, G. (2023). The nerve growth factor-delivered signals in prostate cancer and its associated microenvironment: when the dialogue replaces the monologue. *Cell & Bioscience* 13 (1): 1–18.

Eliasson, R. (1959). Studies on prostaglandin; occurrence, formation and biological actions. *Acta Physiologica Scandinavica* 46(158, suppl.): 1–73.

Fair, W.R., Couch, J., and Wehner, N. (1976). Prostatic antibacterial factor identity and significance. *Urology* 7 (2): 169–177.

Gahankari, D.R. and Golhar, K.B. (1993). An evaluation of serum and tissue bound immunoglobulins in prostatic diseases. *Journal of Postgraduate Medicine* 39 (2): 63.

Gauntner, T.D. and Prins, G.S. (2018). Prostate cell biology and secretion. In: *Encyclopedia of Reproduction* (ed. M. Skinner), 325–333. St Louis, MO: Elsevier.

Goyal, R. and Saxena, N. (2023b). Relationship between androgen, insulin levels, lipid levels, leptin and adiponectin levels in patients suffering with prostate cancer and pre-cancer conditions. *Journal of Vascular Disease Research* 14: 2196–2204.

Heathcote, J.G. and Washington, R.J. (1973). Analysis of the zinc-binding protein derived from the human benign hypertrophic prostate. *Journal of Endocrinology* 58 (3): 421–423.

Hoxha, M., Barbonetti, A., and Zappacosta, B. (2023). Arachidonic acid pathways and male fertility: a systematic review. *International Journal of Molecular Sciences* 24 (9): 8207.

Ješeta, M., Pospíšilová, A., Mekiňová, L. et al. (2023). Non-invasive diagnostics of male spermatogenesis from seminal plasma: seminal proteins. *Diagnostics* 13 (15): 2468.

Jonsson, M., Linse, S., Frohm, B. et al. (2005). Semenogelins I and II bind zinc and regulate the activity of prostate-specific antigen. *Biochemical Journal* 387 (2): 447–453.

Lew, M., Pang, J., and Pantanowitz, L. (ed.) (2023). *Normal Cytology: An Illustrated, Practical Guide*. Cham: Springer Nature.

Ngo, A.N., Murowchick, J., Gounev, A.D. et al. (2023). Physico-chemistry and cytotoxicity of tenofovir-loaded acid phosphatase-responsive chitosan nanoparticles. *AAPS PharmSciTech* 24 (6): 143.

Pitzen, S.P. and Dehm, S.M. (2023). Basal epithelial cells in prostate development, tumorigenesis, and cancer progression. *Cell Cycle* 22 (11): 1303–1318.

Prylutskyi, M.P., Zaletok, S.P., Khrystosenko, R.V. et al. (2023). Optical biosensing analysis of spermine as marker of prostate cancer with help of colloidal gold and anti-spermine antibody modified transducers. *Journal of Biosensors and Bioelectronics Research* 103: 2–4.

Radhi, G.M., Hilal, N.N., and Abdul-Aziz, M.M. (2023). Relationship between PSA and serum zinc in BPH-afflicted Iraqi men. *South Asian Research Journal of Pharmaceutical Sciences* 5 (4): 158–167.

Rodríguez-Díaz, R., Blanes-Zamora, R., Vaca-Sánchez, R. et al. (2023). Influence of seminal metals on assisted reproduction outcome. *Biological Trace Element Research* 201 (3): 1120–1134.

Unuma, K., Sato, H., Wen, S. et al. (2023). The proportion of false-positives in positive Seratec® prostate-specific antigen SemiQuant test results in postmortem screening for seminal fluid. *Legal Medicine* 62: 102243.

Ventura, S., Pennefather, J.N., and Mitchelson, F. (2002). Cholinergic innervation and function in the prostate gland. *Pharmacology & Therapeutics* 94 (1–2): 93–112.

Yun, K.I., Pak, U.G., Han, T.S. et al. (2023). Determination of prostatic fluid citrate concentration using peroxidase-like activity of a peroxotitanium complex. *Analytical Biochemistry* 672: 115152.

Zachary, J.F. and McGavin, M.D. (ed.) (2012). *Pathologic Basis of Veterinary Disease 5*. St Louis, MO: Elsevier Health Sciences.

20

Diseases of the Scrotum

Felix Uchenna Samuel[1,2], *Mojetoluwa S. Afolabi*[2], *Adeniyi Njideka*[2], *Ogunkunle Nathaniel*[2], *Kolawole Jonathan Bamidele*[3], *and Hycinth Ndabatsado Kolo*[4]

[1] *Faculty of Veterinary Medicine, National Animal Production Research Institute, Ahmadu Bello University, Zaria, Nigeria*
[2] *Department of Food and Animal Science, Alabama A&M University, Normal, USA*
[3] *Faculty of Veterinary Medicine, Ahmadu Bello University, Zaria, Nigeria*
[4] *Department of Animal Health and Production, Federal University of Technology, Minna, Nigeria*

20.1 Introduction

The scrotum or scrotal sac is an external male reproductive structure located at the base of the penis that consists of a suspended dual-chambered sac of skin and smooth muscle. It is present in most terrestrial male mammals. The scrotum contains the external spermatic fascia, testes, epididymis, and ductus deferens. It is a distention of the perineum and carries some abdominal tissues into its cavity, including the testicular artery, testicular vein, and pampiniform plexus. The perineal raphe is a small, vertical, slightly raised ridge of scrotal skin under which is found the scrotal septum. It appears as a thin longitudinal line that runs front to back over the entire scrotum. The scrotum is biologically homologous to the labia majora in female animals. It is absent in fusiform marine mammals, such as whales and seals, as well as in some lineages of land mammals, such as the afrotherians, xenarthrans, and numerous families of bats, rodents, and insectivores (Singh et al. 2019).

The scrotum regulates the temperature of the testes and maintains it at two or three degrees below the core body temperature. Higher temperatures affect spermatogenesis. Temperature control is accomplished by the smooth muscles of the scrotum moving the testicles either closer to or further away from the abdomen dependent upon the ambient temperature. This is accomplished by the cremaster muscle in the abdomen and the dartos fascia (muscular tissue under the skin).

The scrotal skin is thin, has few hair follicles and little or no subcutaneous fat, and is richly supplied with sweat glands. Warm arterial blood is cooled as it passes next to venous blood within the pampiniform plexus. Seminiferous tubule temperature needs to be 2–3 °C lower than the body temperature for viable production of spermatozoa (Chaurasia et al. 2023).

The situation of the scrotum and testicles outside the abdominal cavity may provide additional advantages. The external scrotum is not affected by abdominal pressure. This may prevent the emptying of the testes before the sperm have matured sufficiently for fertilization. Another advantage is the it protects the testes from jolts and compressions associated with an active lifestyle. Animals that move at a steady pace – such as elephants, whales, and marsupial moles – have internal testes and no scrotum. Unlike placental mammals, some male marsupials have a scrotum that is anterior to the penis, which is not homologous to the scrotum of placental mammals, although there are several marsupial species without an external scrotum. In humans, the scrotum may provide some friction during intercourse, helping to enhance the activity (Perumal et al. 2023).

20.2 Structure and Anatomy

The external layer of the scrotum is made of skin which is usually darker in color than the neighboring areas of skin. Underneath the skin is the dartos muscle, or tunica dartos. The tunica dartos helps to regulate the temperature of the testicles by contracting to reduce the surface area of the scrotum and decrease heat loss, or relaxing to increase the surface area of the scrotum to help with cooling (Sultan et al. 2023) (Figure 20.1).

Elements of Reproduction and Reproductive Diseases of Goats, First Edition. Edited by Tanmoy Rana.

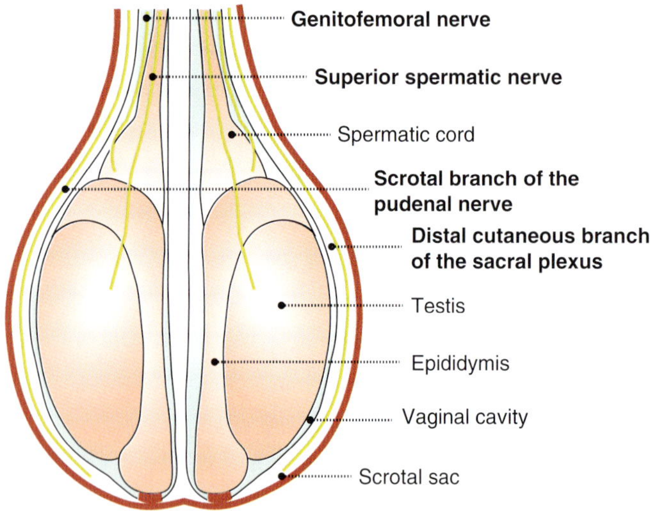

Figure 20.1 Anatomy of the scrotum of small ruminants. *Source:* Mellor and Stafford (2000)/Taylor& Francis.

Another muscle inside the scrotum is the cremaster muscle. There are two such muscles, one on each side. Each of the muscles covers the testes and the spermatic cord and reaches into the pelvis through the inguinal canal. The function of the cremaster muscles is to raise or lower the testicles. This further helps to maintain the testicles at an appropriate temperature (Mohamed et al. 2023).

The cremasteric reflex is a response to light stroking of the inner thigh. It causes the muscle to contract and the testes to elevate. It is also possible for some men to contract the cremaster muscles voluntarily.

The spermatic cord provides blood supply to the testes, vas deferens, and cremaster muscle. It also contains nerves and lymph vessels which connect to the internal structures of the scrotum.

The scrotal septum divides the scrotum into two chambers. It is an extension of the perineal raphe, a line of tissue that extends from the anus through the perineum and upwards through the midline of the penis (Abah et al. 2023).

20.2.1 Anatomy

The scrotum is one of the vital accessory male reproductive organs which is formed by a suspended sac of skin and smooth muscle that has two chambers. It is present in most terrestrial (earthly) males, located under the penis. It is a protective reservoir for the testis and related anatomical structures. Asymmetry of the testis is explicit in that one testis is typically lower than the other, the function of which is to avoid compression in the event of an impact (Husnurrizal et al. 2023).

The perineal raphe is a landmark – a small, vertical, slightly raised ridge of scrotal skin marking the scrotal septum. It is a thin longitudinal line which runs from front to back over the entire scrotum. The contains of the scrotum on the external spermatic fascia, testes, epididymis, and ductus deferens. It is a distention of the perineum, and carries some abdominal tissues such as testicular artery, testicular vein, and pampinform plexus. The scrotum becomes covered with pubic hair at puberty, a secondary sex character. It is biologically homologous to the labia majora in females (Mansour et al. 2023).

- *Nerve supply*: the scrotal surface is divided into the anterolateral portion, supplied by the genital branch of the genitofemoral nerve, anterior portion supplied by the anterior scrotal nerves, a branch of the ilioinguinal nerve, posterior portion supplied by the posterior scrotal nerve, a branch of the perineal nerve, while its inferior surface is supplied by perineal branches of the posterior femoral cutaneous nerve (Husnurrizal et al. 2023).
- *Blood supply*: the blood vessels of the scrotum are the anterior and posterior scrotal artery, and the testicular vein.
- *Integument*: the scrotal integument is relatively thin and has an underlying fascia, the tunica dartos. It is composed of skin-associated tissues, namely hair, sebaceous glands, apocrine sweat glands, and smooth muscles. The skin on the scrotum is pigmented compared to the rest of the body. The septum is a connective tissue membrane dividing the scrotum into two cavities (Mansour et al. 2023).
- *Lymphatic system*: this is formed by lymphatic vessels, namely the superficial inguinal lymph nodes, superficial subinguinal glands, and the deep subinguinal glands.

- *Physiology*: the scrotum regulates the temperature of the testes, and maintains them at 35 °C/95 °F, which is two degrees below the normal body temperature of 37 °C/98.6 °F. Higher temperatures may affect spermatogenesis. Temperature control is accomplished by the smooth muscles of the scrotum moving the testicles either closer to or further away from the abdomen dependent upon the ambient temperature, which is accomplished by the cremaster muscle in the abdomen and the dartos fascia. Furthermore, their situation outside the abdominal cavity provides additional advantage(s) that scrotum is unaffected by abdominal pressure, which may prevent the emptying of the testes before the sperm are matured sufficiently for fertilization. It also protects the testes from jolts and compressions (Mansour et al. 2023).

20.2.2 Anatomical Variations

There are a number of possible anatomical variations of the scrotum. In general, these variations are quite rare (Thobela et al. 2023).

- *Accessory scrotum*: an extra scrotum that develops, usually further down the perineum, toward the anus. The accessory scrotum does not contain testes. It does not generally cause problems with the primary scrotum.
- *Bifid scrotum*: this is when there is a cleft in the middle of the scrotum. It occurs when there is not enough testosterone early in development for the scrotum to fuse. Bifid scrotum often occurs alongside hypospadias.
- *Ectopic scrotum*: where the normal scrotum is located in a different location.
- *Penoscrotal transposition*: where the penis and the scrotum are located incorrectly with respect to each other. The penis can be below the scrotum (complete transposition) or in the middle of the scrotum (partial transposition.)

20.3 Diseases of the Scrotum of Bucks

20.3.1 Orchitis

Orchitis is an inflammatory condition that affects the testicles, which are part of the male reproductive system. In goats, as in other animals, orchitis can be a serious health issue that can lead to discomfort, pain, and potential fertility problems. The following reference provides a more detailed overview of orchitis in goats (Foster 2023).

20.3.1.1 Causes of Orchitis in Goats

20.3.1.1.1 Infections

Orchitis is often caused by bacterial, viral, or fungal infections. In goats, common infectious causes include the following.

- *Bacterial infections*: pathogenic bacteria such as *Brucella melitensis*, which causes brucellosis, can lead to orchitis.
- *Viral infections*: the caprine arthritis encephalitis (CAE) virus, a retrovirus, can also cause orchitis in goats. CAE primarily affects the joints and nervous system but can lead to other complications, including testicular inflammation.
- *Fungal infections*: fungal pathogens can occasionally cause orchitis, especially in environments where fungi thrive.

20.3.1.1.2 Trauma

Physical injury or trauma to the scrotal area can result in inflammation and orchitis.

20.3.1.2 Symptoms of Orchitis

The signs and symptoms of orchitis in goats may include swelling of the scrotum and testicles, pain and discomfort leading to difficulty walking or standing, reluctance to move or lie down, general signs of illness such as fever and loss of appetite, reduced activity and playfulness, changes in the texture and appearance of the scrotal skin, and possible discharge from the penis.

20.3.1.3 Diagnosis

Diagnosing orchitis involves a thorough physical examination, history taking, and diagnostic tests. These tests may include blood tests to identify infectious agents or markers of inflammation, ultrasound or other imaging techniques to assess the extent of inflammation and damage, and testicular biopsy in severe cases to determine the cause and extent of damage.

20.3.1.4 Treatment

Treatment of orchitis depends on the underlying cause. It often involves administering antibiotics or antiviral medications to address infections, providing pain relief and antiinflammatory drugs to alleviate discomfort and swelling, supportive care, such as ensuring proper nutrition and maintaining a clean and comfortable environment.

20.3.1.5 Prevention

Preventing orchitis involves implementing good management practices: maintaining a clean and hygienic environment for goats to minimize the risk of infections, isolating new animals before introducing them to the herd to prevent the spread of potential pathogens, and implementing a vaccination program, where appropriate, to protect against infectious diseases such as brucellosis and CAE (Foster 2023).

20.3.2 Epididymitis

Epididymitis is the inflammation of the epididymis, a coiled tube located on the surface of the testicle. The epididymis plays a crucial role in the maturation and storage of sperm. Epididymitis can occur due to various factors, including infections, trauma, and other underlying conditions. The following reference provides a detailed overview of epididymitis in goats (Monteiro et al. 2023).

20.3.2.1 Causes of Epididymitis in Goats

20.3.2.1.1 Infections

Bacterial, viral, or fungal infections can lead to epididymitis. Common infectious causes include the following.

- *Bacterial infections*: bacteria such as *Brucella melitensis*, which causes brucellosis, can result in epididymitis. Other pathogenic bacteria may also be involved.
- *Viral infections*: the CAE virus, while primarily associated with arthritis and neurological symptoms, can occasionally lead to epididymitis.
- *Fungal infections*: fungi can also infect the epididymis and cause inflammation.
- *Ascending infection*: in some cases, infections may ascend from the urinary tract to the epididymis.

20.3.2.1.2 Trauma

Physical injury or trauma to the scrotal area can lead to epididymitis.

20.3.2.1.3 Other Causes

Conditions such as testicular torsion (twisting of the testicle and spermatic cord) or certain systemic illnesses can indirectly lead to epididymitis.

20.3.2.2 Symptoms of Epididymitis

The signs and symptoms of epididymitis in goats may include swelling and inflammation of the epididymis, leading to a lump or enlargement of the scrotum, pain and discomfort, causing the goat to be restless and exhibit signs of distress, reluctance to walk, stand, or lie down comfortably, changes in behavior, including decreased activity and appetite, possible discharge from the penis, and fever and other signs of illness.

20.3.2.3 Diagnosis and Treatment

Diagnosing epididymitis involves a combination of clinical examination, history, and diagnostic tests, which may include palpation of the scrotum and epididymis to assess swelling and tenderness, blood tests to identify markers of infection and inflammation

ultrasound or other imaging techniques to visualize the epididymis and testicles, aspiration of fluid from the epididymis for laboratory analysis.

Treatment of epididymitis depends on the underlying cause and may include antibiotics or antiviral medications to address the specific infectious agent, pain relief and antiinflammatory drugs to alleviate discomfort and swelling, and supportive care, including rest, proper nutrition, and a clean environment,

20.3.3 Hydrocele

A hydrocele is a build-up of fluid within the scrotum, leading to swelling. It can occur due to trauma, infection, or other underlying conditions. While not typically a serious condition, a large hydrocele may cause discomfort and affect the goat's movement. While hydroceles are more commonly associated with humans, they can also occur in animals, including goats (Balaro et al. 2022).

20.3.3.1 Causes of Hydrocele in Goats

- *Trauma*: physical injury or trauma to the scrotal area can disrupt the blood vessels and lymphatic vessels, leading to the accumulation of fluid.
- *Inflammation or infection*: inflammatory conditions or infections affecting the scrotum or testicles can trigger an abnormal accumulation of fluid.
- *Congenital factors*: some cases of hydrocele in goats may be congenital, meaning they are present at birth due to developmental abnormalities.
- *Lymphatic obstruction*: obstruction or dysfunction of the lymphatic vessels, which play a role in fluid drainage, can result in fluid accumulation.

20.3.3.2 Symptoms of Hydrocele

Hydroceles in goats are characterized by swelling and enlargement of the scrotum, which may vary in size, a fluid-filled, soft, and sometimes fluctuant mass within the scrotum and discomfort or mild pain, which may lead to changes in the goat's behavior or gait.

20.3.3.3 Diagnosis

Diagnosing hydrocele involves a veterinarian's evaluation, which may include palpation and physical examination of the scrotum to assess the size, consistency, and fluid content, and aspiration of fluid from the scrotum for laboratory analysis. In some cases, small hydroceles may resolve on their own without treatment. However, larger or persistent hydroceles may require intervention.

20.3.3.4 Treatment

- *Aspiration*: if the hydrocele is causing discomfort or hindering the goat's movement, the veterinarian may aspirate (draw out) the fluid using a needle and syringe. This is typically a temporary solution as the fluid may reaccumulate.
- *Surgery*: surgical intervention may be considered for larger or recurrent hydroceles. The procedure involves draining the fluid and addressing the underlying cause, such as repairing any damaged blood vessels or lymphatic vessels.

20.3.3.5 Prevention

Hydroceles are often a result of underlying causes such as trauma or infections. Preventive measures include providing a safe and clean environment for goats to minimize the risk of trauma, and implementing good hygiene practices to prevent infections in the scrotal area, It is important to note that the scrotal region is sensitive and important for the goat's reproductive health. If you suspect a hydrocele or notice any changes in your goat's scrotum, it is crucial to consult a veterinarian. Only a veterinarian can accurately diagnose the condition and recommend appropriate treatment options based on the goat's specific situation.

20.3.4 Scrotal Dermatitis

Scrotal dermatitis, also known as "scrotal dermatosis" or "scrotal eczema," refers to skin inflammation and irritation of the scrotum. This can be caused by various factors such as allergies, parasites, fungal or bacterial infections, or physical irritation. It may manifest as redness, itching, hair loss, and scaling of the skin. Scrotal dermatitis can have various causes, and managing the condition typically involves identifying and addressing the underlying factors (Struthers et al. 2022).

20.3.4.1 Causes of Scrotal Dermatitis in Goats

- *Allergies*: contact with allergens, such as certain plants, chemicals, or materials, can lead to an allergic reaction on the scrotal skin.
- *Parasites*: infestations of mites, lice, or other external parasites can cause irritation and inflammation on the scrotum.

- *Fungal infections*: fungal pathogens, such as dermatophytes, can infect the scrotal skin and result in dermatitis.
- *Bacterial infections*: bacterial infections, whether primary or secondary to other skin issues, can contribute to scrotal dermatitis.
- *Environmental factors*: excessive moisture, humidity, and poor hygiene in the scrotal area can create a favorable environment for skin irritation and infections.
- *Trauma*: physical irritation or injury to the scrotal skin can lead to inflammation and dermatitis.

20.3.4.2 Symptoms of Scrotal Dermatitis

Scrotal dermatitis in goats may present with redness, swelling, and inflammation of the scrotal skin, itching and discomfort, leading to scratching or rubbing of the area, formation of lesions, sores, or scabs on the scrotum, hair loss and changes in the texture of the skin and restlessness, irritability, and attempts to alleviate discomfort by licking or biting the scrotum.

20.3.4.3 Diagnosis and Treatment

Diagnosing scrotal dermatitis involves a veterinarian's examination, which may include visual inspection of the scrotal area to assess the extent of inflammation and skin changes and skin scrapings or swabs to identify potential parasites, fungi, or bacteria.

Treatment of scrotal dermatitis depends on the underlying cause and may include the following.

- *Topical treatments*: application of medicated creams, ointments, or sprays to address inflammation, infections, or parasites.
- *Antibiotics or antifungals*: prescription of oral medications to combat bacterial or fungal infections, if present.
- *Pain relief and antiinflammatories*: administration of medications to alleviate discomfort and reduce inflammation.
- *Hygiene and management*: implementing proper hygiene practices, keeping the scrotal area clean and dry, and providing a comfortable environment.

20.3.4.4 Prevention

Maintain a clean and dry living environment to minimize moisture-related issues. Regularly inspect goats for signs of skin irritation or parasites, provide proper grooming and hygiene care for the animals, and avoid exposure to potential allergens or irritants.

20.3.5 Scrotal Hernia

A scrotal hernia occurs when a part of the abdominal contents (intestines, fat, etc.) protrudes into the scrotum through a weakened area or defect in the abdominal wall. This can cause a visible bulge and may lead to complications if not addressed. Scrotal hernias can occur in both humans and animals, including goats. This condition can be serious and may require surgical intervention to correct (Kitessa et al. 2022).

20.3.5.1 Causes of Scrotal Hernia in Goats

Scrotal hernias in goats can have different underlying causes.

- *Congenital*: some scrotal hernias are present at birth and occur due to a failure of the abdominal muscles to close properly during fetal development.
- *Trauma*: injuries or trauma to the abdominal wall can weaken the muscles and create openings through which abdominal contents can protrude.

20.3.5.2 Symptoms of Scrotal Hernia

Symptoms of scrotal hernia in goats may include visible swelling or bulge in the scrotum, often containing abdominal tissue, difficulty walking or moving due to discomfort or pain, behavioral changes such as restlessness or lethargy, and possible complications if the hernia becomes incarcerated (unable to be pushed back in) or strangulated (blood supply to the herniated tissue is compromised).

20.3.5.3 Diagnosis and Treatment

Diagnosing scrotal hernia typically involves a veterinarian's examination, which may include physical inspection and palpation of the scrotum and hernia site to assess the size, location, and content of the hernia, ultrasound or other imaging techniques to evaluate the extent of the hernia and its impact on surrounding structures.

Treatment of scrotal hernia often involves surgical correction, especially if the hernia is large, causing discomfort, or at risk of complications. The surgical procedure aims to reposition the herniated contents back into the abdominal cavity, repair and strengthen the weakened abdominal wall to prevent recurrence, and close any openings through which the hernia protruded.

20.3.5.4 Prevention

Preventing scrotal hernias in goats involves avoiding excessive physical stress or trauma that could weaken the abdominal muscles. If hereditary factors are suspected, selecting breeding animals without a history of hernias may help reduce the risk of passing on this condition.

20.3.6 Tumors

Tumors can also develop in the scrotum, such as testicular tumors. While less common, these growths can affect the health of the goat and may require surgical intervention. Tumors in goats, as in any living organisms, are abnormal growths of cells that can develop in various parts of the body. Tumors can be benign (noncancerous) or malignant (cancerous). They can arise from different types of tissues and can have a range of effects on the goat's health (Muñoz-Salinas et al. 2022).

20.3.6.1 Types of Tumors

- *Benign tumors*: these tumors do not spread to other parts of the body and are generally less aggressive. Examples of benign tumors that can occur in goats include lipomas (fatty tumors), fibromas (connective tissue tumors), and papillomas (wart-like growths).
- *Malignant tumors*: these tumors are cancerous and can invade nearby tissues and potentially spread to other parts of the body through a process called metastasis. Examples of malignant tumors in goats include mast cell tumors, lymphomas, and certain types of sarcomas.

20.3.6.2 Causes and Risk Factors

The exact causes of tumors in goats are often complex and can involve genetic, environmental, and other factors. Some risk factors that might contribute to the development of tumors include the following.

- *Genetic predisposition*: certain breeds or genetic lines may be more prone to specific types of tumors.
- *Exposure to carcinogens*: environmental factors such as exposure to chemicals, radiation, or infectious agents could increase the risk of tumor development.
- *Age*: older goats may have a higher likelihood of developing tumors.

20.3.6.3 Symptoms

The symptoms of tumors in goats can vary widely depending on the type, location, and size of the tumor. Common signs might include swelling or lump under the skin or in internal organs, changes in behavior or activity level, weight loss and decreased appetite and difficulty breathing, swallowing, or moving, depending on the tumor's location.

20.3.6.4 Diagnosis and Treatment

Diagnosing tumors in goats involves a veterinarian's evaluation, which may include physical examination and palpation of the goat's body to locate and assess tumors, imaging tests such as ultrasound, X-rays, or CT scans to visualize the tumor's size and location, and

biopsy, which involves removing a small piece of the tumor for laboratory analysis to determine if it is benign or malignant.

Treatment options for tumors in goats depend on factors such as the tumor type, size, and location.

- *Surgical removal*: benign tumors are often removed surgically if they are causing discomfort or impeding the goat's normal function.
- *Chemotherapy or radiation*: for certain malignant tumors, chemotherapy or radiation therapy might be considered to target and reduce the growth of cancer cells.
- *Supportive care*: managing pain, maintaining proper nutrition, and providing a comfortable environment to support the goat's overall well-being.

20.3.6.5 Prevention

Preventing tumors in goats involves maintaining good herd health practices, which includes proper nutrition, minimizing exposure to potential carcinogens, and regular veterinary care. Additionally, selective breeding and genetic management can play a role in reducing the risk of certain hereditary tumor predispositions.

20.3.7 Trauma

Trauma refers to any physical injury that the goat may experience, whether due to accidents, fights, falls, or other external factors.

20.3.7.1 Scrotal Trauma in Goats

Scrotal trauma specifically involves injuries to the scrotal region, which includes the testicles and surrounding tissues. This can occur in various ways, such as kicks, blows, or accidents that impact the scrotal area. Scrotal trauma can result in the following outcomes.

- *Swelling*: trauma can lead to immediate swelling of the scrotum due to blood pooling or fluid accumulation in the affected area.
- *Bruising*: the force of the impact can cause blood vessels to rupture, leading to bruising (discoloration) of the scrotal skin.
- *Pain*: the goat may experience pain and discomfort due to the injury, leading to behavioral changes such as restlessness, avoidance of movement, or vocalization.
- *Reduced fertility*: severe scrotal trauma can potentially impact the health of the testicles and sperm production, leading to temporary or permanent fertility issues.

20.3.8 Parasitic Infections

Parasites, such as mites or lice, can infest the scrotal skin and cause irritation and inflammation. Parasitic infestations can lead to discomfort, skin problems, and other health issues.

20.3.8.1 Types of Parasites

- *Mites*: mites are tiny arthropods that can infest the skin of goats. They may cause conditions like mange, characterized by intense itching, hair loss, and inflammation. Scabies mites, for instance, can burrow into the skin and cause severe itching and discomfort.
- *Lice*: lice are wingless insects that feed on the goat's blood and can attach to the skin and hair. They cause itching, hair loss, and skin irritation. There are two main types of lice that affect goats: biting lice and sucking lice.

20.3.8.2 Symptoms of Parasitic Infestations

- *Intense scratching*: goats infested with mites or lice will often scratch, rub, or bite at the affected areas in an attempt to alleviate itching.
- *Hair loss*: infestations can lead to patchy hair loss and thinning of the coat.
- *Skin irritation*: affected skin may appear red, inflamed, or scaly.
- *Restlessness*: infested goats may be restless and display abnormal behavior due to the discomfort.
- *Reduced production*: parasitic infestations can affect the overall health of goats, leading to decreased milk production and weight gain.

20.3.8.3 Diagnosis and Treatment

Diagnosing parasitic infestations typically involves a veterinarian's examination, which may include the following.

- *Visual inspection*: a thorough visual examination of the goat's skin and hair to look for signs of parasites or skin irritation.
- *Skin scraping*: a small sample of skin may be scraped and examined under a microscope to identify the presence of mites or lice.

Treatment for parasitic infestations involves the following factors.

- *Topical treatments*: medicated shampoos, sprays, or powders can be used to kill and remove parasites from the skin.
- *Injectable medications*: some parasiticides can be administered through injections.
- *Environmental management*: cleaning and disinfecting the goat's living area can help reduce the risk of reinfestation.
- *Supportive care*: providing proper nutrition, hydration, and comfort can support the goat's recovery.

20.3.8.4 Prevention

Preventing parasitic infestations involves good herd management practices.

- *Regular inspections*: regularly inspect goats for signs of parasites, especially in areas like the scrotum.
- *Quarantine*: quarantine new animals before introducing them to the herd to prevent the spread of parasites.
- *Parasite control*: implement a parasite control program that includes strategic deworming and rotating classes of dewormers to prevent resistance.
- *Hygiene*: maintain a clean and dry living environment to discourage parasites.

20.3.9 Heat Stress

While not a disease, extreme heat can lead to scrotal edema (swelling) due to increased blood flow to the area. This can affect sperm production and fertility (Abioja et al. 2022).

20.3.9.1 Scrotal Edema and Fertility

One of the effects of heat stress in male goats is scrotal edema, which is swelling of the scrotum due to increased blood flow to the area. Scrotal edema can lead to discomfort and affect the goat's fertility. The testicles are sensitive to temperature changes, and excessive heat can lead to decreased sperm production and impaired sperm quality. This can result in reduced fertility and lower breeding success rates.

20.3.9.2 Other Effects of Heat Stress

- *Dehydration*: high temperatures can cause goats to become dehydrated, leading to reduced feed intake, weight loss, and electrolyte imbalances.
- *Respiratory distress*: goats may pant excessively to cool down, leading to respiratory distress and an increased risk of respiratory infections.
- *Reduced milk production*: heat-stressed dairy goats may experience reduced milk production and altered milk composition.
- *Decreased immune function*: heat stress can weaken the immune system, making goats more susceptible to infections and diseases.

20.3.9.3 Prevention and Management

- *Shade*: provide adequate shade and shelter to protect goats from direct sunlight.
- *Water*: ensure access to clean and cool drinking water at all times.
- *Ventilation*: provide good ventilation in barns and shelters to promote air circulation.
- *Cooling methods*: use fans, misters, or sprinklers to help cool the goats and their environment.
- *Time of feeding*: feed goats during the cooler parts of the day to minimize heat generation from digestion.
- *Reduce stress*: minimize handling, transport, and other stressful activities during hot weather.
- *Breeding*: consider breeding practices that take into account heat stress, such as avoiding breeding during the hottest months.

20.4 Conclusion

Diseases of the scrotum in goats pose significant challenges to their reproductive health and overall well-being. By understanding the causes, symptoms, and management strategies for scrotal diseases, goat farmers and livestock managers can take proactive measures to prevent and control these issues. Through proper hygiene, regular health monitoring, and timely veterinary care, goats can lead healthier lives, contributing to the sustainability and success of the livestock industry.

References

Abah, K.O., Fontbonne, A., Partyka, A., and Nizanski, W. (2023). Effect of male age on semen quality in domestic animals: potential for advanced functional and translational research? *Veterinary Research Communications* 47: 1125–1137.

Abioja, M.O., Logunleko, M.O., Majekodunmi, B.C. et al. (2022). Roles of candidate genes in the adaptation of goats to heat stress: a review. *Small Ruminant Research* 218: 106878.

Balaro, M.F.A., Cosentino, I.O., Ribeiro, A.C.S., and Brandão, F.Z. (2022). Ultrasound diagnosis in small ruminants: occurrence and description of genital pathologies. *Veterinary Sciences* 9 (11): 599.

Chaurasia, D.K., Nahak, A.K., Mishra, P.C. et al. (2023). Studies on seasonal variation of scrotal parameters in Ganjam buck. *Pharma Innovation* 12: 2303–2304.

Foster, A.P. (2023). Challenges in the diagnosis and management of skin diseases in alpacas, goats, pigs, and sheep. *Journal of the American Veterinary Medical Association* 261 (S1): S86–S94.

Husnurrizal, H., Akbar, D.G.P., Siregar, T.N. et al. (2023). Comparison of reproductive performance of Gembrong goats and male Boerka goats. *Livestock and Animal Research* 21 (1): 1–8.

Kitessa, J.D., Merga, A.F., Afata, A.W., and Feyisa, C.T. (2022). Inguinal herniorrhaphy in goat: the novel way of using vest-over-pants closure technique. *Veterinary Record Case Reports* 10 (2): e321.

Mansour, M., Wilhite, R., Rowe, J., and Hafiz, S. (ed.) (2023). *Guide to Ruminant Anatomy: Dissection and Clinical Aspects*. Hoboken, NJ: Wiley.

Mellor, D.J. and Stafford, K.J. (2000). Acute castration and/or tailing distress and its alleviation in lambs. *New Zealand Veterinary Journal* 48 (2): 33–43.

Mohamed, R.H., Mohamed, R.S., Abd El-Hamid, I.S. et al. (2023). Semen quality, testicular characteristic, biochemical profile and histopathology of testes of goats under heat stress conditions. *Assiut Veterinary Medical Journal* 69 (176): 76–87.

Monteiro, M.M., de Mello Seal, D.C., de Souza, J.H. et al. (2023). Effect of antifreeze protein type III on frozen/thawed of spermatozoa recover from goat epididymis. *Research in Veterinary Science* 154: 108–112.

Muñoz-Salinas, F., Andrade-Montemayor, H.M., De la Torre-Carbot, K. et al. (2022). Comparative analysis of the protein composition of goat milk from French Alpine, Nubian, and Creole breeds and Holstein Friesian cow milk: implications for early infant nutrition. *Animals* 12 (17): 2236.

Perumal, P., Sunder, J., De, A.K. et al. (2023). Flaxseed oil modulates testicular biometrics, hormone, libido, antioxidant and semen profiles in endangered Teressa goat of Andaman and Nicobar Islands. *Reproductive Biology* 23 (1): 100730.

Singh, M., Kaswan, S., Cheema, R.S. et al. (2019). Effect of scrotal bifurcation on breeding soundness traits in Beetal bucks during summer season. *Tropical Animal Health and Production* 51: 1585–1590.

Struthers, J.D., Chako, C., Ruppert, S. et al. (2022). Diagnostic challenge in veterinary pathology: alopecic crusting dermatitis in a goat. *Veterinary Pathology* 59 (2): 182–185.

Sultan, K.H., Ahmad, W.K., and Mohamed, A.R. (2023). Effect of buck's body weight on some reproductive parameters and it's relation with sexual behavior. *Iraqi Journal of Veterinary Sciences* 37 (3): 733–737.

Thobela, L.T., Mohlabeng, I.M., and Selala, L.J. (2023). Phenotypic relationship between body weight, body condition score and testicular measurement traits in dorper rams raised in Syferkuil farm, Limpopo Province, South Africa. *Pakistan Journal of Zoology* 55 (1): 457.

21

Diseases of the Testes

Felix Uchenna Samuel[1,2], *Peter Ibrahim Rekwot*[3], *Lushaikyaa Allam*[3], *Hycinth Ndabatsado Kolo*[4], *and Aliyu Abdullahi Mohammed*[5]

[1] *Faculty of Veterinary Medicine, National Animal Production Research Institute, Ahmadu Bello University, Zaria, Nigeria*
[2] *Department of Food and Animal Science, Alabama A&M University, Normal, USA*
[3] *Faculty of Veterinary Medicine, Ahmadu Bello University, Zaria, Nigeria*
[4] *Department of Animal Health and Production, Federal University of Technology, Minna, Nigeria*
[5] *Department of Animal Sciences, Usman Danfodio University, Sokoto, Nigeria*

21.1 Introduction

The male goat is called a buck or billy. Many dairy goat owners are offended by the term "billy," and Angora breeders are often confused by "buck" because in many parts of the United States, the ram (male sheep) is referred to as a buck. The buck is frequently described as half of the breeding herd. Many owners find him the more difficult half to control. Because of his size and strength and his distinctive odor, the buck is often skipped when the does are dewormed, vaccinated, given selenium injections, or foot trimmed (Kilgour 2019).

The reproductive functions of the male involve the formation of sperm and the deposition of the sperm into the female. Sperm are produced in the seminiferous tubules of the testes and are then transported through the rete testes to the epididymides, where they are stored and matured. The two testes produce spermatozoa (Walker and Cooke 2023). Although they vary somewhat in size, shape, and location among species, they share a similar structure.

The testicles are suspended away from the body by the pendulous scrotum. The scrotum is composed of undulating epidermis that may or may not be covered by wool, depending on the breed and husbandry practices. A rich plexus of blood vessels, lymphatics, and sweat glands lies beneath the skin. The dartos, a smooth muscle layer, is connected to the vaginal tunics of the testicle by the scrotal fascia (Koziol and Palmer 2023). The scrotal fascia is the connective tissue that is typically broken down when the clinician separates the skin from the testicle during routine castration. The vaginal tunics are outcroppings of the peritoneum and form a protective covering over the testicles. The space between the two layers of vaginal tunic (parietal and visceral) as it reflects around the testicle normally contains a small amount of peritoneal fluid (Koziol and Palmer 2023). The scrotal septum, composed primarily of the dartos muscle, divides the scrotum into two halves.

The seminiferous tubules are convoluted and occupy the greatest portion of each testicle. The spermatozoa are produced within them. The testicle is surrounded by a connective tissue capsule called the tunica albuginea. Support of the seminiferous tubules is provided by connective tissue extensions (septa or trabeculae) into the testis from the tunica albuginea. A cross-section of the testicle shows the relationship of the seminiferous tubules to each other and to their connective tissue support (interstitial tissue).

In addition to spermatozoa in various stages of development, two other important cell types are the Sertoli cell (sustentacular cell) and the Leydig cell (interstitial cell) (Lee et al. 2008). The Sertoli cell provides a "nurse" function for developing spermatozoa. Processes from Sertoli cells surround spermatids and spermatocytes and provide intimate contact with all stages of spermatozoa production; in this respect they are known as sustentacular (supporting) cells. The Sertoli cells have their base at the periphery of the seminiferous tubules and extend toward the center. The basal junction (tight junction) with adjacent Sertoli cells forms a blood–testis barrier that permits control of the environment within the tubule and also prevents spermatozoa from entering the interstitium.

Elements of Reproduction and Reproductive Diseases of Goats, First Edition. Edited by Tanmoy Rana.

The Sertoli cells divide the seminiferous tubules into two compartments: (i) the basal compartment, which communicates with interstitial fluid and provides space for germinal epithelial cells, and (ii) the adluminal compartment, which is the space between Sertoli cells that communicates centrally with the lumen of the tubule. Division of a germinal epithelial cell (spermatogonium) in the basal compartment provides a replacement cell and another cell, which must move through the Sertoli cell junction to enter the adluminal compartment. Here, further divisions occur and spermatozoa are finally formed (Mruk and Cheng 2015). The Sertoli cells secrete a fluid into the adluminal compartment; its composition favors the developing spermatozoa. The seminiferous tubules drain into the rete testes, which in turn are drained by 10–12 efferent ducts. These ducts drain into the head of the epididymis, which is located on the dorsal craniolateral aspect of the testicle. The body of the epididymis curves around the lateral portion of the testes and ends caudomedially as the tail. The tubular structure is reflected dorsally and becomes the vas deferens.

Rams and bucks have a full complement of accessory sex glands. The small bulbourethral glands are located caudally in the pelvic cavity on either side of the pelvic urethra; they can be palpated rectally. They also have lobulated vesicular glands, disseminate prostate gland, and a widening of the vas deferens known as the ampulla.

Spermatogenesis requires about 49–60 days from the start of germ cell division until the sperm are released from the seminiferous tubules. Another 10 days to two weeks are required for the sperm to pass from the seminiferous tubules through the epididymis (Lee et al. 2008).

21.2 Epididymis

The epididymis is a collection and storage tubule for the testis (Figure 21.1). It begins at the pole of the testis in which blood vessels and nerves enter; this is known as the head of the epididymis. The head continues along one side of the testis as the body of the epididymis, which terminates before making a turn upward as the tail of the epididymis. The head of the epididymis receives sperm and adluminal fluid through efferent ducts from the rete testis (the intratesticular network of straight tubules that receives content from the convoluted seminiferous tubules). Spermatozoa move to the epididymis by the flow of fluid into the lumen of the seminiferous tubules from the adluminal spaces (Figure 21.1) (Fietz and Bergmann 2017). Storage in the epididymis allows the spermatozoa to reach maturity and become motile. Reabsorption of much of the seminiferous tubular fluid occurs in the head of the epididymis.

21.3 Ductus Deferens

The ductus deferens, sometimes called the vas deferens, is the continuation of the duct system from the tail of the epididymis to the pelvic urethra. As the ductus deferens leaves the testis, toward the abdomen, it is enclosed along with the testicular artery, vein, and nerve, and lymphatic vessels within the visceral layer of the vaginal tunic. This combination of structures is known as the spermatic cord. The visceral layer of the vaginal tunic also envelops the testis and epididymis. It is derived from abdominal peritoneum of embryonic origin when the testes descended to the scrotum via the inguinal canal.

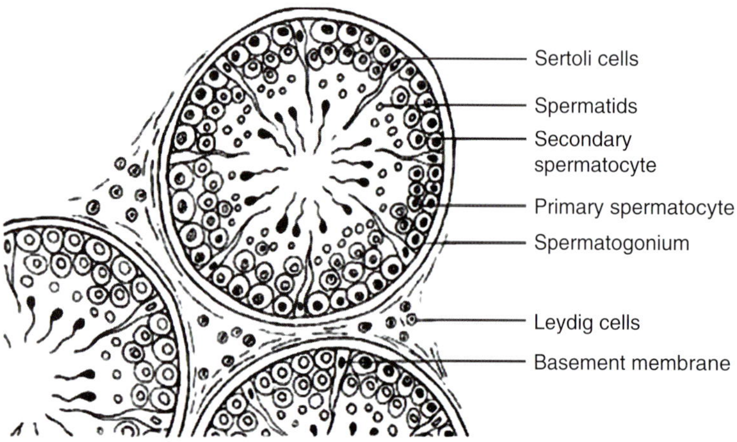

Figure 21.1 Relationship of the seminiferous tubules to each other and to the interstitial tissue.

The inguinal canal is an oblique passage from the abdominal cavity to the exterior of the body that extends from the deep (interior) inguinal ring to the superficial (exterior) inguinal ring. The inguinal rings are slits in the tendinous attachments of the two flat abdominal muscles to the pelvis. After the spermatic cord passes through the inguinal rings, the ductus deferens separates from the spermatic cord to proceed to the pelvic urethra. The ductus deferens terminates with an enlarged, glandular area (variable size among species), known as the ampulla of the ductus deferens (absent in the boar) (Hamada and Saadeldin 2022).

The interstitial tissue is occupied not only by the usual blood vascular network but also by Leydig cells (interstitial cells) and by connective tissue septa (provide support for seminiferous tubules) from the connective tissue capsule (tunica albuginea) of the testis. The rete testis is a network of straight tubules connecting convoluted seminiferous tubules with the highly convoluted epididymal tubule via efferent ducts (extratesticular). The flow of spermatozoa with their fluids is shown by the arrows in Figure 21.2 (Pathak et al. 2022).

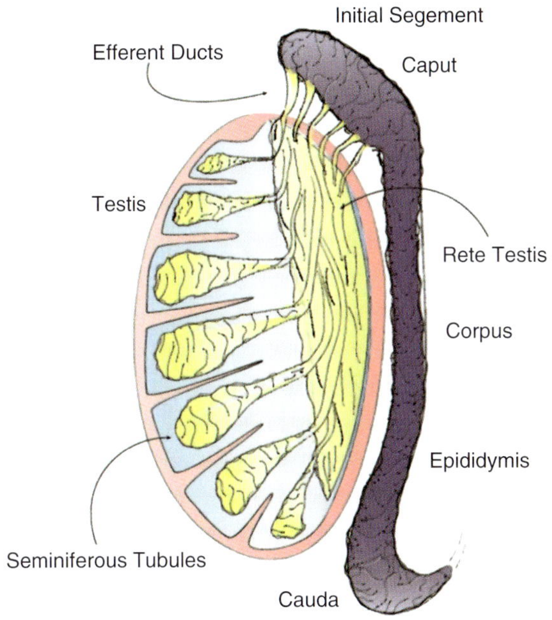

Figure 21.2 Testes showing seminiferous tubules and excurrent ducts.

21.4 Effect of Season on Buck Puberty and Reproduction

Breed, age, and nutrition contribute to the onset of sexual maturity in the buck. The age at puberty depends on the breed, varying from 2–3 months in pygmy breeds to 4–5 months in Nubian and Boer bucks (Rouatbi et al. 2022). Most breeds of goats raised in the temperate environment of the northern hemisphere have sperm in the ejaculate at 4–5 months. However, at this age their semen quality is poor and they are not suitable for breeding.

Nubian and Boer bucks begin exhibiting libido at 10–12 weeks and start producing quality semen at about eight months. Natural adhesions of the urethral process and glans penis to the prepuce make the immature buck incapable of copulation. This attachment begins to separate at three months, and fertile mating is possible at 4–5 months. Fast-growing, well-fed, and well-managed kids are able to breed sooner than starved males of equal age.

Whether bucks are truly seasonal breeders is controversial. Many bucks have depressed libido, reduced pheromones, decreased scrotal circumference (SC), lower semen freezability, and a larger number of abnormal spermatozoa outside the breeding season (Rouatbi et al. 2022). All these changes reflect lower levels of LH and testosterone. LH and testosterone concentration, libido, and odor presence in the buck peak in the fall. Sexual behavior of the buck includes actively seeking does in estrus, courtship (kicking, pawing, muzzling, grunting, and flehmen), mounting, intromission, and ejaculation. Ejaculation occurs spontaneously and is characterized by a strong pelvic thrust with a rapid backward movement of the head. After ejaculation the buck dismounts and shows no sexual arousal for a few minutes to several hours (Shipley 2022).

21.5 Diseases of the Testes

Except for changes induced by fever or malnutrition, most abnormalities are not amenable to treatment.

21.5.1 Procedures for Evaluating Testis and Epididymis

In addition to judging the testicular volume by scrotal circumference or the diameter of each testis by the use of calipers, the consistency of the testes should be evaluated. Normal testicular tissue should feel resilient and approximately as firm as muscle. Its ultrasonographic appearance is uniformly homogeneous with a central hyperechoic line representing the mediastinum testis. The testicular tunics and testicular capsule are also distinct hyperechoic lines, whereas fluid around the testis (hydrocele) is hypoechoic. The tail of the epididymis is more heterogeneous and less echogenic than the testis. The use of ultrasonography for evaluating testicular lesions has also been described for bulls.

Testicular biopsy is not routinely used in goats. In bulls, biopsy procedures have led to decreased semen quality. It is important to avoid highly vascular areas and to suture the incision in the tunica albuginea, or else hemorrhage and infarction may occur.

21.5.2 Varicoceles

A varicocele is defined as a localized dilation and thrombosis of the internal spermatic vein and is recognized as a fluctuant to hard swelling in the spermatic cord. Varicoceles are more common in rams than in bucks. This condition is often manifested as rear limb lameness and awkward posture as the ram tries to relieve pressure on the swollen cords. Affected animals may become weak and susceptible to other diseases as a result of debilitation brought on by an unwillingness to walk to obtain food and water.

Varicoceles can be diagnosed by palpation and diagnostic ultrasound. Abnormalities such as decreased total sperm count, reduced sperm motility, and morphological abnormalities of the sperm are often associated with varicoceles. The exact etiology of the condition is not known but a genetic predisposition is suspected. No easy treatment is available, and affected rams or bucks should be culled (Foster 2016).

21.5.3 Epididymitis

21.5.3.1 Epididymitis in Older Males

Epididymitis is a rare condition in the buck but a clinically important disease in rams. Epididymitis in rams should be considered to be caused by *B. ovis* until proven otherwise. This is especially true of older rams that have been actively breeding in multiple sire units. However, one case report involving an outbreak of *B. ovis* in a group of virgin ram lambs suggests that the disease may be spread *in utero* or neonatally, before any known sexual activity. The primary means of spread is thought to be through contact with mucous membranes, which results in bacteremia. The organism localizes in the epididymis and secondary sex glands. Contact can occur among rams and from recently infected ewes; venereal and oral–nasal transmission routes also are possible.

Swelling of the epididymis is the primary presenting sign, occurring about three weeks after the initial exposure. Grossly, there is localized inflammation followed by hyperplasia and obstruction of the epididymal ducts. This obstruction causes a back-up of spermatozoa, the development of sperm granulomas, and pressure necrosis. The seminal vesicles also are commonly affected, which may account for the large number of infected rams that show no palpable signs of epididymitis. Semen collected from infected rams usually contains a large number of polymorphonuclear neutrophils that can be seen on the motility preparations or on Wright's stained specimens. Serology for *B. ovis* should be considered a routine part of a breeding soundness examination. Both enzyme-linked immunosorbent assay (ELISA) and complement fixation (CF) tests are available.

Herd infections with *B. ovis* can result in a 15–30% reduction in lambing rate depending on the chronicity of the herd problem. This decrease in reproductive efficiency results from lowered fertility in the rams, failure of the ewes to conceive, reabsorption of embryos, abortions, stillbirths, and weak lambs. Recommendations outlined by Bulgin (1990) include the following.

- Buying virgin rams that have been serologically tested for brucellosis.
- Keeping newly purchased rams separate until all rams are tested free from *Brucella*.
- Performing palpation and culling all rams with epididymitis before the breeding season.
- Culling all *B. ovis*-positive rams.
- Retesting all rams in the flock 60 days after any rams are found positive.
- Performing BSEs yearly on all rams. If a large number of serologically positive rams is found after a year of adherence to these guidelines, efforts should be made to determine whether a serologically negative carrier ram is present in the flock by culturing semen from all rams (Sathe and Shipley 2014).

21.5.3.2 Epididymitis in Young Males

In younger rams, and less commonly in bucks, epididymitis can be caused by a number of organisms such as *Histophilus*, *Actinobacillus*, and *Haemophilus* species, as well as *Corynebacterium pseudotuberculosis*. Lamb epididymitis can be spread from ram to ram by the oral or nasal route. The organisms responsible for lamb epididymitis can frequently be cultured from the preputial cavity of rams younger than two years of age and are commonly found in the mucous membranes of the prepuce, penis, mouth, and nasal cavity. Colonization and subsequent disease of the reproductive tract may depend on the hormonal changes that occur during maturation and puberty, along with other unknown differentiating factors that allow most animals to eliminate the bacteria spontaneously while causing others to develop clinical signs.

Diagnosis of lamb epididymitis is made by palpation of the enlarged epididymis and by ruling out *B. ovis* infection. Semen from infected lambs is characterized by a large number of neutrophils and by the morphologically abnormal spermatozoa typical of epididymal disease. Although the signs of most cases of lamb epididymitis are restricted to the reproductive tract, occasionally an associated fever and hindlimb lameness also occur.

Lamb epididymitis can be treated with long-acting oxytetracycline (20 mg/kg intramuscularly or subcutaneously) injections for three treatments at three-day intervals. Inclusion of tetracycline (20 mg/kg by mouth daily) products in the ration may be appropriate in herds experiencing a high incidence of lamb epididymitis. Treatment should be reserved for valuable lambs and cases diagnosed in the early stages because most lambs develop scar tissue in the epididymis that prevents functional recovery (Stapelberg 2022).

21.5.4 Orchitis

Orchitis is a common occurrence in the ram and is occasionally seen in the buck. Scrotal abscesses may be caused by trauma or may be an extension of epididymitis. Whenever testicular trauma or infection is encountered, it should be considered a medical emergency in breeding animals (Crilly et al. 2022). Excessive heat from one testicle can result in possibly irreversible thermal injury to the germinal epithelium of the contralateral testicle. All the organisms discussed in the section on epididymitis can cause orchitis.

The signs include a hot, swollen scrotum (usually unilaterally), inability to move the affected testicle freely in the scrotum, and pain on manipulation of the affected testicle and the scrotum. Some animals may show signs of systemic disease, pain on walking, and decrease in libido. In cases affecting valuable animals, hemicastration in the acute phase may prevent permanent infertility (Stapelberg 2022).

21.5.5 Sperm Granulomas

Although testicular tumors are rare in rams and bucks, granulomatous swellings are occasionally encountered. Sperm granulomas are more common in goats than in sheep, and unlike abscesses or other forms of orchitis, they usually occur bilaterally. Sperm granulomas are often caused by a partial or complete blockage of the efferent ducts draining into the epididymis. As pressure builds, the ducts become distended and may rupture, resulting in a severe inflammation. As fluid accumulates, pressure continues to build and testicular degeneration may occur. Some animals are initially fertile but lose fertility after the efferent ducts become completely occluded. Granulomas are firm swellings found in the head of the epididymis. On palpation, the testicles may be initially edematous but they eventually become hard. The testicles may eventually become small and atrophic. Ultrasonographic evaluation may reveal mineralization of the testicles or the granuloma itself.

No treatment is available for sperm granulomas, and the clinician should be aware of the potential association with the intersex condition (Crilly et al. 2022).

21.5.6 Testicular Atrophy and Degeneration

Testicular hypoplasia and degeneration are difficult to differentiate on initial examination. A common cause of testicular degeneration is debility from malnutrition or parasitism. The chronically recumbent buck might also experience testicular atrophy because of impaired thermoregulation in the scrotum. Sperm granulomas cause progressive testicular degeneration. In rams and bucks out of season, testicular size and palpation characteristics may be difficult to differentiate from subtle cases of testicular atrophy. More extreme differences are encountered in rams than in goats, but in general the testicle in the nonbreeding season is smaller and lacks normal resiliency.

Causes of testicular atrophy include zinc deficiency, hypothyroidism (iodine deficiency, ingestion of goitrogenous plants), starvation diets, systemic disease, and heat and cold stress. Iodine-induced hypothyroidism has been associated with decreased testicular weight, depressed spermatogenesis, and decreased libido. Atrophic or degenerated testicles become elongated, small, and either softer or harder. Normal testicles usually have a homogeneous echogenicity on ultrasound. Atrophic or degenerative testicles tend to have a heterogeneous pattern and more hyperechoic areas. Testicular biopsy can be of value in diagnosis.

Many cases of atrophy and degeneration are not treatable; the exceptions are cases caused by diet or certain diseases. In treating diet-related atrophy, ensuring adequate protein-energy intake and free access to a good-quality trace mineral supplement is essential. If zinc deficiency is suspected, reducing the legume content of the diet and adding a chelated form of zinc (zinc methionine) to the diet or trace mineral mixture is useful. If iodine-induced hypothyroidism is diagnosed, the inclusion of iodine in a trace mineral mixture and the removal of goitrogenous plants from the diet should be undertaken; males should be kept off pastures with goitrogenous plants before and during breeding (Crilly et al. 2022).

Multiple foci of calcinosis are grossly visible on cut surfaces of the testis. Histologically, granuloma formation occurs where masses of dead sperm have accumulated in collecting ducts (Fraser and Wilson 1966). Foci of testicular necrosis or mineralization are hyperechoic during ultrasonographic examination but only the echogenicity of the near-field testis should be assessed, because of attenuation of the far-field ultrasound beam. Firm, mineralized parenchyma, detectable by ultrasound, has been observed in elderly or infertile bucks. These changes are irreversible. Testicular neoplasia, although rare in goats, should also be detectable by ultrasonography. Atrophy and degeneration of the seminiferous tubules have been reported in goats in the Sudan experimentally fed *Acanthospermum hispidum*, which also causes hepatic necrosis and fibrosis. Likewise, the feeding of *Leucaena leucocephala* is reported to cause mild degeneration of the testes, possibly secondary to hypothyroidism.

Experimental hypothyroidism in goats (achieved by feeding thiouracil) was associated with a relative decrease in the weight of the testis and epididymis, a reduction in spermatogenesis, and degenerative changes in the testis and accessory sex glands. There was loss of libido, decreased ejaculate volume, decreased sperm concentration, motility, and viability, and an increase in abnormal spermatozoa. These changes were reversible. Thyroidectomy in young male goats also results in smaller than normal testes. Detrimental effects of naturally occurring hypothyroidism on testicular function in adult goats have not been documented.

21.5.7 Intersex

Caprine intersexes are referred to as *male pseudohermaphrodites* because a majority of them have testes. True hermaphrodites have testicular and ovarian structures and generally constitute a much smaller proportion of intersexes. Intersex is more prevalent in polled dairy goats (Saanen, Toggenburg, Alpine, and Damascus breeds). The polled intersex condition is rare or not reported in some breeds (Nubian and Angora). Cytogenetic evaluations of caprine intersexes clearly show that most polled intersexes are karyotypically female (XX), and the breeding histories of the parents indicate that intersexes are homozygous for the polled trait.

Affected animals are genetically female but may exhibit male, female, or mixed external characteristics. Generally, they are female-appearing at birth but as they reach sexual maturity, they become larger than normal females, with masculine heads and erect hair on their necks. An enlarged clitoris in a doe-like animal or a decreased anogenital distance in a more masculine individual is typical of intersex. Intersexes may start to smell and may act aggressively toward other goats and people during the breeding season. Some dribble urine or stretch out with a concave back and urinate forward between the legs.

Whenever bilateral cryptorchidism is encountered, intersex should be suspected. The testes are generally intraabdominal (in the normal location of the ovaries) but they may be partially or totally descended. Partially descended testes may be mistaken for udders, especially when they begin to enlarge during puberty. Hypospadias (opening of the urethral orifice on the ventral aspect of the penis), sperm granulomas, and hypoplastic testicles should all be considered part of the intersex complex. The principal hormone produced by the gonads in caprine intersexes is testosterone, which accounts for masculine behavior. Intersex goats can be used as teaser animals because they do not produce sperm. Gonadectomy is generally required if the animal is to be used as a pet.

Identifying intersex animals with normal or nearly normal external genitalia is difficult. Failure to exhibit estrus, development of male behavior during the breeding season, a shortened vagina on speculum examination, and smaller than normal teats may be the first signs of the intersex condition. The breeding of phenotypically polled bucks should be avoided.

21.5.8 Testicular Hypoplasia

Abnormally small testes most commonly occur with severe malnutrition (Neathery et al. 1973) or in animals that are actually intersexes (i.e., polled intersexes or freemartins). Hypoplasia is often difficult to distinguish from atrophy, but with either condition, testicular size and function should improve with proper feeding if malnutrition is responsible. Intersexes and freemartins do not produce any sperm at all, even in the breeding season, and generally are less odoriferous than normal bucks. Their testes do not undergo the increase in size that normally occurs at puberty, or else the testes may atrophy at that time (Crilly et al. 2022).

One case of testicular hypoplasia has been reported in a horned buck with chromosomal mosaicism (XXY and XY). Two sterile polled bucks with a Robertsonian translocation were found to have normal seminiferous tubules interspersed with tubules devoid of germinal cells (Ricordeau 1972). Histologically, similar findings have been reported in polled bucks with sperm granulomas obstructing the epididymis but with normal karyotype (Corteel et al. 1969).

Bucks with severe experimental zinc deficiency compounded by reduced feed intake and control bucks with just reduced feed intake in the same trial showed normal tubules adjacent to tubules containing only spermatogonia secondary zinc deficiency, caused by excessive fertilization of fields, resulted in atrophy of the seminiferous tubules, hyperplasia of the germinal epithelium, and thickening of the walls of blood vessels in the testes of young Black Bengal bucks (Ray et al. 1997).

Unilateral testicular hypoplasia (in males producing sperm) has been reported in two goats in India (Mathew and Raja 1978b) and in a polled Saanen XY buck in the United States (Sponenberg et al. 1983). In the Indian bucks, spermatogenesis only progressed to the formation of spermatocytes, while in the latter case, some seminiferous tubules in the affected testis were devoid of sperm cells while others were normal. Three additional bucks (horned feral animals) in Australia with unilateral hypoplasia had small seminiferous tubules lined by Sertoli cells (Tarigan et al. 1990). A unilateral segmental tubular hypoplasia in a testis of normal size but with discrete pale areas on section was been observed in two animals in this Australian slaughterhouse survey of 1000 bucks.

21.5.9 Cryptorchidism

Intersex animals, as discussed previously, may exhibit retained testes or ovotestes. The gonad may be abdominal or inguinal in location. The animals are usually genetic females or freemartins. No sperm are produced. Failure of one testis to descend into the scrotum has been reported frequently in Angora goats. Bilateral cryptorchidism appears to be rare in this breed. The cryptorchid goat is sometimes referred to as a "ridgling."

21.5.9.1 Etiology

Cryptorchidism is hereditary in Angora goats but is not related to the polled intersex condition, which does not occur in this breed. Affected Angoras are genetic males (Skinner et al. 1972). The cryptorchid trait is recessive but controlled by a few pairs of genes (Ruan et al. 2024). In other breeds, cryptorchidism in XY males occurs occasionally, and although less is known about the etiology, a genetic explanation is probable.

21.5.9.2 Clinical Signs and Surgical or Necropsy Findings

The testes normally descend into the scrotum by 12–13 weeks of gestation. Cryptorchidism is detectable at birth. If the condition is bilateral, no scrotum is present. In Texas Angoras and in Indian goats of unspecified breed (Mathew and Raja 1978a), the right testis was retained, whereas in South African Angoras, the left testis was retained (Skinner et al. 1972). In one research farm in India, six out of 89 Tellicherry bucks born during a four-year period were unilaterally cryptorchid. In five of these, the right testis was retained. In a slaughterhouse study in Ethiopia, 22 of 404 (5.5%) horned native breed bucks were cryptorchid; 18 of these were unilateral and 10 involved the right testis (Regassa et al. 2003). The unilaterally affected buck is generally fertile, although semen volume and sperm concentration are reduced. Mohair quality in cryptorchid Angoras is normal.

In the unilateral cryptorchid, the retained testis is often located near the kidney. In two Anglo-Nubian bucks in Brazil with unilateral cryptorchidism, the retained testis (one left, one right) was located at the entrance to the inguinal canal. If castration is required, as for a pet animal, the location of the testis can be confirmed before surgery by ultrasound. The tunica albuginea of the retained testis is echogenic and clearly demarcates it from surrounding tissue (Kaulfuss et al. 2006). This testis is generally smaller than the scrotal testis. The cryptorchid testis resembles a prepuberal testis histologically.

Sertoli cell degeneration has been described in the cryptorchid testis in West African dwarf goats (Ezeasor and Singh 1987), whereas tubular degeneration and Sertoli cell hyperplasia have been reported in two cryptorchid feral goats in Australia (Tarigan et al. 1990).

21.5.9.3 Prevention

The prevalence of the condition in a flock varies with the selection pressure against it, often approximately 2% but as much as 10% in commercial herds and more than 60% when cryptorchids are intentionally bred. Breeders wishing to sell bucks realize that a unilateral cryptorchid is of little commercial value. To decrease the prevalence of the condition, cryptorchid bucks should not be used for breeding and their sires and dams should also be culled. Even stricter selection involves culling all offspring of known carriers (Warwick et al. 1961).

21.5.10 Persistent Müllerian Duct Syndrome

A single male (60, XY) Nubian goat with bilateral cryptorchidism and persistent müllerian duct syndrome has been described (Haibel and Rojko 1990). Hypoplastic testes, rudimentary epididymides, and a bicornuate uterus were present. Vesicular glands, bulbourethral glands, and penis resembled those of a normal male. Similar syndromes are seen in miniature schnauzer dogs and human males and are thought to be associated with a lack of either secretion of or receptors for müllerian inhibiting substance, normally of fetal Sertoli cell origin.

21.6 Infectious Diseases Causing Orchitis and Epididymitis

Bacterial orchitis and epididymitis are far less common in goats than in sheep. Expected clinical findings include swelling, increased heat, and pain on palpation of the testis. The semen may contain pus and the percentage of live spermatozoa drops. In one case report, transrectal ultrasonography also demonstrated changes in the echogenicity of the seminal vesicles.

Coliform bacteria and *Pseudomonas* have been cultured from ejaculates of young bucks. Coliforms have caused both orchitis and epididymitis when injected into the testis. *Actinobacillus seminis* was isolated from four of 40 Angora bucks examined in South Africa, but details as to clinical presentation were not supplied (Van Tonder 1975). When pathological changes are not palpable, they might be suspected based on the presence of increased leukocytes in the semen. The major differential diagnosis is nonsuppurative sperm granuloma originating from a malformation of the epididymis.

In one five-year-old buck, unilateral testicular enlargement progressed to five times the normal size. The animal was inappetent and walked with a stiff, straddling gait. The affected testis was firm and fixed in the scrotum. *Staphylococcus pyogenes* was isolated from a purulent epididymitis at the time of unilateral castration. Involvement of the second testis was obvious within three weeks. In another report, *C. pseudotuberculosis* was associated with epididymitis and orchitis in two bucks in Brazil. *Burkholderia (Pseudomonas) pseudomallei* caused orchitis and periorchitis in a buck (Fatimah et al. 1984). The buck was inappetent and the swollen testes developed pyogranulomas. There was no response to antibiotic therapy. *Mycoplasma putrefaciens* was isolated from the testes of a buck that died during a severe herd outbreak of contagious agalactia with concomitant infection with *Mycoplasma agalactiae* and *M. putrefaciens*. Spermatozoa were absent in seminiferous tubules and there was calcification and loss of germinative epithelium, with only Sertoli cells remaining (Gil et al. 2003).

21.6.1 Brucellosis

Brucella ovis is an important cause of epididymitis and orchitis in sheep. Stamp's stain can be used to demonstrate the organism in semen smears, and white blood cells and detached heads are commonly found in the semen. This organism is not recognized as a cause of natural infections in goats.

Experimental infection of bucks by conjunctival or intrapreputial inoculation of this organism has led to clinical and histological epididymitis, transient infection, and serological response. In a subsequent trial, the organism was isolated from the semen of one of 15 goats (Dadar et al. 2024). In another experiment, inoculation of *B. ovis* onto the preputial epithelium (two yearling goats) and nasal mucosa (two goats) led to an antibody response best detected by ELISA but also (in three animals) by CF testing. One intranasally inoculated buck persistently shed *B. ovis* and white cells in semen. The experiment was concluded at 98 days, when chronic epididymitis and seminal vesiculitis were demonstrated only in the goat that had excreted organisms. Thus, if bucks engage in homosexual activity with infected rams there is some potential for transmission to occur.

Brucella melitensis occasionally causes orchitis in bucks. The Rev 1 vaccine strain has also caused orchitis in a buck kid vaccinated at five months of age (Tolari and Salvi 1980). In South Africa, where the Rev 1 *melitensis* vaccine has been used to control *B. ovis* in sheep, orchitis and epididymitis have developed in Angora bucks soon after vaccination. The authors failed to create clinical disease in bucks by experimental infection with *B. ovis* and concluded that bucks should not be vaccinated unless *B. ovis* has been confirmed on the farm or *B. melitensis* is causing abortions in the herd.

21.6.2 Trypanosomosis

Trypanosoma brucei and *Tabanus vivax* have been associated with inflammatory and degenerative changes in the testis and epididymis of sheep and goats in Africa. After experimental infection with *T. brucei* (in rams), persistent scrotal edema and a nonsuppurative granulomatous periorchitis developed associated with tissue invasion by the parasite. Trypanosomes were readily detected in fluid from the scrotal sac. Secondary degenerative changes in the testis included atrophy and calcification of seminiferous tubules and intertubular sclerosis. In bucks experimentally infected with *T. vivax*, organisms were not seen outside blood vessels in the testes and it was postulated that testicular degeneration occurred because of recurrent fever. Affected animals are expected to have low fertility until some time after the infection has cleared.

Experimental infection of bucks with *Trypanosoma evansi* also caused microthrombi in testicular blood vessels, severe mononuclear cell infiltration in the epididymis and testicular interstitium, and subsequent dystrophic mineralization. The number of abnormal and dead sperm increased greatly, and bucks with clinical orchitis became aspermic. A later experimental infection of bucks with an equine isolate of the same organism caused scrotal edema in 20%, degeneration of spermatogonia and Sertoli cells, and infiltration of the testes with macrophages and lymphoid cells (Dargantes et al. 2005). Experimental infection of bucks with *Trypanosoma congolense*, a plasma parasite that does not invade tissue, also caused testicular degeneration with marked shrinking of seminiferous tubules and epididymides, but the pathogenesis is unknown.

21.6.3 Besnoitiosis

There is one report of a buck in Africa with masses of *Besnoitia* cysts in the wall and lumen of veins and arteries of the pampiniform plexus; parasitic cysts were also present in the epididymis and testis. Thrombosis of vessels, absence of sperm production, and extensive testicular fibrosis were believed to be caused by the parasite. Encrustation of the scrotum and presence of numerous *Besnoitia* cysts in the tunica vaginalis, tunica albuginea, and interstitium of the epididymis were reported from two male wild goats in Iran. The existence of a distinct species, *Besnoitia caprae*, has been proposed in Kenya, where cattle housed with infected goats do not develop besnoitiosis (Figures 21.3 and 21.4).

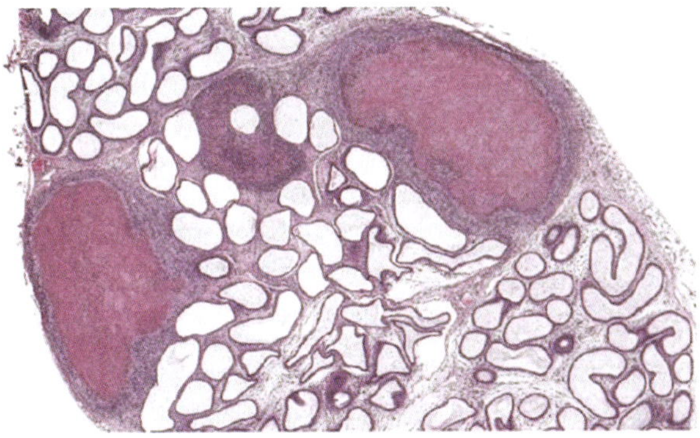

Figure 21.3 Sperm granuloma (epididymis exhibiting multiple sperm granulomas).

(a) (b)

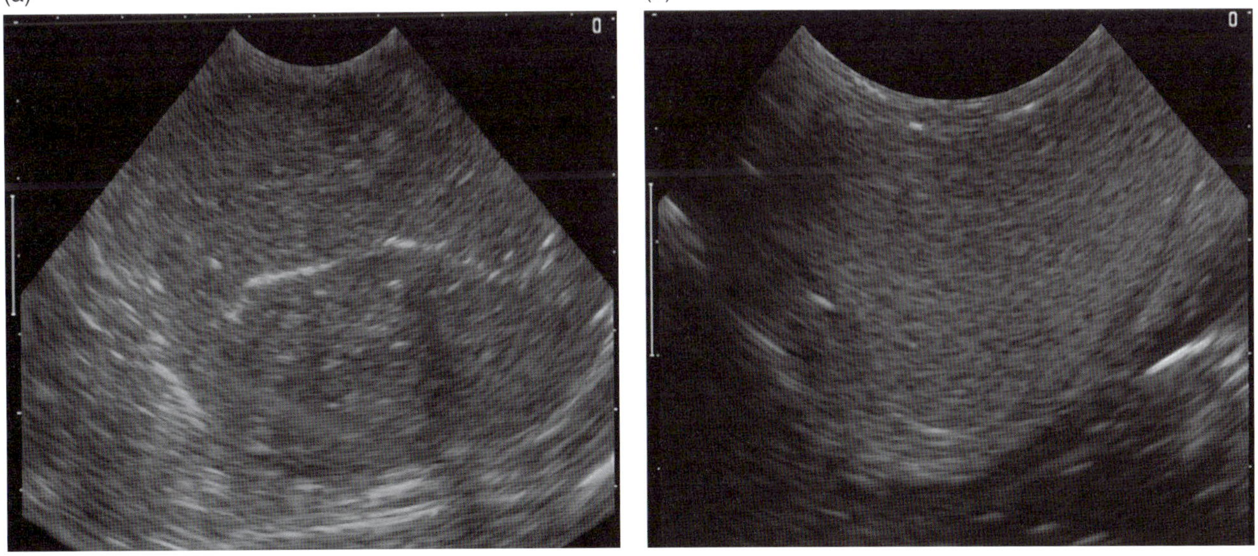

Figure 21.4 Irregular echogenicity indicates testicular pathology such as orchitis, degeneration, or neoplasia (a) and homogeneous appearance of normal testicular tissue (b).

References

Bulgin, M.S. (1990). Brucella ovis epizootic in virgin ram lambs. *Journal of the American Veterinary Medical Association* 196 (7): 1120–1122.

Corteel, J.M., Hulot, F., Courot, M. et al. (1969). Examens morphologiques, caryologiques, physiologiques et pathologiques de boucs stériles sans cornes. *Annales de Génétique et de Sélection Animale* 1: 341.

Crilly, J.P., Wood, M., and Reilly, B. (2022). Such a tease! Production and uses of teaser rams, bucks, boars and bulls. *In Practice* 44 (4): 228–238.

Dadar, M., Bahreinipour, A., Alamian, S. et al. (2024). Serological, cultural, and molecular analysis of Brucella from Buffalo milk in various regions of Iran. *Veterinary Research Communications* 48 (1): 427–436.

Dargantes, A.P., Reid, S.A., and Copeman, D.B. (2005). Experimental Trypanosoma evansi infection in the goat. I. Clinical signs and clinical pathology. *Journal of Comparative Pathology* 133 (4): 261–266.

Ezeasor, D.N. and Singh, A. (1987). Morphologic features of Sertoli cells in the intra-abdominal testes of cryptorchid dwarf goats. *American Journal of Veterinary Research* 48 (12): 1736–1745.

Fatimah, M.Y., Mohsin, A.M., and Kamal, A.M. (1984). Phytoplankton composition and productivity of a shallow tropical lake. *Pertanika* 7 (3): 101–113.

Fietz, D. and Bergmann, M. (2017). Functional anatomy and histology of the testis. In: *Endocrinology of the Testis and Male Reproduction* (ed. M. Simoni and I. Huhtaniemi), 313–341. Cham: Springer International Publishing.

Foster, R.A. (2016). Male genital system. In: *Jubb, Kennedy & Palmer's Pathology of Domestic Animals*, vol. 3 (ed. M. Grant Maxie), 465–510. St Louis, MO: Elsevier.

Fraser, W. and Wilson, M.W. (1966). Remarks on the Clenshaw-Curtis quadrature scheme. *SIAM Review* 8 (3): 322–327.

Gil, G.C., Chang, I.S., Kim, B.H. et al. (2003). Operational parameters affecting the performance of a mediator-less microbial fuel cell. *Biosensors and Bioelectronics* 18: 327–334.

Haibel, G.K. and Rojko, J.L. (1990). Persistent müllerian duct syndrome in a goat. *Veterinary Pathology* 27 (2): 135–137.

Hamada, M.M. and Saadeldin, I.M. (2022). Physiology of the reproductive system. *Advances in Assisted Reproduction Technologies* 5: 1.

Kaulfuss, K.H., Giucci, E., Süss, R., and Wojtowski, J. (2006). An ultrasonographic method to study reproductive seasonality in ewes isolated from rams. *Reproduction in Domestic Animals* 41 (5): 416–422.

Kilgour, R. (2019). *Livestock Behaviour: A Practical Guide*. Boca Raton, FL: CRC Press.

Koziol, J. and Palmer, C. (2023). Pathophysiology, diagnosis, and management of testicular degeneration in the bull. *Clinical Theriogenology* 15.

Lee, J.C., Bhatt, S., and Dogra, V.S. (2008). Imaging of the epididymis. *Ultrasound Quarterly* 24 (1): 3–16.

Mathew, J. and Raja, C.K.S.V. (1978a). Investigation on the incidence of cryptorchidism in goats. *Kerala Journal of Veterinary Science* 9: 47–52.

Mathew, J. and Raja, C.K.S.V. (1978b). Studies on testicular hypoplasia in goats. *Kerala Journal of Veterinary Science* 9: 24–30.

Mruk, D.D. and Cheng, C.Y. (2015). The mammalian blood–testis barrier: its biology and regulation. *Endocrine Reviews* 36 (5): 564–591.

Neathery, M.W., Miller, W.J., Blackmon, D.M., and Gentry, R.P. (1973). Zinc-65 metabolism, secretion into milk, and biological half-life in lactating cows. *Journal of Dairy Science* 56 (12): 1526–1530.

Pathak, D., Kapoor, K., and Gupta, M.K. (2022). Testicular stem cell niche. In: *Stem Cells in Veterinary Science* (ed. R. Choudhary and S. Choudhary), 161–182. Springer Nature Singapore: Singapore.

Ray, T.P., Muxlow, T.W.B., Axon, D.J. et al. (1997). Large-scale magnetic fields in the outflow from the young stellar object T Tauri S. *Nature* 385 (6615): 415–417.

Regassa, F., Terefe, F., and Bekana, M. (2003). Abnormalities of the testes and epididymis in bucks and rams slaughtered at Debre Zeit abattoir, Ethiopia. *Tropical Animal Health and Production* 35: 541–549.

Ricordeau, P. (1972). Accidents de cœlioscopie d'origine anesthésique probable. *Acta Endoscopica* 2: 186–188.

Rouatbi, M., Haile, A., Getachew, T. et al. (2022). *A Review of Goat Reproduction in East and Horn of Africa*. Beirut, Lebanon: ICARDA.

Ruan, L., Gu, M., Geng, H. et al. (2024). Achieving an optimal pregnancy outcome through the combined utilization of micro-TESE and ICSI in cryptorchidism associated with a non-canonical splicing variant in RXFP2. *Journal of Assisted Reproduction and Genetics*, 1–11.

Sathe, S. and Shipley, C.F. (2014). Applied andrology in sheep, goats and selected cervids. In: *Animal Andrology: Theories and Applications* (ed. P. Chenoweth and S. Lorton), 226–253. Wallingford, UK: CABI.

Shipley, C.F. (2022). Applied andrology: ram and buck. In: *Manual of Animal Andrology* (ed. P. Chenoweth and S. Lorton), 108–119. Wallingford, UK: CABI.

Skinner, J.D., van Heerden, J.H.A., and Goris, E.J. (1972). A note on cryptorchidism in Angora goats. *South African Journal of Animal Science* 2: 93–95.

Sponenberg, D.P., Smith, M.C., and Johnson, R.J. Jr. (1983). Unilateral testicular hypoplasia in a goat. *Veterinary Pathology* 20 (4): 503–506.

Stapelberg, W. (2022). The influence of heat stress on the functionality of ovine spermatozoa. MS thesis. Stellenbosch University.

Tarigan, S., Ladds, P.W., and Foster, R.A. (1990). Genital pathology of feral male goats. *Australian Veterinary Journal* 67 (8): 286–290.

Tolari, F. and Salvi, G. (1980). Bilateral orchitis in a kid after vaccination with Rev 1. *Annali della Facolta di Medicina Veterinaria di Pisa* 33: 87–91.

Van Tonder, E.M. (1975). Notes on some disease problems in Angora goats in South Africa. *Veterinary Medical Review* 1 (2): 109–138.

Walker, W.H. and Cooke, P.S. (2023). Functions of steroid hormones in the male reproductive tract as revealed by mouse models. *International Journal of Molecular Sciences* 24 (3): 2748.

Warwick, O.H., Yendt, E.R., and Olin, J. (1961). The clinical features of hypercalcemia associated with malignant disease. *Canadian Medical Association Journal* 85 (13): 719.

Section 3

Diseases of Pregnancy

22

Abortion: General Considerations

Neeti Lakhani[1], Abhijeet Fernandes[2], and Gitesh Saini[2]

[1] Department of Animal Nutrition, College of Veterinary Science, Rampura Phul, Guru Angad Dev Veterinary and Animal Sciences University, Bathinda, India
[2] Department of Veterinary Gynaecology and Obstetrics, College of Veterinary Science, Guru Angad Dev Veterinary and Animal Sciences University, Bathinda, India

22.1 Introduction

Abortion is the premature expulsion of a fetus after completion of organogenesis but before the fetus reaches the viability stage. On the other hand, if pregnancy ends before completion of organogenesis, it is known as early embryonic death. A stillbirth is the delivery of a dead fetus at full term, whereas abortion explicitly refers to the intentional termination of pregnancy before the conclusion of a normal term. In goat breeding, abortion, early embryonic death, and stillbirth are serious issues considering their economic importance. It is important to note that numerous factors leading to abortion can also result in stillbirths and premature birth, as well as the birth of medically or physically compromised neonates, and in some cases even a mummified fetus. The etiology is identified in approximately 47–75% of caprine abortions, with the remaining abortions having idiopathic or unexplained causes (Chanton-Greutmann et al. 2002).

Generally, female goats are distinctly fertile but have a high incidence of abortion compared to other farm animals. Abortion appears to be a major preparturient disorder with incidence ranging between 5% and 8% annually, with a 68.2% incidence in goats (Purohit 2006), and may reach up to 80% in abortion storms, posing a substantial constraint on production systems and impacting productivity and overall efficiency (Smith 1978; Smith and Morrow 1986). As the productivity of goat farming mainly depends on the number of kids produced/fecundity, an increased incidence of abortion greatly affects the economics of farms. The occurrence of abortion not only diminishes the overall productivity of goats globally but also results in detrimental effects such as infertility, reduced milk production, and the need for culling (Figure 22.1). Consequently, these conditions result in substantial economic losses for goat producers as goats suffer from uterine infections, reduced reproductive rates, and prolonged interconception and kidding intervals which cause increased veterinary expenses, decreased milk production, and premature disposal of potentially productive ewes and does (Khair et al. 2013).

Certain conditions occur in caprines which are often mistaken for evidence of abortion. It is important to differentiate these conditions from actual abortion or parturition events.

- *Mammary gland development and premature lactation*: this condition can be observed in both pregnant and nonpregnant animals. It is not necessarily indicative of abortion or occurrence of parturition as it can be triggered by hormonal imbalances, certain medications, or even stress.
- *Bloody vaginal discharge after estrus*: bloody vaginal discharge approximately 2–3 days after estrus is very common. This discharge is a normal part of the reproductive cycle and does not necessarily indicate abortion. It occurs as a result of the shedding of the uterine lining and is typically not a cause for concern.
- *Coccidiosis*: the parasitic infection in animals may exhibit symptoms such as straining, raised tail and bloody feces staining the tail and perineum. While these signs can be alarming, they are not indicative of abortion.

Elements of Reproduction and Reproductive Diseases of Goats, First Edition. Edited by Tanmoy Rana.

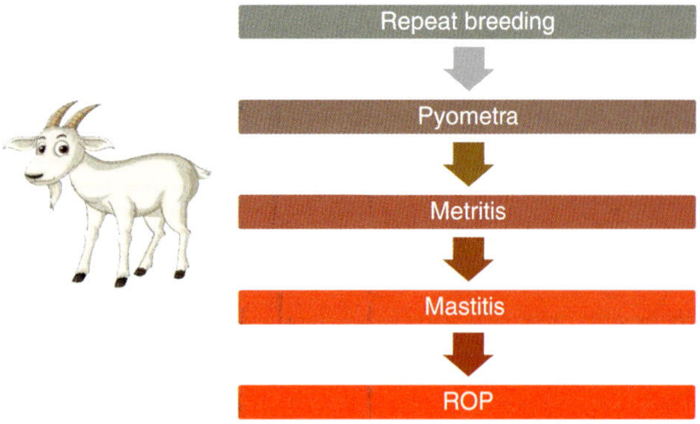

Figure 22.1 Implications of caprine abortion. ROP, retention of placenta.

22.2 Common Causes of Abortion

Etiological factors associated with caprine abortion are numerous and divided into infectious and noninfectious causes (Menzies 2011). Noninfectious causes mainly include management-related factors like trauma, malnutrition, stress, ingestion of certain plant toxins and contaminated feed, pharmaceuticals/drugs, anatomical defect, and neoplasia of reproductive tract (granulosa cell tumor, dysgerminoma of ovaries, uterine tumors, etc.). As pregnancy in goats is dependent on the corpus luteum throughout the pregnancy, any event culminating in luteolysis/luteal insufficiency will lead to abortion. Infectious causes of abortion are much more important as these can spread to a whole herd and include various bacterial, viral, parasitic, and fungal agents (chlamydiosis, toxoplasmosis, leptospirosis, brucellosis, Q fever, mycoplasmosis, campylobacteriosis, salmonellosis, sarcosystosis, akabane virus disease, and listeriosis) (Table 22.1). Moreover, certain causative organisms of infectious abortion are of zoonotic potential and can pose serious public health concerns.

22.3 Noninfectious Causes of Abortion

Reproductive failures in ruminants, including goats, can have significant economic and food implications, in both developing countries and areas with advanced animal husbandry practices. Reproductive failures, which encompass issues such as abortion, stillbirth, premature birth, and infertility, can be attributed to various factors (Ebani 2022). Abortions are often caused by a plethora of infectious agents, but many of the noninfectious agents also contribute to abortion in goats (Borel et al. 2014). Inadequate livestock management practices, nutritional deficiencies and stresses induced by several factors, including transportation, extreme temperature conditions, and high population density, have the potential to cause high abortion rates in goats.

Noninfectious causes of abortion in farm animals pose a considerable challenge for veterinarians and livestock professionals in terms of their diagnosis, often resulting in cases that remain undiagnosed. Noninfectious causes of abortion can be classified as genetic and nongenetic factors (Table 22.2).

Table 22.1 Common causes of abortion.

Infectious	Noninfectious
Bacterial	Nutritional
Viral	Toxic plants
Parasitic	Genetic
	Environmental
	Trauma

Table 22.2 Noninfectious causes of abortion.

Genetic factors	Nongenetic factors
Gene defects	Mineral and vitamin deficiency
Chromosomal abnormality	Stress
	Ingestion of poisonous plants
	Hormonal causes
	Pharmaceutical agents

22.3.1 Genetic Factors

Genetic defects in the fetus may result in abortions, and these usually occur in an individual animal rather than as a herd outbreak. These defects mainly occur due to mutations in genes, chromosomal abnormality, and polygenic defects, resulting in abortion because of the inability of the fetus to develop properly in the uterine environment (Yadav et al. 2021). The fetus experiences noticeable morphological changes as a result of genetic defects, generating congenital deformities and causing fetal death and abortion (Hashiguchi et al. 1979). To establish better breeding programs and management techniques for avoiding such defects, it is necessary to develop advanced tests to identify the biomarker genes associated with such conditions and monitor the prevalence of genetic flaws that cause abortion.

22.3.2 Nongenetic Factors

22.3.2.1 Environmental Factors

Nutrition and stress are the two environmental factors affecting embryo survivability (Lindsay et al. 2019). Stressors such as fluctuations in weather patterns, inadequate nutrition, and increased stock density potentially trigger abortions in does. These stressors activate the hypothalamic-pituitary-adrenal axis, leading to the secretion of adrenocorticotropic hormone and corticoids which can adversely affect the viability of the fetus, ultimately resulting in abortion. The physiology of the reproductive tract may be compromised by heat stress during breeding and the early cleavage stage, which can lead to pregnancy loss through hormonal imbalance, decreased oocyte quality, poor semen quality, interference with protein synthesis, oxidative cell damage, decreased pregnancy recognition, and expression of stress-related genes linked to apoptosis (Krishnan et al. 2017).

Nutritional deficiencies (especially energy and protein along with macro/micronutrients) have been associated with abortion, stillbirth, or birth of weak kids. Abortion from nutritional stress (by providing poor-quality forage, concentrate withdrawal) is mostly seen between 90 and 120 days of gestation (Wentzel et al. 1974; Osuagwuh and Akpokodje 1986). Energy deficiency in late gestation has been associated with the development of periparturient metabolic diseases like pregnancy toxemia (Merrall 1985). Multiple fetuses, displaced rumen, under- and overnutrition, and hypoglycemia are predisposing factors for pregnancy toxemia. Several mineral deficiencies have also been associated with lowered conception rate, embryonic death, and abortion (Table 22.3). Energy and protein should be given as per the physiological needs on and above the maintenance requirement along with area-specific mineral mixtures to combat reproductive disorders.

22.3.2.2 Hormonal Factors

Embryonic death accounts for 6–42% of all pregnancy losses in goats, mostly around 30 days of pregnancy (Bolet 1986; Nancarrow 1994). Loss of genetically abnormal embryos is unavoidable but morphologically normal embryos are lost due to physiological and environmental factors. The maternal environment may be unable to support normal embryo development (Wilmut et al. 1986) due to congenital reproductive tract abnormality, hormonal imbalance or luteal insufficiency. Rate of ovulation also affects the chance of survival (Nancarrow 1994) due to inadequate intrauterine space and compromised nutrition supply to the fetus. Hormonal imbalance and CL insufficiency are estimated using commercial enzyme-linked immunosorbent assay (ELISA) kits and color Doppler ultrasonography respectively.

22.3.2.3 Toxic Plants

The browsing and grazing nature of goats potentially exposes them to a variety of toxic plants (Table 22.4) and fungus-contaminated feed, which can have a significant impact on reproductive health and lead to economic loss owing to reduced

Table 22.3 Minerals and their deficiency symptoms.

Macro/micronutrient	Deficiency symptoms	References
Se	Abortion in the last trimester, necrosis of skeletal muscle and the myocardium in neonates	Gupta et al. (1982)
Zn	Infertility, abortion, and altered myometrial contractibility with prolonged labor	Gupta et al. (1982)
Cu	Enzootic ataxia in kids and lambs, abortion in last trimester, mummification	Corah and Ives (1991)
I_2	Stillbirth, goiter, thyroid hyperplasia	Robert and Moeller (2001)

Table 22.4 Effect of toxic plant ingestion during pregnancy in goats.

Plant	Toxicant	Effect	Duration of gestation	References
1. Teratogenic plants				
Lupines	Alkaloids	Skeletal contracture type malformations and cleft palate	30–60 d of gestation	Panter et al. (1999)
Hemlock Wild tobacco	Alkaloids	Neuromuscular effects	30–60 d of gestation	Panter et al. (1999)
Veratrum californicum	Alkaloids	Early embryonic death	Before 19 d after fertilization	Keeler et al. (1985)
Locoweed (*Oxytropis* and *Astragalus*)	Swainsonine	Tissue necrosis after fetal death may stimulate prostaglandin production	Fetus dies 2–3 days before abortion	James et al. (1981), Welch et al. (2009)
Mimosa tenuiflora	Alkaloids	Arthrogryposis, cleft palate, micrognathia	Embryonic death within 60 d	Dantas (2009)
2. Abortifacient plants				
Aspidosperma pyrifolium	Alkaloid	Embryonic deaths, abortion, and premature birth	Embryonic death before 34 d, abortion during any stage of gestation	Medeiros et al. (2004)
Pinus ponderosa	Isocupressic acid	Premature parturition, constriction of caruncular arterial bed resulting in hypoxic condition in fetal tissue	Abortion may occur 24 hours to up to 3 wks following ingestion	Pfister and Adams (1993)
Nitrate accumulating (oat, sorghum, pigweed, wheat, hay, etc.)	Hemoglobin to methemoglobin (tissue anoxia)	Abortion	Abortion may occur 3–7 days post exposure	Knight and Walter (2003)
Snakeweeds (*Gutierrezia sarothrae* or *microcepha*)	Saponin Terpenoid, flavonids	Abortion when grown on sandy soil, ruminal stasis, jaundice	Abortion in late gestation	Panter et al. (2018)
Western red cedar (*Thuja plicata*)	Isocupressic acid	Abortion, hypoxic condition in fetal tissue		Welch et al. (2009)

fertility rate, increased neonatal mortality, and lower productivity. Additionally, costs associated with veterinary care, diagnosis, and treatment of affected animals can add to the financial burden.

Some toxic plants contain certain teratogenic compounds causing developmental abnormalities in the fetus and can lead to embryonic death or birth of weak or deformed offspring (Smith and Sherman 1994; Panter et al. 1992). Additionally, certain plant toxins have detrimental effects on the placenta, disrupting the transfer of nutrients and oxygen to the developing fetus (Ludders 1988).

Grazing patterns, plant growth cycles, and management practices along with the timing, duration, and amount of exposure to these toxic plants determine the severity of toxins. Exposure to certain toxic plants during early pregnancy results in embryo death or resorption, while exposure during later stages causes abortion or stillbirth. Abortion incidences can be diagnosed by laboratory analysis of metabolites from suspected plants, water, stomach contents, blood and urine of dam and fetus using gas chromatography-mass spectrometry (GCMS)/high-performance liquid chromatography (HPLC) for confirmation of poisoning and detection of pine needle abortion (metabolites like agathic acid, dihydroagathic acid, and tetrahydroagathic acid) from fetal thoracic fluid (Snider et al. 2015). Mycotoxins can be identified in the feed material with the help of thin-layer chromatography, GCMS, and HPLC (Zaki et al. 2012). Various pharmaceutical agents are also known to be abortifacient, such as phenothiazine if given in the last month of gestation (abortion), cambendazole and higher doses of albendazole which may be embryotoxic in early pregnancy but safe in later stages. The use of xylazine or high doses of acetyl promazine in the first half of pregnancy may cause abortion because of their adverse effect on placental perfusion (Ludders 1988).

To mitigate the risks associated with toxic plant exposure, it is crucial for livestock producers to be aware of the toxic plants present in their grazing areas. Implementing proper management strategies such as monitoring and controlling plant populations, providing alternative forage, and ensuring adequate nutrition may help reduce the incidence of reproductive problems caused by toxic plant ingestion (Figure 22.2).

22.3.2.4 Hormonal Causes: Pseudo-pregnancy

This is characterized by persistent corpus luteum, anestrus, and variable accumulation of sterile fluid within the uterus. The accumulation of fluid often results in abdominal distention and the persistence of CL causes elevated progesterone concentrations, mimicking pregnancy. The spontaneous evacuation of accumulated fluid is called a *cloud burst* (Figure 22.3). The doe may search for the nonexistent kid and some may even start lactation. At the end of this period, a bloody vaginal discharge may be seen in a few does. Early embryonic death (≤40 days of gestation) with persistence of CL, late mating after the end of breeding season, and artificial induction of ovulation are possible causes for the development of hydrometra in goats. Diagnosis is based on anestrus and ultrasonographic demonstration of an enlarged, thin-walled, fluid-filled uterus without evidence of a fetus, placenta, or placentomes. Treatment is with a single dose of PGF2-alpha or oxytocin (50 IU IM, BID for four days) (Pieterse and Traverne 1986).

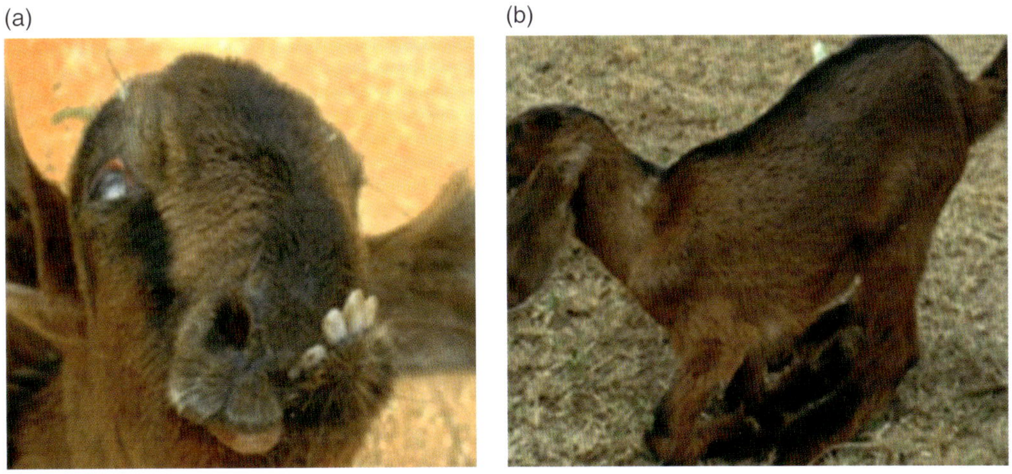

Figure 22.2 Different malformations caused by *Mimosa tenuiflora*: (a) goat with cleft palate owing to aplasia of right incisive bone; (b) permanent flexure of forelimb.

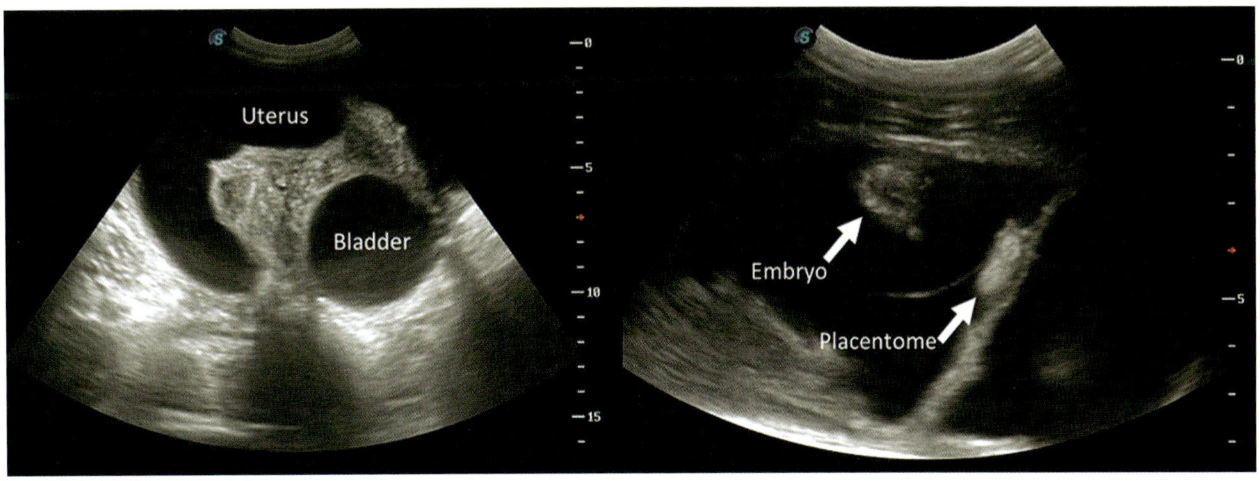

Figure 22.3 Hydrometra and true pregnancy. *Source:* Purohit (2006).

22.4 Infectious Causes of Abortion

Goat herds typically experience an abortion rate of around 2–5% (Menzies 2011). However, it is crucial to note that any percentage exceeding this range is considered a significant issue, as abortions can result in substantial economic losses (Holler 2012). Moreover, when it comes to infectious abortion within a doe herd, it becomes a matter of public health concern due to the potential transmission of zoonotic diseases through infectious agents. In simpler terms, these diseases can be passed from animals to humans. As a result, it is imperative for both the producer and the herd manager to treat infectious abortions with the utmost seriousness.

Abortions can happen days, weeks, or even months after the initial exposure by infectious microorganisms, toxins, stress, or genetic abnormalities, which can affect the developing fetus or placenta (Alemayehu et al. 2021). It is important to note that these factors could have occurred well before the animals entered the export process (Figure 22.4). Several microbial agents have been incriminated as causes of abortion in the goat, but the most common ones are *Chlamydia psittaci*, *Toxoplasma gondii*, *Campylobacter* spp., *Mycoplasma* spp., *Coxiella burnetii*, and *Brucella melitensis* (Table 22.5). Placentitis is the most common lesion observed in all cases of infectious abortion (Yaeger et al. 2021). In some cases, the fetus may die because the impaired placenta fails to facilitate the exchange of nutrients necessary for its survival. Alternatively, the fetus can become infected due to the transfer of infectious agents from the placenta.

22.4.1 Mechanism of Action

Opportunistic bacterial agents that cause abortions in goats may include both commensals of mucous membranes and bacteria commonly found in the environment, e.g., *Bacillus* spp., *Escherichia coli*, *Histophilus somni*, *Pasteurella* spp., *Staphylococcus* spp., and *Streptococcus* spp. Abortions caused by these bacteria are sporadic but their occurrence is widespread (Clothier and Anderson 2016). Mycotic or fungal abortion (*Aspergillus* and *Candida* species) is caused by opportunistic fungal pathogens that are normally present as saprophytes in the environment of the animal (Anderson 2007; Holler 2012; Mee 2020). Infectious agents exert their influence through various mechanisms (Figure 22.5), including the production of toxic metabolic byproducts, fetal or placental infection, chronic endometrial infection, and chorioamnionitis (Nigro et al. 2011).

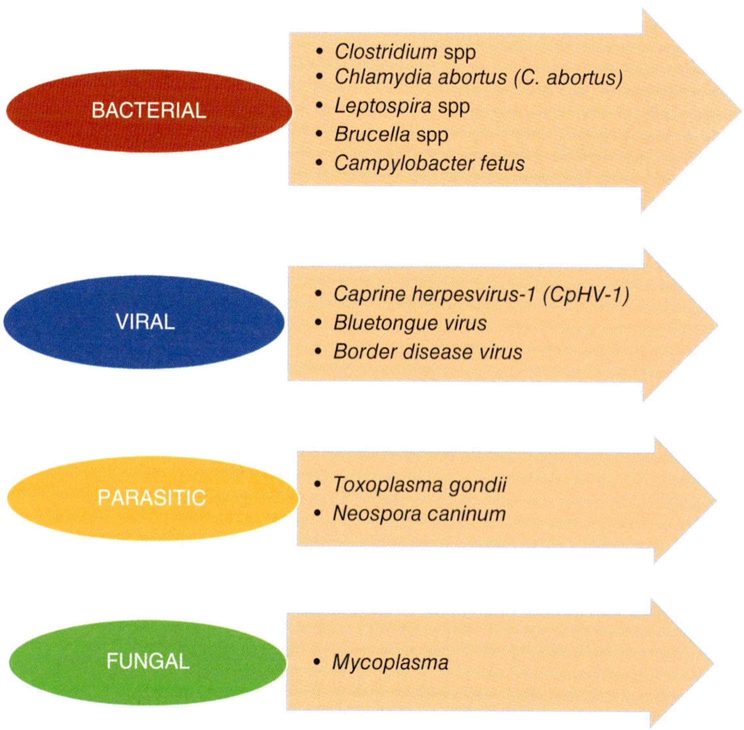

Figure 22.4 Infectious causes of abortion in caprines.

Table 22.5 Infectious causes of abortion and their symptoms.

Name of disease	Causative agent	Stage of abortion	Clinical signs	References
Brucellosis	*Brucella ovis* *B. melitensis* *B. abortus*	Early and late abortion	Abortion, sterility, mastitis, osteoarthritis, synovitis, spondylitis, and orchitis	Ocholi et al. (2005)
Leptospirosis	*Leptospira pomona* *L. grippotyphosa*	Late abortion	Icterus, anemia, hemoglobinuria, high temperature, hemorrhage in brain	Leon-Vizcaino et al. (1987)
Listeriosis	*Listeria monocytogenes*	Late abortion	Unilateral facial paralysis, difficulty in swallowing, fever, blindness, head pressings	Fentahun and Fresebehat (2012)
Ovine genital campylobacteriosis	*Campylobacter fetus* subsp. *fetus*, *C. jejuni*	Abortion in late pregnancy/stillbirth	Infertility, abortion, round necrotic lesion on liver	Sahin et al. (2008)
Enzootic abortion of ewes	*Chlamydia abortus* (*C. psittaci*)	Late pregnancy but early death and mummification can occur	Weak lamb, necrosis of cotyledons	Papp et al. (1993)
Toxoplasmosis	*Toxoplasma gondii*	Early embryonic death	Mummification, abortion, stillbirth, weak kids	Innes et al. (2009)
Neosporosis	*Neospora caninum*	Early embryonic death	Mummification, abortion, stillbirth, weak kids	Dubey and Lindsay (1990)
Q fever	*Coxiella burnetti*	Latter part of pregnancy	High temperature, dystocia, pneumonia, metritis	Kruszewska and Tylewska-Wierzbanowska (1997)
Malignant catarrhal fever	Ovine herpesvirus (OVH-2)	Abortion/stillbirth	Fever, conjunctivitis, nasal discharge	Chénier et al. (2004)
Blue tongue virus (BTV)	Orbi virus of Reoviridae	Abortion/stillbirth	Edema of lips, tongue swollen or cyanotic	Chauhan et al. (2014)
Border disease virus (BDV)	Pestivirus of Flaviviridae	Abortion/mummification	Weak lambs, hair projecting above wool	Nettleton et al. (1998)

- First, production of toxic metabolic byproducts which disrupt normal cellular functions and compromise the overall health of the reproductive system.
- Second, interfering with the normal growth and development of the fetus, impairing nutrient exchange through the placenta and ultimately resulting in abortion.
- Third, chronic endometrial infection, disrupting the uterine environment necessary for successful pregnancy, leading to fetal loss.
- Lastly, chorioamnionitis, which harms the fetus and impairs its viability, potentially resulting in abortion.

22.4.2 Bacterial Causes of Abortion

22.4.2.1 Brucellosis

Brucellosis in goats is caused mainly *by Brucella melitensis* and is a significant concern for goat farmers worldwide. Additionally, *Brucella abortus* can occasionally cause abortion in goats but *Brucella ovis* has never been isolated from cases of caprine abortion. The disease causes significant reproductive losses, including abortion, stillbirth, and birth of weak kids. The bacterium enters the body either through ingestion of products of abortion, infected water, or milk or through inhalation followed by localization in the lymph nodes, udder, uterus, testes, and spleen (Smith and Morrow 1986). Thereafter, the bacterium crosses the placental barrier and infects the fetus, leading to abortion (Godfroid et al. 2010) or mastitis. The organism is excreted in milk, urine, feces, and vaginal discharge for 2–3 months.

22.4.2.1.1 Diagnosis

Isolation of the organism from an aborted fetus, placenta or vaginal discharge. Serological tests such as the Rose Bengal plate test and serum agglutination test are commonly used to diagnose brucellosis in goats (Cetinkaya and Ongör 2000).

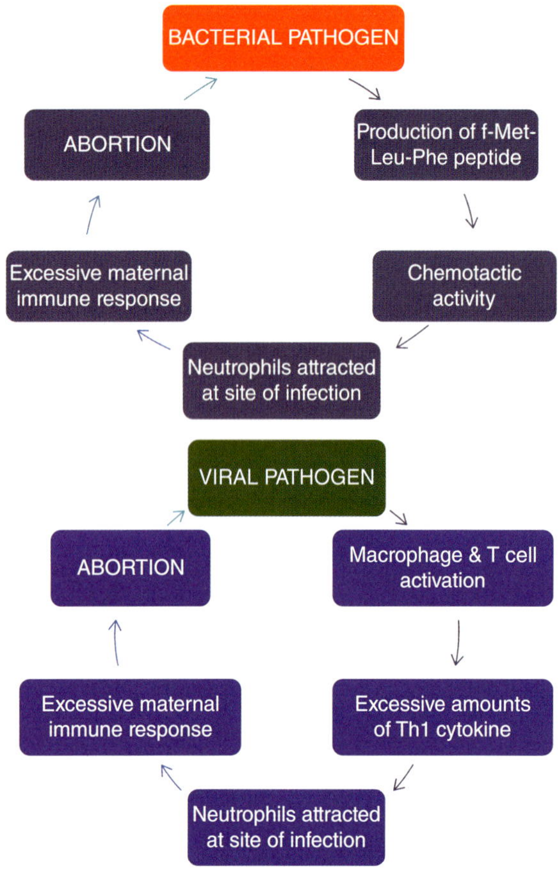

Figure 22.5 Pathogenic mechanisms for induction of abortion in goats.

Postmortem examination can also help in the diagnosis of brucellosis in goats, where characteristic lesions are observed in the reproductive system.

22.4.2.1.2 Prevention and Control

Vaccination against brucellosis (live attenuated strain of *B. melitensis* Rev 1, given to kids and lambs of 3–8 months of age SC) is available and can help prevent the spread of the disease. Biosecurity measures such as quarantine and isolation of infected and newly purchased animals, proper cleaning and disinfection, culling of infected animals, and controlling the movement of people and animals can also help prevent the spread of brucellosis (Wang et al. 2021). Placentas and aborted fetus should be burned/buried deeply to avoid spread of contamination.

22.4.2.2 Campylobacteriosis

This condition, caused by *Campylobacter fetus* (formerly *Vibrio fetus intestinalis*) and *Campylobacter jejuni* (Anderson 1986; Smith and Sherman 1994), is one of the most common causes of abortion in goats (Wassenaar and Newell 2006) that can cause infertility, repeat breeding, and abortion. Moreover, it may result in premature birth or stillbirth as it crosses the placenta and infects the developing fetus, giving rise to severe inflammation and necrosis of cotyledons and fetal liver. A mucopurulent/sanguinopurulent vaginal discharge is reported in all aborting does (Anderson 1986). The severity of the infection and the resulting reproductive problems can vary, depending on the strain of the bacterium and the goat's immune status. Transmission can occur through direct contact with infected animals, ingestion of contaminated feed or water, and vertical transmission from an infected dam to her offspring. The bacterium can survive for prolonged periods in the environment, making it a persistent threat to goat herds (Givens and Marley 2008).

22.4.2.2.1 Diagnosis

Direct microscopic examination and isolation from placenta, fetal abomasal contents, and maternal vaginal discharge (Dennis 1990). Histopathological examination of an aborted fetus is the gold standard for diagnosis. Multiple necrotic foci up to 2 mm diameter may be seen in the liver of aborted fetuses. Serology is of no use for the diagnosis of campylobacteriosis.

22.4.2.2.2 Prevention and Control

Maintaining good hygiene and practicing good biosecurity measures are critical to prevent the spread of infection within the herd and to humans (mild gastroenteritis). Additionally, it is essential to avoid mixing goats from different age groups and to quarantine new animals before introducing them to the herd. Vaccination against *Campylobacter fetus* is an effective method for preventing campylobacteriosis in goats. Several commercial vaccines are available for use in cattle but their efficacy in goats is still under investigation. However, recent studies have reported promising results in using inactivated whole-cell vaccines in goats, indicating their potential use for preventing campylobacteriosis. They should be administered prior to breeding with a booster in 2–3 months followed by annual vaccination before or just after breeding. The antibiotic regimen is penicillin/streptomycin preparation or tetracycline in feed (Anderson 1986).

22.4.2.3 *Chlamydophila* Enzootic Abortion (CEA)

The disease is caused by the Gram-negative intracellular bacterium *Chlamydophila abortus* (formerly *Chlamydia psittaci*), infecting other livestock species and humans. CEA infection in goats is reflected as sudden abortion, premature birth, or stillbirth. Some infected animals may also develop symptoms such as fever, lethargy, loss of appetite, polyarthritis, conjunctivitis, septicemia, and pneumonia (Longbottom and Coulter 2003). Abortion usually occurs during the last four weeks of pregnancy but can occur at any time and the latent period can be as little as two weeks (Wu et al. 2023). Pigeons and sparrows serve as a reservoir and ticks/insects help in transmission of infection (Timoney et al. 1988). Inflammation and necrosis caused by multiplication of chlamydia prevent normal transfer of nutrients across the placenta, leading to fetal death. Does may show a bloody vaginal discharge 2–3 days prior to abortion with autolysis of the fetus. The placenta shows regional to generalized placentitis (whitish-yellow necrotic foci) involving the cotyledons and intercotyledonary space (East 1986).

22.4.2.3.1 Diagnosis

The diagnosis of CEA in goats can be challenging, as the clinical signs can be nonspecific and similar to other reproductive diseases. However, laboratory testing such as serology and polymerase chain reaction (PCR) testing of blood, placenta, and vaginal swabs may be undertaken for confirmation. Histopathology of the placenta can also be helpful in identifying the presence of bacteria (Sachse et al. 2009). Presence of intracellular inclusion bodies in smears from infected fetuses and intercotyledonary areas after Ziehl–Neelsen (ZN) staining can also be used for diagnosis. Serological tests including ELISA and indirect immunofluorescence test (IIFT) are routinely used. Titer in the range of 1:32–1:256 suggests chlamydial infection. Culturing of organisms from placenta or fetal tissue will be helpful in definitive diagnosis (Carter 1986; East 1986). The following samples should be submitted for diagnostic evaluation: fresh placenta and fetus packed in ice, vaginal swab taken within three days of parturition, and paired serum sample from aborting and normal does (Gatewood and Spire 1990).

22.4.2.3.2 Prevention and Control

Vaccination is the most effective means of preventing CEA in goats, with a live attenuated vaccine being the most commonly used. Good management practices, such as separating pregnant animals from nonpregnant ones, regular cleaning, disinfection, and controlling the movement of animals, help to prevent the spread of infection. Long-acting oxytetracycline 20 mg/kg IM should be injected at 6–8 weeks prior to parturition followed by a second injection three weeks after parturition (Timoney et al. 1988). A killed vaccine (combination of *Campylobacter* and *E.coli* bacterin) available in the USA can be given IM or SC eight weeks prior to breeding followed in four weeks with a second dose.

22.4.2.4 Listeriosis

Caused by the Gram-positive, nonacid-fast bacterium *Listeria monocytogenes*, listeriosis is a significant concern for public health with organisms present in soil, water, sewage, and plant litter (Smith and Sherman, 1994). Sudden abortion, stillbirth, and weak or infected kids are noticeable symptoms in listeriosis. Other clinical signs include fever, anorexia, reduced milk yield, lethargy, and neurological symptoms such as head tilt and circling (Barbuddhe et al. 2000). The incubation period is typically 1–3 weeks and abortion usually occurs during the last trimester of pregnancy. Feeding of soil-contaminated, poorly fermented silage is the main source of infection and abortion generally occurs within seven days of silage feeding (Engeland et al. 1997). After entrance to the abdominal cavity, the organism penetrates the gut mucosa leading to septicemia and placentitis causing abortion.

22.4.2.4.1 Diagnosis

Identification of the organism is by culturing samples obtained from placenta, aborted fetus, and vaginal discharge. A fetal liver having gray/white miliary foci of necrosis (sawdust liver) is a typical feature of the disease. Moreover, affected chorion is covered with brownish red exudate and the placenta is necrotic. Bacterial culture and PCR testing of blood, placenta, and fetal tissue can be used to confirm the diagnosis.

22.4.2.4.2 Prevention and Control

Good management practices, such as providing clean water, feeding high-quality forage, and proper disposal of aborted fetuses and placenta, can help reduce the risk of infection. Two doses of attenuated live vaccine before breeding can be given to provide protection.

22.4.2.5 Q Fever

Coxiella burnetii is a highly infectious and zoonotic bacterium that causes Q fever or Queensland fever in humans and animals, including goats. It is primarily transmitted through inhalation of contaminated dust particles but contact with infected animals or their excreta and milk is also reported (Guatteo et al. 2007). Involvement of ticks has also been indicated in spread of Q fever. Once inside the body, the bacterium multiplies within the placenta, causing inflammation and necrosis, leading to abortion in late gestation (Miller et al. 1986; Moore et al. 1991). The bacterium can also cross the placental barrier and infect the fetus, leading to stillbirth or weak kids (Angelakis and Raoult 2010).

22.4.2.5.1 Diagnosis

Laboratory tests such as the indirect fluorescent antibody test (IFAT) in frozen section of placenta and ELISA are commonly used to diagnose Q fever in goats. Agent identification can also be used for diagnosis under strict biosecurity measures (Moore et al. 1991). Antibody titer of ≥1:20 indicates exposure to infection and a fourfold increase in titer between acute and convalescent samples indicates recent infection (Moore et al. 1991).

22.4.2.5.2 Prevention and Control

Vaccination is available and can help prevent spread of the disease but animals infected before vaccination remain chronic carriers. Biosecurity measures such as quarantine and isolation of infected animals, proper cleaning and disinfection, controlling the movement of people and animals help prevent the spread of Q fever. Feeding of 200 mg/animal/day chlortetracycline in the feed for 19 days has prevented abortion in an outbreak (Miller et al. 1986). As it is zoonotic in nature, use of mask and gloves while removing manure and handling an aborted fetus should be practiced.

22.4.3 Viral Causes of Abortion

22.4.3.1 Border Disease Virus (BDV)

Bovine viral diarrhea (BVD) is caused by the *Pestivirus* genus, which also includes the bovine viral diarrhea virus (BVDV) and the classic swine fever virus characterized by abortion, stillbirths, and birth of weak and deformed kids (Ali et al. 2019). Border disease virus (BDV) is transmitted horizontally through direct contact with infected animals or their secretions, or vertically from an infected pregnant dam to her fetus (Mao et al. 2022). Clinical signs depend on the age of the animal, the stage of gestation, and the virulence of the virus strain.

The pathogenesis of BDV infection in pregnant goats is complex, as it crosses the placental barrier and infects the fetus directly, leading to fetal death and abortion. The virus also causes marked placentitis (notable feature of disease), ensuing fetal growth retardation, stillbirths, weak and deformed kids known as hairy shakers or fuzzy lambs due to the exhibition of neurological symptoms like tremors and having coarse fleece (Feknous et al. 2018). The incidence of early abortion, fetal resorption, and mummification is more common than delivery of weak full-term kids in goats. Moreover, immunosuppression in pregnant goats makes them more susceptible to secondary bacterial infections causing abortion.

22.4.3.1.1 Diagnosis

This is challenging, as the clinical signs are not specific to the disease and many infected animals are asymptomatic. ELISA and virus neutralization assays are the most reliable serological tests for diagnosis. PCR-based methods can also be used to detect viral RNA in blood or tissue samples, but are less sensitive than serological tests.

22.4.3.1.2 Prevention and Control

A combination of vaccination, biosecurity measures, and culling of infected animals are common measures that can be followed. Vaccination with inactivated or live attenuated vaccines can provide protection against the disease, but it is important to use a vaccine that matches the local strain of the virus. Biosecurity measures, such as quarantine and testing of new animals before introducing them to the herd, can help prevent the introduction of the virus.

22.4.3.2 Caprine Herpesvirus 1

Caprine herpesvirus 1 (CpHV-1) is a highly contagious virus that causes a range of clinical signs in goats, including abortion, stillbirth, and weak kids. The virus is transmitted through direct contact with infected animals, contaminated fomites, and the respiratory route. CpHV-1 primarily infects the respiratory and reproductive tracts of goats, leading to necrosis, inflammation of placenta, and ultimately abortion (Tempesta et al. 2004).

Diagnosis of CpHV-1 can be made through virus isolation, serology, and PCR. Prevention and control of CpHV-1 involve good management practices, including quarantine, vaccination, and controlling the movement of people and animals (Camero et al. 2016).

22.4.3.3 Akabane Virus

Akabane virus (AKAV) is a bunyavirus that causes abortion, stillbirth, mummification, and congenital malformations (arthrogryposis and hydroencephaly) in goats (Carter 1986; Smith and Sherman 1994). The virus is transmitted through the bite of gnats and infected *Culicoides* mosquitoes (Smith and Sherman 1994). AKAV primarily infects the fetal tissues, leading to necrosis and inflammation, ultimately resulting in abortion or stillbirth.

Diagnosis of AKAV can be made through serology and PCR. Prevention and control involve good management practices, vector control, vaccination in epizootic areas before breeding, and controlling the movement of people and animals (Smith and Sherman 1994; Tang et al. 2019).

22.4.3.4 Bluetongue Virus

Bluetongue virus (BTV) is an orbivirus that causes abortion, stillbirth, and congenital malformations in goats. The virus is primarily transmitted through the bite of infected *Culicoides* mosquitoes. BTV primarily infects the fetal tissues, leading to necrosis and inflammation, ultimately resulting in abortion or stillbirth (Chauhan et al. 2014).

Diagnosis of BTV can be made through serology and PCR. Prevention and control involve good management practices, including mosquito control, vaccination, and controlling the movement of people and animals.

22.4.4 Parasitic Causes of Abortion

22.4.4.1 Toxoplasmosis

Toxoplasmosis is a protozoan parasitic infection caused by *Toxoplasma gondii* and is one of the major causes of abortion in goats worldwide. Goats become infected by ingesting oocysts shed by infected cats or by consuming tissue cysts present in infected tissues (de Oliveira et al. 2022). The incidence varies from region to region, and several factors such as presence of infected cats, type of feeding, age and the immune status of goats influence the prevalence of infection.

After ingestion, oocysts or tissue cysts release the parasite in the gastrointestinal tract, and tachyzoites invade the epithelial cells and disseminate throughout the body. Tissue cysts form in different organs, including the placenta, leading to infection and abortion in pregnant animals. The immune response controls the infection by transforming the tachyzoites into bradyzoites that form tissue cysts, but these cysts can reactivate during pregnancy, invade and multiply in the placenta and fetus, leading to abortion (Dubey 1987; Rodrigues et al. 2022). Additionally, immunity developed against toxoplasmosis is short-lived and the immune animal is also susceptible to new environmental challenge (Dubey 2009).

Abortion usually occurs in the third trimester of pregnancy. Infection between 30 and 90 days after breeding leads to fetal resorption or mummification. Goats that survive the infection can develop immunity whereas others remain carriers and shed oocysts in their feces, contributing to contamination of the environment and other animals. Cotyledons of an affected placenta are bright to dark red in color with multiple small white necrotic foci (1–3 mm in diameter) known as "frosted strawberries" (Dubey 1987).

22.4.4.1.1 Diagnosis

Serology is the most commonly used diagnostic tool, and detection of specific antibodies against *T. gondii* in the serum or fetal fluid is indicative of transplacental infection (Dubey 1990). Sabin and Feldman dye test, IFAT, modified agglutination test, radioimmunoassay, or ELISA can also be used (Dubey 1987, 1990). Elevated titer of a single sample can be indicative of past infection as antibodies remain elevated for years after initial infection. Increasing titer in paired samples at 14-day intervals is indicative of active infection (Rodrigues et al. 2022). PCR, histopathology, and immunohistochemistry can be used to detect the parasite in tissues (fetal brain, lungs, and muscle), placenta or fetal fluids (Dubey 1990). These samples should be shipped on ice but not frozen (Dubey 1987).

22.4.4.1.2 Control

Control measures include prevention of ingestion of oocysts by controlling cat populations, avoiding contact between cats and goats, and using proper hygiene and sanitation practices. Additionally, the use of vaccines (S48) and drugs to prevent or treat the infection can be beneficial, but their use in goats is still not approved.

22.4.4.2 *Neospora caninum*

Neospora caninum is a protozoan parasite that can cause abortion in goats (Dubey and Lindsay 2006). The parasite has a worldwide distribution and infects a variety of host species, including dogs, cattle, and sheep. It is transmitted vertically from an infected dam to her fetus during pregnancy, or horizontally through ingestion of contaminated feed or water. The pathogenesis in pregnant goats is not well understood, but it is believed to cause damage to the placenta and fetal tissues. The parasite can cross the placental barrier and infect the fetus directly, leading to fetal death and abortion. In addition, it can cause placental insufficiency, which results in fetal growth retardation, stillbirths, and weak and deformed kids.

Diagnosis is challenging, as the clinical signs are not specific to the disease and many infected animals are asymptomatic. ELISA and immunofluorescence assays are the most reliable serological tests used for diagnosis. PCR-based methods can also be used to detect parasite DNA in blood or tissue samples, but are less sensitive than serological tests.

22.5 Conclusion

Numerous etiological variables lead to abortion in goats and limit reproductive potential. The current state of abortion in goats necessitates a coordinated global approach by all the stakeholders for improved epidemiological surveillance. This will aid in the development of region- and zone-specific policies and management guidelines to improve farmers' livelihoods and may open new research horizons for the creation of doorstep test kits and indigenous vaccines for the control and eradication of abortion-causing agents. To familiarize farmers with different clinical indicators and diagnostic tests available for early diagnosis, and also to strengthen disease monitoring and reporting systems, extension services/awareness camps can be organized. To help with diagnostic evaluation and care, a detailed history that includes diet and any recent changes in husbandry should be collected.

The best way to prevent abortions and infertility is to keep herds under low stress and take proper biosecurity precautions.

References

Alemayehu, G., Mamo, G., Alemu, B. et al. (2021). Causes and flock level risk factors of sheep and goat abortion in three agroecology zones in Ethiopia. *Frontiers in Veterinary Science* 8: 615310.

Ali, S., Zhao, Z., Zhen, G. et al. (2019). Reproductive problems in small ruminants (sheep and goats): a substantial economic loss in the world. *Large Animal Review* 25: 215–223.

Anderson, K.L. (1986). Campylobacteriosis. In: *Current Therapy in Theriogenology*, 2e (ed. D.A. Morrow), 605. Philadelphia, PA: WB Saunders.

Anderson, M.L. (2007). Infectious causes of bovine abortion during mid- to late-gestation. *Theriogenology* 68 (3): 474–486.

Angelakis, E. and Raoult, D. (2010). Q fever. *Veterinary Microbiology* 140: 297–309.

Barbuddhe, S.B., Malik, S.V.S., Bhilegaonkar, K.N. et al. (2000). Isolation of listeria monocytogenes and anti-listeriolysin O detection in sheep and goats. *Small Ruminant Research* 38: 151–155.

Bolet, G. (1986). Timing and extent of embryonic mortality in pigs sheep and goats: genetic variability. In: *Embryonic Mortality in Farm Animals* (ed. J. Sreenan and M. Diskin), 12–43. Dordrecht: Springer Netherlands.

Borel, N., Frey, C.F., Gottstein, B. et al. (2014). Laboratory diagnosis of ruminant abortion in Europe. *Veterinary Journal* 200 (2): 218–229.

Camero, M., Marinaro, M., Losurdo, M. et al. (2016). Caprine herpesvirus 1 (CpHV-1) vaginal infection of goats: clinical efficacy of fig latex. *Natural Product Research* 30: 605–607.

Carter, G.R. (1986). *Veterinarian's Guide to the Laboratory Diagnosis of Infectious Diseases*. New York: Veterinary Medicine Publishing Co.

Cetinkaya, B. and Ongör, H. (2000). Evaluation of immunocomb in comparison with other serological tests in ovine brucellosis. *Veterinary Record* 147: 632–634.

Chanton-Greutmann, H., Thoma, R., Corboz, L. et al. (2002). Abortion in small ruminants in Switzerland: investigations during two lambing seasons (1996–1998) with special regard to chlamydial abortions. *Schweizer Archiv für Tierheilkunde* 144: 483–492.

Chauhan, H.C., Biswas, S.K., Chand, K. et al. (2014). Isolation of bluetongue virus serotype 1 from aborted goat fetuses. *Revue Scientifique et Technique* 3: 803–812.

Chénier, S., Montpetit, C., and Hélie, P. (2004). Caprine herpesvirus-1 abortion storm in a goat herd in Quebec. *Canadian Veterinary Journal* 45 (3): 241.

Clothier, K. and Anderson, M. (2016). Evaluation of bovine abortion cases and tissue suitability for identification of infectious agents in California diagnostic laboratory cases from 2007 to 2012. *Theriogenology* 85 (5): 933–938.

Corah, L.R. and Ives, S. (1991). The effects of essential trace minerals on reproduction in beef cattle. *Veterinary Clinics of North America: Food Animal Practice* 7: 41–57.
Dantas, A.F.M. (2009). Malformations and embryonic death in ruminants caused by ingestion of Mimosa tenuiflora (black jurema). PhD thesis. Federal Rural University of Pernambuco, Recife, Pernambuco.
De Oliveira, J.M.B., Silva, B.P.E., Ribeiro-Andrade, M. et al. (2022). Toxoplasma gondii infection in goats: serological, pathological, and clinical monitoring during gestation. *Parasitology Research* 121: 3147–3153.
Dennis, S.M. (1990). Campylobacter abortion in sheep. *Laboratory Diagnosis of Livestock Abortion* 3: 82–85.
Dubey, J.P. (1987). Toxoplasmosis in goats. *Agri-practice* 8: 43–52.
Dubey, J.P. (1990). Toxoplasmosis: zoonosis update. *Journal of the American Veterinary Medical Association* 196: 123.
Dubey, J.P. (2009). Toxoplasmosis in sheep – the last 20 years. *Veterinary Parasitology* 163: 1–14.
Dubey, J.P. and Lindsay, D.S. (1990). Neospora caninum induced abortion in sheep. *Journal of Veterinary Diagnostic Investigation* 2 (3): 230–233.
Dubey, J.P. and Lindsay, D.S. (2006). Neosporosis, toxoplasmosis, and sarcocystosis in ruminants. *Veterinary Clinics: Food Animal Practice* 22: 645–671.
East, N.E. (1986). Chlamydiosis. In: *Current Therapy in Theriogenology*, 2e (ed. D.A. Morrow), 603. Philadelphia, PA: WB Saunders.
Ebani, V.V. (2022). Reproductive disorders in domestic ruminants: a one health concern. *Pathogens* 11: 1139.
Engeland, I.V., Waldeland, H., Ropstad, E. et al. (1997). Effect of experimental infection with listeria monocytogenes on the development of pregnancy and on concentrations of progesterone, oestrone sulphate and 15-ketodihydro-PGF2α in the goat. *Animal Reproduction Science* 45: 311–327.
Feknous, N., Hanon, J.B., Tignon, M. et al. (2018). Seroprevalence of border disease virus and other pestiviruses in sheep in Algeria and associated risk factors. *BMC Veterinary Research* 14: 1–11.
Fentahun, T. and Fresebehat, A. (2012). Listeriosis in small ruminants: a review. *Advances in Biology Research* 6 (6): 202–209.
Gatewood, D.M. and Spire, M.F. (1990). Chlamydial abortion in domestic ruminants. *Theriogenology* 6: 202–209.
Givens, M.D. and Marley, M.S.D. (2008). Infectious causes of embryonic and fetal mortality. *Theriogenology* 70: 270–285.
Godfroid, J., Nielsen, K., and Saegerman, C. (2010). Diagnosis of brucellosis in livestock and wildlife. *Croatian Medical Journal* 51: 296–305.
Guatteo, R., Beaudeau, F., Joly, A., and Seegers, H. (2007). Coxiella burnetii shedding by dairy cows. *Veterinary Research* 38: 849–860.
Gupta, R.C., Kwatra, M.S., and Singh, N. (1982). Chronic selenium toxicity as a cause of hoof and horn deformities in buffalo, cattle and goat. *Indian Veterinary Journal* 59: 738.
Hashiguchi, Y., Nanba, K., and Kumagai, T. (1979). Congenital abnormalities in newborn lambs following Akabane virus infection in pregnant ewes. *National Institute of Animal Health Quarterly* 19: 1–11.
Holler, L.D. (2012). Ruminant abortion diagnostics. *Veterinary Clinics: Food Animal Practice* 28: 407–418.
Innes, E.A., Bartley, P.M., Buxton, D., and Katzer, F. (2009). Ovine toxoplasmosis. *Parasitology* 136 (14): 1887–1894.
James, L.F., Hartley, W.J., and Van Kampen, K.R. (1981). Syndromes of Astragalus poisoning in livestock. *Journal of the American Veterinary Medical Association* 178: 146–150.
Keeler, R.F., Young, S., and Stuart, L.D. (1985). Congenital tracheal stenosis in lambs induced by maternal ingestion of Veratrum californicum. *Teratology* 31: 83–88.
Khair, A., Alam, M.M., Rahman, A.K.M.A. et al. (2013). Incidence of reproductive and production diseases of cross-bred dairy cattle in Bangladesh. *Bangladesh Journal of Veterinary Medicine* 11 (1): 31–36.
Knight, A.P. and Walter, R.G. (2003). *A Guide to Plant Poisoning of Animals in North America, 2001*, 194–197. Jackson, WY: Teton New Media.
Krishnan, G., Bagath, M., Pragna, P. et al. (2017). Mitigation of the heat stress impact in livestock reproduction. *Theriogenology* 8: 8–9.
Kruszewska, D. and Tylewska-Wierzbanowska, S. (1997). Isolation of Coxiella burnetii from bull semen. *Research in Veterinary Science* 62 (3): 299–300.
Leon-Vizcaino, L., De Mendoza, M.H., and Garrido, F. (1987). Incidence of abortions caused by leptospirosis in sheep and goats in Spain. *Comparative Immunology, Microbiology and Infectious Diseases* 10 (2): 149–153.
Lindsay, K.L., Buss, C., Wadhwa, P.D., and Entringer, S. (2019). The interplay between nutrition and stress in pregnancy: implications for fetal programming of brain development. *Biological Psychiatry* 85 (2): 135–149.
Longbottom, D. and Coulter, L.J. (2003). Animal chlamydioses and zoonotic implications. *Journal of Comparative Pathology* 128: 217–244.

Ludders, J.W. (1988). Anesthesia for the Pregnant Patient. *Proceedings of the Annual Meeting of the Society of Theriogenology, Annual Meeting*, Orlando, Florida (16–17 September 1988), 36–54. Mathews, AL: Society of Theriogenology.

Mao, L., Li, W., Hao, F. et al. (2022). Research progress on emerging viral pathogens of small ruminants in China during the last decade. *Viruses* 14: 1288.

Medeiros, R.M.T., Neto, S.A.G., Riet-Correa, F. et al. (2004). Mortalidade embrionária e abortos em caprinos causados por Aspidosperma pyrifolium. *Pesquisa Veterinaria Brasileira* 24: 42–43.

Mee, J.F. (2020). Investigation of bovine abortion and stillbirth/perinatal mortality-similar diagnostic challenges, different approaches. *Irish Veterinary Journal* 73 (1): 20.

Menzies, P.I. (2011). Control of important causes of infectious abortion in sheep and goats. *Veterinary Clinics of North America: Food Animal Practice* 27: 81–93.

Merrall, M. (1985). Nutritional and Metabolic Diseases. *Proceedings of a Course in Goat Husbandry and Medicine*, Pub. 106, 126. Veterinarian Continuing Education, Massey University, NZ, 126.

Miller, R.B., Palmer, N.C., and Kierstad, M. (1986). *Coxiella burnetii* infection in goats. In: *Current Therapy in Theriogenology*, 2e (ed. D.A. Morrow), 607. Philadelphia, PA: WB Saunders.

Moore, J.D., Barr, B.C., Daft, B.M., and O'Connor, M.T. (1991). Pathology and diagnosis of Coxiella burnetii infection in a goat herd. *Veterinary Pathology* 28: 81–84.

Nancarrow, C.D. (1994). Embryonic mortality in the ewe and doe. In: *Embryonic Mortality in Domestic Species* (ed. M.T. Zavy and R.D. Geisert), 79–97. Boca Raton, FL: CRC Press.

Nettleton, P.F., Gilray, J.A., Russo, P., and Dlissi, E. (1998). Border disease of sheep and goats. *Veterinary Research* 29 (3–4): 327–340.

Nigro, G., Mazzocco, M., Mattia, E. et al. (2011). Role of the infections in recurrent spontaneous abortion. *Journal of Maternal-Fetal Neonatal Medicine* 24 (8): 983–989.

Ocholi, R.A., Kwaga, J.K.P., Ajogi, I., and Bale, J.O.O. (2005). Abortion due to *Brucella abortus* in sheep in Nigeria. *Revue Scientifique et Technique-Office International Des Epizooties* 24 (3): 973–980.

Osuagwuh, A.I.A. and Akpokodje, J.U. (1986). Outbreak of abortion in West African Dwarf (Fouta Djallon) goats due to malnutrition. *Tropical Veterinarian* 4: 67.

Panter, K.E., Keeler, R.F., James, L.F., and Bunch, T.D. (1992). Impact of plant toxins on fetal and neonatal development: a review. *Rangeland Ecology and Management/Journal of Range Management Archives* 45: 52–57.

Panter, K.E., James, L.F., and Gardner, D.R. (1999). Lupines, poison-hemlock and Nicotiana spp: toxicity and teratogenicity in livestock. *Journal of Natural Toxins* 8: 117–134.

Panter, K.E., Welch, K.D., Gardner, D.R. et al. (2018). Poisonous plants of the United States. In: *Veterinary Toxicology* (ed. R. Gupta), 837–889. New York: Academic Press.

Papp, J.R., Shewen, P.E., and Gartley, C.J. (1993). Chlamydia psittaci infection and associated infertility in sheep. *Canadian Journal of Veterinary Research* 57 (3): 185.

Pfister, J.A. and Adams, D.C. (1993). Factors influencing pine needle consumption by grazing cattle during winter. *Journal of Range Management* 46: 394–398.

Pieterse, M.C. and Taverne, M.A.M. (1986). Hydrometra in goats: diagnosis with real-time ultrasound and treatment with prostaglandins or oxytocin. *Theriogenology* 26: 813–821.

Purohit, G.N. (2006). *Proceedings of the National Seminar on Innovations and Recent Advances in Reproduction for Augmenting Small Ruminant Production*. Avikanagar, Jaipur, India (28–30 December 2006).

Robert, B. and Moeller, J. (2001). Causes of caprine abortion: diagnostic assessment of 211 cases (1991–1998). *Journal of Veterinary Diagnostic Investigation* 13 (3): 265–270.

Rodrigues, A.A., Reis, S.S., da Silva Moraes, E. et al. (2022). A systematic literature review and meta-analysis of toxoplasma gondii seroprevalence in goats. *Acta Tropica* 230: 106411.

Sachse, K., Vretou, E., Livingstone, M. et al. (2009). Recent developments in the laboratory diagnosis of chlamydial infections. *Veterinary Microbiology* 135: 2–21.

Sahin, O., Plummer, P.J., Jordan, D.M. et al. (2008). Emergence of a tetracycline-resistant Campylobacter jejuni clone associated with outbreaks of ovine abortion in the United States. *Journal of Clinical Microbiology* 46 (5): 1663–1671.

Smith, M.C. (1978). Some clinical aspects of caprine reproduction. *Cornell Veterinarian* 68: 200–211.

Smith, M.C. and Morrow, D. (1986). Causes and diagnosis of abortion in goats. In: *Current Therapy in Theriogenology*, 2e (ed. D.A. Morrow). Philadelphia, PA: WB Saunders.

Smith, M.C. and Sherman, D.M. (1994). *Goat Medicine*, 411. Philadelphia, PA: Lea & Febiger.

Snider, D.B., Gardner, D.R., Janke, B.H., and Ensley, S.M. (2015). Pine needle abortion biomarker detected in bovine fetal fluids. *Journal of Veterinary Diagnostic Investigation* 27: 74–79.

Tang, H.B., Ren, P., Qin, S. et al. (2019). Isolation, genetic analysis of the first Akabane virus from goat in China. *Journal of Veterinary Medical Science* 81: 1445–1449.

Tempesta, M., Camero, M., Sciorsci, R.L. et al. (2004). Experimental infection of goats at different stages of pregnancy with caprine herpesvirus 1. *Comparative Immunology, Microbiology and Infectious Diseases* 27: 25–32.

Timoney, J.F., Gillispie, J.H., and Scott, F.W. (1988). The Chlamydiaceae. In: *Hagan and Bruner's Microbiology and Infectious Diseases Of domestic Animals*, 8e, 356. Ithaca, NY: Comstock Publishing Associates.

Wang, Z., Lin, S., Liu, X. et al. (2021). Brucellosis knowledge and personal protective equipment usage among high-risk populations in brucellosis-endemic areas – China, 2019–2020. *China CDC Weekly* 3: 106.

Wassenaar, T.M. and Newell, D.G. (2006). The genus Campylobacter. *Prokaryotes* 7: 119–138.

Welch, K., Davis, T.Z., Panter, K. et al. (2009). The effect of poisonous range plants on abortions in livestock. *Rangelands* 31: 28–34.

Wentzel, D., Morgenthal, J.C., Van Niekerk, C.H., and Roelofse, C.S. (1974). The habitually aborting angora doe. 2. The effect of an energy deficiency on the incidence of abortion. *Agroanimalia* 6: 129–132.

Wilmut, I., Sales, D.I., and Ashworth, C.J. (1986). Maternal and embryonic factors associated with prenatal loss in mammals. *Reproduction* 76: 851–864.

Wu, X.J., Gao, J., Zhang, Q. et al. (2023). Seroprevalence and risk factors of Chlamydia infection in cattle in Shanxi Province, North China. *Animals* 13: 252.

Yadav, R., Yadav, P., Singh, G. et al. (2021). Non-infectious causes of abortion in livestock animals-A. *International Journal of Livestock Research* 11: 1–13.

Yaeger, M.J., Sahin, O., Plummer, P.J. et al. (2021). The pathology of natural and experimentally induced *Campylobacter jejuni* abortion in sheep. *Journal of Veterinary Diagnostic Investigation* 33: 1096–1105.

Zaki, M.M., El-Midany, S.A., Shaheen, H.M., and Rizzi, L. (2012). Mycotoxins in animals: occurrence, effects, prevention and management. *Journal of Toxicology and Environmental Health Science* 4: 13–28.

23

Infectious Abortive Diseases: Chlamydiosis

Chinmoy Maji[1], Kruti Debnath Mandal[2], and Suman Biswas[3]

[1] *Division of Animal Health, North 24 Parganas Krishi Vigyan Kendra, West Bengal University of Animal & Fishery Sciences, Ashokenagar, West Bengal, India*
[2] *Department of Avian Sciences, Faculty of Veterinary & Animal Sciences, West Bengal University of Animal & Fishery Sciences, Nadia, India*
[3] *Teaching Veterinary Clinical Complex, Faculty of Veterinary and Animal Sciences, Institute of Agricultural Science, Banaras Hindu University, Mirzapur, India*

23.1 Introduction

Chlamydiales order members are intriguing Gram-negative, obligatory intracellular bacteria that divide within eukaryotic hosts and share a distinctive biphasic developmental cycle. There are currently nine families that make up the order, and individuals from each family can infect humans, wild and domesticated mammals, reptiles, amphibians, and fish. The elementary bodies (EBs), the extracellular and contagious form of the bacterium (with a diameter of 0.2 mm), infect the host's mucosal epithelial cells to start the biphasic growth cycle. EBs develop inside an inclusion, a membrane-bound endocytic vacuole, which is formed after attachment to and entrance into the host cell. There, EBs evolve into bigger (0.8 mm), metabolically active but noninfectious reticulate bodies (RBs). After several rounds of division, RBs redifferentiate into infectious EBs, mature EBs finish the developmental cycle, and these pathogens leave the host cell either through lysis or the spread of their epidemiology. Moreover, research on novel hosts has revealed new chlamydial species, such as those found in reptile and bird hosts, as well as increased host ranges for current species (Taylor-Brown and Polkinghorne 2017). With over 400 host species documented globally, the majority of which are wild animals, the animal host range of bacteria in the Chlamydiales order is substantially wider than previously imagined (Burnard and Polkinghorne 2016). Recent reports showed that Chlamydiales not only affect wild ungulates and marsupials but also birds, reptiles, amphibians, fish, and eutherians (Burnard and Polkinghorne 2016).

Depending on the chlamydial species involved, chlamydiosis in goats can range from asymptomatic infection to severe infections with life-threatening consequences. Chlamydial infections can cause a variety of illnesses, such as conjunctivitis, which can range in severity from mild symptoms to corneal opacification, rhinitis, pneumonia, mastitis, arthritis and polyarthritis, pericarditis, polyserositis, encephalomyelitis, placentitis, which can result in abortion, stillbirth, or weak newborns, endometritis and metritis, orchitis/epididymitis/urethritis, and infertility in doe and buck. Nonetheless, they may go unnoticed by the pathologist because the lesions are too small to result in the goat's death or because chlamydia is not considered when making a differential diagnosis because there are other more widespread and well-known pathogens. The diagnosis of chlamydial infections can therefore be difficult for pathologists, apart from chlamydial abortion in small ruminants like goat and avian chlamydiosis.

23.2 Etiology

In recent years, there have been numerous changes to the chlamydial nomenclature. In field studies, chlamydiae are detected and species/strain level differences are analyzed using conserved genes like 16S rRNA, 23S rRNA, and genetically variable genes like omp2 and ompA as well as some other targets including GroEL chaperonin, KDO transferase, and ompB (Ababneh et al. 2014). It was also suggested to divide the genus Chlamydia into two genera, *Chlamydia* and *Chlamydophila*, in addition to the creation of new families (Everett et al. 1999). This modification sparked debate. A return to a single genus, *Chlamydia*, was suggested and is now accepted by the chlamydial research community after much debate

Elements of Reproduction and Reproductive Diseases of Goats, First Edition. Edited by Tanmoy Rana.

(Sachse et al. 2015). Chlamydiaceae, Clavichlamydiaceae, Cribchlamydiaceae, Parachlamydiaceae, Parilichlamydiaceae, Piscichlamydiaceae, Rhabdochlamydiaceae, Simkaniaceae, and Waddliaceae are the nine families that now make up the order Chlamydiales (Taylor-Brown et al. 2015). *Chlamydia* (*C*), the sole species in the Chlamydiaceae family, has 11 species: *C. abortus*, *C. avium*, *C. caviae*, *C. felis*, *C. gallinacea*, *C. muridarum*, *C. pecorum*, *C. pneumoniae*, *C. psittaci*, *C. suis*, and *C. trachomatis*, in addition to the three *Candidatus* (Ca.) species: *Ca C. ibidis*, *Ca. C. sanzinia*, and *Ca. C. corallus* (Sachse et al. 2015; Vorimore et al. 2013; Taylor-Brown et al. 2016).

The Chlamydiaceae, which also refers to the *Chlamydia*-related bacteria (CRB), are responsible for various animal diseases, some of which are zoonotic. The most dangerous zoonotic pathogens are *C. abortus* and *C. psittaci*. Abortion is caused by *C. abortus*, which primarily affects goats and sheep. A late-term abortion, a stillbirth, and the delivery of weak neonates which do not survive for more than 48 hours are all caused by *C. abortus* infection in small ruminants like goats, and to a lesser extent in cattle, pigs, horses, and wild ruminants (Longbottom and Coulter 2003).

23.3 Epidemiology

One of the first known ocular illnesses, trachoma, which has a chlamydial origin and causes blindness in people, was first discovered in Egypt in 15 BCE. It is believed that soldiers returning from Napoleon's Egyptian expedition (1798–1802) introduced the illness to Europe, where it spread through contact due to unhygienic conditions (Taylor 2008). Interestingly, a veterinarian from Austria discovered smears from healthy cows with transmissible vaginitis from several farms that were like the so-called "trachoma bodies" and dubbed them "Chlamydozoa" (Blaha 1909).

Chlamydial infections in ruminants have long been known in the Indian subcontinent but in recent years, thanks to the development of better diagnostic tools, chlamydiosis has come to be recognized as one of the most serious health problems affecting livestock (Bandyopadhyay et al. 2009). The disease was found to exist to varying degrees in both sick and healthy animals in recent serological surveys conducted in numerous countries to learn the status of chlamydiosis in local livestock species using various screening techniques (Osman et al. 2012). By using stained smears, antigen tests, immunofluorescence, immunohistochemistry (IHC), or molecular techniques like polymerase chain reaction (PCR), the disease can be identified if a significant number of organisms are present in the infected placental specimens. Other abortogenic agents such as *Toxoplasma*, *Campylobacter*, *Salmonella*, and *Listeria* spp. were also found in most abortion cases (71.6%) where *C. abortus* was present in a goat flock (Longbottom et al. 2013a). A recent PCR and sequencing study in India found *C. abortus* in instances of caprine infectious keratoconjunctivitis, including mixed infections with *C. psittaci* and *Mycoplasma* spp. (Gupta et al. 2015). In addition to epididymitis and pneumonia, *C. abortus* has been isolated from the feces of healthy goats and has been linked to conjunctivitis, arthritis, and conjunctivitis in small ruminants (Rodolakis and Laroucau 2015).

Unlike *C. suis* strains, *C. abortus* strains in Europe have little variation but distinct geographical characteristics (Figure 23.1 and 23.2). They do not contain plasmids and recent research found no evidence of recombination (Seth-Smith et al. 2017). The *C. abortus* strain S26/3, which was isolated from the placenta of a small ruminant that experienced ovine enzootic abortion (OEA) in Scotland, was used in the latter experiment by Longbottom et al. (2013b), whereas strains LLG and POS, which were isolated from aborted goat fetuses in Greece and are genetically distinct from S26/3, were used in a recent comparative study by the same authors (Livingstone et al. 2017). By doing this, they were able to demonstrate that the placental pathology, infection load, and serological response were all noticeably less severe for the *C. abortus* strains LLG and POS than for the strain S26/3.

23.4 Developmental Cycle

All members of the Chlamydiaceae family are Gram negative, nonmotile, obligate intracellular bacterial organisms. All of them possess a unique biphasic developmental cycle. The obligatory intracellular lifestyle is important to know as it is the basis of pathogenesis and treatment procedure.

The characteristic biphasic cycle (Figure 23.3) consists of two chlamydial forms which are functionally and morphologically distinct. One is the infectious EB, around 300 nm in diameter. The EB attaches first to susceptible eukaryotic host cells. After internalization of the EB into the host cell, the infectious form replicates further into the metabolically active noninfectious second form, i.e., RB, around 1–1.6 μm in diameter. RBs reside inside vacuoles named inclusions. This form further multiplies by binary fission and subsequently the affected host cytoplasm becomes completely filled by inclusions. The membrane of these inclusions is made up of sphingomyelin and other host lipids.

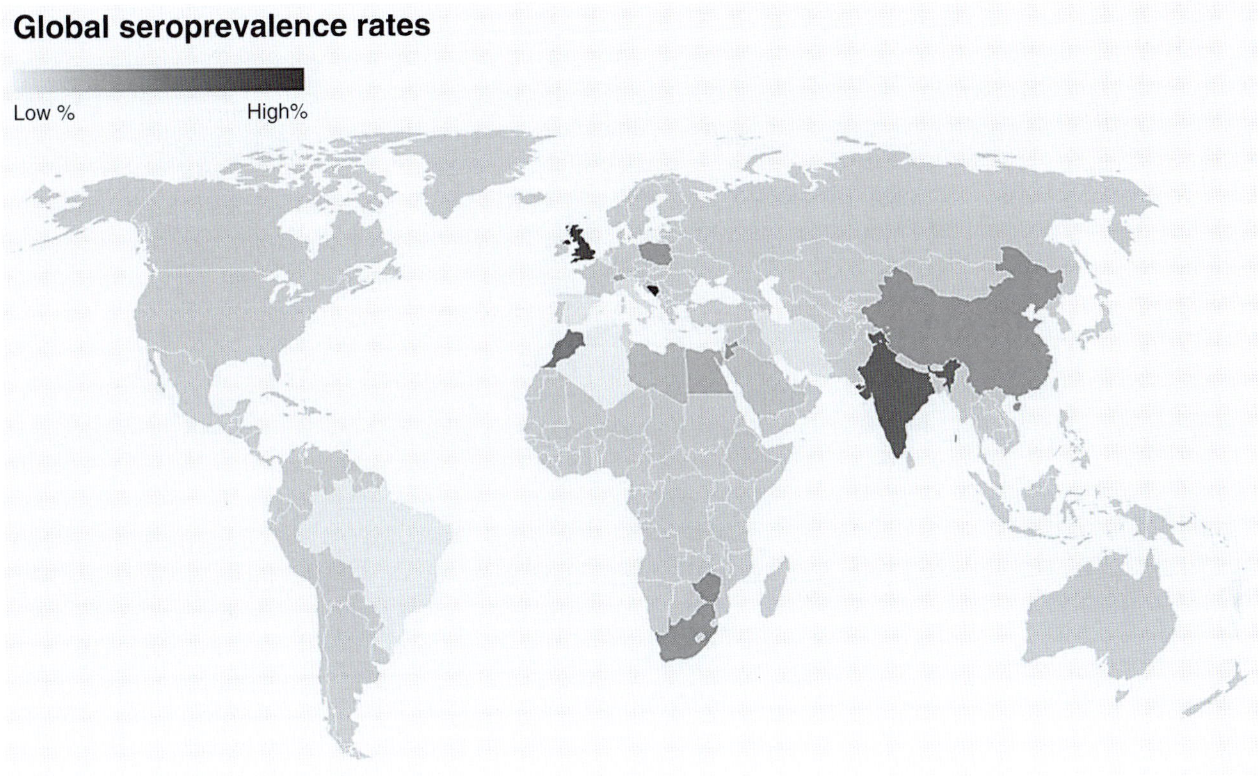

Figure 23.1 Global seroprevalence rate of *C. abortus* (Tourin *et al.*, 2022).

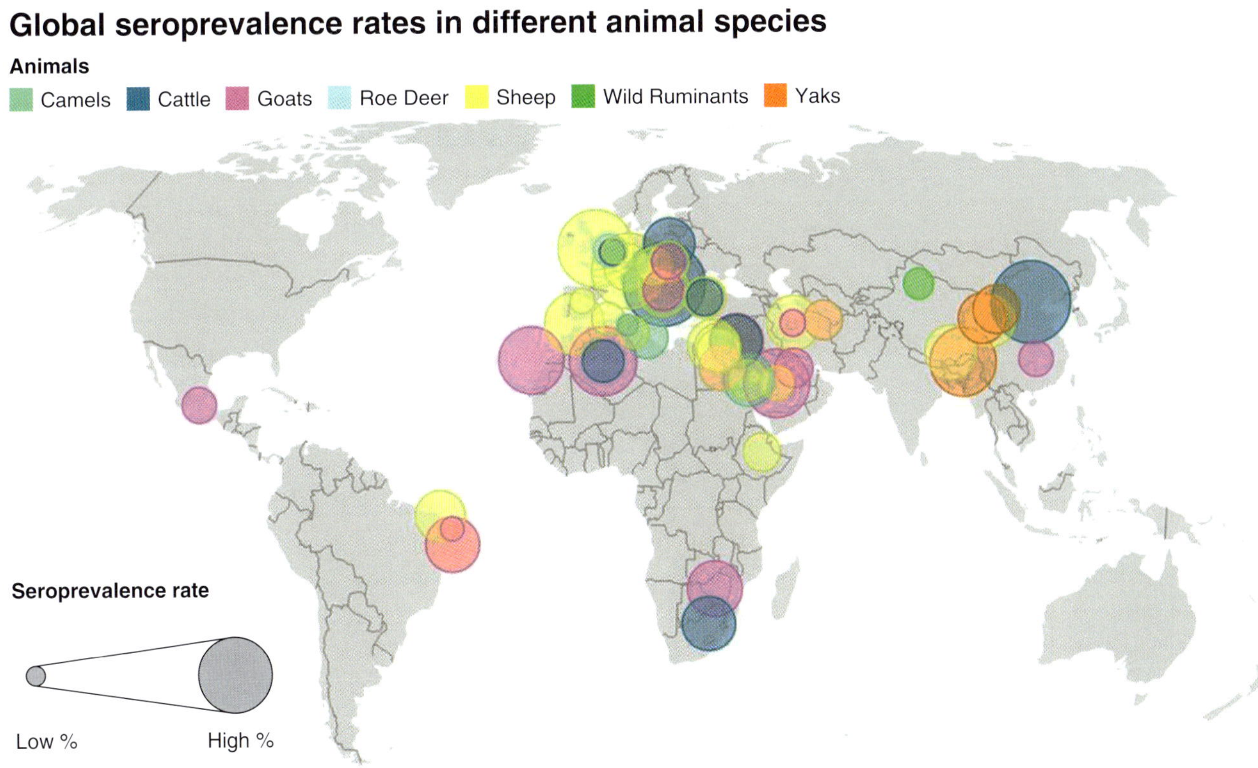

Figure 23.2 Global seroprevalence of *C. abortus* in different animal species (Tourin *et al.*, 2022).

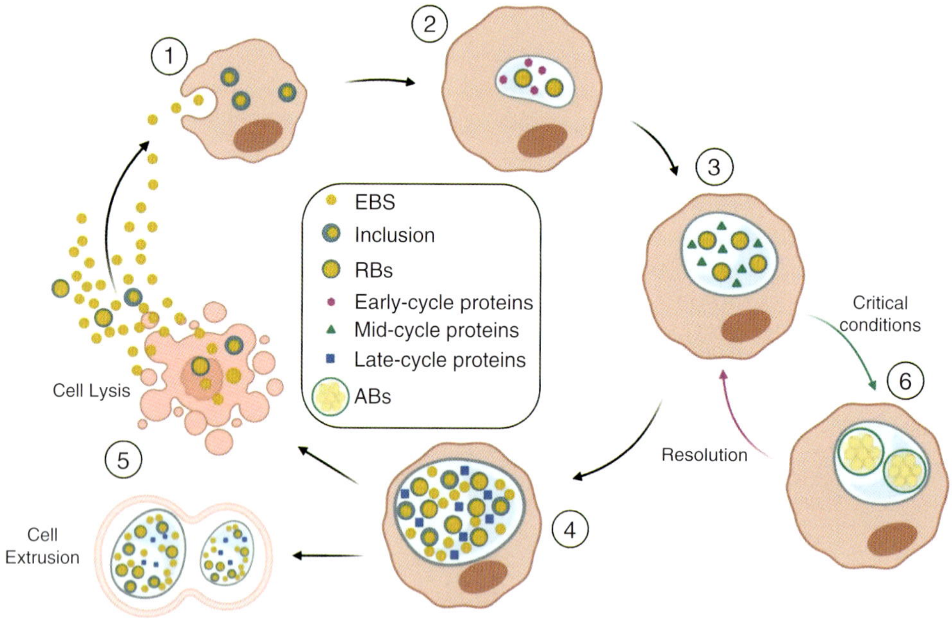

Figure 23.3 Schematic diagram of Chlamydial developmental cycle. EB-Elementary body, RB-reticulate body (Tourin *et al.*, 2022).

Chlamydials do not posses any genome to encode for membrane lipids so it may be postulated that these organisms acquire unique machinery such as exploitation of vesicular and nonvesicular pathways, recruitment of Rab GTPases and Golgi fragmentation (Elwell and Engel 2012) to use host lipids for their own survival. The inclusion membrane is believed to form membrane complexes consisting of multiple tubes with a single bilayered membrane which extends up to 12 μm inside the host cell. Generally, it develops in the middle and last stages of the growth cycle. The exact function of these membrane complexes is still unknown but it is possibly the machinery for utilization of host cell nutrients or protein.

In further development, RBs further differentiate into comparatively smaller infectious EB forms (Wilkat et al. 2014). During this process, different spherical and tubular vesicles (around 55 nm in diameter) appear in the periplasmic spaces of RBs. These vesicles contain chlamydial antigens having the same electron density as the RB. After 48–72 hours, EBs are released from affected host cells and attach to new healthy host cells or are transmitted to the host by aerosol transmission, ingestion or mucosal contact.

23.5 Transmission

Chlamydiaceae family members were once thought to be significant human and animal pathogens with a clearly defined host range and taxonomic diversity. The order Chlamydiales contains at least eight additional families of bacteria that are commonly referred to as *Chlamydia*-related bacteria (CRB) or *Chlamydia*-like organisms (CLO). This paradigm has been challenged by molecular techniques, which have also revealed an expanded host range for some chlamydial species. *C. abortus* has raised new issues regarding the part that crosshost transmission plays in the epidemiology of these infections. Also, following its isolation from nine aborted fetuses, *C. abortus* was hypothesized to contribute to yak abortion in China (Li et al. 2015).

Pregnant women are particularly vulnerable to the zoonotic disease chlamydiosis of small ruminants caused by *C. abortus*. A case of an unusual pneumonia caused by *C. abortus* in a lab worker who had participated in experimental intranasal *C. abortus* infections in sheep was reported (Ortega et al. 2016). Intranasal infection experiments have shown that nonpregnant animals can develop chlamydial latency from relatively low concentrations of infectious organisms (Longbottom et al. 2013b). The infection is asymptomatic in the nonpregnant animals during latency and only becomes visible during a subsequent pregnancy. The infection spreads throughout pregnancy, leading to placental infection and abortion in the animals. The major infection route is thought to be oronasal once organisms are ingested, causing an initial infection in the tonsil from which it may spread by blood or lymph to other organs (Essig and Longbottom 2015).

Massive amounts of *C. abortus* bacteria can be found in the placentas and fetal fluids of infected does. Chlamydiae can be found in the uterine secretions of goats as early as nine days prior to abortion and as late as two weeks following abortion and in ewes from around one day prior to abortion to 2–3 weeks after abortion (Nietfeld 2001). Elementary bodies can spread disease for days or even weeks if the temperature is below freezing during the typical spring weather when lambing usually takes place (Aitken 2000). The most common ways in which grazing animals like goats acquire infections are through ingesting pathogens through contaminated feed or water, licking other animals that have been exposed to reproductive fluids or tissues, or inhaling aerosols produced in contaminated habitats (Wilsmore et al. 1984) (Figure 23.4). Prior to their first pregnancy, when some *C. abortus*-infected kids experience abortion, they are clinically healthy (Wilsmore et al. 1990).

The classic symptoms of an enzootic abortion were reported following initial attempts at venereal transmission, which involved combining *C. abortus* with semen and administering it into the vagina after natural breeding (Appleyard et al. 1985). Because of the management practices utilized in goat farming, it was determined that venereal transmission was feasible but probably not widespread; nevertheless, more recent investigations in goats suggest that venereal transmission may be more significant than previously believed. It is probable that clinically normal does with persistent reproductive tract infections are a source of transmission both within and between flocks. Bucks can carry the infections and shed *C. abortus* in their semen after breeding with an infected doe (Papp and Shewen 1997). *C. abortus* is not known to be spread by sheep milk or colostrum, but it is thought to be spread through goat milk (Matthews 1999). Sometimes *C. abortus* is isolated from ruminant feces, which increases the risk of intestinal infection and fecal–oral transmission in goats (Storz and Kaltenboeck 1993).

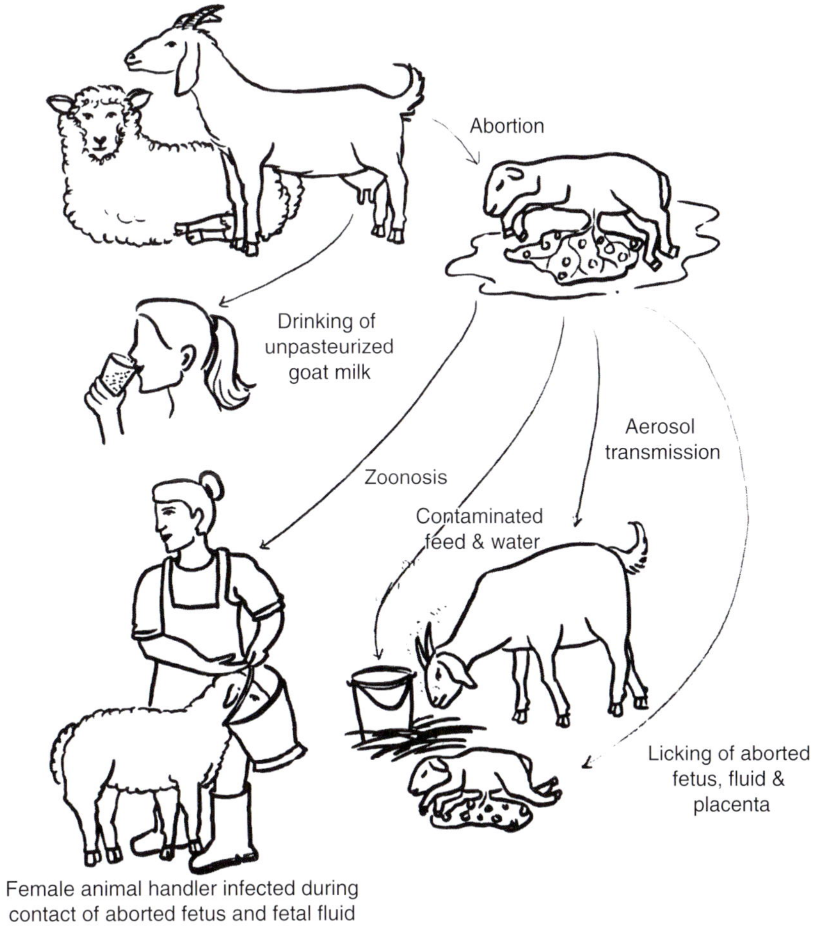

Figure 23.4 Different modes of transmission of *C. abortus* from infected sheep or goat.

23.6 Pathogenesis

Two species of *Chlamydophila* were known to cause infection and diseases in goats. *Chlamydophila abortus* (formerly known as *Chlamydia abortus*) has tropism for the placenta and is well known for causing abortion in goats (Nietfeld 2001) and sheep. It is zoonotic and some women abort in the last trimester through coming into contact with an infected doe while kidding or through drinking unpasteurized milk from an infected doe. The organism does not pass through the milk in sheep. *Chlamydophila pecorum* is isolated from the digestive and reproductive tracts of goats. It causes inapparent clinical signs and arthritis and conjunctivitis depending upon low pathogenic strain or high pathogenic strain infection (Osman et al. 2011). However, there is one reported case of it causing abortion in a Boer goat with pathological lesions in the fetus (Giannitti et al. 2016).

Various theories have been postulated based on experimentation on sheep and goats to define the pathogenesis process of abortion caused by *C. abortus*. It destroys the placentomes upon infection and then moves to the trophoblast cell layer of the placenta. The trophoblast is one of the target tissues where it multiplies (Navarro et al. 2004). The inflammatory response by the fetal trophoblast may be the cause of necrosis, edema, infiltration of neutrophils, macrophages, plasma cells, and lymphocytes. There will be chlamydial inclusion bodies in the uterine endometrium. Damage to the epitheliochorial cells alters the hormonal balance by reduced secretion of progesterone needed for the maintenance of pregnancy. The decrease in the ratio of progesterone to estradiol 17-beta induces prostaglandin E_2 (PGE_2) secretion. PGE_2 in turn initiates uterine contraction and labor (Rodolakis and Laroucau 2015). If pregnancy continues, the fetus is infected, resulting in focal infections of various organs and the possibility of giving birth to a dead or weak fetus (Di Paolo et al. 2019).

The immunological mechanism relating to upregulation or downregulation of different cytokines also plays important role in pregnancy (Figure 23.5). Inflammatory cytokines including tissue necrosis factor (TNF)-alpha, interferon (IFN)-gamma, and interleukin (IL)-2 are considered harmful for pregnancy sustenance whereas regulatory cytokines such as IL-10 and tissue growth factor (TGF)-beta are considered beneficial (Entrican 2002). In normal pregnancy, concentrations of TNF-alpha and IFN-gamma remain low whereas IL-10 and TGF-beta predominate. T-helper lymphocytes secreting different types of cytokines are of T_H1 and T_H2 types. Upon activation, T_H1 releases IFN-gamma and IL-2. Stimulation of T_H2 releases IL-4, IL-5, and IL-13. T_H1 cells are required for immunological control of intracellular parasites including bacteria and protozoan infections via IFN-gamma production. T_H2 cell stimulation controls extracellular parasites like helminths.

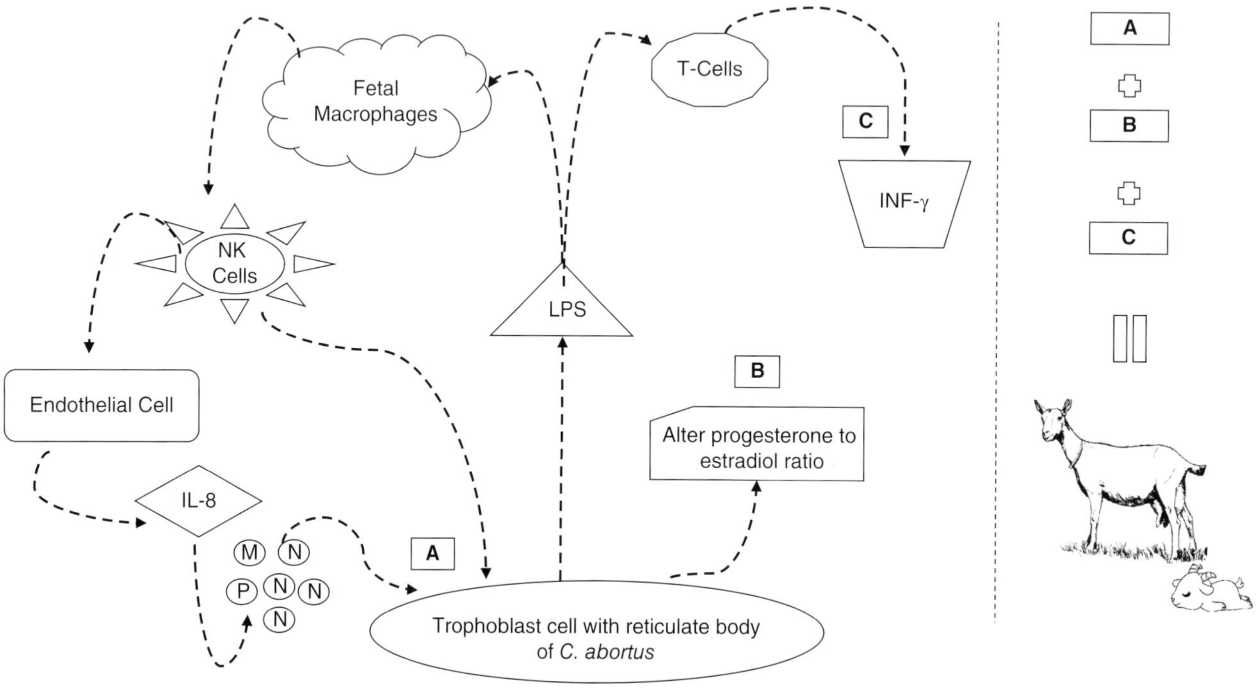

Figure 23.5 Abortion in *C. abortus* infection is the combined effect of inflammation of the placenta, alteration of hormones due to placentitis, and the immunological modulation effect of IFN-gamma. NK, natural killer; IL-8, interleukin 8; LPS, lipopolysaccharides; IFN-gamma, interferon gamma. *Source:* Adapted from Entrican (2002).

In *C. abortus* infection, the EBs multiply in chorionic epithelium of the placenta and lyse the cells upon release. Cell lysis releases lipopolysaccharides (LPS) which in turn activate fetal macrophage secretion of the proinflammatory cytokine TNF-alpha. Natural killer cells are activated by TNF-alpha secretion and destroy the infected trophoblast cells and cause vasoconstriction. Damage to the endothelium cell layer of placental blood vessels releases IL-8, a chemokine interleukin. IL-8 attracts neutrophils, macrophages, and plasma cells to the site and sets up the inflammation process which develops the pathogenic lesions seen on the placenta. LPSs also directly stimulate T lymphocytes to release IFN-gamma. The increase in IFN-gamma level during labor suggests that it has a definitive role in the process of parturition (Veith and Rice 1999). The damage to chorionic epithelium leads to reduced production of progesterone and alteration of the hormonal balance. Wegmann et al. (1993) postulated that in pregnancy in humans or mammals, T_H2 dominates the phase, meaning that the phase dominated by T_H1 is incompatible for successful pregnancy.

Although this phenomenon provides an adequate explanation for the immunological basis of abortion in chlamydiosis, experimentation in sheep suggests that the ability of peripheral blood mononuclear cells does not alter much before and during pregnancy. This suggests that the immune response is not the only factor that determines the abortion time or viable pregnancy. Other factors such as change in hormonal profile and involvement of other T cell types, like regulatory T cells (T_r), have to be taken into consideration (Entrican et al. 2010).

The doe which aborts due to chlamydial infection possesses a high antibody titer and protection from reinfection for 2.5 years. After causing abortion, *C. abortus* remains latent and constantly stimulates the immune system, resulting in high antibody titer. In *in vitro* experiments, it has been shown that the addition of IFN-gamma in low dose limits multiplication of the parasite (Brown et al. 2001). Further, experiments have suggested that tryptophan is an essential amino acid required for maturation and multiplication of the parasite. *C. abortus* lacks all the five gene that comprise the functional operon for synthesis and is therefore dependent on tryptophan host reserves. IFN-gamma limits multiplication of the parasite by modulating activation of the indoleamine 2,3-dioxygenase (IDO) enzyme required for synthesis of tryptophan. So, host control of *C. abortus* infection and maintenance of its latency by IFN-gamma-mediated T_H1 response is well understood (Entrican et al. 2010).

Chlamydophila pecorum has been isolated from the placenta and fetus of goats and sheep but its role in inducing abortion is not well understood. However, there is one report by Giannitti et al. (2016) which isolated *C. pecorum* from aborted twin fetuses of a Boer goat. A detailed description of the placental and fetal lesions was given by the authors. The aborted fetus had anasarca, edema of the hindquarter muscles, and brachygnathia. The cotyledon with placenta expelled during abortion was covered with yellowish white fluid extending to intercotyledonary areas. Suppurative and necrotizing placentitis was observed on histopathology. The organisms (reticulate body) were also observed in the liver and small intestines of the fetus, causing hepatitis and enteritis. This report confirms the abortive potential of *C. pecorum* in natural infections in goats and further warrants epidemiological survey of its prevalence.

23.7 Clinical Signs

Chlamydia abortus is responsible for enzootic abortion in goats and sheep worldwide, except Australia and New Zealand. In an outbreak, more than 60% of naive does may abort or produce stillborn or weak kids. Thereafter, the aborted doe develops protective immunity and rarely aborts again but becomes a carrier for a long period. The subsequent years may see a reduced (less than 10%) abortion rate in new does (Rodolakis and Laroucau 2015).

The most prominent clinical sign of infection is abortion in goats (Figure 23.6). However, severe metritis, pneumonia, and keratoconjunctivitis are also recorded in some cases. The doe may abort at any time during pregnancy, unlike ewes in which most abortions happen in the last two months of pregnancy. The pregnancy in goats is entirely maintained by progesterone produced by the corpus luteum and not the placenta. In ewes, the uteroplacental secretion of progesterone is sufficient to maintain pregnancy. Inflammation of the uterus during infection in goats triggers luteolysis and thus produces abortion. The doe may become infected and abort in the same pregnancy due to the short incubation period.

The most consistent and severe pathological lesions appear on the placenta. The cotyledons and intercotyledonary areas are thickened and covered with reddish brown secretions. The doe continues to pass this inflammatory fluid for several days after abortion. Metritis is the most common complication of infection in this species. The fetus is covered with the reddish exudates and may have excessive abdominal fluid or necrotic foci on the liver. However, in most cases there is no evidence of gross or microscopic lesions recorded in the aborted fetus. Microscopic lesions are generally severe in the placenta and suppurative and necrotizing in nature, with loss of stroma and abundant infiltration of inflammatory cells. In some fetuses, necrotic lesions are observed in the liver and spleen and interstitial pneumonia in the lungs (Nietfeld 2001).

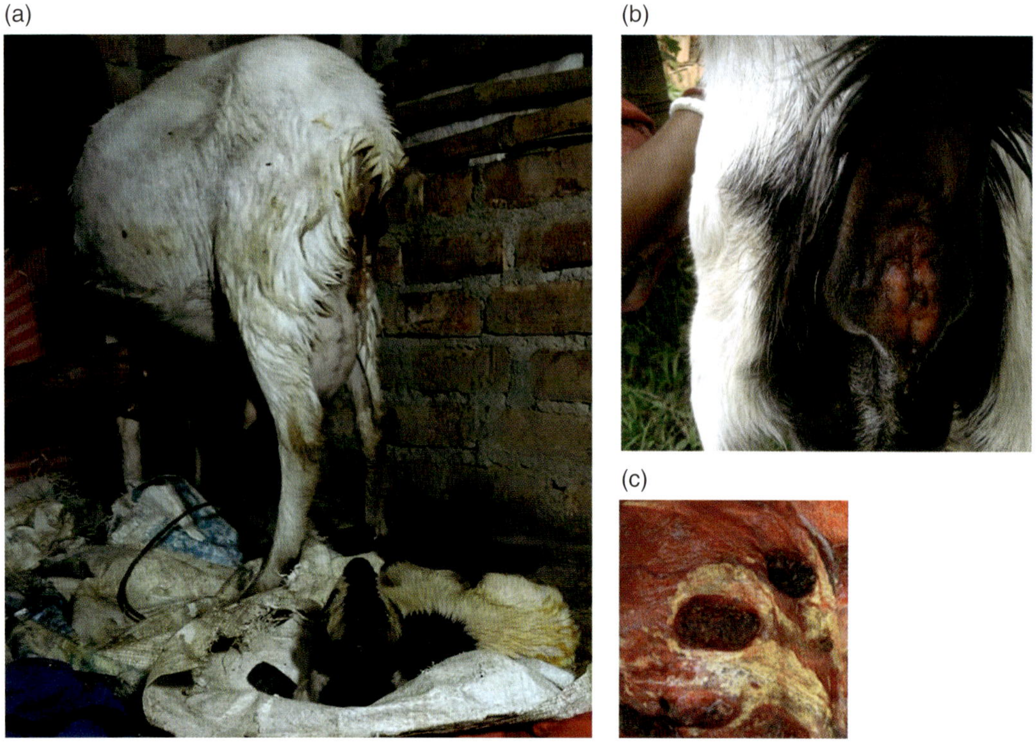

Figure 23.6 A. Almost full time aborted foetus with *C. abortus* infected doe. B. Inflammed and swelled vaginal opening after abortion. C. Characteristic thickened and reddish hyperemic cotyledon in placenta (courtesy Mr. Avishek Barui).

23.7.1 Postmortem Lesions

In one study, the entire aborted fetus and placenta were collected for gross and microscopic pathology observations. Tissue samples from brain, lungs, heart, liver, intestine, skeletal muscles, adrenal and thymus glands, and placenta were collected for histopathology and IHC or molecular diagnosis (Moeller 2001).

Mostly aborted kids are usually fresh with no gross pathology. Sometimes the fetuses may show moderate anasarca, edema of the hindquarters, brachygnathia, and palatoschisis (Giannitti et al. 2016). The placenta is thickened, with extensive multifocal necrotic foci and diffuse yellowish to reddish brown fibrinopurulent exudate on the chorionic surface that extends into the adjacent intercotyledonary areas.

23.8 Histopathology

Diffuse suppurative and necrotizing placentitis with moderate necrotizing vasculitis (arteriolitis) is usually observed. Fetuses show thrombosis, multifocal lymphohistiocytic and neutrophilic hepatitis, and fibrinosuppurative enteritis (Di Paolo et al. 2019).

The chorioallantoic membrane shows diffuse necrosis of the villus and adjacent intercotyledonary epithelium. It is replaced by abundant eosinophilic karyorrhectic debris, abundant extracellular indistinct basophilic bacteria, viable and degenerate neutrophils, fewer lymphocytes, plasma cells and macrophages, and multifocal mineralization. Trophoblasts (mono- and binucleate) are seen scattered throughout the necrotic debris with indistinct granular basophilic bacteria often expanded by many basophilic intracytoplasmic ~1 μm diameter inclusions (chlamydial reticulate bodies). The vascular lumen is occluded by fibrin thrombi. Mural fibrinoid necrosis of deep chorionic arterioles with infiltration of degenerate neutrophils and lytic cellular debris (arteriolitis) may be seen. There can be focal areas of cartilaginous metaplasia in the chorioallantoic stroma (Giannitti et al. 2016).

In the fetal brain, the Virchow–Robin spaces are multifocally distended by a moderate number of lymphocytes and macrophages with fewer neutrophils and necrotic debris. Occasionally central chromatolysis or necrotic neurons can be observed. Hypertrophy of vascular endothelium and inflammatory cell infiltration can also be seen. Surrounding these blood vessels, there is spongiosis and myelin sheaths are dilated surrounding swollen axons. In the fetal liver, small multifocal areas of coagulative necrosis, multifocal moderate histiocytic and neutrophilic portal and periportal hepatitis, sinusoidal leukocytosis, and lymphoplasmacytic chollangiohepatitis are observed. In the lung, diffuse lymphoplasmacytic infiltration is observed in alveolar septae. In the small intestine, there is moderate fibrinosuppurative exudate admixed with necrotic debris filling the lumen. Occasionally, sloughed enterocytes containing abundant intracytoplasmic bacteria morphologically resembling chlamydial reticulate bodies can be seen. Intestinal villi are shortened. Crypts are mildly distended, lined by flattened epithelial cells, and filled with neutrophils (cryptitis).

23.9 Differential Diagnosis

The clinical picture of abortion with necrotzsing placentitis is sufficient to diagnose chlamydial cause of abortion. *Mycoplasma mycoides* subsp. *mycoides* also causes abortion in goats but often systemic involvement causing mastitis, pneumonia, and septicaemia accompanies the infection. *Coxiella burnetii* infection in does causes necrotizing placentitis and is not distinguishable on histopathology. *Campylobacter* and *Listeria* spp. are the other pathogens involved in abortions and produce similar lesions in aborted placenta. The isolation of organisms may confirm the etiology of infection in these cases.

23.10 Laboratory Diagnosis

The diagnosis of chlamydiosis is difficult due to its intracellular viability, unique life cycle inside and outside the host, delayed yet short antibody response during abortion, contamination chances of uterine and fetal materials with other similar organisms, and crossreaction with other chlamydial strains or Gram-negative bacteria. Both direct and indirect methods are used to diagnose *C. abortus* in suspected animals.

23.10.1 Direct Methods

23.10.1.1 Direct Smear Method

The organism can be detected macroscopically in stained smears of affected chorionic villi or adjacent chorion or exudates or feces or in impression smears of liver and spleen. Smears are stained according to modified Machiavello, Giemsa, Brucella differential, or modified Ziehl–Neelsen, Stamp and modified Giménez stains, using carbolfuchsin and malachite green (Stamp et al. 1952). After staining, in positive cases the organism appears red to purple against a blue background in modified ZN stain. This method may be useful initially but due to its lower sensitivity and specificity, other molecular methods are highly recommended. Care must be taken as *Coxiella* or *Brucella* appear similar with similar staining.

23.10.1.2 Isolation of Causative Agent by Cell Culture or Using Chicken Embryo

Tissue samples, such as cotyledons, placental membranes, fetal lung or liver, or vaginal swabs may be used for microbiological cell culture and isolation of *Chlamydia*. McCoy, Buffalo Green Monkey (BGM) or baby hamster kidney (BHK) cells are most commonly used.

Similarly test samples in nutrient broth and antibiotic are inoculated into the yolk sac of 6–8-day-old embryos for further incubation. Infected embryos die between four and 13 days after inoculation. Smears from yolk sac membranes reveal the organism.

23.10.2 Indirect Methods

23.10.2.1 Detection of DNA by PCR Methods

Due to its high sensitivity and specificity, conventional PCR amplification of chlamydial DNA for detection of the presence of chlamydiae in suspected samples is the method of choice. For *C. abortus* detection in conventional PCR protocols, 16S–23S rRNA region (Everett and Andersen 1999) or pmp genes (Laroucau et al. 2001) are generally targeted. With real-time PCR, sequences of the outer membrane protein (ompA) (Livingstone et al. 2009) are preferred due to their high specificity, rapidity, high throughput, and ease of standardization. DNA microarray hybridization assays have also been validated for the detection and identification of *Chlamydia* organisms from clinical or suspected samples.

23.10.2.2 Detection by Molecular Typing

Molecular typing of *C. abortus* strains using multiple-locus variable-number tandem repeat (VNTR) analysis (MLVA) based on the analysis of five VNTR loci, as well as a different approach using a multilocus sequence typing (MLST) system targeting seven house-keeping genes, is being used. These techniques may provide additional information about the origins and evolutionary pattern of *C. abortus* (Selim 2016).

23.10.3 Detection by Serological Methods

Goats suspected of chlamydial infection should be screened serologically within three months of abortion or parturition. As the organism acquires the potential for active placental invasion in the last month of gestation, the presence of *C. abortus*-specific antibody during bacteremia or abortion ensures detection.

23.10.3.1 Detection by ELISA

Commercial ELISA kits for *Chlamydia* diagnosis in samples from aborting sheep and goats are available care must be taken as LPS or EB antigen-based ELISAs cannot differentiate between *C. abortus* and *C. pecorum*. More sensitive results may be achieved with ELISAs based on synthetic peptides of MOMP, recombinant MOMP or POMP90 (polymorphic outer membrane protein). Indirect ELISA using POMP90 has shown more sensitivity and specificity in recent years. The best samples of ELISA tests are placenta or vaginal swabs from infected abortive animals within three days of abortion.

23.10.3.2 Detection by Complement Fixation Test (CFT)

The CFT is the most widely used serological test though it has some limitations. The target chlamydial antigen is LPS which is an immunodominant component but common to all Chlamydiaceae species. While CFT detects the antibodies to this antigen, it cannot differentiate between titers of *C. abortus*, *C. pecorum* or *C. psittaci* as well as some Gram-negative bacteria (e.g., *Acinetobacter*). Other chlamydiales occasionally infect small ruminants but *C. abortus* is more dominant and detectable during termination of pregnancy at 14–21 days. CFT is best used with paired sera samples taken at the time of abortion and at about 2–3 weeks. Due to these limitations, CFT is now not recommended as the method of choice for serological diagnosis, but it can be used for herd diagnosis when other methods are not available.

23.11 Prevention and Control

Chlamydial abortion is the most common contagious abortion in small ruminants worldwide. Long incubation period and late abortion are two important characteristics of this infection. Improper handling of abortive materials and other management factors enhance the spread of the organism within herds. Pregnant animals infected in late gestation, but not aborted, may show further abortion in subsequent gestations as they became carriers.

The following preventive measures may be taken.

- Pregnant animals should be isolated in separate pens. The pen should be regularly disinfected and cleaned.
- Antibody investigation should be performed when introducing new animals to an existing herd.
- Placentas, aborted fetuses, stillborn animals, and bedding materials should be properly destroyed to prevent carnivore ingestion.
- Due to the zoonotic potential of the disease, the animal keeper should wear gloves, boots, masks, and protective clothing. Healthy animals should be managed daily before treating suspected or infected goats.
- Proper housing, balanced feed, and clean drinking water are extremely important.

Inactivated and live attenuated vaccines are available against *C. abortus*. These vaccines should be administered intramuscularly or subcutaneously at least four weeks before breeding. While live attenuated vaccines are prepared from a chemically induced temperature-sensitive mutant strain of the organism, inactivated vaccines are prepared by using infected yolk sacs or cell cultures. Inactivated vaccines may be used during pregnancy but live vaccines should not be used in pregnant animals. Immunocompromised people and pregnant women should take care when handling live vaccines. Live vaccine should not be used in animals being treated with antibiotics, especially of the tetracycline group.

Both inactivated and live attenuated vaccines significantly decrease the rate of abortion and shedding of organism. However, no vaccine can completely ensure complete protection against *C. abortus*. Revaccination is advised every 1–3 years depending upon the infection.

For control measures, if infected, long-acting oxytetracycline (20 mg/kg, IM) may be given at 95–100 days of gestation. The dose may be continued at two-week intervals up to lambing to suppress the multiplication of organisms. Some successful findings have been observed with oral tylosin (200 mg/head/day). However, these treatments do not ensure eradication of the organism and in heavy infections the affected animal may still abort.

23.12 Economic and Zoonotic Importance

Economic loss can be severe if chlamydial abortion occurs in a flock. In a new flock, about 30–60% of goats may abort and the abortion process continues in a cyclic way for 3–4 years until all the primiparous goats have aborted.

Chlamydia abortus possess considerable zoonotic potential. The kidding season and handling of placenta or uterus or aborted flesh should be avoided by pregnant women. Transmission of *C. abortus* from goats to humans may also take place through inhalation of infectious dust and aerosols at the time of abortions and kiddings (Figure 23.7). In pregnant infected women, spontaneous abortion, stillbirth, septicemia, mild to medium fever and flu-like illness may present as initial symptoms (Roberts et al. 1967; Pospischil et al. 2002). An elevated C-reactive protein, leukopenia and thrombocytopenia,(Meijer et al. 2004), coagulopathy, pneumonia, and liver disease may occur. In advanced cases, septicemic shock, acute renal failure, disseminated intravascular coagulation, pulmonary edema, and respiratory distress (Walder et al. 2005) are also observed in affected women. There are also reports of conjunctivitis (Tontis and Zwahlen 1991) and urogenital symptoms (Stěpánek et al. 1983). There are a few reports of laboratory-acquired *C. abortus* infection in humans with mild respiratory signs but in general, except for pregnant women working with infected small ruminants, no other humans are reported to develop clinical illness (Aitken 2000).

In most zoonotic chlamydial cases, proper antibiotic and supportive treatment is successful in promoting complete and uneventful recovery of affected humans except in one case when the patient died (Beer et al. 1982).

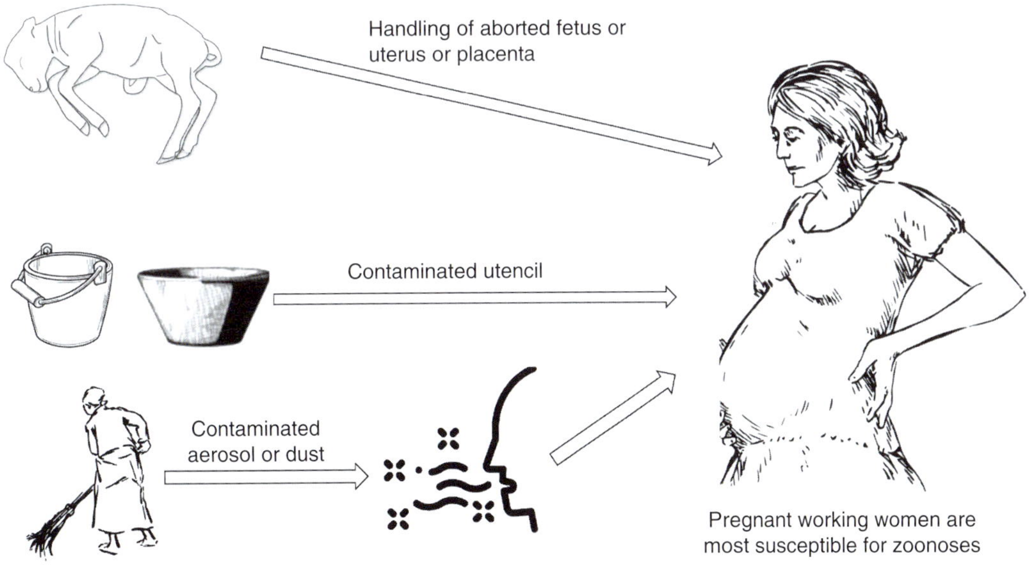

Figure 23.7 Schematics diagram showing zoonotic transmission modes of *C. abortus*. Pregnant women handling infected animal or aborted material or contaminated inanimate sources are most susceptible.

References

Ababneh, H.S., Ababneh, M.M.K., Hananeh, W.M. et al. (2014). Molecular identification of chlamydial cause of abortion in small ruminants in Jordan. *Tropical Animal Health and Production* 46: 1407–1412.

Aitken, I.D. (2000). Chlamydial abortion. In: *Diseases of Sheep*, 3e (ed. W.B. Martin and I.D. Aitken), 81–86. Oxford: Blackwell Science.

Appleyard, W.T., Aitken, I.D., and Anderson, I.E. (1985). Attempted venereal transmission of *Chlamydia psittaci* in sheep. *Veterinary Record* 116: 535–538.

Bandyopadhyay, S., Sasmal, D., Biswas, T.K. et al. (2009). Serological evidences of antibodies against Chlamydophila abortus in free-ranging yak (*Poephagus grunniens*) in Arunachal Pradesh, India. *Revue Scientifique et Technique* 28: 1051–1055.

Beer, R.J., Bradford, W.P., and Hart, R.J. (1982). Pregnancy complicated by psittacosis acquired from sheep. *British Medical Journal (Clinical Research Ed.)* 284 (6323): 1156–1157.

Blaha, E.A. (1909). Ansteckender Scheidenkatarrh der Rinder und "Trachomkorperchen" bzw. ProwazekscheKorper (Chlamydozoa) beidemselben (article in German). *Berl Tierärztl Wschr* 25: 879–881.

Brown, J., Howie, S.E., and Entrican, G. (2001). A role for tryptophan in immune control of chlamydial abortion in sheep. *Veterinary Immunology and Immunopathology* 82 (1–2): 107–119.

Burnard, D. and Polkinghorne, A. (2016). Chlamydial infections in wildlife – conservation threats and/or reservoirs of "spill-over" infections? *Veterinary Microbiology* 196: 78–84.

Di Paolo, L.A., Alvarado Pinedo, M.F., Origlia, J. et al. (2019). First report of caprine abortions due to *Chlamydia abortus* in Argentina. *Veterinary Medicine and Science* 5 (2): 162–167.

Elwell, C.A. and Engel, J.N. (2012). Lipid acquisition by intracellular Chlamydiae. *Cellular Microbiology* 14 (7): 1010–1018.

Entrican, G. (2002). Immune regulation during pregnancy and host–pathogen interactions in infectious abortion. *Journal of Comparative Pathology* 126 (2–3): 79–94.

Entrican, G., Wattegedera, S., Wheelhouse, N. et al. (2010). Immunological paradigms and the pathogenesis of ovine chlamydial abortion. *American Journal of Reproductive Immunology* 64 (4): 287–294.

Essig, A. and Longbottom, D. (2015). Chlamydia abortus: new aspects of infectious abortion in sheep and potential risk for pregnant women. *Current Clinical Microbiology Reports* 2: 22–34.

Everett, K.D. and Andersen, A.A. (1999). Identification of nine species of the Chlamydiaceae using PCR-RFLP. *International Journal of Systematic and Evolutionary Microbiology* 49 (2): 803–813.

Everett, K.D.E., Bush, R.M., and Andersen, A.A. (1999). Emended description of the order Chlamydiales, proposal of Parachlamydiaceae fam. nov. and Simkaniaceae fam. nov., each containing one monotypic genus, revised taxonomy of the family Chlamydiaceae, including a new genus and five new species, and standards for the identification of organisms. *International Journal of Systematic Bacteriology* 49 (pt 2): 415–440.

Giannitti, F., Anderson, M., Miller, M. et al. (2016). Chlamydia pecorum: fetal and placental lesions in sporadic caprine abortion. *Journal of Veterinary Diagnostic Investigation* 28 (2): 184–189.

Gupta, S., Chahota, R., Bhardwaj, B. et al. (2015). Identification of *Chlamydiae* and *Mycoplasma* species in ruminants with ocular infections. *Letters in Applied Microbiology* 60 (2): 135–139.

Laroucau, K., Souriau, A., and Rodolakis, A. (2001). Improved sensitivity of PCR for Chlamydophila using pmp genes. *Veterinary Microbiology* 82 (2): 155–164.

Li, Z., Cao, X., Fu, B. et al. (2015). Identification and characterization of Chlamydia abortus isolates from yaks in Qinghai, China. *Biomed Research International* 2015: 658519.

Livingstone, M., Wheelhouse, N., Maley, S.W., and Longbottom, D. (2009). Molecular detection of Chlamydophila abortus in post-abortion sheep at oestrus and subsequent lambing. *Veterinary Microbiology* 135 (1–2): 134–141.

Livingstone, M., Wheelhouse, N., Ensor, H. et al. (2017). Pathogenic outcome following experimental infection of sheep with Chlamydia abortus variant strains LLG and POS. *PLoS One* 12 (5): e0177653.

Longbottom, D. and Coulter, L.J. (2003). Animal chlamydioses and zoonotic implications. *Journal of Comparative Pathology* 128 (4): 217–244.

Longbottom, D., Entrican, G., Wheelhouse, N. et al. (2013a). Evaluation of the impact and control of enzootic abortion of ewes. *Veterinary Journal* 195 (2): 257–259.

Longbottom, D., Livingstone, M., Maley, S. et al. (2013b). Intranasal infection with Chlamydia abortus induces dose-dependent latency and abortion in sheep. *PLoS One* 8 (2): e57950.

Matthews, J. (1999). Abortion. In: *Diseases of the Goat*, 22. Oxford: Blackwell Science.

Meijer, A., Brandenburg, A., De Vries, J. et al. (2004). Chlamydophila abortus infection in a pregnant woman associated with indirect contact with infected goats. *European Journal of Clinical Microbiology and Infectious Diseases* 23: 487–490.

Moeller, R.B. Jr. (2001). Causes of caprine abortion: diagnostic assessment of 211 cases (1991–1998). *Journal of Veterinary Diagnostic Investigation* 13 (3): 265–270.

Navarro, J.A., Garcia de la Fuente, J.N., Sanchez, J. et al. (2004). Kinetics of infection and effects on the placenta of *Chlamydophila abortus* in experimentally infected pregnant ewes. *Veterinary Pathology* 41: 498–505.

Nietfeld, J.C. (2001). Chlamydial infections in small ruminants. *Veterinary Clinics of North America. Food Animal Practice* 17 (2): 301–314.

Ortega, N., Caro, M.R., Gallego, M.C. et al. (2016). Isolation of Chlamydia abortus from a laboratory worker diagnosed with atypical pneumonia. *Irish Veterinary Journal* 69: 8.

Osman, K.M., Ali, H.A., El Jakee, J.A., and Galal, H.M. (2011). *Chlamydophila psittaci* and *Chlamydophila pecorum* infections in goats and sheep in Egypt. *Revue Scientifique et Technique* 30 (3): 939.

Osman, K.M., Ali, H.A., ElJakee, J.A., and Galal, H.M. (2012). Chlamydiaceae in riverine buffalo (*Bubalus bubalis*) and cows (*Bos taurus*) in Egypt with and without signs of reproductive disease. *New Zealand Veterinary Journal* 60 (4): 228–233.

Papp, J.R. and Shewen, P.E. (1997). Chlamydia psittaci infection in sheep: a paradigm for human reproductive tract infection. *Journal of Reproductive Immunology* 34: 185–202.

Pospischil, A., Thoma, R., Hilbe, M., and Grest, P. (2002). Abortion in woman caused by caprine Chlamydophila abortus (Chlamydia psittaci serovar 1). *Swiss Medical Weekly* 132 (0506): 64–66.

Roberts, W., Grist, N.R., and Giroud, P. (1967). Human abortion associated with infection by ovine abortion agent. *British Medical Journal* 4 (5570): 37.

Rodolakis, A. and Laroucau, K. (2015). Chlamydiaceae and chlamydial infections in sheep or goats. *Veterinary Microbiology* 181 (1–2): 107–118.

Sachse, K., Bavoil, P.M., Kaltenboeck, B. et al. (2015). Emendation of the family Chlamydiaceae: proposal of a single genus, Chlamydia, to include all currently recognized species. *Systematic and Applied Microbiology* 38 (2): 99–103.

Selim, A. (2016). Chlamydophila abortus infection in small ruminants: a review. *Asian Journal of Animal and Veterinary Advances* 11 (10): 587–593.

Seth-Smith, H.M.B., Busó, L.S., Livingstone, M. et al. (2017). European Chlamydia abortus livestock isolate genomes reveal unusual stability and limited diversity, reflected in geographical signatures. *BMC Genomics* 18 (1): 344.

Stamp, J.T., Watt, J.A.A., and Cockburn, R.B. (1952). Enzootic abortion in ewes. Complement fixation test. *Journal of Comparative Pathology* 62: 93–101.

Stěpánek, O., Jindrichova, J., Horacek, J., and Krpata, V. (1983). Chlamydiosis in cattle and in man: an epidemiologic and serologic study. *Journal of Hygiene, Epidemiology, Microbiology, and Immunology* 27 (4): 445–459.

Storz, J. and Kaltenboeck, B. (1993). Diversity of chlamydia-induced diseases. In: *Rickettsial and Chlamydial Diseases of Domestic Animals* (ed. Z. Woldehiwet and M. Ristic), 363–393. New York: Pergamon Press.

Taylor, H. (2008). *Trachoma: A Blinding Scourge from the Bronze Age to the Twenty-First Century*. Melbourne, Australia: Centre for Eye Research Australia.

Taylor-Brown, A. and Polkinghorne, A. (2017). New and emerging chlamydial infections of creatures great and small. *New Microbes New Infections* 18: 28–33.

Taylor-Brown, A., Vaughan, L., Greub, G. et al. (2015). Twenty years of research intro Chlamydia-like organisms: a revolution in our understanding of the biology and pathogenicity of members of the phylum Chlamydiae. *FEMS Pathogens and Disease* 73 (1): 1–15.

Taylor-Brown, A., Bachmann, N.L., Borel, N. et al. (2016). Culture-independent genomic characterisation of *Candidatus* Chlamydia sanzinia, a novel uncultivated bacterium infecting snakes. *BMC Genomics* 17: 710.

Tontis, A. and Zwahlen, R. (1991). Chlamydia infections in sheep and goats. With a reference to its significance as a zoonosis. *Tierärztliche Praxis* 19 (6): 617–623.

Veith, G.L. and Rice, G.E. (1999). Interferon gamma expression during human pregnancy and in association with labour. *Gynecologic and Obstetric Investigation* 48 (3): 163–167.

Vorimore, F., Hsia, R.C., Huot-Creasy, H. et al. (2013). Isolation of a new chlamydia species from the feral sacred ibis (*Threskiornis aethiopicus*): *Chlamydia ibidis*. *PLoS One* 8 (9): e74823.

Walder, G., Hotzel, H., Brezinka, C. et al. (2005). An unusual cause of sepsis during pregnancy: recognizing infection with: Chlamydophila abortus. *Obstetrics & Gynecology* 106 (5 Part 2): 1215–1217.

Wegmann, T.G., Lin, H., Guilbert, L., and Mosmann, T.R. (1993). Bidirectional cytokine interactions in the maternal-fetal relationship: is successful pregnancy a TH2 phenomenon? *Immunology Today* 14 (7): 353–356.

Wilkat, M., Herdoiza, E., Forsbach-Birk, V. et al. (2014). Electron tomography and cryo-SEM characterization reveals novel ultrastructural features of host-parasite interaction during Chlamydia abortus infection. *Histochemistry and Cell Biology* 142: 171–184.

Wilsmore, A.J., Parsons, V., and Dawson, M. (1984). Experiments to demonstrate routes of transmission of ovine enzootic abortion. *British Veterinary Journal* 140: 380–391.

Wilsmore, A.J., Izzard, K.A., Wilsmore, B.C. et al. (1990). Breeding performance of sheep infected with Chlamydia psittaci (avis) during their preceding pregnancy. *Veterinary Record* 126: 40–41.

24

Infectious Abortive Diseases: Toxoplasmosis

K. Justin Davis and K. Athira

Department of Veterinary Epidemiology and Preventive Medicine, College of Veterinary and Animal Sciences, Mannuthy, India

24.1 Introduction

Goats, the "poor man's cow," are the main livelihood of many poor and marginalized farmers in developing countries (Ajith 2012). The profit from goat farming mainly relies on production of kids. Abortion rates of 2–5% are acceptable, but any loss above this can result in severe economic hardship.

The most common infectious causes of abortions in goats are brucellosis, leptospirosis, listeriosis, toxoplasmosis, chlamydiosis, and Q fever, contributing to a loss of 25–30% in a season. Among these, toxoplasmosis occurring as a benign form in most animals is considered as one of the most important infectious causes of ovine and caprine abortion worldwide with both medical and veterinary importance (Dubey 2004; Buxton et al. 2007; Steffen et al. 2021).

Toxoplasmosis caused by the protozoan parasite *Toxoplasma gondii* is a cosmopolitan zoonotic parasitic infection prevalent throughout the world, affecting all warm-blooded animals, including birds (Dubey and Beattie 1988; Shahbazi et al. 2019; Karthika et al. 2021). It is one of the most common neglected zoonotic diseases affecting one-third of the world's human population (Montoya and Liesenfeld 2004; Innes 2010; Fatmawati et al. 2020; Celi et al. 2022). Following infection, oocysts are shed in the feces of definitive hosts (felids), whereas the infection is often asymptomatic in intermediate hosts (goats) (Frenkel et al. 1970; Ahmed et al. 2008; Giadinis et al. 2011). Herbivores become infected when they feed on pastures, concentrates or drinking water contaminated with *T. gondii* oocysts. The rapidly replicating abortion-causing invasive forms (tachyzoites) enter the bloodstream to reach the brain, heart, and lungs, where they form slowly replicating or quiescent (bradyzoites) cystic aggregates that remain latent throughout the life of the host. This intracellular protozoan parasite is responsible for the clinical signs of fetal resorption, mummification, abortion, stillbirth, neonatal mortalities or weak and nonviable newborns in small ruminants (Ahmed et al. 2008; Dechicha et al. 2015).

Human toxoplasmosis is transmitted by consumption of undercooked meat, improper handling of cat feces and through blood transfusion. Even though most people are infected in early childhood, clinical signs will not appear in healthy individuals. This has serious implications in HIV-infected patients and causes miscarriages and birth defects in pregnant women (Garcia et al. 2012).

24.2 History

In 1908, Charles Nicolle and Louis Manceaux discovered the *Toxoplasma gondii* parasite within the liver of a North African rodent named the common gundi (*Ctenodactylus gundi*) (Innes et al. 2009). *Ctenodactylus gundi* was primarily used for leishmaniasis research in the laboratory of Charles Nicolle at the Pasteur Institute in Tunis (Innes et al. 2009). The researcher initially thought the parasite was a member of the *Leishmania* genus but soon realized that he had discovered a new organism and named it *T. gondii* based on the morphology and the host (toxon = arc or bow, plasma = shape, form).

In 1917, Chatton and Blanc reported that gundis acquired the infection in captivity and were not infected naturally (Dubey 2009a). Nicolle and Manceaux had incorrectly identified the host as *Ctenodactylus gondii,* otherwise the correct name for the parasite should have been *T. gundi*. Despite the worldwide distribution and the widest host range, there is only

Elements of Reproduction and Reproductive Diseases of Goats, First Edition. Edited by Tanmoy Rana.

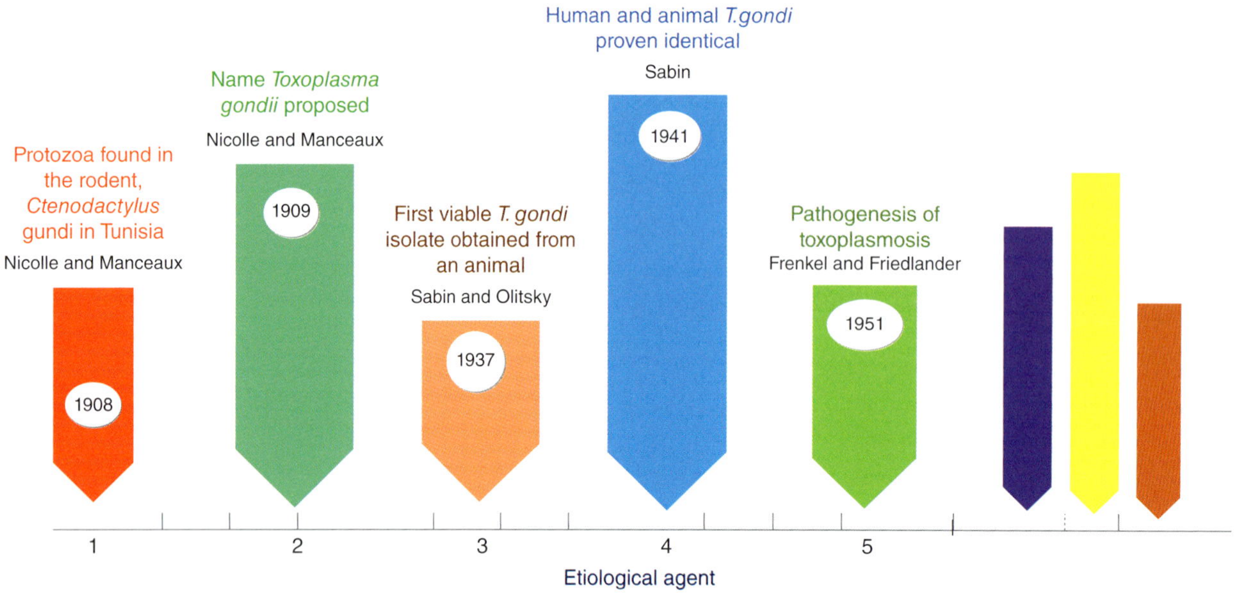

Figure 24.1 Landmarks in the discovery of *Toxoplasma gondii*. *Source:* Adapted from Dubey (2008).

one species, *gondii*, in the genus *Toxoplasma* (Dubey 2008). The first conclusive identification of a congenital route of transmission of toxoplasmosis was done in an infant girl on May 23, 1938 at Babies Hospital, New York, by the pathologists Wolf, Cowen, and Paige (Dubey 2008, 2009a). Discovery of toxoplasmosis in sea otters indicates the contamination of seas with *T. gondii* oocysts washed from land (Cole et al. 2000). Ovine toxoplasmosis was first reported to be an important pathogen in sheep in the 1950s with a series of abortion reports from Bill Hartley and colleagues in New Zealand (Innes et al. 2009). The landmarks in the discovery of *T. gondii* are depicted in Figure 24.1.

24.3 Taxonomy

Toxoplasma gondii is placed in the kingdom Chromista, subkingdom Harosa, infrakingdom Halvaria, superphylum Alveolata, phylum Myozoa, infraphylum Apicomplexa, superclass Sporozoa, class Coccidiomorphea, family Sarcocystidae, genus *Toxoplasma*, species *gondii* (Delgado et al. 2022). It can be grouped into three molecular genotypes or lineages (types I, II, and III, XII and haplotypes X and A) (Attias et al. 2020). The genetic lineages type II and III are associated with toxoplasmosis in animals while type II is the predominant form identified in human infections (Howe and Sibley 1995; Sibley et al. 2009; Khan et al. 2006; World Organisation for Animal Health 2022).

Samples obtained from Europe and North America were used for the initial characterization of *T. gondii* populations (Delgado et al. 2022). This led to the identification of a highly clonal population structure grouped as types I, II, and III strains (Howe and Sibley 1995). Type I strains (e.g., RH and GT1) are the more virulent clonal lineage with high morbidity and mortality, mostly found in Europe and America (Robert-Gangneux and Darde 2012). Type I and II strains predominate in Europe and North America, while type III strains have a worldwide distribution (Delgado et al. 2022; Robert-Gangneux and Darde 2012). Type III (e.g., CTG and VEG) strains are slightly more virulent than type II (e.g., ME49 and Prugniaud) strains, but generally considered to be avirulent with low morbidity and high rates of chronic infection with tissue cyst formation (Delgado et al. 2022; Robert-Gangneux and Darde 2012).

24.4 Epidemiology

Toxoplasmosis is an emerging and reemerging, life-threatening zoonosis of global public health importance (Muhie and Kebkes 2014; Pal et al. 2021). This intracellular apicomplexan protozoan is found worldwide, capable of infecting almost any cell type with an exceptionally broad host range, including humans, livestock, companion animals, and wildlife (Dubey 2010), making it one of the most successful protozoan parasites on earth (Ferguson 2009; Webster 2010). The worldwide seroprevalence of *T. gondii* infection has been estimated as 33.86% in sheep and 31.78% in goats (Ahaduzzaman

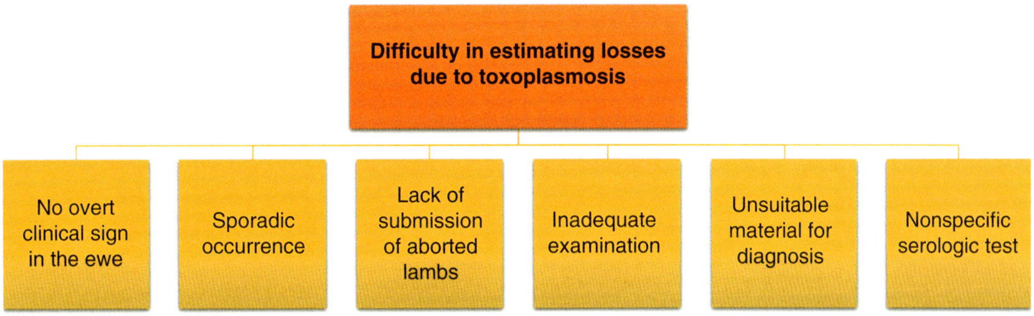

Figure 24.2 Difficulties in estimating losses due to toxoplasmosis. *Source:* Dubey (1982)/American Veterinary Medical Association.

and Hasan 2022). The higher activity in goats increases the probability of contact with contaminated sources and makes them more susceptible to toxoplasmosis than sheep. The risk factors that have a positive correlation with development of toxoplasmosis are large flock size and improper disposal of aborted fetuses. There was a fourfold increase in risk of toxoplasmosis on farms that left fetuses on the ground compared to those farms that fed aborted fetuses to dogs (Abu-Dalbouh et al. 2012). The difficulties faced in field conditions to estimate losses due to toxoplasmosis are depicted in Figure 24.2.

24.4.1 Geographic Distribution

The worldwide prevalence of goat abortions due to toxoplasmosis is estimated as 3.3–27.2% (Dubey et al. 2021). There are also reports of highly variable seroprevalence of toxoplasmosis in sheep and goat populations worldwide (Dubey 2022). The climatic conditions of the temperate sheep-rearing countries are favorable for oocyst survival (Aitken 2007). Meat-producing animals like pigs, sheep, and goats in India pose a threat to human health owing to their high prevalence of toxoplasmosis (Khan et al. 2017). A high seroprevalence of 56.94% was reported in recently aborted goats in south India, which is attributed to repeated exposure to oocyst-contaminated pastures (Karthika et al. 2021).

The parasite prefers a humid and damp climate rather than dry and hot environmental conditions. In highly humid areas, oocysts are protected against desiccation, thereby enabling their survival and sporulation (Singh and Nautiyal 1991; Dubey et al. 1993). In Switzerland, a protective factor for seropositivity to *T. gondii* infections in sheep and goats was considered to be alpine grazing in summer. This was due to the lower density of cats in mountain regions, leading to a lower environmental contamination with *T. gondii* oocysts. Apart from this, factors with negative influence on oocyst survival were altitude, extreme low temperatures, and exposure to ultraviolet rays (Basso et al. 2022).

24.4.2 Transmission

Toxoplasma gondii is adapted to be transmitted biologically by carnivorism in cats and by ingesting oocysts (fecal–oral route) in nonfeline hosts (Dubey 2022). Oocysts shed by cats are the important source of infection for herbivores (Dubey 2022). Vertical transmission of *T. gondii* can also occur in small ruminants by both exogenous transplacental transmission (ExTT) and endogenous transplacental transmission (EnTT) mechanisms. The exogenous route is the most frequent mechanism during pregnancy and the endogenous route occurs after the recrudescence of a latent infection acquired *in utero* (Sanchez-Sanchez et al. 2018) (Figure 24.3).

The important source of *Toxoplasma* infection for humans is ingestion of raw or undercooked meat from infected sheep, goats, pigs, and gamebirds (Basso et al. 2022; Cook et al. 2000; Edelhofer and Prossinger 2010). Consumption of raw milk or unpasteurized dairy products from infected sheep and goats represents a risk of infection for humans and animals (Dubey 2022; Basso et al. 2022). The intermediate hosts can be infected via different pathways including ingestion of non-pasteurized milk or milk products, water, vegetables and fruits contaminated with viable oocysts, improperly cooked meat and meat products containing viable tissue cysts, congenital transmission from the mother through the placenta, blood transfusion, and organ transplantation where the organs may contain cysts or tachyzoites (Attias et al. 2020). Both horizontal and vertical routes of transmission are reported for ovine toxoplasmosis, but the main route of infection for herbivores is ingestion of infective oocysts (Dubey 2010) (Figure 24.4).

Pigs, humans, and mice can be infected by ingesting even one oocyst, whereas 100 oocysts may not infect cats (Dubey 2006). Even after ingesting only one bradyzoite, cats could shed millions of oocysts, while ingestion of hundreds of bradyzoites might not infect mice orally (Kniel et al. 2002). Sporulated oocysts survive on fruits and vegetables for long

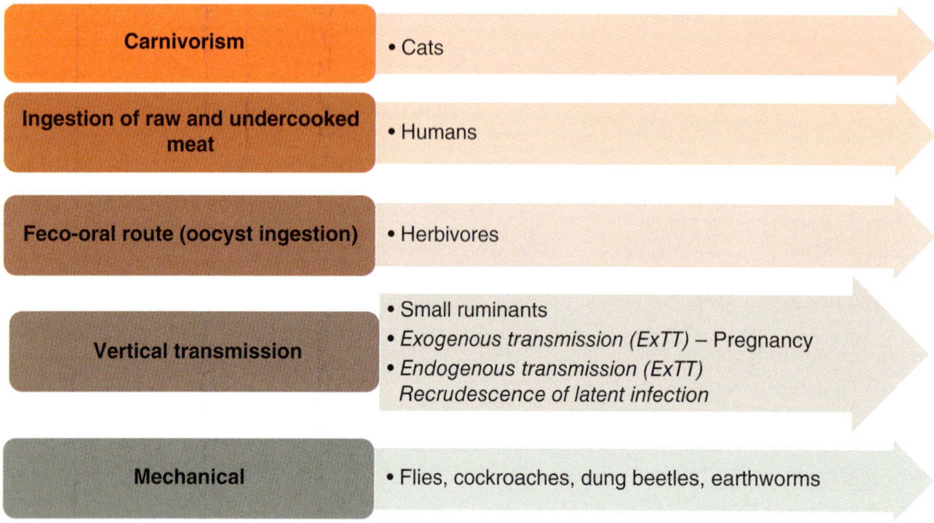

Figure 24.3 Routes of transmission.

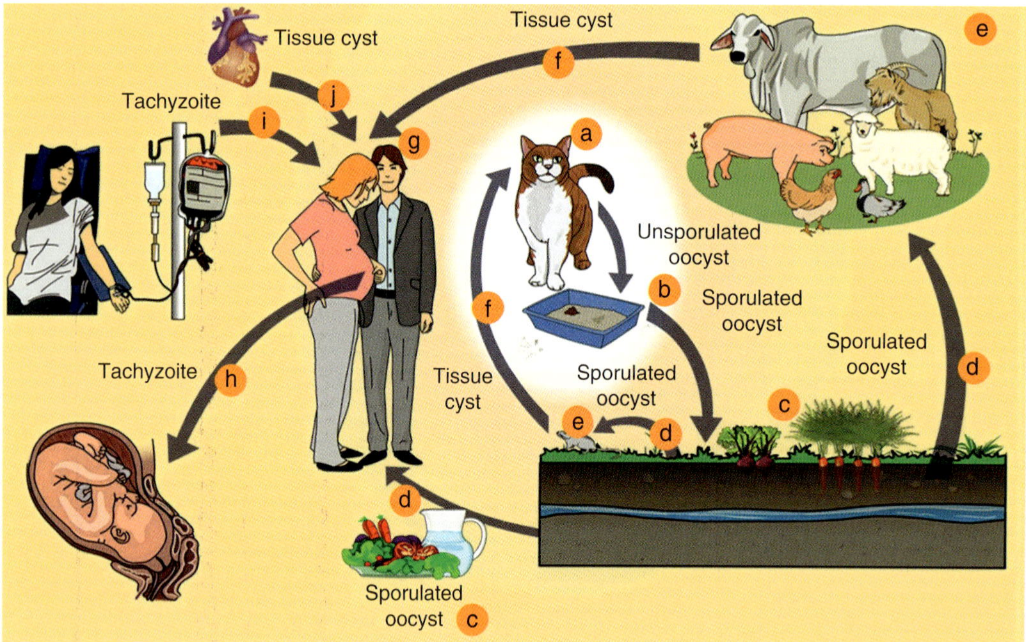

Figure 24.4 The pathways of transmission of *T. gondii* are (a) cats (definitive host), (b) unsporulated oocysts (cat feces), (c) food contaminated with sporulated oocysts, (d) ingestion of oocysts by intermediate hosts through water or raw vegetables, (e) cattle, sheep, poultry, and swine (intermediate hosts), (f) ingestion of tissue cysts in uncooked meat, (g) humans (intermediate hosts), (h) tachyzoites transmitted through the placenta to the fetus, (i) transmission by blood transfusion and (j) organ transplant. *Source:* Reproduced from Attias et al. (2020) under a Creative Commons Attribution 4.0 International License.

periods under moderate environmental conditions and can be spread by erosion of topsoil and mechanically by flies, cockroaches, dung beetles, and earthworms (Kniel et al. 2002; Lindsay and Dubey 2020).

24.4.3 Hosts

Toxoplasma gondii is capable of crossing all geographical boundaries (Dubey 2019), affecting a wide range of hosts including felids, dogs, pigs, cattle, horses, humans, small ruminants, poultry, nonhuman primates, Australian marsupials, sea otters (Delgado et al. 2022), wild canids, deer, bears, rodents, small mammals and miscellaneous animals like antelopes (dik-dik, Saiga antelope, nilgais), musk ox, bats, and Rocky Mountain bighorn sheep (Webster 2010; Muralikrishna et al. 2017). Cattle and chickens are mostly resistant to clinical toxoplasmosis, and free-range chickens, due to their ground feeding activity, act as sentinels of environmental contamination with *Toxoplasma* oocysts (Delgado et al. 2022).

Domestic cats may shed oocysts only during a limited period of time of 2–3 weeks, when they lost their passive immunity and had started to hunt or to eat raw meat containing the tissue cysts. Most of the spontaneous excretors of oocysts are kittens younger than six months of age. Thus, they act as the major source of contamination of the environment (Lindsay and Dubey 2020; Knapen and Overgaauw 2008). Humans might acquire infection by grooming dogs that have rolled in infected cat feces (Sharif et al. 2006). Estimating the *Toxoplasma* infection in the prey population such as local avians and rodents will be helpful in determining the seroprevalence of the same in cats (Lindsay and Dubey 2020; Sharif et al. 2006).

Among domestic species, sheep and goats are most commonly affected, leading to acute infection in goats and infective abortions in sheep (Delgado et al. 2022). Ewes of all ages are susceptible to *T. gondii*-induced abortions but maiden ewes are mostly affected (Dubey 2019). Older small ruminants and sheep (compared to goats) had a higher risk of being seropositive to *T. gondii*. The difference in the grazing habits of these small ruminants is responsible for this. Sheep are grazers that are more likely to ingest oocysts contaminating grass and soil while eating short plants near to the ground, whereas goats are mainly browsers that prefer leaves, shrubs, and vines (Nahar et al. 2020; Basso et al. 2022). The highest prevalence of *T. gondii* infection was reported in the age group of 6–18 months and more than 18 months in goats and sheep respectively (Ferguson and Dubremetz 2014).

24.5 *Toxoplasma gondii*: An Apicomplexan Parasite

The defining hallmark features of Apicomplexan parasites are an apicoplast, apical complex, intracellular parasitic life style, and a glideosome. Apart from this, *T. gondii* presents highly specialized structures such as secretory organelles, inner membrane complex (IMC), and apical and basal complexes (Delgado et al. 2022).

24.5.1 Parasite Morphology

In most of its life cycle, *T. gondii* exhibits a permanently polarized crescent-shaped cell (merozoites, tachyzoites, bradyzoites, and sporozoites) in the motile or invasive zoite stages and develops nonmotile cells (micro- and macrogamonts) during sexual development to produce gametes (Delgado et al. 2022; Ferguson and Dubremetz 2014; Harding and Frischknecht 2020). The three different infectious stages of *T. gondii* seen in all hosts are tachyzoites, bradyzoites (in tissue cysts), and sporozoites (in oocysts) (Sukthana et al. 2003) (Figure 24.5). Each microgamont can produce 15–30 mature

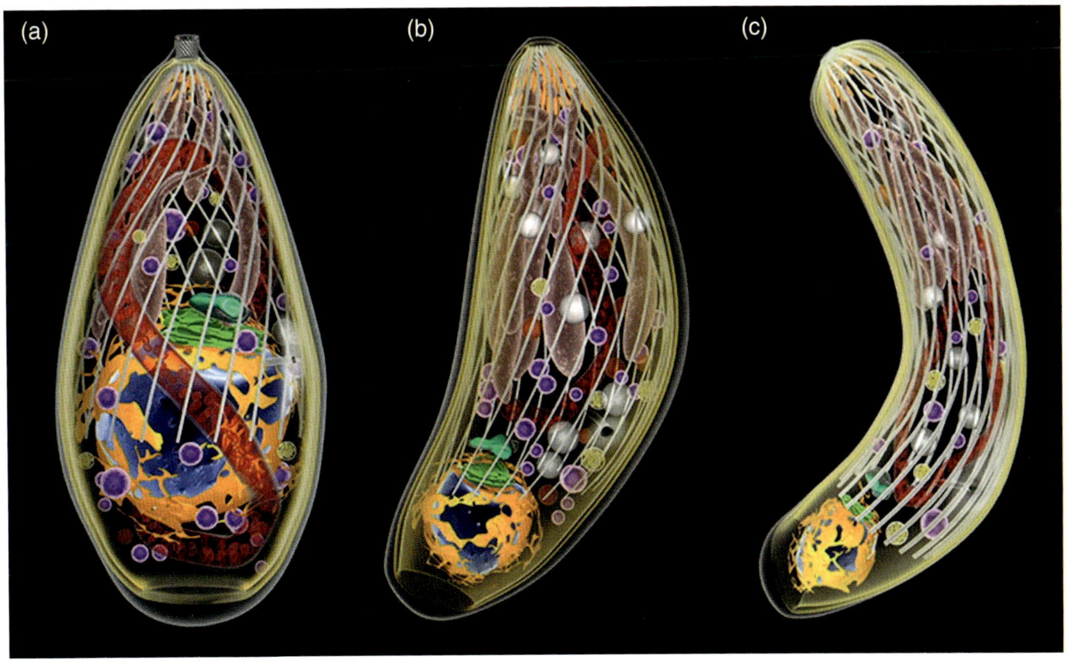

Figure 24.5 The three infective stages of *T. gondii* are tachyzoite (a), bradyzoite (b), and sporozoite (c). *Source:* Reproduced from Attias et al. (2020) under a Creative Commons Attribution 4.0 International License.

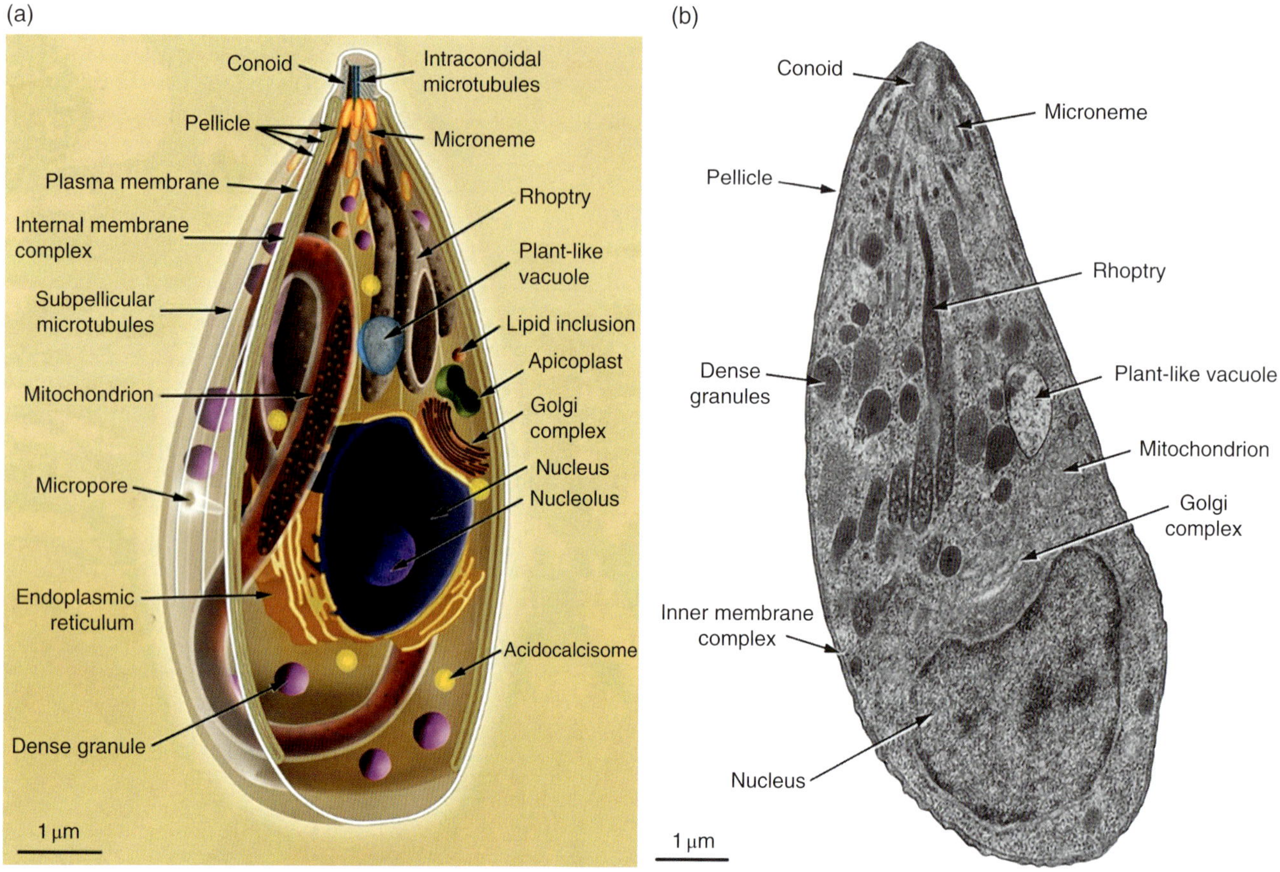

Figure 24.6 (a) Longitudinal section view of the tachyzoite form of *Toxoplasma gondii* (3D animation view). (b) Transverse section of a tachyzoite of *Toxoplasma gondii* observed by transmission electron microscopy (TEM). *Source:* Reproduced from Attias et al. (2020)/ Springer Nature/CC BY 4.0/CC0 1.0.

microgametes and a macrogamont will synthesize only one mature macrogamete. After fertilization, the unsporulated oocyst is formed with a single sporont. During sporulation, the sporont forms two sporocysts, each containing four sporozoites, originating the sporulated oocyst (Delgado et al. 2022; Attias et al. 2020).

24.5.1.1 Tachyzoites

The tachyzoite (tachos = speed) or endozoite is the rapidly multiplying, proliferative and feeding form with a crescent/moon shape. It is the stage which Nicolle and Manceaux found in the gundi. The tachyzoite is often 2×6 µm in size with a pointed anterior end and a rounded posterior end (Figure 24.6). It consists of various organelles and inclusion bodies. It enters the host cell by active penetration of the cell membrane and becomes surrounded by a parasitophorous vacuole that protects it from host defense mechanisms. The tachyzoite multiplies asexually by repeated binary divisions until the host cell ruptures (Dubey 2004). Tachyzoites divide into two by a specialized form of reproduction called endodyogeny, in which two progenies are formed within the parent parasite, consuming it (Dubey 2008). The parasite nucleus becomes horseshoe-shaped and the ends of the nucleus move into dome-shaped anterior ends of the developing progeny (Dubey 2010).

24.5.1.2 Bradyzoites and Tissue Cysts

Bradyzoites (brady = slow) or cystozoites are the stage seen in tissues and the name was proposed by Frenkel in 1973. After an unknown number of divisions, tachyzoites give rise to another stage called a tissue cyst which grows and remains intracellular with an elastic, thin (<0.5 µm), argyrophilic wall (Dubey 2004). They may enclose hundreds of crescent-shaped slender bradyzoites each measuring 7×1.5 µm. Tissue and organ cysts are 10–100 µm in diameter; the cysts have a clear wall in which hundreds of slim parasites without significant metabolism are piled up (rest phase or latent toxoplasmosis) (Figure 24.7) (Knapen and Overgaauw 2008).

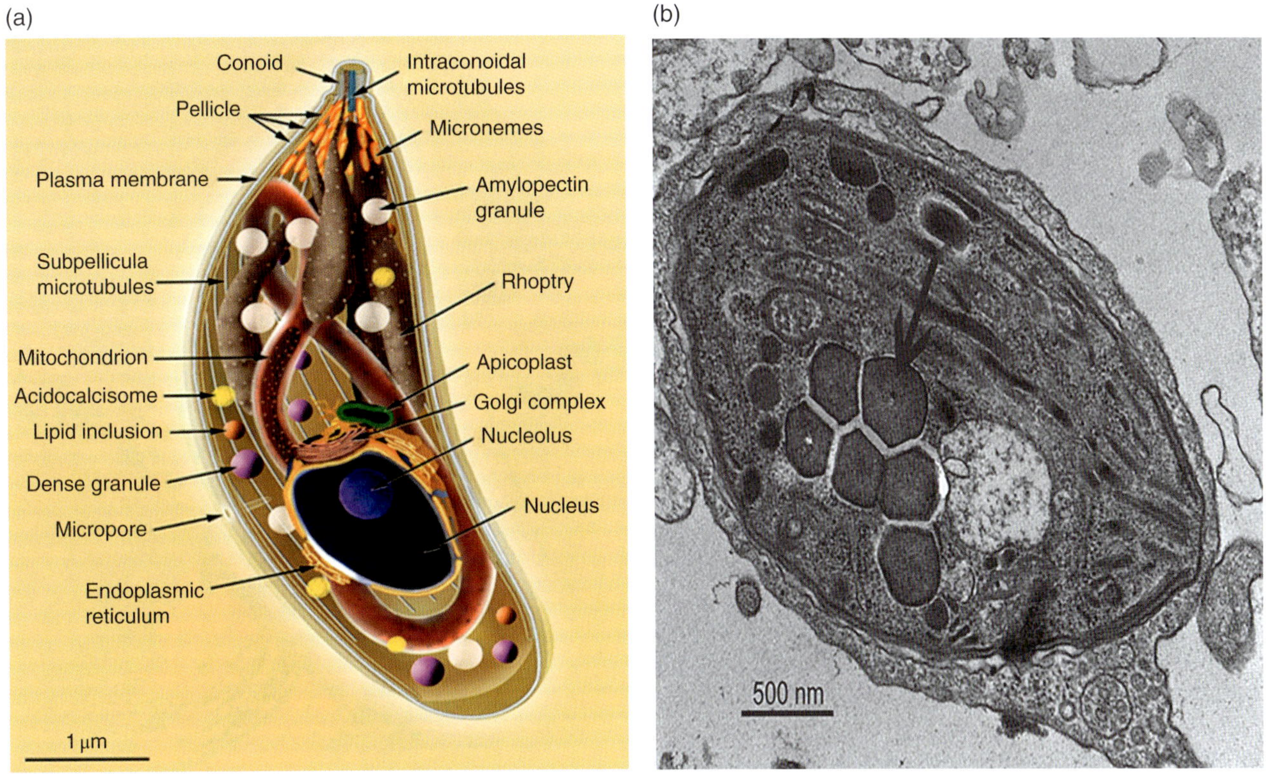

Figure 24.7 (a) Longitudinal section view of the bradyzoite form of *Toxoplasma gondii* (3D animation). (b) Bradyzoite inside a parasitophorous vacuole. Amylopectin granules are indicated by the arrow (transmission electron microscopy view).
Source: Reproduced from Attias et al. (2020)/Springer Nature/CC BY 4.0/CC0 1.0.

Tissue cysts are important in the life cycle of *Toxoplasma* spp. because carnivorous hosts can ingest infected meat. Intact tissue cysts are harmless and can persist lifelong in the visceral organs (lungs, liver, and kidneys) of the host, with a greater prevalence in the muscular (skeletal and cardiac muscle) and neural tissues of brain and eye (Dubey et al. 2021; Dubey 2022). Bradyzoites appear plump and small, with only two bradyzoites and fewer organelles in younger tissue cysts than in older tissue cysts that may contain thousands of organisms (Dubey 2010). Bradyzoites differ only slightly from tachyzoites in having a nucleus situated toward the posterior end whereas the nucleus in tachyzoites is more central. Also, bradyzoites are slenderer than tachyzoites and less susceptible to destruction by proteolytic enzymes (Dubey 2010) (Figures 24.8 and 24.9).

24.5.2 Life Cycle

Toxoplasma, an obligate intracellular parasite, has a sexual life cycle in the enteroepithelial cells of felids and a two-stage asexual cycle in all warm-blooded animals (World Organisation for Animal Health 2022). During the life cycle of *T. gondii*, three developmental stages can infect cells: tachyzoite (rapid proliferative form in acute infections), bradyzoite (slow multiplication form in chronic infection), and sporozoite (seen only in the definitive host during the sexual reproduction and released as oocysts in felid feces) (Attias et al. 2020). Cats can shed oocysts after ingesting any of the infectious stages (Dubey 2010).

Following a primary infection, oocysts are shed in cat feces for several days. The oocysts sporulate in the environment over the next 2–5 days, depending on aeration, humidity, and temperature. Sporulated oocysts contain four sporozoites in each of two sporocysts and remain infectious for two years in garden soil (Knapen and Overgaauw 2008). The prepatent periods in the cat after ingesting tissue cysts and oocysts are 3–10 days and more than 18 days respectively, irrespective of the dose (Dubey 2022).

In an acute infection, when a susceptible animal ingests sporulated oocysts, the sporozoites are released to penetrate the intestinal lining and establish an infection as tachyzoites. The tachyzoites actively penetrate and multiply in the host

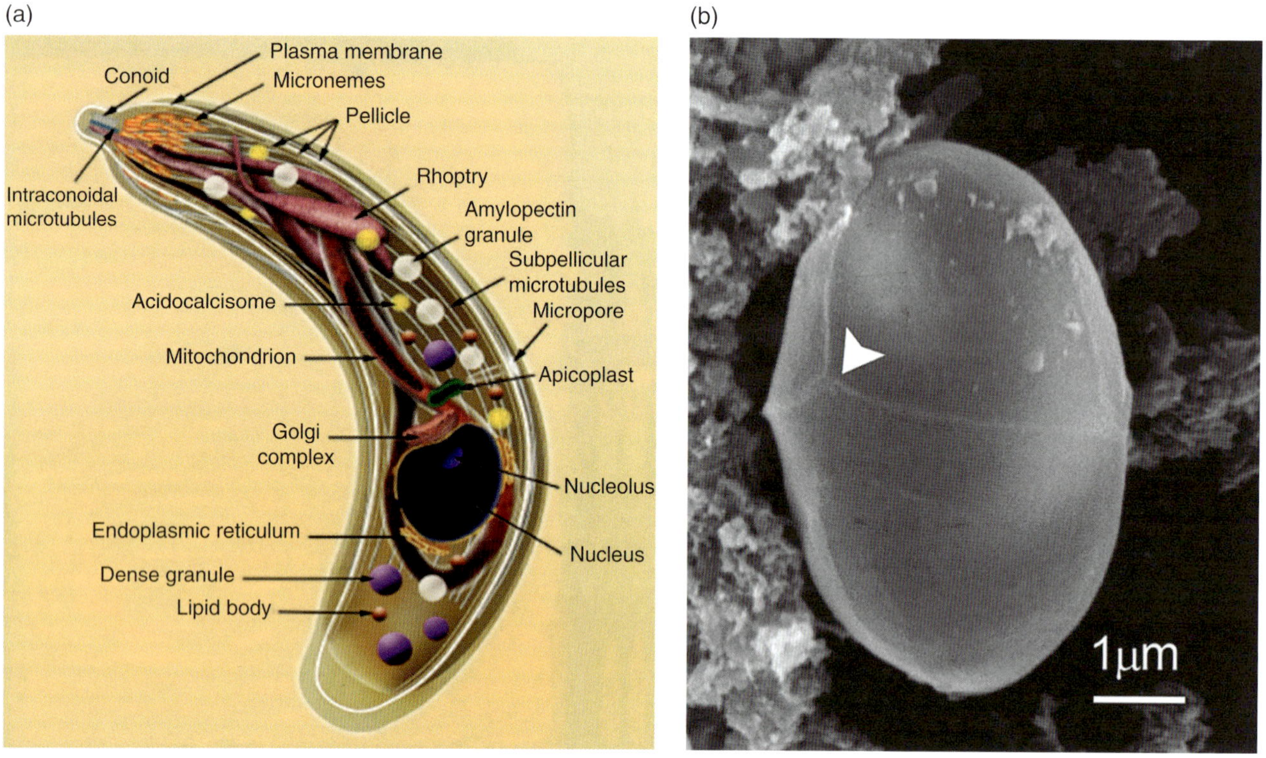

Figure 24.8 (a) Longitudinal section view of the sporozoite form of *Toxoplasma gondii* (3D animation). Sporozoites have amylopectin granules like bradyzoites and are more elongated than tachyzoites and bradyzoites, (b) Suture lines (arrowhead) of the sporocyst wall are visible under the scanning electron micrograph. *Source:* Reproduced from Attias et al. (2020)/Springer Nature/CC BY 4.0/CC0 1.0.

intestinal cells, leading to rupture and release of organisms both locally and into the bloodstream. Further, when the host develops immunity, the parasite retains its overall size and shape to establish a persistent infection by transforming into a slow multiplying chronic form, i.e., bradyzoite stage, within tissue cysts. These tissue cysts are capable of lifelong infections in sheep, goats, pigs, horses, and humans (World Organisation for Animal Health 2022).

24.5.3 Host–Parasite Relationship

The pathogenicity of *T. gondii* is determined by the innate susceptibility of the host, virulence of different genotypes and the stage at which the infection is acquired by the host. It can multiply in most of the nucleated cell types in the body. The oocysts are less infective and less pathogenic for cats than for mice and adapted to both an oocyst–oral cycle in herbivores and tissue cyst–oral cycle in carnivores and omnivores for the efficient transmission of the infection. In response to a host stimulus, tachyzoites are converted to bradyzoites and develop into tissue cysts. In immunosuppressed individuals the infection can be reactivated, which leads to dissemination of infection in the host (Lindsay and Dubey 2020).

24.6 Pathogenesis

Toxoplasmosis is frequently a silent infection, causing mild or no signs in immunocompetent hosts upon primary infection. Tachyzoite–bradyzoite conversion privileges the formation of tissue cysts that remain viable in the host; however, these do not cause disease unless the host immune system becomes compromised. Persistent infection is a concern mainly due to the risk of recrudescence (Delgado et al. 2022).

Toxoplasmosis can have a serious impact on the fertility and overall production of ewes, with an abortion percentage ranging from 5% to 100%. Abortions and neonatal mortality occur when sheep and goats suffer a primary infection during pregnancy.

Upon ingestion of sporulated oocysts by susceptible sheep, the organism multiplies in the intestinal submucosa and associated lymph nodes and spreads quickly to other organs via lymph and blood. Upon reaching the mesenteric lymph

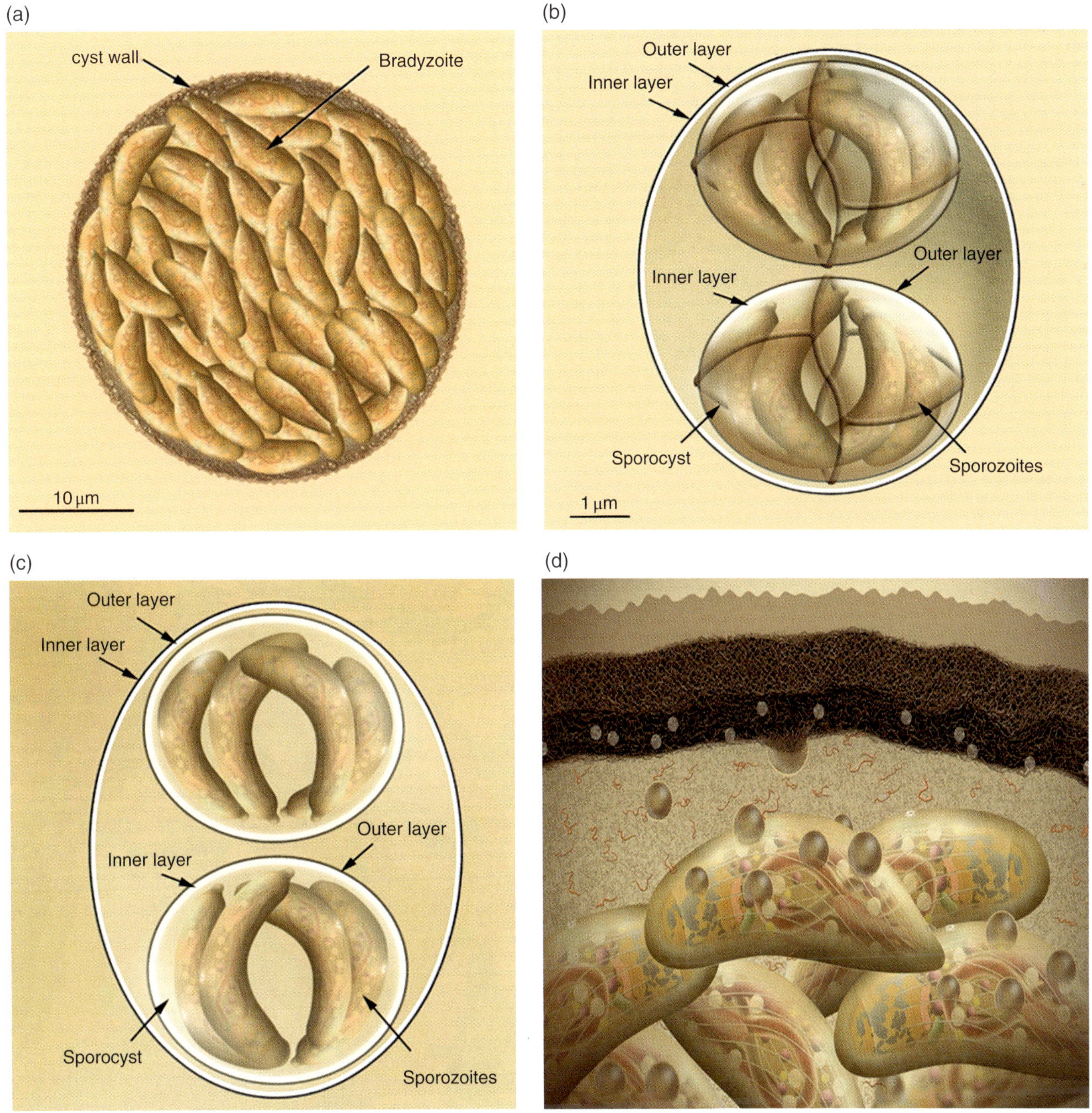

Figure 24.9 (a) Tissue cyst of *Toxoplasma gondii* (3D animation), with a thick and filamentous wall and each bradyzoite contains hundreds of bradyzoites. (b) Sporulated oocyst containing two sporocysts and four sporozoites inside each one. (c) Cross-sectional view of a sporulated oocyst of *Toxoplasma gondii*, each sporocyst containing four sporozoites. (d) Magnified view of the tissue cyst. *Source:* Reproduced from Attias et al. (2020)/Springer Nature/CC BY 4.0/CC0 1.0.

nodes, they multiply there, causing marked lymphadenopathy and focal necrosis within four days post infection. The tachyzoites are released from the oocysts by day 5 and are responsible for the parasitemia in intermediate hosts which lasts up to day 12. Around day 6 or 7, the parasitemia in ewes will be displayed as a febrile response which exceeds 105.8 °F. With the exception of the gravid uterus, the infection persists within the tissue cysts as bradyzoites and an effective maternal immune response will further decrease the parasitemia. Ewes may suffer from diarrhea, nasal discharge, and respiratory distress but usually recover by 14 days post infection (Dubey 2019).

The gravid uterus is the "immunologically privileged" site in pregnant ruminants (Buxton 1990). Fetal death was found to be caused by the multiplication of *T. gondii* in the placenta, rather than invasion of the fetus by the parasite. The immaturity of the fetal immune system and local suppression of immune mechanism in the maternal placenta lead to the continuous multiplication of the parasite in the placenta and fetus (Karthika et al. 2021; Ahmed et al. 2008). Fertilization of the ovum and implantation occur in ewes by around two weeks and the earliest effects of toxoplasmosis are expected after implantation. Tachyzoites circulate in the blood during the first two weeks after ingestion of oocysts and infection of the fetus occurs after the end of parasitemia (Dubey 2019).

Infection of the ewe during midpregnancy leads to abortion and mild disease in lambs during the last month of pregnancy. The immunocompetency of ovine fetuses acquired at 60 days of gestation was not sufficient to protect the animal throughout the pregnancy. *T. gondii* infections are lethal to a one-month-old fetus and infections prior to 40 days of gestation (fetuses less than 100 g) cause embryonic death and fetal resorption. Infections during midpregnancy (between 40 and 120 days of gestation) results in fetal maceration, mummification or abortion. Infections after 120 days of gestation produce stillbirth or birth of weak lambs. The synthesis and release of prostaglandin F2-alpha induced by inflammatory reactions in the placenta are luteolytic, leading to decreased progesterone level and subsequent abortions in ovine toxoplasmosis (Ahmed et al. 2008).

24.7 Clinical Signs

Toxoplasmosis is one of the main causes of infectious reproductive failure in small ruminants across the world, with a greater severity in goats compared to sheep. It causes fetal resorption, early embryonic mortality, mummification, abortion, stillbirth, neonatal deaths and birth of congenitally infected weak kids or lambs, resulting in great economic losses (Ahmed et al. 2008; Lindsay and Dubey 2020). The stage of gestation when transplacental transmission of *T. gondii* to the developing fetus occurs is critical in determining the clinical outcome (Innes et al. 2009). The chances of abortions in *Toxoplasma* infections in subsequent pregnancies are negligible. Infection in midgestation is more likely to cause abortion and birth of weak kids, while infection in late gestation results in the birth of live, infected, and immune kids (Buxton et al. 1991).

24.7.1 Clinical Signs in Adult Nonpregnant Sheep and Goats

Toxoplasma gondii infection in nonpregnant ewes and goats is generally asymptomatic, or with unspecific clinical signs such as fever, nasal discharge, cough, tachypnea, and loss of appetite (Glor et al. 2013). In acute cases, clinical signs may include lymphadenopathy, hepatomegaly, interstitial pneumonia, and neural signs (World Organisation for Animal Health 2022). Sometimes, the only evident clinical sign associated with acquired toxoplasmosis (horizontal transmission) is a brief episode of fever and lack of appetite about 3–6 days after infection and lasting usually for about 4–5 days or even up to 10 days (Stelzer et al. 2019).

24.7.2 Clinical Signs in Pregnant Ewes and Does

The clinical manifestations of ovine toxoplasmosis vary from early embryonic death with reabsorption to stillbirth or neonatal death, or even the birth of transplacentally infected lambs, depending upon the stage of pregnancy at which the primary infection occurred (Jackson-O'Brien 2010; Fernandez-Escobar et al. 2020). Affected ewes were clinically normal at the time of abortion, except there was some difficulty in lambing as a result of uterine inertia due to dead fetuses. Ewes that have aborted due to toxoplasmosis return to heat and conceive normally (Dubey 2019).

In pregnant does, *T. gondii* can invade and multiply in the placenta and pass to the fetus, causing fetal death, mummification, stillbirth, or the birth of weak kids. Lambs might be mummified, macerated, aborted, stillborn, born weak or die within a week of birth. Infection of goats with *T. gondii* in early gestation may cause death and reabsorption of the fetus (Pavlovic and Ivanovic 2005). In such cases the ewes may appear barren, which in turn can mimic a flock infertility problem (World Organisation for Animal Health 2022; Dubey 2010; Johnston 1988; Rodger et al. 2006). In a typical case of abortion, a ewe or doe infected in midgestation produces a stillborn lamb or kid a few days earlier than the predicted end of pregnancy. The aborted fetus is often accompanied by either a weak sibling or a mummified fetus (Aitken 2007; Buxton 2000). A proportion of lambs born alive are weak and die within the first few days of life despite careful nursing (Buxton and Brebner 1998). Those lambs that survive the first week generally grow normally to adulthood, producing *T. gondii*-free lambs (Dubey 2019). Abortions from this microorganism occurring in the last trimester of pregnancy usually progress normally by giving birth to a normal kid and this might happen in successive pregnancies (Leite-Browning 2006; Azimi et al. 2021).

24.7.3 Clinical Signs in Congenitally Infected Lambs

Congenitally infected lambs may be uncoordinated, weak and unable to nurse, and often die. Some animals may have signs of disseminated disease, such as fever and dyspnea. Lambs infected late in gestation are less likely to be affected and may be asymptomatic. Reproductive losses are generally not thought to recur during subsequent pregnancies (Stelzer et al. 2019; Spickler 2017).

24.7.4 Clinical Signs in Chronically Infected Ewes

Transplacental transmission due to reactivation of an endogenous infection is thought to be infrequent in sheep, thus the chances of chronically infected ewes transmitting the infection to future generations are scarce (Buxton 2000; Dubey 2009b). However, repeated abortions associated with *T. gondii* infection have been observed in goats (Basso et al. 2022; Dubey 1982). Infected goats remain protected for life and as the disease is not spread laterally, they do not present a risk to other animals (Pavlovic and Ivanovic 2005; Dubey and Kirkbride 1989).

24.7.5 Clinical Signs in Other Intermediate Hosts

Toxoplasma does not usually cause clinical illness in cattle, camelids or deer, but can cause fatal disease in New World monkeys, marsupials and certain other animals including hares, Arctic fox, some birds, and marine mammals (World Organisation for Animal Health 2022). There are no confirmed reports of clinical toxoplasmosis in cattle and water buffalo, which are considered to be more resistant to acute infections (Lindsay and Dubey 2020). It causes fever, respiratory distress, nasal discharge, and conjunctival hyperemia in experimentally infected calves (Stelzer et al. 2019; Spickler 2017).

24.8 Pathological Findings

The ewe or doe remains clinically normal. At postmortem examination, there might be splenomegaly, hepatomegaly, and lymphadenopathy with pale foci (World Organisation for Animal Health 2022). Necrosis of the placental cotyledons is characteristic (Dubey 2019). There may be a typical speckled appearance of the placental cotyledons with a white chalky nodule around 2–3 mm in diameter with a normal appearance of the intercotyledonary membranes (World Organisation for Animal Health 2022; Dubey 2010; Rodger et al. 2006).

Macroscopic lesions in the fetus are not pathognomonic (Dubey 2019). Pathological examinations of *Toxoplasma*-affected aborted fetuses' brains showed hyperemia and edema as the most common lesions in pathological examinations, followed by encephalomalacia, meningitis, leukomalacia, meningoencephalitis, demyelination, and gliosis (Shahbazi et al. 2019). Postmortem examination of late-gestation aborted fetuses revealed generalized subcutaneous edema (anasarca) associated with accumulation of moderate quantities of blood-tinged fluids in the thoracic and abdominal cavities, and an enlarged, congested and friable liver with rounded borders. Sections of aborted fetus heart revealed several dark purple banana-shaped tachyzoites with apical nuclei in between cardiac muscles (Ahmed et al. 2008). Myocarditis, interstitial nephritis, nonsuppurative encephalitis, hepatitis, and diffuse interstitial pneumonia were the predominant histopathological changes of aborted fetuses (Ahmed et al. 2008).

24.9 Differential Diagnosis

Abortion in sheep and goats due to *T. gondii* must be differentiated from that caused by other infectious agents, including infections with *Chlamydophila abortus*, *Coxiella burnetii*, *Brucella melitensis*, *Campylobacter fetus*, *Salmonella* spp., border disease, and the viruses that cause bluetongue and Akabane disease (World Organisation for Animal Health 2022).

24.10 Diagnosis

Diagnosis of small ruminant toxoplasmosis can be made by biological, serological, animal inoculation, or histological methods or by combination of these methods (Dubey 2019; Azimi et al. 2021). Due to the presence of multiple etiological agents and the advanced stages of autolysis in the fetuses submitted for diagnosis, the accurate diagnosis of abortion is often difficult. Molecular assays such as polymerase chain reaction (PCR) are a specific and sensitive tool to diagnose small quantities of target DNA (Azimi et al. 2021). Rapid diagnosis of toxoplasmosis can be made by examination of impression smears from the lesions. Further, the diagnosis might be established based on serum antibody detection, placental and fetal brain histopathology, immunohistochemistry, and PCR (Giadinis et al. 2011).

24.10.1 Sample Collection

Diagnosis of *Toxoplasma* infection is generally carried out using one or more of the following samples: vaginal mucosa, saliva, nasal secretion, urine, etc. collected from experimentally infected goats and milk, placental material, brains from aborted fetuses, fetal fluids, blood (blood from aborted ewes, precolostral blood from live lambs) from naturally infected goats (Buxton and Brebner 1998; Leite-Browning 2006).

24.10.2 Identification of the Agent

Toxoplasma gondii can be isolated from placental cotyledons, brain, pleural and peritoneal fluids and heart blood from aborted fetuses that are not too autolyzed. Isolation of *T. gondii* from samples is expensive and slow but, if required, is best achieved by inoculation of mice with tissue homogenate derived from fetal brain or placenta.

24.10.2.1 Histopathology

Focal mononuclear inflammation with or without focal necrosis is seen in the liver, heart, and lungs of animals that die with acute toxoplasmosis. Placental cotyledons collected from aborted ewes typically contain large foci of coagulative necrosis with mineralization. Neuropathological changes characteristic of *Toxoplasma* infection include focal leukomalacia and focal lymphoid meningitis. These changes are due to fetal anoxia in late gestation caused by advanced lesions in the placentome and a fetal immune response to direct damage by local parasite multiplication respectively. Confirmation of the identity of *T. gondii*-like structures in tissue sections can be achieved by immunohistochemistry (World Organisation for Animal Health 2022).

24.10.2.2 Nucleic Acid Recognition Methods

Molecular methods rely on PCR for the specific detection or analysis of *T. gondii* DNA. These methods can be divided into two groups. The first group deals with specific detection of *T. gondii* DNA in biological samples, e.g., conventional PCR, nested PCR (n-PCR), and quantitative real-time PCR (qPCR) of repetitive DNA sequences (Halonen and Weiss 2013; Pal et al. 2014). The second group of molecular methods includes multilocus PCR-RFLP, microsatellite, and multilocus sequence typing (MLST) of single copy DNA sequences which is based on high-resolution identification of *T. gondii* isolates (Fernandez-Escobar et al. 2020; Halonen and Weiss 2013).

Polymerase chain reaction is an extremely sensitive, reliable diagnostic test for the detection of nucleic acids from *T. gondii*. Parasite DNA can be extracted and purified from several tissues, including placenta, central nervous system, heart, and skeletal muscle. The main target regions are the B1 repetitive sequence, P30 (SAG1) gene, and 18SrRNA (Ahmed et al. 2008). Real-time PCR allows simultaneous quantification and amplification of DNA from the *T. gondii* B1 gene (Costa et al. 2000; Lin et al. 2000). This quantification of parasite DNA can be used to determine the number of parasites in tissues and fluids (Nagy et al. 2007).

24.10.2.3 Serological Tests

Serological tests widely used for detection of IgG and IgM antibodies to *T. gondii* include the Sabin–Feldman dye test (DT), indirect hemagglutination (IHA), indirect fluorescent antibody test (IFAT), modified agglutination test (MAT), latex agglutination (LA), enzyme-linked immunosorbent assay (ELISA), and complement fixation test (CFT). Of these, the IFAT, ELISA, and MAT have been modified to detect IgM antibodies, which appear sooner after infection than IgG and disappear faster than IgG after recovery (Lindsay and Dubey 2020).

The Sabin–Feldman dye test is the gold standard serological test for detecting *Toxoplasma* infections in humans. The test uses live, virulent *Toxoplasma* tachyzoites and is both specific and sensitive in humans, but may be unreliable in other species. It is expensive, requiring expert staff, and in addition is potentially hazardous as live parasite is used.

The IFAT is a simple serological test widely used to diagnose toxoplasmosis in small ruminants (Dubey 2010). The IFAT is safer, gives titers comparable with the dye test and can be used to differentiate IgM and IgG antibodies. Evaluating the antibody titer in paired samples (2–4 weeks) is recommended to evaluate potential seroconversion and identify an active or chronic infection (Dubey 2019). A 4–16-fold increase in anti-*T. gondii* titers has been associated with acute infection, reinfection or reactivation (Steffen et al. 2021; Dubey et al. 2021; Lindsay and Dubey 2020).

The IHA test is simple in principle but acute infections are often missed. The direct agglutination test (DAT) and the latex agglutination test are both relatively rapid and neither requires complex laboratory facilities. The MAT is widely used for the diagnosis of toxoplasmosis in animals (Dubey 2019).

Clinically, there is a need to distinguish acute recent infections from long-standing infections. The CFT detects antibodies during acute infection, but is not considered as a test of choice because of its complex procedures and lack of standardization of antigens and reagents. A soluble antigen preparation made from *Toxoplasma* RH strain tachyzoites is used for ELISA test. The assay is simple and easy to perform and can readily test a large number of samples. With the conventional ELISA, the detection of *Toxoplasma*-specific IgG and IgM antibodies along with IgA may permit a degree of discrimination between acute and chronic toxoplasmosis. An assay to define the avidity of IgG for the P30 antigen of *T. gondii* in sheep is a good diagnostic tool for discriminating relatively recent infections from more established ones.

24.11 Treatment

The most devastating economic effects due to toxoplasmosis are due to epidemic abortion storms rather than losses due to endemic cases (Castano et al. 2016; Sanchez-Sanchez et al. 2018). Toxoplasmosis can be controlled effectively with the use of live vaccines applied before the mating period. However, the use of vaccines in flocks with an abortion storm due to toxoplasmosis is not effective. In such cases, the administration of appropriate treatment is necessary to stop the abortions.

The treatment of small ruminant toxoplasmosis should be focused on three main levels: chemotherapy or chemoprophylaxis in infected ewes and goats (Table 24.1), treatment of newborn congenitally infected lambs and kids, and treatment of definitive hosts in order to reduce environmental contamination with *T. gondii* oocysts (Sanchez-Sanchez et al. 2018).

Sulfadimidine at a higher dose rate of 33 mg/kg with four injections, every 48 hours, was found to be effective in reducing the abortion rate, normal length of gestation, and milk production in sheep (Giadinis et al. 2011). Feeding goats orally continuously during pregnancy with anticoccidial drugs such as monensin (15–30 mg/head/day) produced more live heavier lambs, but the drug was not licensed for use in goats. Decoquinate (2 mg/kg bw/day) is a safer and palatable anticoccidial drug compared to monensin, licensed for use in sheep and goats (Leite-Browning 2006). Combination drugs like sulfamezathine and pyrimethamine had been shown to reduce severity of acute toxoplasmosis, but not to eradicate the infection in small ruminants (Pavlovic and Ivanovic 2005). Sulfamezathine and pyrimethamine act synergistically by blocking the metabolic pathway involving p-aminobenzoic acid and the folic–folinic acid cycle respectively. Spiramycin,

Table 24.1 Treatment of toxoplasmosis in small ruminants.

Drug			
Class	**Compounds**	**Treatment**	**References**
Macrolide antibiotics	Spiramycin	100 mg/kg PO from 3 weeks after infection until parturition	Dubreuil (1972)
Polyether ionophore antibiotics	Monensin	15 mg/day PO from day 80 of pregnancy until parturition	Buxton et al. (1987)
		15–30 mg/day PO from day 80 of pregnancy until parturition	Buxton et al. (1988)
	Lasalocid	30 g/day PO from day 55 of pregnancy until parturition	Kirkbride et al. (1992)
Folate inhibitors	Sulfamezathine and pyrimethamine	Sulfamezathine (83–166 mg/kg SC). Pyrimethamine (1–2 mg/kg IP) on days 100, 115, and 130 of gestation, each of three consecutive days	Buxton et al. (1993)
	Sulfadimidine	20–33 mg/kg IM, 4 times every 48 hours	Giadinis et al. (2011)
Quinolones	Decoquinate	1–2 mg/kg PO from day 80 of pregnancy until parturition	Buxton et al. (1996)
Triazinones	Toltrazuril	20–40 mg/kg PO twice, once every week, beginning 15 days post infection	Kul et al. (2013)

PO, per os (oral administration); SC, subcutaneous; IP, intraperitoneal.

clindamycin, atovaquone, azithromycin, roxithromycin, clarithromycin, dapsone, ponazuril, and several other drugs are available for treatment of toxoplasmosis, but none of them are approved in food animals (Lindsay and Dubey 2020).

24.12 Prevention and Control

Toxoplasmosis was recognized as the parasitic zoonosis with highest human incidence by the European Food Safety Authority (EFSA), affecting 25–50% of the population, in spite of the underdetection and underreporting of cases (Olivier et al. 2007). For control of toxoplasmosis on farms, a combination of different approaches is the optimal strategy. For reducing the level of environmental contamination of *T. gondii* oocysts via feces, implementation of farm biosecurity, hygiene, and management practices are suggested. Biosafety measures include control of wild cat populations and rodents, proper disposal of dead livestock, placenta and fetal materials, restricting cat access to pregnant ruminants, areas of food and water storage, etc. (Sanchez-Sanchez et al. 2018).

In the farm environment, young cats that were weaned recently are more likely to pass *T. gondii* oocysts in feces than older cats (Lindsay and Dubey 2020). Neutering of farm cats also reduces the levels of infection (Glor et al. 2013). Proper disposal of aborted fetuses by incineration or burying significantly decreases the risk of toxoplasmosis seropositivity in sheep and goats by 8% (Abu-Dalbouh et al. 2012). Proper diagnosis of abortion storms in flocks with the assistance of a veterinary laboratory is useful for the control of infections on farms (Pavlovic and Ivanovic 2005). To minimize the risks of prenatal infection, pregnant women should be educated about consuming raw milk or undercooked meat from farm animals (Garcia et al. 2012).

24.12.1 Vaccination

Vaccination is considered as the most promising and economically viable solution for controlling toxoplasmosis in small ruminants. A live attenuated strain (S48) of *T. gondii* was developed in New Zealand in the 1980s for sheep vaccination. In immunized sheep, it caused a mild, short-lived infection and protected them from the clinical disease and chronic infections (Pavlovic and Ivanovic 2005). Ewes vaccinated with the S48 strain vaccine retain immunity for at least 18 months but it is not recommended in pregnant ewes (Lindsay and Dubey 2020).

24.12.1.1 Live Vaccines in Livestock Animals and Cats

Most of the live attenuated *T. gondii* vaccines utilize tachyzoites, which are the only stage which allows *in vitro* production in large quantities (Mevelec et al. 2020). Toxovax® (S48 strain) was the first commercially available vaccine for protection against congenital toxoplasmosis in sheep. The S48 strain has lost the ability to differentiate into bradyzoite and tissue cysts as a result of being passaged for many years in laboratory mice. In ewes, subcutaneous inoculation of 10^5 tachyzoites of the S48 strain induced both cellular and humoral responses and conferred significant protection against abortion after oral challenge with *T. gondii* oocysts (Buxton et al. 1993; Mevelec et al. 2020). A chemically induced mutant *T. gondii* strain (T-263) was found to be effective in inducing immunity in cats after ingesting tissue cysts. It lacked the capacity to form oocysts in cats but undergoes both schizogony and gametogony in the intestine of cats (Mevelec et al. 2020; Dubey 2017).

In recent years, with the availability of the complete *T. gondii* genome sequence and genetic engineering methods, new attenuated *T. gondii* strains have been created by gene deletions. These newer strains are safer than the S48 and T263 strains. The first to be tested in sheep and cats was the strain called Mic1-3KO obtained by deletion of MIC1 and MIC3 genes in the *T. gondii* RH strain (Cerede et al. 2005). A transmission blocking vaccine based on the HAP2-deficient *T. gondii* strain was created recently using CRISPR/Cas9 technology. Oral administration of HAP2-deficient *T. gondii* tissue cysts to cats totally prevented oocyst excretion that failed to produce sporozoites, after an oral infection with tissue cysts from wild-type *T. gondii* (Mevelec et al. 2020; Ramakrishnan et al. 2019).

24.13 Public Health Importance

Toxoplasmosis is a major cause of death among patients with AIDS and considered as one of the five neglected zoonotic parasitic diseases. *T. gondii* is transmitted to humans by organ transplantation, ingestion or handling of undercooked or raw meat containing tissue cysts or water or food containing oocysts excreted in the feces of infected cats (Pavlovic and Ivanovic 2005). Vertical transmission of toxoplasmosis can cause serious disease in the fetus with a prevalence of 1–10 per

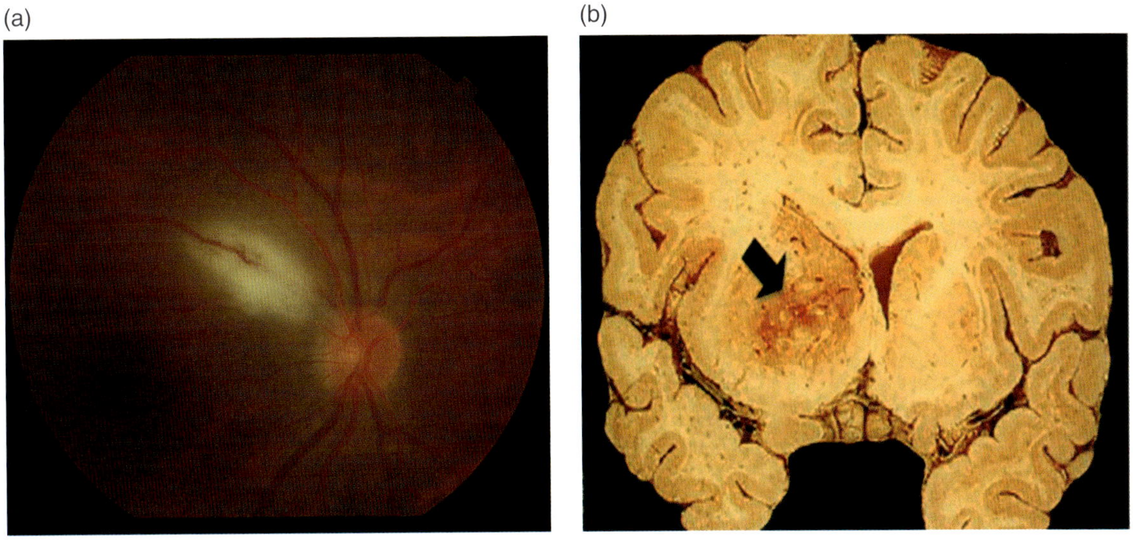

Figure 24.10 (a) Acquired ocular toxoplasmosis characterized by retinochoroiditis and necrosis. *Source:* Courtesy of Prof. Rubens Belfort Jr. (b) Expansive necrosis, leading to compression of the ventricular space and deviation of the septum pellucidum. *Source:* Reproduced from Attias et al. (2020)/Springer Nature/CC BY 4.0/CC0 1.0. Courtesy of Prof. C. Basilio-de-Oliveira.

10 000 livebirths (Montoya and Liesenfeld 2004; Remington et al. 2001). Clinical manifestations of toxoplasmosis in humans are classified into primary (postnatally acquired form) and secondary/congenital (prenatally transmitted) toxoplasmosis. It is more commonly reported in boys and young women than in girls and young men, possibly due to hormonal reasons (Dubey 2019).

In congenitally infected infants, the severity of fetal damage is related inversely to the stage of pregnancy when maternal infection occurs and the most severe damage to the fetus is reported in the first trimester (Pavlovic and Ivanovic 2005; Mihu et al. 2022). Lymphadenitis and ocular disease were the most frequently observed conditions in acquired and congenital forms of toxoplasmosis in humans, respectively (Dubey 2019). Lymphadenopathy may be associated with fever, excessive sweating, myalgia, fatigue, muscle pain, sore throat, maculopapular rash, and headache. Encephalitis was the most clinically important manifestation of toxoplasmosis in immunosuppressed patients. A wide spectrum of clinical disease occurs in congenitally infected children, with a slightly diminished vision in mild disease and full tetrad of signs (retinochoroiditis, hydrocephalus, convulsions, and intracerebral calcification) (Figure 24.10) in severely diseased children. This condition is unique to congenitally acquired toxoplasmosis in humans and not reported in other animals (Montoya and Liesenfeld 2004).

Pregnant women should avoid direct contact with cats, raw meat, and cat litter. Vegetables should be washed thoroughly before eating and gloves should be worn while gardening because the soil may have been contaminated with cat feces. People should avoid drinking unfiltered water from lakes, ponds, and rivers and access to water reservoirs by cats should be prevented (Dubey 2004).

References

Abu-Dalbouh, M.A., Ababneh, M.M., Giadinis, N.D., and Lafi, S.Q. (2012). Ovine and caprine toxoplasmosis (*Toxoplasma gondii*) in aborted animals in Jordanian goat and sheep flocks. *Tropical Animal Health and Production* 44: 49–54.

Ahaduzzaman, M.D. and Hasan, T. (2022). Seroprevalence of *Toxoplasma gondii* infection in sheep and goats from different geographical regions of the world: Systematic review and meta-analysis. *Transboundary and Emerging Diseases* 69: 1–33.

Ahmed, Y.F., Sokkar, S.M., Desouky, H.M., and Soror, A.H. (2008). Abortion due to toxoplasmosis in small ruminants. *Global Veterinaria* 2 (6): 337–342.

Aitken, I.D. (2007). *Diseases of Sheep*, 4e, 137–142. Oxford: Blackwell.

Ajith, Y. (2012). Gateway to dairy production and products. Food and Agriculture Organization of the United Nations. www.fao.org/dairy-production-products/resources/photo-gallery (accessed 1 August 2023).

Attias, M., Teixeira, D.E., Benchimol, M. et al. (2020). The life-cycle of *Toxoplasma gondii* reviewed using animations. *Parasites and Vectors* 13: 588.

Azimi, K., Amouei, A., Mehdi Sharif, M. et al. (2021). Diagnosis of toxoplasmosis in ruminants aborted foetuses in Northern Iran using molecular and bioassay techniques. *Iranian Journal of Parasitology* 16 (2): 229–235.

Basso, W., Holenweger, F., Schares, G. et al. (2022). *Toxoplasma gondii* and *Neospora caninum* infections in sheep and goats in Switzerland: seroprevalence and occurrence in aborted foetuses. *Food and Waterborne Parasitology* 28: e00176.

Buxton, D. (1990). Ovine toxoplasmosis: a review. *Journal of the Royal Society of Medicine* 83: 509–511.

Buxton, D. (2000). Toxoplasmosis and neosporosis. In: *Diseases of Sheep* (ed. W.B. Martin and I.D. Aitken), 86–94. Oxford, UK: Blackwell Science.

Buxton, D. and Brebner, J. (1998). Toxoplasmosis. In: *Manual for Laboratory Diagnosis of Infectious Abortions in Small Ruminants* (ed. A. Rodolakis, P. Nettleton, and A. Benkirane), 97–109. Rome: FAO.

Buxton, D., Donald, K.M., and Finlayson, J. (1987). Monensin and the control of experimental ovine toxoplasmosis: a systemic effect. *Veterinary Record* 120: 618–619.

Buxton, D., Blewett, D.A., Trees, A.J. et al. (1988). Further studies in the use of monensin in the control of experimental ovine toxoplasmosis. *Journal of Comparative Pathology* 98: 225–236.

Buxton, D., Thomson, K., Maley, S. et al. (1991). Vaccination of sheep with a live incomplete strain (S48) of *Toxoplasma gondii* and their immunity to challenge when pregnant. *Veterinary Record* 129: 89–93.

Buxton, D., Thomson, K.M., and Maley, S. (1993). Treatment of ovine toxoplasmosis with a combination of sulphamezathine and pyrimethamine. *Veterinary Record* 132: 409–411.

Buxton, D., Brebner, J., Wright, S. et al. (1996). Decoquinate and the control of experimental ovine toxoplasmosis. *Veterinary Record* 138: 434–436.

Buxton, D., Maley, S.W., Wright, S.E. et al. (2007). *Toxoplasma gondii* and ovine toxoplasmosis: new aspects of an old story. *Veterinary Parasitology* 149: 25–28.

Castano, P., Fuertes, M., Regidor-Cerrillo, J. et al. (2016). Experimental ovine toxoplasmosis: influence of the gestational stage on the clinical course, lesion development and parasite distribution. *Veterinary Research* 47: 1.

Celi, K., Guzman, L., and Rey-Valeiron, C. (2022). Apicomplexans in goat: prevalence of *Neospora caninum, Toxoplasma gondii, Cryptosporidium* spp., *Eimeria* spp. and risk factors in farms from Ecuador. *Animals* 12: 2224.

Cerede, O., Dubremetz, J.F., Soête, M. et al. (2005). Synergistic role of micronemal proteins in Toxoplasma gondii virulence. *Journal of Experimental Medicine* 201 (3): 453–463.

Cole, R.A., Lindsay, D.S., Howe, D.K. et al. (2000). Biological and molecular characterizations of *Toxoplasma gondii* strains obtained from southern sea otters (*Enhydra lutris nereis*). *Journal of Parasitology* 86: 526–530.

Cook, A.J.C., Gilbert, R.E., Buffolano, W. et al. (2000). Sources of Toxoplasma infection in pregnant women: European multicentre case-control study. *British Medical Journal* 321: 142–147.

Costa, J.M., Pautas, C., Ernault, P. et al. (2000). Real-time PCR for diagnosis and follow-up of Toxoplasma reactivation after allogeneic stem cell transplantation using fluorescence resonance energy transfer hybridization probes. *Journal of Clinical Microbiology* 38: 2929–2932.

Dechicha, A.S., Bachi, F., Gharbi, I. et al. (2015). Sero-epidemiological survey on toxoplasmosis in cattle, sheep and goats in Algeria. *African Journal of Agricultural Research* 10 (20): 2113–2119.

Delgado, I.L.S., Zuquete, S., Santos, D. et al. (2022). The Apicomplexan parasite *Toxoplasma gondii*. *Encyclopedia* 2: 189–211.

Dubey, J.P. (1982). Repeat transplacental transfer of *Toxoplasma gondii* in dairy goats. *Journal of the American Veterinary Medical Association* 180: 220–1221.

Dubey, J.P. (2004). Toxoplasmosis – a waterborne zoonosis. *Veterinary Parasitology* 26: 57–72.

Dubey, J.P. (2006). Comparative infectivity of oocysts and bradyzoites of *Toxoplasma gondii* for intermediate (mice) and definitive (cats) host. *Veterinary Parasitology* 140: 69–75.

Dubey, J.P. (2008). The history of *Toxoplasma gondii* – the first 100 years. *Journal of Eukaryotic Microbiology* 55 (6): 467–475.

Dubey, J.P. (2009a). History of the discovery of the life cycle of *Toxoplasma gondii*. *International Journal for Parasitology* 39: 877–882.

Dubey, J.P. (2009b). Toxoplasmosis in sheep – the last 20 years. *Veterinary Parasitology* 163: 1–14.

Dubey, J.P. (2010). General biology. In: *Toxoplasmosis in Animals and Humans*, 2e, 1–47. Boca Raton, FL: CRC Press/Taylor & Francis Group.

Dubey, J.P. (2017). Schizogony and gametogony of oocyst-deficient T-263 strain of *Toxoplasma gondii*. *Veterinary Parasitology* 245: 160–162.

Dubey, J.P. (2019). Toxoplasmosis in sheep and goats. In: *Toxoplasmosis in Animals and Humans*, 2e, 7–89. Boca Raton, FL: CRC Press/Taylor & Francis Group.

Dubey, J.P. (2022). Biology of *Toxoplasma gondii*. In: *Toxoplasmosis in Animals and Humans*, 3e, 7–89. Boca Raton, FL: CRC Press/Taylor & Francis Group.

Dubey, J.P. and Beattie, C.P. (1988). *Toxoplasmosis of Animals and Man*. Boca Raton, FL: CRC Press.

Dubey, J.P. and Kirkbride, C.A. (1989). Economic and public health considerations of congenital toxoplasmosis in lambs. *Journal of the American Veterinary Medical Association* 195: 1715–1716.

Dubey, J.P., Somvanshi, R., Jithendran, K.P., and Rao, J.R. (1993). High seroprevalence of *Toxoplasma gondii* in goats from Kumaon region of India. *Journal of Veterinary Parasitology* 7: 17–21.

Dubey, J.P., Murata, F.H.A., Cerqueira-Cezar, C.K., and Kwok, O.C.H. (2021). Recent epidemiologic and clinical *Toxoplasma gondii* infections in wild canids and other carnivores: 2009–2020. *Veterinary Parasitology* 290: 109337.

Dubreuil, G. (1972). Trial of spiramycin in the prevention of experimental toxoplasmosis. PhD thesis. University of Lyon, France.

Edelhofer, R. and Prossinger, H. (2010). Infection with *Toxoplasma gondii* during pregnancy. Seroepidemiological studies in Austria. *Zoonoses and Public Health* 57 (1): 18–26.

Fatmawati, M., Laili, M., Padaga, M.C. et al. (2020). Risk factors of toxoplasmosis in goat and sheep at Batu city. *Veterinary Practitioner* 21 (2): 345–349.

Ferguson, D.J.P. (2009). *Toxoplasma gondii*: 1908–2008, homage to Nicolle, Manceaux and Splendore. *Memórias do Instituto Oswaldo Cruz* 104: 133–148.

Ferguson, D.J.P. and Dubremetz, J.F. (2014). The ultrastructure of *Toxoplasma gondii*. In: *Toxoplasma gondii* (ed. L.M. Weiss and K. Kim), 19–59. Dordrecht, The Netherlands: Elsevier.

Fernandez-Escobar, M., Calero-Bernal, R., Benavides, J. et al. (2020). Isolation and genetic characterization of *Toxoplasma gondii* in Spanish sheep flocks. *Parasites and Vectors* 13: 396.

Frenkel, J.K., Dubey, J.P., and Miller, N.L. (1970). *Toxoplasma gondii* in cats: faecal stages identified as coccidian oocysts. *Science* 167: 893–896.

Garcia, G., Sotomaior, C., Nascimento, A.J. et al. (2012). Toxoplasma gondii in goats from Curitiba, Paraná, Brazil: risk factors and epidemiology. *Revista Brasileira de Parasitologia Veterinária* 21 (1): 42–47.

Giadinis, N.D., Terpsidis, K., Diakou, A. et al. (2011). Massive toxoplasma abortions in a dairy sheep flock and therapeutic approach with different doses of sulfadimidine. *Turkish Journal of Veterinary and Animal Sciences* 35 (3): 207–211.

Glor, S.B., Edelhofer, R., Grimm, F. et al. (2013). Evaluation of a commercial ELISA kit for detection of antibodies against *Toxoplasma gondii* in serum, plasma and meat juice from experimentally and naturally infected sheep. *Parasites and Vectors* 6: 85.

Halonen, S.K. and Weiss, L.M. (2013). Toxoplasmosis. In: *Handbook of Clinical Neurology*, Neuroparasitology and Tropical Neurology, vol. 114 (ed. H.H. Garcia, H.B. Tanowitz, and O.H. Del Brutto), 125–145. St Louis, MO: Elsevier.

Harding, C.R. and Frischknecht, F. (2020). The riveting cellular structures of apicomplexan parasites. *Trends in Parasitology* 36: 979–991.

Howe, D.K. and Sibley, D. (1995). *Toxoplasma gondii* comprises three clonal lineages: correlation of parasite genotype with human disease. *Journal of Infectious Diseases* 172: 1561–1566.

Innes, E.A. (2010). A brief history and overview of *Toxoplasma gondii*. *Zoonoses and Public Health* 57: 1–7.

Innes, E.A., Bartley, P.M., Buxton, D., and Katzer, F. (2009). Ovine toxoplasmosis. *Parasitology* 136: 1887–1894.

Jackson-O'Brien, D. (2010). Toxoplasmosis: common cause of abortion in sheep and goats. Delaware State University Cooperative Extension. https://cast.desu.edu/sites/cast/files/document/16/toxoplasmosis_fact_sheet_djo.pdf (accessed 18 December 2023).

Johnston, W.S. (1988). An investigation into toxoplasmosis as a cause of barrenness in ewes. *Veterinary Record* 122: 283–284.

Karthika, R., Devada, K., Lakshmanan, B. et al. (2021). Seroprevalence of *Toxoplasma gondii* in aborted goats in Kerala. *Journal of Veterinary and Animal Sciences* 52 (2): 166–170.

Khan, A., Bohme, U., Kelly, K.A. et al. (2006). Common inheritance of chromosome Ia associated with clonal expansion of *Toxoplasma gondii*. *Genome Research* 16: 1119–1125.

Khan, M.U., Rashid, I., Akbar, H. et al. (2017). Seroprevalence of *Toxoplasma gondii* in south Asian countries. *Revue Scientifique et Technique* 36: 3.

Kirkbride, C.A., Dubey, J., and Libal, M.C. (1992). Effect of feeding lasalocid to pregnant ewes experimentally infected with *Toxoplasma gondii*. *Veterinary Parasitology* 44: 299–303.

Knapen, F. and Overgaauw, P.A.M. (2008). Toxoplasmosis. *European Journal of Companion Animal Practice* 18 (3): 242–245.

Kniel, K.E., Lindsay, D.S., Sumner, S.S. et al. (2002). Examination of attachment and survival of *Toxoplasma gondii* oocysts on raspberries and blueberries. *Journal of Parasitology* 88: 790–793.

Kul, O., Yildiz, K., Ocal, N. et al. (2013). In-vivo efficacy of toltrazuril on experimentally induced *Toxoplasma gondii* tissue cysts in lambs: a novel strategy for prevention of human exposure to meat-borne toxoplasmosis. *Research in Veterinary Science* 94: 269–276.

Leite-Browning, L. M. (2006). Causes of infectious abortions in goats. Alabama Cooperative Extension System, 1–7.

Lin, M.H., Chen, T.C., Kuo, T. et al. (2000). Real-time PCR for quantitative detection of *Toxoplasma gondii*. *Journal of Clinical Microbiology* 38: 4121–4125.

Lindsay, D.S. and Dubey, J.P. (2020). Neosporosis, toxoplasmosis, and sarcocystosis in ruminants: an update. *Veterinary Clinics of North America: Food Animal Practice* 36: 205–222.

Mevelec, M.N., Lakhrif, Z., and Dimier-Poisson, I. (2020). Key limitations and new insights into the *Toxoplasma gondii* parasite stage switching for future vaccine development in human, livestock, and cats. *Frontiers in Cellular and Infection Microbiology* 10: 607198.

Mihu, A.G., Lupu, M.A., Nesiu, A. et al. (2022). Screening for the detection of *Toxoplasma gondii* IgG, IgM and IgA in females of reproductive age from western Romania. *Life* 12: 1771.

Montoya, J.G. and Liesenfeld, O. (2004). Toxoplasmosis. *Lancet* 363: 1965–1976.

Muhie, Y. and Kebkes, S. (2014). Toxoplasmosis: emerging and re-emerging zoonosis. *African Journal of Applied Microbiology Research* 3: 1–11.

Muralikrishna, P., Sunil, B., Savita, R.K. et al. (2017). Toxoplasmosis – the public health significance. *International Journal of Science, Environment and Technology* 6 (5): 2752–2758.

Nagy, B., Lazar, L., Nagy, G. et al. (2007). Detection of *Toxoplasma gondii* in amniotic fluid using quantitative real-time PCR method. *Orvosi Hetilap* 148: 935–938.

Nahar, S.F., Sah, R.P., Ashfia, K.M. et al. (2020). Seroprevalence of zoonotic protozoa *Toxoplasma gondii* infection in food animals of Chattogram division. *Research in Agriculture Livestock and Fisheries* 7 (2): 275–281.

Olivier, A., Herbert, B., Sava, B. et al. (2007). Surveillance and monitoring of Toxoplasma in humans, food and animals: a scientific opinion of the panel on biological hazards. *EFSA* 583: 1–64.

Pal, M., Alem, B., Gari, G., and Tuli, G. (2014). Toxoplasmosis in animals and humans – its diagnosis, epidemiology and control. *International Journal of Livestock Research* 4 (2): 1–10.

Pal, M., Berhanu, G., Steinmetz, C.H.D., and Durglishvili, N. (2021). Toxoplasmosis: an emerging and re-emerging zoonosis of global public health concern. *American Journal of Infectious Diseases and Microbiology* 9 (2): 32–38.

Pavlovic, I. and Ivanovic, S. (2005). Toxoplasmosis of goats and its role and importance in pathology of goat production. *Biotechnology in Animal Husbandry* 21 (5): 123–126.

Ramakrishnan, C., Maier, S., Walker, R.A. et al. (2019). An experimental genetically attenuated live vaccine to prevent transmission of *Toxoplasma gondii* by cats. *Scientific Reports* 9 (1): 1474.

Remington, J.S., McLeod, R., Thulliez, P. et al. (2001). Toxoplasmosis. In: *Infectious Diseases of the Foetus and Newborn Infant* (ed. J.S. Remington and J.O. Klein), 205–346. Philadelphia, PA: W. B. Saunders.

Robert-Gangneux, F. and Darde, M.L. (2012). Epidemiology of and diagnostic strategies for toxoplasmosis. *Clinical Microbiology Reviews* 25: 264–296.

Rodger, S.M., Maley, S.W., Wright, S.E. et al. (2006). Role of endogenous transplacental transmission in toxopasmosis in sheep. *Veterinary Record* 159: 768–772.

Sanchez-Sanchez, R., Vazquez, P., Ferre, I., and Ortega-Mora, L.M. (2018). Treatment of toxoplasmosis and neosporosis in farm ruminants: state of knowledge and future trends. *Current Topics in Medicinal Chemistry* 18: 1304–1323.

Shahbazi, G., Hoghooghi Rad, N., Madani, R. et al. (2019). *Toxoplasma gondii* in aborted fetuses of sheep in Ardebil Area, North-West of Iran. *Iranian Journal of Parasitology* 14 (3): 430–435.

Sharif, M., Gholami, S.H., Ziaei, H. et al. (2006). Seroprevalence of Toxoplasma gondii in cattle, sheep and goats slaughtered for food in Mazandaran province, Iran, during 2005. *Veterinary Journal* 174: 422–424.

Sibley, L.D., Khan, A., Ajioka, J.W., and Rosenthal, B.M. (2009). Genetic diversity of *Toxoplasma gondii* in animals and humans. *Philosophical Transactions of the Royal Society B* 364: 2749–2761.

Singh, S. and Nautiyal, B. (1991). Seroprevalence of toxoplasmosis in Kumaon region of India. *Indian Journal of Medical Research* 93: 247–249.

Spickler, A. R. 2017. Toxoplasmosis. Centers for Disease Control and Prevention. www.cfsph.iastate.edu/Factsheets/pdfs/toxoplasmosis.pdf

Steffen, K.D., Gos, M.L., Gortari, L. et al. (2021). Eleven years of *Toxoplasma gondii* serological follow-up in a goat herd and association of toxoplasmosis with reproductive losses. *Veterinary Parasitology: Regional Studies and Reports* 25: 100599.

Stelzer, S., Basso, W., Silvan, J.B. et al. (2019). *Toxoplasma gondii* infection and toxoplasmosis in farm animals: risk factors and economic impact. *Food and Waterborne Parasitology* 12: e00037.

Sukthana, Y., Waree, P., Pongponratn, E. et al. (2003). Pathologic study of acute toxoplasmosis in experimental animals. *Southeast Asian Journal of Tropical Medicine and Public Health* 34 (1): 1–17.

Webster, J.P. (2010). Review of "Toxoplasmosis of Animals and Humans (Second Edition)" by J.P. Dubey. *Parasites and Vectors* 3: 112.

World Organisation for Animal Health (2022). Toxoplasmosis. www.woah.org/fileadmin/Home/fr/Health_standards/tahm/3.10.08_TOXO.pdf (accessed 18 December 2023).

25

Infective Abortive Diseases: Q Fever

Bhavanam Sudhakara Reddy and Sirigireddy Sivajothi

College of Veterinary Science, Sri Venkateswara Veterinary University, Proddatur, Andhra Pradesh, India

25.1 Introduction

In goats, abortions at different stages of gestation are caused by either infectious or noninfectious agents. Noninfectious causes of abortion in goats include plant toxins (broom weed or locoweed poisoning), dietary deficiencies (copper, selenium, vitamin A, magnesium), and certain drugs (estrogen, glucocorticoids, phenothiazine, carbon tetrachloride, levamisole). Major infectious causes of abortions in goats are chlamydiosis, toxoplasmosis, leptospirosis, brucellosis, listeriosis, Q fever, and caprine herpes virus infection.

Brucella melitensis is the organism involved in abortions in animals with brucellosis. Abortions are sometimes accompanied by other systemic conditions like mastitis and lameness. In infected animals the placenta is grossly normal but in chronic cases it may develop uterine lesions (Megid et al. 2010; Ashenafi et al. 2007). Adult animals with infection are a source of infection lifelong and shed the organisms in milk. This can be controlled by the test and slaughter method (Tsehay et al. 2014; Ebrahimi et al. 2014). Caprine herpes virus 1 infection can cause vulvovaginitis, balanoposthitis, and respiratory disease in adult goats; enteric and systemic diseases in neonatal goats. Aborted fetuses are normal or sometimes autolyzed but it will not contain diagnostic gross lesions (Elhazary et al. 1984; Six et al. 2001). Microscopic identification of necrosis with the presence of intranuclear inclusion bodies in the liver, lungs, and other organs provides the initial diagnosis. All infected adult goats shed the virus and the infection remains latent (Williams et al. 1997; Tempesta et al. 1999).

Chlamydia abortus causes enzootic abortion of ewes and is the most common cause of abortion in goats. In a farm around 60% of pregnant does can abort or give birth to stillborn or weak kids if they have chlamydial infection. Abortions can occur at any stage of pregnancy but most are seen in the last month (Heidari et al. 2018). In addition to reproductive failure, concurrent respiratory disease, polyarthritis, conjunctivitis, and retained placentas are noticed. Aborted fetuses do not have any gross pathology changes but inflammation of the placenta with reddish brown exudate covering the cotyledons and intercotyledonary areas is present. *C. abortus* is zoonotic, occasionally causing serious disease in pregnant women (Kalender et al. 2013; Masala et al. 2005).

The most common serovars of *Leptospira* involved in caprine abortion are *grippotyphosa*, *pomona*, *icterohaemorrhagiae*, and *autumnalis*. Although sheep are relatively resistant to leptospirosis, goats are susceptible, with abortions occurring at the time of leptospiremia. Sometimes goats may have anemia, icterus, and hemoglobinemia in association with abortions. Leptospirosis is diagnosed by serology or identification of *Leptospira* spp. in the dam's urine, the placenta, or fetal kidney.

Listeria monocytogenes is a pathogen which can cause sporadic abortions in goats. There are no specific fetal lesions, and the fetus is often autolyzed, and goats may develop severe metritis after abortion. Diagnosis is by isolation from the placenta, abomasal contents, or uterine discharge (Barbuddhe et al. 2000; Kumar et al. 2007).

Toxoplasmosis is caused by the obligate intracellular protozoan *Toxoplasma gondii* which leads to abortion in goats. It is transmitted by ingestion of feed which may be contaminated with cat feces (Caldeira et al. 2011). Goats may exhibit the signs of fever, diarrhea, cough, dyspnea, icterus, seizures, and death. The agent causes abortions, mummification, stillbirths, and weak kids (Rahman et al. 2015; Tzanidakis et al. 2012).

In 1935, Q fever was first noticed in Queensland, Australia, as a febrile outbreak with unknown origin (query fever) among abattoir workers (Angelakis and Raoult 2010). Q fever is an OIE notifiable zoonotic disease and is poorly reported.

Elements of Reproduction and Reproductive Diseases of Goats, First Edition. Edited by Tanmoy Rana.

Domestic ruminants including cattle, sheep, and goats are the main reservoirs for the disease and it is also reported in humans, dogs, cats, birds, fish, reptiles, and arthropods (EFSA 2010).

The causal agent of Q fever is *Coxiella burnetii*, an obligate intracellular Gram-negative bacterium of the Legionellales order whose target cells are the macrophages located in body tissues (e.g., lymph nodes, spleen, lungs, liver) and the monocytes circulating in the bloodstream. Two different antigenic forms of *Coxiella burnetii* can be distinguished. The difference between phase I and phase II bacterial forms resides in the variation of the surface lipopolysaccharide (LPS) as classically described for enterobacteria (Amano and Williams 1984). Only phase I bacteria have a complete LPS on their surface and are virulent. Phase I bacteria can be isolated from a naturally infected individual or from animals infected in a laboratory (Krt 2003). On the other hand, phase II bacteria have an incomplete LPS due to a spontaneous genetic deletion of 25 992 bp and are nonvirulent (Setiyono et al. 2005). Phase II bacteria occur during serial passage in an immunologically incompetent host, such as cell cultures or fertilized eggs (Thompson et al. 2003). The deleted chromosomal region comprises a high number of genes that are predicted to function in LPS or lipooligosaccharide biosynthesis, as well as in general carbohydrate and sulfur metabolism (Hoover et al. 2002).

Antigenic variation of *Coxiella burnetii* is important for serological diagnosis and elaboration of vaccines. Indeed, serologically, anti-phase II antibodies (IgG and IgM) are found at high levels in acute Q fever, whereas anti-phase I antibodies (IgG and IgA) are found at high levels only during chronic infection. Moreover, host factors seem to be more important than genomic variation for development of acute or chronic infection (Scola et al. 1998). According to a recent report by the OIE, no specific genotype is associated with acute or chronic infection, with a particular clinical outcome, or with a specific host.

25.2 Transmission and Spread

Coxiella burnetii is shed in the milk, urine, and feces of infected goats. Most importantly, during parturition, huge concentrations of bacteria, up to a billion per cubic centimeter, are found in the amniotic fluids and placenta which will contaminate the environment. When the agent occurs outside the animal, it becomes a small, dense, long-lasting spore-like form which is able to resist hot environmental conditions. In later stages, it contaminates the air and mixes with dust particles and is therefore further spread by the wind for long distances (Amano and Williams 1984). The organisms are highly contagious and can be inhaled which can cause clinical illness in affected living beings.

Most disease outbreaks occur immediately following abortions in which the environment is contaminated with amniotic fluids and uterine discharges. The agent is also spread by tick bites which pass the bacteria from an infected animal to other susceptible animals, and whose feces contain the bacteria, thus also contaminating the environment. Since it is also shed in the milk of an infected animal, it can be contracted by drinking unpasteurized infected milk (Figures 25.1 and 25.2) (Scola et al. 1998).

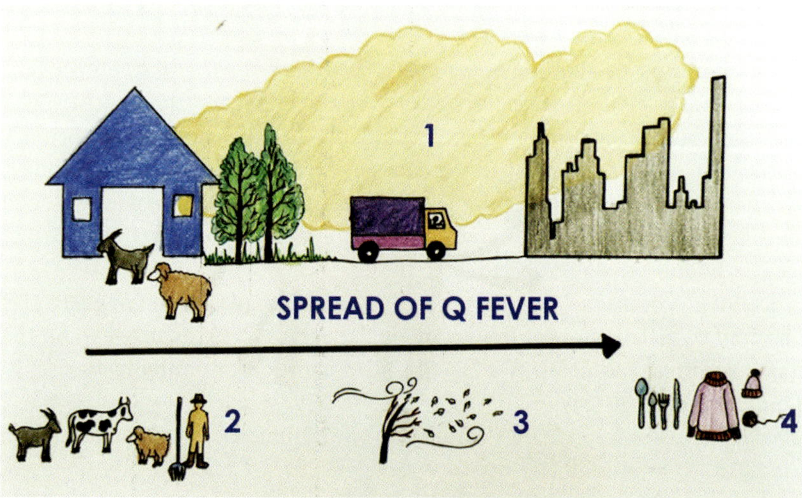

Figure 25.1 Spread of Q fever among the population. 1. Aerosol. 2. Human contacts. 3. Contact with plants. 4. Instrumentations.

25.3 Routes of Infection

Inhalation is the most common route of infection in both animals and humans (Russell-Lodrigue et al. 2006). Infected animals contaminate the environment by shedding *C. burnetii* in milk, feces, urine, saliva and, very importantly, in vaginal secretions, placenta, amniotic fluids, and other products of conception (Guatteo et al. 2007). *Coxiella burnetii* also spreads by the wind, causing infections at a distance from the initial source of bacteria. In domestic ruminants, milk is the most frequent route of pathogen shedding. The OIE advises not to drink raw milk originating from infected farms. If infection by the oral route is proven to be efficient, the sufficient number of pathogens capable of causing Q fever should be determined. Currently, risk of transmission through blood transfusion is considered negligible (Delsing and Kullberg 2008). Transplacental transmission, intradermal inoculation, and postmortem examinations have been associated with sporadic cases of Q fever (Bildfell et al. 2000).

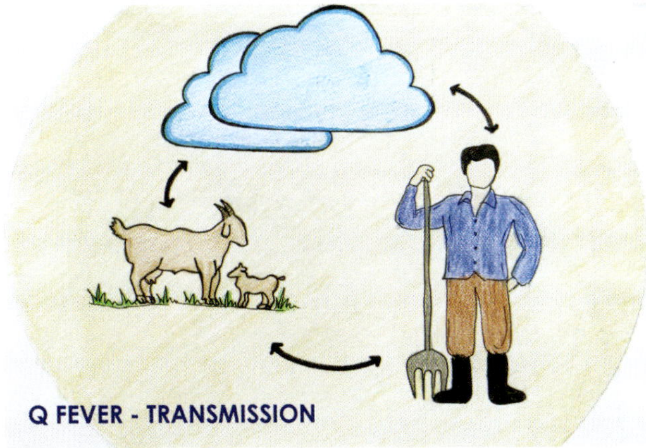

Figure 25.2 Transmission of Q fever (humans–animals–aerosol).

In many countries, goats are the most common source of human infection due to their extensive close contact with humans. Q fever in goats can induce pneumonia, abortions, stillbirth, and delivery of weak kids, the latter two clinical signs being the most frequently observed (Vaidya et al. 2008). Commonly, abortions are reported in the last month of gestation (Berri et al. 2005). Most goats with natural infection are limited to shedding the organisms in the kidding season following infection. In some experimental studies, organisms were shed during two successive kidding seasons in vaginal mucus and milk (Berri et al. 2007). Moreover, shedding in milk can be maintained for a long period. Milk has been considered the major route of bacteria excretion for this species (Figure 25.3).

25.4 Pathogenesis

The most important route of infection is inhalation of bacteria-contaminated dust, while the oral route is considered of secondary importance. Once inhaled or ingested, the extracellular form of *C. burnetii* attaches itself to a cell membrane and is internalized into the host cells. Phagolysosomes are formed after the fusion of phagosomes with cellular acidic lysosomes. The multiple intracellular phagolysosomes eventually fuse together, leading to the formation of a large unique vacuole (Rousset et al. 2009). *Coxiella burnetii* has adapted to the phagolysosomes of eukaryotic cells and is capable of multiplying in the acidic vacuoles. Multiplication of *C. burnetii* can be stopped by raising the phagolysosomal pH using lysosomotropic agents such as chloroquine (Raoult et al. 1990).

Hill and Samuel (2011) analyzed *C. burnetii*'s genome and identified two acid phosphatase enzymes. They demonstrated experimentally that both a recombinant acid phosphatase (rACP) enzyme and *C. burnetii* extracts had a

Figure 25.3 Different routes of infection in goats.

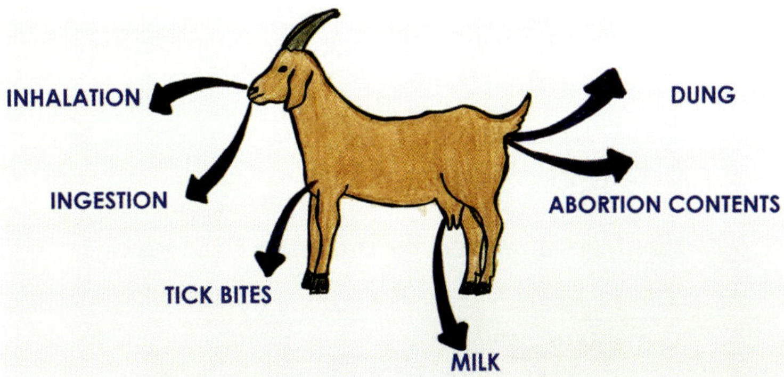

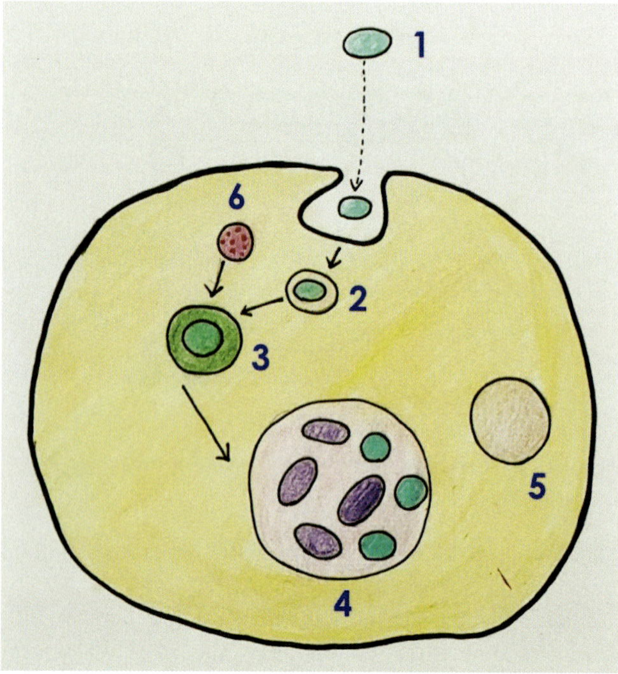

Figure 25.4 Pathogenesis of Q fever. 1. *C. burnetii* organisms. 2. Nascent *Chlamydia*-containing vacuole (CCV). 3. Maturation of CCV. 4. Mature CCV. 5. Nucleus. 6. Lysosomes.

pH-dependent acid phosphatase activity. Inhibition of the assembly of the NADPH oxidase complex was found to be the mechanism involved. The intracellular cycle of *C. burnetii* leads to the formation of two developmental stages of the bacterium known as small-cell variant (SCV) and large-cell variant (LCV). SCV is the extracellular form of the bacterium. SCVs are considered to be metabolically inactive and capable of resisting extreme conditions such as heat, desiccation, high or low pH, disinfectants, chemical products, osmotic pressure, and UV rays (Samuel 2000). SCVs of *C. burnetii* are reversible. Indeed, once inhaled or ingested, the SCV attaches itself to a cell membrane and is internalized. After phagolysosomal fusion, the acidity of the newly formed vacuole induces activation of SCV metabolism and its development into the LCV (Coleman et al. 2004). LCVs are considered to be the metabolically active intracellular form of *C. burnetii* which are more pleomorphic than SCVs. Their cell wall is thinner and they have a more dispersed filamentous nucleoid region. Intracellular growth is relatively slow with a doubling time of approximately 8–12 hours. LCVs can differentiate into spore-like bacteria by binary asymmetrical division. The endogenous spore-like forms can undergo further development and metabolic changes until finally reaching the SCV form. Finally, cell lysis, or possibly exocytosis, releases the resistant bacteria into the extracellular media.

Most natural infections by *C. burnetii* are probably due to SCV or pseudospores present in the environment. Studies on the immune reaction in naturally or experimentally infected individuals have suggested that cellular immunity and the synthesis of IFN-γ are essential for control of *C. burnetii* infection (Shannon et al. 2009). In chronic infections, peripheral blood lymphocytes do not proliferate when exposed to *C. burnetii* antigens despite proliferating when exposed to other antigens or mitogens which were not observed in acute infection (Koster et al. 1985) (Figure 25.4).

25.5 Clinical Signs

In livestock, the infection is usually subclinical. It may produce abortion in late pregnancy, stillbirths, retained placenta, inflammation of the lining of the uterus, infertility, and small or weak offspring. Most animals are asymptomatic but goats will have decreased appetite and may be depressed for one or two days before an abortion. However, disease occurs most frequently in the form of abortion outbreaks in goats. Susceptible pregnant females develop necrotizing placentitis, which results in late-term abortion. Some ewes and does abort without apparent clinical signs, whereas others show anorexia and depression one to two days before aborting (Figures 25.5 and 25.6).

25.6 Diagnosis

25.6.1 Direct Visualization of the Organisms on Smears

Direct visualization of *C. burnetii* on smears or frozen tissue is the most simple method for Q fever diagnosis. Placenta of aborted goats and/or stomach contents of the fetus should be collected from suspected cases with Q fever. *Coxiella burnetii* does not stain reliably with Gram stain but needs special staining (Macc staining – Stamp/Macchiavello)

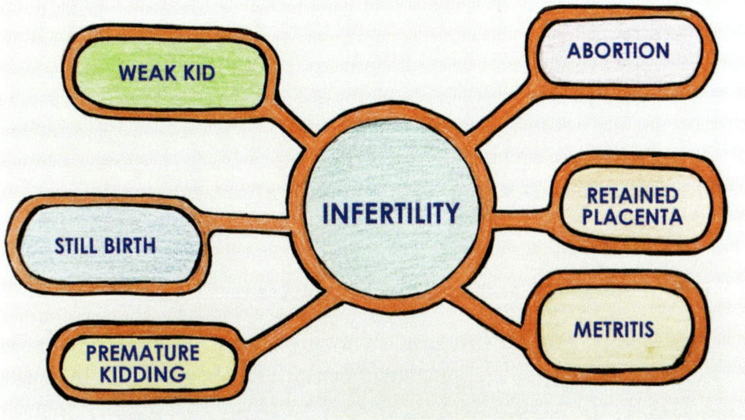

Figure 25.5 Clinical signs in goats with Q fever.

(Hogerwerf et al. 2011). The specificity and sensitivity of direct visualization by bacterioscopic examination are very low and there can be similarity with pathogens such as *Brucella* spp., *Chlamydophila* spp., or *Chlamydia* spp.

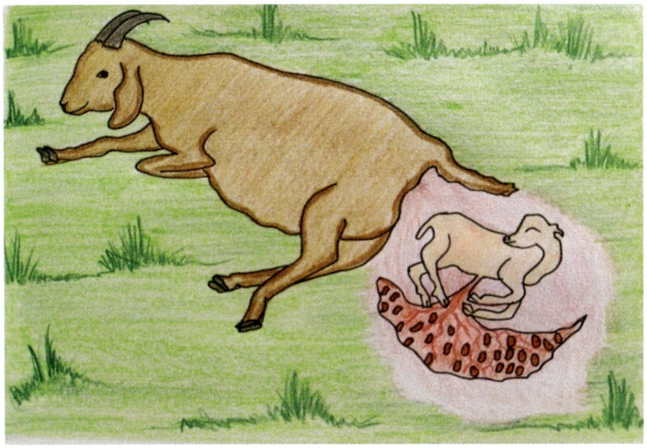

Figure 25.6 Goat with Q fever showing the aborted kid with changes in the placenta and cotyledons.

25.6.2 Immunohistochemistry (IHC)

Immunohistochemistry has been performed for the diagnosis of subclinical or chronic cases of Q fever in small ruminants. It is used to detect *C. burnetii* in tissue samples fixed in paraffin or acetone smears. Dilbeck and McElwain (Omsland et al. 2009) developed an avidin-biotin-peroxidase complex IHC staining method for diagnosis and routine screening of ovine and caprine placental tissues after abortion. This method is rapid and does not require live organisms or fresh tissues for diagnosis but it is not useful for screening of large samples in suspected outbreaks.

25.6.3 Bacterial Culture

The gold standard diagnostic method for diagnosis of Q fever is bacterial culture. *Coxiella burnetii* can be cultured efficiently in the yolk sac of chicken embryos or human embryonic lung fibroblasts, mosquito cells, and green monkey kidney (Vero) cells (Scola et al. 1998). Sensitivity of the culture is limited and it is a difficult process which requires a level 3 biosafety laboratory for the isolation studies. In one study, *C. burnetii* was grown outside a host cell in a cell-free laboratory medium composed of the organism's metabolic requirements in the phagolysosome (Hogerwerf et al. 2011). As a result of the difficulty, culture is rarely performed, especially in veterinary medicine (Fournier et al. 1998).

25.6.4 Polymerase Chain Reaction (PCR)

Polymerase chain reaction is useful in the diagnosis of early clinical stages of illness (Frangoulidis et al. 2009). This method can be used to detect the DNA of *C. burnetii* in various clinical samples and experimental study samples (Ughetto et al. 2009). However, quantification of bacteria is limited. To quantify the bacteria present in the samples, real-time quantitative PCR was developed and can be used to screen the large-scale studies. Negative serology is most frequent in Q fever cases where sampling has been performed within two weeks of illness (Hou et al. 2011). PCR and RTq PCR are considered the methods of choice for DNA detection in different types of samples. However, PCR and RTq PCR are incapable of distinguishing bacterial DNA from live and/or dead bacteria. The disadvantage is that interpretation of positive results in fresh samples can be difficult (Tatsumi et al. 2006).

25.6.5 Complement Fixation Test (CFT)

The complement fixation test is the most preferred indirect test for serological diagnosis of Q fever in small ruminants. It is capable of detecting approximately 65% of infected subjects during the second week after initial clinical signs and 90% during the fourth week. the CFT is more laborious, less specific, and less sensitive than indirect immunofluorescence assay (IFA) or enzyme-linked immunosorbent assay (ELISA). Rousset et al. (2007) suggested that the CFT should not be used for serological animal screening because of its low sensitivity.

25.6.6 Enzyme-Linked Immunosorbent Assay

This method is more sensitive and easier to perform and to standardize than the CFT (Frangoulidis et al. 2009). Moreover, a strong association was reported between strongly positive ELISA results and the occurrence of abortion in goats (Tatsumi et al. 2006).

25.6.7 Immunofluorescence Assay

The immunofluorescence assay is commonly considered the reference diagnostic test as it is accurate, highly sensitive, and specific and is the most frequently used test worldwide (Shannon et al. 2009). One study reported that IFA results obtained on sera of aborting and nonaborting goats were significantly different and were associated with occurrence of abortion (Rousset et al. 2007). Moreover, the IFA is capable of detecting the two antigenic variants of *C. burnetii* (phase I and phase II). As mentioned previously, in acute infections, anti-phase II antibodies are detected. In chronic infections, anti-phase I and anti-phase II antibodies are present but anti-phase I antibodies predominate (Shannon et al. 2009).

The preferential use of the IFA instead of CFT in veterinary medicine would be advantageous for diagnosis and control of Q fever. The IFA is currently the gold standard test for serology. The dependence of CFT, IFA, and ELISA on the presence of antibodies limits their diagnostic value. Indeed, specific antibodies are often absent during the first two to three weeks of infection, making early diagnosis by serology difficult, if not impossible (Fournier et al. 1998). In Q fever, phase II antibodies can be detected within two weeks of infection in most cases and within three weeks 90% are seropositive. The global clinical and epidemiological context must be taken into account as well as the limitations of diagnostic assays. Bacteriological analyses are necessary to confirm any suspicion of Q fever (Rousset et al. 2007).

25.6.8 Skin Test

A skin test method was proposed to investigate the cellular response and to improve detection of infected cows at herd level (Shannon et al. 2009). The skin test consists of an intradermal injection of extremely diluted inactivated vaccine which induces an antigenic reaction. If the animal has previously been infected by Q fever, a nodule of variable size will appear at the site of injection. This test could easily be applied by rural practitioners.

25.6.9 Diagnosis by Histopathology

In acute cases of hepatitis, the presence of doughnut granulomas can be visualized in histopathology hepatic specimens but they are not pathognomonic of Q fever. However, in chronic infections, granulomas are less organized but bacteria can be detected in large vacuoles (Frangoulidis et al. 2009). As mentioned above, in bovids, placentitis was found to be significantly associated with *C. burnetii* infection. Placental necrosis is significantly associated with the presence of *C. burnetii*. Chorionic epithelial cells and villus tips are the most frequently affected. Infected trophoblasts are distended and contain basophilic granular to foamy material. The cytoplasm of infected cells appears bright red with Macc stain, and their nuclei are commonly eccentric. A modified Koster's acid-fast (MAF) staining of fresh placenta smears is considered a good screening test, but confirmation by immunohistochemical techniques remains necessary (Koster et al. 1985). In endocarditis lesions, *C. burnetii* is visible as a voluminous intracytoplasmic mass within infected mononuclear cells (Frangoulidis et al. 2009).

25.7 Control Methods and Vaccination

During a Q fever outbreak, sanitary and prophylactic measures should be applied at herd level, in order to limit disease transmission. Early diagnosis and treatment are essential to prevent the development of chronic infections and secondary complications. There is a possibility to spread the infection from manure of infected herds until 90 days after suspicion of infection. The effectiveness of this measure must be evaluated and modified if necessary (Brouqui et al. 1994). Adding 0.5% of calcium to contaminated dung is an effective disinfectant. Milk from the remainder of the flock can be used for transformation, unless it is highly suspected that dairy products originating from these animals are dangerous for human consumption. In the latter case, the milk must be pasteurized at 72 °C for 15 minutes or by an equivalent thermal treatment (Cerf and Condron 2006). Guidelines suggest the use of 2% formaldehyde, 1% lysol, 5% hydrogen peroxide, 70% ethanol, or 5% chloroform for decontamination of surfaces, and spills of contaminated material should be dealt with immediately using hypochlorite, 5% peroxide, or phenol-based solutions. High-risk material (contaminated bedding, placenta, aborted fetuses) should be buried with lime or incinerated. Vaccination should be scheduled in herds presenting a PCR-positive BTM result, and pools of 10 individual milk samples should be tested by PCR to identify shedding animals.

In goats, the inactivated phase I vaccine protects efficiently against abortion and has been shown to prevent bacterial shedding in vaginal mucus, feces, and particularly in milk. However, vaccination proved more effective in nulliparous animals than in parous animals. Furthermore, vaccination did not clear infection in previously infected goats. Vaccination of previously infected animals and of native animals during pregnancy proved ineffective.

New vaccines, such as recombinant vaccines, have been developed. Several of these vaccines have proven to be antigenic but nonprotective. Others still require an investigation of their effectiveness in field conditions (Waag 2007). An inactivated phase II vaccine, Chlamyvax FQ®, has also been tested on animals but was not effective (Rousset et al. 2009).

Gefenaite et al. (2011) concluded that generalization of the results to the general population or to a specific risk group was not possible. The authors advised more blinded, randomized, and unbiased research on Qvax effectiveness. Development of recombinant protein subunit vaccines has proven disappointing (Zhang et al. 1994).

Before initiating a vaccination program, epidemiological knowledge of the area is necessary. Indeed, in endemic regions, vaccination is impossible for practical reasons (screening) and noneffective as a preventive measure. However, vaccination could be beneficial for at-risk individuals such as pregnant or immunocompromised individuals, farmers, veterinarians, abattoir workers, and research and reference laboratory personnel in contact with *C. burnetii* (Cerf and Condron 2006).

25.8 Perspectives for the Future

A better knowledge of Q fever would improve diagnostic procedures, control, and prevention of the disease in the future. A better understanding of the bacterium and its pathogenesis (entry into the cell, "sporulation-like" phenomenon, metabolism, mechanism of resistance to acidic conditions, infectivity of the bacterium, survival time in the environment under different management practices) is essential. The veterinary aspects of Q fever also necessitate further investigations. Indeed, the effect of antibiotic treatment on shedding of bacteria in ruminants has been insufficiently studied.

25.9 Conclusion

Q fever is an underestimated disease that remains poorly understood. The lack of awareness of this disease leads to underdiagnosing and underreporting of Q fever cases. Q fever is ubiquitous, and the potential hosts for the infectious bacteria are extremely numerous. Q fever infections can have a significant economical impact on animal reproduction, animal trade, and the production and commercialization of animal products. In small ruminant flocks, the consequences of Q fever can be disastrous.

Its zoonotic potential renders Q fever even more important. Human infections can lead to death. Furthermore, with advances in human medicine, the number of immunosuppressed, premature, elderly, and chronically ill individuals has greatly increased in recent years. Thus, the population predisposed to infection, and especially to chronic infection, has also greatly increased. Chronic infections can lead to severe consequences that necessitate intense medical treatment, increasing public health costs and patient suffering. Early diagnosis and early initiation of treatment are essential to improve prognosis by preventing the development of a chronic infection or other potential complications associated with coxiellosis.

References

Amano, K.I. and Williams, J.C. (1984). Chemical and immunological characterization of lipopolysaccharides from phase I and phase II *Coxiella burnetii*. *Journal of Bacteriology* 160 (3): 994–1002.

Angelakis, E. and Raoult, D. (2010). Q fever. *Veterinary Microbiology* 140 (3): 297–309.

Ashenafi, F., Teshale, S., Ejeta, G. et al. (2007). Distribution of brucellosis among small ruminants in the pastoral region of Afar, eastern Ethiopia. *Revue Scientifique et Technique* 26: 731–739.

Barbuddhe, S.B., Malik, S.V.S., Bhilegaonkar, K.N. et al. (2000). Isolation of *Listeria monocytogenes* and anti-listeriolysin O detection in sheep and goats. *Small Ruminant Research* 38: 151–155.

Berri, M., Rousset, E., and Hechard, C. (2005). Progression of Q fever and *Coxiella burnetii* shedding in milk after an outbreak of enzootic abortion in a goat herd. *Veterinary Record* 156 (17): 548–549.

Berri, M., Rousset, E., Champion, J.L. et al. (2007). Goats may experience reproductive failures and shed *Coxiella burnetii* at two successive parturitions after a Q fever infection. *Research in Veterinary Science* 83 (1): 47–52.

Bildfell, R.J., Thomson, G.W., Haines, D.M. et al. (2000). *Coxiella burnetii* infection is associated with placentitis in cases of bovine abortion. *Journal of Veterinary Diagnostic Investigation* 12 (5): 419–425.

Brouqui, P., Dumler, J.S., and Raoult, D. (1994). Immunohistologic demonstration of *Coxiella burnetii* in the valves of patients with Q fever endocarditis. *American Journal of Medicine* 36 (5): 451–458.

Caldeira, F.H.B., Ubiali, D.G., de Godoy, I. et al. (2011). Outbreak of caprine abortion by *Toxoplasma gondii* in Midwest Brazil. *Pesquisa Veterinaria Brasileira* 31: 933–937.

Cerf, O. and Condron, R. (2006). *Coxiella burnetii* and milk pasteurization: an early application of the precautionary principle. *Epidemiology and Infection* 134 (5): 946–951.

Coleman, S.A., Fischer, E.R., Howe, D. et al. (2004). Temporal analysis of *Coxiella burnetii* morphological differentiation. *Journal of Bacteriology* 186 (21): 7344–7352.

Delsing, C.E. and Kullberg, B.J. (2008). Q fever in the Netherlands: a concise overview and implications of the largest ongoing outbreak. *Netherlands Journal of Medicine* 66 (9): 365–367.

Ebrahimi, A., Milan, J.S.K., Mahzoonieh, M.R., and Khadije, K. (2014). Shedding rates and seroprevalence of *B. melitensis* in lactating goats of Shahrekord, Iran. *Jundishapur Journal of Microbiology* 7: 93–94.

EFSA (2010). Development of harmonized schemes for the monitoring and reporting of Q-fever in animals in the European Union. www.efsa.europa.eu/en/supporting/pub/en-48 (accessed 14 December 2023).

Elhazary, M.A.S.Y., Silim, A., and Dea, S. (1984). Prevalence of antibodies to bovine respiratory syncytial virus, bovine viral diarrhea virus, bovine herpesvirus-1, and bovine parainfluenza-3 virus in sheep and goats in Quebec. *American Journal of Veterinary Research* 45: 1660–1662.

Fournier, P.E., Marrie, T.J., and Raoult, D. (1998). Diagnosis of Q fever. *Journal of Clinical Microbiology* 36 (7): 1823–1834.

Frangoulidis, D., Rodolakis, A., Heiser, V. et al. (2009). DNA microarray-chip based diagnosis of Q-fever (*Coxiella burnetii*). *Clinical Microbiology and Infection* 15 (2): 165–166.

Gefenaite, G., Munster, J.M., Houdt, R.V., and Hak, E. (2011). Effectiveness of the Q fever vaccine: a meta-analysis. *Vaccine* 29 (3): 395–398.

Guatteo, R., Beaudeau, F., Ledoux, D. et al. (2007). Risk of false-negative results when delaying PCR from sampling for *Coxiella burnetii* detection in dairy cows. *Revue de Médecine Vétérinaire* 158 (12): 641–644.

Heidari, S., Derakhshandeh, A., and Firouzi, R. (2018). Molecular detection of *Chlamydophila abortus*, *Coxiella burnetii*, and *Mycoplasma agalactiae* in small ruminants' aborted fetuses in southern Iran. *Tropical Animal Health and Production* 50 (4): 779–785.

Hill, J. and Samuel, J.E. (2011). *Coxiella burnetii* acid phosphatase inhibits the release of reactive oxygen intermediates in polymorphonuclear leukocytes. *Infection and Immunity* 79 (1): 414–420.

Hogerwerf, L., Brom, R., and Roest, H.I.J. (2011). Reduction of *Coxiella burnetii* prevalence by vaccination of goats and sheep, The Netherlands. *Emerging Infectious Diseases* 17 (3): 379–386.

Hoover, T.A., Culp, D.W., Vodkin, M.H. et al. (2002). Chromosomal DNA deletions explain phenotypic characteristics of two antigenic variants, phase II and RSA 514 (crazy), of the *Coxiella burnetii* nine mile strain. *Infection and Immunity* 70 (12): 6726–6733.

Hou, M.Y., Hung, M.N., and Lin, P.S. (2011). Use of a single-tube nested real-time PCR assay to facilitate the early diagnosis of acute Q fever. *Japanese Journal of Infectious Diseases* 64 (2): 161–162.

Kalender, H., Kilic, A., and Eroksuz, H. (2013). Identification of *Chlamydophila abortus* infection in aborting ewes and goats in eastern Turkey. *Revue de Médecine Vétérinaire* 164 (6): 295–301.

Koster, F.T., Williams, J.C., and Goodwin, J.S. (1985). Cellular immunity in Q fever: specific lymphocyte unresponsiveness in Q fever endocarditis. *Journal of Infectious Diseases* 152 (6): 1283–1289.

Krt, B. (2003). The influence of *Coxiella burnetti* phase I and phase II antigens on the serological diagnosis of Q fever in cattle. *Slovenian Veterinary Research* 40: 203–207.

Kumar, H.B., Singh, B., Bal, M.S. et al. (2007). Pathological and epidemiological investigations into listerial encephalitis in sheep. *Small Ruminant Research* 71: 293–297.

Masala, G., Porcu, R., and Sanna, G. (2005). Role of *Chlamydophila abortus* in ovine and caprine abortion in Sardinia, Italy. *Veterinary Research Communications* 29: 117–123.

Megid, J., Mathias, L.A., and Robles, C.A. (2010). Clinical manifestations of brucellosis in domestic animals and humans. *Open Veterinary Science Journal* 4: 119–126.

Omsland, A., Cockrell, D.C., and Howe, D. (2009). Host cell free growth of the Q fever bacterium *Coxiella burnetii*. *Proceedings of the National Academy of Sciences of the United States of America* 106 (11): 4430–4434.

Rahman, M., Alauddin, M., Hossain, K.M.M. et al. (2015). Prevalence and dynamics of antibodies against *Toxoplasma gondii* in kids born from naturally infected goats. *Parasitology International* 64: 389–391.

Raoult, D., Drancourt, M., and Vestris, G. (1990). Bactericidal effect of doxycycline associated with lysosomotropic agents on *Coxiella burnetii* in P388D1 cells. *Antimicrobial Agents and Chemotherapy* 34 (8): 1512–1514.

Rousset, E., Durand, B., and Berri, M. (2007). Comparative diagnostic potential of three serological tests for abortive Q fever in goat herds. *Veterinary Microbiology* 124 (3): 286–297.

Rousset, E., Berri, M., and Durand, B. (2009). *Coxiella burnetii* shedding routes and antibody response after outbreaks of Q fever-induced abortion in dairy goat herds. *Applied and Environmental Microbiology* 75 (2): 428–433.

Russell-Lodrigue, K.E., Zhang, G.Q., McMurray, D.N., and Samuel, J.E. (2006). Clinical and pathologic changes in a guinea pig aerosol challenge model of acute Q fever. *Infection and Immunity* 74 (11): 6085–6091.

Samuel, J.E. (2000). Developmental cycle of *Coxiella burnetii*. In: *Procaryotic Development* (ed. Y.V. Brun and L.J. Shimkets), 427–440. Washington, DC: ASM Press.

Scola, B.L., Lepidi, H., Maurin, M., and Raoult, D. (1998). A guinea pig model for Q fever endocarditis. *Journal of Infectious Diseases* 178 (1): 278–281.

Setiyono, A., Ogawa, M., Cai, Y. et al. (2005). New criteria for immunofluorescence assay for Q fever diagnosis in Japan. *Journal of Clinical Microbiology* 43 (11): 5555–5559.

Shannon, J.G., Cockrell, D.C., Takahashi, K. et al. (2009). Antibody-mediated immunity to the obligate intracellular bacterial pathogen *Coxiella burnetii* is Fc receptor- and complement-independent. *BMC Immunology* 10–16.

Six, A., Banks, M., Engels, M. et al. (2001). Latency and reactivation of bovine herpesvirus 1 (BHV-1) in goats and of caprine herpesvirus 1 (CapHV-1) in calves. *Archives of Virology* 146: 1325–1335.

Tatsumi, N., Baumgartner, A., Qiao, Y. et al. (2006). Detection of *Coxiella burnetii* in market chicken eggs and mayonnaise. *Annals of the New York Academy of Sciences* 1078: 502–505.

Tempesta, M., Pratelli, A., Corrente, M., and Buonavoglia, C. (1999). A preliminary study on the pathogenicity of a strain of caprine herpesvirus-1. *Comparative Immunology, Microbiology and Infectious Diseases* 22: 137–143.

Thompson, H.A., Hoover, T.A., Vodkin, M.H., and Shaw, E.I. (2003). Do chromosomal deletions in the lipopolysaccharide 14 International Journal of Microbiology biosynthetic regions explain all cases of phase variation in *Coxiella burnetii* strains? An update. *Annals of the New York Academy of Sciences* 990: 664–670.

Tsehay, H., Getachew, G., Morka, A. et al. (2014). Seroprevalence of brucellosis in small ruminants in pastoral areas of Oromia and Somalia regional states, Ethiopia. *Journal of Veterinary Medicine and Animal Health* 6 (11): 289–294.

Tzanidakis, N., Maksimov, P., Conraths, F.J. et al. (2012). *Toxoplasma gondii* in sheep and goats: seroprevalence and potential risk factors under dairy husbandry practices. *Veterinary Parasitology* 190: 340–348.

Ughetto, E., Gouriet, F., Raoult, D., and Rolain, J.M. (2009). Three years experience of real-time PCR for the diagnosis of Q fever. *Clinical Microbiology and Infection* 15 (2): 200–201.

Vaidya, V.M., Malik, S.V.S., Kaur, S. et al. (2008). Comparison of PCR, immunofluorescence assay, and pathogen isolation for diagnosis of Q fever in humans with spontaneous abortions. *Journal of Clinical Microbiology* 46 (6): 2038–2044.

Waag, D.M. (2007). *Coxiella burnetii*: host and bacterial responses to infection. *Vaccine* 25 (42): 7288–7295.

Williams, N.M., Vickers, M.L., Tramontin, R.R. et al. (1997). Multiple abortions associated with caprine herpesvirus infection in a goat herd. *Journal of the American Veterinary Medical Association* 211: 89–91.

Zhang, Y.X., Zhi, N., Yu, S.R. et al. (1994). Protective immunity induced by 67 K outer membrane protein of phase I *Coxiella burnetii* in mice and guinea pigs. *Acta Virologica* 38 (6): 327–332.

26

Infectious Abortive Diseases: Brucellosis

Shivangi Udainiya[1], *Amita Tiwari*[2], *Brejesh Singh*[2], *and Manoj Kumar Ahirwar*[3]

[1] *Veterinary Polytechnic College, Nanaji Deshmukh Veterinary Science University, Bhopal, India*
[2] *Department of Veterinary Medicine, College of Veterinary Science and Animal Husbandry, Jabalpur, India*
[3] *Department of Veterinary Surgery and Radiology, College of Veterinary Science and Animal Husbandry, Jabalpur, India*

26.1 Introduction

Brucellosis is also known as caprine brucellosis, undulant fever, Malta fever, Mediterranean fever, contagious abortion or Bang disease. In humans, it is known as undulant fever, because of the severe intermittent fever accompanying human infection, or Malta fever because it was first recognized as a human disease on the island of Malta. Brucellosis is the common name used for the animal and human infections caused by several species of the genus *Brucella*, mainly *Brucella abortus*, *B. melitensis*, and *B. suis*. *Brucella melitensis* is the main causative agent of infection with *Brucella* in sheep and goats. Sporadic infections caused by *B. abortus* or *B. suis* have been observed in goats, but such cases are extremely rare. *B. melitensis* infection in goats is very similar to *B. abortus* infection in cattle. *Brucella melitensis* occurs naturally in sheep and goats and is highly pathogenic for humans, causing one of the most serious zoonoses in the world.

The disease is responsible for considerable economic losses to the small ruminant industry (OIE 2009). It is a serious disease of livestock that has significant animal health, public health, and international trade consequences. Considering the damage done by the infection in animals – decreased milk production, weight loss, loss of young, infertility, and lameness – this disease is a formidable threat to livestock. The fact that this disease can spread rapidly and be transmitted to humans makes it all the more serious. Sheep and goat brucellosis is endemic in most countries of the Mediterranean basin, the Middle East and Central Asia (Al-Majali 2005), Latin America, and parts of Africa (Benkirane 2006).

Clinically, infection with *Brucella* in goats is characterized by one or more of the following signs: abortion, infertility, retained placenta, orchitis, epididymitis, and, rarely, arthritis, with excretion of the organisms in uterine discharges, milk, urine, and semen. Unequivocal diagnosis depends on the isolation of *Brucella* from abortion material, udder secretions or tissues removed at postmortem. *Brucella abortus*, *B. melitensis*, and *B. suis* are highly pathogenic for humans, and potentially contaminated tissues, cultures, and materials must be handled under appropriate containment conditions.

In most circumstances, the primary transmission routes of *Brucella* are the placenta, fetal fluids, and vaginal discharges expelled by infected ewes and goats at and up to several months following abortion or parturition. Shedding of *Brucella* is also common in udder secretions and semen, and *Brucella* may be isolated from various tissues, such as lymph nodes from the head, spleen, and organs associated with reproduction (uterus, epididymides and testes), and from arthritic lesions (Alton et al. 1988).

26.2 Etiology

The disease is caused by a group of bacteria known scientifically as the genus *Brucella*. Brucellosis caused by *B. melitensis* in goats is an infectious bacterial disease that can affect most domestic animals. *Brucella melitensis* is a Gram-negative coccobacillus which belongs to the family Brucellaceae and class Alphaproteobacteria. The organisms of *Brucella* are

Elements of Reproduction and Reproductive Diseases of Goats, First Edition. Edited by Tanmoy Rana.

facultatively intracellular bacteria. *In vivo*, they often occur within the cytoplasm of cells in closely packed clusters (Corbel and Brinley-Morgan 1984).

They are partially acid fast as they are not decolorized by 0.5% acetic acid in the modified Ziehl–Neelsen (MZN) stain (Alton et al. 1988). Flagella, endospore, and capsule are absent although capsule-like structures have been reported in preparations treated with antiserum. Most strains require anaerobic conditions, optimal temperature of 37 °C, and supplemented CO_2 for growth. All strains lose viability at 56 °C. Optimal pH conditions are from 6.6 to 7.4. *Brucella* strains are fairly resistant to drying and can survive in biological material for long periods, especially at low temperatures. They are sensitive to a wide variety of disinfectants including formaldehyde, hypochlorite, iodophors, and phenols provided that excess organic matter is not present. The organisms are killed by heat under pasteurization conditions.

Nearly all strains of *Brucella* are susceptible to gentamicin, tetracycline, and rifampicin. Additionally, many strains are susceptible to ampicillin, chloramphenicol, erythromycin, kanamycin, streptomycin, and trimethoprim. Susceptibility to antibiotics can differ among species, biovars, and even strains (Vemulapalli 2000). There are three biovars, 1–3. *B. abortus* and *B. suis* have been found occasionally in small ruminants, but clinical cases caused by these organisms seem to be rare. At one time, the genus *Brucella* was reclassified into a single species, *B. melitensis*, based on the genetic and immunological evidence that all members of this genus are closely related. Under this system, the various species of *Brucella* were considered to be biovars. This proposal was controversial and has fallen out of favor for practical reasons.

The bacteria cause a severe debilitating disease in people and are the leading cause of brucellosis in humans globally. The primary hosts for *B. melitensis* are sheep and goats but infections have also been reported in cattle, yaks (*Bos grunniens*), water buffalo, Bactrian and dromedary camels, alpacas, dogs, horses, and pigs. Among wildlife, it has been found in wild Alpine ibex (*Capra ibex*), chamois (*Rupicapra rupicapra*), Iberian wild goats (*C. pyrenaica*), impala (*Aepyceros melampus*), and sable antelope (*Hippotragus niger*), as well as in a captive Arabian oryx (*Oryx leucoryx*).

26.3 Geographical Distribution

Brucella melitensis infection mostly occurs in the Middle East, some southern and eastern European countries, and parts of Asia and Latin America, including Mexico. It has been found in sub-Saharan Africa, particularly East Africa, but its distribution on that continent is still unclear. This organism is absent from domesticated animals in northern and central Europe, Canada, the US, Australia, New Zealand, Japan, and some other countries. Sporadic cases are occasionally reported in travelers and immigrants in *B. melitensis*-free nations.

26.4 Zoonotic Importance

Brucellosis is an important zoonotic disease and some *Brucella* species, most notably *B. melitensis*, *B. abortus*, *B. suis*, and, probably to a lesser extent, *B. canis*, are readily transmissible to humans (Figure 26.1). It is a well-characterized occupational disease in shepherds, abattoir workers, veterinarians, dairy industry professionals, and laboratory personnel who handle infected animals/carcases and aborted fetuses or placentas (Agasthya et al. 2007).

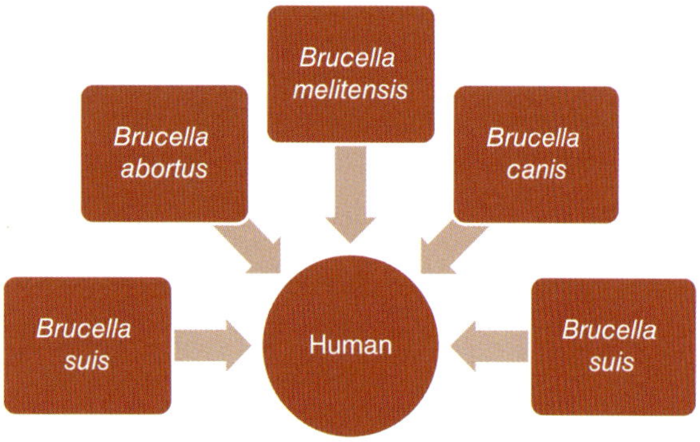

Figure 26.1 The various zoonotic *Brucella* species affecting humans.

Humans mainly acquired infection due to direct animal contact or ingestion of contaminated dairy products, causing acute febrile illness – undulant fever – which may progress to a more chronic form and can produce serious complications affecting the musculoskeletal, cardiovascular, and central nervous systems (Mantur et al. 2007).

Precautions should be taken to prevent human infection. *B. melitensis* spreads to people from infected animals through raw milk, unpasteurized dairy products, processing meat from infected goats, and contact with aborted kids or infective reproductive tissues and/or secretions. Pasteurized milk products and cooked meats do not spread disease. Inhaling contaminated dust and aerosols, contact with carcases, or handling wool from infected animals can also infect people. Milkers can be infected through the skin and by milk that may contact mucous membranes. People exposed to infected animals should take precautions to prevent disease. It is one of the most easily acquired laboratory infections. People who do not work with animals or tissues usually become infected by ingesting unpasteurized dairy products.

The Rev-1 *B. melitensis* vaccine is also pathogenic for humans and must be handled with caution to avoid accidental injection or contamination of mucous membranes or abraded skin.

Asymptomatic infections can occur in humans. In symptomatic cases, the disease is extremely variable and clinical signs may appear insidiously or abruptly.

26.5 Transmission of *B. melitensis*

In animals, *B. melitensis* is usually transmitted by contact with the placenta, fetus, fetal fluids, and vaginal discharges from infected animals. Small ruminants are infectious after either abortion or full-term parturition. Goats usually shed *B. melitensis* in vaginal discharges for at least 2–3 months. This organism can also be found in the milk and semen; shedding in milk and semen can be prolonged or lifelong, particularly in goats. Kids and lambs that nurse from infected dams may shed *B. melitensis* in the feces.

Most animals become infected by ingestion or through the mucous membranes of the oropharynx, upper respiratory tract, and conjunctiva, but *Brucella* can also be transmitted through broken skin. Although the mammary gland is usually colonized during the course of an infection, it can also be infected by direct contact, with subsequent shedding of the organisms in the milk. *In utero* infections also occur. Transmission during breeding is possible but seems to be uncommon during natural mating. *B. melitensis* can be spread on fomites, and could be disseminated mechanically by carnivores that carry away infected material (Moreno et al. 2002).

In conditions of high humidity, low temperatures and no sunlight, *Brucella* can remain viable for several months in water, aborted fetuses, manure, wool, hay, equipment, and clothes. *Brucella* species can withstand drying, particularly when organic material is present, and can survive in dust and soil. Survival is longer when the temperature islow, particularly when it is below freezing. Cattle and other species can be infected with *B. melitensis* after contact with infected sheep and goats (Tibary et al. 2006). The incubation period, i.e., the period between infection and abortion or other reproductive signs, is variable.

Brucella melitensis is highly pathogenic for humans and is considered to be the most severe human pathogen in the genus. Occupational exposure is seen in laboratory workers, farmers, veterinarians, and others who contact infected animals or tissues (Yongqun 2012).

26.6 Pathogenesis and Immune Response

Brucella is a facultative intracellular parasite of the reticuloendothelial system. The virulence of *Brucella* varies considerably according to species, strain, and the size of infecting inoculum. Host susceptibility is also variable and is associated with reproductive status. Thus, in the field, all intermediate stages between typical acute infection and complete resistance may be observed. In addition, vaccinal immunity may modify the parasite–host relationship. Usually it is found that *B. melitensis* infection in sheep and goats is similar to *Brucella* infection in cattle. Nevertheless, differences are significant, and each species of *Brucella* causes a different disease (OIE 1996).

The infection in female goats follows a course very similar to *B. abortus* infection in cattle and the most common route of infection appears to be through the mucous membranes of the oropharynx and upper respiratory tract or the conjunctiva. Other potential routes of infection are through the mucous membranes of the male or female genital tract.

When the infective organisms enter the body, they encounter the cellular defenses of the host but generally succeed in arriving via the lymph channels at the nearest lymph node. Usually, the fate of invading bacteria is mainly determined by the cellular defenses of the host, chiefly macrophages and T lymphocytes, though specific antibodies undoubtedly play a part. Prognosis mainly depends on the ruminant species infected, age, immune status of the host, pregnancy status, and the virulence and number of the invading *Brucella*.

When the bacteria prevail over the body defenses, a bacteremia is generally established and this is detectable after 10–20 days and persists from 30 days to more than two months. In case of pregnancy, bacteremia often leads to invasion of the uterus. At the same time, infection becomes established in various lymph nodes and organs, often the udder and sometimes the spleen. During this first stage of infection, the major clinical sign is abortion but other signs due to localization of *Brucella* may be observed (luteinizing hormone, orchitis, epididymitis, hygroma, arthritis, metritis, subclinical mastitis, etc.). However, numerous animals develop self-limiting infections or become asymptomatic latent carriers and potential excretors. Abortion generally does not occur if the female becomes infected at the end of pregnancy.

The second stage is characterized by either elimination of *Brucella* or, more frequently, persistent infection of mammary glands and supramammary and genital lymph nodes (Fensterbank et al. 1987) with constant or intermittent shedding of the organisms in the milk and genital secretions. Animals generally abort once, during the mid third of gestation, but reinvasion of the uterus occurs in subsequent pregnancies with shedding in fluids and membranes. The pregnancy can also continue to full term. The proportion of newly infected females that abort varies with the circumstances. The percentage of infected females lambing/kidding in a flock may reach 40%. Females that are born into an infected environment and subsequently become infected generally abort less than others. This explains the high level of abortions in newly infected flocks and the relatively low frequency in flocks where infection is enzootic.

The udder is a very important predilection site for *B. melitensis*. Infection in lactating nonpregnant goats is likely to lead to colonization of the udder with excretion of *B. melitensis* in the milk (Renoux et al. 1953). In goats, about two-thirds of acute infections acquired naturally during pregnancy lead to infection of the udder and excretion of bacteria in milk during the subsequent lactation (Alton 1985). In some goats, excretion may cease during this lactation, but in many it persists and often continues during the next (Alton 1962). Greatly reduced milk yield follows abortion, and infection of the udder following a normal birth also leads to a considerable reduction in yield. In spite of this, clinical signs of mastitis are seldom detectable in naturally infected goats (Alton 1990).

26.7 Clinical Signs

The most important clinical signs in goats are abortions (most often during the last trimester), stillbirths, and the birth of weak offspring. Most of the animals abort only once and subsequent pregnancies are usually normal. The period between infection and reproductive losses is variable, as animals can be infected at any time (including before they become pregnant), but abortions usually occur late in gestation.

A huge drop in milk yield is common. While mastitis has been reported in small ruminants experimentally infected with large doses of *B. melitensis*, clinically apparent mastitis is uncommon in the field.

Uncomplicated reproductive losses are not usually accompanied by signs of illness; however, retention of the placenta and secondary metritis are possible complications. Acute orchitis and epididymitis are sometimes seen in males, and may result in infertility.

Many nonpregnant sheep and goats remain asymptomatic but arthritis and hygromas have been reported. Hygromas are reported to be most common at the carpal joint. Deaths are rare except in the fetus or newborn.

Brucella melitensis is a significant problem in small ruminants, particularly in developing nations where infections can be widespread. The relative importance of *B. melitensis* for sheep and goats varies with geographical region, and can be influenced by husbandry practices and the susceptibility of sheep breeds in the region. Management practices and environmental conditions significantly influence the spread of infection. Lambing or kidding in dark, crowded enclosures favors the spread of the organism, while open air parturition in a dry environment results in decreased transmission (Yilma et al. 2016). The abortion rate is high when *B. melitensis* enters a previously unexposed and unvaccinated flock or herd, but much lower in flocks where this disease is enzootic.

Ruminants usually abort only during the gestation when they are first infected. Inflammatory changes in infected mammary glands usually reduce milk yield by a minimum of 10% (Tibary et al. 2006). Fertility in males can be permanently impaired. Deaths are rare except in the fetus (Figure 26.2).

26.8 Postmortem Lesions

Granulomatous inflammatory lesions in the reproductive tract, udder, supramammary lymph nodes, other lymphoid tissues, and sometimes in the joints and synovial membranes are important necropsy findings in brucellosis in goats. Other important findings include necrotizing orchitis, epididymitis, seminal vesiculitis, and prostatitis. The fetus may be

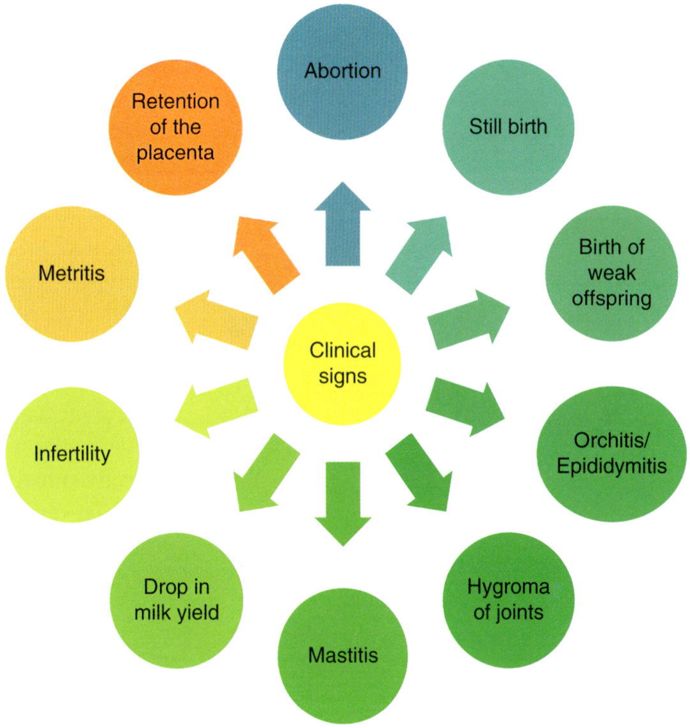

Figure 26.2 The various clinical signs in goats with *Brucella* infection.

autolyzed, normal, or have an excess of blood-stained fluid in the body cavities and an enlarged spleen and liver. Placentitis with edema and/or necrosis of the cotyledons and a thickened and leathery intercotyledonary region can be seen. These lesions are not pathognomonic for brucellosis (Xavier et al. 2009).

26.9 Diagnosis

Tentative diagnosis of brucellosis is mainly done on the basis of history and clinical sign and symptoms. All the cases of abortion as well as orchitis in goats and in other animals should be considered as suspected brucellosis and should be investigated through the herd/flock history and submission of specimens for laboratory testing. In case of brucellosis, the clinical signs are not pathognomonic and the confirmatory diagnosis of *Brucella* infections can be made only by the isolation and identification of *Brucella* organism, but in situations where bacteriological examination is not practicable, diagnosis must be based on molecular or immunological methods.

There are various methods for the detection of *Brucella* including detection of the agent by staining methods, sampling and culturing of organism, identification and typing, nucleic acid recognition methods and identification of vaccine strains, various serological methods, and tests for cellular immunity.

Detection of *B. melitensis* can be done by microscopic examination of stained smears from tissues, secretions, and exudates (e.g., placenta, reproductive discharges or contents of the fetal stomach), using MZN (Stamp) staining (Figure 26.3). This procedure provides a presumptive diagnosis of brucellosis, especially if supported by serology. It is said that the *Brucella* organisms are not truly acid fast, but they are resistant to decolorization by weak acids and stain red. They appear as coccobacilli

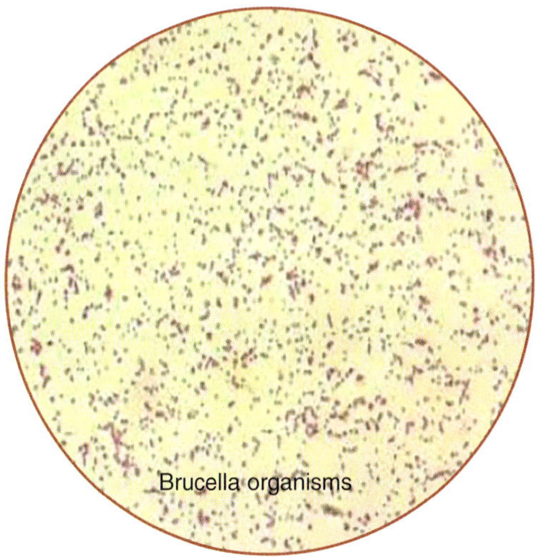

Figure 26.3 Gram-stained *Brucella* under light microscopy. *Source:* Bayu MD, et al. (2013)/ Reproduced with permission from AVENS Publishing Group/CC BY 4.0.

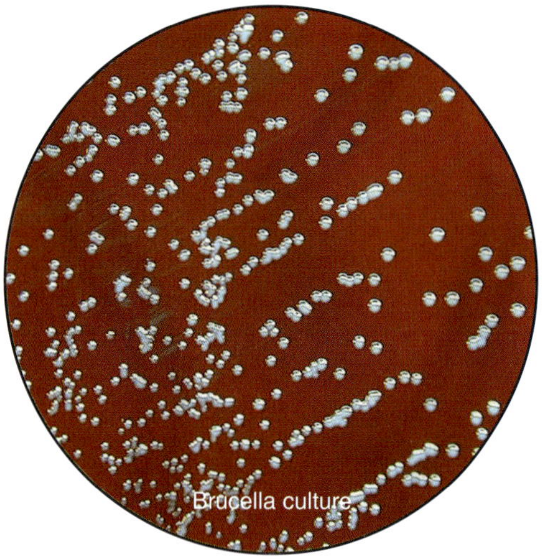

Figure 26.4 *Brucella* species colony characteristics showing pinpoint, smooth, entire translucent, and nonhemolytic colonies on blood agar. *Source:* Bayu MD, et al. (2013)/Reproduced with permission from AVENS Publishing Group/ CC BY 4.0.

or short rods, usually arranged singly but sometimes in pairs or small groups. Organisms such as *Chlamydia* spp. and *Coxiella burnetii* can resemble *Brucella*. If available, immunostaining may be helpful.

Confirmatory diagnosis requires culture and/or detection of nucleic acids by PCR or other genetic techniques. Isolation of *B. melitensis* can be done from aborted fetuses (e.g., stomach contents, spleen, lung), placenta, vaginal swabs, milk, colostrum, semen, testis or epididymis, and sites of clinical localization such as infected joints and hygroma fluids. In case of necropsy, recommended samples include the spleen, various lymph nodes (e.g., supramammary and genital lymph nodes), the pregnant or early postparturient uterus, the udder and male reproductive organs.

Culturing of *B. melitensis* organisms can be done on a variety of nonselective media, or on selective media such as Farrell's, Thayer-Martin's or CITA medium. Some isolates of *B. melitensis* do not grow well on certain selective media, and the use of more than one medium is often recommended (Figure 26.4). Enrichment techniques can also be employed. Care must be taken during culturing as certain treatment with antibiotics or bacterial overgrowth in nonsterile samples can interfere with culture. A modified *Brucella* selective medium (named MBS) has been developed to select *B. abortus* strains, including the RB51 vaccine strain, more effectively than previously described media but needs further validation studies to confirm performance (Her et al. 2010). Contrary to the situation with several *B. abortus* biovars as well as *B. ovis*, the growth of *B. melitensis* or *B. suis* is not dependent on an incubating atmosphere containing 5–10% CO_2, but such a CO_2-enriched atmosphere is optimal for the culture of all *Brucella*.

Animal inoculation is another method for detection of brucellosis in goats. *B. melitensis* can also be isolated by inoculation into guinea pigs or mice, but this is rarely done. Use of laboratory animals should be avoided unless absolutely necessary, but sometimes they provide the only means of detecting the presence of *Brucella*, especially when samples have been shown to be heavily contaminated or are likely to contain a low number of *Brucella* organisms. Animal inoculation may be intravenous or intraperitoneal in mice or intramuscular, subcutaneous or intraperitoneal in guinea pigs. This work must be carried out under appropriate biosafety conditions. The spleens of inoculated animals are cultured at seven days (mice) or 3–6 weeks (guinea pigs) after inoculation. Serum samples can be collected by intracardiac puncture before necropsy from guinea pigs and subjected to buffered *Brucella* antigen tests (BBAT); a positive serological result is highly suggestive of brucellosis (Alton et al. 1988).

Species identification can be done by various methods. *B. melitensis* can be identified to the species and biovar level by phenotypical methods (phage typing and cultural, biochemical, and serological characteristics) or genetic techniques. On the basis of growth characteristics and sensitivity to antibiotics and other additives, as well as by genetic tests, the Rev-1 vaccine strain can be distinguished from field strains. Species identification is often done at reference laboratories, as it is complicated by the high genetic similarity between brucellae and the possibility of ambiguous phenotypical tests. Most of the PCR tests only identify *Brucella* to the genus level but a few *B. melitensis*-specific PCRs have been published. Multiplex PCR assays that can identify more than one species of *Brucella* (e.g., the Bruceladder assay or the older AMOS test) are also used. Other tests that can be employed for species identification, such as single nucleotide polymorphism (SNP) typing and matrix-assisted laser desorption/ionization time-of-flight mass spectrometry (MALDI-TOF MS), have been described.

For epidemiological investigations, techniques such as multiple-locus variable number tandem repeat analysis (MLVA) can be used in case of outbreaks. The *Brucella* PCR tests are mainly used to identify organisms in culture but some laboratories may use these tests directly on clinical samples. Loop-mediated isothermal amplification (LAMP) assays have been published.

There are various antigen detection techniques, such as immune staining/immune histochemistry, which can be used for diagnosis. Usually these tests are used for research purposes and not for diagnosis.

For diagnosis of clinical cases or herd screening, serological tests are mostly performed but they cannot distinguish reactions to any of the *Brucella* species that have "smooth" LPS in the cell wall, including *B. melitensis*, *B. abortus*, and *B. suis*. Assays that were originally developed for cattle and contain *B. abortus* antigens are generally assumed to be adequate for diagnosing *B. melitensis* infections in sheep and goats; however, some tests may need to be optimized for these species.

Commonly used assays in small ruminants include the buffered *Brucella* agglutination tests (e.g., buffered plate agglutination and rose bengal tests) fluorescence polarization assay, complement fixation, and indirect or competitive enzyme-linked immunosorbent assay (ELISA). To improve sensitivity and specificity, combinations of serological tests are often used. Antibodies to *Brucella* in sheep and goat milk can be detected with ELISA.

26.9.1 Procedure for Rose Bengal Test

This is a simple spot agglutination test using antigen stained with rose bengal and buffered to a low pH, 3.65 ± 0.05 (Morgan et al. 1969).

1) Bring the serum samples and antigen to room temperature (22 ± 4 °C).
2) Place 25–30 μl of each serum sample on a white tile, enamel or plastic plate, or in a WHO hemagglutination plate.
3) Shake the antigen bottle well, but gently, and place an equal volume of antigen near each serum spot.
4) Immediately after the last drop of antigen has been added to the plate, mix the serum and antigen thoroughly (using a clean glass or plastic rod for each test) to produce a circular or oval zone approximately 2 cm in diameter.
5) The mixture is agitated gently for four minutes at room temperature (22 ± 4 °C) on a rocker or three-directional agitator (if the reaction zone is oval or round, respectively).
6) Read for agglutination immediately after the four-minute period is completed. Any visible colored agglutination is considered to be a positive reaction. A control serum that gives a minimum positive reaction should be tested before each day's tests are begun to verify the sensitivity of test conditions. This test is very sensitive and appears to be adequate as a screening test for detecting infected herds or to guarantee the absence of infection in brucellosis-free herds or flocks

26.9.2 Procedure for Buffered Plate Agglutination Test

Antigen for the BPAT is prepared from *B. abortus* S1119-3 according to the procedure described by Angus and Barton (1984).

1) Bring the serum samples and antigen to room temperature (22 ± 4 °C).
2) Shake the sample well. Place 80 μl of each serum sample on a glass plate marked in 4 × 4 cm squares
3) Shake the antigen bottle well, but gently, and place 30 μl of antigen near each serum spot.
4) Immediately after the last drop of antigen has been added to the plate, mix the serum and antigen thoroughly (using a clean glass or plastic rod for each test) to produce a circular zone approximately 3 cm in diameter.
5) After the initial mixing, the plate should be rotated three times in a tilting motion to ensure even dispersal of the reagents, and then incubated for four minutes in a humid chamber at ambient temperature.
6) The plate should be removed and rotated as above, and then returned for a second four-minutes incubation.
7) Read for agglutination immediately after the eight-minute period is completed. Any visible reaction is considered to be positive. A control serum that gives a minimum positive reaction should be tested before each day's tests are begun to verify the sensitivity of test conditions.

Like the rose bengal test, the BPAT is very sensitive in cattle, especially for detection of vaccine-induced antibody, and positive samples should be retested using a confirmatory or complementary test(s). False-negative reactions may occur, usually due to prozoning, which may be overcome by diluting the serum or retesting after a given time. While the BPAT has been extensively used with apparent good results in small ruminants and pigs in some countries, its diagnostic value in these species has not been reported at international level (Figure 26.5).

Vaccine-induced antibodies may sometimes need to be distinguished from infections. Sera from sheep and goats vaccinated with Rev-1 are reported to be less likely to react in the native hapten-based gel precipitation tests (gel diffusion or radial immunodiffusion tests) than in some other serological tests.

To test unvaccinated sheep and goats for exposure to *B. melitensis*, the brucellin skin test has also been used. It is carried out by injecting the allergen into the lower eyelid. Skin tests can be useful as herd tests, but are not sensitive enough to be used for detecting infections in individual animals.

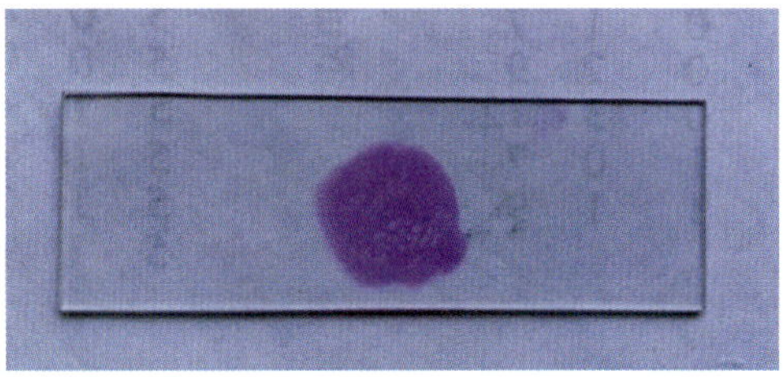

Figure 26.5 RBPT testing of sera from animals suspected of brucellosis showing positive test results.

26.10 Biomarkers of *Brucella* and Brucellosis

In the absence of a single accurate serodiagnostic test for brucellosis based on antibody detection, efforts are ongoing to identify a specific biomarker of brucellosis for correct diagnosis.

A biomarker is a characteristic that is objectively measured and evaluated as an indicator of normal biological processes, pathogenic processes, or pharmacological responses to a therapeutic intervention or other healthcare intervention. The biomarker is produced either by the diseased organ or by the body in response to disease. Biomarkers are potentially useful along the whole spectrum of the disease process. Before diagnosis, markers could be used for screening and risk assessment. During diagnosis, markers can determine staging, grading, and selection of initial therapy. Genetics, genomics, proteomics, and modern imaging techniques and other high-throughput technologies allow us to measure markers. However, there are few studies on biomarkers in the diagnosis of brucellosis.

Diagnosis of brucellosis is currently performed with serological techniques that mainly detect antibodies against lipopolysaccharide. However, antibodies against lipopolysaccharide are also induced in animals vaccinated with *Brucella* sp. attenuated strains. Therefore, an important goal in brucellosis research is the identification of protein antigens that induce an intense antibody response during infection and that are not essential for the induced protective immunity or for survival of the bacterium.

In a study by Al-Garadi (2011), cluster of differentiation (CD) markers and their combination in different populations of peripheral blood mononuclear cells (PMNC) were measured in detail, in different stages of *B. melitensis* infection and in experimentally infected mice and goats by using specific monoclonal antibody. The CD biomarkers, namely CD14, CD4, and CD25, were identified as good markers for the different stages of *B. melitensis* infection.

Ahmed et al. (2015) conducted a study in which omp25, omp28, and omp31 of *B. melitensis* were cloned and expressed using a prokaryotic pET-32 Ek/LIC system and their respective recombinant outer membrane proteins (rOMPs) were combined as one coating antigen to develop a rOMPs I-ELISA. The production of rOMP25, rOMP28, and rOMP31 of *B. melitensis* was achieved and Western immunoblotting analysis demonstrated their reactivity.

Liang et al. (2010) conducted a study to better understand the antibody responses that develop after *B. melitensis* infection. A protein microarray was fabricated containing 1406 predicted *B. melitensis* proteins. The array was probed with sera from experimentally infected goats and naturally infected humans from an endemic region in Peru. The assay identified 18 antigens differentially recognized by infected and noninfected goats, and 13 serodiagnostic antigens that differentiated human patients proven to have acute brucellosis from syndromically similar patients. There were 31 crossreactive antigens in healthy goats and 20 crossreactive antigens in healthy humans.

Wareth et al. (2015) carried out a study to identify immunodominant proteins of two species of *Brucella* using antibodies present in the serum of naturally infected ruminants to gain insight into the mechanism of their infection in different hosts. In the study, whole-cell protein extracts of *B. abortus* and *B. melitensis* were separated using sodium dodecyl-sulfate polyacrylamide gel electrophoresis (SDS PAGE) and Western blotting was performed using field sera from cows, buffalo, sheep, and goats.

Rolan et al. (2008) studied the vir B proteins as potential biomarkers. The *Brucella* species type IV secretion system, encoded by the virB1-12 locus, is required for intracellular replication and persistent infection *in vivo*. VirB proteins are expressed *in vivo* and may therefore represent serological markers of infection. Purified recombinant VirB1, VirB5, VirB11, and VirB12 were tested for their recognition by antibodies in sera from experimentally infected mice and goats by using an indirect ELISA. The results suggested that VirB12 may be a useful serodiagnostic marker for brucellosis.

26.11 Treatment

There is no effective treatment for brucellosis. Antibiotics can mitigate the clinical signs, and a few studies have reported that treatment may have eliminated brucellae from small ruminants or cattle. However, even when the organisms seem to have disappeared, they might persist in lymph nodes or other tissues and reemerge. In addition, none of the published treatments have been extensively evaluated. For these reasons (as well as the zoonotic risks), treatment is generally discouraged. It is also unlikely to be cost-effective in many herds.

Some sources have recommended castrating males and not breeding females if owners refuse to euthanize animals and treatment is attempted.

26.12 Control

Prevention and control of brucellosis are very important because it is a disease of major economic and zoonotic importance, so a strategy for its control in small ruminants is essential in endemic areas.

Some of the common points which need to be considered for prevention of disease are purchasing goats or sheep from known sources, avoiding mixing animals with other flocks, testing new purchases before adding to the flock, not using dogs that have been exposed to infected sheep and goats in countries where the disease is endemic, pasteurizing milk, and proper hygiene.

The initial aim of the strategy selected will be the reduction of infection in the animal population to such a level that the impact of the disease on human health, animal health, and production will be minimized (Kaplan 1966). Subsequent steps can include eradication from a region by test and slaughter and, following successful eradication, measures to prevent reintroduction of the disease. It is accepted that before a zoonosis control program is designed and implemented, a well-functioning surveillance system, which should be fed with valid data collected from the field, must be established. Disease-reporting veterinarians who encounter or suspect brucellosis should follow their national and/or local guidelines for disease reporting. A selection can be made from the following strategies, which are implemented for the control of brucellosis (Figure 26.6).

26.12.1 Immunization

According to Nicoletti and Tanya (1993), vaccination practically eliminates the clinical signs of brucellosis and is accompanied by reduced contamination of the environment as well as decreased exposure of the population at risk to the infectious agent. By using vaccination, control of brucellosis can be achieved to increase the population's resistance to the disease.

The initial campaigns to control brucellosis in small ruminants were based on vaccination of young animals, kept as replacements, with the Rev.1 vaccine. This approach was based on the hypothesis that the Rev.1 vaccine offered life-long immunity and that after implementing the vaccination program for 5–7 years (the productive lifespan of sheep and goats), the whole population would be vaccinated and fully protected against brucellosis. This method was also recommended to minimize postvaccinal diagnostic problems and avoid abortions (Blasco 1997). However, in many countries, where the animals were kept under extensive conditions with nomadic or seminomadic husbandry, this approach was impractical

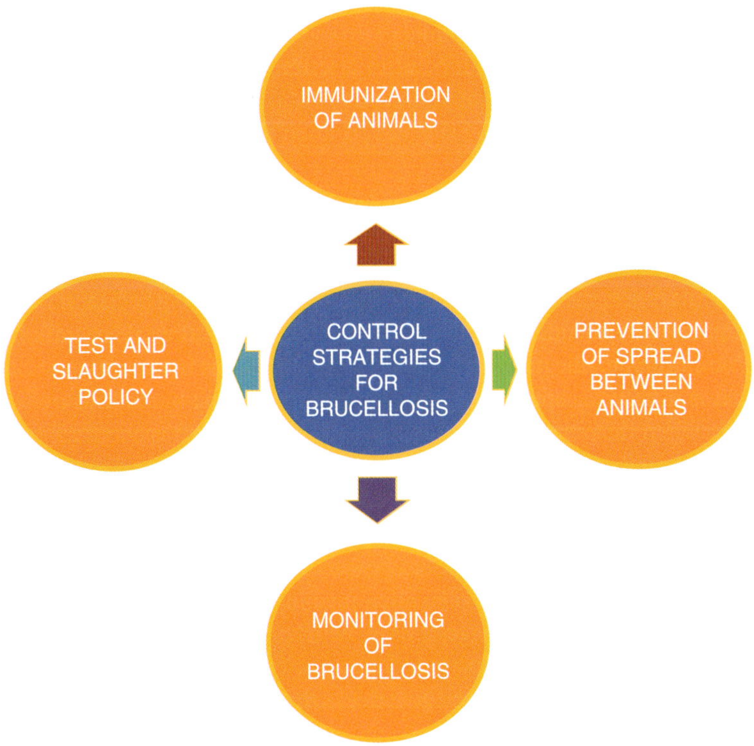

Figure 26.6 Various control strategies for brucellosis.

and failed to reduce the incidence and prevalence of the disease, because the development of herd immunity was very slow (Blasco 1997). In addition, unvaccinated adult animals remain unprotected and the infection can spread (Kolar 1995).

Vaccination of all animals (young and adults) in a flock or region is an alternative approach for the control of brucellosis in small ruminants. Mass immunization of small ruminants has been applied with success in many countries under different socioeconomic conditions. In general, mass immunization is indicated where the prevalence of infected animals is high. It should be based on knowledge of the prevalence in the flock or region. Mass vaccination of a flock helps to rapidly establish a relatively immune stock, and reduces the level of abortions and excretors of *Brucella*, thus reducing contamination of the environment and disease transmission (Kolar 1995). However, this strategy has the limitation that pregnant animals cannot be vaccinated because the vaccine is not innocuous enough for pregnant animals, and the efficacy of the strategy depends on the continuous availability of the vaccine (WHO 1986).

Provided that the prevalence of disease is moderate, financial resources are available, and a well-functioning surveillance by the veterinary service is in place, vaccination of young animals can be combined with a test and slaughter policy in a long-term action to control brucellosis in small ruminants (WHO 1998).

26.12.1.1 Adverse Effect of Vaccination

In young replacement stock, i.e., animals 3–6 months old, when Rev.1 is administered by the standard method ($1–2 \times 10^9$ CFU SC), it induces a solid and durable immunity but also a long-lasting serological response, complicating the interpretation of serological tests conducted after vaccination (Díaz-Aparicio et al. 1994). This causes obvious problems for the application of combined vaccination and test and slaughter eradication programs.

In adult animals when the Rev.1 vaccine is used exhaustively in high-prevalence situations, it reduces the transmission process and, in the medium term, leads to a substantial decrease in the prevalence of brucellosis in both small ruminants and humans (Elberg 1996), then allowing the application of test and slaughter policies for definitive eradication of the disease.

However, the Rev.1 mass vaccination strategy has two main drawbacks.

- The vaccination of pregnant animals with standard Rev.1 doses administered subcutaneously is followed by vaccine-induced abortion in many animals (Blasco 1997). It has been stated that the ability of the Rev.1 strain to induce abortion depends on dose and stage of pregnancy when the females are vaccinated: a reduction of the dose increases the degree of safety, and the risk of abortion is minimized when animals are vaccinated at the end of pregnancy or during lactation (Elberg 1996).
- The vaccination of adult animals with standard Rev.1 doses administered subcutaneously induces a long-lasting serological response, making it difficult to discriminate the serological response evoked, when test and slaughter eradication programs are operated simultaneously (Marín et al. 1999). In general, the residual immune response induced by the vaccination is of less intensity and duration when the dose is reduced and/or the conjunctival route is used.

26.12.2 Test and Slaughter Policy

A brucellosis control and eradication plan based on a test and slaughter strategy can be either voluntary or compulsory. Voluntary schemes, which apply to individual flocks, may be useful in the early stages of the campaign but may need to be supported by adequate incentives such as a bonus on the sale of milk from brucellosis-free herds or per capita payments. Compulsory eradication is required in the final stages but is often advisable from the start (WHO 1986).

It is usually accepted that a program of eliminating brucellosis by test and slaughter is justified on economic grounds only when the prevalence of infected animals in an area is about 2% or less. For the implementation of such a program, it is essential that the flocks are under strict surveillance and movement control. Animals must be individually identified and an efficient and well-organized veterinary service for surveillance and laboratory testing must be in place (Nicoletti and Tanya 1993).

Flock size and the prevalence of brucellosis are the most important factors of this strategy, which has been shown to be ineffective and unreliable when attempted in large flocks with a high prevalence of brucellosis (Kolar 1995). The limited reliability of the diagnostic tests used, which are unable to reveal all infected animals and which may give false-negative results due to incubation period, latency, or criteria used to interpret the results, must also be considered. These drawbacks apply more to sheep and goat flocks than to cattle herds, where a test and slaughter strategy has been more effective (Nicoletti and Tanya 1993).

Before embarking on the implementation of such a strategy, it is necessary to ensure that the epidemiological situation is favorable, the necessary facilities and financial resources are available, a pool of healthy replacement animals is ready, and the resources exist for continuing surveillance for a considerable period. Full cooperation of farmers is also essential as slaughter of seropositive animals can be resisted by owners because of lack of clinical signs, inadequate compensation or lack of replacement animals (Nicoletti and Tanya 1993).

26.12.3 Prevention of Spread Between Animals and Monitoring of Brucellosis-free Herds and Zones

In areas where the brucellosis-free status has been established or where such a status is suspected on epidemiological grounds, the risk of importing the disease by means of animal movement must be curtailed. Movement of potentially infected animals into such areas must be prohibited or importation permitted only from certified brucellosis-free farms or areas. This applies to the transport of animals and of certain animal products within countries as well as between countries, following the general principles and procedures as specified in the International Zoo-sanitary Code of the OIE which also describes the essential testing of animals and quarantine measures. It should be noted that there have been incidents of spread of brucellosis by serologically negative animals originating from inadequately certified and supervised sources (Schnurrenberger et al. 1987).

References

Agasthya, A.S., Isloor, S., and Prabhudas, K. (2007). Brucellosis in high risk group individuals. *Indian Journal of Medical Microbiology* 25: 28–31.

Ahmed, I.M., Khairani-Bejo, S., Hassan, L. et al. (2015). Serological diagnostic potential of recombinant outer membrane proteins (rOMPs) from *Brucella melitensis* in mouse model using indirect enzyme-linked immunosorbent assay. *BMC Veterinary Research* 11: 275.

Al-Garadi, M.A.M. (2011). Detection of infection and determination of biomarkers for *Brucella melitensis* infection in goats. PhD thesis. Universiti Putra, Malaysia.

Al-Majali, A.M. (2005). Seroepidemiology of caprine brucellosis in Jordan. *Small Ruminant Research* 58: 13–18.

Alton, G.G. (1962). The reactions of goats naturally infected with *Brucella melitensis* to vaccination with living attenuated vaccine. *Research in Veterinary Science* 3: 326.

Alton, G.G. (1985). The epidemiology of *Brucella melitensis* in sheep and goats. In: *Brucella melitensis, A CEC Seminar* (ed. J.M. Verger and M. Plommet), 187–196. Dordrecht: Martinus Nijoff.

Alton, G.G. (1990). *Brucella melitensis*. In: *Animal Brucellosis* (ed. K. Nielsen and J.R. Duncan), 383–409. Boca Raton, FL: CRC Press.

Alton, G.G., Jones, L.M., Angus, R.D., and Verger, J.M. (1988). *Techniques for the Brucellosis Laboratory*. Paris: INRA.

Angus, R.D. and Barton, C.E. (1984). The production and evaluation of a buffered plate antigen for use in a presumptive test for brucellosis. *Developments in Biological Standardization* 56: 349–356.

Benkirane A. (2006). Ovine and caprine brucellosis: world distribution and control/eradication strategies in West Asia/North Africa region. *Small Rumin Res.* 62 (1–2): 19–25.

Blasco, J.M. (1997). A review of the use of *B. melitensis* Rev 1 vaccine in adult sheep and goats. *Preventive Veterinary Medicine* 31 (3–4): 275–283.

Corbel, M.J. and Brinley-Morgan, W.J. (1984). Genus Brucella Meyer and Shaw 1920, 173AL. In: *Bergey's Manual of Systematic Bacteriology*, vol. 1 (ed. N.R. Krieg and J.G. Holt), 377–388. Baltimore, MD: Williams & Wilkins.

Díaz-Aparicio, E., Marín, C., Alonso, B. et al. (1994). Evaluation of serological tests for diagnosis of *Brucella melitensis* infection of goats. *Journal of Clinical Microbiology* 32: 1159–1165.

Elberg, S.S. (1996). Rev 1 *Brucella melitensis* vaccine. Part III 1981–1995. *Veterinary Bulletin* 66: 1193–1200.

Fensterbank, R., Verger, J.M., and Grayon, M. (1987). Conjunctival vaccination of young goats with *Brucella melitensis* strain Rev 1. *Annales de Recherches Vétérinaires* 18 (4): 397–403.

Her, M., Cho, D.H., Kang, S.I. et al. (2010). The development of a selective medium for the *Brucella abortus* strains and its comparison with the currently recommended and used medium. *Diagnostic Microbiology and Infectious Disease* 67: 15–21.

Kaplan, M. (1966). *The Problems of Choice between Control and Eradication*, 6–12. Geneva: Joint WHO/FAO Expert Committee on Zoonoses.

Kolar, J. (1995). Some Experience from Brucellosis Control with Rev.1 Vaccine in a Heavily Infected Country – Mongolia. FAO/WHO/OIE Round Table on the Use of Rev.1 Vaccine in Small Ruminants and Cattle. CNEVA, Alfort, France.

Liang, L., Leng, D., Burk, C. et al. (2010). Large scale immune profiling of infected humans and goats reveals differential recognition of *Brucella melitensis* antigens. *PLoS Neglected Tropical Diseases* 4 (5): e673.

Mantur, B.G., Amarnath, S.K., and Shinde, R.S. (2007). Review of clinical and laboratory features of human brucellosis. *Indian Journal of Medical Microbiology* 25: 188–202.

Marín, C.M., Moreno, E., Moriyón, I. et al. (1999). Performance of competitive and indirect ELISAs, gel immunoprecipitation with native Hapten polysaccharide and standard serological tests in diagnosis of sheep brucellosis. *Clinical and Diagnostic Laboratory Immunology* 6: 269–272.

Moreno, E., Cloeckaert, A., and Moriyo'n, I. (2002). Brucella evolution and taxonomy. *Veterinary Microbiology* 90: 209–227.

Morgan, W.J.B., Mackinnon, D.J., Lawson, J.R., and Cullen, G.A. (1969). The rose bengal plate agglutination test in the diagnosis of brucellosis. *Veterinary Record* 85: 636–641.

Nicoletti, P. and Tanya, V. (1993). Comparison of enzyme-labeled immunosorbent assay and particle concentration fluorescence immunoassay with standard serologic methods and bacteriologic culture for detection of Brucella sp-infected cows in herds with brucellosis. *Journal of the American Veterinary Medical Association* 202 (12): 1975–1977.

OIE (1996). Caprine and ovine brucellosis. In: *Manual of Standards for Diagnostic Tests and Vaccines*, 3e, 350–362. Paris, France: Office International des Epizooties.

OIE (2009). Bovine brucellosis. In: *Manual of the Diagnostic Tests and Vaccines for Terrestrial Animals*, 5e, vol. 1, 1–35. Paris, France: Office International des Epizooties.

Renoux, G., Alton, G.G., and Sacquet, E. (1953). Etudes sur la brucellose ovine et caprine. X. Elimination de *B. mellitensis* par le lait de chevres suedises artificiellement infectess. *Archives de l'Institut Pasteur de Tunis* 33: 413.

Rolán, H.G., Den Hartigh, A.B., Kahl-McDonagh, M. et al. (2008). VirB12 is a serological marker of Brucella infection in experimental and natural hosts. *Clinical and Vaccine Immunology* 15 (2): 208–214.

Schnurrenberger, P., Sharman, R., and Wise, G. (1987). *Attacking Animal Diseases. Concepts and Strategies for Control and Eradication*. Ames, IA: Iowa State University Press.

Tibary, A., Fite, C., Anouassi, A., and Sghiri, A. (2006). Infectious causes of reproductive loss in camelids. *Theriogenology* 66: 633–647.

Vemulapalli, T.H. (2000). Genetic and immunological analyses of a *Brucella abortus* protein exhibiting lectin-like properties. Thesis. Virginia Polytechnic Institute and State University.

Wareth, G., Melzer, F., Weise, C. et al. (2015). Proteomics-based identification of immunodominant proteins of Brucellae using sera from infected hosts points towards enhanced pathogen survival during the infection. *Biochemical and Biophysical Research Communications* 456: 202–206.

WHO (1986). *Joint FAO/WHO Expert Committee on Brucellosis, Technical Report 740*, 86–88. Geneva: WHO.

WHO/MZCP (1998). Human and Animal Brucellosis. *Report of a WHO/MZCP workshop*. Damascus, Syrian Arab Republic, 4–5 May.

Xavier, M.N., Paixao, T.A., Poester, F.P. et al. (2009). Pathological, immunohistochemical and bacteriological study of tissues and milk of cows and fetuses experimentally infected with Brucella abortus. *Journal of Comparative Pathology* 140 (2–3): 149–157.

Yilma, M., Mamo, G., and Mammo, B. (2016). Review on brucellosis sero-prevalence and ecology in livestock and human population. *Achievements in the Life Sciences* 10 (1): 80–86.

Yongqun, H.E. (2012). Analyses of Brucella pathogenesis, host immunity, and vaccine targets using systems biology and bioinformatics. *Frontiers in Cellular and Infection Microbiology* 2: 2.

27

Infectious Abortive Diseases: Campylobacteriosis

Ashok Baindha[1], *Rashmi Singh*[1], *Prerna Yadav*[1], *Akanksha Choudhary*[1], *Amitava Roy*[2], *and Tanmoy Rana*[3]

[1] *Post Graduate Institute of Veterinary Education & Research, Jaipur, India*
[2] *Department of Livestock Farm Complex, West Bengal University of Animal & Fishery Sciences, Kolkata, India*
[3] *Department of Veterinary Clinical Complex, West Bengal University of Animal & Fishery Sciences, Kolkata, India*

27.1 Etiology

Microaerophilic, Gram-negative bacteria include *Campylobacter jejuni* and *C. fetus*. Some sheep and other farmed and wild animals that exhibit no symptoms of illness can harbor the germs in their intestinal tracts (Yamzaki-Matsune et al. 2007). The intestinal carrier stage of *C. fetus* is not well understood. *C. jejuni* can be found in sheep and cattle but its prevalence seldom rises above 50%. When compared to animals on pastures, there appears to be a larger prevalence in young animals than in older animals, as well as in animals kept in environments with higher stocking densities (such as feed lots and saleyards).

27.2 The Genus *Campylobacter*

Theodore Escherich is thought to have observed and described noncultivable spiral-shaped bacteria in 1886, which is when the first report of *Campylobacter* is thought to have been made (Vandamme et al. 2010). Following this, two British veterinarians discovered "large numbers of a peculiar organism" in the uterine fluid of a pregnant sheep, leading to the discovery of *Campylobacter* for the first time in 1906 (Zilbauer et al. 2008). These bacteria were isolated in 1913 by McFadyean and Stockman from caprine fetuses that had been aborted. Later, Skirrow (2006) gave the bacterial strain *Vibrio jejuni*'s name after isolating it from the feces of cattle with diarrhea.

Doyle identified a distinct vibrio from the feces of pigs with diarrhea in 1944, and labeled them as *Vibrio coli* (Vandamme et al. 2010). The genus *Campylobacter* was first proposed by Sebald and Véron in 1963, separating them from the "true" *Vibrio* spp. due to their low DNA base composition, nonfermentative metabolism, and need for microaerophilic development. Following that, a study by Butzler and Oosterom (1991) increased interest in *Campylobacter* by highlighting its high prevalence in cases of human diarrhea.

The taxonomic structure of the *Campylobacter* genus has undergone significant alterations since its origin, and even some aspects of the current genus taxonomy are still debatable and need more research (Debruyne et al. 2005). There are 14 *Campylobacter* species that have been legitimately characterized, according to Debruyne et al. (2005). The genus consists of 20, according to Fernández et al. (2008), who published their findings more recently. However, according to other scientists (Foster et al. 2004), the genus *Campylobacter* contains 16 species and an additional six subspecies.

Since 1909, campylobacters have been known to cause disease in animals but only recently have they been widely accepted as a source of illness in people. The two genera *Campylobacter* and *Arcobacter*, which make up the family Campylobacteraceae, are most frequently found as commensals in humans and domestic animals (Vandamme 2000).

Small (0.2–0.8 ×0.5–5 m) Gram-negative, slender spirally curled rods make up the *Campylobacter* genus. Bacterial cells can create a "S" or "V" shaped gull's wing when they are gathered together in groups of two or more. The majority of

Elements of Reproduction and Reproductive Diseases of Goats, First Edition. Edited by Tanmoy Rana.

species move in a corkscrew-like fashion at one or both ends of the cell using a single polar unsheathed flagellum. The only exceptions are the nonmotile *C. gracilis* and the numerous flagellated *C. showae* (see Debruyne et al. 2005 for a detailed discussion of the taxonomy of Campylobacteraceae). All species, with the exception of *C. gracilis,* exhibit oxidase activity. They do not oxidize or ferment carbohydrates but rather get their energy from amino acids, which are intermediates in the tricarboxylic acid cycle (Vandamme 2000).

In addition to reducing nitrate, *C. jejuni* hydrolyzes hippurate and indoxyl acetate. The majority of strains have been shown to be resistant to cephalothin and fluoroquinolones, a class of antibiotics typically used to treat both human and animal illnesses (Koenraad et al. 1995). These microbes can develop viable but nonculturable cells when growing conditions are unfavorable (Portner et al. 2007). According to Cappelier (1997), *Campylobacter* strains isolated from the soil near a broiler house may have undergone transformation into viable but uncultivable (VBNC) forms that may have changed into cultivable forms after passing through chickens' intestines. Numerous issues have been raised regarding the relationship between nonculturability and viability (McKay 1992), the feasibility of converting the VBNC form into a culturable form, and the existence of a VBNC form of *Campylobacter* (ACMSF 2010).

27.3 Detection, Isolation, and Confirmation

The invention of various selective media containing one or more oxygen scavengers, such as blood, ferrous iron, pyruvate, etc., and selective agents, particularly antibiotics, was prompted by the sensitivity of *Campylobacter* spp. to oxygen and oxidizing radicals. Preenrichment in a liquid medium is a common step before plating on agar. In some protocols, the initial suspension of samples is produced in a basal broth without selective agents, with the latter being gradually added after a brief period of incubation, in order to alleviate the inhibitory effects of the selective agents on potentially injured cells. The incubation temperature can also be gradually raised from 37 °C to the final incubation temperature of 41.5 °C to allow for the recovery of injured cells. One of the ISO standard procedures is based on this methodology (ISO 2006a). The use of a selective broth followed by plating on selective agars allowed for the greatest number of chicken samples to be acquired, negating the need for such a technique (Mason et al. 1999).

Bolton broth (BB), *Campylobacter* enrichment broth (CEB), and Preston broths (PB) are a few of the selective broths that have had their effectiveness compared (Baylis et al. 2000). *Campylobacter* spp. can more easily be isolated from naturally contaminated samples when the enzyme oxyrase is added to selective broths, according to research by Abeyta et al. (1997). However, it has been demonstrated that a blood-free enrichment broth that does not call for the addition of oxyrase or unique environments outperforms other, more sophisticated isolation techniques (Tran 1998). The effectiveness of various selective agars in isolating campylobacters has been studied. For instance, it has been discovered that Preston, charcoal cefoperazone deoxycholate (CCDA), and Butzler agars are all similarly efficacious. Since it enables the separation of more *Campylobacter* strains, the methodology of choice is typically the use of CCDA and incubation at 42 °C as opposed to 37 °C (Zanetti et al. 1996).

Charcoal cefoperazone deoxycholate was modified by Corry and Atabay (2001) to create CAT agar, which allowed for the development of a variety of *Campylobacter* spp. strains, including *C. upsaliensis*. After enriching a large number of samples from a variety of sources in either Preston or Park and Sanders broths, Federighi et al. (1999) compared the results and found that Park and Sanders broth followed by isolation on Karmali agar was the more efficient combination. mCCDA is used as the selective agar in both the most recent standard method (ISO 2006a) for detection and isolation and a direct plating approach (ISO 2006b) for counting campylobacters. The enrichment step makes use of Bolton broth, and the suspension is then incubated at 37 °C for 4–6 hours in a microaerophilic environment before being heated to 41.5 °C for 40–48 hours and being plated on mCCDA and another agar medium of the operator's choosing. Because the organisms are challenging to grow and maintain in reference cultures, *Campylobacter* spp. methods are not frequently employed in everyday laboratories.

Since phenotypic results are frequently unusual and challenging to read, procedures based on polymerase chain reaction (PCR) reactions may be the most useful for confirmation. One example is the hippurate hydrolysis test for separating *C. coli* from *C. jejuni*. With some success (Waller and Ogata 2000), the PCR reaction has been paired with immunoseparation to identify minute amounts of the organism in just six hours. But some elements of both food samples and particular broths can stymie PCR reactions. The use of molecular typing methods like PCR, random amplification of polymorphic DNA (RAPD), and pulsed field gel electrophoresis (PFGE) has been beneficial for epidemiological studies (such as epidemic investigations).

27.4 Clinical Signs

The normal condition comprises term delivery of poor goats or abortion during the final eight weeks of pregnancy. The majority of the time, there are no signs of impending abortion, but some does may exhibit previous vaginal discharge. On rare occasions, metritis and the ewe's mortality come after an abortion. The severity of an abortion outbreak in a flock may be significantly influenced by the timing of infection. In an experimental model, when infected at 105 days of gestation, almost all of the does miscarried, whereas at 126 days, only 20% did. This may be due to the fetus's developing immunocompetence (Grogono-Thomas et al. 2000).

27.5 Pathology

27.5.1 Gross Pathology

Aborted fetuses may merely exhibit subcutaneous edema but occasionally blood-stained fluid may enlarge bodily cavities, giving the appearance of having a pot belly. Gross lesions are seen in the placenta and/or the aborted fetus in such circumstances. Although there are not many placental diseases, the fetal cotyledons could develop necrotic plaques and yellow or dark brown exudate, and edema could develop in the intercotyledonary regions. White foci in the cotyledons of the fetus are indicative of *Toxoplasma*-induced placentitis, in contrast. Gross liver lesions with extensive yellow-brown multifocal necrosis up to 2–3 cm in diameter and uneven borders are present in 10–30% of fetuses or deceased neonatal kids. The liver is more frequently enlarged, friable, and diffusely necrotic.

Differentiating between liver lesions brought on by *C. fetus* and *C. jejuni* and those brought on by *Listeria monocytogenes*, *Yersinia pseudotuberculosis*, and *Fusobacterium necrophorum* is important. Neonatal and older kids, typically 2–4 weeks old, have necrocaseous lesions in their livers when exposed to *F. necrophorum*, but not aborted lambs. Pleomorphic *F. necrophorum* can produce long filamentous Gram-negative rods or short coccoid forms in smears collected from lesions. Multiple tiny focal abscesses in the liver and occasionally in other organs are a hallmark of postnatal septicemia brought on by *L. monocytogenes* or *Y. pseudotuberculosis*, which is the cause of abortion, as well as these conditions.

27.5.2 Histopathology

Polymorphonuclear leukocyte infiltration and severe necrosis of the chorionic epithelium characterize the placental lesion. Numerous *Campylobacter* organisms may be present in the chorionic villi's terminal vessels. There may also be a purulent bronchopneumonia in the oetus. Ovine campylobacteriosis does not display the distinct focal necrosis found in *Toxoplasma* placentitis. The liver lesions are zones of necrosis that occasionally contain small patches of healthy liver tissue. Infiltration of polymorphonuclear and mononuclear leukocytes is prevalent. Bacteria in the liver lesions are difficult to see. Compared to necrosis, the liver lesions caused by listeriosis are substantially smaller and are made up of thick cellular infiltration. Although the abortions in these cases were attributed to *Flexispira rappini*, an anaerobic flagellated bacterium that has not been classified, the gross and microscopic lesions on aborted kids in the United States were indistinguishable from those produced in *Campylobacter* abortions (Dewhirst et al. 2000).

27.6 Epidemiology and Transmission

The organisms are common in the environment because they are a natural component of the gut flora of several species, such as sheep, cattle, and birds. Disease outbreaks are often managed intensively, and it is believed that carrier goats are mostly to blame. Sexual transmission and infertility do not occur; instead, transmission occurs when contaminated feed, water, or aborted material is consumed. Usually, 10–20% of pregnancies end in abortion but in severe outbreaks, 50% of does have abortions. Aborted does and other goats in the sick flock develop acquired immunity. The majority of does recover quickly and subsequent years' fertility is unaffected. However, carrier goats persist and can infect freshly introduced susceptible animals.

Microaerophilic Gram-negative bacteria *C. jejuni* and *C. fetus* both exist. The organisms are present in certain sheep's gastrointestinal tracts, as well as those of wild and domesticated animals that are otherwise healthy. Little is currently

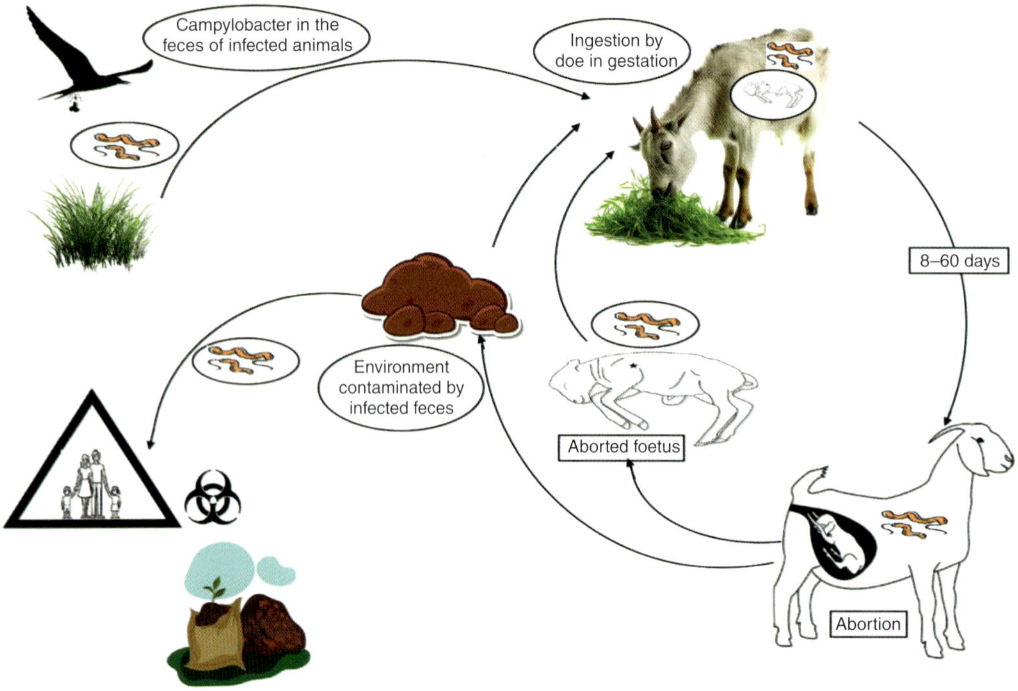

Figure 27.1 Contamination by *Campylobacter* spp.

known about the intestinal carrier stage of *C. fetus* (Figure 27.1). Although the prevalence of *C. jejuni* in cattle and sheep fluctuates, it rarely rises above 50% (Mearns 2007). Higher stocking densities have been linked to younger animals appearing to be more at danger than older animals.

Campylobacter fetus is spread by ingestion. Crows and magpies can become infected for several months and serve as vectors. Following consumption of infected kids or placentas, foxes and crows have been shown to excrete the organism for a number of weeks. Stressful situations, in this example a cold, rainy winter and recently implemented management practices, cause increased *Campylobacter* shedding, which spreads throughout the flock. Abortion happens 7–25 days after infection, usually during the third, fourth, or fifth month of pregnancy. Campylobacteriosis can also cause weak, nonviable lambs and stillbirths. Two to three weeks after the first sporadic abortion, abortion storms may happen. The incidence is usually between 10% and 20%, although outbreaks can reach 50%.

The pathogen spreads during an outbreak mostly through contamination of pasture with uterine fluids and discharge following birth or abortion. Does can release the organism through uterine discharge for up to six weeks. Infected does typically do not show any signs of abortion, while some may display vaginal discharge. Sometimes those affected do experience metritis and pass away. In an experiment, it was discovered that although does infected at 105 days had a 100% abortion rate, does infected after 126 days only had a 20% abortion rate, demonstrating the immunocompetence of the fetal gestation (Grogono-Thomas et al. 2000). Subcutaneous edema and dilated abdominal cavities that give a pot-bellied look are examples of gross pathological lesions. In such circumstances, gross lesions may be visible in the fetus or placenta. Necrotic plaques or edema may be present in the intercotyledonary regions, and the fetal cotyledons may be covered with yellow or dark brown exudate. Large yellow-brown multifocal necrosis up to 2–3 cm in diameter with uneven edges makes up liver lesions. The liver is frequently large and fragile with different degrees of necrosis. Additionally, diseases like pneumonia and lung consolidation (seen through histology) may be present in fetuses that have been aborted.

27.7 Occurrence and Distribution

The illness, which is contagious everywhere, has been documented in all Australian and New Zealand states and territories. According to West (2002), the disease is frequently linked to certain management techniques such as heavy stocking, strip/block grazing, or grain feeding. Caprine camplyobacteriosis is the most common cause of identified goat miscarriages in different countries (West 2002).

27.8 Diagnostic Tests and Specimens

Campylobacter organisms from the placenta or fetus can be used to demonstrate or isolate caprine campylobacteriosis. *C. fetus* and *C. jejuni* have similar morphology and motility, therefore the diagnosis is most easily made by demonstrating the presence of curved, S-shaped or spiral rods measuring $0.2–0.9 \times 0.5–5.0\,\mu m$ in abomasal smears, or by the observation of rapidly motile organisms with characteristic darting or corkscrew motion in abomasal content, body fluid or cotyledonary scrapings using dark-field or phase contrast microscopy. However, isolation and identification of *C. fetus* or *C. jejuni* are necessary for a conclusive diagnosis.

27.8.1 Diagnostic Sampling in Abortion Cases

The entire fetus and placenta may be submitted, but it is important to be aware that doing so would result in a postmortem and corpse disposal fee for the fetus. In its stead, samples of the placenta, fetal fluid, fetal stomach contents, liver preserved in formalin, and lung preserved in formalin can all be used. For the purpose of culture, samples of the fetal fluid and stomach contents should be collected using a sterile needle and syringe and deposited in a sterile container. All of these are representative samples and will help in excluding or diagnosing various causes of abortion in investigations. Additionally, Coopers provides a limited number of goat growers with complimentary laboratory testing. With this testing program, flocks with significant unexplained losses between scanning and kid marking or flocks whose maiden does have significantly lower kid marking rates than their older does cohorts are the target. Ten blood samples will be taken from each property in accordance with the following rules.

- On approved properties, a mob of first kidding does (or a mob identified as having unexplained losses) with low kid marking percentages will be chosen.
- A random sample of 10 does will have blood drawn for testing, and dry does will be recognized at kid marking. (While does can be checked at any time, kid marking is frequently the quickest and easiest, because at this point dry and wet does can be distinguished. Although some wet does could also be examined for comparison if preferred, dry does will most obviously indicate exposure.)
- Blood will be drawn from each doe into a 10 ml red-topped Vacutainer® tube.

27.9 Zoonotic Potential

The zoonotic illness camplyobacteriosis exists. As a result, proper hygiene precautions must be followed. This entails handling aborted fetuses and the materials related to them with gloves and thoroughly cleaning hands with soap and water before consuming anything. After handling any hazardous substance, clothing, footwear, and equipment should all be washed. It is not advisable for pregnant people or those with impaired immune systems to handle aborted fetuses.

27.10 Campylobacteriosis and Abortion Storms in Goats

Active *Campylobacter* spp. infection in pregnant does can result in full-term abortions or the birth of sick or deceased kids. The cotyledons easily split from the caruncles due to the disease's ability to cause placentitis. Abortions typically take place between seven and 25 days after infection and are more prevalent after the 12th week of pregnancy (Mearns 2007). Healthy does may be exposed to high concentrations of *Campylobacter* bacteria through contact with aborted fetuses, placentas, and uterine secretions once abortions begin (Sahin et al. 2008). Serosanguinous fluid may be present throughout the abdomen and thorax, as well as specific liver abnormalities, in *Campylobacter* abortions. The illness is self-limiting because the flock acquires immunity as a result of interaction with carriers.

According to Dewhirst et al. (2000), an outbreak is often limited to a single kidding season but could return after a 5–7-year interval. In Britain, seasonal variation in *Campylobacter* spp. recovery from cattle and goats has been noted. Although intestinal infection is likely near to 100%, *Campylobacter* spp. can be carried in the intestines and gallbladder of healthy goats without developing clinical illnesses (Mearns 2007). It is the amount of *Campylobacter* spp. shed that varies with season and food. According to various studies, *Campylobacter* spp. was intermittently shed by grazing goats in lowland farmlands, saltmarshes, and highland fells regions depending on the season. When goats were fed hay and silage instead of pasture, *Campylobacter* spp. shedding was at its lowest (0%) in November and December (Dewhirst et al. 2000). The highest shedding rates (100%) were related to higher stress levels brought on by kidding, weaning, and moving to new pastures.

27.11 Treatment, Prevention, and Control

To stop transmission of infection among the flock, aborted tissues, fetal membranes, and secretions are all contagious. Avoiding contamination of water sources is crucial. Little can be done to prevent losses once the virus has spread across the flock. Effective single- or multiple-strain *C. fetus* vaccinations are available and frequently used for prevention and control, as is a vaccine that also contains *C. jejuni*. Abortions brought on by *C. jejuni* or certain field strains of *C. fetus* with different antigenic compositions from the vaccine strain are not prevented by *C. fetus*-containing vaccines.

Additionally, a significant challenge may outweigh the immunity provided by vaccination. Although few vaccine breakdowns have been documented in New Zealand, immunization of yearly replacement does and of does that have never been exposed to the bacteria is advised in endemic areas to prevent eventual losses (Docherty et al. 1996). Different nations have lately received a vaccination. It has a single *C. fetus* strain that has demonstrated crossprotection against a number of field strains.

Early diagnosis is crucial if vaccine is to be administered during an outbreak, and immunization must begin as soon as the diagnosis is made.

References

Abeyta, C., Trost, P.A., Bark, D.H. et al. (1997). The use of bacterial membrane fractions for the detection of *Campylobacter* species in shellfish. *Journal of Rapid Methods and Automation in Microbiology* 5: 223–247.

ACMSF (2010). *Foodborne Outbreaks of Campylobacter Associated with Consumption of Chicken Liver Pâté/parfait*. London: Advisory Committee on the Microbiological Safety of Food.

Baylis, C.L., MacPhee, S.A., Martin, K.W. et al. (2000). Comparison of three enrichment media for the isolation of *Campylobacter* spp. from foods. *Journal of Applied Microbiology* 89: 884–891.

Butzler, J.P. and Oosterom, J. (1991). *Campylobacter*: pathogenicity and significance in foods. *International Journal of Food Microbiology* 12: 1–8.

Cappelier, J. M. (1997). Létat viable non cultivable chez une bacterie responsable de toxi-infections alimentaires: *Campylobacter jejuni*. PhD thesis. Université de Nantes.

Corry, J.E.L. and Atabay, H.I. (2001). Poultry as a source of *Campylobacter* and related organisms. *Journal of Applied Microbiology* 90: 96S–114S.

Debruyne, L., Gevers, D., and Vandamme, P. (2005). Taxonomy of the family Campylobacteraceae. In: *Campylobacter*, 3e (ed. I. Nachamkin and M.J. Blaser), 3–27. Washington, DC: ASM.

Dewhirst, F.E., Fox, G.J., Mendes, E.N. et al. (2000). '*Flexispira rappini*' strains represent at least 10 *Helicobacter* taxa. *International Journal of Systematic and Evolutionary Microbiology* 50: 1781–1787.

Docherty, L., Adams, M.R., Patel, P., and McFadden, J. (1996). The magnetic immuno-polymerase chain reaction assay for the detection of *Campylobacter* in milk and poultry. *Letters in Applied Microbiology* 22: 288–292.

Federighi, M., Magras, C., Pilet, M.F. et al. (1999). Incidence of thermotolerant *Campylobacter* in foods assessed by NF ISO 10272 standard: results of a two-year study. *Food Microbiology* 16: 195–204.

Fernández, H., Vera, F., Villanueva, M.P., and García, A. (2008). Occurrence of *Campylobacter* species in healthy well-nourished and malnourished children. *Brazilian Journal of Microbiology* 39: 1–3.

Foster, G., Holmes, B., Steigerwalt, A.G. et al. (2004). *Campylobacter insulaenigrae* sp. nov., isolated from marine mammals. *International Journal of Systematic and Evolutionary Microbiology* 54: 2369–2373.

Grogono-Thomas, R., Dworkin, J., Blaser, M.J., and Newell, D.G. (2000). Roles of the surface layer proteins of *Campylobacter fetus* subsp. *fetus* in ovine abortion. *Infection and Immunity* 68: 1687–1691.

ISO (2006a). *Microbiology of Food and Animal Feeding Stuffs – Horizontal Method for Detection and Enumeration of Campylobacter spp. Part 1: Detection Method. ISO 10272-1:2006*. Geneva: International Organization for Standardization.

ISO (2006b). *Microbiology of Food and Animal Feeding Stuffs – Horizontal Method for Detection and Enumeration of Campylobacter spp. Part 2: Colony Count Technique. ISO/TS 10272-2:2006*. Geneva: International Organization for Standardization.

Koenraad, P.M., Jacobs-Reitsma, W.F., van der Laan, T. et al. (1995). Antibiotic susceptibility of *Campylobacter* isolates from sewage and poultry abattoir drain water. *Epidemiology and Infection* 115: 475–483.

Mason, M.J., Humphrey, T.J., and Martin, K.W. (1999). Isolation of sublethally injured campylobacters from poultry and water sources. *British Journal of Biomedical Science* 56: 2–5.

McKay, A.M. (1992). Viable but non-culturable forms of potentially pathogenic bacteria in water. *Letters in Applied Microbiology* 12: 129–135.

Mearns, R. (2007). Other infectious causes of abortion. In: *Diseases of Sheep* (ed. I.D. Aitken), 131–132. Oxford: Blackwell.

Portner, D.C., Leuschner, R.G.K., and Murray, B.S. (2007). Optimising the viability during storage of freeze-dried cell preparations of *Campylobacter jejuni*. *Cryobiology* 54: 265–270.

Sahin, O., Plummer, P.J., Jordan, D.M. et al. (2008). Emergence of a tetracycline-resistant *Campylobacter jejuni* clone associated with outbreaks of ovine abortion in the United States. *Journal of Clinical Microbiology* 46: 1663–1671.

Skirrow, M.B. (2006). John McFadyean and the centenary of the first isolation of *Campylobacter* species. *Clinical Infectious Diseases* 43: 1213–1217.

Tran, T.T. (1998). A blood-free enrichment medium for growing *Campylobacter* spp. under aerobic conditions. *Letters in Applied Microbiology* 26: 145–148.

Vandamme, P. (2000). Taxonomy of the family Campylobacteraceae. In: *Campylobacter* (ed. I. Namchamkin and M.J. Blaser), 3–27. Washington, DC: ASM.

Vandamme, P., Debruyne, L., DeBrandt, E., and Falsen, E. (2010). Reclassification of Bacteroides ureolyticus as *Campylobacter ureolyticus* comb. nov., and emended description of the genus *Campylobacter*. *International Journal of Systematic and Evolutionary Microbiology* 60: 2016–2022.

Waller, D.F. and Ogata, S.A. (2000). Quantitative immunocapture PCR assay for detection of *Campylobacter jejuni* in foods. *Applied and Environmental Microbiology* 66: 4115–4118.

West, D.M. (2002). Ovine abortion in New Zealand. *New Zealand Veterinary Journal* 50 (supplement): 93–95.

Yamzaki-Matsune, W., Taguchi, M., Seto, K. et al. (2007). Development of a multiplex PCR assay for identification of *Campylobacter coli*, *Campylobacter fetus*, *Campylobacter hyointestinalis* subsp. *hyointestinalis*, *Campylobacter jejuni*, *Campylobacter lari* and *Campylobacter upsaliensis*. *Journal of Medical Microbiology* 56: 1467–1473.

Zanetti, F., Varoli, O., Stampi, S., and DeLuca, G. (1996). Prevalence of thermophilic *Campylobacter* and *Arcobacter butzleri* in food of animal origin. *International Journal of Food Microbiology* 33: 315–321.

Zilbauer, M., Dorrell, N., Wren, B.W., and Bajaj-Elliott, M. (2008). *Campylobacter jejuni* mediated disease pathogenesis: an update. *Transactions of the Royal Society of Tropical Medicine and Hygiene* 120: 123–129.

28

Noninfectious Abortive Diseases: Toxic Plants, Nutritional, and Genetic

Manoj Kumar Kalita[1], *Himangshu Baruah*[2], *Laishram Sanathoi Khuman*[3], *and Prerona Patowary*[4]

[1] *Department of Animal Reproduction Gynaecology and Obstetrics, Lakhimpur College of Veterinary Science, Assam Agricultural University, North Lakhimpur, India*
[2] *Department of Veterinary Pharmacology and Toxicology, Lakhimpur College of Veterinary Science, Assam Agricultural University, North Lakhimpur, India*
[3] *Department of Extension Education, Lakhimpur College of Veterinary Science, Assam Agricultural University, North Lakhimpur, India*
[4] *Department of Veterinary Clinical Medicine, Ethics and Jurisprudence, Assam Agricultural University – Goat Research Station, Burnihat, India*

28.1 Introduction

A key element in ensuring profitable animal production is reproductive efficiency. Increasing production performance will depend upon the successful measures taken for eliminating infertility. Understanding the normal reproductive process and possible associated problems is the first step toward improving reproductive efficiency (Amin et al. 2001).

The goat is clearly superior to other ruminants in tropical areas due to its status as the "poor man's cow" for landless labor and socially unprivileged members of society (Rajpal and Kaushal 2021). The goat is a multipurpose animal that is important to the financial security and nutrition of small, marginal, and landless farmers. A significant portion of the population in rural areas has engaged in the enterprise of raising goats for their dairy and agricultural subsistence. The unorganized backyard system that was once common in India is rapidly changing, and organized goat farming on a commercial basis is becoming more and more significant.

However, a major drawback in rearing goats and sheep is that they frequently experience malformations or abortions due to noninfectious causes. Noninfectious reasons are frequently undiagnosed because they are difficult to identify. Implementing efficient disease control measures for infectious causes of abortion necessitates quick diagnosis at diagnostic laboratories. There is a lack of literature on abortion in does and ewes owing to noninfectious reasons.

Physical, genetic/chromosomal, nutritional, pharmacological, drug-induced, hormonal, and other agents are examples of noninfectious causes (Roberts 1986). According to Thurmond and Picanso (1990), pregnancy losses are more common in bovines during the first and second trimesters than in the middle of pregnancy. This is likely true for other livestock animal species. According to Essawi et al. (2021), in bovines parity significantly affects the incidence of abortion, which is highest in the second parity (5.11–10.60%) and lowest in the first parity. According to Vidic et al. (2007), abortions in sheep typically happen during the last trimester, and this is most likely in the goat also. Bovines and small ruminants have the highest rates of abortion owing to noninfectious causes, followed by mares.

In small ruminants, nutrition is crucial for fertility and reproduction and a lack of feed resources may result in a decline in reproductive performance. High feed consumption can boost reproductive output while in goats, undernutrition may have a deleterious long- and short-term impact on ovarian activity (Tanaka et al. 2004). To extend the seasonal breeding time, the feed flushing system has been used in sheep and goat management systems (Seegers et al. 2011).

A basic principle for maximizing reproductive effectiveness is the link between diet and ovarian function. Additionally, small ruminants sometimes suffer from reproductive dysfunction, including infertility, abortion, and fetal abnormalities, as a result of grazing poisonous plants or consuming feed that has been tainted by toxic plants.

It can be difficult to pinpoint the exact cause of reproductive disease because there are many management aspects involved in addition to reproductive xenobiotic poisons, such as plant toxins (Riet-Correa et al. 2011). To make an accurate diagnosis, create intervention strategies, and enhance reproductive performance, it is necessary to use all diagnostic tools, including field studies, clinical signs, gross, and microscopic pathology, as well as chemical identification of plant and plant

Elements of Reproduction and Reproductive Diseases of Goats, First Edition. Edited by Tanmoy Rana.

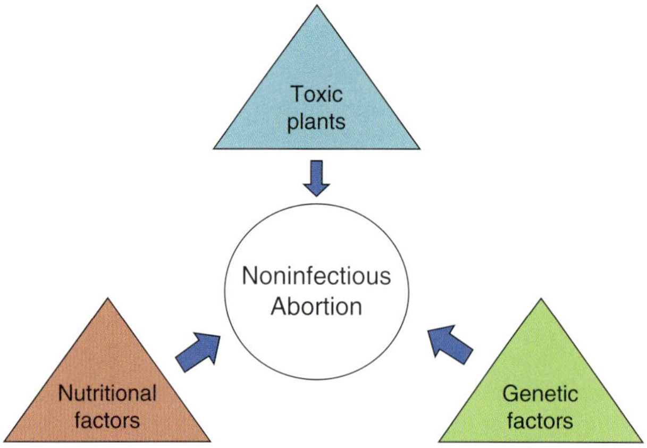

Figure 28.1 Basic factors for noninfectious abortion in small ruminants.

toxins in animal samples. This chapter discusses a number of likely noninfectious causes of abortion in does and ewes, mainly pertaining to toxic plants, nutrition, and genetics factors as well as their adverse effects on the reproductive system (Figure 28.1).

28.2 Toxic Plants

28.2.1 Abortifacient Plants

28.2.1.1 *Aspidosperma pyrifolium*

In the semiarid region of northern Brazil, a tree belonging to the Apocynaceae family, called *Aspidosperma pyrifolium* (Figure 28.2), causes embryonic deaths, abortions, and premature births in goats. Sheep and cattle are also likely affected. Poisoning mostly happens in the first few months of the dry season, when fodder is scarce due to a lack of rain. When pregnant goats are moved to plant-infested areas, abortions are also seen. According to earlier research, inexperienced goats have a higher rate of abortion than experienced goats (Lima and Soto-Blanco 2010). *A. pyrifolium* consumption has also been linked to abortion in sheep and cattle (Silva et al. 2006). Goats, however, were the only animals to experience abortion in outbreaks that affected flocks of sheep and goats (Lima and Soto-Blanco 2010). The most common clinical symptom of *A. pyrifolium* poisoning is abortion at any stage of pregnancy or the premature birth of kids that die shortly after birth.

Although the monoterpenoid indole alkaloids aspidofractinine, 15-demethoxypyrifoline, and N-formylaspidofractine have been previously found in the plant (Araújo et al. 2007), the poisonous component of *A. pyrifolium* is currently unknown. Isocupressic acid, a recognized abortifacient in pine needles, was not found in the plant's leaves (Riet-Correa et al. 2009b).

It is important to confirm the diagnosis of plant-caused abortion in sheep and goats and to distinguish it from other causes of abortion, such as toxoplasmosis. There are no known infectious disease-related causes of abortion in sheep or goats found in north-east Brazil's semiarid regions. Leptospirosis and brucellosis are additional conditions that result in abortions in cattle in this area.

28.2.1.2 *Ateleia glazioveana* and *Tetrapterys* spp.

According to several studies (Tokarnia et al. 1989; Stolf et al. 1994; Gava and Barros 2001), the Malpighiaceae plants *Ateleia glazioveana* (Leg. papilionoideae; Figure 28.2), *T. acutifolia*, and *T. multiglandulosa* (Figure 28.3) cause abortions and neonatal death in cattle. *A. glazioveana* has occasionally been reported to cause abortion in sheep (Gava et al. 2003), and

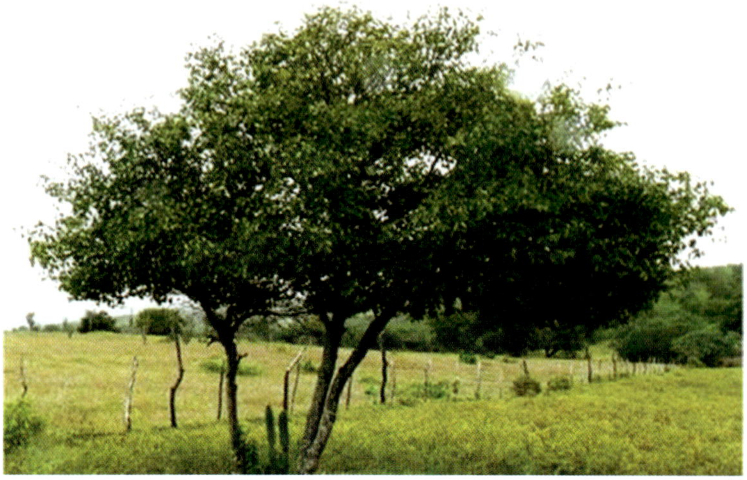

Figure 28.2 *Aspidosperma pyrifolium* tree. *Source:* F. Riet-Correa et al. (2011)/Journal of Applied Toxicology 32: 245–254.

experimentally induced abortion and neonatal mortality have been observed in cattle, sheep, and goats (Gardner et al. 2011; Riet-Correa et al. 2009a). These plants can also lead to cardiac disease, which involves heart fibrosis and can result in sudden death or congestive heart failure, as well as a condition of the neurological system that causes vacuolation (status spongiosus) of the central nervous system.

The most significant toxic plant in western Santa Catarina and north-western Rio Grande do Sul is *Ateleia glazioveana*. It can grow as tall as 15 m but usually stands between 5 and 10 m. The winter season, which runs from June to August, is when this deciduous tree is leafless. Animals eat the leaves because they are tasty, although they typically do so when there is a paucity of food due to drought or overgrazing (Gava and Barros 2001; Gava et al. 2001). Cattle, sheep, and horses who consume this plant experience abortions. Cattle can have abortions at any point in the gestation period, although they typically happen between November and May when the animals are eating green foliage. When livestock consume autumn tree litter, abortions can occasionally happen if the leaves are mixed with grasses. According to Gava and Barros (2001) and Gava et al. (2001), 10–40% of pregnant cows abort their calves.

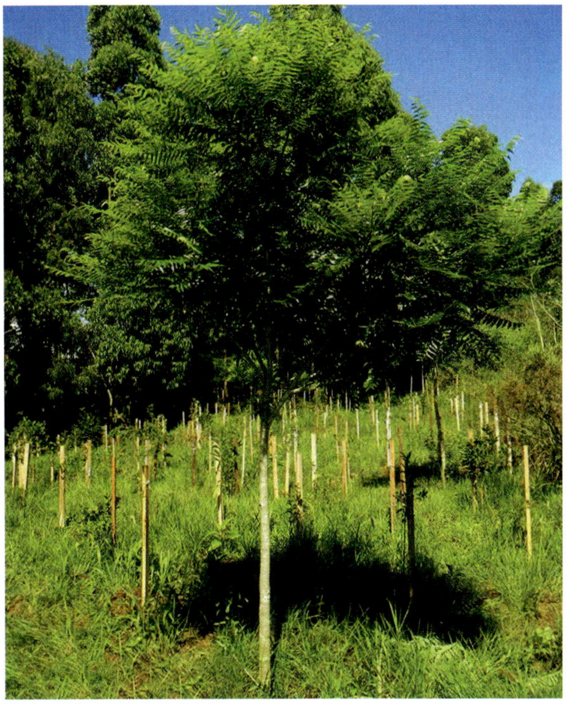

Figure 28.3 *Ateleia glazioveana* tree. *Source:* F. Riet-Correa et al. (2011)/Journal of Applied Toxicology 32: 245–254.

28.2.1.3 *Tetrapterys acutifolia* and *Tetrapterys multiglandulosa*

Both *Tetrapterys multiglandulosa* and *T. acutifolia* are categorized as shrubs or vines. *T. multiglandulosa* is found in the states of Rio de Janeiro, São Paulo, and Mato Grosso do Sul, while *T. acutifolia* is found in the states of Minas Gerais and Esprito Santo. These plants can cause abortions, but the frequency of those abortions varies. Seven cows died from cardiac insufficiency and 230 out of 290 cows (or 79%) either had abortions or delivered weak calves during an outbreak of *T. multiglandulosa* poisoning (Figure 28.4) (Carvalho et al. 2006). Similar clinical symptoms and lesions are seen in animals poisoned by *Tetrapterys* spp. and *A. glazioveana*.

Abortions can happen at any stage of pregnancy (Riet-Correa et al. 2009b), although various studies have shown that the incidence of abortions in cattle is highest between the sixth and ninth months of gestation (Peixoto et al. 2011). Some cows go through a stage of lethargy for 1–3 days before giving birth. Other cows spend a lot of time in lying down and occasionally show signs of blindness. Most of the lambs that aborted after ingesting *A. glazioveana* or *Tetrapterys* spp. in one experiment did not exhibit clinical signs (Raffi et al. 2004; Riet-Correa et al. 2009b). Cattle have been known to have retained placentas and bloody vaginal discharge (Stolf et al. 1994).

Calves and lambs can survive birth when consumption occurs near the end of pregnancy and at lower dosages, but newborns may be weak and unable to stand or suckle normally, sometimes dying in a few hours or days (Gardner et al. 2011; Raffi et al. 2004; Riet-Correa et al. 2009a). The newborns that are able to stand may be weak and lethargic. Although some of these animals do survive, the majority pass away soon after birth (Riet-Correa et al. 2009a; Stolf et al. 1994).

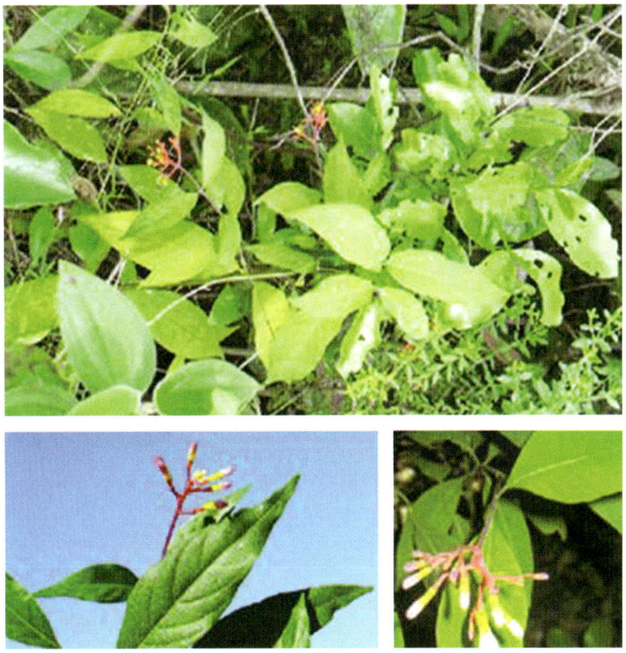

Figure 28.4 *Tetrapterys multiglandulosa. Source:* F. Riet-Correa et al. (2011)/Journal of Applied Toxicology 32: 245–254.

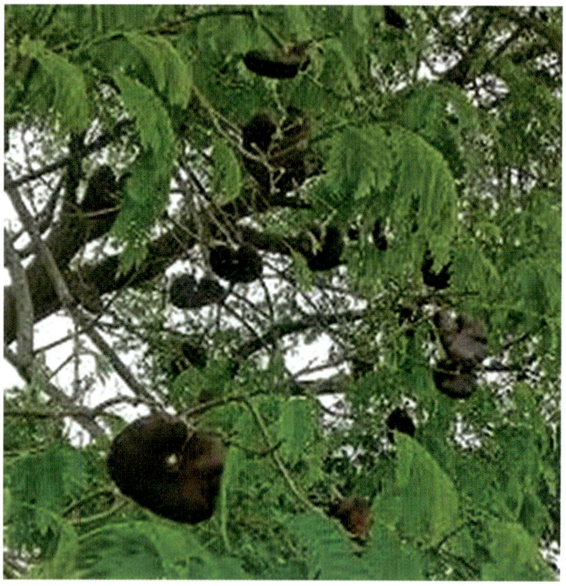

Figure 28.5 *Enterolobium timbouva. Source:* F. Riet-Correa et al. (2011)/Journal of Applied Toxicology 32: 245–254.

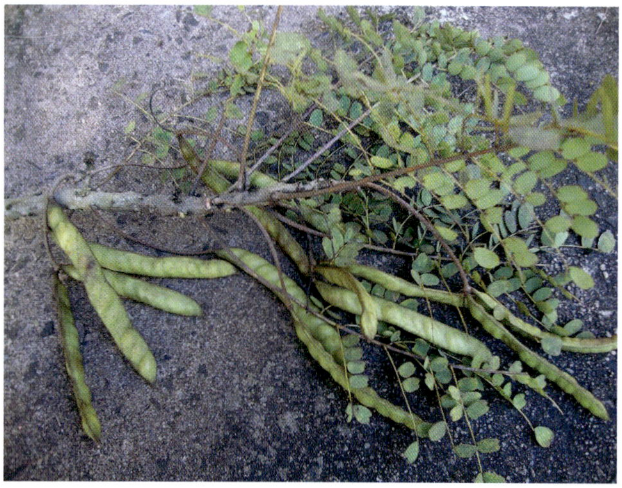

Figure 28.6 *Stryphnodendron obovatum. Source:* Reginaldo Baiao/Flickr/Public domain/.

28.2.1.4 *Enterolobium contortisiliquum, Stryphnodendron obovatum*, and *Stryphnodendron fissuratum*

Leguminous trees from the family Fabaceae and subfamily Mimosoideae can be found in Brazil. This group includes *Enterolobium contortisiliquum* (= *Enterolobium timbouva*) (Figure 28.5) (Grecco et al. 2002; Mendonça et al. 2009; Dobereiner and Canella 1956; Tokarnia et al. 1991), *Stryphnodendron obovatum* (Figure 28.6) (Tokarnia et al. 1998), and *Stryphnodendron fissuratum* (Figure 28.7) (Ferreira et al. 2009). These trees yield pods that, when eaten, have been linked to gastrointestinal symptoms, photosensitivity, and calf abortion. *E. contortisiliquum* has also been linked to photosensitivity in sheep (Bezerra 2011) and diarrhea and abortion in goats (Benício et al. 2005). Despite numerous poisoning incidents involving these plants that are linked to abortion, only *S. obovatum* in cattle (Tokarnia et al. 1998), *S. fissuratum* in goats (Albuquerque et al. 2011), and *E. contortisiliquum* in guinea pigs (Bonel-Raposo et al. 2008) have been shown to have abortive properties. Retained placenta and endometrial bacterial infection have been seen to potentially worsen the toxicosis in the case of abortion caused by *S. fissuratum* (Albuquerque et al. 2011).

28.2.2 Teratogenic Plants

28.2.2.1 Lupines

The *Lupinus* genus has approximately 150 species in North America, many of which are closely related and challenging to categorize taxonomically. Though hundreds of sheep are poisoned by lupine poisoning, the more frequent side-effect of lupines nowadays is cow teratogenesis, also known as crooked calf disease. Lupines are regarded as very nutritious legumes and play a significant role in the diets of both livestock and wildlife in many habitats. However, they are also abundant in a wide variety of teratogenic and poisonous alkaloids.

When calves are born with cleft palates and skeletal contracture-type abnormalities, they are said to have crooked calf disease. Axial lesions, such as scoliosis, lordosis, torticollis, and kyphosis, are among the musculoskeletal contractures. Along with permanent contractures, rotational faults, significant joint deformation, ankyloses, and bony deformation, it also causes appendicular contractures, which most frequently affect the front legs. Crooked calf disease has been linked to specific lupine populations and, later, specific lupine alkaloids. As the disease depends on pregnant cows grazing toxic lupines between days 40 and 100 of pregnancy, exposure time and duration are crucial (Panter et al. 1999a; Shupe et al. 1967).

The severity of birth abnormalities brought on by lupine ingestion depends on poison dose and duration. Some severe calf abnormalities can cause dystocia and make vaginal delivery impossible. Some calves can be unable to stand and nurse. Others may just have insignificant lesions that eventually go away. A cleft palate is a common development that is sometimes disregarded, but it is still a severe lesion since it makes it harder for kids to suckle and raises the risk of inhalation pneumonia. Despite the fact that clinical lupine-induced teratogenesis most frequently affects cattle, comparable birth abnormalities have been replicated in several rodent and animal species, indicating that many species are susceptible (Panter et al. 1999a).

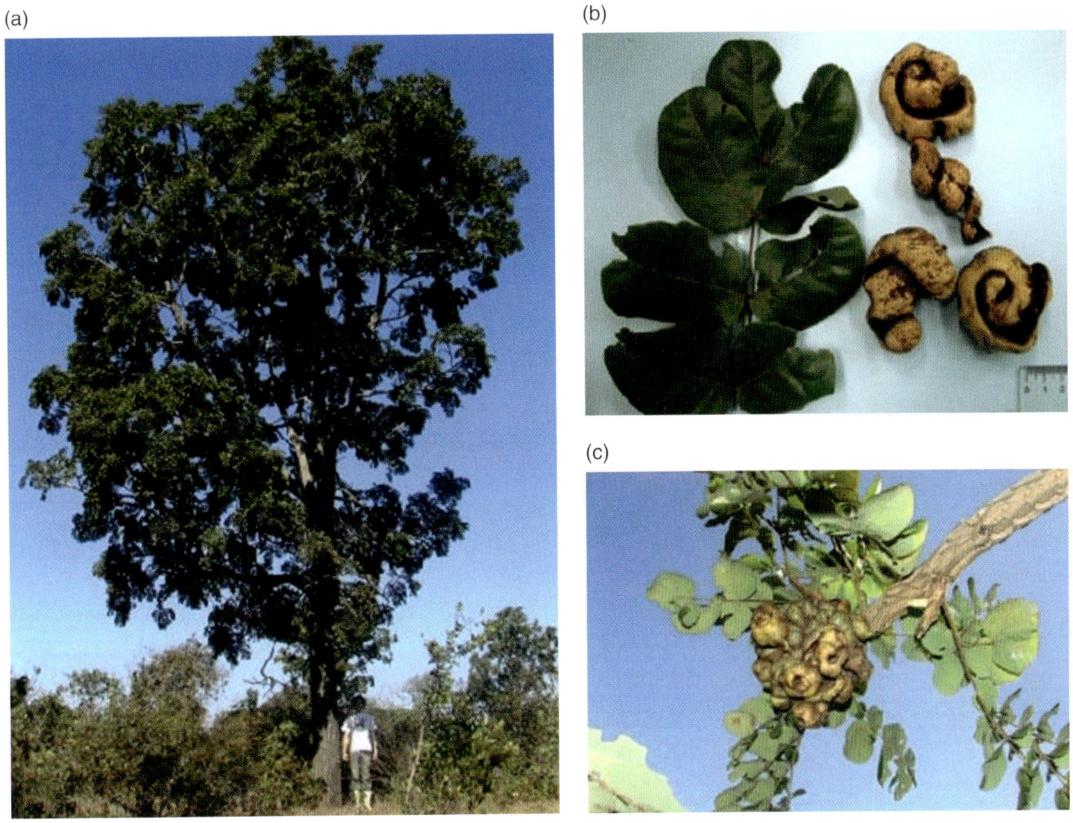

Figure 28.7 *Stryphnodendron fissuratum*. (a) Tree. (b) Leaves. (c) Seeds. *Source:* F. Riet-Correa et al. (2011)/Journal of Applied Toxicology 32: 245–254.

For instance, the yellow lupine *Lupinus sulphureus*, which is native to Oregon, Washington, and British Columbia, has seven distinct populations, each of which has a different alkaloid profile and teratogen concentration that affect the incidence of disease and relative risk. Anagyrine (Keeler 1973) and ammodendrine (Keeler and Panter 1989) are lupine teratogens. According to physiological research, the restriction in fetal movement caused by alkaloids during the crucial periods of gestation is the cause of the harmful effect (Panter et al. 1990). The skeletal muscle nicotinic acetylcholine receptors have become desensitized as a result. Other plants that generate comparable contracture abnormalities, such as poison hemlock (*Conium maculatum*) and wild tree tobacco (*Nicotiana glauca*), have been found to have similar processes. As mentioned, there are various other plants that can result in cleft palates and skeletal deformities similar to contractures.

28.2.2.2 *Conium maculatum, Nicotiana glauca*, and *Nicotiana tabacum*

Tobacco stalks (*Nicotiana tabacum*), wild tobacco (*N. glauca*), and poison hemlock (*Conium maculatum*) have all been linked to birth malformations in cattle and pigs, though less frequently than lupine-induced teratogenesis. Cattle, pigs, lambs, and goats have all undergone experimental induction of these birth abnormalities. The congenital malformations include cleft palate, arthrogryposis, scoliosis, torticollis, and angular limb deformities. The neuromuscular effects of plant toxins, which limit fetal movement during crucial gestational developmental phases, have also been demonstrated to contribute to the teratogenic consequences (Lee et al. 2019). The sensitive period of gestation lasts 30–60 days in pigs, sheep, and goats (Panter et al. 1999a). When pregnant goats were exposed to plant or refined toxins on days 32–41 of gestation, a nearly 100% incidence of cleft palate was produced in the fetuses (Panter et al. 1999a). As with lupines, the association of these terata with exposure during vulnerable gestation phases allows for the identification of plant-induced arthrogyroposis with these plants.

28.2.2.3 *Veratrum californicum* (*False Hellebore* or *Corn Lily*)

Veratrum californicum grows predominantly in damp, open meadows and marshes, or along the edges of streams, ponds, and lakes in western North America's high mountain ranges. It is an upright plant with leaves that range in shape from oval to lanceolate and are about 30 cm long. It can grow as tall as 2.5 m.

In pregnant sheep that grazed on *V. californicum*, craniofacial birth abnormalities were first found to be caused by the bacterium. In the flock, over 25% of the pregnant ewes experienced high rates of morbidity. From mild superior brachygnathism to severe cyclopia with anencephaly, these birth defects vary in severity (Welch et al. 2009). Due to these spectacular malformations, producers began calling the syndrome "monkey-faced lamb disease" (Binns et al. 1965). Since these first studies, teratogenic *Veratrum* toxins have been found as well as the susceptible gestation time in different species.

There are numerous neurotoxins, poisons that bind to sodium channels and cause cardiotoxic and respiratory effects, but the teratogens cyclopamine and jervine, which both cause congenital cyclopia, are among the more than 50 complex steroidal alkaloids that have been observed (Binns et al. 1965). As the cyclopic deficiency only manifests in pregnant sheep who consume the plant after the 14th day of gestation, these teratogenic consequences are gestation age specific. Before the 19th day of pregnancy, exposure may result in death of the embryo. Phocomelia and tracheal stenosis are frequently caused by exposure between days 28 and 33 of pregnancy (Keeler et al. 1986). The sonic hedgehog signaling system, which is crucial for development of the craniofacial embryo, is disrupted by both jervine and cyclopamine (Gaffield and Keeler 1984).

28.2.2.4 *Mimosa tenuiflora*

In sheep, goats, and cattle, *Mimosa tenuiflora* (Figure 28.8) and most likely *M. ophthalmocentra* (Fabaceae, Mimosoideae) induce deformities and embryonic mortality. According to Riet-Correa et al. (2007), 273 120 kids as well as 259 582 lambs are lost annually in north-eastern Brazil as a result of abnormalities. Goats that solely consumed *M. tenuiflora* as green forage throughout all stages of gestation were shown to have a number of abnormalities (Pimentel et al. 2007). Goats have had a significant rate of embryonic mortality after receiving *M. tenuiflora* as their sole supply of green fodder during the first 60 days of pregnancy (Dantas 2010). In areas of Brazil where deformities in goats and sheep are common, *M. ophthalmocentra* is a common plant; in contrast, *M. tenuiflora* is either uncommon or nonexistent. Malformations seen in ruminants in the semiarid region of Brazil are also caused by *M. ophthalmocentra* poisoning (Pessoa et al. 2011). Malformations caused by *M. tenuiflora* frequently affect both sheep and goats, but less frequently affect cattle. In regions where *M. tenuiflora* has spread, higher incidence rates have been seen in sheep and goats fed diets supplemented with grain or byproducts near the end of the dry season.

Lambs, young kids, and calves may be born with a wide range of bone abnormalities, including permanent forelimb flexion (arthrogryposis), which may also be shortened or twisted; malformations of the head and face, such as micrognathia, primary cleft lip associated with hypoplasia, or unilateral or bilateral aplasia of the incisive bone and secondary cleft palate (palatoschisis). Animals can be born blind in some cases, with variable degrees of corneal opacity and/or microphthalmia, whereas in other cases they may have ocular dermoids. Acephaly, bicephaly, hydranencephaly, hypoplasia of the tongue, meningocele, and syringocele are further possible anomalies. Variations of these deformities can be seen in several animals. However, many animals that just have forelimb flexion are able to survive with this abnormality (Medeiros et al. 2005; Nóbrega et al. 2005; Dantas et al. 2007). In contrast, the majority of animals with head and spine deformities die.

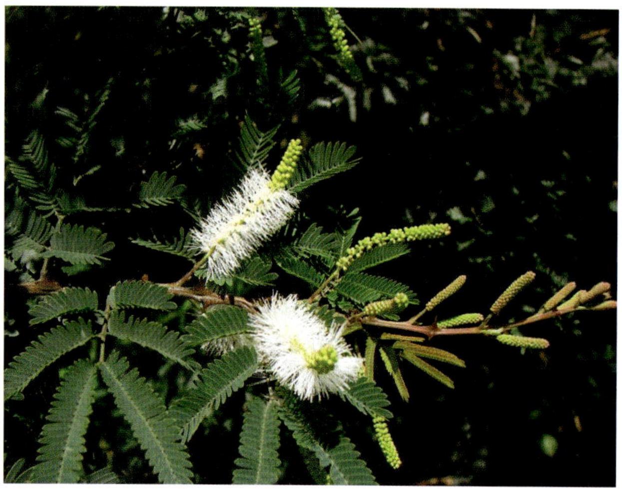

Figure 28.8 *Mimosa tenuiflora. Source:* João Medeiros/Wikimedia Commons/CC BY 2.0.

Although the principal toxin in *M. tenuiflora* is currently unknown, tryptamine-derived alkaloids have been found in the plant's leaves and seeds (Gardner et al. 2011). Animal abnormalities in *M. tenuiflora* or *M. ophthalmocentra* growing regions are indicative of poisoning.

28.2.3 Reproductive Toxins

Often, poisonous plants have an impact on reproductive function, but the more apparent lesions and diseases overshadow these reproductive alterations. Locoweeds, for instance, are typically thought of as neurotoxins because they frequently cause spectacular neurological damage but in specific circumstances (dosage, duration, and frequency of poisoning), reproductive failure may be the first symptom of locoweed poisoning. Strong endocrine disruptors, locoweeds change spermatogenesis and spermatic maturation, and reduce libido, all of which leads to male reproductive failure when consumed (Panter et al. 1999b). Female reproduction is also negatively impacted by poisoning, which can cause abortion, fetal myocardial dysfunction with placental injury, hydrops amnii, and cystic ovaries with altered estrus. Neonatal victims of locoweed poisoning struggle to walk and stand, and some are unable to suckle. Small calves or lambs with phocomelia are examples of locoweed-related birth abnormalities.

Reproductive failure has also been linked to chronic selenium toxicity. Animals which graze or consume contaminated feeds containing seleniferous plants become sick. Acute myocardial necrosis and sudden death are the most common symptoms of acute selenium overdose. With loss of condition, lesions on the hair and hooves, and anecdotal accounts of infertility, chronic poisoning is very different. Recent research has shown that chronically poisoned rams exhibit substantial motility impairments due to impaired spermatic maturation (Davis and Stegelmeier 2019). According to preliminary investigations, bulls are not similarly influenced by the same doses and periods of time. Ewes that have been poisoned repeatedly may experience lower conception rates and early embryonic death. To more fully understand these alterations and identify whether cattle are similarly impacted, more research is required.

Numerous other poisonous plants harm particular organ systems, which may afterwards impair fertility. For instance, plant-induced liver disease affects a person's ability to reproduce. Similar to humans, animals plagued by significant plant-induced photosensitivity would struggle to maintain body condition, breed, and conceive on schedule.

28.2.3.1 Nitrate Poisoning

Nitrate poisoning occurs primarily in cattle and at a lower frequency in sheep and goats. Numerous plant species can build up lethal amounts of nitrates. Nitrate build-up varies greatly amongst fodder species, although these levels are frequently correlated with environmental conditions like dryness, particularly when plant growth is constrained while nitrate intake is unaffected (Worth et al. 1997). At the end of a dry season, particularly in the flush of new growth following the first rains, high amounts of nitrates may be present. In soils that have been highly fertilized with nitrogen-based fertilizer or organic matter derived from animals, nitrate concentrations may also be raised (Hintz and Thompson 1998).

All plant parts acquire nitrates, although stalks and leaves may have very high levels. In general, seeds and grains are exempt. Oats, beets, rape, turnips, soybeans, barley, flax, alfalfa, millet, rye, sorghum, Sudan grass, Johnson grass, wheat, and corn are examples of crops that frequently develop lethal nitrate concentrations (>0.5%). Ragweed, pigweed, wild oats, cudweeds, sunflowers, fireweed, cheese weed, sweet clover, smart weed, and golden eye are typical nitrate-accumulating weeds. Abortions have been linked to nitrate poisoning in cattle grazing on ryegrass (*Lolium multiflorum*) and/or oats (*Avena sativa*) in the state of Santa Catarina (Jonck et al. 2011).

Nitrate can enter the placenta and produce fetal methemoglobinemia, which is followed by fetal anoxia and death, leading to abortions. Nitrites are easily absorbed, and once in the bloodstream, they attach to hemoglobin and oxidize it to produce methemoglobin. Due to its inability to bind oxygen, methemoglobin is ineffective. According to Knight and Walter (2001), methemoglobinemia also affects how oxygen is transported through the placenta, which can lead to fetal hypoxia, abortion, and death.

28.3 Nutritional Effects on Reproduction

Serious nutritional shortages of trace metals like copper, cobalt, selenium, iodine, manganese, and zinc are regularly experienced by livestock animals. It is thought that concurrent infertility in these animals is related to enzymatic dysfunctions brought on by these deficits. It is challenging to identify which nutrient shortage results in abortion since several processes are engaged in the fetomaternal axis's nutrient exchange. The probability of estrus disorders (prolonged estrus) and early embryonic death or abnormality because of ovum aging rises when the animal is fed primarily with roughage (hay) (Uçar et al. 2004, 2008). Additionally, it is crucial to supply supplemental nutrition (for at least 2–3 months) to dairy Saanen does and twin-lambing ewes during the lactation phase (Aytug et al. 1990). If this is not done, there may be a higher chance of metabolic abnormalities and reproductive diseases in the mother as well as a higher risk of weakness or growth retardation in lambs and kids (Uçar et al. 2004, 2008).

Deficits in vitamin A, some minerals (manganese and iodine), and energy lower fertility and, in cases of chronic shortage, may be linked to abortion (Hurley and Doane 1989). According to Corah and Ives (1991), a copper deficit in farm animals is linked to infertility and embryo mortality. According to Duffy et al. (1977), low zinc levels have been linked to altered myometrial contractibility during prolonged labor, decreased fertility, and abortion. In his review on trace element deficiencies and ruminant fertility, Hidiroglou (1979) suggested that there was a close connection between the plasma levels of some elements and vitamins and the reproductive performance and abortion in ruminants. He also explains the role of various minerals and vitamins on the reproductive performances of ruminants. Giadinis et al. (2016) verified in cows what had long been hypothesized – that low selenium level is associated with abortion.

The effects of an energy-deficient diet have not been observed in large ruminants or other livestock animals, but they may cause pregnant toxemia in small ruminants carrying twins or multiple fetuses (Hidiroglou 1979). According to Waldhalm et al. (1979), protein deficiency in late pregnancy may contribute to newborn mortality.

In ewes that had abortions as well as in healthy controls, Aytekin and Aypak (2011) measured the serum levels of calcium, phosphorus, magnesium, copper, zinc, iron, nitric oxide, retinol, and beta-carotene. Retinol, carotene, phosphorus, and zinc concentrations were considerably lower in aborted ewes compared to healthy controls, but calcium and nitric oxide concentrations were higher. The control and aborted ewes did not have significantly different serum levels of iron, copper, or magnesium. In three of 211 abortions in caprines, thyroid hyperplasia was found (Moeller 2001). Iodine levels were not tested, despite the fact that thyroid hyperplasia may be caused by an iodine deficit and is likely a cause of abortion. In six and two out of 211 entries respectively, selenium and copper deficiency were mentioned as potential causes of abortion. Small ruminants are more likely to experience miscarriages due to trace element deficiencies.

28.3.1 Selenium/Vitamin E Deficiency (Nutritional Muscular Dystrophy or White Muscle Disease)

Nutritional muscular dystrophy (NMD), also known as stiff lamb disease, is a type of muscular dystrophy brought on by a lack of vitamin E, selenium (Se), or both in young ruminants. Together, selenium and vitamin E work as antioxidants to prevent oxidative damage to cell membranes. The enzyme glutathione peroxidase, which transforms hydrogen peroxide into water and other harmless substances, requires selenium as a cofactor. Loss of membrane integrity arises from a deficiency in one or both nutrients (Sobiech and Kuleta 2002).

Clinically, the condition has been divided into cardiac and skeletal types. The cardiac type usually develops quickly in newborns and is most frequently detected in severely disabled or dead animals (Ramírez-Bribiesca et al. 2001). A sign suggesting damage to the cardiac, diaphragmatic, and intercostal muscles is respiratory difficulty. In elderly animals, respiratory symptoms may be accompanied by locomotor dysfunction and/or circulatory failure. Clinically, animals may exhibit abrupt death, paresis, stiffness, or the inability to stand (Larsen 1988). Young calves, lambs, and kids who are growing quickly can develop Se deficit and NMD.

Se-deficient soils are widespread both globally and in many parts of the United States, including the North-east, North-west, and Great Lakes regions. If the mineral is not supplemented, diets based on foods produced in these regions will lead to Se insufficiency. Supplemental Se is only allowed in complete ruminant diets at a maximum level of 0.3 ppm (no more than 0.7 mg/day for adult sheep and 3 mg/day for adult cattle). The use of injectable sources is required to prevent clinical deficits since this level of supplementation is frequently insufficient in poor areas (Aziz et al. 1984).

The determination of plasma vitamin E levels (1.1 ppm) and whole-blood levels of selenium (>0.07 ppm selenium is normal) serves as the basis for the final diagnosis. Red blood cell levels of glutathione peroxidase can be assessed indirectly (Ramírez-Bribiesca et al. 2001).

Petechial hemorrhages and muscular edema are necropsy lesions. The damaged skeletal and cardiac muscle, diaphragm, and tongue will have pale white streaking as a hallmark. However, juvenile ruminants' muscles are often quite pale, thus lesions could not be obvious without a histological investigation (Cuesta et al. 1995). The differential diagnoses for neonatal ruminants with respiratory and cardiac dysfunction include pneumonia and congenital heart abnormalities.

Considering that many diseases are asymptomatic, awareness of regional selenium deficits is crucial. Supplementing with vitamin E and selenium is a method of control, especially for pregnant cows and/or young animals in locations with low levels of the nutrients. In areas with severe selenium deficiency, injectable selenium supplements are necessary to prevent clinical disease (Gabryszuk and Klewiec 2002). Affected animals may be treated by administering vitamin E and selenium injections.

28.3.2 Pregnancy Toxemia

The nutrition of the unborn lamb or kid is a significant component in the nutrition of the pregnant ewe or doe. Compared to many other animals, sheep and goats have a short gestation period, and the last two months of pregnancy are when fetal need for nutrients and glucose is highest. In actuality, the final six weeks of pregnancy are when the fetus grows by roughly 80%; if twins are present, the total weight gain is significant (Fthenakis 2022).

Although there is still much to understand about pregnancy toxemia, good management and a nutritious diet can reduce the risk of the disease (Van Saun 2000). During late pregnancy, the overall metabolic rate rises by at least 50%. It has been demonstrated that late-pregnant ewes and goats require approximately 50% more feed when delivering a single lamb and approximately 75% more feed when producing twins. However, the increased feed intake occasionally surpasses the sheep's ability to digest it unless some of the hay is replaced with grain. The digestive system of the animal will be crowded with several fetuses, which will limit intake; in this situation, concentrates can be useful (Lima et al. 2012).

During the last six weeks of pregnancy, one pound of corn or the equivalent in high-energy concentrate should be provided every day.

Affected ewes frequently lack nourishment, stand aside from the rest of the flock, walk haphazardly, and appear dull. They may have compromised vision and exhibit minimal fear of people or dogs. Blindness is frequently the end outcome, and convulsions, teeth grinding, difficult breathing, and typically mucus flow from the nostrils can follow. The mortality rate is roughly 80%, and deaths often take place within 2–10 days. Eventually, a shock-like condition develops.

Ewes or goats that are pregnant should have a body condition score of 3.5 and be in medium condition. Excess fat should be decreased throughout the first half of pregnancy, and weight increase should only be permitted in the six weeks leading up to lambing or kidding. Ewes and does that are excessively overweight appear to be more vulnerable than normal ewes and does to the stress syndrome of pregnancy toxemia. Ewes and does that are late in their pregnancies should always be handled carefully to reduce any potential physical or emotional stress. Never withhold food and if at all possible, avoid transportation (Al-Qudah 2011).

Other options for treating pregnancy toxemia in ewes and does besides feeding concentrates include administering oral propylene glycol or corn syrup as quick sources of energy at a rate of 200 ml four times per day along with 3–4 l of an electrolyte solution made for livestock dehydration (Schlumbohm and Harmeyer 2008).

28.3.3 Milk Fever

A metabolic disorder known as parturient paresis affects pregnant and lactating ewes and does and is characterized by acute-onset hypocalcemia, fast development of hyperexcitability and ataxia, and eventual mortality. In contrast to parturient paresis in dairy cattle, which typically develops within a few days of calving, the condition in ewes and does typically develops prior to parturition and less frequently later. This condition may be underdiagnosed in some situations (Fthenakis 2022).

Parturient paresis results from a decrease in calcium intake when calcium requirements are elevated, typically during late gestation. This causes a low serum calcium content, especially in animals carrying numerous kids. Pregnancy toxemia that is present concurrently can worsen some situations. Ewes with both hyperketonemia and hypocalcemia run the risk of more severe disease because they may not be able to create endogenous glucose as quickly as ewes with only hyperketonemic symptoms (Fthenakis 2022).

The greatest requirement for calcium due to mineralization of the fetal skeleton occurs 1–3 weeks prior to delivery, especially when several fetuses are present *in utero*. Parturient paresis can occur at any time between six weeks before and 10 weeks following parturition (Fthenakis 2022).

Every time there is a sudden decrease in calcium intake, the body needs 24–72 hours to start the metabolic processes required to release calcium from storage. In older ewes and does, animals with chronic calcium shortage, and those whose diets are low in calcium, the mobilization of stored calcium may be insufficient to meet the animal's demands (Fthenakis 2022).

Low-quality green hays, corn silage, cereal hays, and pasture are a few examples of forages with low calcium contents. The majority of grains have low calcium contents but high phosphorus concentrations as well, creating an inverse calcium:phosphorus ratio that raises dietary risk. During the winter, vitamin D deficiency in housed ruminants reduces calcium absorption from the GI tract.

Parturient paresis typically occurs in epidemics, with the majority of instances taking place in the final few weeks of pregnancy, while it is not unusual for individual animals to be affected. Typically, only about 5% of the animals are affected but in extreme outbreaks, up to 30% of the flock may be afflicted.

Parturient paresis should be treated as soon as possible, typically with calcium borogluconate IV (50–150 ml of a 23% solution). Products with calcium that also include phosphorus, magnesium, and dextrose probably have extra medicinal potential. Relapse can be avoided by administering a calcium solution orally or subcutaneously. Calcium solution should be heated to between 35 and 40 °C before delivery. Intravenous administration needs to be done gradually over a period of 5–7 minutes (Fthenakis 2022).

28.4 Genetic Effects

High milk production is a trademark of the Saanen goat breed, which is well suited for intensive breeding (Elmas 2013; Yarsan 2020). In general, the genetic characteristic affects the offspring yield about 15% (Ileri 2007). Indigenous goats are projected to have fewer reproduction issues due to their superior tolerance to all circumstances, but lower output levels than culture breeds. However, despite their high levels of yield (kids and milk), culture breeds also experience increased stress as a result of their high levels of output (Dwyer 2020; Uçar et al. 2020). It is critical to monitor culture breeds' male and female fertility rates in particular. In dairy breeds with twinning traits and adaption sensitivity, episodes of infertility brought on by extreme stress can occur more frequently (Elmas 2013).

28.4.1 Breed

Indigenous breeds may also vary in fertility (Aytug et al. 1990; Elmas 2013; Yarsan 2020). According to Sonmez (2012) and Elmas (2013), twin-lambing Chios and Romanov breeds are more vulnerable to pregnancy toxemia. Low-yielding but resilient native breeds, like Morkaraman sheep and Hair goats, may experience fertility issues less frequently than high-yielding but fragile varieties.

The main cause of the rise in infertility is that not enough is being done to prevent the welfare of animals from declining when productivity rises (Uçar et al. 2020; Dwyer 2020). High-yielding female breeders may experience hoof, udder, and gastrointestinal issues, as well as early culling, infertility, pregnancy toxemia, and abortus instances, in intensive dairy farms if they are not adequately handled and nourished (Aytug et al. 1990; Arthur et al. 1993; Elmas 2013).

28.4.2 Anatomy and Structural Defects

Rarely hymens are seen in fleshy pillars caused by the cervix in sheep and goats, and anatomical anomalies or developmental arrests such as unicornuate uterus, uterus didelphys, persistence of the medial wall of the müllerian duct, and the hymen are also associated with these species. In sheep genitalia from abattoirs, ovine infertility can occasionally be caused by hydrosalpinx and oviduct occlusion.

Goats and cows are nearly identical in terms of anatomical make-up and physiological processes. Adoption of some clinical techniques is made difficult or impossible by the reduced size of does. Although sheep are thought to be generally productive animals, Britain reports annual infertility losses of 5–10%. Ewes that refuse to mate are typically sold for slaughter. At the conclusion of each mating season, a harsh culling helps to get rid of unhealthy animals and control genetic sterility (Jost 1955). The rams are allowed to roam freely with the ewes throughout the breeding season and sheep are raised in a natural environment. The majority of infectious infertility in sheep is caused by abortions, and it can be inherited, congenital, or acquired due to environmental, dietary, and viral causes (Hashiguchi et al. 1979).

Intersex development as a result of abnormal sexual differentiation during embryological and fetal development is relatively prevalent in goats, particularly breeds like the Alpine, Saanen, and Toggenburg. It is far more common among polled animals, which have "polledness" as a straightforward dominant trait with full penetrance as well as a recessive hermaphrodite effect with partial penetrance. Freemartinism, in which twins of different sexes experience placental fusion, can also result in intersex births; cases of goat freemartinism have been documented. In this species, hermaphroditism appears to be more common than freemartinism, which is substantially less prevalent in goats than in cattle (Hashiguchi et al. 1979).

The majority of intersex goats have a female karyotype and are male pseudohermaphrodites. "Hermaphroditism is hereditary, showing close to 100% linkage to hornlessness, which is hereditary," (Haugen 1960). A recessive trait called hermaphroditism is passed down through heterozygous parents. Caprine hermaphrodites' external genitalia range from appearing to be normal male to appearing to be normal female. As a result, in some animals, the disease cannot be identified at a young age.

Eaton (1943) documented a group of 29 instances at the age of 10 days and, based on external appearance, categorized 15 as female types and 14 as male types. One goat, which appeared to be a healthy female, had one uterine horn, ovotestes, and aplasia of the uterine tubes. Ovotestes and male internal reproductive organs were present in another apparent female. The other 13 female-type individuals had testicles, bulbous vulvas, and varied degrees of clitoral hypertrophy. The clitoris protruded more noticeably from the vulvar cleft and started to resemble a glans penis as the defect's severity worsened. Except for the goat that from the outside appeared to be normal, every female goat had vesicular glands (seminal vesicles). Five of the 14 goats with male appearance on the outside appeared to be typical males. The penis of the others was malformed to varied degrees, ranging from a short penis to a large penile clitoris. In four cases, hypospadias was visible. The other nine had two testes, while three were monorchids. Vesicular glands were present in all of the animals, and four out of the 14 had some degree of uterine development. The degree of internal organ development was closely connected with the outside appearance. Externally, the animal looked to be of the female type when the paramesonephric ducts were more highly developed, and vice versa.

Hamerton et al. (1969) researched 35 polled intersex goats, comprising 15 Saanens, three Toggenburgs, five British Alpines, and 12 crossbreeds. Thirty-two goats, 31 of which were 60,XX and one of which was a 60,XX/60, XY mixoploid freemartin, were used in the chromosome research. Their anatomical research mostly concurred with that of Eaton (1943). In those older than 20 days, the anogenital distance was used as a quantitative indicator of maleness or femaleness. According to the authors, "The normal male anogenital distance ranges between 30 and 40 cm, whereas the normal female anogenital distance is approximately 2 cm." Intraabdominal gonads, suboptimal mesonephric duct development, and well-developed paramesonephric duct development were all present in hermaphrodites with an anogenital distance of 2–2.5 cm. The anogenital distance correlated with both the outward and internal masculinization of the reproductive system. When the anogenital distance was 7.0 cm or greater, scrotal or inguinal testes were present. Three of the animals had internal genitalia asymmetry that matched the gonad anatomy. When there was a neighboring testis, the ductus deferens and epididymis were both fully grown. With an ovary or ovarian tumor, there was a well-formed uterus but a poorly developed ductus deferens and no epididymis.

According to Hamerton et al. (1969), all gonads, except for those in two animals having both ovarian and testicular tissue, resembled testes. The other two had one gonadal tumor (of ovarian or ovariotesticular origin) and one testis, and one had bilateral ovotestes. The tumors could not be positively recognized. Three diagnoses were given for a single gonad: ovotestis with interstitial cell tumor (hilar cell tumor), ovotestis with granulosa cell tumor, or testis with sustentacular (Sertoli) cell tumor. This serves as an example of the diagnostic uncertainty. Interstitial gland and sustentacular (Sertoli) cell hyperplasia could have been the "tumors" in question. The gonads, which were thought to be testes, had sustentacular cells lining the seminiferous tubules but no germinal cells. Two adults had sustentacular cell hyperplasia visible on their bodies. The seminiferous tubules were frequently atrophied and hyalinized, while the interstitial (Leydig) cells were hyperplastic in animals with just testicular tissue.

A male pseudohermaphrodite goat's testicular tumor was reported by McGeady and Fitzpatrick (1978). The goat's uterine horns, uterine body, tiny cervix, vagina, vestibule, and enlarged clitoris were all kept on both sides of the goat. It also possessed bilateral retained testes and epididymides. In the right testis, a small encapsulated tumor was observed. It was challenging to determine the tumor's type, although it was probably a Leydig cell tumor. An intersex polled Saanen goat was described by Basrur and Coubrough (1964) as having "testicular tissue that showed all stages of meiosis and fully formed sperm indicating normal spermatogenesis." The goat was phenotypically female but she had abdominal testes, a well-developed uterus, and a large clitoris; 950 cc of clear, straw-colored fluid filled the uterus.

28.5 Conclusion

For sustainable small ruminant breeding, necessary precautions against noninfectious low fertility, management, and nutrition should be taken into consideration. Protective and preventive measures are to be favored over problem-solving techniques. The sustainable individual reproductive yields of candidate dams increase when their welfare is prioritized. Additionally, males which are used heavily throughout specific seasons should be well cared for to allow for normal breeder performance. Careful management of feeding techniques in accordance with the typical level of welfare is necessary for perfect production in order to prevent infertility or any disease risk and to manage disease in all animals. Also, selecting an animal that is ideal for breeding can significantly improve fertility success and operating profits by lowering operating costs and flock health issues.

Unfavorable environmental factors should be avoided, such as the presence of noise (airport, railway, highway, bridge), high-voltage lines (power plant), excessive wind (peak, slope), and heavy smoke (factory, heating chimneys), as well as stress-inducing activities (being pursued by dogs, traveling, inclement weather), as well as the consumption of toxic plants.

References

Albuquerque, R.F., Evêncio-Neto, J., Freitas, S.H. et al. (2011). Abortion in goats after experimental administration of Stryphnodendron fissuratum (Mimosoideae). *Toxicon* 58: 602–605.

Al-Qudah, K.M. (2011). Oxidant and antioxidant profile of hyperketonemic ewes affected by pregnancy toxemia. *Veterinary Clinical Pathology* 40: 60–65.

Amin, M.R., Hussain, S.S., and Islam, A.B.M.M. (2001). Reproductive peculiarities and litter weight in different genetic groups of Black Bengal does. *Asia Australia Journal of Animal Science* 14: 197–301.

Araújo, C. Jr., Antheaume, R.C.P., Trindade, R.C.P. et al. (2007). Isolation and characterization of the monoterpenoid indole alkaloids of Aspidosperma pyrifolium. *Phytochemical Reviews* 6: 183–188.

Arthur, G.H., Noakes, D.E., and Pearson, H. (1993). *Veterinary Reproduction and Obstetrics*, 6e. London: Baillière Tindall.

Aytekin, I. and Aypak, S.U. (2011). Levels of selected minerals, nitric oxide, and vitamins in aborted Sakis sheep raised under semitropical conditions. *Tropical Animal Health and Production* 43 (2): 511–514.

Aytug, C.N., Alaçam, E., Ozkoç, U. et al. (1990). *Koyun-Keçi Hastalıkları ve Yetiştiriciliği. Tüm Vet. Hayvancılık Hizmetleri Yayını. No. 2*. İstanbul, Turkey: Teknografik Matbaası.

Aziz, E.S., Klesius, P.H., and Frandsen, J.C. (1984). Effect of selenium on polymorphonuclear leukocyte function in goats. *American Journal of Veterinary Research* 45: 1715–1718.

Basrur, P.K. and Coubrough, R.I. (1964). Anatomical and cytological sex of a Saanen goat. *Cytogenetics* 3: 414–426.

Benício, T.M.A., Nardelli, M.J., Nogueira, F.R.B. et al. (2005). Intoxication by the pods of Enterolobium contortisiliquum in goats. In: *Poisonous Plants: Global Research and Solutions* (ed. K.E. Panter, T.L. Wierenga, and J.A. Pfister), 80–85. Wallingford, UK: CABI Publishing.

Bezerra, C.W.C. (2011). Plantas toxicas para ruminantes e eqüideos da Microrregião Cariri Cearense. Master's thesis. Federal University of Campina Grande.

Binns, W., Shupe, J.L., Keeler, R.F., and James, L.F. (1965). Chronologic evaluation of teratogenicity in sheep fed Veratrum californicum. *Journal of the American Veterinary Medical Association* 147: 839–842.

Bonel-Raposo, J., Riet-Correa, F., Guim, T.N. et al. (2008). Acute poisoning and abortions in Guinea pigs by the pods of Enterolobium contortisiliquum (Leg. Mimosoideae). *Pesquisa Veterinaria Brasileira* 28 (12): 593–596.

Carvalho, N.M., Alonso, L.A., Cunha, T.G. et al. (2006). Intoxicação por Tetrapterys multiglandulosa em bovinos em Mato Grosso do Sul, Brasil. *Pesquisa Veterinaria Brasileira* 26: 139–146.

Corah, L.R. and Ives, S. (1991). The effects of essential trace minerals on reproduction in beef cattle. *Veterinary Clinics of North America: Food Animal Practice* 7: 41–57.

Cuesta, P.A., Mcdowell, L.R., Kunkle, W.E. et al. (1995). Effects of high-dose prepartum injections of Se and vitamin E on milk and serum concentrations in ewes. *Small Ruminant Research* 18: 99–103.

Dantas, A.F. (2010). Malformações e morte embrionaria em ruminantes causadas pela ingestão de Mimosa tenuiflora (jurema preta). PhD thesis. Federal Rural University of Pernambuco.

Dantas, A.F.M., Riet-Correa, F., Gardner, D.R. et al. (2007). Swainsonine-induced lysosomal storage disease in goats caused by the ingestion of Turbina cordata in Northeastern Brazil. *Toxicon* 49: 111–116.

Davis, T.Z. and Stegelmeier, B.L. (2019). Characterization of the effects of high selenium feed on spermatogenesis in rams. *Journal of Animal Science* 97: 449–450.

Dobereiner, J. and Canella, C.F.C. (1956). Intoxicação de bovinos pela fava do "barbatimão" (Stryphnodendrom coriaceum Bth.). *Bolm Revista Brasileira de Medicina Veterinari* 24: 49–69.

Duffy, J.H., Bingley, J.B., and Cove, L.Y. (1977). The plasma zinc concentration of nonpregnant, pregnant and parturient Hereford cattle. *Australian Veterinary Journal* 53: 519–522.

Dwyer, C.M. (2020). Can improving animal welfare contribute to sustainability and productivity. *Black Sea Journal of Agriculture* 3 (1): 61–65.

Eaton, O.N. (1943). An anatomical study of hermaphrodism in goats. *American Journal of Veterinary Medicine* 4: 333.

Elmas, M. (2013). *Koyun-Keçi El Kitabı*. Konya, Turkey: Billur Yayınevi.

Essawi, W.M., El-Raghi, A.A., Ali, F. et al. (2021). The association of the potential risk factors and nutrition elements with abortion and calving rates of Egyptian buffaloes (*Bubalus bubalis*). *Animals* 11 (7): 2043.

Ferreira, E.V., Boabaid, F.M., Arruda, L.P. et al. (2009). Intoxicação pelas favas de Stryphnodendron fissuratum (Mimosoideae) em bovinos. *Pesquisa Veterinaria Brasileira* 29 (11): 951–957.

Fthenakis, G. (2022). *Parturient Paresis in Sheep and Goats (Milk Fever, Hypocalcemia, Lambing Sickness). MSD-MerckVeterinary Manual*. Rahway, NJ: Merck & Co.

Gabryszuk, M. and Klewiec, J. (2002). Effect of injecting 2- and 3-year-old ewes with selenium and selenium-vitamin E on reproduction and rearing of lambs. *Small Ruminant Research* 43: 127–132.

Gaffield, W. and Keeler, R.F. (1984). Structure and stereochemistry of steroidal amine teratogens. *Advances in Experimental Medicine and Biology* 177: 241–251.

Gardner, D.R., Riet-Correa, F., and Panter, K.E. (2011). Alkaloid profiles of Mimosa tenuiflora and associated methods of analysis. In: *Poisoning by Plants, Mycotoxins, and Related Toxins* (ed. F. Riet-Correa, J. Pfister, A.L. Schild, and T. Wierenga), 600–605. London: CAB International.

Gava, A. and Barros, C.S.L. (2001). Field observations of Ateleia glazioveana poisoning in cattle in southern Brazil. *Veterinary and Human Toxicology* 43: 37–41.

Gava, A., Barros, C.S.L., Pilati, C. et al. (2001). Intoxicação por Ateleia glazioveana (Leg. Papilionoideae) em bovinos. *Pesquisa Veterinaria Brasileira* 21: 49–59.

Gava, D., Reis, R.N., Rocha, T.S. et al. (2003). Intoxicação natural por Ateleia glazioveana em ovinos. *Anais Encontro Nacional de Patologia Veterinária* 11: 60.

Giadinis, N., Loukopoulos, P., Petridou, E. et al. (2016). Abortions in three beef cattle herds attributed to selenium deficiency. *Pakistan Veterinary Journal* 36: 145–148.

Grecco, F.B., Dantas, F.A.M., Riet-Correa, F. et al. (2002). Cattle intoxication from Enterolobium contortisiliquum pods. *Veterinary and Human Toxicology* 44: 160–162.

Hamerton, J.L., Dickson, J.M., Pollard, C.E. et al. (1969). Genetic intersexuality in goats. *Journal of Reproduction and Fertility* 7: 25–51.

Hashiguchi, Y., Nanba, K., and Kumagai, T. (1979). Congenital abnormalities in newborn lambs following Akabane virus infection in pregnant ewes. *National Institute of Animal Health Quarterly* 19 (1–2): 1–11.

Haugen, E. (1960). Tvekjonn hos geit (Hermaphroditism in goats). *Med. Norg. Landr. Hogsk.* 39 (10): 1–33.

Hidiroglou, M. (1979). Trace element deficiencies and fertility in ruminants; a review. *Journal of Dairy Science* 62: 1195–1206.

Hintz, H.F. and Thompson, L.J. (1998). Nitrate toxicosis in horses. *Veterinary Clinical Nutrition* 5: 4–5.

Hurley, W.L. and Doane, R.M. (1989). Recent developments in the roles of vitamins and minerals in reproduction. *Journal of Dairy Science* 72: 784–804.

Ileri, I.K. (2007). Suni tohumlama ve gebelik şansını artırıcı uygulamalar. IV. Ulusal Reprodüksiyon ve Suni Tohumlama Bilim Kongresi. Manavgat-Antalya, Türkiye.

Jonck, F., Gava, A., Furlan, F. et al. (2011). Spontaneous nitrate/nitrite poisoning in cattle fed with oats (Avena sativa) and ryegrass (Lolium multiflorum) in the state of Santa Catarina, Brazil. In: *Poisoning by Plants, Mycotoxins, and Related Toxins* (ed. F. Riet-Correa, J. Pfister, A.L. Schild, and T.(e.). Wierenga), 469–472. London: CAB International.

Jost, A. (1955). *Modalities in the Action of Gonadal snd Gonad Stimulating Hormones in the Foetus*, vol. 4, 237. Cambridge, UK: Cambridge University Press.

Keeler, R.F. (1973). Lupin alkaloids from teratogenic and nonteratogenic lupins. II. Identification of the major alkaloids by tandem gas chromatography-mass spectrometry in plants producing crooked calf disease. *Teratology* 7: 31–35.

Keeler, R.F. and Panter, K.E. (1989). Piperidine alkaloid composition and relation to crooked calf disease-inducing potential of Lupinus formosus. *Teratology* 40: 423–432.

Keeler, R.F., Stuart, L.D., and Young, S. (1986). When ewes ingest poisonous plants: the teratogenetic effects [*Veratrum californicum*]. *Veterinary Medicine* 81: 449.

Knight, A.P. and Walter, R.G. (2001). *A Guide to Plant Poisoning of Animals in North America*, 18–19. Jackson Hole, WY: Teton New Media.

Larsen, H.J. (1988). Influence of selenium on antibody production in sheep. *Research in Veterinary Science* 45: 4–10.

Lee, S.T., Stonecipher, C.A., Dos Santos, F.C. et al. (2019). An evaluation of hair, oral fluid, earwax, and nasal mucus as noninvasive specimens to determine livestock exposure to teratogenic lupine species. *Journal of Agricultural Food Chemical* 267: 43–49.

Lima, M.C.J.S. and Soto-Blanco, B. (2010). Poisoning in goats by Aspidosperma pyrifolium Mart.: biological and cytotoxic effects. *Toxicon* 55: 320–324.

Lima, M.S., Pascoal, R.A., and Stilwell, G.T. (2012). Glycaemia as a sign of the viability of the foetuses in the last days of gestation in dairy goats with pregnancy toxaemia. *Irish Veterinary Journal* 65: 1.

McGeady, T.A. and Fitzpatrick, E. (1978). Anatomical, histological and cytogenetic studies on an intersex goat. *Irish Veterinary Journal* 32 (11): 191–195.

Medeiros, J.M., Tabosa, I.M., Simões, S.V.D. et al. (2005). Mortalidade perinatal em cabritos no semi-árido da Paraíba. *Pesquisa Veterinaria Brasileira* 25: 201–206.

Mendonça, F.S., Evêncio-Neto, J., Baratella Evêncio, L. et al. (2009). Natural and experimental poisoning of cattle by Enterolobium contortisiliquum pods (Fabaceae-Mimosoideae) in Central-Western Brazil. *Acta Veterinaria Brno* 78 (4): 621–625.

Moeller, R.B. Jr. (2001). Causes of caprine abortion: diagnostic assessment of 211 cases (1991–1998). *Journal of Veterinary Diagnostic Investigation* 13: 265–270.

Nóbrega, J., Riet-Correa, F., Medeiros, J. et al. (2005). Mortalidade perinatal em ovinos no semi-árido da Paraíba. *Pesquisa Veterinaria Brasileira* 25: 171–178.

Panter, K.E., Keeler, R.F., Bunch, T.D., and Callan, R.J. (1990). Congenital skeletal malformations and cleft palate induced in goats by ingestion of Lupinus, Conium and Nicotiana species. *Toxicon* 28: 1377–1385.

Panter, K.E., James, L.F., and Gardner, D.R. (1999a). Lupines, poison-hemlock and Nicotiana spp: toxicity and teratogenicity in livestock. *Journal of Natural Toxins* 8: 117–134.

Panter, K.E., James, L.F., Stegelmeier, B.L. et al. (1999b). Locoweeds: effects on reproduction in livestock. *Journal of Natural Toxins* 8: 53–62.

Peixoto, P.V., Caldas, S.A., França, T.N. et al. (2011). Chronic heart failure and abortion caused by Tetrapterys spp. in cattle in Brazil. In: *Poisoning by Plants, Mycotoxins, and Related Toxins* (ed. F. Riet-Correa, J. Pfister, A.L. Schild, and T. Wierenga), 256–263. London: CAB International.

Pessoa, C.R.M., Pessoa, A.F.M., Dantas, A.F.M. et al. (2011). Recently diagnosed poisonous plants in the Cariri region, State of Paraiba, Brazil. In: *Poisoning by Plants, Mycotoxins, and Related Toxins* (ed. F. Riet-Correa, J. Pfister, A.L. Schild, and T. Wierenga), 91–95. London: CAB International.

Pimentel, L.A., Riet-Correa, F., Gardner, D.R. et al. (2007). Mimosa tenuiflora as a cause of malformations in ruminants in the Northeastern Brazilian Semiarid Rangelands. *Veterinary Pathology* 44: 928–931.

Raffi, M.B., Barros, R.R., Bragança, J.F.M. et al. (2004). The pathogenesis of reproductive failure induced in sheep by the ingestion of Ateleia glazioveana. *Veterinary and Human Toxicology* 46: 233–238.

Rajpal, K. and Kaushal, M. (2021). Goat rearing: a way of self-employment and economic enhancement of rural people. *Science World* 1: 13–17.

Ramírez-Bribiesca, J.E., Tórtora, J.L., Huerta, M. et al. (2001). Diagnosis of selenium status in grazing dairy goats on the Mexican plateau. *Small Ruminant Research* 41: 81–85.

Riet-Correa, F., Medeiros, R.M.T., Tokarnia, C.H., and Döbereiner, J. (2007). Toxic plants for livestock in Brazil: economic impact, toxic species, control measures and public health implications. In: *Poisonous Plants: Global Research and Solutions* (ed. K.E. Panter, T.L. Wierenga, and J.A. Pfister), 2–14. Wallingford, UK: CAB International.

Riet-Correa, G., Riet-Correa, F., Schild, A.L. et al. (2009a). Abortion and neonatal mortality in sheep poisoned with Tetrapterys multiglandulosa. *Veterinary Pathology* 46: 960–965.

Riet-Correa, F., Medeiros, R.M.T., Pfister, J. et al. (2009b). *Poisonings by Plants, Mycotoxins and Related Substances in Brazilian Livestock*, 246. Santa Maria, RS: Editora Pallotti.

Riet-Correa, F., Medeiros, R.M.T., and Schild, A.L. (2011). A review of poisonous plants that cause reproductive failure and malformations in the ruminants of Brazil. *Journal of Applied Toxicology* 32: 245–254.

Roberts, S.J. (1986). *Veterinary Obstetrics and Genital Diseases*. New Delhi: CBS Publishers.

Schlumbohm, C. and Harmeyer, J. (2008). Twin-pregnancy increases susceptibility of ewes to hypoglycaemic stress and pregnancy toxaemia. *Research in Veterinary Science* 84: 286–299.

Seegers, H., Taurel, A., and Joly, A. (2011). Prevalence of Coxiella burnetii infection in domestic ruminants: a critical review. *Veterinary Microbiology* 149: 1–16.

Shupe, J.L., Binns, W., James, L.F., and Keeler, R.F. (1967). Lupine, a cause of crooked calf disease. *Journal of the American Veterinary Medical Association* 151: 198–203.

Silva, D.M., Riet-Correa, F., Medeiros, R.M.T., and Oliveira, O.F. (2006). Plantas tóxicas para ruminantes e eqüídeos no Seridó Ocidental e Oriental do Rio Grande do Norte. *Pesquisa Veterinaria Brasileira* 26: 223–236.

Sobiech, P. and Kuleta, Z. (2002). Usefulness of some biochemical indicators in detection of early stages of nutritional muscular dystrophy in lambs. *Small Ruminant Research* 45: 209–215.

Sonmez, M. (2012). Reprodüksiyon, Suni Tohumlama ve Androloji Ders Notları. Fırat Üniversitesi Veteriner Fakültesi, Elazığ, Turkey.

Stolf, L., Gava, A., Varaschin, M.S. et al. (1994). Aborto em bovinos causado pela ingestão de Ateleia glazioveana (Leg.-papilionoideae). *Pesquisa Veterinaria Brasileira* 14: 15–18.

Tanaka, T., Fujiwara, K., Kim, S. et al. (2004). Ovarian and hormonal responses to a progesterone-releasing controlled internal drug releasing treatment in dietary-restricted goats. *Animal Reproduction Science* 84: 35–46.

Thurmond, M.C. and Picanso, J.P. (1990). A surveillance system for bovine abortion. *Preventive Veterinary Medicine* 8: 41–53.

Tokarnia, C.H., Peixoto, P.V., Döbereiner, J. et al. (1989). Tetrapterys spp. (Malpighicieae), a causa de mortandades em bovines mcaracterizadas por alterações cardíacas. *Pesquisa Veterinaria Brasileira* 9: 23–44.

Tokarnia, C.H., Peixoto, P.V., Gava, A., and Döbereiner, J. (1991). Intoxicação experimental por Stryphnodendron coriaceum (Leg. Mimosoideae) em bovinos. *Pesquisa Veterinaria Brasileira* 11: 25–29.

Tokarnia, C.H., Brito, M.F., Driemeier, D. et al. (1998). Aborto em vacas na intoxicação experimental por pelas favas de Stryphnodendron obovatum (Leg. Mimosoideae) em bovinos. *Pesquisa Veterinaria Brasileira* 18: 35–38.

Uçar, O., Unal, Y., and Yıldız, S. (2004). Ruminantlarda yetersiz beslenmenin sindirimsel ve metabolik adaptasyonlar ve üreme üzerine etkileri (Çeviri). *Kafkas Üniversitesi Veteriner Fakültesi Dergisi* 10: 227–241.

Uçar, O., Çenesiz, M., Kaya, M., and Yıldız, S. (2008). Koyunlarda vücut kondisyon skorunun üreme üzerine etkileri (Derleme). *Bültendif Veterinay Bülten* 29: 2–5.

Uçar, O.T., Bulbul, A., and Saatci, M. (2020). The effects of insufficient management and nutrition on reproductive performance in dairy cows: struggle between modern and traditional breeding. International Congress on Domestic Animal Breeding, Genetics and Husbandry. İzmir, Turkey.

Van Saun, R.J. (2000). Pregnancy toxemia in a flock of sheep. *Journal of the American Veterinary Medical Association* 217: 1536–1539.

Vidic, B., Savic, S., Grgic, Z. et al. (2007). Infectious abortion in sheep. *Biotechnology in Animal Husbandry* 23: 383–389.

Waldhalm, D.G., Hall, R.R., and Delong, W.J. (1979). Restricted dietary proteins in pregnant beef cows. The effect on length of gestation and calfhood mortality. *Theriogenology* 12: 61–68.

Welch, K.D., Panter, K.E., Lee, S.T. et al. (2009). Cyclopamine-induced synophthalmia in sheep: defining a critical window and toxicokinetic evaluation. *Journal of Applied Toxicology* 29: 414–421.

Worth, A.J., Ainsworth, S.J., Brocklehurst, P.J. et al. (1997). Nitrite poisoning in cats and dogs fed a commercial pet food. *New Zealand Veterinary Journal* 45: 193–195.

Yarsan, E. (2020). Koyun ve Keçi Hekimliği, Güncellenmiş 2. Baskı. Güneş Tıp Kitabevleri, Ankara, Turkey.

29

Management of Abortive Diseases

Jigar Raval[1], *Sunant Raval*[2], *and Tanmoy Rana*[3]

[1] *National Dairy Development Board, Anand, India*
[2] *College of Veterinary Science and Animal Husbandry, Kamdhenu University, Anand, India*
[3] *Department of Veterinary Clinical Complex, West Bengal University of Animal and Fishery Sciences, Kolkata, India*

29.1 Introduction

Goats play an important role in agriculture, providing communities around the world with meat, milk, and fiber. Abortive diseases, also known as reproductive disorders, can result in premature pregnancy loss, which has a negative impact on herd productivity and profitability. To ensure the well-being and sustainability of goat herds, these diseases must be effectively managed and prevented. Abortive diseases in goats can result in significant financial losses for farmers. When goats have abortions, their expected production of kids or marketable products is jeopardized, resulting in lower income. Furthermore, repeated abortions in a herd can have a negative impact on breeding success, fertility rates, and the herd's overall genetic potential. Additionally, it can be extremely difficult for goat farmers to meet market demands and contractual obligations when they are dealing with abortive diseases. In addition to affecting livestock industries and trade, these disease outbreaks may also have broader economic repercussions at regional or national levels (Ali et al. 2019; Orskov 2011).

Abortive diseases not only affect the economic aspect of goat farming but also impact the health and welfare of individual animals. The stress and strain caused by these diseases can lead to weakened immune systems, making goats more susceptible to other infections. In some cases, goats may experience severe illness or die as a result of complications arising from abortive diseases. Moreover, reproductive health is essential for sustaining the goat population. Any disruption in the reproductive cycle due to abortive diseases can lead to decreased fertility rates and increased interkidding intervals, reducing the number of offspring born per year and hindering the growth and expansion of the herd (Alemayehu et al. 2021).

The management of abortive diseases in goats is a critical aspect of goat farming that requires careful attention. Abortive diseases are those that lead to the premature termination of pregnancy, resulting in significant economic losses, reduced reproductive efficiency, and potential long-term impacts on the overall health and productivity of the goat herd. It is essential that a goat farmer or breeder understands the causes, prevention, and management strategies for abortive diseases to safeguard the herd's health and maximize its productivity (Wodajo et al. 2020; Holler 2012).

29.2 Causes of Abortion in Goats

Abortion causes can be divided broadly into infectious and noninfectious causes. Infectious agents include microorganisms like *Brucella*, *Campylobacter*, *Coxiella*, and others that can infect goats and possibly cause abortion. Noninfectious causes, such as dietary factors and environmental factors, can still cause goats to lose their pregnancies even though they are unrelated to microorganisms (Figure 29.1).

Elements of Reproduction and Reproductive Diseases of Goats, First Edition. Edited by Tanmoy Rana.

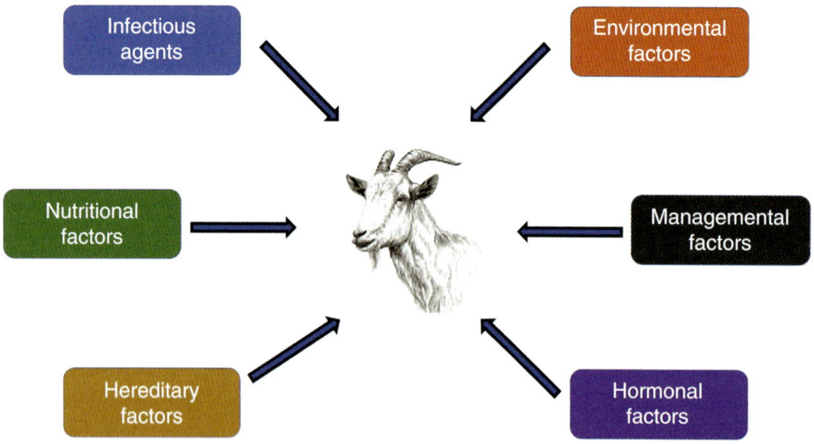

Figure 29.1 Causes of abortion in goats. *Source:* BigJoy/Adobe Stock Photos.

29.2.1 Infectious Causes

For goat breeders and farmers, infectious diseases that cause abortion in goats are a serious concern. Abortion can lead to significant financial losses, decreased herd productivity, and higher veterinary costs. A healthy and productive goat-breeding operation depends on knowing the typical infectious agents that cause goat abortion, their symptoms, prevention, and management. Let's look at a few of the main infectious diseases that can cause abortion in goats.

29.2.1.1 Leptospirosis

The pathogenic spirochete *Leptospira interrogans* is the source of the zoonotic disease known as leptospirosis. According to DNA related species, the genus *Leptospira* includes pathogenic and nonpathogenic species. *Leptospira* colonies are excreted in urine from the kidneys of various animals. Leptospiremia is followed by a 7–10-day localization and persistence period in renal tubules. Leptospirosis is spread through direct contact with infected rodents, ruminants, swine, and dogs as well as through exposure to water or soil contaminated by their urine (Adler and de la Peña Moctezuma 2010). In tropical climates, the environment is also thought to be a source of leptospirosis maintenance. Additionally, transmission happens when an animal comes in contact with standing water, such as in a lake or pond.

Small ruminants are susceptible to leptospirosis, which can manifest acutely as increased body temperature, anorexia, depression, jaundice, and anemic or hemorrhagic syndrome, as well as chronically as impaired fertility, neonatal death, abortions, and decreased milk production that occur more frequently and result in significant financial losses. A subclinical infection is marked by stillbirths, weak lambs, abortion, and repeat breeding. Because leptospirosis is a neglected condition, it is unknown how it affects animals (Lilenbaum et al. 2009).

Leptospirosis in animals has not been studied extensively, and research on outbreaks and surveys has also been scarce. It has been determined that leptospirosis is the most common cause of abortion in goats, with severe symptoms of the disease. The urine of infected animals contains the disease and spreads it. Avoid isolating and immunizing animals that have been through an abortion with contaminated water. According to serological research, goat infections with *Leptospira* are widespread throughout the world. For many years, small ruminants were thought to be incidental hosts of leptospirosis, affected only by incidental serovars carried by other domestic and wild species. Small ruminant leptospirosis is frequently linked to strains from the serogroup Hardjo serovar (Desvars et al. 2002).

Leptospirosis is a serious infectious disease that affects the reproduction of small ruminants. *Leptospira* infection in animals may occur as a result of numerous risk factors. There has never been a thorough study with adequate analysis of those factors regarding infection in sheep, even though leptospirosis is most common in cattle. Serological techniques are used in many nations to determine whether sheep and goats are infected with *Leptospira*. Seropositivity for leptospirosis is 25.9% in goats. The most significant application of leptospirosis worldwide is the agglutination test. An aborted dam, placenta, and fetus urine test can also be used to make the diagnosis. Vaccination is critical for controlling leptospirosis in the herd (Pacheco dos Santos et al. 2011).

29.2.1.1.1 Preventive Measures for Leptospirosis

Leptospira-contaminated water should not be used as drinking water. Isolate sick or aborting animals from vaccinated animals. The use of vaccines can greatly lower the occurrence of clinical signs (abortions) in a herd and help control leptospirosis. Leptospirosis control in small ruminants entails locating and treating carriers and other sources of infection.

Quarantine is required for new flocks and herds. Aborted products should be burned or buried. While handling tissues and fluids, wear rubber gloves. Educate veterinarians, public health workers, and farmers regarding the impact of disease on animal as well as human health.

29.2.1.2 Brucellosis

During the Crimean War, the British first introduced "Malta fever," now known as brucellosis. Brucellosis is a zoonotic disease with a substantial impact on rural livelihoods that is underestimated in terms of febrile sickness. The biggest issue in developing nations is the impact of brucellosis on the economy and public health. Abortion, reduced herd fertility, stillbirths, and low milk production are all substantial production losses brought on by this disease. The zoonotic effect causes morbidity as a result; it is regarded as the most prevalent zoonotic disease that exists worldwide.

The most prevalent bacterial disease in the world is brucellosis (Germeraad et al. 2016; Dean et al. 2013). The Gram-negative intracellular coccobacillus species known as *Brucella* can infect a wide range of animal species, including humans. *Brucella melitensis* infects goats, which are found in many areas. The primary clinical consequence of brucellosis is connected to goat production. Although it can infect goats, *B. abortus* primarily affects cattle. The agent can be transmitted to other related animals in a herd through milk and vaginal discharge (McDermott et al. 2002). *B. abortus* has been linked to both small ruminants and cattle in several nations. *B. suis* and *B. abortus* are the next most dangerous for human health, while others are virulent. This illness results in late-gestational abortions, placental retention, and possibly some frail newborn animals (Rahman et al. 2006; Bekele et al. 2011).

Serological assays such as complement fixation, agar gel immunodiffusion (AGID), and indirect ELISA are the most frequently used diagnostic methods. While seroreactivity to a substance does not always imply that the animal was clinically harmed by that pathogen, it does not exclude it either. Furthermore, we deduced that these infections contributed to the decreased production of these animals. A new herd should be placed in quarantine until additional serological testing reveals no fresh illnesses. In general, brucellosis results in significant production losses due to miscarriage, stillbirth, and reduced milk production. Improved diagnosis can be useful for adequate treatment if brucellosis is widespread in a nation. According to research, small ruminants that have antibodies against brucellosis have a higher probability of contracting *B. melitensis* infection due to age, a history of abortion, and party number. Seroprevalence in people and small ruminants in Nigeria is reported to range from 0% to 74%.

Although brucellosis primarily affects livestock, it can potentially harm people if they consume tainted milk or meat or come into close contact with diseased animals. Direct contact with vaginal and placental fluid, tissue, and aborted fetuses of infected animals as well as intake of raw milk or unpasteurized dairy products from these animals are two ways in which animal-to-human transmission can happen. In European Mediterranean nations, brucellosis is endemic. Northern and eastern Africa, India, Central Asia, Mexico, and South America are also affected (Pappas et al. 2006).

29.2.1.2.1 Preventive Measures for Brucellosis

Avoid consumption of unpasteurized foods or coming into close contact with sick animals. In government-owned farms, vaccination was used to prevent widespread caprine abortions. Additionally, a "test and kill" policy was put into place. By using this approach, brucellosis has been eradicated in several nations.

Separate aborted animals from healthy animals. Manure, soiled bedding, and the aborted fetus and placenta should be cleaned up and burned. Keep all tissues and fluids from aborted animals away from dogs and birds. Floors, feed bunks, structures, and equipment should be cleaned and sanitized. Use serological tests to detect sick animals, and if brucellosis testing is positive, send the animals to slaughter and quarantine the new arrivals for 30 days.

29.2.1.3 Listeriosis

Listeriosis is caused by the bacterium *Listeria monocytogenes*. Small, Gram-positive rod-shaped *Listeria* species measure between one and two microns in length and 0.5 μm in breadth. These bacteria thrive best at temperatures between 30 and 37 °C. However, organisms can also develop and reproduce under aerobic or microaerophilic conditions between −0.4 and 45 °C with a pH range of 4.5–9.6. Goats are frequently affected, although sheep can also be.

As a global organism, *L. monocytogenes* relies on soil as its main passageway for animal transmission and persistence. The winter season and the use of silage are connected with risk factors for listeriosis. While some pathogens cannot grow at low temperature, *Listeria* can (Vivant et al. 2013). The incidence rate for this can reach 9%, but it is more likely to be as low as 2%.

Listeria monocytogenes is primarily found in animal environments, feces, and dirt. It can become very pathogenic and cause significant sickness under specific circumstances. Clinical signs include abortion, a deteriorated fetus, necrosis of cotyledons, and foci of necrosis in the liver and lungs. Abortion usually happens during late pregnancy, and the agent spreads via rotten silages with dirt and rat contamination. This can result in a serious uterine infection. Septicemia, abortion, mastitis, and gastroenteritis are other clinical indicators of listeriosis. The pathogen can be excreted by the sick animal in its milk and feces (Hurtado et al. 2017; Esteban et al. 2009).

Because the agent is also zoonotic, contamination via milk and meat is a serious concern. Most abortions occur in the final stages of pregnancy. The animal may also experience metritis, depression, and fever. Bilateral or unilateral nerve system dysfunction is the predominant clinical symptom. An outbreak of listeriosis can also happen when cattle are fed low-quality pasture or vegetation instead of silage. Goats are among the most often infected ruminants, with symptoms such as encephalitis, septicemia, miscarriage, mastitis, and gastroenteritis. By managing silage or other forages properly during storage, the disease can be avoided. Antibiotics might be given for a long time and result in a recovery time of approximately a month. Compared to goats, cattle have a higher prevalence of the bacterium.

Since *L. monocytogenes* can thrive in extremely severe environmental circumstances, getting rid of it is an unattainable goal. However, effective management and control strategies can lessen food contamination (Dhama et al. 2015).

29.2.1.3.1 Preventive Measures for Listeriosis

Silages and forages should be handled and stored properly because they are sources of infectious agents.

29.2.1.4 Campylobacteriosis

Campylobacter is the primary infectious agent that causes campylobacteriosis. Small ruminants are not as well studied as other agricultural animals when it comes to *Campylobacter*. It is possible to isolate *Campylobacter* from goat meat, liver, carcases, guts, and feces. The percentage of carcase contamination varies according to the age of the animal – 94% for lambs, 63% for goats, 78% for kids, and 72% for sheep. On average, 30% of the intestinal contents and 70% of the surface of the carcase and liver exhibited *Campylobacter*. Abortion and stillbirth occur in late pregnancy, with *Campylobacter fetus* subsp. *fetus* being the main cause (Horrocks et al. 2009). To prevent contaminating the food and water of other animals who are not affected, remove the entire aborted fetus and placenta. In late-term pregnancy, *C. fetus* causes stillbirths and abortions. It results in an inflamed placenta, necrotic cotyledons, and a leathery region between cotyledons. It spreads through tissues, all discharges, and the aborted fetus (Figure 29.2). Additionally, the digestive system likely serves as a long-term reservoir.

The European Union frequently receives reports of this gastrointestinal bacterial pathogen in humans. The presence of 72–78% *Campylobacter* in the carcase and liver of goats provides evidence that humans can contract the disease. Consuming contaminated undercooked food greatly increases the risk of contracting human campylobacteriosis.

Once exposed to a contaminated external environment, the animal's carcase and liver become colonized by *Campylobacter*, but they largely remain asymptomatic intestinal carriers. Since no surveillance has been carried out thus far, the majority of the information that is currently available on *Campylobacter* in goats comes from clinical investigations, according to the European Food Safety Authority. Additionally, the EU has the fourth largest sheep population and the largest goat population. At the time of slaughter, the majority of goats had liver- and meat-borne *Campylobacter*. This suggests that a diverse population of thermophilic campylobacters is frequently present in meat and offal of goat origin, and that they can infect humans. Tetracycline (47.9%), streptomycin (22.9%), ciprofloxacin, and nalidixic acid (18.3%) all showed resistance. Only 2.5% of the isolates were resistant to erythromycin, and they were susceptible to gentamicin (Lazou et al. 2014; Humphrey et al. 2007).

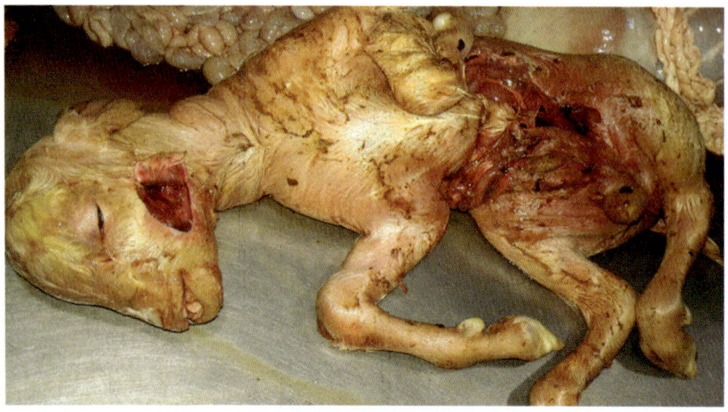

Figure 29.2 Aborted fetus of goat.

29.2.1.4.1 Preventive Measures for Campylobacteriosis

There are now vaccines on the market to stop *Campylobacter* infections. Ovine vaccines are available but they should be used in advance of exposure and might not offer protection against all strains. Tetracycline, 100 mg/head/day, can be administered as a preventive dose of antibiotics during pregnancy. To prevent feed and water being contaminated by the aborted remains of infected animals, place food in mangers and water in troughs. Remove the placenta, fetus, and aborting female from the kidding area. Oxytetracycline (an antibiotic) administered via parenteral injection, followed by additional injections, will reduce abortion loss.

29.2.1.5 Q Fever

A common zoonotic disease called Q fever, which is brought on by the pathogen *Coxiella burnetii*, causes abortion, anorexia, and lesions in goats, among other acute and chronic clinical symptoms. The three main reservoirs are cattle, sheep, and goats. Worldwide, *C. burnetii* is a common small, obligate intracellular Gram-negative pathogen. Based on gene sequence analysis, the genus *Coxiella* was placed in the Legionellales family Coxiellaeceae alongside Rickettsia and Aquicella (Bøtner et al. 2010). This substance is extremely osmotic resistant.

Ranch animals and pets are the main sources of infection, and humans can contract the disease by inhaling contaminated aerosols. This bacterium is also shed in milk, urine, feces, placental debris, and amniotic fluid, and it can cause illness with a wide range of clinical symptoms, from asymptomatic to fatal disease (Van Brom et al. 2015; Roest et al. 2013). Most bacterial introduction to farm animals occurs via aerosol. Milk must be pasteurized before use in order to protect humans from oral *C. burnetii* infection. It mainly causes late-pregnancy abortion and stillbirth in small ruminants without clinical signs.

The trophoblast cells of the allantochorion are the primary target cells for *C. burnetii* when it is injected into pregnant goats. The base of the cotyledonary villi and the trophoblasts of the inner-cotyledon allantochorion are almost always affected. Metritis incidence increases the risk of abortion in dairy goats. Most abortions happen without any prior clinical symptoms (Roest et al. 2012).

Numerous studies show that living close to a farm and having a history of abortions caused by *C. burnetii* are higher risk factors for human Q fever. Abortion, stillbirth, and premature birth have all been reported in small ruminants. Rarely, *C. burnetii* infection is also linked to chronic fatigue. It is still unclear whether or not *C. burnetii* is present in tissues other than the placenta. *C. burnetii* aids in the induction of a durable immune response against many diseases. Although goats have been studied more thoroughly than sheep when it comes to the immune response to *C. burnetii* infection, results from work in goats may also be applicable to sheep. IgM and IgG antibodies against *C. burnetii* can be detected two weeks after inoculation and can persist for up to 13 weeks (Schimmer et al. 2010; Kennerman et al. 2010).

On the basis of the examination of various bodily fluids and tissues, the prevalence of *C. burnetii* in sheep or goats has been described. Seroprevalence data have been reported for many nations, but these are difficult to compare due to variations in study design. Cattle, sheep, and goats are frequent hosts, but many other species are susceptible to infection. The agent is excreted in high concentrations in fetal membranes and birth fluids, as well as in milk, urine, and feces. Ticks can act as a reservoir for the disease and spread it as well. Tick bites or contact with contaminated excrement can also spread *C. burnetii* to sheep, goats, cats, cattle, and dogs (Woldehiwet 2004). Animals kept in small spaces are almost always infected.

By performing routine serum checks on research flocks and eliminating any infected animals, the level of infection can be brought down. A wide variety of domestic and wild animals are affected by this disease, which is present on a global scale. Except for New Zealand, *C. burnetii* is present everywhere. Rural outbreaks of Q fever are common in many nations, and it is endemic among workers. Small ruminant herds in urban areas are a source of concern for the European Commission due to the high risk of human Q fever. The incidence and prevalence of Q fever are still unknown (Vellema and van den Brom 2014).

Increased kidding rate during the kidding season leads to an increase in the pathogen's introduction and transmission to small ruminants. Additional factors, such as visiting and employed professionals and animal supplies, also contribute to an increase in the pathogen's transmission on farms. Milk tanks from dairy goats with the reproduction issue are used for *C. burnetii* DNA detection by PCR.

For a variety of reasons, including chronic infection in a small number of animals, the presence of shedding, and the fact that test-negative animals are potentially carriers of the agent, eliminating Q fever from a herd is currently not an easy task (Kennerman et al. 2010; Clemente et al. 2009).

29.2.1.5.1 Preventive Measures for Q Fever

A phase 1 *C. burnetii* vaccine for animals has been shown to reduce excretion, but the effectiveness of the vaccine may depend on the herd's level of infection and the timing of the vaccination. Animals must be vaccinated along with frequent testing in order to reduce risks to human health. To strengthen laboratory analysis, it is first necessary to train healthcare professionals and laboratory staff. Vaccination is a good way to prevent shedding and abortion. Some vaccines claim to stop abortions and reduce shedding in milk, feces, and vaginal discharge. Vaccination appears to work best when given to small ruminants which are not infected before they become pregnant. To avoid human oral infection, pasteurization of milk from infected farms is advised. Fetuses and placentas should be collected, stored safely, and then destroyed. Protective clothing should be worn, though it has been shown that this does not entirely shield humans from infection. The exposure of animals to the infectious agent can also be decreased by general hygiene practices.

29.2.1.6 Toxoplasmosis

The blood protozoan *Toxoplasma gondii*, which causes toxoplasmosis, is common in animal species and has been linked to numerous countries and climatic conditions. Goats are more commonly affected than sheep, and females are more likely to be affected than males. Males have also been noted to have a higher incidence than females.

Toxoplasmosis is a protozoal, parasitic blood disease that affects small ruminants all over the world and has a serious negative impact on reproduction as well as economic losses. It is now known that *T. gondii* is a significant contributor to livestock losses and food safety risks. Toxoplasmosis prevalence varies from nation to nation and from state to state due to climate changes. Goats have a 15% global seroprevalence of toxoplasmosis. The prevalence of toxoplasmosis is also influenced by the age of the animal. *T. gondii* prevalence is highest in the age group of 16–28 months and lowest in the age group of 68–80 months. The body weight of the animal is also a significant determinant of prevalence (Van der Puije et al. 2000; Buxton et al. 2007).

Toxoplasma gondii is a common cause of abortion in goats. It may also have an impact on the fetus. Although infection has been reported in cattle, goats are more susceptible to *T. gondii* infection. Additionally, because humans consume the meat and milk of infected animals, goats that have *T. gondii* infections are a significant source of human disease. Infection late in gestation may result in resorption or a mummified fetus, abortion or stillbirth. Following abortion, females are immune. Cats are the main reservoir and host, and they typically only spread the disease for a short time when they are kittens. While abortions are most common later in pregnancy, early infection can result in the fetus being reabsorbed. The disease and method of abortion are distinct from the bacterial cause of abortion (Oncel and Vural 2006; Dubey 2004).

29.2.1.6.1 Preventive Measures for Toxoplasmosis

Keep cats away from areas where food is stored and served. Some farmers have discovered that keeping just one adult, neutered cat works best because it deters younger, stray cats from the area. Aborted products should be burned. When handling tissues and aborted fluid, wear rubber gloves.

29.2.2 Noninfectious Causes

Numerous noninfectious factors can cause abortion in goats. These causes are linked to various environmental, nutritional, and management elements that may have an impact on a pregnant doe's general health and well-being. To reduce the risk of abortion and keep a healthy breeding herd, goat farmers and breeders must be aware of these noninfectious causes.

29.2.2.1 Nutritional Deficiencies

Abortion may result from inadequate nutrition, especially during the crucial stages of pregnancy. Vitamin and mineral deficiencies, such as vitamin E and selenium, as well as copper and zinc, can affect fetal viability and development. Provide pregnant does with a well-balanced diet that meets their specific nutritional requirements during all stages of pregnancy.

29.2.2.2 Stress

Extreme weather conditions, travel, abrupt dietary changes, and crowding are just a few examples of environmental stressors that can affect pregnant does and possibly result in abortion. Create a low-stress environment for pregnant does by providing adequate space, shelter, and proper management practices.

29.2.2.3 Toxic Plants

Goats may be affected by ingesting poisonous plants, including larkspur, locoweed, and specific species of oak. Identify any poisonous plants and remove them from the goats' grazing areas and food sources.

29.2.2.4 Trauma

If the pregnant doe experiences significant trauma, physical harm or accidents, such as falls or attacks by predators, this can lead to abortion. Preventing physical harm and shielding them from predators will help to ensure the safety of pregnant does.

29.2.2.5 Hereditary Factors

The risk of abortion in the offspring can be raised by certain genetic anomalies or hereditary diseases in either the doe or the buck. To prevent hereditary problems, breeding decisions should take into account both the doe and the buck's health and genetic background.

29.2.2.6 Mycotoxins

Pregnant does may experience abortion if they consume feed that has been tainted with mycotoxins, which are poisonous compounds produced by mold. Feed should be stored carefully to avoid the growth of mold.

29.2.2.7 Hormonal Imbalances

Abortion can result from hormonal imbalances in pregnant women. Numerous things, such as underlying medical conditions or improper hormonal therapy use, can result in hormonal imbalances. Avoid using hormonal treatments improperly and ask a veterinarian how to use them.

29.2.2.8 Fetal Abnormalities

Abnormalities in the developing fetus, either genetic or developmental, can lead to spontaneous abortion.

29.2.2.9 Medication or Chemical Exposure

Abortion may occur if certain drugs, substances, or pesticides are encountered or used improperly during pregnancy. Pregnant does should not be exposed to chemicals or medications without veterinary supervision.

29.2.2.10 Summary

Farmers can improve the general reproductive health and breeding herd success by being proactive in identifying and addressing noninfectious factors that may cause abortion in goats. The key to maintaining a healthy and effective goat breeding operation is regular monitoring and early intervention, along with appropriate nutrition and management.

29.3 General Approach for the Management of Abortion in Goats

Prevention of abortion in goats requires a multifaceted strategy that includes biosecurity precautions, wholesome feeding, vaccination, and careful management techniques. If miscarriages still happen despite precautions, quick and efficient management techniques can help lessen the burden on the goat herd. Here are some key preventive measures and management strategies for abortive diseases.

29.3.1 Biosecurity

Strict biosecurity controls must be put in place to stop the introduction and spread of infectious agents. Limit visitor access to the goat facility, quarantine new animals, and refrain from mixing goats from various sources without conducting necessary testing.

29.3.2 Vaccination

Develop a vaccination schedule in close consultation with a veterinarian that is specific to the diseases which are common in your area. The danger of outbreaks can be considerably reduced by vaccinations against prevalent abortive infections.

29.3.3 Nutrition

Make sure your goats eat a balanced diet that satisfies their unique nutritional needs. Maintaining reproductive health requires getting enough vitamins and minerals.

29.3.4 Herd Health Monitoring

Keep a close eye on your herd's health and run diagnostic tests if any unusual symptoms are noticed. The risk of abortion can be decreased and illness transmission slowed with early diagnosis of infectious agents.

29.3.5 Isolation and Diagnosis

To stop the infectious agent from spreading, isolate the infected animals. Together with a veterinarian, carry out rigorous diagnostic procedures to pinpoint the underlying cause and choose the best course of therapy or preventive action.

29.3.6 Sanitation

By routinely cleaning and sanitizing barns, equipment, and feeding places, owners can keep the surroundings clean and hygienic. By doing this, pathogen accumulation and transmission will be reduced.

29.3.7 Record Keeping

Keep thorough records of the times of each breeding, the history of each vaccine, and any anomalies that are noticed. It will be easier to spot trends and potential risk factors for abortive illnesses with reliable records.

29.3.8 Culling

Consider culling sick animals if the situation is serious or if there have been repeated abortions in order to stop the spread of disease and maintain the herd's general health.

29.3.9 Educating Goat Farmers

The effective management of abortive diseases depends heavily on education and knowledge exchange. The warning signs and symptoms of these illnesses should be made known to goat farmers, along with the best methods for early detection and prevention. Workshops, training courses, and instructional materials are excellent instruments for educating goat producers and promoting the use of ethical management techniques.

29.4 Conclusion

Managing abortive disorders in goats necessitates a proactive and comprehensive approach that takes into account all the elements that influence reproductive health. Goat farmers and breeders can reduce the number of abortions, safeguard the health of their herd, and guarantee sustained productivity in their goat farming operations by being aware of the causes of abortive diseases, putting preventive measures in place, and applying efficient management techniques. A good abortive disease management program must include regular consultations with a veterinarian as well as knowledge of the most recent findings and recommended procedures.

References

Adler, B. and de la Peña Moctezuma, A. (2010). Leptospira and leptospirosis. *Veterinary Microbiology* 140: 287–296.

Alemayehu, G., Mamo, G., Alemu, B. et al. (2021). Causes and flock level risk factors of sheep and goat abortion in three agroecology zones in Ethiopia. *Frontiers in Veterinary Science* 8: 615310.

Ali, S., Zhao, Z., Zhen, G. et al. (2019). Reproductive problems in small ruminants (sheep and goats): a substantial economic loss in the world. *Large Animal Review* 25: 215–223.

Bekele, M., Mohammed, H., Tefera, M. et al. (2011). Small ruminant brucellosis and community perception in Jijiga district, Somali regional state, Eastern Ethiopia. *Tropical Animal Health and Production* 43: 893–898.

Bøtner, A., Broom, D., Doherr, M.G. et al. (2010). Scientific opinion on Q fever. *Wiley Online Library* 8 (5): 1595.

Buxton, D., Maley, S., Wright, S. et al. (2007). Toxoplasma gondii and ovine toxoplasmosis: new aspects of an old story. *Veterinary Parasitology* 149 (1–2): 25–28.

Clemente, L., Barahona, M., Andrade, M.F. et al. (2009). Diagnosis by PCR of Coxiella burnetii in aborted fetuses of domestic ruminants in Portugal. *Veterinary Record* 164 (12): 373.

Dean, A., Bonfoh, B., Kulo, A. et al. (2013). Epidemiology of brucellosis and Q fever in linked human and animal populations in northern Togo. *PLoS One* 8 (8): e71501.

Desvars, A., Naze, F., Benneveau, A. et al. (2002). Endemicity of leptospirosis in domestic and wild animal species from Reunion Island (Indian Ocean). *Epidemiology and Infection* 141 (6): 1154–1165.

Dhama, K., Karthik, K., Tiwari, R. et al. (2015). Listeriosis in animals, its public health significance (food-borne zoonosis) and advances in diagnosis and control: a comprehensive review. *Veterinary Quarterly* 35 (4): 211–235.

Dubey, J.P. (2004). Toxoplasmosis – a waterborne zoonosis. *Veterinary Parasitology* 126 (1–2): 57–72.

Esteban, J., Oporto, B., Aduriz, G. et al. (2009). Faecal shedding and strain diversity of listeria monocytogenesin healthy ruminants and swine in northern Spain. *BMC Veterinary Research* 5: 1–10.

Germeraad, E., Hogerwerf, L., Faye-Joof, T., and Goossens, B. (2016). Low seroprevalence of brucellosis in humans and small ruminants in the Gambia. *PLoS One* 11 (11): e0166035.

Holler, L.D. (2012). Ruminant abortion diagnostics. *Veterinary Clinics of North America: Food Animal Practice* 28 (3): 407–418.

Horrocks, S., Anderson, R., Nisbet, D. et al. (2009). Incidence and ecology of Campylobacter jejuni and coli in animals. *Anaerobe* 15 (1–2): 18–25.

Humphrey, T., O'Brien, S., and Madsen, M. (2007). Campylobacters as zoonotic pathogens: a food production perspective. *International Journal of Food Microbiology* 117 (3): 237–257.

Hurtado, A., Ocejo, M., and Oporto, B. (2017). Salmonella spp. and Listeria monocytogenes shedding in domestic ruminants and characterization of potentially pathogenic strains. *Veterinary Microbiology* 210: 71–76.

Kennerman, E., Rousset, E., Gölcü, E., and Dufour, P. (2010). Seroprevalence of Q fever (coxiellosis) in sheep from the Southern Marmara Region, Turkey. *Comparative Immunology, Microbiology and Infectious Diseases* 33 (1): 37–45.

Lazou, T., Houf, K., Soultos, N. et al. (2014). Campylobacter in small ruminants at slaughter: prevalence, pulsotypes and antibiotic resistance. *International Journal of Food Microbiology* 173: 54–61.

Lilenbaum, W., Varges, R., Ristow, P. et al. (2009). Identification of Leptospira spp. carriers among seroreactive goats and sheep by polymerase chain reaction. *Research in Veterinary Science* 87: 16–19.

McDermott, J., John, J., and Arimi, S.M. (2002). Brucellosis in sub-Saharan Africa: epidemiology, control and impact. *Veterinary Microbiology* 90 (1–4): 111–134.

Oncel, T. and Vural, G. (2006). Occurrence of toxoplasma gondii antibodies in sheep in Istanbul, Turkey. *Veterinarski Arhiv* 76 (6): 547–553.

Orskov, E.R. (2011). Goat production on a global basis. *Small Ruminant Research* 98 (1–3): 9–11.

Pacheco dos Santos, J., Monteiro Correia Lima, A., Ferreira Júnior, Á., and Medeiros, A. (2011). Seroprevalence and risk factors for leptospirosis in goats in Uberlândia, Minas Gerais, Brazil. *Tropical Animal Health and Production* 44 (1): 101–106.

Pappas, G., Papadimitriou, P., Akritidis, N. et al. (2006). The new global map of human brucellosis. *Lancet Infectious Diseases* 6: 91–99.

Rahman, M., Han, J., Park, J. et al. (2006). Prevalence of brucellosis and its association with reproductive problems in cows in Bangladesh. *Veterinary Record* 159 (6): 180.

Roest, H., van Gelderen, B., Dinkla, A. et al. (2012). Q Fever in pregnant goats: pathogenesis and excretion of Coxiella burnetii. *PLoS One* 7: e48949.

Roest, H., Post, J., van Gelderen, B. et al. (2013). Q fever in pregnant goats: humoral and cellular immune responses. *Veterinary Research* 44: 1–9.

Schimmer, B., Ter Schegget, R., Wegdam, M. et al. (2010). The use of a geographic information system to identify a dairy goat farm as the most likely source of an urban Q-fever outbreak. *BMC Infectious Diseases* 10 (1): 1–7.

Van den Brom, R., Van Engelen, E., Roest, H.I. et al. (2015). Coxiella burnetii infections in sheep or goats: an opinionated review. *Veterinary Microbiology* 181 (1–2): 119–129.

Van der Puije, W., Bosompem, K., Canacoo, E.A. et al. (2000). The prevalence of anti-Toxoplasma gondii antibodies in Ghanaian sheep and goats. *Acta Tropica* 76 (1): 21–26.

Vellema, P. and van den Brom, R. (2014). The rise and control of the 2007–2012 human Q fever outbreaks in the Netherlands. *Small Ruminant Research* 118 (1–3): 69–78.

Vivant, A., Garmyn, D., and Piveteau, P. (2013). Listeria monocytogenes, a down-to-earth pathogen. *Frontiers in Cellular and Infection Microbiology* 3: 87.

Wodajo, H., Gemeda, B., Kinati, W. et al. (2020). Contribution of small ruminants to food security for Ethiopian smallholder farmers. *Small Ruminant Research* 184: 106064.

Woldehiwet, Z. (2004). Q fever (coxiellosis): epidemiology and pathogenesis. *Research in Veterinary Science* 77 (2): 93–100.

Section 4

Metabolic Diseases

30

Ketosis/Pregnancy Toxemia

Amita Tiwari, Shivangi Udainiya, Varsha Mishra, and Aditya Pratap

Department of Veterinary Medicine, College of Veterinary Science and Animal Husbandry, Jabalpur, India

30.1 Introduction

Pregnancy toxemia, also known as "twin lamb disease," "gestational toxemia," and "pregnancy-associated ketosis," is a metabolic disorder of small ruminants occurring in late gestation, most commonly during the last 4–6 weeks of pregnancy, as a result of inappropriate metabolism of carbohydrates and fats, characterized by low circulating levels of blood glucose and high levels of ketone bodies caused by negative energy balance (NEB). Pregnancy toxemia and ketosis poses a threat to goat health during late gestation and early lactation. These diseases are often (though not exclusively) seen in dairy goats, especially in higher producing animals. Although many animals are able to cope and recover from a NEB by metabolizing body fat, albeit with a negative impact on productivity at the subclinical stage, some metabolize too much fat, become overwhelmed with the associated byproducts (ketone bodies), and develop pregnancy toxemia (before kidding) and ketosis (after kidding). Pregnancy toxemia occurs frequently within 1–3 weeks from kidding, and is associated with prepartum mortality in a doe herd.

The first signs of pregnancy toxemia are little or no appetite, depression, lethargy or sluggishness, muscular imbalance or poor coordination, known as ataxia, grinding of teeth, and blindness. Does become so weak that they are forced to lie down and in most cases will not be able to rise again; legs are usually tucked underneath the body. They also have sweet- or foul-smelling breath when there is a high level of ketones or toxins in the blood. These symptoms may occur within a few hours to two days from the onset of signs. If symptoms persist, does could progress to coma or even death. A doe's death is attributed to reduced liver and kidney function. When the doe dies, the fetus or fetuses also die. However, if a fetus dies and is not removed quickly, septicemia will occur, carrying the pathogen throughout the doe's bloodstream.

An increase in blood and urine ketone concentrations is used to confirm the diagnosis. Compared to blood concentrations, urine concentrations are more accurate and precise. Cases of pregnancy toxemia can be diagnosed using Rothera's qualitative test from urine samples.

A good feeding management practice is needed in the late stage of pregnancy. During the last six weeks of gestation, provide grain as it is an essential source of carbohydrates. Does carrying multiple fetuses should be fed adequate energy with total digestible nutrient (TDN) levels. Producers should be mindful that levels of energy in the diet might vary depending on forage quality and availability, doe body weight and condition score, and the number of fetuses the doe is carrying.

30.2 Etiology

Before discussing the actual cause of pregnancy toxemia in goats, we will look at NEB. The final stages of pregnancy and the onset of milk production (lactation) require a lot of energy, this high demand usually being met by feed intake and topped up by body reserves. If the (metabolizable) energy from feed intake and body reserves is less than required for the fetus to grow or to produce milk, the body is in NEB. NEB is considered the norm in high-yielding animals during early lactation, but stress can cause further reduction in feed intake and lead to the onset of subclinical or clinical ketosis. NEB is a detrimental consequence of human selection for high-yielding animals, hence the emerging trends in dairy cattle and reduction in milk yield and gain in animal welfare.

Elements of Reproduction and Reproductive Diseases of Goats, First Edition. Edited by Tanmoy Rana.

Pregnancy toxemia and ketosis in goats typically occur during late-term pregnancy and at the onset of lactation. During this life stage, dairy goats need considerable energy. Energy requirements are compounded in a doe carrying multiple fetuses because the kids compress the rumen, and the doe simply cannot physically eat enough to meet energy needs. Consequently, the dairy goat must call on body fat reserves for energy. The breakdown of large amounts of fat can result in compounds called ketones in the blood. Ketones can have a toxic effect in large concentrations.

Early symptoms of pregnancy toxemia and ketosis in goats include apathy, poor appetite, a decrease in milk production (if the goat is milking), a rough hair coat, and disorientation. Ketosis or pregnancy toxemia is a multifactorial negative energy metabolic disorder with hypoglycemia and hyperketonemia as primary disturbances observed in pregnant goats. Females with body conditioning score of <2 and obese ewes or does with body conditioning score of >5, carrying multiple fetuses, are at higher risk of developing the disease primarily because of the insufficient energy density in rations required for the rapid fetal development during late gestation and limited space for adequate intake of feed due to compression of the rumen by the fetus.

The primary predisposing cause of pregnancy toxemia is inadequate energy intake in late pregnancy of does with more than one fetus. The body weight of the fetuses, the dam's physical condition, the number of lactations, age and breed, food, and stresses are some predisposing variables (Hefnawy et al. 2011).

30.3 Risk Factors for Pregnancy Toxemia in Goats

Various factors are responsible for the onset and progression of this metabolic disease and they may be categorized under nutritional, management, and metabolic headings.

- Risk factors for pregnancy toxemia include carriage of multiple fetuses, age, and extreme body condition score (BCS), fat or thin (Rook 2000). Obese animals carrying multiple fetuses are at highest risk of developing disease.
- Clinical signs of pregnancy toxemia are usually nonspecific at the onset of disease and may include anorexia, isolation from herd mates, swollen lower limbs, tremors, recumbency, blindness, ataxia, coma, and death (Rook 2000).
- In dairy goats the final month of pregnancy is a critical period for the management of energy balance because approximately 60–80% of fetal growth occurs during this period, and because dry matter intake declines simultaneously (Rook 2000).
- Pregnancy toxemia can be fatal in does and ewes if not diagnosed in a timely manner, therefore early identification of goats at risk of developing pregnancy toxemia increases the chances of recovery (Rook 2000).

30.4 Risk Factors for Ketosis in Goats

- As the energy requirements of does considerably increases with the onset of lactation, most does will develop mild or lactational ketosis. Goats in early lactation lose excessive body weight if the feed quantity and quality are not adequate to meet the energy requirements of producing milk, hence animals are in NEB.
- In dairy goats, clinical ketosis manifests predominantly in early lactations carrying multiple fetuses; undernourished or overweight animals are likely to develop clinical ketosis (Rook 2000).
- Clinical signs include anorexia, recumbency, lethargy, muscle spasm of the head and neck (opisthotonos), dropped head, convulsion, sweet-smelling breath, apparent blindness, bloat, teeth grinding, and frothy salivation (Vasava et al. 2016).

30.5 Epidemiology

Although many factors relating to the occurrence of pregnancy toxemia are yet to be determined, one of the major factors is that the gestation period of the goat/sheep is comparatively short compared to many animals and fetal demand for nutrition is greatest in the last two months of pregnancy. In late gestation while the fetus is rapidly growing, the total metabolic rate and energy requirement increase during the last 4–6 weeks of pregnancy causing development of hypoglycemia; hence, increased gluconeogenesis by the liver is initiated to facilitate rapid fetal growth in the situation of NEB.

Thus mobilization of fat stores is increased by the liver to assure adequate energy for increased demands. Excessive lipid mobilization causes elevated concentration of serum beta-hydroxybutyrate >1.7 mmol/l, thus developing ketosis which causes further suppression of endogenous glucose production and promotes the development of hyperketonemia.

Classification of pregnancy toxemia can be undertaken by cause or by clinical manifestations.

30.5.1 Cause

- *Primary pregnancy toxemia*: this is the most common manifestation observed, which occurs due to either a fall in the plane of nutrition during the later part of pregnancy or thin body conditioning of ewes or does due to inadequate feeding or intake of low-energy density feed. It is more often seen in pastoral flocks.
- *Secondary pregnancy toxemia*: secondary stress generating conditions of disease, lameness, dental problems, traveling and parasitic infestation which drain additional glucose reserves of the body, caused sporadically.
- *Fat ewe pregnancy toxemia*: this develops in ewes or does that are overconditioned during the early stages of pregnancy. As time passes, due to the enlarging uterus and massive intraabdominal fat deposits, these pregnant ewes or does may experience a drop in nutrition during late gestation.
- *Starvation pregnancy toxemia*: extremely thin sheep and goats can experience starvation pregnancy toxemia due to lack of food after periods of drought, heavy snowfall, or flooding, or because of an inability to fulfill increasing demands of the growing fetus.
- *Stress-induced pregnancy toxemia*: this is the least common cause of the disease and occurs in ewes or does which are transported during pregnancy, given altered nutrition, and close housing of pregnant ewes in late gestation. In sheep, it can occur by mishandling while shearing.

30.5.2 Clinical Manifestations

- *Clinical pregnancy toxemia*: pregnancy toxemia, also known as pregnancy-associated ketosis, may develop in does or ewes in the late stages of pregnancy in nations with intensive goat or sheep breeding, particularly during the winter. Pregnancy-related ketosis is seen in sheep during the final 4–6 weeks of gestation (Van Saun 2000). The disease is driven by the NEB, which develops as a result of the developing fetuses' increased demand for glucose (Van Saun 2000; Schlumbohm and Harmeyer 2008). Anorexia, recumbency, lethargy, opisthotonos, dropped head, periodic convulsion, sweetish fruity odor from breath, apparent blindness, bloat, grinding of teeth, and foamy salivation were the most notable clinical findings seen in naturally affected goats with pregnancy toxemia (Pough 2002). In terms of biochemical parameters, goats with pregnancy toxemia had markedly lower levels of glucose (30.89 ± 0.38 mg/dl) and calcium (8.10 ± 0.20 mg/dl) and significantly higher levels of serum glutamic pyruvic transaminase (SGPT) (216.01 ± 4.07 IU/l), serum glutamic oxaloacetic transaminase (SGOT) (84.23 ± 1.44 IU/l), blood urea nitrogen (BUN) (22.24 ± 0.31 mg/dl), creatinine (2.13 ± 0.09 mg/dl), beta-hydroxybutyric acid (BHBA) (0.46 ± 0.83 mmol/l), and nonesterified fatty acid (NEFA) (1.67 ± 0.71 mmol/l) compared to healthy goats (Vasava et al. 2016).
- *Subclinical pregnancy toxemia*: subclinical pregnancy toxemia is frequently linked to the death of lambs and dams in intensively farmed flocks and occurs at a high incidence of 20%, without visible clinical symptoms (Feijó et al. 2016). Hence the disease is considered to be of significant economic importance (Moghaddam and Hassanpour 2008). Early subclinical phases of the disease are marked by steadily rising rates of hypoglycemia and hyperketonemia in the absence of clinical indications (Barbagianni et al. 2015; Cal-Pereyra et al. 2015). Since the initial clinical cases of clinical pregnancy toxemia signal the presence of a far more serious metabolic issue in the flock as a whole, subclinical diagnosis is of the utmost importance (Rook 2000; Marteniuk and Herdt 1988). Does with subclinical pregnancy toxemia had significantly lower glucose concentrations and significantly higher urea ($P = 0.042$) and total protein ($P = 0.048$) concentrations compared to pregnant does (Bani Isail et al. 2008).

30.6 Pathophysiology

Pregnancy toxemia can occur even in properly conditioned ewes/does on an adequate ration, but it is most common in females with a poor body condition score (BCS 2/5) or who are overconditioned (BCS 4/5) and carrying multiple fetuses.

When blood glucose levels are dangerously low during pregnancy, brain function is impaired, which can escalate to dehydration, kidney failure, or even death in late pregnant does compared to ones in early gestation. According to Herdt (2000), when the supply of precursors for glucose is high, glucose production may exceed metabolic needs and any extra glucose is stored as glycogen in the liver. Bergman (1993) claimed that body stores of glucose and glycogen can only maintain the animal for a few hours since the amount of glucose stored in the liver is small compared to metabolic demands.

The body's initial response to hypoglycemia is a decrease in insulin secretion, an increase in glucagon, and stimulation of the hypothalamus to boost adrenaline secretion. Glycerol and NEFA are mobilized from adipose tissue as a result of these mechanisms, which also result in an increase in glycogenolysis in the liver. Additionally, muscle is stimulated to release amino acids, which increases the amount of glucose precursors that are accessible for gluconeogenesis (Bergman 1993). NEFA can undergo the following oxidation processes in the liver: (i) total oxidation to CO_2, (ii) partial oxidation to ketones, and (iii) reesterification to triglycerides.

Transporting fatty acids to mitochondria is necessary for their oxidation, and as a result, mitochondria are where NEFA are transformed into ketone bodies. Untransported fatty acids (NEFA) are reesterified to create triglycerides, which must then be integrated into very low-density lipoproteins in order to be excreted from the liver. The main triglyceride carriers in blood are lipoproteins (Herdt 2000). Ruminants' inefficient transit of lipoproteins from the liver to adipose tissue overwhelms the organ's capacity to deal with this huge build-up, resulting in a fatty liver (Pough 2002).

While each fetus needs 30–40 g of glucose per day (Edmondson and Pugh 2009), which is a significant portion of the ewe's glucose output and is preferentially used to maintain the fetuses rather than the sheep, in order to ensure sufficient energy for the increased demands of the developing fetuses and imminent lactation, mobilization of fat stores is enhanced in late gestation. The amount of metabolizable energy required increases significantly in the last 4–6 weeks of pregnancy. For instance, a 70 kg sheep bearing a single lamb needs 2.8 Mcal/day of energy in early gestation versus 3.45 Mcal/day in late gestation – a 23% increase. This rise is more pronounced in ewes carrying twins, whose energy requirements increase from 3.22 Mcal/day in early gestation to 4.37 Mcal/day in late gestation (36% increase). Similar variations in energy requirements apply to dairy goats (Edmondson and Pugh 2009).

This enhanced mobilization, however, may be too much for the liver to handle in a situation of NEB, leading to ketone body production and hepatic lipidosis and a consequent impairment of function. When glucose is not readily available, the liver produces ketone bodies, which are then used peripherally as an energy source. Acetoacetate and beta-hydoxybutyrate are two major ketone bodies alongside acetone. Ketone body production causes the formation of free radicals, which transform into hydroxyl radicals. Besides causing membrane phospholipid peroxidation and an accumulation of the byproducts of lipid peroxidation, these free radicals also cause cytotoxicity.

While healthy cells have the ability to detoxify superoxide radicals using antioxidant enzymes like superoxide dismutase (SOD), glutathione peroxidase (GSH-Px), glutathione reductase (GR), and catalase (CAT), which help maintain the intracellular concentration of reduced glutathione and nicotinamide adenine dinucleotide phosphate (NADPH), these products are known to crosslink membrane components (Jain et al. 2006). Furthermore, twin-bearing ewes seem to have more trouble generating glucose and removing ketone bodies, which makes them more vulnerable to pregnancy toxemia.

In contrast, animals which are overconditioned may have diminished appetites and rapidly mobilize adipose tissue, which overwhelms the liver's capacity and causes hepatic lipidosis. When dietary intake is insufficient, there can also be a population of animals that is less susceptible to the generation of insulin. If feed intake is abruptly reduced by circumstances like inclement weather, transportation, handling for shearing or preventive medicine, or other concurrent disease, ewes meeting these criteria may quickly transition from subclinical ketosis to clinical pregnant toxemia (foot rot, pneumonia, etc.). The development of ketosis due to lack of feed intake is depicted in Figure 30.1.

These pregnancy toxemia variations include estate ketosis (overconditioned sheep), primary pregnancy toxemia (thin ewes and inadequate nutrition), and secondary pregnancy toxemia (ewes suffering from other disease). When kidding occurs, dairy animals frequently go into ketosis (serum BHBA >1.7 mmol/l), which may or may not be related to pregnant ketosis before kidding. After kidding, ketosis seems to occur more frequently in herds fed a complete pelleted meal.

30.7 Clinical Findings

Early detection of pregnancy toxemia is very important for successful treatment. The last 2–4 weeks of gestation are when pregnancy toxemia is most prevalent. Early in the course of the disease, very few clinical indications may be visible. The paucity of metabolic symptoms especially in goats may mislead the diagnosis.

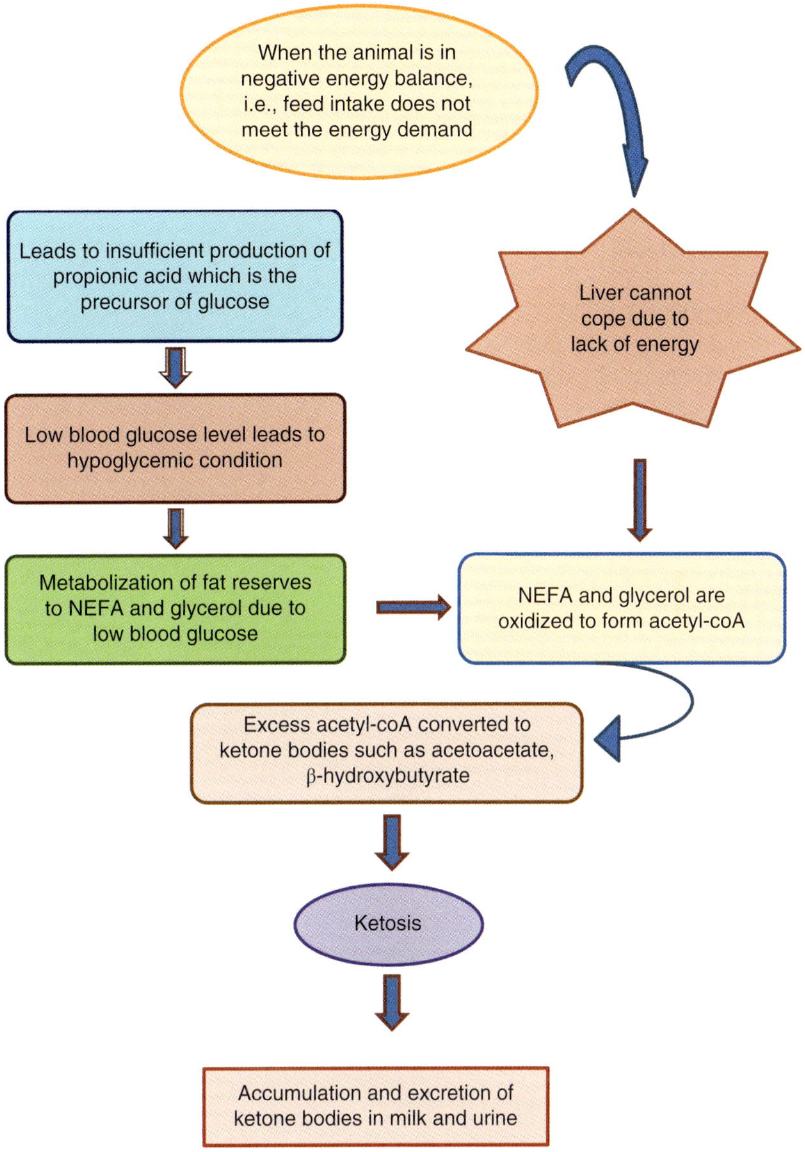

Figure 30.1 Process of development of ketosis due to lack of feed intake.

Vital parameters like rectal temperature and respiration rate are normal in ailing animals but sometimes heart rate is increased. Lowering of feed intake before kidding is one of the major contributory factors for the disease. The sweetish odor typical of ketone bodies along with frothy salivation are observed by many scientists. Chewing movement of jaws and tooth-grinding behavior are commonly seen in pregnancy toxemia in does. Furthermore, dropped head, extension of head, and stargazing posture are some of the symptoms observed due to hypoglycemia, ketonemia, and neurodegeneration. As the toxemia worsens, neurological involvement is visible characterized by despondency, recumbency, the emergence of tremors, staring into space, lack of coordination, circling, and tooth grinding. The clinical symptoms are caused by elevated ketones and low glucose concentrations.

Mild clinical symptoms typically go unreported in the early stages of the disease. Initially the animal may refuse to eat concentrate but may continue to eat grass and hay (Clarkson 2000). When moving to feeding or watering locations, affected animals often lag behind the flock or herd and appear sluggish. As the illness worsens, affected animals become isolated from the pack, exhibit signs of blindness or confusion, stray into objects or remain in one spot, or fail to get away from oncoming humans, dogs, or machinery. Constipation and tooth grinding are typical symptoms of the condition. Weakness and mental drowsiness worsen in the final stages of the illness, resulting in recumbency and death. Due to maternal and fetal deaths caused by pregnancy toxemia, sheep and goat farmers suffer enormous economic losses.

Anorexia (100.00%), recumbency (100.00%), lethargy (86.67%), opisthotonos (73.33%), dropped head (62.22%), periodic convulsion (57.78%), sweetish fruity odor from breath (51.11%), apparent blindness (42.22%), bloat (40.00%), grinding of teeth (37.78%), and frothy salivation (24.44%) were the most notable clinical findings in naturally affected goats with pregnancy toxemia (Vasava et al. 2016).

Recumbency (lateral is more detrimental than sternal), drooping ears, and neurological symptoms, particularly opisthotonus or "star gazing," incoordination, and muscle tremors are the clinical indicators most frequently linked to a bad prognosis (Lima et al. 2016).

Lateral deviation of the neck in a pregnant doe is shown in Figure 30.2 (a–d).

Less than 1–2% of a mature ewe flock usually suffer from pregnancy toxemia-related morbidity, which is typically relatively modest. However, mortality rates in infected animals frequently surpass 80–86%, particularly if treatment is neglected (Rook 2000). Even when kidding was induced or a caesarean was performed, and medical interventions (fluids, electrolytes, glucose, propylene glycol) were vigorously administered, an 86% case fatality rate has been seen in animals

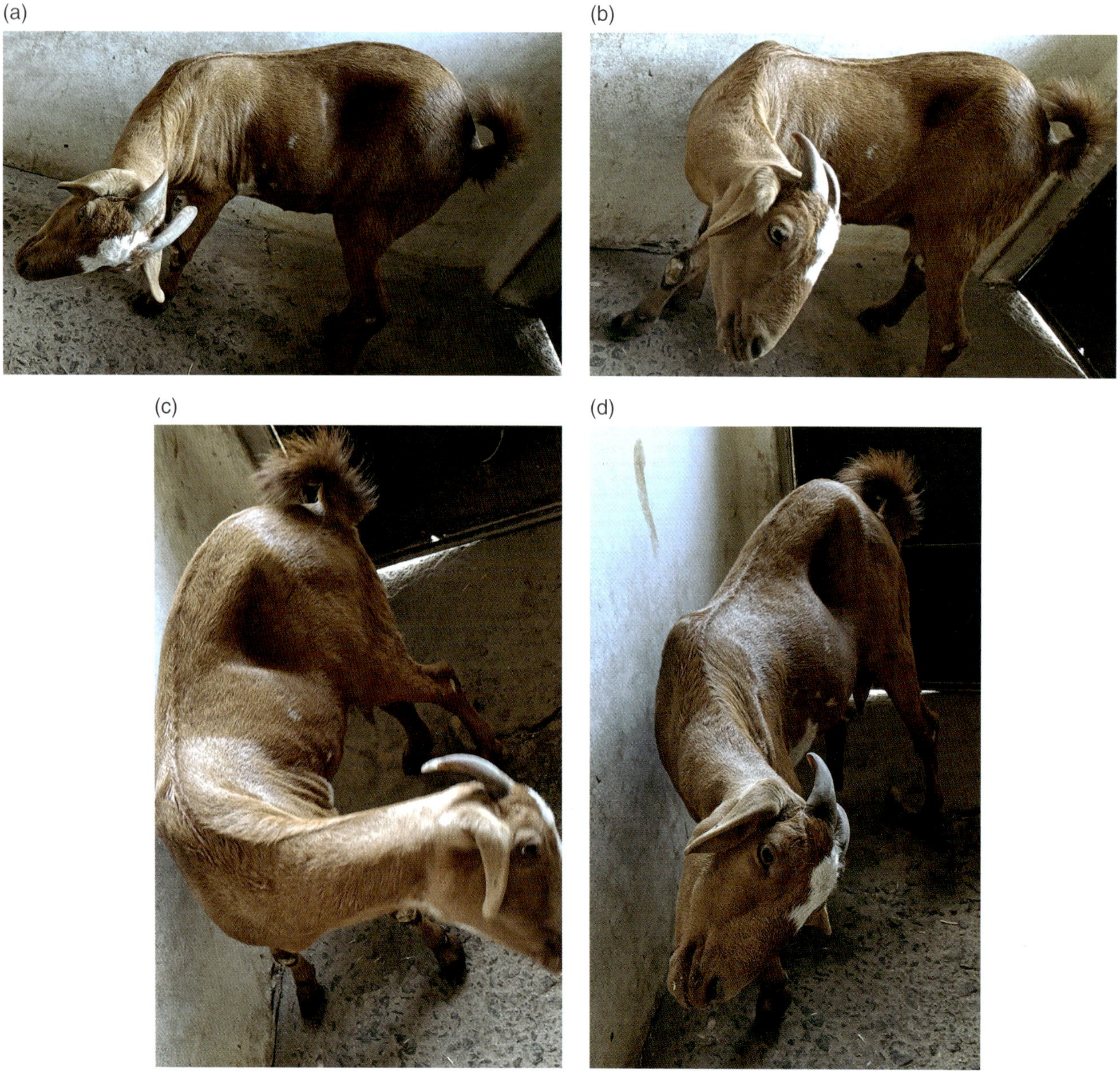

Figure 30.2 (a–d) Lateral deviation of the neck in a pregnant doe.

(Lima et al. 2016). Given the high mortality rate, predicting how a disease will turn out is a crucial tactic for reducing financial loss (Lima et al. 2016). Due to the complexity of pregnancy toxemia, infected animals might be challenging to recognize at first, and once the condition has been diagnosed, it may proceed quickly. Therefore, clinical decisions about management and therapy must be put into action quickly throughout the course of the disease as postponement can be fatal.

30.8 Diagnosis

Pregnancy toxemia occurs due to disturbances in carbohydrate metabolism. Characteristic biochemical patterns associated with pregnancy toxemia in goats showed that there is a decreased level of glucose and calcium in the blood and increased levels of ketone bodies (Vasava et al. 2016). As glucose is an essential component for proper brain functioning, its deficiency may lead to nervous disturbances, coma, and death.

Increased concentrations of BHBA and/or low blood glucose during the late stage of pregnancy and early lactation are associated with pregnancy toxemia and ketosis. In dairy cows, dipsticks can be used to detect BHBA in urine or milk, however in goats these semiquantitative tests are not as accurate as blood tests. An increase in blood and urine ketone concentrations confirms the diagnosis. Compared to blood concentrations, urine concentrations are more accurate and precise. Cases of pregnancy toxemia can be diagnosed using Rothera's qualitative test from urine samples. Details of the procedure of Rothera's test are given in Figure 30.3 and the results are shown in Figure 30.4. Other results include lower levels of serum calcium and potassium, higher BUN, higher levels of free fatty acids (more than 500 g/ml), and higher levels of BHBA (>1 mmol/l) (Pough 2002).

For an accurate diagnosis of pregnancy toxemia, a differential diagnosis is important to distinguish this metabolic disorder from other disorders with similar signs such as hypocalcemia or hypomagnesemia, resulting from low calcium or magnesium levels in the blood. Other disorders with similar symptoms include diseases that affect the nervous system such as polioencephalomalacia, enterotoxemia, rabies, listeriosis, and lead poisoning. When possible, a quick laboratory analysis is important to diagnose and treat pregnancy toxemia.

While hypoglycemia, hypocalcemia, and/or hypomagnesemia are related to pregnancy toxemia in sheep and may aggravate the clinical picture (Vania and Plamen 2017), low blood glucose and elevated amounts of NEFA, which can be partially or fully oxidized to ketone bodies by the Krebs cycle, are also the results of NEB (Drackley et al. 2001). Even though the kidney makes relatively fewer contributions, the liver is crucial for the metabolism of blood sugar, for the delivery of glucose to the tissues, and because it is the only organ in which gluconeogenesis occurs, so it is important to evaluate liver function parameters (Harmeyer and Schlumbohm 2006).

Laboratory findings in pregnant does and other small ruminants include hypoglycemia (often <2 mmol/l), elevated urine ketone levels, elevated serum BHBA levels (normal <0.8 mmol/l, subclinical ketosis ≥0.8 mmol/l, clinical disease >3 mmol/l), and occasionally hypocalcemia (Rook 2000). Even when BHBA readings are normal, decreased serum fructosamine may serve as a helpful early warning sign of probable pregnancy toxemia (Rook 2000). Since up to 40% of cases with hypoglycemia have normal glucose levels and up to 20% have hyperglycemia, BHBA is a more trustworthy diagnostic of disease than blood glucose levels.

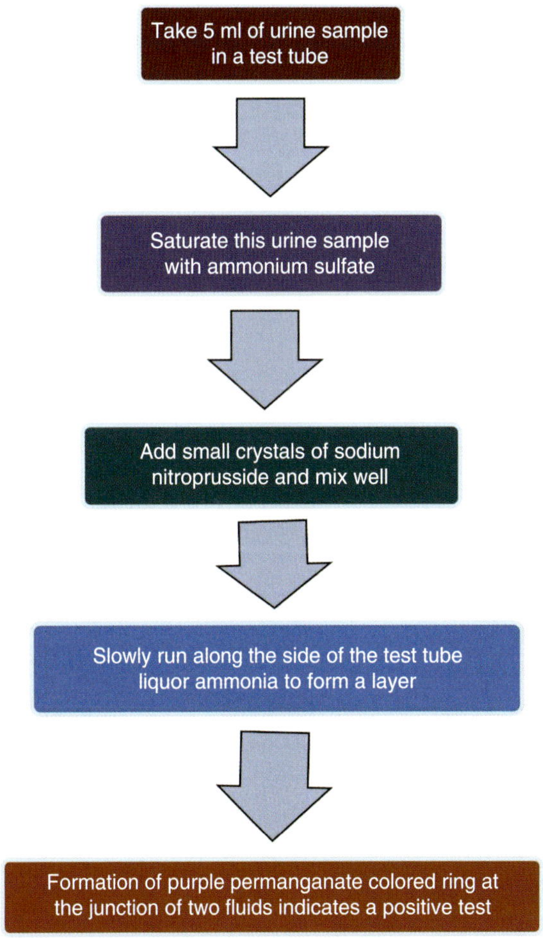

Figure 30.3 Procedure of Rothera's test for detection of ketone bodies in urine.

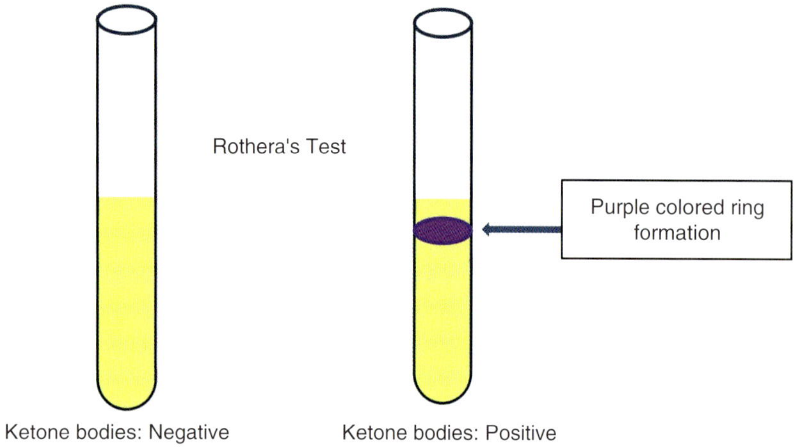

Figure 30.4 Results of Rothera's test.

Cerebrospinal fluid glucose levels, which remain low even as serum glucose rises in severe cases following fetal death, may be more accurate than blood glucose levels in circumstances when the diagnosis needs to be confirmed (Scott and Woodman 1993). Increase in NEFA exceeding 0.4 mmol/l is another sign of possible hepatic lipidosis and decreased liver function.

Low blood potassium and magnesium concentrations were found in pregnancy toxemia by Marteniuk and Herdt (1988), and these findings were later supported by Edmondson and Pugh (2009) and Hefnawy et al. (2011). Sodium and potassium ions are lost as a result of the prolonged urine excretion of ketone bodies in ewes, which lowers the plasma alkali reserve (Sargison 2007). Blood potassium levels may also have fallen in a study by Lima et al. (2016) which also found a significant decrease in blood sodium concentration.

Hefnawy et al. (2011) replicated Marteniuk and Herdt's (1988) observation of lower blood calcium blood concentrations in pregnancy toxemia. According to Marteniuk and Herdt (1988), one of the ways to diagnose pregnancy toxemia with primary hypocalcemia is total calcium concentrations which are normally above 6 mg/dl. According to Sargison (2007), 20% of sheep with pregnancy toxemia also show mild hypocalcemia as measured by serum calcium concentration below 1.9 mmol/l.

This may be related to sheep with extensive hepatic fatty degeneration having inadequate vitamin D hydroxylation. In ewes with pregnancy toxemia, Anoushepour et al. (2014) found elevated levels of NEFA, cortisol, and ceruloplasmin together with lower calcium and glucose levels. In goats, Rani et al. (2015) discovered a significant reduction in the serum levels of sodium, potassium, magnesium, and calcium in pregnancy toxemia. This finding may be explained by the stress of starvation, dehydration, and renal involvement in the pathogenesis of caprine pregnancy toxemia, as well as by enhanced lipolysis that can result in hypomagnesemia and hypocalcemia (Sakha et al. 2013).

30.9 Treatment

Treatment of ketosis is relatively simple – administer a readily usable form of energy (usually glucose) and get the doe eating on her own again (usually with the help of anabolic steroids). Unfortunately, response to treatment is usually not very good; however, it is worth the effort of trying especially if the affected doe is valuable. Once pregnancy toxemia is in advanced stages (doe lying down unable to rise), no treatment is highly effective. A common treatment is oral administration of propylene glycol three times a day. Thiamin supplementation may also be suggested to help jump-start carbohydrate metabolism. Always consult with your veterinarian for advice on treatment options and dosage recommendations. If the doe recovers sufficiently to begin eating on her own again, add an energy supplement to increase energy intake. Cesarean section or induced abortion will usually lead to recovery of the doe if ketosis is caught early enough. If the kids are near term, they may also be saved.

Treatment should focus on two aspects.

- Management of energy sources and elimination of elements contributing to decreased energy availability.
- Better care for neonates.

Different therapies have been suggested, including dosage with glycerol, glucose, propylene glycol, adrenocorticotropic hormone (ACTH), synthetic glucocorticoids, or anabolic steroids. According to Buswell et al. (1986), the majority of treatments raise blood glucose levels and are, to varying degrees, effective in treating the condition. According to Andrews (1997), early diagnosis of the condition is crucial to ensuring a speedy return to normal appetite since a decreased appetite further reduces nutrient intake, which in turn hastens the onset of the disease and raises morbidity.

When sheep are treated very early in the disease course, they often respond well but once they have become recumbent, their response to therapy is weak, and giving them an IV dose of 50% dextrose at this point could expedite their demise. Along with glucose replacement therapy, treatment calls for the correction of fluid, electrolyte, and acid–base abnormalities.

30.9.1 Parenteral Medication

Individual sheep should ideally undergo metabolic testing before receiving fluids, electrolytes, and dextrose over an extended length of time as part of corrective therapy. One approach for glucose therapy is the delivery of 20–40 units of zinc protamine insulin given IM every other day for three days together with the infusion of 5–7 g of glucose IV 6–8 times per day. Because of accessibility issues, financial constraints, or the volume of infected sheep in many sheep-raising regions, rigorous laboratory monitoring and therapy are not feasible.

In the absence of biochemical monitoring, glucose therapy should be combined with an IV infusion of lactated Ringer's solution or isotonic sodium bicarbonate, as well as stomach tube administration of additional fluids. Even though corticosteroids are frequently used, they have minimal therapeutic benefit in sheep, so treatment with them is not advised. In ewes that are still able to stand, very large doses are successful but the efficacy is likely due to elimination of the glucose drain through the inducement of premature parturition.

Treatment with recombinant bovine somatotropin (0.15 mg/kg body weight) along with dextrose and electrolytes may shorten treatment time, enhance ewe survival, and increase the viability of newborn lambs, although the results so far have not been very promising.

30.9.2 Oral Therapy

Previously, parenteral glucose therapy has been supported by oral administration of propylene glycol or glycerin (110 g/d). Propylene glycol or glycerin alone can be used as a less intensive therapy and has had good results for some farmers but not all.

A concentrated oral rehydration solution for diarrheal calves that contains 45 g of glucose, 8.5 g of sodium chloride, 6.17 g of glycine, and electrolytes is commercially available and has been shown to be effective when administered orally every 4–8 hours.

In the UK, this treatment is currently widely utilized. When nonpregnant sheep are drenched with this solution, their blood glucose levels are higher than when they are drenched with glycerol or propylene glycol. Pregnancy toxemia has shown recovery rates of 90% in early instances and 55% in later cases. Vasopressin has been used in conjunction with the oral intake of glucose to cause the esophageal groove to close. Compared to treatment with oral glucose precursors and electrolytes alone, medication with insulin coupled with oral glucose precursors and electrolytes revealed a considerably greater survival rate (87%).

30.10 Prevention

Since treatment is not generally effective, avoiding conditions that lead to ketosis is best. First, avoid overconditioning does in early pregnancy. This includes preventing does from becoming too fat and also slimming down does that are already fat. Next, be sure to feed high-quality forages in addition to supplements that are very palatable during the last two months of pregnancy. This allows does to receive adequate energy even though rumen volume is decreased. If adequate and suitable feed is not available for the whole herd during late pregnancy, gentle driving can identify early cases of ketosis. Ketotic does can be recognized by the symptoms outlined above. These does can then be separated from the rest of the herd and given special care.

One of the guiding principles of sustainable livestock production is to feed high levels of roughage in the diet so as to promote good rumen digestion. However, as the doe progresses in the late stage of pregnancy, the energy density of the ration should increase to accommodate the inevitable reduction in dry matter intake. Anecdotally, there is evidence that in intensively reared small ruminants, access to external paddocks and grazing during the late stage of pregnancy will help to reduce the onset of pregnancy toxemia. Feed more energy to the late-term pregnant and early lactation doe to help address ketosis or pregnancy toxemia. When fed at the right amounts, grains are much higher in energy compared to forages and will take up less room in the rumen. Gradually increase the grain portion of the diet and reduce the hay portion. If this is done too quickly, the rumen pH could change rapidly and lead to more problems. Feeding some of the forage in pelleted form and providing more frequent, smaller meals will help to maintain dietary fiber levels in a lower volume of goat feed. A small amount of fat (such as corn oil) in the feed will also help increase energy intake. Some producers give their does a little honey or molasses right after they give birth to provide immediate carbohydrate energy.

Remember to consult your veterinarian before administering this type of feeding program to ensure optimal goat nutrition. Keep good records, so you know which does are prone to ketosis or pregnancy toxemia. Some does sail through pregnancy and lactation without problems and might put on unneeded fat if given extra energy in their feed. Providing a healthy diet and reducing stressors like higher workloads and parasitism are key to preventing pregnant toxemia. Niacin and ionophores may be included as additional treatment options for this illness.

Shearing pregnant sheep is advantageous because the increased body heat loss that results may encourage the consumption of dry materials. The ewe has to labor harder because of the weight of the fleece coat. Additionally, late-pregnant does/ewes bearing multiple fetuses have a tendency to be bigger and less graceful than the rest of the flock. Management procedures must guarantee that these animals are given access to food and have enough space to sleep.

A doe's nutritional state can be predicted by serum BHB concentrations. When values are higher than 0.7 mmol/l, it means that the herd animals are in NEB, and the producer should prevent pregnancy toxemia immediately rather than waiting for clinical instances to show up. Goats bearing twins are separated using ultrasonography so caregivers can provide for their extra dietary requirements.

Although they are less frequent, overconditioned females (BCS 4–5) can be seen in small hobby flocks. Owners should be advised on how to prevent the issue through good food management because overweight and obese females are far less susceptible to treatment. However, in overconditioned females, late pregnancy is not the time to reduce body condition.

To identify flocks at risk of pregnancy toxemia, a flock screening test based on serum BHBA content can be used. For the purpose of identifying animals that are more likely to contract the disease, a concentration of 0.8 mmol/l should be taken into consideration if the number of fetuses in the pregnancy has not been established. Otherwise, only animals having multiple fetuses should have their blood BHBA concentration evaluated; in this scenario, the cut-off value utilized to identify animals at risk is 1.1 mmol/l. Keep good records, so you know which does are prone to ketosis or pregnancy toxemia.

Effective anthelmintic therapy would further aid in disease prevention, particularly in farms with high parasite burdens.

30.11 Conclusion

Pregnancy toxemia in sheep and goats is a metabolic disorder which occurs principally due to faulty carbohydrate metabolism and low blood sugar levels. However, the disease is often triggered by many contributory factors like stress which may either be nutritional or physiological due to two or more lambs/kids. The disease is prevalent in almost all parts of the world and is more likely to occur during the last two months of gestation. Excessively fat or extremely thin animals are more likely to suffer from the disease. Prevention is better than treatment and the best preventive measure is to feed high-energy concentrates during the last two months of pregnancy.

References

Andrews, A. (1997). Pregnancy toxemia in the ewe. *In Practice* 19: 306–312.

Anoushepour, A., Mottaghian, P., and Mehdi, S. (2014). The comparison of some biochemical parameters in hyperketonemic and normal ewes. *European Journal of Experimental Biology* 4 (3): 83–87.

Bani Isail, Z., Al-Majali, A., Amireh, F., and Al-Rawashdeh, O. (2008). Metabolic profiles in goat does in late pregnancy with and without subclinical pregnancy toxemia. *Veterinary Clinical Pathology* 37: 434–437.

Barbagianni, M.S., Spanos, S.A., Ioannidi, K.S. et al. (2015). Increased incidence of peri-parturient problems in ewes with pregnancy toxaemia. *Small Ruminant Research* 132: 111–114.

Bergman, E.N. (1993). Disorders of carbohydrate and fat metabolism. In: *Dukes' Physiology of Domestic Animals*, 11e (ed. M.J. Swenson and W.O. Reece), 412–421. Ithaca, NY: Cornell University Press.

Buswell, J.F., Haddy, J.P., and Bywater, R.J. (1986). Treatment of pregnancy toxaemia in sheep using a concentrated oral hydration solution. *Veterinary Record* 118: 208–209.

Cal-Pereyra, L., Benech, A., González-Montaña, J.R. et al. (2015). Changes in the metabolic profile of pregnant ewes to an acute feed restriction in late gestation. *New Zealand Veterinary Journal* 63: 141–146.

Clarkson, M.J. (2000). Pregnancy toxaemia. In: *Diseases of Sheep*, 3e (ed. W.B. Martin and L.D. Aitken), 315–317. Oxford, UK: Blackwell Science.

Drackley, J.K., Overton, T.R., and Dowlen, H.H. (2001). Adaptations of glucose and long-chain fatty acid metabolism in liver of dairy cows during the peri-parturient period. *Journal of Dairy Science* 84: 100–112.

Edmondson, M.A. and Pugh, D.G. (2009). Pregnancy toxemia in sheep and goats. In: *Food Animal Practice*, 5e (ed. D. Anderson and M. Rings), 144–145. St Louis, MO: Elsevier.

Feijó, J.O., Oliveira, A.M., Pereira, R.A. et al. (2016). Protocolo de indução de cetose subclínica e seu efeito sobre parâmetros bioquímicos em ovelhas gestantes. *Science and Animal Health* 4: 21–34.

Harmeyer, J. and Schlumbohm, C. (2006). Pregnancy impairs ketone body disposal in late gestating Ovisaries: implications for onset of pregnancy toxaemia. *Research in Veterinary Science* 81 (2): 254–264.

Hefnawy, A.E., Shousha, S., and Youssef, S. (2011). Hemato-biochemical profile of pregnant and experimentally pregnancy toxemic goats. *Journal of Basic and Applied Chemistry* 1: 65–69.

Herdt, T.H. (2000). Ruminant adaptation to negative energy balance. Influences on the etiology of ketosis and fatty liver. *Veterinary Clinics of North America: Food Animal Practice* 16 (2): 215–229.

Jain, S.K., McVie, R., and Bocchini, J.A. (2006). Hyperketonemia (ketosis), oxidative stress and type 1 diabetes. *Pathophysiology* 13: 163–170.

Lima, M.S., Cota, J.B., Vaz, Y.M. et al. (2016). Glucose intolerance in dairy goats with pregnancy toxemia: lack of correlation between blood pH and beta hydroxybutyric acid values. *Canadian Veterinary Journal* 57: 635–640.

Marteniuk, J.V. and Herdt, T.H. (1988). Pregnancy toxemia and ketosis of ewes and does. *Veterinary Clinics of North America: Food Animal Practice* 4: 307–315.

Moghaddam, G. and Hassanpour, A. (2008). Comparison of blood serum glucose, beta hydroxybutyric acid, blood urea nitrogen and calcium concentrations in pregnant and lambed ewes. *Journal of Animal and Veterinary Advances* 7: 308–311.

Pough, D.G. (2002). *Sheep and Goat Medicine*, 1e. Philadelphia, PA: Saunders.

Rani, R.U., Palanichamy, V., and Muruganandan, B. (2015). Clinical and serobiochemical studies on pregnancy toxaemia in does. *International Journal of Current Innovation Research* 1 (4): 102–104.

Rook, J.S. (2000). Pregnancy toxemia of ewes, does, and beef cows. *Veterinary Clinics of North America: Food Animal Practice* 16: 293–317.

Sakha, M., Anoushepour, A., Nadalian, M.G., and Khaki, Z. (2013). Liver copper and serum ceruloplasmin concentrations in hyperketonemic pregnant ewes. *European Journal of Experimental Biology* 3 (4): 57–60.

Sargison, N.D. (2007). Pregnancy toxaemia. In: *Diseases of Sheep*, 4e (ed. I.D. Aitken), 359–363. Ames, IA: Blackwell Publishing.

Schlumbohm, C. and Harmeyer, J. (2008). Twin-pregnancy increases susceptibility of ewes to hypoglycaemic stress and pregnancy toxaemia. *Research in Veterinary Science* 84: 286–299.

Scott, P.R. and Woodman, M.P. (1993). An outbreak of pregnancy toxaemia in a flock of Scottish blackface sheep. *Veterinary Record* 133: 597–598.

Van Saun, R.J. (2000). Pregnancy toxemia in a flock of sheep. *Journal of the American Veterinary Medical Association* 217: 1536–1539.

Vania, M. and Plamen, M. (2017). Clinical and hematological studies in sheep with subclinical and clinical ketosis. *Tradition and Modernity in Veterinary Medicine* 2 (3): 37–44.

Vasava, P.R., Jani, R.G., Goswami, H.V. et al. (2016). Studies on clinical signs and biochemical alteration in pregnancy toxemic goats. *Veterinary World* 9 (8): 869–874.

31

Hypocalcemia

Gowdaiahnadoddi K. Chetan Kumar, Ashok Ashwini, and Rayala S. Sagar

Department of Veterinary Medicine, Veterinary College, Hassan, India

31.1 Introduction

Goat farming has attracted great commercial interest globally. India has the world's largest goat population. According to the Livestock Censuses carried out by the Government of India, the goat population expanded from 47.2 million in 1951 to 148.2 million in 2019.

Healthy animals will have metabolic balance, in which a substance's intake or synthesis equals its excretion. The term "metabolism" refers to the collection of all physical, chemical, and metabolic activities that take place within a live cell or organism in relation to the assimilation, disintegration, or synthesis of essential organic components. In order for the body to function normally, energy must be extracted from nutrients during metabolism. Metabolic disease is caused by metabolic process dysfunction or disruption. Disorders in one or more of the organism's metabolic systems are associated with metabolic diseases.

Hypocalcemia, commonly known as "milk fever," "parturient paresis," "paresis puerperalis," and "parturient apoplexy," is a production and metabolic disorder. When an animal develops hypocalcemia as a result of failure to maintain calcium homeostasis, it is classified as a metabolic disease. The deficiency here is not in the diet but rather within the animal due to some physiological failure in adjustment. Similarly, hypocalcemia becomes a production disease when an animal's potential to meet its requirements of high output is compromised by inadequate food. This is primarily owing to poor husbandry.

31.2 Calcium in Goats

Calcium is a significant macromineral. The skeleton contains 99% of calcium in its bound state, which works in conjunction with phosphorus to aid in bone production (Ca:P = 2.2:1). For several physiological processes, including neuromuscular stimulation, muscle contraction, blood coagulation, heart contraction, and enzyme activation, the calcium component is crucial. There are three main fractions of calcium in the plasma: 50% is free, 40% is protein bound, and 10% is complexed with anions such as lactate, citrate, inorganic phosphate, and bicarbonate. Only calcium in the ionized state is physiologically active.

Mature goats weighing 50–100 kg require around 3.5–6 g of calcium per day for maintenance (Morand-Fehr and Sauvant 1978; Kessler 1991). When food supplies are insufficient/deficient of calcium during pregnancy, the goat will rely on its bone reserves. Goat milk has about 1.4 g of calcium per kilogram (NRC 1981).

31.3 Regulation of Calcium Homeostasis

The three main factors in calcium homeostasis are parathormone, calcitriol, and calcitonin. Parathyroid hormone (PTH; parathormone) enhances calcium mobilization into the circulation. 1,25 Dihydroxycholecalciferol/vitamin D_3/calcitriol increases calcium absorption from the gut, whereas calcitonin inhibits calcium absorption from the gut and enhances bone mineralization.

Elements of Reproduction and Reproductive Diseases of Goats, First Edition. Edited by Tanmoy Rana.

When serum calcium levels fall, the parathyroid gland releases PTH, which then works on the bones to cause osteoclastic activity and bone resorption. In order to normalize the level of calcium in the serum, parathormone acts on the kidneys to secrete vitamin D_3, which in turn acts on the intestine to aid in calcium absorption from the gut. When the level of plasma calcium rises, the thyroid gland releases calcitonin, which stimulates the activity of osteoblasts and causes more calcium to deposit in the bones. Thus, the normal plasma/serum calcium level is preserved.

High-yielding lactating does will experience a brief phase of hypocalcemia, but most of them will adjust to the increased calcium demand within 48 hours of kidding by raising their plasma parathormone and vitamin D_3 concentrations. Goats that are unable to acclimatize to this endocrine-mediated mechanism experience milk fever. Most of the time, deficiency is caused by an animal's slow rate of adaption to a high calcium demand, not by their food.

31.4 Factors Influencing Absorption of Calcium

Calcium metabolism and absorption are influenced by a variety of dietary, animal, and environmental variables. Some of the essential factors that have a critical role are described below.

- One of the key factors in the development of hypocalcemia is age. The rate of calcium absorption varies between 90% and 99% in young animals and 45–55% in adults, making adult animals more susceptible to hypocalcemia.
- The level of vitamin D_3 is also crucial because a healthy level of vitamin D_3 encourages calcium absorption from the intestines. This lessens the likelihood of hypocalcemia in goats.
- The optimum calcium to phosphorus ratio for absorbing food-based calcium is 2:1 because low levels of calcium to phosphorus can interfere with homeostasis of calcium and accelerate bone resorption. Low dietary Ca consumption has detrimental effects on bones as well, while excessive dietary P intake alone can damage bones by increasing PTH secretion. Phosphorus levels in the blood may impede the activity of the renal 25-hydroxycholecalciferol 1-alpha hydroxylase enzyme which is required for the production of 1,25 dihydroxycholecalciferol.
- The pH of the gastrointestinal system is particularly crucial because alkaline pH inhibits calcium absorption from the gut while acidic pH favors it.
- Dietary anion–cation balance is a major determinant in the development of hypocalcemia. Systemic acidification is caused by anions such as sulfate and chloride (metabolic acidosis). This activates the Ca transport mechanism. As a result, the level of plasma 1,25 $(OH)_2$ D will rise. Vitamin D_3 has a dual mechanism for boosting the plasma pool of calcium from bone and enhancing calcium absorption from the gut. Most forage, particularly legumes and grasses, are high in potassium, which causes metabolic acidosis and inhibits the calcium transport pathway.
- Excess magnesium, oxalates, or phytates in the diet reduce calcium absorption. A drop in serum magnesium levels has two effects on calcium metabolism: by lowering parathormone secretion and by lowering tissue sensitivity to parathormone.
- Protein levels in the diet also influence calcium absorption. A low-protein diet reduces calcium absorption from the intestine, resulting in a sudden spike in serum PTH and secondary hyperparathyroidism.

31.5 Calcium Deficiencies

31.5.1 Nutritional Secondary Hyperparathyroidism

When there is a chronic dietary shortage of calcium and vitamin D, the amount of calcium absorbed across the intestine into the extracellular space is reduced. As a result, the level of calcium in the blood decreases, stimulating PTH release. Because the diet is poor in calcium, the activity of PTH cannot effectively boost intestinal calcium absorption. PTH's only action in this scenario is on the bones, resulting in osteoclastic activity. Fibrous osteodystrophy is caused by the constant elimination of bone calcium without replenishment. This phenomenon is more typical in young animals.

31.5.2 Renal Secondary Hyperparathyroidism

Kidney failure causes renal secondary hyperparathyroidism. This ailment has been recorded on occasion in elderly animals. Pyelonephritis during late gestation has been described in dairy cows and may be a cause in goats as well. The renal tissue will be destroyed as a result of this disorder. The compromised kidney is unable to eliminate phosphorus efficiently, leading to hyperphosphatemia. The increasing blood phosphorus content will lower the blood's ionized calcium content. This is because high phosphate levels in animals with renal failure produce calcium precipitation in the blood. Second, elevated phosphate levels will have an effect on the remnant renal tissues. It inhibits the activity of the enzyme 1-alpha-hydroxylase, which catalyzes the conversion of 25-dihydroxycholecalciferol to the active form of 1,25 dihydroxycholecalciferol. As a result, even while PTH stimulates this conversion, hypophosphatemia prevents it from occurring.

31.5.3 Hypocalcemia

The contraction of skeletal, cardiac, and smooth muscles depends on calcium. Low calcium concentration promotes vulnerability to various metabolic and viral illnesses and decreases feed intake, rumen contractions, uterine and intestinal motility. The "gateway disease" label is applied to hypocalcemia as numerous additional disorders may be triggered by it. Due to ineffective myometrial muscle contractions, hypocalcemia is thought to be the primary cause of dystocia in small ruminants. Animals with hypocalcemia are more likely to experience immunological suppression, uterine prolapse, delayed uterine involution, puerperal metritis, pregnancy toxemia, and mastitis as a result of improper teat sphincter closure.

The health of the animal and a positive economic impact depend on effective care and management of the doe during the transition phase. The 4–6-week period centered on parturition is known as the transition phase or periparturient period. The doe is susceptible to multiple metabolic problems due to failure to meet her nutritional needs in late gestation and early lactation because many metabolic changes and adaptations to the new physiological status occur during this crucial phase (Figure 31.1). The transition phase is absolutely essential for maintaining the health and productivity of dairy goats (Huang et al. 2021). In intensive dairy goat farms, subclinical hypocalcemia and subclinical hyperketonemia are metabolic diseases that frequently arise during the periparturient phase (Roche 2003). Due to lower milk production and increased veterinary costs for the treatment of diseased goats, the frequency of these two diseases has resulted in financial losses for the dairy goat sector.

The nonfebrile acute or subacute metabolic disease condition known as hypocalcemia affects cattle, sheep, and goats. It most frequently manifests around the time of parturition and is characterized by generalized muscular weakness, recumbency circulatory collapse, depression of consciousness, shock, and death. At kidding, the periparturient doe goes from not lactating to nursing and thus faces great difficulties in preserving calcium homeostasis. The animals that fail to preserve calcium homeostasis may develop parturient paresis, a clinical illness that puts the doe's life in danger and puts her at risk for a number of additional diseases. Goats have a somewhat lower frequency of hypocalcemia than dairy cattle (Oetzel 1988).

Unlike goats, in which the disease is widespread during both the late gestation and early lactation periods, more than 91% of occurrences of the syndrome in cattle happen within 24–48 hours of parturition. Hypocalcemia in goats can happen at any time between six weeks before and 10 weeks after parturition. Animals bearing multiple fetuses are more vulnerable since the developing fetuses will require a lot of calcium for bone calcification. Moreover, goats with a high potential for milk production, such as Alpine, Saanen, and Jamunapari, have a susceptibility to experience postpartum hypocalcemia (Allen and Sansom 1986). An exogenous reserve of diet/nutrition or an endogenous reserve of body/tissue is used to meet this higher demand.

Animals become susceptible to hypocalcemia when their dietary needs are not met throughout the late stages of pregnancy and early stages of lactation. Goats with a high milk production capacity and a propensity for multiple fetuses have greater fetoplacental needs and are more prone to hypocalcemia. Concurrent pregnancy toxemia complicates the hypocalcemia in certain goats (Ramsey 1945).

Pre- or postpartum hypocalcemia in a doe is possible. The parturient type of hypocalcemia will predominate when goats are kept intensively just for milk production, such as in systems like zero grazing. The prepartum variant of hypocalcemia is typical in goats that are extensively grown and carry multiple fetuses and not stressed for high milk output. Importantly, a doe's milk has a higher calcium loss rate than cow's milk.

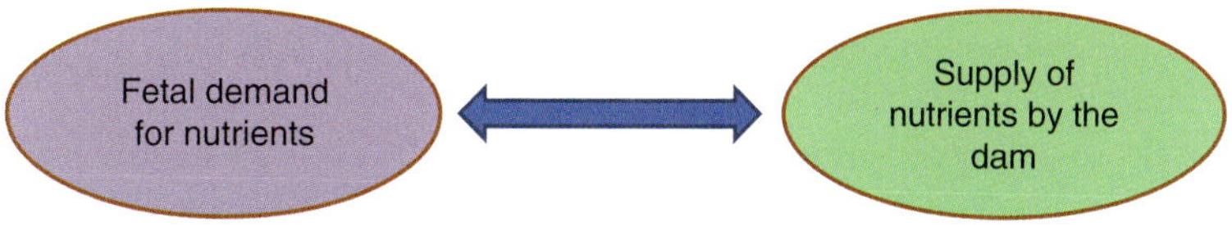

Figure 31.1 Failure to meet nutritional requirements during the transition phase/ periparturient period makes the animals susceptible to many metabolic diseases.

Research done on 45 polyparous native goats showed that during times of transition, hypocalcemia has led to both metabolic and oxidative stress. Moreover, It delayed uterine involution throughout the postpartum period (Bayoumi et al. 2021). Both nursing and pregnancy are physiologically stressful times. Significant metabolic and endocrine changes are its defining characteristics. In contrast to milk fever in cattle, the illness in goats is frequently misdiagnosed and undertreated.

Hypocalcemia, which is unrelated to pregnancy or kidding, can occur in goats and generally goes unreported or unnoticed. As the level of estrogen in the blood rises during the estrus phase, calcium ionization levels fall, resulting in subclinical hypocalcemia. This is quite important for the action of the forestomach. The reticulorumen motility is inhibited by the drop in calcium, which causes ruminal stasis and anorexia.

31.6 Epidemiology of Hypocalcemia in Goats

The condition of hypocalcemia is sporadic. Goat breeds that produce a lot of milk, such as Alpine, Saanen, and Jamunapari, among others, are more vulnerable because of the increased calcium loss through the milk. The frequency of periparturient hypocalcemia is highest in older (over three years) and greater parity does. Osteoblasts are the only form of bone cells that express the 1,25 $(OH)_2$ D receptor protein. The ability of bone to supply calcium to the plasma calcium pool could be delayed by the age-related decline in osteoblast numbers.

31.7 Predisposing Factors for Hypocalcemia in Goats

- As extensive or semiintensive goat husbandry is the norm in India, an abrupt feed restriction lasting longer than 24 hours may cause hypocalcemia in the animal.
- Due to a lack of good-quality roughage, prevalence is higher in colder climates.
- The doe is predisposed to hypocalcemia by grazing on oxalate-rich plants such as alfalfa hay, beetroot pulp, sesame meal, or green cereal crops. Oxalates are calcium chelators that generate indigestible calcium complexes. Cereals grown in green are often poor sources of calcium.
- Drugs: some aminoglycosides (neomycin, gentamicin), as well as sulfonamides, reduce the degree of ionization of serum calcium when administered intravenously. Tetracyclines are thought of as chelators for calcium. Studies have indicated a significant decrease in serum calcium levels following oral zinc oxide treatment for the prevention of facial eczema. Hence, caution is advised in utilizing these medications during the transition phase in does.

31.8 Etiology for Hypocalcemia in Goats

The basic biochemical abnormality is a decrease in ionized calcium levels in the extracellular area, including plasma. This decline is primarily due to a breakdown in calcium homeostasis. Hypocalcemia is caused by a sudden decrease in calcium intake mixed with precipitating conditions such as forced exercise, long-distance transportation, feed deprivation, exposure to inclement weather, and grazing on oxalate-rich plants or green grain. Hypocalcemia is also caused by inadequate dietary calcium and vitamin D supplementation, as well as an incorrect Ca:P ratio. Hypocalcemia during the prepartum period is caused by increased fetal demand, whereas postpartum hypocalcemia is caused by increased calcium loss in the milk (Figure 31.2).

31.9 Pathogenesis of Hypocalcemia in Goats

Calcium is important in the following processes:

- cell membrane stability
- muscular contractility
- release of acetylcholine.

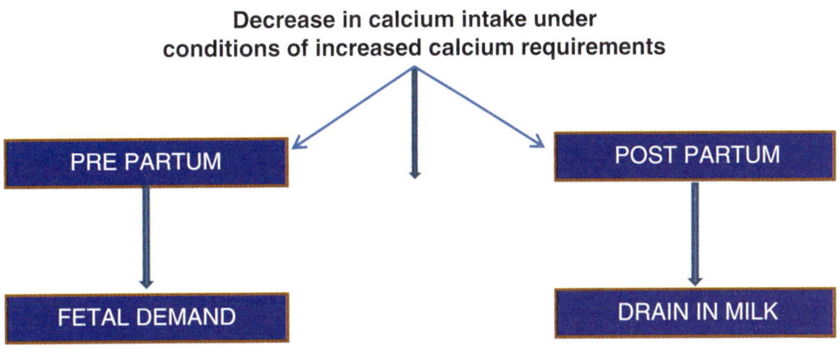

Figure 31.2 Reasons for hypocalcemia in the pre- and postpartum periods.

31.9.1 Cell Membrane Stability

Calcium linked to the cell membrane helps to maintain membrane stability. Reduced ionized calcium promotes cell membrane permeability, making the nerve cell more excitable.

31.9.2 Muscular Contractility

Calcium is essential for myosin to attach to the actin molecule. The basis for muscle contraction is the crossbridge between actin and myosin. As a result, reduced calcium leads to poor muscle contractility.

31.9.3 Release of Acetylcholine

Calcium is essential for the release of acetylcholine into the neuromuscular junction's synaptic cleft. Reduced calcium inhibits acetylcholine release, impairing signal transmission at the neuromuscular endplate. As a result, ruminal stasis and subsequent bloat are common symptoms of hypocalcemia.

Apart from these effects, a low calcium level lowers ruminal and abomasal contractility, resulting in decreased feed intake. There is a negative energy balance, which causes adipose tissue mobilization and a rise in the concentration of nonesterified fatty acids (NEFA) in the blood circulation. This metabolic state may put the animal at risk for pregnancy toxemia.

31.10 Clinical Signs of Hypocalcemia in Goats

The main clinical manifestations in hypocalcemic goats are hyperesthesia, tetany, and flaccid paralysis. In comparison with dairy cattle, dairy does with classic parturient paresis have less severe clinical symptoms (Guss 1977). At first, hyperexcitability, restlessness (Figure 31.3), stiff and jerky gait, ataxia, salivation, urine stasis, constipation, and muscle twitching more evident in the lips, eyelids, and ears are observed, extending to other muscles of the body. Only an attentive animal caretaker or an on-site veterinarian will detect these clinical indications.

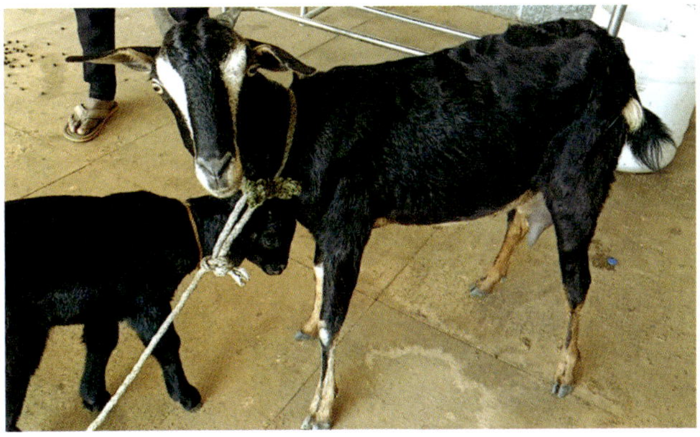

Figure 31.3 Hyperexcitability and restlessness.

Other clinical signs include decreased rectal temperature, decreased ruminal motility, anorexia, and recumbency, bloat, and relaxed rectal mucosa with loss of anal reflex and retained fecal pellets, and ruminal stasis followed by tympany, which causes salivation and tachypnea. Later, affected does exhibit sternal recumbency with a frog posture with extended hind legs and head resting on the ground, subnormal temperature, and tachycardia with feeble heart sounds, and sluggish pupillary response. Because of the lowered venous pressure, the pulse becomes impalpable and veins are

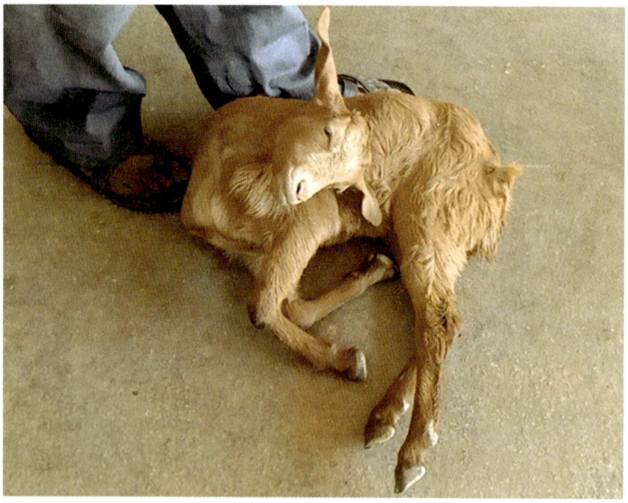

Figure 31.4 Doe in lateral recumbency.

difficult to rise. There will be drowsiness and significant mental depression. The doe eventually succumbs to lateral recumbency (Figure 31.4) and coma. If therapy is not initiated within 6–12 hours, death is unavoidable (Pugh and Baird 2012).

If a doe develops hypocalcemia just before or during parturition, the second stage of parturition may be delayed, resulting in dystocia. Vaginal examination usually indicates a completely dilated cervix and normal fetal presentation. A common consequence of hypocalcemia is uterine prolapse. As a result, intravenous calcium is often used to treat cases of uterine prolapse.

Muscle twitching, early agitation and nervousness, tetany that usually begins in the hind limbs, hypersensitivity, and convulsive movements of the head and limbs are the most common clinical indications of hypocalcaemic tetany in nonruminant monogastric species. However, in the case of ruminants, when the owner presents the doe, the animal is already in a comatose state with flaccid paralysis. Hypocalcemia is frequently more severe in pregnant goats than in lactating goats, presumably due to the presence of hypomagnesemia and pregnancy toxemia at the same time (Radostits et al. 2006). Several pregnant goats on high-grain diets developed hypocalcemia, which was followed by intestinal and vaginal prolapses.

31.11 Diagnosis of Hypocalcemia in Goats

A detailed history, clinical symptoms, physical examination, and laboratory testing are essential for identifying hypocalcemia in goats. A doe's history of pregnancy or parturition, transportation, exposure to inclement weather, or forced exercise all contribute to the suspicion of hypocalcemia. The clinical manifestations of hypocalcemia have already been described. The disease usually has a short course. It could persist anywhere from 12 to 24 hours.

The presence of neutrophilia, lymphopenia, and eosinophilia points to a stress leukogram, which is brought on by an overactive adrenal cortex. Dehydration is shown by hematopathology to increase pack cell volume and hemoglobin (Pugh et al. 2020). Goats typically have blood calcium concentrations of 10–12.8 mg/dl and 4.3–5.1 mg/dl for serum ionized calcium (Smith and Sherman 2009). Hypocalcemia is the term used to describe the condition when the serum calcium level is below 9.8 mg/dl (Quader et al. 2017).

The fundamental biochemical problem is a decrease in the level of total and ionized calcium below the normal range. This decrease typically varies in intensity with the clinical condition. Ca:P ratio falls to 1:1 (normal 2:1). The Ca:Mg ratio falls to 2:1 (normal 4:1). Blood glucose levels in dairy cattle are normal or slightly raised after parturient paresis. Acute stress may be to blame for this since it promotes gluconeogenesis and the production of endogenous glucocorticoids. Insufficient calcium availability also affects insulin release, which causes hyperglycemia. For the pancreas to secrete insulin, calcium is necessary. Calcium is not detected by the Sulkowitch test in urine analysis. Calcium excretion in the urine will stop as a compensatory response as serum calcium levels drop.

Upon making a diagnosis, if laboratory assistance is unavailable, an immediate response with intravenous calcium therapy is recommended in the hypocalcemic doe.

31.12 Differential Diagnosis of Hypocalcemia in Goats

Toxic septic metritis, polioencephalomalacia, grain overload, acute or subacute coliform mastitis, botulism, enterotoxemia, pregnancy toxemia, aspiration pneumonia, hypomagnesemia, acute diffuse peritonitis, and hypophosphatemia should all be distinguished from hypocalcemia in goats because their clinical symptoms are similar.

31.12.1 Polioencephalomalacia/Cerebrocortical necrosis

Thiamine or vitamin B_1 deficiency is the root cause of this condition. It is more prevalent in young kids and is linked to abrupt dietary changes or excessive carbohydrate intake. Amprolium and sulfonamide, two coccidiostats, also increase the risk of developing polioencephalomalacia. Clinical signs of polioencephalomalacia in goats include cortical blindness, edema, cerebellar herniation, and the loss of brain cells governing motor and visual skills. Convulsions happen every 2–5 minutes. Laboratory investigation of these animals reveals that thiaminase, pyruvate in urine, blood pyruvate, lactate levels, and pyruvate kinase levels are all elevated; transketolase activity values are lower in affected animals. Intravenous administration of thiamine HCl at a dose of 4.5–10 mg/lb results in improvement within minutes or a few hours. Full clinical recovery may be impossible in cases of delayed diagnosis and therapy.

31.12.2 Grain Overload/Acute Carbohydrate Engorgement/Lactic Acidosis

There will be a recent history of consuming a high-fermentability carbohydrate diet. An enlarged abdomen can be detected upon examination. Fluid splashing sounds in the rumen can be heard during ballottement and auscultation. On percussion and auscultation of the left flank, a positive steelband sound and splashing sound are audible above the rumen. Ruminal fluid analysis for color, odor, pH, and motility helps distinguish this condition from hypocalcemia. The cardinal symptom of hypocalcemia is solid pellet-like feces held in the rectum, whereas the predominant sign of ruminal acidosis is semisolid to loose feces. Physical examination of the ruminal fluid reveals a sour odor, a milky gray color, and a pH of 5. After staining, microscopic analysis of ruminal fluid reveals the absence of living motile protozoa and the prevalence of Gram-positive bacteria.

31.12.3 Acute or Peracute Coliform Mastitis

A wide range of bacterial infections have been identified as the cause of caprine mastitis. Physical examination of the mammary gland as well as microbiological investigation of the milk will aid in the diagnosis. Additional clinical symptoms include early-stage pyrexia, which is followed by hypothermia, tachycardia, dehydration, and depression, later accompanied by watery diarrhea brought on by septicemia and toxemia. Mastitis-afflicted goats may have clearly swollen, inflamed mammary glands that exude fluid or serous-like substances. Animals suffering from hypocalcemia are more likely to develop mastitis.

Calcium is required for effective muscular contraction. The teat sphincter is made up of smooth muscle that must contract in order for the teat end to close. If low blood calcium inhibits teat sphincter contraction, the teat canal may remain open, allowing pathogens from the environment to access the mammary gland. If the animal suffers from mastitis on a regular basis, calcium imbalance must be estimated or corrected.

31.12.4 Botulism

Clostridium botulinum causes this condition, which is most common in animals that have a pica habit and live near poultry farms. Botulism causes flaccid ascending paralysis progressing from the hindquarter, widespread weakness and hyporeflexia in muscles innervated by the cranial nerves (e.g., reduced jaw and tongue tone). Diagnosis is based on clinical findings that rule out other causes of neuromuscular problems, as well as the absence of internal lesions found during postmortem examination. Laboratory confirmation is often required since clinical signs alone are insufficient to establish an accurate diagnosis.

31.12.5 Enterotoxemia

Clostridium perfringens is the culprit behind this disease. In overfed, well-nourished animals, enterotoxemia is a regular occurrence that can cause violent convulsions, diarrhea, and even death. Enterotoxemia can cause glucosuria and severe hypoglycemia.

31.12.6 Pregnancy Toxemia/Kidding Sickness/Pregnancy Ketosis

This is an often fatal goat metabolic disorder induced by disruption in carbohydrate and fat metabolism, primarily due to negative energy balance. Severe nervous signs will predominate in this condition, including tonic-clonic convulsions, head pressing, circling, opisthotonus, forehead raising, star gazing posture, and a sweetish acetone odor in the breath. These symptoms will aid in distinguishing pregnancy toxemia from hypocalcemia, in which the animal will be comatose. Only pregnant animals with cerebral involvement are affected by this condition. The presence of ketone bodies in the urine and the serum concentration of beta-hydroxybutyric acid can be used to detect pregnancy toxemia. Calcium treatment will have no effect. Hypocalcemia is associated with an increased risk of incurring ketosis due to decreased gut motility and digestion.

31.12.7 Aspiratory Pneumonia

One of the complications linked with hypocalcemia is aspiration of rumen contents, which is caused by regurgitation or faulty drenching of calcium suspension. Fever, dyspnea, and expiratory grunt are common clinical symptoms, as are anxiety and severe depression. When the animal is lying on one side with ruminal contents regurgitating from the nostrils, aspiration pneumonia should always be suspected, especially if there is a history of drenching. Even if atypical auscultatory sounds are present, they may not be heard until the second day. Because the mortality rate is high, early diagnosis is critical if the animal is to be rescued.

31.12.8 Hypomagnesemia

When hypomagnesemia coexists with hypocalcemia, hyperesthesia, tetany, and convulsions are observed for an extended period of time instead of depression and flaccid paralysis. Tachycardia and loud heart sounds are common clinical indications of hypomagnesemia. Nonetheless, in hypocalcemia, tachycardia may occur; heart sounds are quieter than normal.

31.12.9 Hypophosphatemia

Low serum phosphorus levels have been explored as a cause of persistent recumbency in cows with hypocalcemia (Radostits et al. 2006). Nevertheless, parturient paresis in goats has yet to be examined. Ionized calcium estimation is the gold standard for diagnosing hypocalcemia.

31.12.10 Acute Diffuse Peritonitis

This happens when the uterus or abomasum is traumatized and perforated. Severe depression, tachycardia, dehydration, ruminal stasis, fever, weakness, recumbency, and moaning or grunting are all signs of acute peritonitis. Assessment of peritoneal fluid will help with diagnosis.

31.12.11 Toxic Septic Metritis/Metritis/Puerperal Metritis

Systemic or toxic metritis can be fatal and is characterized by a foul-smelling, watery uterine discharge that is frequently followed by a sharp decrease in milk production and fever. This condition develops a few days following parturition. Depression, fever, tachycardia (100–200 bpm), and anorexia are its hallmarks. During vaginal examination, uterine discharge with a bad odor is discovered. Septicemia and toxemia may result from uterine rupture. Calcium salts may induce ventricular fibrillation and mortality if given to a toxemic patient.

31.13 Treatment of Hypocalcemia in Goats

In general, timely treatment works effectively for hypocalcemia (Oetzel 1988). As the clinical signs become clear, every effort must be made to treat the affected animal as quickly as possible. The likelihood of recovery decreases the longer there is between presentation of an animal and treatment. The value of early therapy must be made clear to goat owners. Attempts should be made to keep the goat in sternal recumbency until treatment is started if it is lying on its side. If the goat regurgitates, this will make eructation easier and lessen the chance of aspiration.

31.13.1 Calcium Therapy

Calcium salt infusion by the parenteral route is the norm. The intravenous form of calcium administration is particularly efficient and fast recovery from treatment has been observed (Constable et al. 2016). Intravenous administration of Ca gluconate or Ca borogluconate solutions is commonly utilized because they cause less tissue irritation.

The addition of boric acid raises the calcium gluconate level. Cows with milk fever can be successfully treated with Ca salt solutions with 8–10 g of Ca (Ca borogluconate has 8.3% Ca) (Goff 2008). A reclined periparturient dairy cow's projected Ca deficit is 4 g Ca; additional Ca should be supplied to compensate for continued milk losses (Constable 2014). In goats, a rapid intravenous infusion of 23% calcium borogluconate at 1 g/45 kg body weight (1–1.5 ml/kg) produced good results.

Many workers have discovered that an ARD approach of dose fixing is convenient while treating cows with milk fever. ARD stands for A – Appetite, R – Ruminal motility, and D – Defecation. Normal ARD animals that are somewhat hypocalcemic – 2 g calcium, IV; animals lacking one or two ARD functions – 6 g calcium, IV; significantly depressed ARD animals – 6 g, IV. Use of the ARD system in caprine hypocalcemia has not been determined.

Slow IV calcium administration is recommended, as is regular heart auscultation. If arrhythmias are detected, the infusion should be discontinued immediately and resumed only when the heart rate returns to normal. Calcium underdosing results in an inadequate response to therapy where the animal fails to rise or hypocalcemia may relapse, whereas calcium overdose may result in possibly deadly cardiac toxicity. The calculated dose of Ca borogluconate is typically administered during a 15-minute period.

Subcutaneous calcium administration is preferred to avoid relapse by creating a calcium reservoir (depot preparation). Salt solutions comprising Ca gluconate or Ca borogluconate are appropriate for SC administration but salt solutions containing Ca chloride should be avoided because of their strong causticity. Calcium oral formulations are frequently based on Ca chloride ($CaCl_2$) and Ca propionate. Calcium chloride formulations have the advantage of being low in cost and requiring only a little amount. Oral Ca formulations should only be given to animals with normal swallowing abilities. In clinical situations, they cannot be utilized as the first line of treatment. Drenching calcium gel preparations is not recommended since it increases the risk of aspiration.

31.13.2 Typical Favorable Response to Intravenous Ca Borogluconate

- Belching (eructation).
- Sweating of muzzle and salivation.
- Muscle tremor, extending to the whole body.
- Improvement in the amplitude and pressures of the pulse.
- Decrease of the heart rate and increase in intensity of heart sounds.
- Defecation of firm fecal ball covered with mucus.
- Animal stands up quickly with balance.
- Urination once the animal stands.
- A slight transitory tetany of the limbs still persists.

Many animals will eat and drink within minutes after successful treatment if offered feed and water. In general, 60% cases respond immediately, 15% cases respond within two hours, 10% cases are complicated but recover, and 15% cases either die or require disposal. Unlike in cattle, recurrence is more common in goats; hence there is an obvious need to repeat the treatment after eight hours with subcutaneous or oral calcium preparation.

31.13.3 Calcium Toxicity

Calcium toxicity could be caused by human errors such as overdosing/calculated dosage, rapid calcium administration, and repetitive calcium administration. It can also develop as a result of animal variables such as toxemia or excessive excitation during calcium administration. Calcium toxicity is marked by significant elevation in heart rate (up to 180 beats per minute), respiratory distress, trembling, collapse, and death within a few minutes due to ventricular fibrillation in toxemic animals. Acute cardiac block can cause sudden death in an otherwise healthy animal. Due to sensitivity to adrenaline, frightened or aroused animals may die suddenly following calcium administration.

31.13.4 Failure to Respond to Treatment

When an animal fails to respond well to treatment, it may be due to a misdiagnosis, incomplete diagnosis, inadequate diagnostic, or inappropriate treatment. To maximize success, every effort should be made to diagnose and treat hypocalcemia as soon as possible.

31.14 Prevention and Control

The Metabolic Profile Test (MPT), which evaluates calorie, protein, and macromineral status in commercial dairy cattle, should be implemented on dairy goat farms as well. Ultrasonography can be used in advanced goat farms to identify does carrying twins and triplets. The dietary needs of goats carrying twins and triplets should be considered when feeding them. Minerals should be administered in predictable proportions during the periparturient phase in the form of a grain mixture or a total mixed ration (TMR). Feeding pregnant ewes vegetable oil (soya bean oil) during the last 2–3 weeks of pregnancy will enhance calcium absorption and reduce susceptibility to fasting-induced hypocalcemia (Constable et al. 2016).

Oxalates chelate calcium and impede absorption so special care must be taken with feed stuffs containing them. Minimize management stressors such as transportation and forced exercise during late gestation since they increase the risk of hypocalcemia in prepartum animals.

Due to a negative feedback mechanism, providing high-calcium diets to cattle prepartum has resulted in a high prevalence of milk fever. Cattle fail to maintain calcium homeostasis, resulting in clinical milk fever (Constable et al. 2016). Further research is needed to determine whether the same is true in small ruminants.

The negative feedback mechanism stimulates:

- the secretion of PTH, which increases calcium reabsorption from the renal system within seconds
- calcium resorption from the bones within hours to days
- conversion of vitamin D to 1,25 $(OH)_2$ D, which facilitates active transport of calcium across the intestinal epithelial cells. Hence, it is advocated to feed a low-Ca diet at least 14 days before parturition to minimize the incidence of clinical hypocalcemia.

31.14.1 Level of Phosphorus

Dietary phosphorus levels greater than 0.5% kg dry matter have been linked to an increase in the prevalence of milk fever in cows. High dietary phosphorus causes hyperphosphatemia, which inhibits renal enzymes involved in catalyzing vitamin D_3 bioactivation. Calcium absorption in the intestine is reduced when levels of bioactive vitamin D_3 are low. Phosphorus-rich foods should be avoided.

31.14.2 Calcium to Phosphorus Ratio in Diet

The Ca:P ratio has little importance in ruminants, unlike in monogastric animals, provided that minimum nutritional demands of both minerals are met. The probable explanation for this difference from monogastric animals is that there is a high concentration of phosphorus in the saliva along with large volumes of saliva entering the rumen every day. This phosphorus content in the saliva will distort the Ca:P ratio in the ingested feed.

31.14.3 Dietary Cation/Anion Balance

Dietary cation/anion difference (DCAD) manipulation during the prepartum period has proven to be a more reliable method of controlling parturient paresis in cows (Constable et al. 2016). Diets rich in cations, such as potassium and sodium, are more likely to produce hypocalcemia through limiting calcium absorption. Milk fever can be reduced by feeding animals a diet high in anions like chloride and sulfur. The increasing cation concentration in the diet raises the plasma strong ion difference (SID), resulting in metabolic alkalosis. Increased concentrations of dietary anions, on the other hand, reduce plasma SID, resulting in metabolic acidosis (Blanc et al. 2014).

In the presence of mild metabolic acidosis, PTH-mediated bone resorption and PTH-dependent renal synthesis of 1,25 $(OH)_2$ D are increased (low DCAD). Hence, generating mild to moderate acidosis during late pregnancy with low DCAD will surely minimize the risk of postpartum hypocalcemia. Anionic salts are often obtained from chloride and sulfate salts of calcium, ammonium, and magnesium. Magnesium sulfate is the most often used anionic salt supplement. Ammonium chloride is also an excellent acidifier. This has been extensively researched in the field of cow nutrition but urther research is needed to see whether it is applicable to small ruminants.

31.14.4 Supplementation of Vitamin D_3 During Late Gestation

Stall-fed goats have limited access to sunlight, which increases the likelihood of vitamin D insufficiency. As a result, there is a need for vitamin D supplementation in the gestational stage of stall-fed animals.

31.14.4.1 Parenteral Vitamin D_3 Administration

The hydroxylation of vitamin D_3 into 25,hydroxycholecalciferol takes place at the liver. 25,Hydroxycholecalciferol is metabolized into 1,25 dihydroxycholecalciferol (calcitriol). This is the active form of vitamin D_3 with a hypercalcemic effect. 1-alpha-hydroxycholecalciferol is the analogue of 1,25 dihydroxycholecalciferol which is easy to prepare when compared to 1,25 $(OH)_2$ D_3 and is used pharmacologically. A parenteral dose of 1 million units per 45 kg body weight of vitamin D_3 given intramuscularly 2–8 days before parturition has given better results.

31.14.4.2 Oral Vitamin D_3 Administration

The oral administration of 20 million IU of vitamin D_2/day for five days to cows prior to five days of calving reduced the incidence of milk fever significantly. Similar research has not been undertaken in periparturient goats.

31.14.5 Supplementation of Calcium During Late Gestation

Calcium supplementation is required for goats kept in a large-scale production system. This is because cereal grains and hay are low in calcium.

31.14.5.1 Oral Calcium Administration

The oral administration of easily absorbable calcium salts such as calcium chloride or calcium propionate 12–24 hours before and 24 hours following parturition is a management strategy that will considerably boost plasma calcium concentrations. Calcium chloride is extremely soluble and causes an increase in plasma Ca concentration within 30 minutes; nevertheless, $CaCl_2$ is caustic and causes epithelial lesions of the mucosa of the oral, pharyngeal, esophageal, forestomach, or abomasum area.

31.14.5.2 Parenteral Calcium Administration

Calcium administration in the form of Ca gluconate or Ca borogluconate to animals around parturition may raise plasma Ca concentrations to supraphysiological levels, disrupting the endocrine circuits that regulate calcium homeostasis. As a result, parenteral calcium administration should be used only to address clinical hypocalcemia and not as a regular regimen for preventing goat milk fever.

References

Allen, W.M. and Sansom, B.F. (1986). Parturient paresis (milk fever) and hypocalcemia (cows, ewes, and goats). *Current Veterinary Therapy: Food Animal Practice* 2: 311–320.

Bayoumi, Y.H., Behairy, A., Abdallah, A.A., and Attia, N.E. (2021). Peri-parturient hypocalcemia in goats: clinical, hematobiochemical profiles and ultrasonographic measurements of postpartum uterine involution. *Veterinary World*, 2021 14 (3): 558–568.

Blanc, C.D., Van der List, M., Aly, S.S. et al. (2014). Blood calcium dynamics after prophylactic treatment of subclinical hypocalcemia with oral or intravenous calcium. *Journal of Dairy Science* 97 (11): 6901–6906.

Constable, P.D. (2014). *Proceedings of the XXVIII World Buiatrics Congress* (1 August 2014). Cairns, Australia: World Association for Buiatrics.

Constable, P.D., Hinchcliff, K.W., Done, S.H., and Grünberg, W. (2016). *Veterinary Medicine: A Textbook of the Diseases of Cattle, Horses, Sheep, Pigs and Goats*. St Louis, MO: Elsevier Health Sciences.

Goff, J.P. (2008). The monitoring, prevention, and treatment of milk fever and subclinical hypocalcemia in dairy cows. *Veterinary Journal* 176 (1): 50–57.

Guss, S.B. (1977). *Management and Diseases of Dairy Goats*. Arizona, USA: Dairy Goat Journal Publishing Corporation.

Huang, Y., Wen, J., Kong, Y. et al. (2021). Oxidative status in dairy goats: periparturient variation and changes in subclinical hyperketonemia and hypocalcemia. *BMC Veterinary Research* 17: 1–12.

Kessler, J. (1991). Mineral nutrition of goats. *Goat Nutrition* 46: 104–119.

Morand-Fehr, P. and Sauvant, D. (1978). Nutrition and optimum performance of dairy goats. *Livestock Production Science* 5 (2): 203–213.

National Research Council (1981). *Nutrient Requirements of Goats: Angora, Dairy, and Meat Goats in Temperate and Tropical Countries*, vol. 15. New York: National Academies Press.

Oetzel, G.K. (1988). Parturient paresis and hypocalcemia in ruminant livestock. *Veterinary Clinics of North America: Food Animal Practice* 4 (2): 351–364.

Pugh, D.G. and Baird, N.N. (2012). *Sheep & Goat Medicine-E-Book*. St Louis, MO: Elsevier Health Sciences.

Pugh, D.G., Baird, N.N., Edmondson, M., and Passler, T. (2020). *Sheep, Goat, and Cervid Medicine-E-Book*. St Louis, MO: Elsevier Health Sciences.

Quader, N., Islam, K.M.F., Jalal, S. et al. (2017). Investigation of clinical hypocalcemia in cattle and goats at the selected veterinary hospitals in Bangladesh and India. *Journal of Dairy Veterinary Animal Research* 5 (1): 33–36.

Radostits, O.M., Gay, C., Hinchcliff, K.W., and Constable, P.D. (ed.) (2006). *Veterinary Medicine: A Textbook of the Diseases of Cattle, Horses, Sheep, Pigs and Goats*. St Louis, MO: Elsevier Health Sciences.

Ramsey, F. (1945). Caprine acetonemia complicated with parturient paresis. *Iowa State University Veterinarian* 8 (1): 13.

Roche, J.R. (2003). The incidence and control of hypocalcemia in pasture-based systems. *Acta Veterinaria Scandinavica* 97 (suppl.): 141–144.

Smith, M.C. and Sherman, D.M. (2009). *Goat Medicine*. Hoboken, NJ: Wiley.

Section 5

Postpartum Disorders

32

Uterine and Rectal Prolapse

Prakash M. Chauhan[1], Ankit S. Prajapati[2], Rajesh Kumar[3], and Ravi D. Prajapati[4]

[1] Department of Clinics, College of Veterinary Science and Animal Husbandry, Kamdhenu University, Sardarkrushinagar, Gujarat, India
[2] Department of Veterinary Medicine, College of Veterinary Science and Animal Husbandry, Kamdhenu University, Sardarkrushinagar, India
[3] Department of Veterinary Gynaecology and Obstetrics, College of Veterinary Science and Animal Husbandry, Acharya Narendra Deva University of Agriculture and Technology, Ayodhya, India
[4] Department of Veterinary Gynaecology and Obstetrics, College of Veterinary Science and Animal Husbandry, Kamdhenu University, Sardarkrushinagar, India

32.1 Uterine Prolapse

Uterine prolapse is an eversion of the uterus, defined as part of the uterus extruding from its normal anatomical position through the vaginal orifice. Uterine prolapse is a common complication of the third stage of parturition in all domestic animals when the fetus has been expelled and the fetal cotyledons have separated from maternal caruncles (Roberts 1986; Bodner-Adler et al. 2007; Noakes et al. 2009; Wachida and Kisani 2011). Goats are susceptible to uterine prolapse (Kabir et al. 2010) but the occurrence is infrequent (Lucky et al. 2016), with an incidence of 19.9% among periparturient diseases (Majeed 1994). It is more frequently observed at first kidding in young goats suffering from dystocia and having triplets.

Prolapse of the uterus generally occurs immediately after or a few hours after kidding when the cervix is open and the uterus lacks tone (Hanie 2006; Gupta et al. 2018). It rarely occurs more than 24 hours after kidding due to partial closure of the cervix, but in rare cases, it may occur 48–72 hours after kidding (Roberts 1986; Fubini and Ducharme 2006). The prolapsed uterus is usually atonic and slowly expelled from the vulvar lips rather than forcefully expelled by straining. In goats, uterine prolapse may be complete with both the uterine horns protruding from the vulva (Figure 32.1) or occasionally limited to the uterine body (Figure 32.2). Immediately after prolapse, the tissues appear almost normal but become enlarged and edematous within a few hours.

This is an emergency condition that needs immediate treatment. Otherwise, interference with the blood supply may result in edema, cyanosis, and, later on, gangrene (Noakes et al. 2009; Kapadiya et al. 2015). Some animals will develop hypovolemic shock secondary to internal blood loss, prolapsed organ laceration, or abdominal viscera incarceration (Potter 2008).

32.1.1 Predisposing/Risk Factors

The exact etiology of uterine prolapse is unknown, but certain predisposing factors have been associated with uterine prolapse in goats (Jackson 2004; Hanie 2006). Uterine prolapse is made more likely by long mesometrial attachment, violent or intense tenesmus, atonic and flaccid uterus, retention of placenta, especially at the ovarian pole of the gravid uterus and weight of retained placenta, excessive traction at assisted parturition, endocrine imbalance, closed confinement, lack of exercise, inadequate secretion of prostaglandin F2-alpha and oxytocin, and by extreme relaxation of the pelvic and perineal region (Roberts 1971; McDowell 1992; Drost and Thomas 1996; Youngquist 1997; Gallentine and Cespedes 2001; Noakes et al. 2009). In dystocia, forced extraction will likely result in prolapse when the uterus is contracted tightly around a dry fetus.

Uterine prolapse may occur after kidding due to forced extraction of the kid, excessive traction on the fetal membrane, and severe relaxation in the perineum and vulvar lips (Noakes et al. 2001). Dystocia, hypocalcemia, and

Elements of Reproduction and Reproductive Diseases of Goats, First Edition. Edited by Tanmoy Rana.

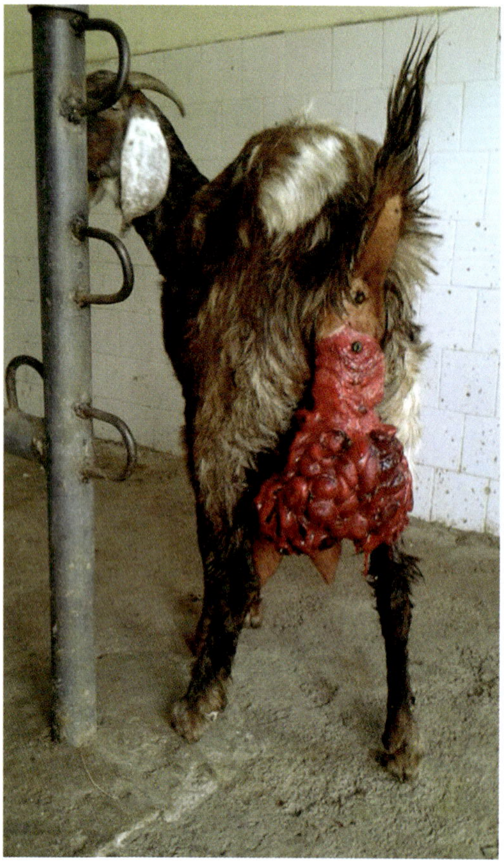

Figure 32.1 Complete uterine prolapse. *Source:* Courtesy of Prakash M. Chauhan (chapter author).

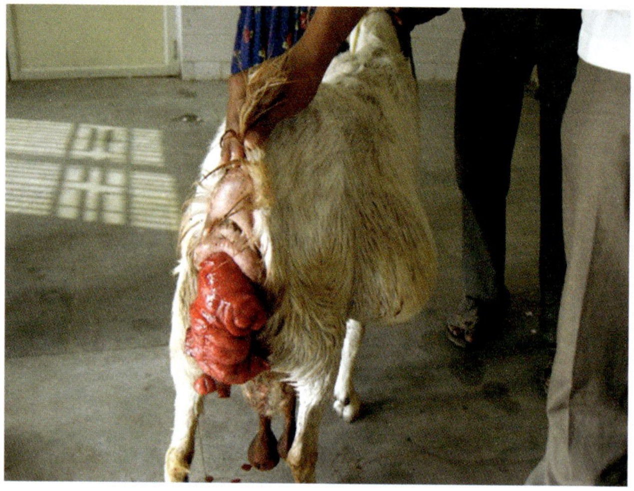

Figure 32.2 Incomplete uterine prolapse. *Source:* Courtesy of Prakash M. Chauhan (chapter author).

confinement without exercise during gestation can all increase the risk of this relatively uncommon problem (Engum and Lyngset 1970; Franklin 1986; Majeed and Taha 1991). High estrogenic content in the feed can act as a cause of uterine prolapse. Multiparous goats are more prone to uterine prolapse than uniparous goats (65% vs 35%) due to excessive relaxation of pelvic ligaments and weakness in the uterine musculature (Bhatti et al. 2006; Mosa and Faraj 2021). Goats with retained placental membranes may be predisposed to uterine prolapse by around 70%, and goats without retained placental membranes have a 30% chance of uterine prolapse (Mosa and Faraj 2021). Scarcity of nutrition and poor quality of feed can act as predisposing factors (Constable et al. 2016). Low serum calcium, phosphorus, and magnesium are also associated with uterine prolapse (Pandey et al. 2007). Significantly, hypocalcemia may contribute to the atony of genitalia, predisposing to uterine prolapse (Pandit et al. 1982). Nutritionally poor, thin, debilitated, aged goats are more prone to uterine prolapse.

Prolapse of the uterus is not hereditary, although occasionally it may be seen in the dam and daughter. However, the condition can reoccur at subsequent kidding in goats. Recently, the various risk factors of uterine prolapse in goats have been described by Mosa and Faraj (2021).

32.1.2 Symptoms and Clinical Observations

The symptoms of uterine prolapse are apparent. The uterine prolapse is visible as a large, pear-shaped mass protruding from the vulva and hanging down to the hock joint. The fundamental characteristic of uterine prolapse is that cotyledon and endometrium can be visible (Figure 32.3). The goat hunches her back and may try to urinate. The goat is usually exhausted and recumbent but may stand with the uterus hanging. Initially, the prolapsed mass is bright red in appearance. As time passes, uterine tissues become enlarged, edemated, cyanotic, and contaminated with dung, dirt, debris, and straw (Noakes et al. 2009; Chauhan et al. 2013). Later, the prolapsed mass may be injured, and lacerations and various bleeding points may be seen (Singh et al. 2018).

Both uterine horns (gravid and nongravid) are usually everted in goats. Sometimes, the nongravid horn does not evert completely and lies inside the peritoneal surface of the prolapsed gravid horn due to the strong intercornual ligament and is found as a slit or oval-shaped opening. If the gravid horn prolapses sufficiently, the cervix is presented at the vulva. The fetal membranes are likely to be attached to the everted uterine horns (Roberts 1986; Velladurai and Alagar 2017). Several researchers have recorded the clinical features of uterine prolapse in goats, which are tabulated in Table 32.1.

Prolapse of the intestine may occur through a rupture or laceration in the uterus, cervix, or cranial portion of the vagina at the time of parturition or during handling for uterine prolapse. Tooth grinding may be observed due to severe pain (Senthilkumar et al. 2017).

32.1.3 Prognosis

The prognosis in immediate cases is almost always favorable, and the goat recovers without complications. However, in delayed cases, the prognosis is unfavorable due to tearing of the mesovarium and severe internal bleeding causing hypovolemic shock. Further, the condition may be complicated with septic metritis and death may occur (Noakes et al. 2009). Prostration and shock make the prognosis poor to hopeless.

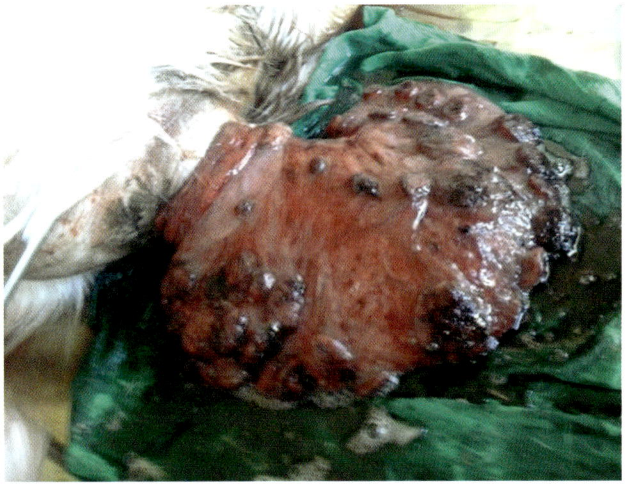

Figure 32.3 Uterine prolapse with visible cotyledon and endometrium. *Source:* Courtesy of Prakash M. Chauhan (chapter author).

32.1.4 Obstetrical Management and Treatment

Uterine prolapse is an emergency that needs prompt attention and immediate treatment; otherwise, it may lead to edema, ischemia, laceration, and severe internal hemorrhage (Noakes et al. 2009). The success of treatment depends on the type and duration of the case, the degree of damage, and the contamination. The main aim of treatment is to replace the prolapsed genitalia properly.

The goat should be secured before initiating treatment. Caudal epidural anesthesia is achieved by infiltrating 0.5–2 ml of 2% lignocaine solution into the lumbosacral, sacrococcygeal or intercoccygeal space to prevent straining during replacement (Chauhan et al. 2013; Katare and Sharma 2014; Senthilkumar et al. 2017; Singh et al. 2018). The most common site for epidural anesthesia in goats is the intersacrococcygeal space (Noakes et al. 2009). The everted uterus is carefully examined,

Table 32.1 Clinical features of uterine prolapse in goats.

Breed	No. of kids delivered	After kidding (h)	Placenta	Partial or complete	Retention suture	References
West African dwarf goat	–	72	Without	Complete	Horizontal mattress	Wachida and Kisani (2011)
Nondescript	–	3	With	Complete eversion	Rope truss	Katare and Sharma (2014)
Nondescript	Single	14	Detached from a prolapsed uterus	Complete	Horizontal mattress	Singh et al. (2016)
Nondescript	Single	24	Tightly adhered to the uterus	–	No retention suture	Senthilkumar et al. (2017)
Nondescript	Single	7	Attached	Total	Vulval retention suture	Velladurai and Alagar (2017)
Nondescript	–	>24	Without	Complete	Horizontal mattress	Kumar et al. 2017
Korean black goat	–	Within 1–2	–	–		Oh and Shin (2017)
Nondescript	Twin	18	–	–	Buhner suture	Hanumantha Raju et al. (2018)
Nondescript	Twin	48	–	–	Buhner suture	Singh et al. (2018)
Nondescript	Twin	3	Without	Complete	No vulval suture	Gupta et al. (2018)
Nondescript	Twin	24	Without	Complete	Horizontal mattress	Singh et al. (2020)
Nondescript	Twin	5	Attached	Complete	No suture	Pasha et al. (2021)

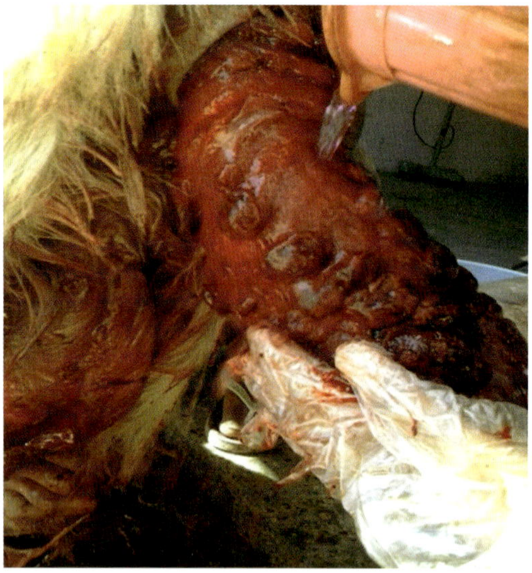

Figure 32.4 Antiseptic washing of prolapsed uterus. *Source:* Courtesy of Prakash M. Chauhan (chapter author).

and gross debris and contaminations are gently removed using a mild antiseptic solution, either 1% potassium permanganate (1:1000) or a povidone-iodine solution (Figure 32.4), followed by flushing with metronidazole solution (Singh et al. 2011; Oh and Shin 2017). The fecal-contaminated prolapsed uterus may increase the risk of toxemia, and vigorous attempts to remove external contaminants also increase toxin uptake (Scott and Gessert 1998). If it is attached, the placenta should be separated manually from the maternal caruncle. If the placenta is firmly attached, then it should left as such. The mass should be gently washed with a mild potassium permanganate solution to clear debris and blood clots. If the uterus becomes hard in consistency, ice packs are applied for 20–30 minutes to soften it.

The "triple R" concepts – reduction, replacement, and retention – are used to correct uterine prolapse (Roberts 1971). To reduce the size of the mass, it should be lifted to the level of the ischial arch, and urine should be removed from the urinary bladder either by catheterizing with an artificial insemination sheath or pressing the prolapsed part (Singh et al. 2016), followed by the application of an ice pack to reduce the edema. Uterine edema can be reduced by pressing the genitalia with the palm, and the prolapsed uterus can be covered with sugar. Pop-in spray can be applied to the prolapsed genitalia, reducing the mass to a reasonable size within 10 minutes. A 200 g paste of *Mimosa pudica* leaves can be used on the prolapsed uterus to exert its tocolytic effect (Hanumantha Raju et al. 2018).

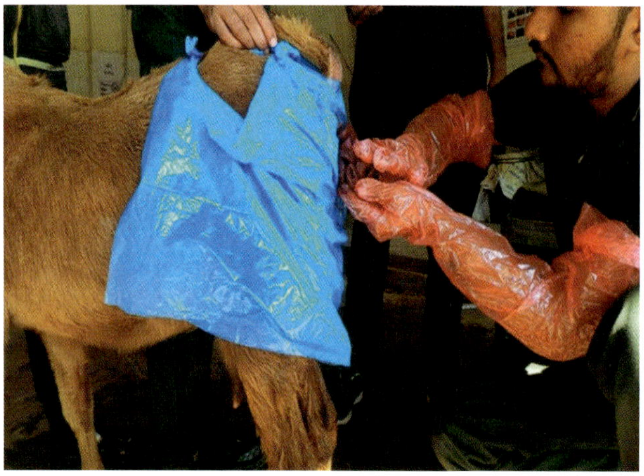

Figure 32.5 Repositioning of prolapsed uterine mass. *Source:* Courtesy of Prakash M. Chauhan (chapter author).

The prolapsed mass should be gently cleaned with mild antiseptic solutions and well lubricated with lignocaine jelly and liquid paraffin, or 2% sodium carboxy methyl cellulose or Soframycin® ointment, before its replacement in the abdominal cavity. The replacement procedure can be aided by raising the goat's hindquarters off the ground, which leads to correct intraabdominal positioning of the prolapsed uterus. The body of the uterus near the vulva is first pushed forward with the palms of both hands, alternatively from each side, followed by the horns (Figure 32.5) (Chauhan et al. 2013). Using the fingers, the uterus and uterine horns are placed in their normal anatomical position, starting from the tips of the prolapsed uterus after proper lubrication using obstetrical gel (Chauhan et al. 2013; Velladurai and Alagar 2017).

Once the uterus is replaced, the hand should be inserted up to the tip of the uterine horn to invaginate the remaining part of both uterine horns (Fubini and Ducharme 2006). The prolapse is unlikely to reoccur if the uterine horns are entirely and correctly replaced (Hanie 2006). The complete replacement of the uterus up to the tips can be achieved by passively infusing warm fluid into the uterus to reduce the inverted uterine horns. A small pessary or a blunt round object can be inserted into the vagina to avoid reprolapse (Katare and Sharma 2014), which may induce straining. Uterine or cervical laceration should be sutured using a simple interrupted suture with chromic catgut no. 2.

After adequately replacing the prolapsed uterus, a retention suture should be applied to hold the uterus in place, but this depends on the straining tendency. Many techniques have been described for retention of the prolapsed mass, including Buhner's suture, horizontal or cross mattress suture, boot lace suture, paravaginal stents, Caslik's suture, and rope slings. All these techniques are used to maintain the position of the genitalia within the vaginal vault. Suture techniques in goats are at high risk of tearing through perineal tissue. Buhner sutures should be placed using a Buhner needle inserted via a 1 cm incision made approximately at the level of the ischium (4 cm width proximal to the ventral commissure of the vulva) and exiting a 1 cm incision made on the midline of the perineum (4 cm dorsal to the dorsal commissure of the vulva).

Then, 6.4 mm width umbilical tape is inserted in the eye part of the needle, and the suture is pulled back through as the needle is withdrawn. The same procedure is repeated on the contralateral side, and the knot is tied as needed. Hanumantha Raju et al. (2018) modified the Buhner suture for easy postoperative care by adjusting the dorsally and ventrally knots when the suture area is severely inflamed. Horizontal mattress sutures using nylon (no. 0) can be placed in the vulva alone (Wachida and Kisani 2011) or by placing 6 to 12 mm diameter rubber stents parallel to the vulva to prevent a vulval tear.

Immediately after repositioning, the goat is stabilized by infusing dextrose normal saline solution intravenously. Broad-spectrum antibiotics and analgesics should be given intramuscularly for at least 3–5 days to prevent secondary bacterial infection and pain (Hosie 1993; Plunkett 2000; Borobia 2006). IM injection of dexamethasone can be administered to control shock. Most goats suffering from uterine prolapse are hypocalcemic (Fubini and Ducharme 2006; Mosa and Faraj 2021)so calcium borogluconate should be administered in recommended doses; 10–20 IU of oxytocin is also given IM (Wachida and Kisani 2011; Hanumantha Raju et al. 2018) to hasten uterine involution. The vulval retention suture should be removed within 3–7 days.

The amputation of part or all of the uterus is occasionally indicated in some cases of uterine prolapse in which the uterus has severe necrosis or circumferential lacerations (Arthure and Savage 1957).

32.1.5 Complications

A goat with uterine prolapse treated promptly recovers without any complications. However, a delay in treatment could result in the death of an animal within a few hours due to severe internal hemorrhage caused by the weight of the uterus leading to tears in the mesovarium (Noakes et al. 2009). The common complications of uterine prolapse include hemorrhage, shock, septic metritis, suckling problems, infertility, and death. Prolapse of the intestine may occur through a rupture or laceration in the uterus or cranial portion of the vagina during handling. Protrusion of the involuted uterus may occur through vaginal tears during the handling of goats after a few hours to days (Figure 32.6). However, if appropriately managed, goats can conceive again without a problem.

32.2 Rectal Prolapse

Rectal prolapse is defined as one or more layers of the rectum protruding outside the anus due to persistent tenesmus associated with intestinal, anorectal, or urogenital diseases. It can occur in all domestic animals (Anderson and Miesner 2008) but is rare in goats (John 2016), and less common in goats compared to sheep. It is neither as serious nor as extensive in goats compared to mares. Goats of any breed, age, or sex may be involved. The protruded rectal mass is sausage-shaped.

Rectal prolapse may occur with prepartum cervicovaginal prolapse in goats due to severe tenesmus and expulsive straining (Collins and Gary 1989; Anya et al. 2016; Raja et al. 2020). Slight eversion of the rectum at the time of parturition is common but severe prolapse is rare. Rectal prolapse associated with cervicovaginal prolapse in twin pregnant WAD goats has been reported (Anya et al. 2016). Viable triplet kids have also been delivered normally following the replacement of rectal prolapse without recurrence (Kumar et al. 2020). Eviscerated intestines and mesentery through the torn rectal wall can be successfully managed surgically (Chacko et al. 2015).

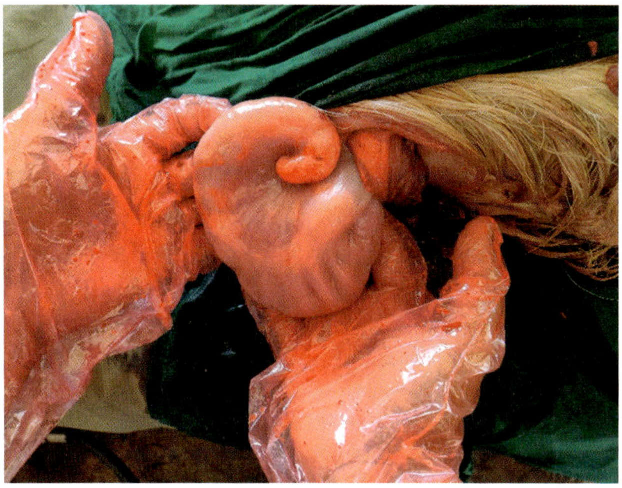

Figure 32.6 Uterine prolapse through vaginal tear exposing the serosal layer. *Source:* Courtesy of Prakash M. Chauhan (chapter author).

32.2.1 Classification

Rectal prolapse may be categorized as incomplete, in which only the rectal mucosa is everted, or complete, in which all the layers are protruded (Chakrabarti 2004). Further, rectal prolapse may be classified as class I to IV based on

Table 32.2 Classification of rectal prolapse by tissue layer.

Classification	Description	Frequency
I	Prolapse of rectal mucosa only. These are small and usually intermittent	Common
II	Complete prolapse of all layers of rectal tissue (mucosa to the serosa). Length is variable and occurrence can be intermittent	Common
III	Type II prolapse with the addition of prolapse of the colon (intussusception of the colon into the rectum). These prolapses are longer and more painful, and clinical signs progress rapidly	Uncommon
IV	Type III prolapse except that the anal sphincter is intact, causing constrictions of the rectum and colon (intussusception of rectum and colon through the anus)	Rare

Table 32.3 Classification of rectal prolapse by severity.

Classification	Description	Frequency
I	Tear of mucosa and submucosa only	Common
II	Disruption of muscular layers with mucosa and submucosa intact (causes diverticulum formation)	Uncommon
III	Tear through mucosa, submucosa, and muscular layer. Serosa remains intact	Uncommon
	a) Tear in any location other than the dorsal midline	–
	b) Tear in dorsal midline at the attachment of mesorectum	–
IV	Tear through the mucosa, submucosa, muscular layer, and serosa	Rare

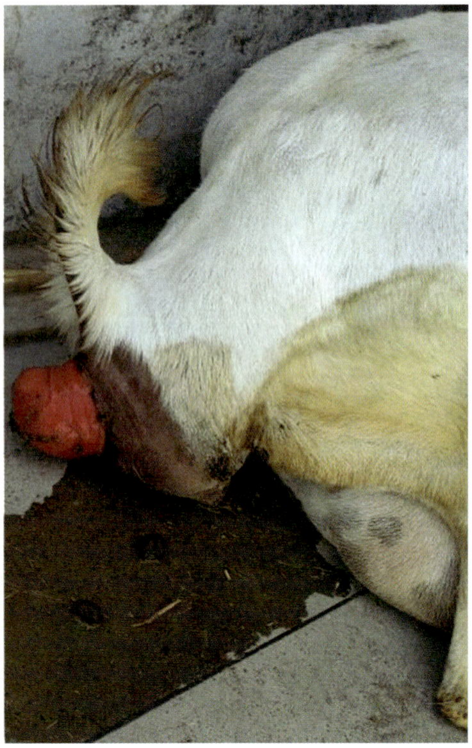

Figure 32.7 Class II rectal prolapse in goat. *Source:* Courtesy of Prakash M. Chauhan (chapter author).

involvement of the tissue layer (Table 32.2) and severity (Table 32.3), as per Haskell (2004) and Anderson and Miesner (2008). Class II prolapses are the most common prolapses presented to veterinarians for correction (Figure 32.7) (Kumar et al. 2020).

32.2.2 Causative and Predisposing Risk Factors

Rectal prolapse is a complicated problem with many causative factors, such as sex, age, diet, condition, tail docking length, coughing, chronic diarrhea, and as a result of severe tenesmus. Prolapse of the rectum occurs following straining, which may be associated with tenesmus; with coccidiosis, colitis, dysuria, and other conditions; as a complication of cystitis, urolithiasis, dystocia, neoplasia, and other conditions; neuropathy, chronic constipation coughing or genetics (Haskell 2004; Steiner 2004; Arulkumar et al. 2022). Perineal hernia or other interruption of normal innervations of the external anal sphincter may cause prolapse.

Rectal prolapse may be predisposed by conditions that increase intrapelvic pressure or abdominal straining, such as persistent riding behavior, coughing, coccidiosis, and chronic diarrhea (Radostits et al. 2009). It can be a sequel to lesions of the pelvic musculature or anal sphincter (Amand 1974). Persistent and severe tenesmus can also cause rectal prolapse (Collins and Gary 1989). Cervicovaginal or vaginal prolapse in females and urinary tract obstruction (urolithiasis) in males may predispose to rectal prolapse (Roberts 1986). Multiple fetuses *in utero* and concurrent hypocalcemia in advanced pregnant goats can also lead to rectal prolapse (Anya et al. 2016; Kumar et al. 2020). Rectal prolapse can occur following the strained delivery of a kid (Chacko et al. 2015). Any partial or intermittent prolapse may lead to rectal mucosal injury and irritation, more straining, and eventually complete prolapse (Arthur et al. 1996; Kumar et al. 2020). A high estrogenic feed also predisposes to rectal prolapse (Tyagi and Singh 2002). Moreover, hereditary predisposition is also reported.

32.2.3 Symptoms and Clinical Observations

Rectal prolapse is very easy to recognize by its clinical features. The symptoms of rectal prolapse vary according to severity and the anatomical involvement of rectal layers (Anderson and Miesner 2008).

The exposed tissue of the rectum is usually short, elongated, cylindrical, nonulcerated, inflamed, and bright to cherry red initially. Later, the mucosal surface is darkened, dried, and hardened, and cracks on the protruded part cause more irritation and straining. Finally, it may be marked by necrosis (Fubini and Ducharme 2006; Gallagher 2020; Kumar et al. 2020; Arulkumar et al. 2022). Other common signs include ulcerations, inflammation, and congestion of the rectal mucosa. The intestines and mesentery can be eviscerated through a 270° tear on the prolapsed rectum (Chacko et al. 2015).

Rectal prolapse must be differentiated from ileocolic intussusception by inserting a probe, blunt object, or finger between the prolapsed mass and the inner rectal wall. The above items cannot be inserted in rectal prolapse because of the fornix.

If untreated, rectal prolapse can become life-threatening, and animals may die cruelly due to prolapse of the entire intestinal tract, leading to shock.

32.2.4 Treatment

Rectal prolapse management includes immediate resolution of the prolapse, often requiring one of the following treatments: (i) replacement of prolapse and placement of purse-string suture; (ii) amputation using prolapse ring; (iii) submucosal resection; or (iv) resection and anastomosis (Freeman 2012; Anderson and Miesner 2008; Hartnack and Jones 2017).

The treatment of rectal prolapse comprises nonsurgical and surgical means, including replacement, retention, and amputation (Oconnor 2005). Treatment method selection depends on the type of rectal prolapse and the severity of damage to the exposed tissue. Class I and II prolapses are generally managed nonsurgically. In contrast, recurrent and refractory Class II and all Class III and IV prolapses require either rectum resection or amputation (Kumar et al. 2020). In very mild, early Class I cases, frequent topical application of hemorrhoidal ointment and replacement of the everted tissue may be successful and preclude using a purse-string suture. Another quick and inexpensive treatment option for mild cases is the injection of counterirritants (e.g., Lugol's iodine) in the retroperitoneal, perirectal space, either alone or in conjunction with a purse-string suture (Parish 1979).

Replacement and purse-string suture (nonsurgical correction) is indicated for mild rectal prolapses Class I and II. Caudal epidural anesthesia can be achieved by using 0.5–2 ml of 2% lignocaine or 0.5 ml/45 kg body weight of 2% lignoocaine in the sacrococcygeal space to minimize pain and straining. Combining xylazine (0.01–0.03 mg/kg) with 2% lignocaine may provide more extensive analgesia and reduced straining than that obtained by lignocaine anesthesia alone. The hair in the perineum region is closely clipped.

The prolapsed part is thoroughly washed with clean water, a mild antiseptic solution, and a warm hypertonic solution of 50% dextrose to reduce the edema. Elevation of the hindquarters of the goat can also facilitate prolapse reduction. The prolapsed part of the rectum is adequately replaced into the anus after proper washing and lubricating with liquid paraffin oil or petroleum jelly. The prolapsed mass can be retained by applying a rope truss (Figure 32.8) or purse-string suture using heavy nylon material or silk (2/0) around the anus (Borobia 2006; Kumar et al. 2020; Arulkumar et al. 2022). To minimize fecal contamination, the bow-knot should be dorsal or lateral to the anus. The purse-string suture is tightened sufficiently to prevent reprolapse but allow easy passage of feces. The purse-string suture ideally should be removed within a week of placement to minimize suture tract infection.

Recently, a prolapse retention device has been suggested to allow a rectal prolapse to be retained *in situ* (Figure 32.9) (Anya et al. 2016). This device comprises a 10 or 20 ml sterile plastic syringe with the plunger removed . The needle end of the syringe is cut to ensure a wider diameter to allow loose feces through it. The cut end must be smoothed to prevent trauma and irritation to the rectal mucosa, and two holes must be made at the other free end of the syringe to place into the rectum with two stay sutures at the ano-cutaneous junction. The prolapse retainer is removed after a week. If the intestines or mesentery have protruded through the rectal tear, this could be managed by replacing the viscera followed by suturing the torn edges from the luminal side to the serosal side using a simple continuous pattern (Chacko et al. 2015).

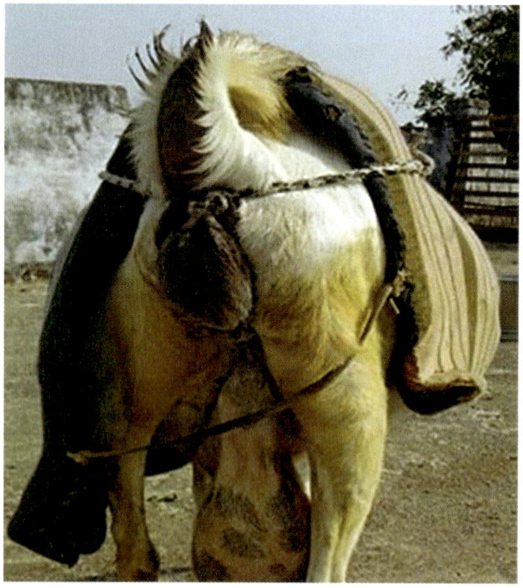

Figure 32.8 Goat with applied truss. *Source:* Courtesy of Prakash M. Chauhan (chapter author).

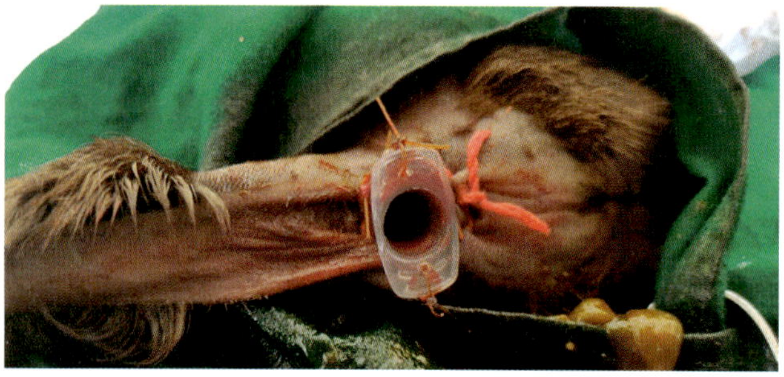

Figure 32.9 Improvised retainer suture. *Source:* Courtesy of Prakash M. Chauhan (chapter author).

The goat is given fluids, analgesic, and calcium therapy for 3–5 days and are fed with mineral oil or mild laxative daily to keep the feces soft. Broad-spectrum antibiotics, analgesics, and antihistamines are infused at appropriate doses for 3–5 days to avoid postoperative complications.

Rectal amputation using a prolapse ring is often used in field conditions where a surgical procedure is impossible economically or logistically. Placement of a prolapse ring is also considered a salvage procedure. The prolapse ring is inserted into the rectum and the elastrator band or ligature is placed. The elastrator band and ligature serve as vascular compromisers, leading to necrosis of the rectal part, which is sloughed off. So, healing may be started by forming fibrotic bands anterior to the elastrator or ligature, and mucosa grows across the area. In this technique, complications may occur, including premature dislodgment of the prolapse ring, rectal stricture, peritonitis, and abscess formation (Anderson and Miesner 2008).

Submucosal resection is indicated in rectal prolapse with a necrotic or traumatized mucosa with healthy underlying tissue. The advantages of this technique over full-thickness resection (amputation) and anastomosis are faster healing time, less postoperative straining, minimum constriction of luminal diameter, salvage of healthy tissue, maintenance of blood supply, nonexposure of the serosa, and reduced chances of peritonitis and perirectal abscess formation. However, submucosal resection requires more surgical time. The perineum and prolapsed tissue are prepared surgically. Epidural anesthesia can be achieved as described earlier. An appropriate size flexible tube is inserted into the lumen and fixed by two spinal needles (18 gauge, 15 cm long) or similar sized stylets at 90° to each other in crosspinning fashion. The needles are placed through the external anal sphincter and approximately 2–4 mm cranial to the healthy prolapsed tissue. Two complete circumferential incisions are created through the mucosa on either side of healthy tissue to be removed. A longitudinal incision is put at the same tissue depth to connect earlier circumferential incisions. Dissection of necrotic mucosa and submucosa is performed by elevating a strip of tissue to be removed and leaving a deep layer of healthy tissue. Bleeding is controlled by ligating individual vessels. The mucosa is apposed with four simple interrupted sutures around the circumference of the prolapse to prevent twisting of the closure. The four quadrants are then apposed separately in a simple continuous suture pattern using 2-0 to 3-0 monofilament absorbable suture material. The spinal needles are removed and the tissue is replaced in the rectum (Anderson and Miesner 2008). A retention suture is placed as described earlier to prevent prolapse of the surgical site. Postoperative management is also carried out, as described earlier, to control pain, inflammation, and secondary bacterial infections.

Resection and anastomosis are adopted in Class III and IV rectal prolapse, in which the prolapsed tissue is devitalized and cannot be reduced and replaced. The surgical preparation and procedure can be performed as for submucosal resection, including the fixation of pins for stabilizing tissue during dissection. Full-thickness circumferential incisions are made in the inner and outer walls of healthy tissue with removal of necrotic tissue along with serosa instead of only the submucosa dissection in the submucosal resection technique. Alternatively, a stairstep amputation can be performed to maximize the length of the inner mucosal and submucosal layers, which facilitates easier adaptation of mucosal apposition of the respective segments (Ducharme et al. 2017). Mesenteric blood loss is minimized by ligating the blood vessels of prolapsed tissue during resection. The proximal and distal edges of the resected prolapse tissue are apposed by interrupted horizontal mattress sutures circumferentially, including full-thickness monofilament absorbable suture material. The mucosal edges are aligned with a simple continuous suture pattern using a 2-0 monofilament absorbable suture, divided into interrupted quadrants (Hartnack and Jones 2017). The crosspins are removed and a routine purse-string suture is applied.

Postoperative care is similar to that described for other techniques. Antibiotic coverage should be extended up to 7–10 days. The goats are closely monitored for postoperative complications such as peritonitis, sepsis, mucosal stricture formation, site dehiscence, intestinal evisceration, adhesion formation, and abscessation of the perirectal tissues.

32.2.5 Prevention

Predisposing factors should be taken care of to prevent the incidence of rectal prolapse. Diarrhea, pneumonia, coccidiosis, urinary calculi, etc. should be treated as early as possible. Proper care should be given to advanced pregnant goats suffering from cervicovaginal prolapse. Adequate nutrition should be provided along with hygiene maintenance.

References

Amand, W.B. (1974). Nonneurogenic disorders of the anus and rectum. *Veterinary Clinics of North America* 4 (3): 535–550.

Anderson, D.E. and Miesner, M.D. (2008). Rectal prolapse. *Veterinary Clinics of North America: Food Animal Practice* 24 (2): 403.

Anya, K.O., Nnaji, T.O., and Udegbunam, S.O. (2016). Cervico-vaginal prolapse in two West African Dwarf (WAD) goats in Nsukka, Nigeria: a case report. *Nigerian Veterinary Journal* 27 (3): 105–108.

Arthur, G.H., Noakes, D.E., Peterson, H., and Parkinson, T.J. (1996). *Veterinary Reproduction and Obstetrics*, 7e. London: WB Saunders.

Arthure, H.G. and Savage, D. (1957). Uterine prolapse and prolapse of the vaginal vault treated by sacral hysteropexy. *Journal of Obstetrics and Gynaecology of the British Empire* 64 (3): 355–360.

Arulkumar, S., Arunkumar, R., Ragulraj, S., and Priyadharsini, R. (2022). Correction and management of rectal prolapse in indigenous goat: a case report. *Pharma Innovation Journal* 11 (8): 698–699.

Bhatti, M.S., Ahmed, I., Ahmad, N. et al. (2006). Epidemiological survey of genital prolapse in buffaloes kept under different systems and serum micro-mineral contents. *Pakistan Veterinary Journal* 26 (4): 197–200.

Bodner-Adler, B., Shrivastava, C., and Bodner, K. (2007). Risk factors for uterine prolapse in Nepal. *International Urogynecology Journal and Pelvic Floor Dysfunction* 18 (11): 1343–1346.

Borobia, B.J. (2006). Replacement of rectal prolapse in sows. *Veterinary Record* 158 (11): 380.

Chacko, L., Shuhaib, P., and Sooryadas, S. (2015). Prolapse and 270° tear of rectum with bowel evisceration in a goat. *International Journal of Advanced Research* 3 (8): 807–809.

Chakrabarti, A. (2004). *Text Book of Clinical Veterinary Medicine*, 233. New Delhi: Kalyani Publishers.

Chauhan, P.M., Sutaria, T.V., Maheswari, V.K., and Sharma, V.K. (2013). Post-parturient complete uterine eversion in a Surti goat: a case report. *Ruminant Science* 2 (2): 223–224.

Collins, F.B. and Gary, V.E. (1989). Recto-anal diseases. In: *Textbook of Veterinary Internal Medicine*, 3e (ed. S. Ettinger), 1563. Philadelphia, PA: W.B. Saunders.

Constable, P.D., Hinchcliff, K.W., Done, S.H., and Gruenberg, W. (2016). *Veterinary Medicine: A Textbook of the Diseases of Cattle, Horses, Sheep, Pigs and Goats*. Oxford: Elsevier Health Sciences.

Drost, M. and Thomas, P.G.A. (1996). Female reproductive disorders. In: *Large Animal Internal Medicine*, 2e (ed. B.P. (e.) Smith), 1519–1565. St Louis, MO: Mosby.

Ducharme, N.G., Desrochers, A., and Fubini, S.L. (2017). Surgery of the bovine digestive system. In: *Farm Animal Surgery*, 2e (ed. S.L. Fubini and N.G. Ducharme), 223–343. Philadelphia, PA: Elsevier.

Engum, J. and Lyngset, O. (1970). Gynaecology and obstetrics in the goat. *Iowa State University Journal* 120: 120–124.

Franklin, J.S. (1986). Dystocia and obstetrics in goats. In: *Current Therapy in Theriogenology*, 2e (ed. D.A. Morrow), 590–592. Philadelphia, PA: W.B. Saunders.

Freeman, D.E. (2012). *Equine Surgery*, 4e, 494–505. Philadelphia, PA: W.B. Saunders.

Fubini, S.L. and Ducharme, G.N. (2006). *Farm Animal Surgery*. St Louis, MO: Elsevier.

Gallagher, A. (2020). *Rectal Prolapse in Animals*. Department of Small Animal Clinical Sciences, College of Veterinary Medicine, University of Florida.

Gallentine, M.L. and Cespedes, R.D. (2001). Occult stress urinary incontinence and the effect of vaginal vault prolapse on abdominal leak point pressures. *Urology* 57 (1): 40–44.

Gupta, S., Sharma, A., and Singh, M. (2018). Post-partum uterine eversion and its management in a doe: a case report. *Dairy and Veterinary Science Journal* 8 (2): 555731.

Hanie, E.A. (2006). *Large Animal Clinical Procedures for Veterinary Technicians*. St Louis, MO: Elsevier.

Hanumantha Raju, N.S., Naresh, M., Tajunnisa, M., and Mayakkannan, T. (2018). Reduction and reposition of uterine prolapse by using *Mimosa pudica* leaves paste in non-descriptive goat. *Journal of Entomology and Zoology Studies* 6 (6): 573–575.

Hartnack, A. and Jones, M. (2017). Surgery of the sheep and goat digestive system. In: *Farm Animal Surgery*, 2e (ed. S.L. Fubini and N.G. Ducharme), 561–567. Philadelphia, PA: Saunders.

Haskell, S.R. (2004). Surgery of the sheep and goat digestive system. In: *Farm Animal Surgery*, 2e (ed. S.L. Fubini and N.G. Ducharme), 521–526. Philadelphia, PA: Saunders.

Hosie, B. (1993). Treatment of vaginal prolapse in ewes. *Practice* 15: 10–11.

Jackson, P.G.G. (2004). *Hand Book of Veterinary Obstetrics*, 2e. Oxford, UK: Elsevier Saunders.

John, M. (2016). *Diseases of the Goat*, 4e, 116. Oxford, UK: Wiley Blackwell.

Kabir, M.H., Reza, M.A., Razi, K.M. et al. (2010). A report on clinical prevalence of diseases and disorders in cattle and goat at the Upazilla Veterinary Hospital, Ulipur, Kurigram. *International Journal of Biological Research* 2 (11): 17–23.

Kapadiya, P.S., Chauhan, P.M., Nakhashi, H.C. et al. (2015). Recurrent post-partum uterine prolapse in a primiparous Mehsana buffalo – a case report. *Journal of Livestock Science* 6: 109–112.

Katare, B. and Sharma, R. (2014). Management of uterine prolapse in goat – a case report. *International Journal of Livestock Research* 4 (8): 27–29.

Kumar, K., Shukla, S.N., Inwati, P., and Bisen, A. (2017). Uterine prolapse in a doe goat: a case report. *Indian Journal of Applied Research* 7 (8): 503–504.

Kumar, R., Diwakar, R.P., Ramakant et al. (2020). A rare case of antepartum rectal prolapse in a goat and its management: a case report. *Journal of Entomology and Zoology Studies* 8 (2): 1285–1287.

Lucky, N.S., Hossain, M.K., Roy, A.C. et al. (2016). A longitudinal study on clinical diseases and disorders of cattle and goats in Sylhet, Bangladesh. *Journal of Advanced Veterinary and Animal Research* 3 (1): 24–37.

Majeed, A.F. (1994). Obstetrical problems and their management in Iraqi goats. *Small Ruminant Research* 13: 73–78.

Majeed, A.F. and Taha, M.B. (1991). Ringwomb in relation to serum calcium, inorganic phosphorus and magnesium in Iraqi goats. *Mesopotamia Journal of Agriculture* 23: 65–58.

McDowell, L.R. (1992). *Minerals in Animal and Human Nutrition*. London: Academic Press.

Mosa, F.A. and Faraj, A.A. (2021). Most common risk factors of uterine prolapse in local goat breeds. *Biochemical Cellular Archives* 21: 1987–1990.

Noakes, D.E., Parkinson, T.J., and England, G.C.W. (2001). *Arthur's Veterinary Reproduction and Obstetrics*, 8. London: Saunders.

Noakes, D.E., Parkinson, T.J., and England, G.C.W. (2009). *Veterinary Reproduction and Obstetrics*, 9e. London: Harcourt Publishers.

Oconnor, J.J. (2005). *Dollar's Veterinary Surgery*, 4e, 699–707. New Delhi: CBS Publisher & Distributors Pvt. Ltd.

Oh, A. and Shin, S.T. (2017). Uterine prolapse in Korean black goat. *Journal of Veterinary Clinics* 34 (4): 307–309.

Pandey, A.K., Shukla, S.P., and Nema, S.P. (2007). Certain haematobiochemical alterations during post-partum uterine prolapse in buffaloes (*Bubalus bubalis*). *Buffalo Bull* 26 (1): 20–22.

Pandit, R.K., Gupta, S.K., and Pattabirman, S.R. (1982). A clinical study of vagina and uterus in buffaloes. *Indian Veterinary Journal* 59: 975–980.

Parish, S.M. (1979). A method for nonsurgical correction of rectal prolapse in lambs. *Veterinary Medicine Small Animal Clinician* 74: 871–872.

Pasha, M.M., Venkanagouda, D., Bijurkar, R.G., and Malashri, G. (2021). Successful management of uterine prolapse in a non-descriptive goat: a case report. *Pharma Innovation Journal* 10 (12): 93–94.

Plunkett, S.J. (2000). *Emergency Procedure for the Small Animal Veterinarian*. Oxford, UK: Elsevier Health Sciences.

Potter, T. (2008). Prolapse of the uterus in the cow, UK. *Veterinary Journal* 13: 1–3.

Radostits, O.M., Gay, C.C., Hinchcliff, K.W., and Constable, P.D. (2009). *Veterinary Medicine: A Textbook of the Diseases of Cattle, Horses, Sheep, Pigs and Goats*, 10e, 279. St Louis, MO: W.B. Saunders.

Raja, S., Jayaganthan, P., Prabaharan, V., and Satheshkumar, S. (2020). Concurrent occurrence of vagino-cervical and rectal prolapse in a doe and its successful management. *Journal of Food and Animal Sciences* 1 (2): 136–139.

Roberts, S.J. (1971). *Veterinary Obstetrics and Genital Diseases*, 2e. New Delhi: CBS Publisher & Distributors Pvt. Ltd.

Roberts, S.J. (e.) (1986). *Veterinary Obstetrics and Genital Diseases*, 3e. Woodstock, VT: David & Charles.

Scott, P. and Gessert, M. (1998). Management of ovine vaginal prolapse. *Practice* 20: 28–34.

Senthilkumar, A., Balamurugan, P., Sribalaji, N. et al. (2017). Post-partum total uterine prolapse in a goat. *International Journal of Environment and Technology* 6: 770–773.

Singh, G., Pandey, A.K., Kumar, R., and Kumar, S. (2011). Post-parturient uterine prolapse in a goat – a case report. *Veterinary Practitioner* 12 (2): 192–193.

Singh, G., Pandey, J., Kavita, A.K. et al. (2016). Clinical management of post partum uterine prolapse in doe: a case report. *Haryana Veterinarian* 55 (1): 114–115.

Singh, K.P., Singh, B., Singh, R.V. et al. (2018). Management of post-partum uterine prolapse in a goat with vulval lip suture technique. *Indian Journal of Animal Health* 57 (2): 225–228.

Singh, B., Singh, K.P., Kumar, R. et al. (2020). Postpartum uterine prolapse in a goat and its successful management. *Indian Journal of Veterinary Science and Biotechnology* 16 (1): 73–74.

Steiner, A. (2004). Surgery of the colon. In: *Farm Animal Surgery* (ed. S.L. Fubini and N.G.(e. Ducharme), 257–262. Philadelphia, PA: Saunders.

Tyagi, R.P.S. and Singh, J. (2002). *A Text Book of Ruminant Surgery*, 1e. New Delhi: CBS Publishers.

Velladurai, C. and Alagar, S. (2017). Successful clinical management of total uterine prolapse in a non descriptive goat – a case report. *Asian Journal of Science and Technology* 8 (11): 6455–6456.

Wachida, N. and Kisani, A.I. (2011). Uterine prolapse in a doe goat: a case report. *International Journal of Animal and Veterinary Advances* 3: 135–137.

Youngquist, R.S. (1997). *Current Therapy in Large Animal Theriogenology*. Philadelphia, PA: WB Saunders, pp 429–444. .

33

Retained Placenta and Fetal Membranes

Jeetendra S. Rajoriya[1], Rajesh Kumar[2], Abhiyuday P. Singh[1], and Prakash M. Chauhan[3]

[1] Department of Veterinary Gynaecology and Obstetrics, College of Veterinary Science and Animal Husbandry, Jabalpur, India
[2] Department of Veterinary Gynaecology and Obstetrics, College of Veterinary Science and Animal Husbandry, Acharya Narendra Deva University of Agriculture and Technology, Ayodhya, India
[3] Department of Clinics, College of Veterinary Science and Animal Husbandry, Kamdhenu University, Sardarkrushinagar, India

33.1 Introduction

The third stage of kidding consists of expulsion of the placenta after birth. Failure of expulsion leads to retention of fetal membranes (RFM). RFM is one of the major periparturient complications in dairy goats which causes considerable economic losses in the herd due to decreased milk production, treatment cost, and decreased market value of the animal and negatively influences the animal's health, reproductive efficacy, and welfare (Djuricic et al. 2015).

The reported incidence of RFM ranges from 2% to 11% depending on herd (Durrani and Kamal 2009; Mude et al. 2010; Ameen and Ajayi 2013; Alenyorege and Mensah 2015; Djuricic et al. 2015). Predisposing factors such as body condition score, nutritional deficiencies such as selenium and vitamin A deficiencies or hypocalcemia (Islam et al. 2012), lack of fresh forage and feeding grains, abortions, stillbirths, dystocia or caesarean section, metritis, oversized fetus, etc. have been reported as causes of RFM. Furthermore, listeriosis, toxoplasmosis, and chlamydiosis infections can lead to premature fetal death and subsequent RFM.

A ewe/doe may normally take up to 12–18 hours to expel the placenta. If the placenta is still attached after 12 hours, there is a problem and the placenta is considered retained. Retention for over three days, especially in the absence of appropriate treatment, can seriously affect the animal's health. As a consequence of the access of atmospheric air, putrefaction of the afterbirth sets in, and this is also affected by the surrounding temperature and how strongly the fetal envelopes are saturated with fluids. The portion of afterbirth hanging from the vulva becomes longer and more discolored, is easily torn, frequently trails on the ground, and exhales a highly offensive odor. A discolored, dirty red or grayish, putrid, strongly stinking fluid, containing decomposed parts of the afterbirth, flows from the dirty vulva and fouls the tail, thighs, and hocks. This discharge is particularly obvious during urination and defecation. Animals show febrile symptoms, elevated rectal and vaginal temperature, increased frequency of the pulse, diminished appetite, and diminished milk secretion. They lose condition, the skin becomes closely adherent to the ribs, the hair coat becomes lusterless and rough, and stiffness of the hindquarters sets in.

The afterbirth, as a rule, is expelled from the ninth to the tenth days and, indeed, almost always entire. Usually the animals recover somewhat rapidly, but in some considerable and lasting uterine catarrh sets in. Should the afterbirth not be expelled by day 11 or 12, it separates into fragments, which in part are discharged, in part retained in the uterus. There is escape of a discolored, putrid, highly offensive fluid from the vagina usually during urination and defecation. Moreover, this discharge frequently continues for a long time and the animals become more and more emaciated. If no treatment or insufficient treatment is applied, pyrexia, septic metritis, and fatal illness ensue due to resorption of the septic uterine contents.

Fortunately, the majority of animals can be saved by administration of proper medication. In appropriately treated cases, the discharge gradually loses its foul smell and assumes a whitish mucopurulent character. The appetite improves, milk secretion gradually increases, and the animals recover after a variable period but generally remain sterile. If cases of RFM

Elements of Reproduction and Reproductive Diseases of Goats, First Edition. Edited by Tanmoy Rana.

are accompanied by injuries of the birth canal, cotyledons, or uterine mucous membrane, the putrefying afterbirth frequently causes a per-acute, often fatal septicemia and gangrenous inflammation of the uterus and vagina. This consequent disease as a rule sets in from the fourth to the seventh day after parturition.

Verma and Singh (2009) reported that medicinal herbs as potential therapeutic aids have attained a significant role in health systems all over the world not only for diseased animals but also as potential material for maintaining proper health.

Tardy uterine involution and RFM is one of the leading causes of delayed resumption of cyclicity. Normally, the fetal membranes are expelled 1–4 hours after kidding. Immediate veterinary attention is essential if expulsion has not happened within 12 hours as contraction of the uterus and closure of the cervix will soon prevent manual removal of the RFM (Matthews 2009).

The expulsion of fetal membranes in the third and final stage of parturition depends on various factors, mainly hormonal. The hormonal processes that lead to normal placental separation are multifactorial and begin before parturition (Beagley et al. 2010). Collagenases are proteolytic enzymes that have a crucial role in fetal membrane release, by breaking the peptide bonds in collagen (Noakes et al. 2009).

Several authors have recommended different therapies for RFM although the efficacy of many of these treatments is questionable. Current evidence does not support manual removal as an effective treatment for RFM, but it is still commonly practiced (Peters and Laven 1996; Drillich et al. 2006, 2007).

The appearances found at necropsy vary according to the length of the disease. In general, the vaginal mucous membrane is dirty red, in places showing a diphtheritic infiltration, and covered with a croupous deposit, diphtheritic scurf, products of necrosis, and ulcers of a dirty greenish appearance. The uterus is a dirty brownish-red to greenish-black color, thickened and in places caseation, suppuration, excoriation, and crust formation of the mucous membrane may be seen. There is serous and purulent infiltration of the uterine mucous membrane, purulent centers in the lymphatic vessels, and thrombi in the uterine veins. In many cases, there is more or less extensive loss of substance of the mucous membrane, especially the cotyledons, and also discolored but not entirely degenerated cotyledons. The flaccid uterus contains a collection of brownish-red, putrid, fetid fluid, mixed with shreds of mucous membrane and putrid fragments of the afterbirth. In persisting pyemia, metastatic infarcts and abscesses are found in the lungs, liver, kidneys, and other organs.

33.2 Structural Components of Placenta

The caprine placenta, characterized by the development of restricted areas of interdigitation between fetal and maternal tissues known as placentomes, is classified as cotyledonary.

Histologically, the placentome is composed of caruncular (maternal) tissue with crypts filled with ramified projections of the chorion, known as chorionic villi. In the placentomes, the maternal blood circulation is separated from the fetal circulation by six tissue layers: maternal vascular endothelium, maternal connective tissue, syncytium, trophoblastic epithelium, fetal mesenchyma, and fetal vascular endothelium, so that the caprine placenta is also classified as epitheliochorial (Wooding 1992). Some workers have proposed that the ruminant placenta be classified as synepitheliochorial due to the migration of fetal cells through the maternal–fetal junction and fusion of these cells with the maternal epithelial cells.

The maternal epithelium of the caruncular crypts persists throughout gestation as a syncytium, which is the result of binucleate chorionic cell fusion (Wooding 1983, 1992). The trophoblastic epithelium is composed of columnar epithelium intermixed with binucleate chorionic cells, which migrate through the maternal–fetal interface and fuse with the syncytial cells (Wooding 1992). The binucleate cells correspond to 15–20% of the epithelial trophoblastic cells and approximately 1/7 of these cells are seen migrating to the caruncular maternal tissue (Wooding 1983). Although ruminant placentomes have been a subject for research, and many workers have studied morphometric parameters and their relation to fetal development in sheep (Derivaux et al. 1988; Hradecky et al. 1988; Wooding 1992), there is no histometric evaluation of the main histological components of the caprine placentome, and no information about changes in its structural components throughout gestation. Moreover, the maturation process of the caprine placenta, including morphological changes at the end of gestation, is not well understood.

In other ruminant species, mainly bovines, it is known that many structural changes occur in the placentomes at the end of gestation and these changes are related to normal delivery of the placenta, including decrease in the number of binucleate cells (Williams et al. 1987) and in the number of epithelial cells in the caruncular crypts (Stegeman 1974). It was found that the average ratio between maternal and fetal tissues in the ovine placentome ranges from 0.44 to 0.73, and that the fetal connective tissue decreases, even with the increase in the degree of branching in the chorionic villi throughout gestation. Moreover, the degree of vascularization of the chorionic villi increases after the tenth week of gestation.

33.3 Basic Features of Placenta

In the ruminant placenta, the intimate fetomaternal contact is restricted to multiple discrete structures named placentomes. These are formed during placentation by interactions of the chorion with preformed placentation sites of the endometrium, whose number and placement vary considerably between ruminant species (Hradecky et al. 1988). Placentomes are composed of fetal chorionic villi cotyledon and the maternal caruncle. In the placentomes, fetal villi arising from the chorionic plate of the cotyledon interdigitate with a corresponding system of widely ramified caruncular crypts.

Based on initial histomorphological studies, the bovine trophoblast was described as being composed of uninucleated cells (UTCs) and larger binucleated cells (BNCs). Later, it was realized that in the bovine trophoblast throughout gestation, terminally differentiated trophoblast giant cells (TGCs) differentiate continuously from UTCs. The TGCs, which generally possess two octaploid nuclei, become binucleate and subsequently polyploid by a series of acytokinetic mitoses. Several stages of TGC development can be observed, which differ in size, location within the trophoblast epithelium, and presence of cytoplasmic granules. As during bovine TGC differentiation binucleated intermediates with lower ploidy levels occur, in this chapter the term TGC refers to mature trophoblast giant cells. TGCs may fuse with cells of the maternal caruncular epithelium. This fusion leads to short-lived trinucleate fetomaternal hybrid cells and to larger syncytial plaques in sheep and goats (Wooding 1992). The function of this fusion is thought to be the exocytotic release of fetal-derived mediator substances into the maternal compartment. Due to this fusion, the ruminant placental barrier is now classified as synepitheliochorial (Wooding 1992).

33.4 Physiology of Expulsion of Placenta

The proximate cause of the detachment of the placenta lies partly in the contractions of the uterus itself. Immediately after the birth of the fetus, the womb contracts and to an important extent diminishes its capacity. Since the fetal envelopes can shrink to only a slight extent and are not at all contractile, they cannot follow these contraction movements of the uterus. In proportion, as the uterus contracts, the fetal envelopes become wrinkled and folded together in its cavity. The relationship of the two contacting surfaces of the chorion and uterine mucous membrane changes from moment to moment. These surfaces glide on one another, and by this gliding movement the villi of the fetal placenta are torn out of the follicles of the uterine mucous membrane and separation of the fetal and maternal cotyledons occurs. The strong contractions of the uterus bring about detachment of the placenta in most domestic animals immediately.

In consequence of the extreme branching and strong development of the villus stems of the cotyledons, the connection of the fetal and maternal placenta is very intimate, and this might be the chief cause of the frequent retention of the afterbirth. The strong contraction of the uterus at the same time creates anemia of the cotyledons, and this appears to be an essential factor in placental detachment. Apparently in consequence of the anemia, paralysis of the muscular strands of the cotyledons sets in, and fatty degeneration of these will favor detachment of the fetal membrane.

According to these two theories, which supplement each other and which doubtless are correct for normal anatomical and physiological conditions, everything that causes a weakening of the uterine musculature must hinder placental detachment and, with that, expulsion of the fetal membrane. A weakening of the uterine musculature may be determined directly by any condition which produces overdistension of the uterus. The uterine musculature is indirectly weakened by all factors that weaken the organism as a whole. One of the chief factors of this nature is insufficient or unsuitable nourishment of the animal during pregnancy. Indeed, retention of the fetal membrane is frequently observed after wet summers, in which the fodder formed is poor in nutritive material.

Difficult labors, more or less marked exhaustion of the mother, and fatigue of the uterus are frequent causes of delayed expulsion of the fetal membrane. A further frequent cause of nonexpulsion of the afterbirth is inflammatory conditions of the uterus, determined by difficult labors and the consequent injuries to the uterus and genital passages.

Retention of the afterbirth is especially frequent as a consequence of abortion; indeed, it is the rule. In such cases, the fetal and uterine placenta are still very firmly united. Even after normal births, a too intimate abnormal connection of some or the majority of the fetal placental villi with the cotyledons is a frequent cause of delayed expulsion of the afterbirth.

Anyone who has tried to separate the placenta manually knows with what great difficulty that operation is often associated, and that sometimes it cannot be effected without dangerous wounding of the cotyledons and the production of more or less dangerous hemorrhage. However, the changes in the texture of these organs which determine this abnormal connection of the fetal and uterine placenta are not yet understood. Further causes of retention of afterbirth include premature partial or complete occlusion of the uterine neck, coiled envelopes, fleshy bands in the uterine neck or the womb itself, large fatty tumors developing between the envelopes, and a fold of the membranes around the stalk of a cotyledon. However, these abnormal conditions are found only seldom.

33.5 Clinical Signs

A doe normally takes up to 12–18 hours to expel the placenta. If the placenta is still attached after 12 hours, there is a problem and the placenta is considered retained (Figures 33.1). A doe which has retained the placenta will often have some of the placenta hanging out of the vagina. This can vary in length from a few inches to more than a foot. In some cases, none of the retained placenta can be seen from the outside and the entire placenta is still contained within the uterus and vagina. When infection is present, does with a retained placenta will sometimes have a fever, act sick, and not want to eat. As the placenta decomposes and infection sets in, a very foul odor can be noticed and a dark, blood-tinged fluid may come out of the vagina. Most cases of retained placenta can be diagnosed by observing the doe.

33.6 Therapeutic Management

Verma and Singh (2009) concluded that medicinal herbs as potential therapeutic aids have attained a significant role in health systems all over the world not only for diseased animals but also as potential material for maintaining proper health. Herbal uterine tonics are scientifically proven to be uterine cleansers that increase uterine tone and the involution process, thus mimicking PGF_2-alpha activity. It has been documented that absence of proper involution in the postparturient period, in cases of retained placenta, interferes with timely reestablishment of reproductive cyclicity. Moreover, mineral supplementations along with polyherbal uterine cleanser and heat inducer therapy is efficacious in induction of postpartum estrus and the induced ovulatory estrus can suitably improve conception rate in small ruminants (Patil et al. 2011).

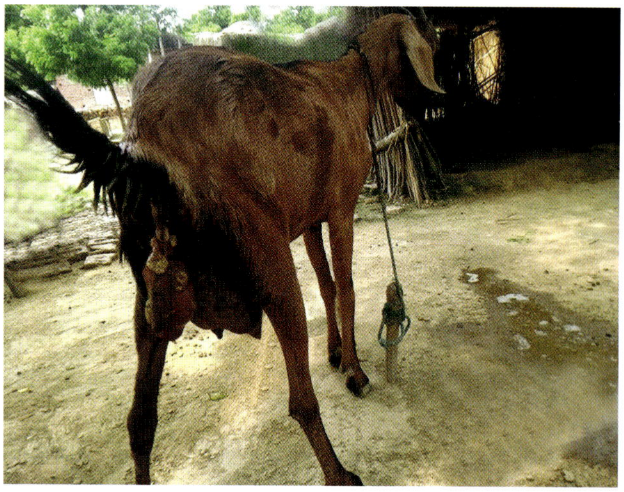

Figure 33.1 Goat with retained fetal membrane. *Source:* Courtesy of Rajesh Kumar (chapter author).

Internal administration of medicinal substances for the purpose of bringing about expulsion of the afterbirth is very uncertain in action. Very little reliance is to be placed on any of the medicinal substances recommended and employed, such as ergot, rue leaves, laurel, juniper, carbonate of potash, and bicarbonate of soda. In the majority of cases, administration of these medicaments does not promote expulsion of the afterbirth and they may, on the contrary, in consequence of their irritant action on the uterus, aggravate the condition. It is only in the entire absence of inflammatory or irritant conditions of the uterus, in pronounced weakness of the mother, when marked loosening or extensive detachment of the fetal placenta has already taken place that pain-exciting media can be usefully employed. In such cases, however, slight traction on the dependent parts of the membranes, since it is more successful, is preferable to these means.

Local antiseptic treatment can be helpful. This consists of thorough washing out of the organ by introducing into it large quantities of warm water, either simple or mixed with antiseptic substances. The introduction of large quantities of lukewarm water determines weak uterine contractions, in consequence of which a great part of the fluid is expelled. These uterine contractions and the warm irrigation of the placenta loosen the connection of the latter. Repeated abundant introduction of warm water frequently brings about detachment of the membranes in a short time. It is useful at first to add antiseptic substances to the warm water, in order to retard decomposition of the membranes, and thus to prevent the danger of infection (Meyer et al. 1989).

A dull, depressed, weak, and anorexic doe should first be stabilized with an antihistamine normal saline drip. After stabilization, the treatment can be further planned after keen observation of the exposed fetal membranes. The perineal region and exposed fetal membranes should be cleaned with 1% $KMnO_4$ solution and the region dried using soft cotton to prevent microbial invasion into the uterus. If the fetal membranes are adhered loosely to the uterine portion, slight manual traction can be applied to remove the fetal membrane remnants. Following removal of the retained fetal membranes, intrauterine preparations should be placed pervaginally into the uterus to avoid secondary bacterial contamination and eliminate uterine debris which could lead to metritis (Kipjen Singh et al. 2018). The doe should be further treated with nonsteroidal antiinflammatory drugs, antiexudative, analgesic, and broad-spectrum antibiotics for five days to combat the current infection and prevent further bacterial multiplication, along with uterine cleansers or ecbolics and mineral mixture to expel uterine remnants and supplement lost minerals.

33.7 Discussion

Retention of placenta (RP) in farm animals is a serious postpartum disorder which occurs when the final stage of parturition is delayed. Although there are several methods to treat RP, i.e., manual and hormonal therapy in cattle and goats (Paisley et al. 1986; Majeed et al. 1991; Majeed 1994), studies have not supported the use of hormones as a general treatment for RFM (Garcia et al. 1992; Stevens and Dinsmore 1997; Drillich et al. 2005). RFM has been associated with increased risk for endometritis, metritis, ketosis, and mastitis in animals where the fetal membrane is not removed (Schukken et al. 1989; Bruun et al. 2002; Melendez et al. 2003). Manual removal of fetal membranes remains a common practice despite numerous studies failing to demonstrate a beneficial effect on reproductive performance (Drillich et al. 2006, 2007).

Proper nutrition and management can resolve the problem of RFM in farm animals, thus preventing economic losses and promoting better health and fertility of the animals.

33.8 Preventive Measures

- Minimization of stressful conditions during the prelambing/kidding period.
- Prevention of metabolic disorders and problems such as dystocia, abortions, and milk fever.
- Vaccination of all animals for potential reproductive diseases (listeriosis, toxoplasmosis, etc.).
- Ensuring proper nutrition by supplementation of rations containing calcium, selenium, phosphorus, magnesium, vitamins A and E, or carotene.

33.9 Conclusion

Retention of fetal membranes is uncommon in goats and is usually associated with malnutrition, birth of a mummified or rotten fetus, or a difficult delivery. However, an increased incidence has been reported in dairy goats which causes negative effects on the health and welfare of the animals and huge economic losses for farmers due to treatment cost and reduced market value of the animals. Retained fetal membranes are the most common complication after C-section in small ruminants. Veterinarians and clients should take necessary precautions in handling fetal membranes in cases where an infectious cause is suspected because many infectious causes of abortion in small ruminants are zoonotic. Systemic treatment to guard against infection and gentle traction on exposed membranes may be used.

References

Ahmed, W.M., El-khadrawy, H. H., and Abel Hameed, A. R. (2006). Applied investigation on ovarian inactivity in buffalo heifers.

Alenyorege, B. and Mensah, K. (2015). Incidence of retained placenta in ruminants and its treatment by rural farmers in Northern Ghana. *Indian Journal of Applied Research* 5: 7.

Ameen, S.A. and Ajayi, J.A. (2013). Studies on influence of seasonality on clinical conditions of small ruminants in Ogbomoso areas of Oyo State. *International Journal of Applied Agriculture and Apiculture Research* 9: 18–27.

Beagley, J.C., Whitman, K.J., Baptiste, K.E., and Scherzer, J. (2010). Physiology and treatment of retained fetal membranes in cattle. *Journal of Veterinary Internal Medicine* 24: 261–268.

Bruun, J., Ersbll, A.K., and Alban, L. (2002). Risk factors for metritis in Danish dairy cows. *Preventive Veterinary Medicine* 54: 179–190.

Derivaux, J., Ectors, F., and Beckers, J.F. (1988). *The Ruminant Placenta: Structure and Endocrine Function*. Brussels: State University of Liege.

Djuricic, D., Valpotic, H., and Samardzija, M. (2015). The intrauterine treatment of the retained foetal membrane in dairy goats by ozone: novel alternative to antibiotic therapy. *Reproduction in Domestic Animals* 50: 236–239.

Drillich, M., Schroder, A., and Tenhagen, B.A. (2005). Efficacy of a treatment of retained placenta in dairy cows with prostaglandin F2a in addition to a local antibiotic treatment. *Deutsche Tierärztliche Wochenschrift* 112: 174–179.

Drillich, M., Mahistedt, M., and Reichert, U. (2006). Strategies to improve the therapy of retained fetal membranes in dairy cows. *Journal of Dairy Science* 89: 627–635.

Drillich, M., Klever, N., and Heuwieser, W. (2007). Comparison of two management strategies for retained fetal membranes on small dairy farms in Germany. *Journal of Dairy Science* 90: 4275–4281.

Durrani, A.Z. and Kamal, N. (2009). Prevalence of genital tract problems in clinical cases of various species of animals. *Journal of Animal and Plant Sciences* 19: 160–162.

Garcia, A., Bath, A.D., and Mapletoft, R.J. (1992). The effects of treatment with cloprostenol or dinoprost within one hour of induced parturition on the incidence of retained placenta in cattle. *Canadian Veterinary Journal* 33: 175.

Hradecky, P., Mossman, H.W., and Stott, G.G. (1988). Comparative development of ruminant placentomes. *Theriogenology* 29 (3): 715–729.

Islam, M.H., Sarder, M.J.U., Rhaman, M. et al. (2012). Incidence of retained placenta in relation with breed, age, parity and body condition score of dairy cows. *International Journal of Natural Sciences* 2 (1): 15–20.

Kipjen Singh, L., Pipelu, W., Mishra, G.K., and Patra, M.K. (2018). Retention of foetal membranes in a non-descript doe: a case report. *International Journal of Current Microbiology and Applied Sciences* 7 (3): 2405–2409.

Majeed, A.F. (1994). Obstetrical problems and their management in lraqi goats. *Small Ruminant Research* 14: 73–78.

Majeed, A.F., Taha, M.B., and Azawi, O.I. (1991). Hormonal treatment of retained placenta in local breed of cattle. *Iraqi Journal of Veterinary Sciences* 4: 61–72.

Matthews, J.G. (2009). *Diseases of the Goat*, 3e. Oxford: Blackwell Publishing.

Melendez, P., Risco, C.A., and Donovan, G.A. (2003). Effect of calcium-energy supplements on calving-related disorders, fertility and milk yield during the transition period in cows fed anionic salts. *Theriogenology* 60: 843–854.

Meyer, H.H., Enzenhofer, G., and Feck, H. (1989). Improvement of radioimmunoassays for prostaglandinsin bovine blood plasma and their application to monitor reproductive functions. *Theriogenology* 31: 701–720.

Mude, S.W., Waghmare, S.P., Mode, S.G. et al. (2010). Effect of mineral supplementation on post-parturient diseases in pregnant goats. *Veterinary World* 3: 109–110.

Noakes, D.E., Timothy, J.P., England, G.C.W., and Arthur, G.H. (2009). *Arthur's Veterinary Reproduction and Obstetrics*, 408–415. New York: W. B. Saunders.

Paisley, L.G., Mickelseno, W.D., and Anderson, P.B. (1986). Mechanisms and therapy for retained fetal membranes and uterine infections of caws: a review. *Theriogenology* 25: 353–381.

Patil, A.D., Raghuwanshi, D.S., Kumbhar, U.B., and Shivi, M. (2011). Effect of herbal durgs and minerals on fertility in postpartum anestrus Osmanabadi goats. *Indian Journal of Animal Reproduction* 32 (1): 57–58.

Peters, A.R. and Laven, R.A. (1996). Treatment of bovine retained placenta and its effects. *Veterinary Record* 139: 539–541.

Schukken, Y.H., Erb, H.N., and Scarlett, J.M. (1989). A hospital-based study of the relationship between retained placenta and mastitis in dairy cows. *Cornell Veterinarian* 79: 319–326.

Stegeman, J.H.J. (1974). Placental development in the sheep and its relation to fetal development. *Bijdragen tot de Dierkunde* 44 (1): 3–72.

Stevens, R.D. and Dinsmore, R.P. (1997). Treatment of dairy cows at parturition with prostaglandin F2α or oxytocin for prevention of retained fetal membranes. *Journal of the American Veterinary Medical Association* 21: 1280–1284.

Verma, S. and Singh, S.P. (2009). Current and future status of herbal medicines. *Veterinary World* 1 (11): 347–350.

Williams, W.F., Margolis, M.J., Manspeaker, J. et al. (1987). Peripartum changes in the bovine placenta related to fetal membrane retention. *Theriogenology* 28 (2): 213–223.

Wooding, F.B.P. (1983). Frequency and localization of binucleate cells in the placentomes of ruminants. *Placenta* 4 (2): 527–539.

Wooding, F.B.P. (1992). The synepitheliochorial placenta of ruminants: binucleate cell fusions and hormone production. *Placenta* 13 (2): 101–113.

34

Metritis

Annadurai Thangamani, Abdul Reshma, Sakthivel Manokaran, Ramasamy Rajkumar, Tulasiraman Sarath, and Ayyasamy Elango

Department of Veterinary Gynaecology and Obstetrics, Veterinary College and Research Institute, Tamil Nadu Veterinary and Animal Sciences University, Salem, India

34.1 Introduction

Uterine infections are common disorders affecting goats during the postpartum period. Prospective studies suggest that uterine infections decrease subsequent reproductive performance (Fuquay et al. 1975; Bartlett et al. 1986; Gilbert 1992; Dohmen et al. 1995). In these reports, however, no differentiation was made among the types of infection, and uterine infection was classified as a disease complex with clinical manifestations ranging from minimal or none to life-threatening sepsis (Fuquay et al. 1975; Hartigan 1980; Etherington et al. 1984). Consequently, a divergence of opinion continues to exist among veterinarians regarding diagnosis and treatment of uterine infections (Hussain et al. 1990).

34.2 Definition

The uterus is normally protected from bacterial contamination by the vulva, vestibular sphincter, and cervix. During and immediately after parturition, these mechanical barriers are breached and the uterus normally is contaminated by a variety of pathogenic and nonpathogenic microorganisms (Watson 1989).

Metritis is a severe inflammation involving all layers of the uterus (endometrial mucosa and submucosa, muscularis, and serosa). It generally develops during the first week after kidding and is associated with dystocia, retention of fetal membranes (RFM), and kidding trauma (Markusfeld and Ezra 1993). Affected goats may be septic and present with fever, depression, and anorexia. In addition, a copious fetid vaginal discharge may be present.

34.3 Diagnosis

34.3.1 Clinical Signs

Clinical signs of uterine infection vary with the virulence of the causative organism and the presence of factors that predispose to the disease. Lochia normally is expelled from the reproductive tract during the first few weeks after kidding, and the discharge may persist for up to 30 days if uterine involution is delayed. Normal discharges range in color from dark brown to red to white; discharge usually should not be considered abnormal unless the fluid is fetid (Figure 34.1) or clinical signs of sepsis are present.

Elements of Reproduction and Reproductive Diseases of Goats, First Edition. Edited by Tanmoy Rana.

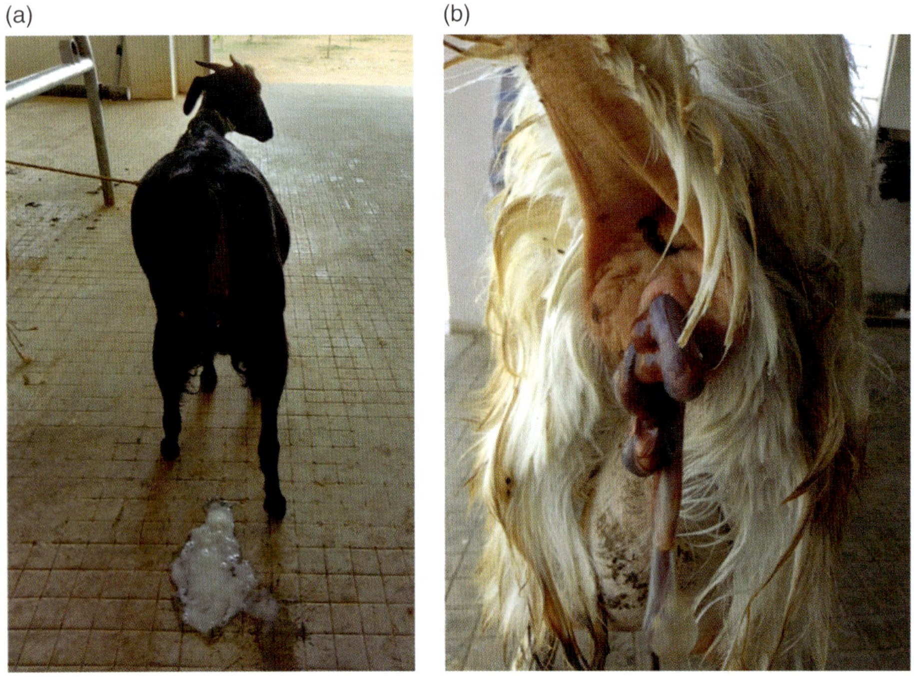

Figure 34.1 (a) Abnormal vaginal discharge in goat. (b) RFM in goat.

34.3.2 Vaginoscopy

Observation of purulent exudate with the aid of a vaginal speculum has been reported to be a useful tool for diagnosis of subacute and chronic endometritis and for evaluation of response to treatment (Lourens 1995). Unfortunately, the requirements for sterile and disposable specula and for aseptic preparation of the perineum and external genitals make this procedure cumbersome when goat are examined in free-stalls or lock-up stanchions.

34.3.3 Ultrasonography

Real-time ultrasonography has been used to demonstrate uterine changes associated with postpartum infections. The intrauterine fluid associated with uterine infections contained echogenic particles and was easily distinguished from clear nonechogenic fluid associated with estrus and pregnancy (Olson et al. 1987). In addition, the uterine wall of goats affected with uterine infections was variably thickened.

34.3.4 Bacterial Culture

Guarded culture instruments can be passed up to the cervix and samples obtained for bacterial culture. Samples should be cultured in both aerobic and anaerobic environments. Under most circumstances, however, samples from individual animals are rarely submitted for bacterial culture because a decision to treat usually is made before results of culture are available. The cost of the procedure can only rarely be justified. *Streptococcus pyogenes* and Gram-negative anaerobes are usually assumed to be the most likely causative organisms (Rajala and Grohn 1998). Bacterial culture and antibiotic sensitivity tests may be indicated on farms that have an unusually high incidence of uterine infection.

34.4 Treatment

Few topics are more controversial among clinicians than appropriate treatment for uterine infections, perhaps because of the lack of precise diagnostic criteria and lack of controlled trials in which various therapeutic options have been rigorously compared. Therapy for uterine infection has fallen into the broad categories of intrauterine therapy (antibiotics and antiseptic chemicals), systemic antibiotics, and supportive therapy and hormone therapy (Watson 1989).

34.5 Conclusion

Goats affected by periparturient abnormalities such as pregnancy toxemia, dystocia, and RFM are more likely to contract uterine infections than those that kidded normally. Thus, management of sanitation, nutrition, population density, and stress to prevent or reduce the incidence of these predisposing factors should be impeccable. The most sanitary environment possible should be provided for kidding, and strict attention paid to asepsis when relief of dystocia is necessary.

References

Bartlett, P.C., Kirk, J.C., Wilke, M.A. et al. (1986). Metritis complex in Michigan Holstein-Friesian cattle: incidence, descriptive epidemiology and estimated economic impact. *Preventive Veterinary Medicine* 4: 235.

Dohmen, M.J.W., Lohuis, J.A.C.M., Huszenicza, G. et al. (1995). The relationship between bacteriological and clinical findings in cows with subacute/chronic endometritis. *Theriogenology* 43: 1379.

Etherington, W.G., Bosu, W.T.K., Martin, S.W. et al. (1984). Reproductive performance in dairy cows following postpartum treatment with gonadotropin-releasing hormone and/or prostaglandin: a field trial. *Canadian Journal of Comparative Medicine* 48: 245.

Fuquay, J.W., Harris, R.A., McGee, W.H. et al. (1975). Routine postpartum treatment of dairy cattle with neomycin sulfate boluses. *Journal of Dairy Science* 58: 1367.

Gilbert, R.O. (1992). Bovine endometritis: the burden of proof. *Cornell Veterinarian* 82: 11.

Hartigan, P.J. (1980). Fertility management in the dairy herd: the need to control bacterial contamination in the environment. *Irish Veterinary Journal* 34: 43.

Hussain, A.M., Daniel, R.C.W., and O'Boyle, D. (1990). Postpartum uterine flora following normal and abnormal puerperium in cows. *Theriogenology* 34: 291.

Lourens, D.C. (1995). A comparative observational study on the reproductive performance of dairy cows with metritis and normal cows. *South African Journal of Animal Science* 25: 21.

Markusfeld, O. and Ezra, E. (1993). Body measurements, metritis, and post-partum performance of first lactation cows. *Journal of Dairy Science* 76: 3771.

Olson, J.D., Ball, L., Oetzel, G.R. et al. (1987). Metritis and pyometra. *Journal of the Society for Theriogenology* 14: 65.

Rajala, P.J. and Grohn, J.T. (1998). Effects of dystocia, retained placenta and metritis on milk yield in dairy cows. *Journal of Dairy Science* 81: 3172.

Watson, E.D. (1989). In vitro function of bovine neutrophils against actinomyces pyogenes. *American Journal of Veterinary Research* 50: 455.

35

Pyometra

Jitumoni Das[1], Manoj Kumar Kalita[1], Prerona Patowary[2], Parimita Dutta[3], and Tanmoy Rana[4]

[1] *Department of Animal Reproduction, Gynaecology and Obstetrics, Lakhimpur College of Veterinary Science, Assam Agricultural University, North Lakhimpur, India*
[2] *Department of Veterinary Clinical Medicine, Ethics and Jurisprudence, Assam Agricultural University-Goat Research Station, Burnihat, India*
[3] *Krishi Vigyan Kendra (KVK), Tirap, India*
[4] *Department of Veterinary Clinical Complex, West Bengal University of Animal and Fishery Sciences, Kolkata, India*

35.1 Introduction

Reproductive performance is one of the most imperative economic traits in terms of livestock production (Alexandre et al. 2012; Arguello 2011). The most common parameters used to estimate reproductive performance in goat are the kidding rate, twinning ability, abortion rate, and the number of kids born alive or dead (Arguello 2011). Particularly in developing countries, many people's survival, economic security, and social livelihoods depend heavily on small ruminants like sheep and goats (Kosgey and Okeyo 2007). A significant portion of the rural population, notably landless, small and marginal farmers, engage in goat rearing that directly or indirectly helps them to improve their socioeconomic status. In commercial goat farms, reproductive efficiency is the major determining factor for productivity and economic viability. Reproductive abnormalities have been described as the largest single cause of loss of livestock production (McDowell 1972). They have a negative impact on meat production since pregnancy and parturition are prerequisites for reproduction. The reproduction of goats has an effect on successful fertility (Sattar and Khan 1988). Gynaecoobstetrical disorders like dystocia, abortion, and retention of placenta and other miscellaneous abnormalities such as metritis, pyometra, and vaginitis are vital factors causing economical losses to the sheep and goat industry.

Fertility in healthy goat herds is influenced by prepubertal and postpartum nutrition (Bocquier et al. 1996), age of the dam at kidding (Erasmus and Fourie 1985), and body score (Absy et al. 2001). Goats can tolerate moderate weight loss at breeding but still become pregnant (Goonewardene et al. 1997). More severe changes in energy intake during pregnancy markedly affect fetal development and survival, so abortion and stillbirth are significant sources of economic loss for the goat industry under intensive (Engeland et al. 1998) and extensive (Mellado et al. 2001) production systems. Moreover, uterine infections severely affect the productive and reproductive performance of the animal that lead to severe economic losses for farmers and may force them to cull infertile or sterile animals.

Pyometra is a chronic uterine infection that develops as a sequel to uterine infections such as metritis or endometritis and is characterized by the accumulation of purulent or mucopurulent material in the uterine lumen with persistent corpus luteum and closed cervix (Sheldon et al. 2006).

In cows, pyometra is frequently diagnosed during the postpartum period due to early ovulation with formation of the corpus luteum that can take place before uterine clearance of bacteria during the physiological involution process (Olson et al. 1984). Increased levels of progesterone secreted by the persistent corpus luteum make the uterus susceptible to infection. However, in small ruminants, pyometra is a rare disease and has been described secondary to metritis or endometritis and ovulation during anestrus periods that causes a persistent corpus luteum (Pugh and Baird 2012).

Elements of Reproduction and Reproductive Diseases of Goats, First Edition. Edited by Tanmoy Rana.

35.2 Incidence

Pyometra in goat is infrequent. Authors worldwide have reported its incidence in goats as 0.58% (Lyngset 1968) or 0.05% (Timurkaan and Karadas 2000). However, Agarwal et al. (2015) identified pyometra in 1.34% caprine specimens while studying the histopathology of genital tract diseases after collecting 341 female genitalia from local abattoirs.

However, the incidence of hydrometra or mucometra in goats is far more common than pyometra. Pyometra in goats may often be confused with hydrometra or mucometra due to similarities of some clinical signs including cessation of cyclical activity and variable degree of abdominal distension. Mucometra or hydrometra is a uterine pathological condition associated with accumulation of thin to viscid mucus in the uterus. These two conditions are similar except for the degree of hydration of the mucin present in the uterus which may vary from watery fluid to thick viscid mucus. So, mucometra is characterized by accumulation of thick mucus in the uterus while hydrometra is characterized by accumulation of aseptic watery fluid in the uterine lumen and presence of persistent corpus luteum in the ovaries of goats (Pieterse and Taverne 1986), also referred to as pseudopregnancy or "cloud-burst" condition in goats. In temperate areas, the incidence of hydrometra in goats varies between 3.0% and 20.8% (Hesselink 1993b). However, reports of this pathological condition from the tropics are scarce (Lopes Junior et al. 2004).

35.3 Pathogenesis of Postpartum Uterine Infection

Development of postpartum uterine infection and disease is dependent on adherence of pathogenic organisms to the uterine mucosa, colonization or penetration of the epithelium, and/or release of bacterial toxins that lead to establishment of uterine disease (Janeway et al. 2001).

During parturition, the mammalian uterus may be contaminated with a wide range of microbes. Mostly, aerobic and anaerobic Gram-positive andGram-negative bacteria such as *E. coli*, *Corynebacterium pyogenes*, *Streptococcus*, *Staphylococcus*, *Pseudomonas*, and *Bacillus* are found to be present in the uterus during the early postpartum period (Sheldon et al. 2008). In addition, other microbes including virus, fungi, and mycoplasma were also found to be responsible for uterine infections postpartum. However, this microbial contamination need not necessarily indicate infection or development of uterine disease.

Microbial contamination or load in the uterine lumen decreases substantially in the majority of healthy animals during the physiological process of involution of the uterus. Most of the bacteria contaminate the uterine lumen and are removed by host defense mechanisms. Failure of the defense mechanism and aggravated infection by these organisms are the major contributors to postparturient disorders such as metritis, endometritis, and infertility (Farin et al. 1989; Bonnett et al. 1993) (Figure 35.1).

Furthermore, development of postpartum uterine infection or disease is also dependent on the pathogen (bacterial strain and its load), the pathogenicity of bacteria, and the immune status of the animal (Sheldon et al. 2002; LeBlanc et al. 2011; Jeon et al. 2016). However, during and after parturition this balance can be tipped in favor of disease by several risk factors (Grohn and Rajala-Schultz 2000; Kim and Kang 2003).

35.3.1 Risk Factors Associated with Uterine Diseases

Different risk factors that favor the development of uterine infection or disease during postpartum period are illustrated in Figure 35.2.

- *Factors associated with uterine trauma and damage at parturition*, such as dystocia, retained fetal membrane (RFM), stillbirth, etc., may delay the normal uterine involution process. Out of these factors, RFM is the most important risk factor for development of postpartum uterine disease because the necrotic materials associated with RFM provide a suitable environment for bacterial growth in the uterine lumen. Additionally, the RFM obstructs the physical barrier provided by the cervix and finally delays the involution process. Incidence of RFM is higher in goats carrying a dead fetus or as a result of medical termination of pregnancy in order to remove a dead fetus (Pugh and Baird 2012), and due to inappropriate methods of induction of parturition. The prevalence of RFM among goats is high, ranging from 10.6% to 11.8% based on previous studies (Durrani and Kamal 2009; Sultan et al. 2015).
- *Parity* is also associated with postpartum uterine disease. Occurrence of postpartum uterine infections is more prevalent either in the first parity or in higher parities, i.e., in older animals.

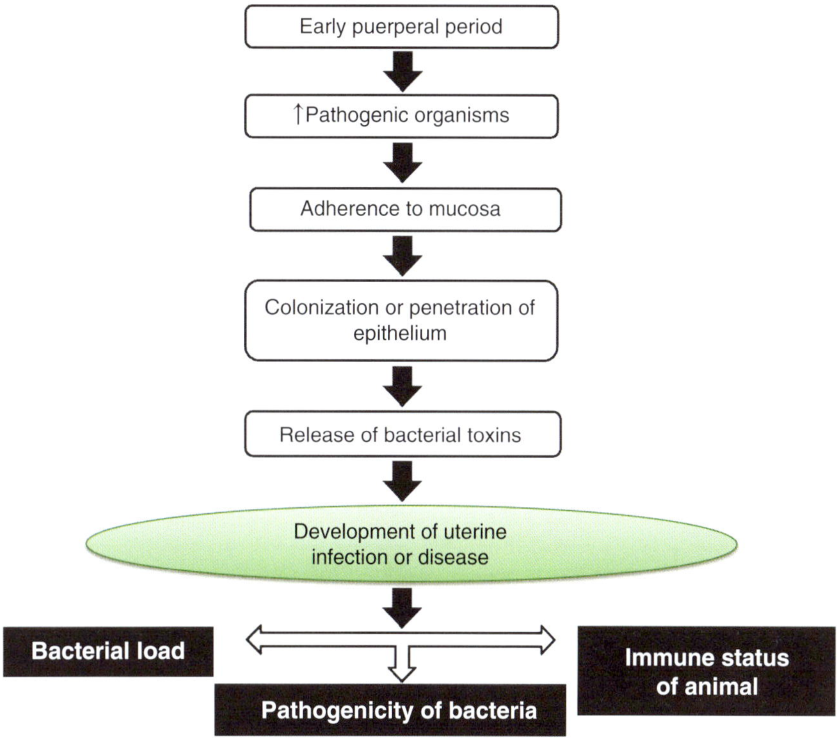

Figure 35.1 Schematic representation of the development of postpartum uterine disease.

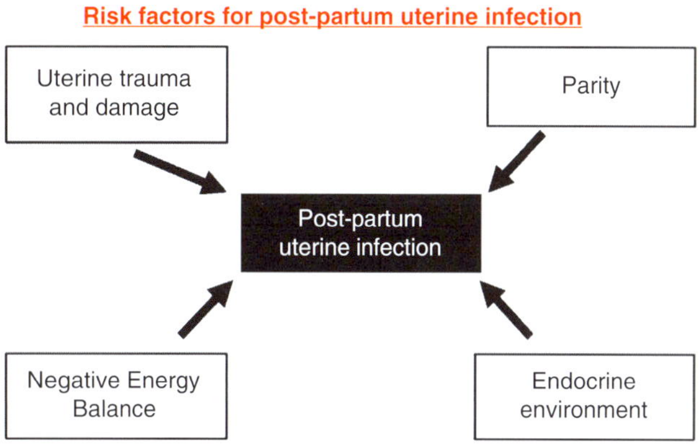

Figure 35.2 Risk factors for postpartum uterine infection.

- *Negative energy balance (NEB) following parturition* is also an important risk factor for the onset and development of postpartum uterine infection. Periparturient metabolic disorders and lack of energy or reduced feed intake after parturition are important risk factors for the development of metritis, endometritis, and subclinical endometritis (Kim and Kang 2003). Moreover, there is increasing demand of energy for milk synthesis during early lactation. If this fails, the animal may face a period of negative energy balance.

  Energy homeostasis and metabolism are closely associated with the effectiveness of the immune system to combat infections (Mathis and Shoelson 2011). In cattle, studies have given weight to the argument that cows with markers of more exacerbated tissue catabolism because of negative energy balance are more likely to develop uterine diseases (Silvestre et al. 2011; Giuliodori et al. 2013; Ribeiro et al. 2013).

  Hammon et al. (2006) also reported that cows in greater NEB have more pronounced impairment of immune functions and become more likely to develop metritis or endometritis.
- *Endocrine environment:* establishment of uterine bacterial infection may depend in part on the endocrine environment, particularly on progesterone level, as it seems to suppress uterine immune defenses. Formation of the first corpus luteum after parturition and secretion of progesterone often precede the onset of uterine disease.

35.4 Etiology

The uterus generally does not harbour any bacterial infections, but it can become infected during mating and at parturition.

Postservice pyometra is mostly due to *Trichomonas fetus*, a flagellate protozoan which is transmitted via coitus and colonizes the uterus. It does not prevent fertilization but causes embryonic death at early stages of gestation; sometimes early embryonic death is followed by pyometra with persistent corpus luteum.

Genital infections in female domestic ruminants are often caused by opportunistic secondary invaders, especially *E. coli*, which has frequently been isolated in ewes (Manes et al. 2010; Martins et al. 2009; Sargison et al. 2007) and goats (Ababneh and Degefa 2006). Under stress conditions, different opportunist bacteria may cause genital infection that can lead to reproductive failure in ruminants (Levinson and Jawetz 1994; Shallali et al. 2001). However, the development of uterine disease depends on the immune response of the animals, as well as the species and number of bacteria.

Pyometra can arise from an ongoing specific bacterial infection such as campylobacterosis (Morrow 1986), *E. coli* and *Proteus* with fetid odor or nonspecific uterine infections especially during the puerperal period. Other than the ubiquitous *E. coli*, Rind and Shaikh (2000) reported three different species of *Staphylococcus*, *S. aureus*, *S. intermedius*, and *S. epidermidis*, as major pathogens in the uterus of goats in Pakistan.

Some Nubian and dwarf goats resume estrous cycles shortly after parturition and may develop pyometra. During the breeding season, cervical damage or bacterial infections introduced at breeding may progress to pyometra.

35.5 Clinical Signs

Does with pyometra show few or no signs of ill health (Kahn and Line 2010); the main reason for them being examined is the absence of cyclical activity or perhaps the presence of an intermittent vaginal discharge. A common presenting sign in affected does is anestrus due to persistent corpus luteum (PCL). In most cases of postpartum pyometra, the cervix is relaxed so that some of the pus may escape through the vulva, particularly when the doe lies down, urinates or defecates. According to Jainudeen and Hafez (1987) and Hasnain (1985), the pus is typically thick, mucoid, creamy, and yellow or greenish-gray in color. Systemic signs of endotoxemia are not reportedly associated with pyometra in sheep and goats (Castillo et al. 2017).

35.6 Diagnosis

Diagnosis can be made by observing clinical signs such as prolonged anestrus, abdominal distension, and presence of an intermittent purulent vaginal discharge. However, vaginal examination using a speculum or vaginoscope, or ultrasonographic examination of the uterus is essential for confirmatory diagnosis. Additionally, the condition must be differentiated from pregnancy and hydrometra.

35.6.1 Vaginal Examination Using a Vaginoscope

The endoscopic examination of the vagina and its surrounding structures, such as the vestibule, vaginal fornix, external os cervix, etc., using a rigid or flexible fiberoptic vaginoscope is called vaginoscopy. Vaginoscopy is an effective tool for genital tract disease diagnosis, particularly for inspection of the vaginal cavity to determine the presence of pus or evaluate the nature and extent of disease in the vestibule, vagina, and external os cervix. It can also be used for biopsy material collection, reproductive tract fluid aspiration, and vaginal sample collection for cellular examination and culture.

A flexible fiberoptic endoscope is ideal to examine almost any animal because it provides cool lighting and excellent visualization. However, a pediatric proctoscope less than 12 mm in diameter can also be used as it has the advantage of easy passage through the vagina of the goat, as well as lower cost, greater durability, and easier maintenance (Figure 35.3).

35.6.1.1 Vaginoscopic Examination Procedure in Goats

1) The perineal region including the vulva should be washed and cleaned before insertion of the vaginoscope.
2) All instruments used for vaginoscopy should be sterilized. Chemical sterilization is not recommended if swabs for culture are to be obtained.
3) Prior to insertion, the vaginoscope should be well lubricated using sterile nonirritating lubricant.
4) Insert the vaginoscope through the vulva and examine the area to be investigated.

35.6.1.2 Pathological Findings During Vaginoscopy Indicating Uterine Infection

Presence of pus in the external os cervix or on the floor of the anterior vagina in the absence of any visible lesions may suggest endometritis or uterine infection.

35.6.2 Ultrasonographic Diagnosis

Real-time ultrasonography is an accurate, reliable, and efficient method for detecting uterine pathology in non-pregnant goats. It is a very useful aid by which pregnant and nonpregnant does with any kind of uterine pathology can easily be diagnosed.

In small ruminants like sheep and goats, ultrasonographic examination of the female reproductive tract is carried out by the transcutaneous method from the right side of the abdomen. Abdominal ultrasonography is the preferred technique for examination of the female reproductive tract of small animals. The animal should be properly restrained either in dorsal or lateral recumbency by attendants. Standing position is mostly preferred and used in goats and sheep. The abdominal area must be shaved or clipped properly before commencement of the ultrasonography technique, so that the skin in that area is bare, and then allowed to air dry. A linear array transducer with 3.5 or 5 MHz frequency is mostly used for the transabdominal approach in sheep and goats. The transducer face must be well lubricated with a suitable coupling medium and it should be pressed firmly over the abdominal wall in order to effect ultrasound transmission.

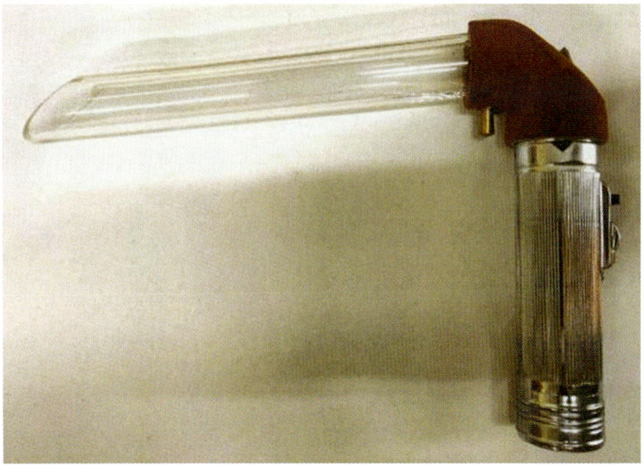

Figure 35.3 Vaginoscope for use in sheep and goats. *Source:* J.M. Das (chapter contributor).

35.6.2.1 Ultrasonographic Findings in Goats Affected with Hydrometra and Pyometra

In hydrometra, a no echogenic (i.e. black) fluid-filled compartmentalized uterus is demonstrated, no fetal parts or placentomes are seen (Ahmed et al. 2010).

In pyometra, a hypoechoic fluid-filled compartmentalized uterus is demonstrated with a highly echogenic material which represents inflammatory cells.

35.6.3 Histopathology of Naturally Occurring Pathological Uterine Conditions

Histologically, the uterus of normal nonpregnant animals, particularly sheep and goats, reveals normal architecture comprising a uniform layer of surface epithelium, dense endometrial stroma, and well-distributed endometrial glands (Agarwal et al. 2015). However, the gravid/pregnant uterus shows an increase in the size and number of endometrial glands, sparse stromal cell population, and increased cellularity of the surface epithelium.

Uterus with pyometra shows dilated and hyperplastic endothelial glands variably filled with pus. In acute cases, the neutrophil is the predominant cell present in the stroma and lumen of the endometrial glands. However, in subacute to chronic pyometra cases, the surface epithelium of the uterus is variably hyperplastic or hypertrophied in nature, a large number of lymphocytes, plasma cells, and occasional macrophages are present, and areas of infiltrated inflammatory cells are noted frequently in the endometrial stroma.

Uterus with hydrometra shows an unevenly dilated lumen with a thin wall and variable sized areas in the endometrial stroma filled with serous fluid, which is comparatively reduced in size. The endometrium is comparatively thin and flat in appearance and the endometrial glands are decreased in number and size due to variable pressure atrophy caused by the fluid accumulated in the uterine lumen.

Uterus with mucometra shows a variably dilated lumen with a thin wall and flat appearance and there is an increase in the number and size of endometrial glands with increased epithelial activity. Excessive mucin or mucinous substances are present within and between the stromal cell population of the endometrium. The luminal epithelial cells are comparatively taller, columnar, and hypertrophied with vacuolated cytoplasm.

35.7 Prognosis

Early diagnosis and proper treatment have a good prognosis. However, in long-standing cases, the endometrium is destroyed and the uterine wall undergoes fibrotic changes resulting in permanent sterility.

35.8 Treatment

The treatment goal for pyometra is to lyze the retained corpus luteum so that the cervix will dilate, the uterus will contract, and pus will be evacuated with timely clearance of the infection and return of the animal to a normal reproductive state. Treatment of goats with pyometra generally involves hormonal and antibiotic therapy, either alone or in combination.

35.8.1 Hormonal Therapy

Different hormonal preparations either alone or in combination can be used with variable success rates, such as:

- estrogen therapy
- estrogen and oxytocin therapy
- estrogen and glucocorticoid therapy
- PGF2-alpha or its analogue – safer and with better results than estrogen.

Estradiol has been recommended by some workers as it stimulates myometrium contractions, phagocytosis, and mucus production (Roberts 1986). However, Overton et al. (2003) and Risco and Hernandez (2003) concluded that administration of estradiol did not have beneficial effects on reproductive performance.

Among different hormonal preparations, PGF2-alpha or its analogue is safer and the best choice for treatment of pyometra in goats. Its single injection causes regression of the corpus luteum, dilation of the cervix, and expulsion of pus within 5–7 days along with subsequent onset of estrus.

Recommended dose and route of natural and syntheticPGF2-alpha or its analogue drugs in goats are:

- dinoprost, 5–10 mg, by intramuscular (IM) or subcutaneous (SC) route, or
- clorprostenol, 62.5–125 μg, by intramuscular (IM) or subcutaneous (SC) route.

In some cases, a single administration of prostaglandin may not be sufficient for complete evacuation of uterine pus. According to Hesselink (1993a), a second dose of prostaglandin within an interval of 12 days significantly increases reproductive performance.

35.8.2 Antibiotic Therapy

The effectiveness of antibiotic treatment in clearing uterine infection can be improved only after complete evacuation of pus. Based on the severity of the condition, both parenteral and intrauterine antibiotics are recommended for the treatment of pyometra in does.

Parenteral antibiotics should be administered during hormonal treatment, mainly to prevent the spread of infection from the uterus to the oviduct due to uterine contraction. Ceftiofur 2.2 mg/kg body weight daily for five days is effective against both Gram-positive and Gram-negative bacteria and has been useful in the treatment of caprine pyometra. Local or intrauterine (IU) antibiotics should be infused only after evacuation of pus. Penicillin is the antibiotic of choice for IU administration.

Al-Hamedawi (2011) recommended PGF2-alpha (Estrumate™, 250 μg, IM) in combination with IU Lugols iodine (0.5%, 25 ml) infusion in the treatment of postpartum pyometra in does.

35.8.3 Supportive Therapy

- Calcium preparation in oral or injectable form should be prescribed to increase the tonicity of the uterine musculature.
- Vitamin A, D, and E preparation should be prescribed to help in regeneration of damaged endometrium, and enhance immunity and calcium absorption.

35.8.4 Sexual Rest

It is important not to bred the doe naturally or artificially during the first posttreatment estrus.

35.9 Managing Female Goats to Prevent Uterine Diseases

Uterine infections or diseases in goats can be best prevented by adopting the principles of hygiene and sanitation at the time of breeding and parturition, good management practices, and appropriate nutritional management. Suboptimal nutrition and management can make the female goat more susceptible to postpartum uterine disease.

An obvious way to avoid postpartum uterine disease is by controlling the various risk factors. The predominant risk factors for postpartum uterine disease are trauma to the genital tract followed by colonization with pathogenic bacteria. Trauma to the genital tract is more likely in the first parity, after induction of parturition, or following dystocia, stillbirths, twins, male calves, or retained placenta.

Selection of easy-calving breeds and easy-calving sires within a breed can reduce the risk of parturient trauma to the genital tract. So, controlled selective breeding of the doe with appropriate sized and healthy bucks in a clean and hygienic environment must be adopted. Primiparous does should be mated for the first time with a young buck which has not previously been exposed to trichomoniasis. It is vitally important to carry out a detailed physical examination of the doe before breeding. Precautions must be taken to remove any infected buck from the herd to reduce the chances of infertility conditions. Artificial insemination should be carried out by well-trained and skilled technicians in a clean environment and hygienic way. Regular ultrasonography is of crucial importance for intensive farm reproductive management in large dairy goat farming enterprises, particularly after breeding to diagnosis pregnancy or fetal abnormalities.

Prevention of uterine disease also requires appropriate nutritional management, particularly during the transition period in dairy goat breeds. Pregnant does should be dried off at the target body condition score, fed a prepartum diet that provides the appropriate fiber, vitamins, and minerals, and then fed a postpartum diet with sufficient energy and protein to satisfy the metabolic requirements for lactation.

At the time of parturition, the animal should be kept in a clean and hygienic environment. In case of any emergency during kidding such as dystocia, retention of fetal membrane, etc., immediate consultation with a veterinary practitioner is essential. If there is need for intervention during parturition, farmers and veterinarians should ensure that they use clean techniques, are gentle, and maintain the cleanliness of the environment to prevent postpartum genital tract infection and diseases. After parturition, it is important to monitor the animal's health carefully, particularly those animals that experience risk factors for uterine disease. Veterinary examination of the reproductive tract is important to identify animals with disease and decide on their treatment.

Encouraging an early return to ovarian cyclic activity by appropriate nutrition and reproductive management during the transition period also helps to counter uterine disease.

35.10 Conclusion

Goats are extremely prolific creatures that often have two kiddings per year and attain sexual maturity at an early age. However, numerous studies have suggested that uterine lesions, including infection in female goats, induces infertility or sterility, which incurs heavy economic losses to the producers and may force farmers to cull such animals. In order to save the animals and maintain their productivity, it is necessary to screen the animals for various diseases that can affect the reproductive tract, particularly the uterus, and to take necessary preventive and control measures. Early and precise diagnosis of pregnancy, determination of fetal number and gestational age in goats is crucial for improving farm economy.

The lack of an overview of reproductive performance is a major setback in the implementation of strategic plans to improve food animal production. Furthermore, evaluation of factors affecting reproductive performance has received little attention in the field. However, in the worst cases, the treatment cost of reproductive disorders is high. For this reason, farmers may lose interest in rearing goats and sheep. It is important to diagnose reproductive disorders properly for the improvement of reproductive and productive efficiency.

References

Ababneh, M.M. and Degefa, T. (2006). Bacteriological findings and hormonal profiles in the postpartum Balady goats. *Reproduction in Domestic Animals* 41: 12–16.

Absy, G., Abuzead, S.M.M., and Zeidan, A.E. (2001). Resumption of postpartum ovarian activity in goats as affected by kidding season and body condition score under Egyptian conditions. *Indian Journal of Animal Sciences* 71: 922–926.

Agarwal, J.K., Vashistha, N.K., Sharma, A. et al. (2015). Histopathological study of naturally occurring pathological conditions of uterus affecting reproduction in small ruminants. *Indian Journal of Veterinary Science and Biotechnology* 11 (2): 19–22.

Ahmed, B.H., Hamad, R.J., and Abdelghafar, R.M. (2010). Ultrasonography for diagnosis of hydrometra and pyometra (two case reports). *Assiut Veterinary Medicine Journal* 56 (124): 1–6.

Alexandre, G., Gonzalez-Garcia, E., Lallo, C.H.O. et al. (2012). Genetic diversity of Ardi goat based on microsatellite analysis. *African Journal of Biotechnology* 11: 16539–16545.

Al-Hamedawi, T.M. (2011). Post partum pyometra in Iraqi goats: clinical and therapeutical study. *Iraqi Journal of Veterinary Medicine* 35 (2): 36–39.

Arguello, A. (2011). Trends in goat research: a review. *Journal of Applied Animal Research* 39 (4): 429–434.

Bocquier, F., Leboeuf, B., Guedon, L., and Chilliard, Y. (1996). Reproductive performances of artificially inseminated prepubertal goat: effects of feeding level and body weight. 33emes rencotres autours des rech.

Bonnett, B.N., Martin, S.W., and Meek, A.H. (1993). Associations of clinical findings, bacteriological and histological results of endometrial biopsy with reproductive performance of postpartum dairy cows. *Preventive Veterinary Medicine* 15: 205–220.

Castillo, J.M., Dockweiler, J.C., Cheong, S.H. et al. (2017). Pyometra and unilateral uterine horn torsion in a sheep. *Reproduction in Domestic Animals* 53: 274–277.

Durrani, A.Z. and Kamal, N. (2009). Prevalence of genital tract problems in clinical cases of species of animals. *Journal of Animal and Plant Science* 19 (3): 160–162.

Engeland, I.V., Waldeland, H., Andersen, O. et al. (1998). Foetal loss in dairy goats: an epidemiological study in 22 herds. *Small Ruminant Research* 30: 37–48.

Erasmus, J.A. and Fourie, A.J. (1985). Influence of age on reproductive performance of the improved Boer goat doe. *South African Journal of Animal Science* 15: 5–7.

Farin, P.W., Ball, L., Olson, J.D. et al. (1989). Effect of actinomyces pyogenes and gram-negative anaerobic bacteria on the development of bovine pyometra. *Theriogenology* 31: 979–989.

Giuliodori, M.J., Magnasco, R.P., Becu-Villalobos, D. et al. (2013). Metritis in dairy cows: risk factors and reproductive performance. *Journal of Dairy Science* 96: 3621–3631.

Goonewardene, L.A., Whitmore, W., Jaeger, S. et al. (1997). Effect of prebreeding maintenance diet on subsequent reproduction by artificial insemination in Alpine and Saanen goats. *Theriogenology* 48: 151–159.

Grohn, Y.T. and Rajala-Schultz, P.J. (2000). Epidemiology of reproductive performance in dairy cows. *Animal Reproduction Science* 60–61: 605–614.

Hammon, D.S., Evjen, I.M., Dhiman, T.R. et al. (2006). Neutrophil function and energy status in Holstein cows with uterine health disorders. *Veterinary Immunology and Immunopathology* 113: 21–29.

Hasnain, H.U. (1985). *Sheep and Goats in Pakistan. FAO Animal Production and Health Paper 56.*, 102–103. Rome: FAO.

Hesselink, J.W. (1993a). Hydrometra in dairy goats: reproductive performance after treatment with prostaglandins. *Veterinary Record* 133 (8): 186–187.

Hesselink, J.W. (1993b). Incidence of hydrometra in dairy goats. *Veterinary Record* 132: 110–112.

Jainudeen, M.R. and Hafez, E.S.E. (1987). Sheep and goats. In: *Reproduction in Farm Animals*, 3e (ed. E.S.E. (e.) Hafez), 135–146. Philadelphia, PA: Lea and Febiger.

Janeway, C.A., Travers, P., Walport, M., and Shlomchik, M.J. (e.) (2001). Infectious agents and how they cause disease. In: *Immunobiology: The Immune System in Health and Disease*, 382–388. New York: Garland Publishing.

Jeon, S.J., Cunha, F., Ma, X. et al. (2016). Uterine microbiota and immune parameters associated with fever in dairy cows with metritis. *PLoS One* 11 (11): e0165740.

Kahn, C.M. and Line, S. (2010). *The Merck Veterinary Manual*, 10e. Whitehouse Station, NJ: Merck and Co., Inc.

Kim, I.H. and Kang, H.G. (2003). Risk factors for postpartum endometritis and the effect of endometritis on reproductive performance in dairy cows in Korea. *Journal of Reproduction and Development* 49: 485–491.

Kosgey, I.S. and Okeyo, A.M. (2007). Genetic improvement of small ruminants in low-input, smallholder production systems: technical and infrastructural issues. *Small Ruminant Research* 70: 76–88.

LeBlanc, S.J., Osawa, T., and Dubuc, J. (2011). Reproductive tract defense and disease in postpartum dairy cows. *Theriogenology* 76: 1610–1618.

Levinson, W.E. and Jawetz, E. (1994). *Medical Microbiology and Immunology*, 3e, 20–23. Englewood Cliffs, NJ: Prentice Hall International Inc.

Lopes Junior, E.S., Cruz, J.F., Teixeira, D.I. et al. (2004). Pseudopregnancy in Saanen goats (Capra hircus) raised in Northeast Brazil. *Veterinary Research Communications* 28: 119–125.

Lyngset, O. (1968). Pathological conditions and malformations of the genital organs of the goat. *Acta Veterinaria Scandinavica* 9: 364–375.

Manes, J., Fiorentino, M.A., Kaiser, G. et al. (2010). Changes in the aerobic vaginal flora after treatment with different intravaginal devices in ewes. *Small Ruminant Research* 94: 201–204.

Martins, G., Figueira, L., Penna, B. et al. (2009). Prevalence and antimicrobial susceptibility of vaginal bacteria from ewes treated with progestin-impregnated intravaginal sponges. *Small Ruminant Research* 81: 182–184.

Mathis, D. and Shoelson, S.E. (2011). Immunometabolism: an emerging frontier. *National Review Immunology* 11 (2): 81.

McDowell, R.E. (1972). *Improvement of Livestock Production in Warm Climates*, 3e. San Francisco, CA: W.H. Freeman.

Mellado, M., Gonzalez, H., and Garcia, J.E. (2001). Body traits, parity and number of fetuses as risk factors for abortion in range goats. *Agrociencia* 35: 124–128.

Morrow, D.A. (1986). *Current Therapy in Veterinary Theriogenology: Diagnosis, Treatment and Prevention of Reproductive Diseases in Small and Large Animals*, 2e. Philadelphia, PA: W. B. Saunders.

Olson, J.D., Ball, L., Mortimer, R.G. et al. (1984). Aspects of bacteriology and endocrinology of cows with pyometra and retained fetal membranes. *American Journal of Veterinary Research* 45: 2251–2255.

Overton, M.W., Sischo, W.M., and Reynolds, J.P. (2003). Evaluation of the effect of estradiol cypionate administered prophylactically to post parturient dairy cows at high risk for metritis. *Journal of the American Veterinary Medical Association* 223: 846–851.

Pieterse, M.C. and Taverne, M.A.M. (1986). Hydrometra in goats: diagnosis with real time ultrasound and treatment with prostaglandin or oxytocin. *Theriogenology* 26 (5): 813–821.

Pugh, D.G. and Baird, N. (2012). *Sheep and Goat Medicine*, 216–238. St Louis, MO: Elsevier Health Sciences.

Ribeiro, E.S., Lima, F.S., Greco, L.F. et al. (2013). Prevalence of periparturient diseases and effects on fertility of seasonally calving grazing dairy cows supplemented with concentrates. *Journal of Dairy Science* 96: 5682–5697.

Rind, R. and Shaikh, S.N. (2000). Bacteriological studies on the uteri of slaughtered goats. *Pakistan Journal of Biological Sciences* 3: 1944–1947.

Risco, C.A. and Hernandez, J. (2003). Comparison of ceftiofur hydrochloride and estradiol cypionate for metritis prevention and reproductive performance in dairy cows affected with retained fetal membranes. *Theriogenology* 60: 47–58.

Roberts, S.J. (1986). *Veterinary Obstetrics and Genital Diseases*, 3e, 381–359. Woodstock, NY: S.J. Roberts.

Sargison, N.D., Howie, F., Mearns, R. et al. (2007). Shiga toxin-producing *Escherichia coli* as a perennial cause of abortion in a closed flock of Suffolk ewes. *Veterinary Record* 160: 875–876.

Sattar, A. and Khan, M.Z. (1988). Incidence and pathology of ovarian diseases of goats. *Pakistan Veterinary Journal* 3: 18–21.

Shallali, A.A., Hussein, A.M., Salih, M.M., and Dafalla, E.A. (2001). A preliminary report on bacteria isolated from the female genital tract of Sudanese sheep and goats. *Sudan Journal of Veterinary Research* 17: 55–63.

Sheldon, I.M., Noakes, D.E., Rycroft, A.N. et al. (2002). Influence of uterine bacterial contamination after parturition on ovarian dominant follicle selection and follicle growth and function in cattle. *Reproduction* 123: 837–845.

Sheldon, M., Lewis, G.S., LeBlanc, S., and Gilbert, R.O. (2006). Defining postpartum uterine disease in cattle. *Theriogenology* 65: 1516–1530.

Sheldon, I.M., Willians, E.J., Miller, A.N.A. et al. (2008). Uterine diseases in cattle after parturition. *Veterinary Journal* 176 (3): 115–121.

Silvestre, F.T., Carvalho, T.S., Crawford, P.C. et al. (2011). Effects of differential supplementation of fatty acids during the peripartum and breeding periods of Holstein cows: II. Neutrophil fatty acids and function, and acute phase proteins. *Journal of Dairy Science* 94: 2285–2301.

Sultan, A., Islam, M.R., Yadav, R.K. et al. (2015). Prevalence of different reproductive disorders of small ruminants in five upazillas of Mymensingh district. *Asian Journal of Medical and Biological Research* 1 (1): 74–79.

Timurkaan, N. and Karadas, E. (2000). Morphological investigations on the pathological changes of the female reproductive organs in goat. *Saglik Bilimleri Dergisi Firat Universitesi* 14 (1): 209–220.

36

Mastitis

Anil Kumar[1], Pardeep Sharma[2], Ankesh Kumar[1], and Tanmoy Rana[3]

[1] *Department of Veterinary Clinical Complex, Bihar Veterinary College, Bihar Animal Sciences University, Patna, India*
[2] *Department of Veterinary Medicine, Dr G.C. Negi College of Veterinary and Animal Sciences, Palampur, India*
[3] *Department of Veterinary Clinical Complex, West Bengal University of Animal and Fishery Sciences, Kolkata, India*

36.1 Introduction

Dairy goat farmers suffer significant economic losses as a result of intramammary infections (IMI). Mastitis losses result from poor milk quality, reduced milk yield, increased treatment costs, milk discard after treatment, and, in some cases, death due to the disease or culling of affected livestock (Mahlangu et al. 2018). Having a significant impact on human nutrition, goat milk and its byproducts are frequently utilized to feed starving and undernourished people in developing countries.

Mastitis is a complicated condition that causes inflammation of the mammary glands as a result of infection or physical trauma and, less commonly, allergy and neoplasm, ultimately leading to changes in intramammary tissues and related anatomical structures such as nipples, mammary areolas, and milk ducts. Mastitis is largely influenced by host, pathogen, and environmental predisposing factors. In the majority of small ruminants, cases of mastitis are caused by bacterial IMI, which are typically infections brought on by bacterial agents carried in the mammary and cutaneous tissues and/or disseminated during the milking process (Kahinda 2022). Apart from bacterial pathogens, viruses like lentivirus or caprine arthritis encephalitis and fungi also cause mastitis in goats (Machado 2018). The disease can develop in any type and breed of doe regardless of its milk yield.

Mastitis in goats is classified as either clinical or subclinical. Animals with clinical mastitis may exhibit edema, increased temperature, hardening and pain in the mammary gland, as well as the presence of lumps, pus, or other changes in the physical characteristics of the milk, and systemic alterations that may result in loss of the mammary gland and the animal's death (Machado 2018). In animals with subclinical mastitis, macroscopic changes do not occur in the milk but milk composition changes occur, with no signs of inflammation in the mammary halves. Subclinical mastitis is important because it serves as a reservoir for microorganisms and spreads infection to other animals in the herd (Shearer and Harris 2003). So, unless further diagnostic methods are applied, subclinical mastitis will go undetected. Cases of clinical mastitis can occur at any time of lactation or during the dry period.

36.2 Etiology

Several different groups of pathogens are responsible for IMI in goats, but *Staphylococcus* spp. are the most frequently diagnosed causal microorganisms in goats and sheep (Contreras et al. 2007). *Escherichia coli* is the main environmental pathogen. Apart from this, other pathogens, such as *Streptococcus* spp., the Enterobacteriaceae family, *Pseudomonas aeruginosa*, *Mannheimia haemolytica*, *Corynebacterium* spp., and fungi, can produce IMI in small ruminants (Polveiro et al. 2022).

Udder infections are classified into contagious or environmental-associated mastitis (Hogan and Smith 1987). Contagious bacteria can be found in the microbiota of the skin of the mammary, mucosal, and conjunctival parts of animals, as well

Elements of Reproduction and Reproductive Diseases of Goats, First Edition. Edited by Tanmoy Rana.

Table 36.1 Different groups of pathogens as causative agents of caprine mastitis.

Pathogens	References
Bacterial	
Staphylococcus spp.	Mahlangu et al. (2018), Shearer and Harris (2003), Ferdous et al. (2018), Danmallam et al. (2018), Bourabah et al. (2013), Najeeb et al. (2013), Danmallam and Pimenov (2019), Ahmed et al. (2020)
Escherichia coli	Mahlangu et al. (2018), Ferdous et al. (2018), Danmallam et al. (2018), Bourabah et al. (2013), Najeeb et al. (2013), Danmallam and Pimenov (2019)
Streptococcus spp.	Shearer and Harris (2003), Danmallam et al. (2018), Bourabah et al. (2013), Najeeb et al. (2013), Danmallam and Pimenov (2019)
Pseudomonas spp.	Ferdous et al. (2018), Danmallam et al. (2018), Bourabah et al. (2013), Najeeb et al. (2013)
Klebsiella spp.	Mahlangu et al. (2018), Ferdous et al. (2018), Danmallam et al. (2018), Bourabah et al. (2013), Danmallam and Pimenov (2019)
Bacillus spp.	Ferdous et al. (2018), Danmallam et al. (2018), Najeeb et al. (2013)
Corynebacterium spp.	Mahlangu et al. (2018), Shearer and Harris (2003), Bourabah et al. (2013), Ahmed et al. (2020)
Proteus spp.	Mahlangu et al. (2018), Danmallam et al. (2018), Danmallam and Pimenov (2019)
Serratia spp	Mahlangu et al. (2018), Danmallam and Pimenov (2019)
Citrobacter spp.	Mahlangu et al. (2018), Danmallam et al. (2018)
Micrococcus spp.	Mahlangu et al. (2018), Bourabah et al. (2013), Danmallam and Pimenov (2019)
Providencia spp.	Mahlangu et al. (2018), Danmallam and Pimenov (2019)
Micrococcus spp.	Mahlangu et al. (2018), Danmallam and Pimenov (2019)
Morganella spp.	Mahlangu et al. (2018), Danmallam et al. (2018), Danmallam and Pimenov (2019)
Mycoplasma spp.	Mahlangu et al. (2018), Shearer and Harris (2003)
Fungal	
Aspergillus niger, *A. nidulens*, and *A. fumigatus*	Bourabah et al. (2013), Ilhan et al. (2016), Ahmed et al. (2020)
Candida spp.	Ilhan et al. (2016), Khalaf et al. (2020), Ahmed et al. (2020)
Cryptococcus neoformans	Ilhan et al. (2016), Eunice (1999)
Nocardia spp.	Ilhan et al. (2016)
Penicillium spp.	Ilhan et al. (2016)
Scopulariopsis brevicaulis	Ilhan et al. (2016)

as on milking equipment, cleaning and drying cloths, and milkers' hands. Flies may act as mechanical vectors of contagious agents, which is important in properties with a high infestation and contributes to the transmission of microorganisms to goats and sheep (Anderson et al. 2004). Contagious agent infections are most common during milking, and microorganisms opportunistically invade the mammary gland, causing a rapid inflammatory response. Among the most common contagious pathogens, *S. aureus* and *S. agalactiae* are prevalent and usually cause subclinical mastitis with a high somatic cell count (SCC) (Hortet and Seegers 1998). *Staphylococcus aureus* is considered to be the primary causative agent of the inflammations. Several authors have reported different groups of pathogens of IMI in goats around the world as presented in Table 36.1.

36.3 Udder Immunity

The occurrence of mastitis increases when the mammary gland's defense mechanisms are impaired. Mammary gland immune defense varies throughout lactation in dairy animals and is typically suppressed with stress and around drying off and parturition, increasing susceptibility to mastitis.

The mammary gland's immune system provides both specific and nonspecific defenses to the newborn and to itself. Nonspecific defense mechanisms involve the gland's anatomical structure, the integrity of the teat canal, humoral factors, phagocytic cells, and food supplements, whereas specific defense mechanisms involve the release of species-specific immunoglobulins (Eunice 1999). Innate host defenses are based on germline-encoded receptors that recognize conserved structures expressed by a variety of microbes, as well as early induced cellular and soluble defenses.

When pathogens infect the mammary gland, the innate immune system reacts by infiltrating leukocytes and producing cytokines at the infection site (Ahmed et al. 2020; Hill et al. 1994). The teat end is regarded as the first line of defense against invading pathogens. Mastitis occurs when bacteria enter the mammary gland through the teat canal. Sphincter muscles in the teat maintain a tight closure between milking and prevent bacterial penetration (Zecconi et al. 2000). Furthermore, the teat duct's stratified squamous epithelium produces keratin, a waxy material that lines the teat canal and traps invading bacteria while preventing microorganism migration into the gland cistern. Keratin also contains antimicrobial agents that aid in the fight against infection (Paulrud 2005).

The canal of a teat may remain partly open for 1–2 hours after milking, and pathogens may freely enter the teat canal during this time from the environment, in particular from dirty bedding. Bacterial pathogens that can pass through the opening of the teat end avoid the antibacterial activity of the teat canal and start the disease process in the mammary gland, the host's second line of defense. Therefore, it is recommended that ruminants be moved to clean areas after milking and fed to avoid lying down and being exposed to contaminating environmental microbial organisms until teat ends close.

The mammary gland in dairy animals has a simple system consisting of teats and udder, where bacteria multiply and produce toxins, enzymes, and cell wall components that stimulate the production of inflammatory mediators that attract phagocytes. However, the severity of the inflammatory response is determined by both host (parity, lactation stage, age, and immune status, as well as SCC) and pathogen (species, virulence, strain, and inoculum size of bacteria) factors (Khan and Khan 2006).

In colostrum and milk, various types of innate immune components have been identified, including cellular defense components, which contain leukocytes, neutrophils, macrophages, and humoral defense components which contain complement system, immune-modulating factors, cytokines, lactoferrin, transferrin, and lysozyme. The components of the lactoperoxidase/myeloperoxidase systems, oligosaccharides, gangliosides, reactive oxygen species, acute-phase proteins, ribonucleases, and a wide range of antimicrobial peptides and proteins also play an important role in the innate immune response. These components are tightly integrated with the adaptive immune system and respond quickly to microbes during the early stages of infection (Stelwagen et al. 2009; Zigo et al. 2021).

36.4 Risk Factors Associated with Mastitis

Clinical and subclinical mastitis increase with increasing age, parity, and litter size. Prevalence is also higher in the early lactation stage (Islam et al. 2011). The higher occurrences in second and third lactations may be attributed to chronic infections from the previous lactation that had not been eliminated during the dry period, rather than solely to higher rates of new infection in older animals (Moroni et al. 2005). A late state of milk production (>90 days), number of births (>3), poor body condition, size of teats (>2 cm) and lack of premilking teat cleaning programs are associated with increased prevalence of subclinical mastitis in dairy herds (Tarazona-Manrique et al. 2022).

The main risk factor for increased mastitis prevalence is poor body condition (malnutrition or parasitic infection and old age compounded with reproduction stresses), which could be due to the animals' reduced defense status, which makes them more susceptible to udder infections by opportunistic organisms. In dairy cattle, a link between poor body condition and increased mastitis prevalence has been established (Tarazona-Manrique et al. 2022). Mastitis is more common during the wet season than during the dry season due to suitable microenvironmental conditions for mastitis microbes' maintenance and transmission. When, a dirty teat becomes wet due to rain or excessive discharge, the risk of infection increases. Wetness or water allows bacteria to move into the teat end, resulting in udder infection (Tarazona-Manrique et al. 2022; Megersa et al. 2010). Decreased teat end to floor distance in the mastitic doe increases the prevalence of mastitis. Goats with inverted or pointed teat ends are more prone to mastitis than goats with normal teat end shapes (Ameh and Tari 2000).

Milking technique and equipment are associated with mastitis, including poor udder preparation, cleanliness and milk let-down; dirty hands; cracked and worn teat liners; high vacuum levels; inadequate vacuum reserve; incorrect pulsation rate and ratio; overmilking; and failure to dip teats properly. Nutritional factors like low energy, selenium, and vitamin E also play a part (Menzies 2018). Therefore, farmers can improve their production processes by analyzing relevant risk factors and thus increase their income and improve their quality of life (Tarazona-Manrique et al. 2022).

36.5 Clinical Signs

Clinical mastitis can occur at any time during lactation or the dry period. The most severe clinical or per-acute mastitis seems to occur 2–4 weeks after lambing or kidding, and again shortly after weaning, but evidence to support this impression is lacking. Mastitis that develops during the dry period or late lactation is frequently overlooked until the following kidding (Menzies and Ramanoon 2001). Mastitis in does may be per acute (Menzies and Ramanoon 2001), acute, subclinical, or chronic (Ahmed et al. 2020). The clinical picture of per acute mastitis is typically dominantly presented by depression, an initial fever that may be followed by hypothermia, dehydration, anorexia, and a swollen, discolored gland (Figure 36.1). Lameness can be an important presenting sign in some cases. The affected gland's skin may turn reddish to purple and become cold to the touch. The discoloration frequently spreads beyond the gland to the belly wall and groin. The secretions are serum-like and reddish in color, and some time may contain gas (Menzies and Ramanoon 2001).

Acute mastitis is characterized by abnormal appearance and composition of milk, heat, pain, and swelling in the mammary gland with systemic signs including pyrexia, anorexia and altered milk secretion from affected halves. The most consistent clinical sign observed is abnormal secretion in the form of clots, flakes, or watery milk (Ahmed et al. 2020). There may be fibrotic lesions within the mammary tissues with a range of secretions from purulent to cheesy or no milk because of teat occlusion with fibrous tissue (Menzies and Ramanoon 2001).

Subclinical mastitis in goats is considered a major threat because it reduces milk production and is not readily detected clinically. It causes kid mortality due to mastitis milk feeding (Basavashree et al. 2022). Subclinical mastitis is difficult to detect because there are no visible signs in the mammary glands or milk (Mohammadian 2011). The presence of the subclinical form in the herd serves as a reservoir for microorganisms that cause infection of other animals. This form of the disease is important because it is 15–40 times more prevalent than the clinical form, and usually precedes the clinical form. It is of long duration, difficult to detect, reduces milk production, and adversely affects milk quality (Shearer and Harris 2003).

36.6 Diagnosis

Mastitis is the most common infection in dairy goats, affecting milk production and quality. Bacterial cultures and SCCs are the best diagnostic methods for detecting IMI in goats (Paterna et al. 2014) and are widely accepted as the gold standard by many authors (Contreras et al. 2007). Aside from microbial culture, identifying macroscopic changes in milk and signs of inflammation in the udder is critical for determining clinical mastitis in goats (Bergonier et al. 2003). It is usually detected by visual inspection and palpation of the mammary gland. Clinical mastitis is relatively easy to detect but animals with subclinical mastitis are frequently difficult to locate due to a lack of reliable diagnostic methods, particularly at farm level. The presence or absence of external inflammation distinguishes clinical and subclinical mastitis. In the absence of signs of inflammation, indirect methods of diagnosis based on the measurement of inflammation indicators, with a focus on SCCs, are the primary tools for subclinical mastitis diagnosis.

Subclinical forms of the disease are common, which lack the typical clinical signs but are still associated with reduced milk production and safety for human consumption, with a high bacterial count (Matuozzo et al. 2020). As a result, subclinical forms necessitate a wide range of diagnostic techniques, both on the farm and in the laboratory. The presence of inflammatory markers in the milk and microbiological isolation of the causative agent are used to diagnose subclinical mastitis. Mastitis causes changes in milk SCCs as well as physical and chemical properties (Hristov et al. 2015; Dimitrov et al. 2018). Clinical mastitis is uncommon in goats but subclinical mastitis is much more common, and SCC is more common in goats than cows (Contreras et al. 2007; Paape et al. 2007; Koop et al. 2012; Paterna et al. 2014).

The traditional diagnosis of clinical or subclinical mastitis using microbiological cultures is simple and does not necessitate complex laboratory procedures. Aerobic blood agar is typically used for bacterial culture, in accordance with the protocols of the US National Mastitis Council (Oliver et al. 2004; Paterna et al. 2014). Plate count agar (PCA) is used to determine total bacterial growth in accordance with ISO 4833:2003 (Koop et al. 2011), and these procedures necessitate collecting milk under aseptic conditions and after removing the first jets of milk. The samples are cultured and incubated for 24–72 hours according to the methodology, and the result is a count of observable colonies expressed in colony-forming units (CFU) per ml (Contreras et al. 2007). The infection threshold utilized in the diagnosis of subclinical IMI, with certain

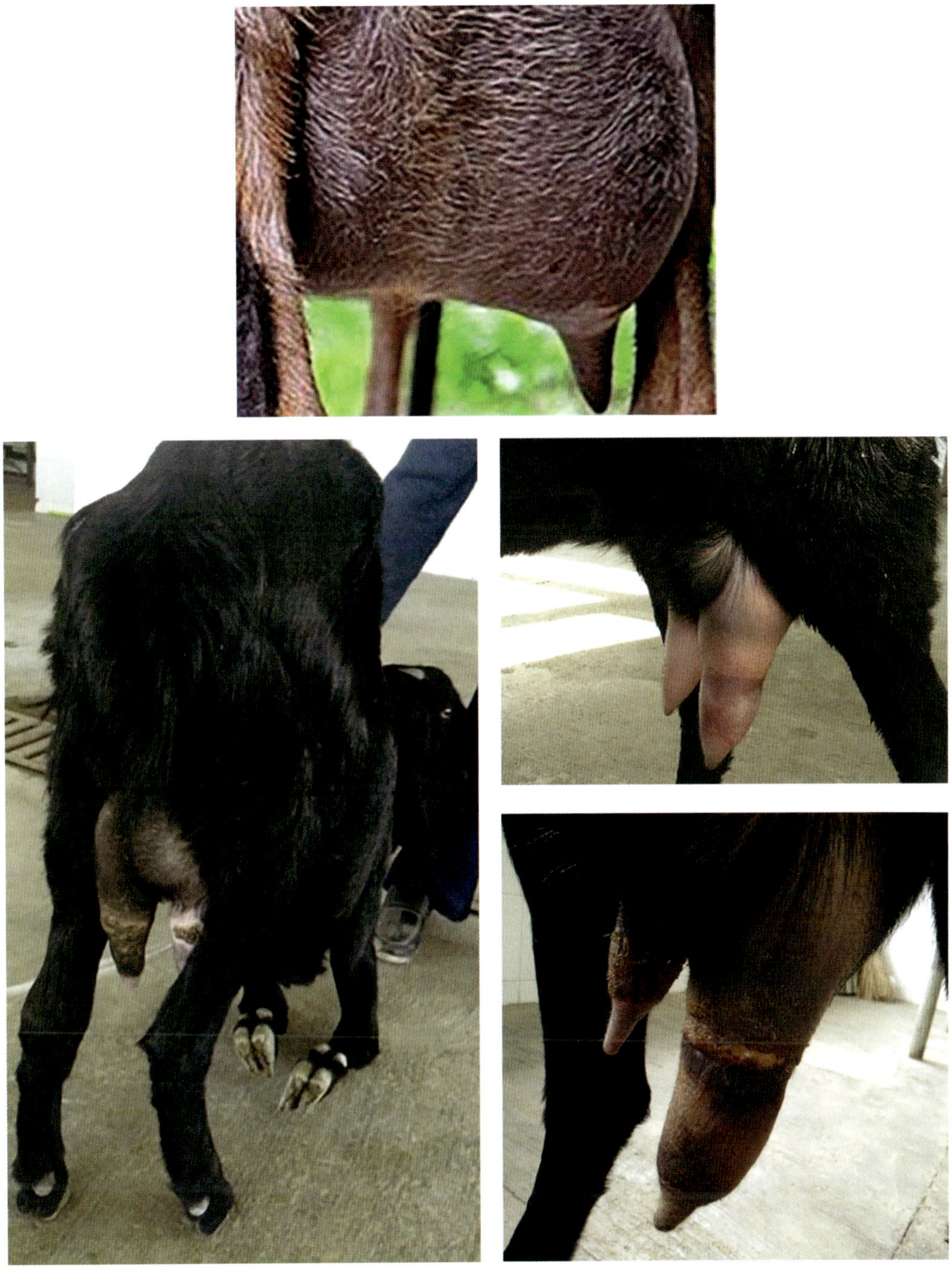

Figure 36.1 Mastitis in a goat.

exceptions (such as *Staphylococcus aureus* and *Mycoplasma* spp.), varies from 250 to 500 CFU/ml (Oliver et al. 2004). Bacterial contamination of the sample can result in false-negative results due to the inhibition of bacterial growth by lowering pH which is caused by fermentation of the contaminating flora, which decreases the test's sensitivity. Moreover, it has limitations in terms of identifying mastitis caused by *S. aureus* (Koop et al. 2011, 2012).

Techniques based on the detection of particular DNA fragments by PCR can be a supplement to bacterial culture. Due to the high specificity gained, the use of PCR has advantages over conventional approaches, such as the capacity to detect infections that have been altered by storage conditions (such as freezing) or chemical preservatives quickly and with fewer false negatives (Schwaiger et al. 2012). Because the sample may contain multiple bacterial species or produce false-positive results in animals without inflammation, the interpretation of PCR data should be undertaken with caution (Koskinen et al. 2009).

Somatic cells are white blood cells in milk, as well as a small number of epithelial cells from milk-secreting tissues, measured at gland level, at animal level, or at herd level. The SCC at herd level (bulk milk SCC) is a weighted average of the SCCs of all animals contributing to the milk in the bulk tank. Similarly, animal-level SCC (composite SCC) is a weighted average of the SCC of both udder glands of a goat. Because of dilution with milk from the uninfected udder half, the composite SCC of an infected animal will generally be lower than the gland-level SCC of an infected gland (Koop et al. 2012).

These cells play an important role in the goat's natural defense system. When udder tissue is damaged or infected, a large number of white blood cells accumulate in the milk. Normal goat milk contains more cells than normal cow milk. The higher cell count of goat milk is caused in part by an increase in the rate of sloughing of these epithelial cells and the presence of cytoplasmic masses as a result of the apocrine secretory process. Epithelial cell sloughing is a normal physiological process in the mammary gland. It is important to note that excessive cell sloughing is also found due to infection with the caprine-arthritis-encephalitis virus (Shearer and Harris 2003). Therefore, standards for SCC in milk established for cows are not appropriate for goats. The SCC test in goats is still not widely recognized as a standard diagnostic test, because of the biological specifics of these animals. Large numbers of inflammatory cells are found in milk from both infected and culture-negative goats, and SCC appears to be affected by both infectious and noninfectious factors. Noninfectious factors should be considered when using SCC as a diagnostic tool to assess the udder health status of a goat or goat herd (Koop et al. 2012).

A reliable direct method of measuring SCC is to use an automatic cell counter, either at the farm with a portable cell counter or by sending milk samples to a laboratory for measurement. An automatic cell counter has the advantage of being objective and accurate. The disadvantages are that it can be time consuming if sent to a laboratory or costly if used on the farm due to the expensive equipment required (Persson and Olofsson 2011).

The California Mastitis Test (CMT) can be used to perform SCCs on milk samples from individual goats with reasonable accuracy. The CMT reagent forms a gel by reacting with the genetic material of somatic cells found in milk. This reaction leads to changes in the milk viscosity so the higher the cell content, the higher the viscosity change. Guidelines to interpretation of CMT and SCC results are presented in Tables 36.2 and 36.3 (Shearer and Harris 2003).

The scores are roughly proportional to the number of somatic cells in milk. SCCs in milk tend to rise during milking and remain elevated for a few hours afterwards. Tests should be performed just before milking, after stimulating the milk and discarding the foremilk, for reliable results. The use of milk electrical conductivity is not widely accepted yet in dairy goat practice compared to dairy cattle, and is still to be developed. This is due to the absence of research and evidence in goat practice. Significant correlation between electrical conductivity and SCC, as has been established in cow's milk, has not been described in goats (Park 1991).

Table 36.2 Scores from the California Mastitis Test on goat milk.

CMT score	Reaction	Mean no. neutrophils per ml
0	No reaction	68 000
Trace	Slight slime, and tends to disappear with continued swirling	268 000
1	Distinct slime but without gel	800 000
2	Immediate gel formation, moves as a mass during swirling	256 000
3	Gel develops a convex surface and adheres to the bottom of the cup	≥10 000 000

Table 36.3 Interpretation of somatic cell count (SCC) from individual goat milk samples.

SCC/ml	Interpretation
<1000	Healthy glands
2000 to 500 000	Infection by weak pathogens
Over 1 500 000	Significant infection

In mastitis, the inflammation increases the concentration of some hydrolytic enzymes like NAGase and beta-glucoronidase, which are normally stored in lysosomes. Another nonlysosomic enzyme that also increases is lactate dehydrogenase which could be used as a diagnostic characteristic of the mastitic gland (Dimitrov et al. 2018). Increased level of lactoferrin (LF) can serve as an indicator for mastitis diagnosis. It is a nonspecific immune factor, having antimicrobial activity against bacteria, fungi, and some viruses. LF is not affected by the season or lactation stage so can be used to diagnose mastitis at any stage of the reproductive cycle (Dimitrov et al. 2018).

Mastitis causes an increase in milk lysozyme concentration, especially in clinical forms. Lysozyme is a glycoprotein that can be found in large quantities in egg whites and other biological fluids from both humans and animals. It acts on peptidoglycan, a substance found in bacterial cell walls of Gram-positive bacteria. It can lyze Gram-negative bacteria with synergistic interaction with some basic proteins released by neutrophilic granulocytes, which makes it easier for them to pass through the bacterial cell wall. Due to the following immunological characteristics of the products of peptidoglycan destruction, lysozyme also has an immunomodulatory function: it induces humoral and cellular immune responses; activates lymphocytes and macrophages through the release of cytokines; and increases neutrophil granulocytes' bactericidal activity (Cannas et al. 2019). A protein called amyloid A, which is found in milk after mammary gland inflammation, has been proposed as a biomarker for mastitis diagnosis (Winter et al. 2006; Miglio et al. 2013).

36.7 Treatment and Control

In small ruminants, no detailed protocols for treatment of mastitis are available, as have been developed in cows. As soon as the first symptoms of the disease are noticed, treatment should begin immediately and efficient antibiotic drugs should be used. Rapid disease progression and consequent gland damage occur, and histological lesions in the mammary gland become visible two days after infection. Thus, early treatment initiation is crucial to reduce mammary lesions and restore the health of affected does. Although clinical cure occurs, bacteriological cure is not always possible. Bacteria in the mammary gland may thus result in decreased production, the development of mammary abscesses, or the recurrence of clinical disorders (Mavrogianni et al. 2011).

Very few drugs are approved for use in lactating dairy sheep and goats, and frequently off-label drugs are prescribed. The veterinarian must ensure that residues do not enter the food chain. There is little research on the right withdrawal times for dairy sheep and goat milk. The animal's attitude, appetite, and the presence of fever should be used as the first indicators of whether there is severe systemic involvement. One may continue with treatment if the mastitis looks to be contained to the udder by first "milking out" the affected gland. On rare occasions, this process can be assisted by injecting 2 IU of oxytocin (avoid using oxytocin if the animal is in the second part of gestation), followed by the infusion of an intramammary infusion product into the affected gland (Figure 36.2). It is sufficient to use half of a tube of bovine mastitis medicine (Shearer and Harris 2003).

Many errors can occur when infusing intramammary tubes, leading to treatment failure. The most common error is inadequate cleansing of the teat orifice prior to insertion of the tube, which can result in the introduction of new bacteria, fungi, or yeasts into the teat, potentially leading to more severe disease, so the area around the teat orifice should be thoroughly cleaned and disinfected with an alcohol solution before inserting the antibiotic tube. Administration of half an intramammary tube (when using cow tubes) can lead to underdosing with two consequences: treatment failure and promotion of resistance development among causal bacteria.

The above described technique for treating local inflammation involving the udder should also be used in cases where the infection is systemic (affecting the entire body), along with intramuscular administration of medicines like penicillin, ampicillin, erythromycin, or tetracycline. In extreme cases, hydration treatment, antihistamines, and antiinflammatory medications may be necessary. Owners are advised to consult their local veterinarian for specific advice on therapy under such circumstances (Shearer and Harris 2003).

Numerous antibiotics are used in field conditions for treating mastitis in goats in Bangladesh. Commonly used antimicrobials include gentamicin, gentamicin+ amoxicillin, amoxicillin, benzylpenicillin, streptomycin + procaine penicillin, ceftriaxone, sulfadimidine, gentamicin + sulfadimidine + trimethoprim, gentamicin + amoxicillin + sulfadimidine, and tetracycline. Gentamicin + colistin has greater efficacy for the treatment of coliform mastitis caused by *E. coli* (Rudra and Dutta 2018). A broad-spectrum antibiotic, ceftriaxone, was found to be effective in mastitis following single-dose intravenous administration in cows and goats (Sar et al. 2006). Treatment should include the use of effective antimicrobial agents. To preserve pathogen susceptibility to available drugs, treatment should ideally be performed with a narrow-spectrum drug that is specifically

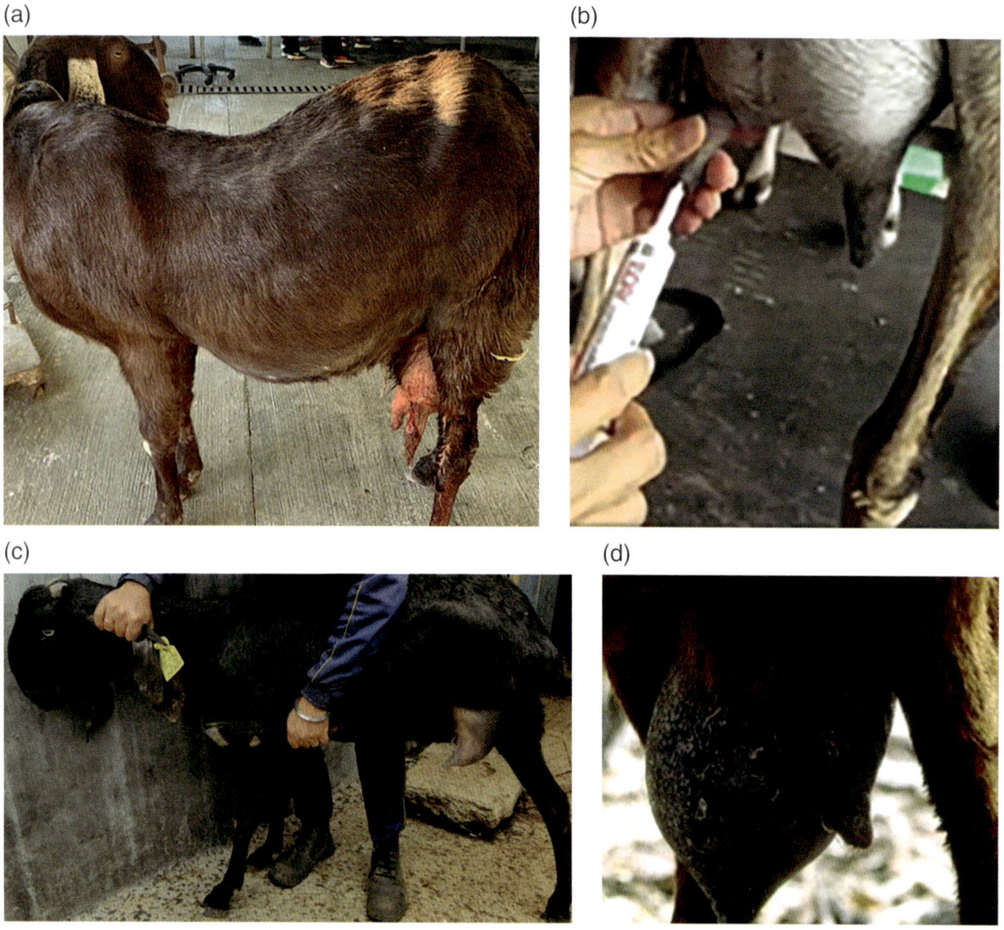

Figure 36.2 (a) Inflamed udder. (b) Intramammary infusion. (c) Examination of inflamed udder. (d) Inflamed sloughing udder.

effective against the causal agent of each case. The drug should be administered after the causal agent has been identified and its susceptibility profile established. This may not always be possible due to two competing factors: (i) the need for prompt treatment at early investigation, and (ii) the time required to conduct a thorough bacteriological examination including bacterial isolation, identification, and susceptibility testing. Therefore, treatment can be initiated blindly with a broad-spectrum product that is effective against the disease's major causal agents.

Treatment is also important for reducing sources of infection in the rest of the flock (Kiossis et al. 2007). When the disease progresses quickly or is accompanied by systemic symptoms, systemic administration of injectable antibiotics is indicated. In these situations, the resulting bacteremia cannot be treated by intramammary administration of antibiotics alone. In addition, systemic administration of injectable antibiotics is indicated in cases of long-lasting, subacute mastitis when inflammatory debris clogs the mammary gland's duct system, preventing full diffusion of intramammary antibiotics (Mavrogianni et al. 2011). Nonsteroidal antiinflammatory drugs have been recommended as a supportive treatment for mastitis to reduce the disease's clinical symptoms and raise the animal's welfare standards. For this reason, flunixin meglumine has been found to help by improving clinical signs, especially those of the mammary gland, and by restoring normal body temperature.

Electrolytes and intravenous dextrose administration can be recommended in severe disease cases and should be continued until the animal has fully recovered. With effects on antibody production, cell proliferation, cytokine production, prostaglandin metabolism, and neutrophil functions, vitamin E supplementation is crucial for the immune system's proper operation. The antioxidant effect of this vitamin, which helps to protect phagocytic cells and tissues from oxidative attacks of free radicals caused by the neutrophil and macrophage respiratory burst during phagocytosis, is thought to be the mechanism by which it improves the body's defense against infections (Machado 2018).

In areas with low levels of selenium, it is strongly advised to supplement programmes to prevent clinical mastitis and enhance milk quality with selenium from any source (Sanchez et al. 2007).

Treatment during the drying-off period is an efficient method for the cure of subclinical mastitis and for control of somatic cell counting. Mastitis treatment failure is a common event. The following are the main causes of treatment failure: (i) a delayed start to treatment; (ii) the use of an inappropriate or ineffective medication (i.e., one that is inappropriate or ineffective when used to treat the specific mastitis case at issue); (iii) using an improper route of administration (for instance, an abscess within the parenchyma prevents an antimicrobial agent infused into the mammary gland from reaching bacteria); (iv) ceasing treatment at the first sign of clinical improvement – an improvement in clinical symptoms does not mean that all bacteria have been killed, which could result in a subsequent recurrence of the illness; (v) using a full intramammary tube rather than the recommended dosage at each treatment site; (vi) using products that are out of date, which have decreased efficacy; (vii) using products that have been contaminated due to improper handling or storage; and (viii) contamination of the mammary gland while inserting the intramammary tube to an inadequately cleaned teat orifice, which can result in the simultaneous entry of other organisms that can cause mastitis (Mavrogianni et al. 2011).

The fundamental principles of mastitis control are to decrease the exposure of the teat to potential pathogens and increase resistance of dairy animals to infection. As there are few specific drugs available for treatment of mastitis in goats and resistance to antibiotics needs to be considered, prevention is essential in the management of mastitis. The main goal of prevention is knowing the risk factors that favor the onset and spread of udder diseases and taking action against them (De Vliegher et al. 2012). Therefore, maintaining proper farming practices and respecting animal needs are necessary to prevent mastitis.

In particular, hygiene and health procedures associated with the implementation of biosecurity measures represent the necessary tools to prevent mastitis and its spread, as well as minimizing the use of antibiotics. Attention must be paid to the milking routine, as well as to management of the milking machine and milking parlor, because milking is a crucial stage for the onset and spread of mastitis (Cannas et al. 2019). Udder health and milk quality are influenced by the milking routine. It must be performed in a clean environment. Small ruminants are particularly sensitive to stressful situations like noises and sudden movements, which must be minimized. To detect any milk abnormalities, the first milk jets must be examined (strip test) for indications of clinical mastitis). It is advised to change the milking entry order during a mastitis outbreak to give the healthy animals priority or to manually milk the infected animals.

Teat dipping is the action of cleaning the teats after each milking, intended to keep bacterial contamination of the teats under control. Reducing the amount of bacteria on the teat skin is essential for preventing udder infections, which reduces the risk of mastitis developing and spreading, as well as its direct effect on milk quality (Cannas et al. 2019). There are various methods of applying disinfectants, including sprinklers and teat immersion. Immersion ensures that the teat is completely cleaned but it also raises the possibility of contamination, necessitating the replacement of the disinfectant when this happens. Teat spraying is quicker and less prone to contamination, although less accurate. Improving udder and teat cleanliness should be the main goal of managing environmental diseases. Prior to cluster attachment, animals should be checked for hygiene both in and out of the milking parlor, i.e., in housing or the field. The management of bedding, increased ventilation, and premilking practices are all likely to be crucial in preventing an environmental mastitis outbreak. To encourage animals to stand for 30 minutes after milking to facilitate teat sphincter closure, good access to feed and water is crucial. In comparison to cattle, goats and sheep carry a higher percentage of milk in the milk cistern as opposed to the alveoli. This indicates that prior to milking, teat cleaning is more crucial for maintaining teat cleanliness than milk letdown. Gross contamination must be eliminated since it can result in higher bacterial counts in bulk milk or environmental mastitis. To save time, clusters are frequently administered fast and without foremilking.

It is important to ensure that the milking machines are correctly set up for different species. In comparison to cattle, a system vacuum of 37–38 Pa and a pulsation rate of 90–120 pulses per minute are recommended in goats. Farms that use an automatic cluster removal system need to calibrate it for a lower milk flow rate than dairy cattle. Starting rates of 200 g/min + 10 second delay for goats and 150 g/min + 10 second delay for sheep are advised, though settings should be assessed on a farm-by-farm basis. Moreover, postmilking teat cleaning is advised in herds, especially those with an infectious etiology. Small ruminant dairies hardly ever utilize it, despite evidence that it lowers the rate of new infections.

Animals with palpable lesions or other signs of irreversible udder damage should be culled because they pose a risk to other animals by acting as reservoirs of pathogens and because they are less productive. Animals that are chronically infected and relapse frequently should also be culled (Manning et al. 2021). Startvac® (Hipra), a vaccine that is used in cattle, contains inactive *Escherichia coli* and *S. aureus* and prevents development of the staphylococcal slime factor and the capsule formation of coliform bacteria. This vaccine could increase treatment success in gangrenous mastitis cases in sheep and goats when administered as a single dose at the beginning of treatment in addition to the classic clinical treatment.

In order to provide protection from the start of the lactation period (i.e., when the mammary gland starts to be at risk for developing mastitis), the full immunization schedule should be finished before the anticipated parturition. Many studies have demonstrated milder clinical symptoms and a decrease in the incidence risk of infection. When compared to unvaccinated controls, vaccinated does show a decrease in SCC and infection rate and an increase in the rate of spontaneous cure (Kautz et al. 2014).

Thus, it can be concluded that the administration of the mastitis vaccine in addition to the standard clinical treatment could increase the effectiveness of treatment (Yesilmen et al. 2017). In any case, vaccination should not be viewed as the exclusive method of mastitis management. To better control the infection, other udder health management strategies should be included (Manning et al. 2021).

References

Ahmed, Y., Ezzo, O.H., and Ahmed, S.M. (2020). Some udder problems associated with productivity in goats. *Egyptian Journal of Veterinary Science* 51 (1): 1–9.

Ameh, J.A. and Tari, I.S. (2000). Observations on the prevalence of caprine mastitis in relation to predisposing factors in Maiduguri. *Small Ruminant Research* 35: 1–5.

Anderson, D.E., Hull, B.H., and Pugh, D.G. (2004). Enfermidades da glândula mamária. In: *Clínica de Ovinos e Caprinos* (ed. D.E. Anderson, L.H. Bruce, and D.G. Pugh), 379–399. Roca, Sao Paulo: Capitulo.

Basavashree, K., Patil, N.A., Halmandge, S.C. et al. (2022). Prevalence and therapeutic management of subclinical mastitis in goats. *Pharma Innovation Journal* SP-11 (8): 2041–2042.

Bergonier, D., de Cremoux, R., Rupp, R. et al. (2003). Mastitis of dairy small ruminants. *Veterinary Research* 34: 689–716.

Bourabah, A., Ayad, A., Boukraa, L. et al. (2013). Prevalence and etiology of subclinical mastitis in goats of the Tiaret region, Algeria. *Global Veterinaria* 11 (5): 604–608.

Cannas, E.A. et al. (2019). *Mastitis in Small Ruminants*. Sardinia: Istituto Zooprofilattico Sperimentale Della Sardegna.

Contreras, A., Sierra, D., Sánchez, A. et al. (2007). Mastitis in small ruminants. *Small Ruminant Research* 68: 145–153.

Danmallam, F.A. and Pimenov, N.V. (2019). Study on prevalence, clinical presentation, and associated bacterial pathogens of goat mastitis in Bauchi, Plateau, and Edo states, Nigeria. *Veterinary World* 12 (5): 638–645.

Danmallam, F.A., Pimenov, N.V., Ngulukun, S.S., and Mwankon, S.E. (2018). Prevalence and bacterial etiology of mastitis in small ruminants in Toro local government area, Bauchi state, Nigeria. *Russian Journal of Agricultural and Socio-Economic Sciences* 7 (79): 341–345.

De Vliegher, S., Fox, L.K., Piepers, S. et al. (2012). Mastitis in dairy heifers: nature of the disease, potential impact, prevention and control. *Journal of Dairy Science* 95 (3): 1025–1040.

Dimitrov, D., Stoimenov, G., and Morrison, O. (2018). Diagnosis of subclinical mastitis in dairy goats (review). *MedInform* 1: 702–707.

Eunice, N.N. (1999). Prevalence of dairy goat mastitis in Central Kenya Highlands. MSc thesis. University of Nairobi.

Ferdous, J., Rahman, M.S., Khan, M.I. et al. (2018). Prevalence of clinical and subclinical caprine mastitis of northern region in Bangladesh. *Progressive Agriculture* 29 (2): 127–138.

Hill, A.W., Finch, J.M., Field, T.R., and Leigh, J.A. (1994). Immune modification of the pathogenesis of *Streptococcus uberis* mastitis in the dairy cow. *FEMS Immunology and Medical Microbiology* 8 (2): 109–117.

Hogan, J.S. and Smith, K.L. (1987). A practical look at environmental mastitis. *Compendium on Continuing Education for the Practicing Veterinarian* 9: 341–346.

Hortet, P. and Seegers, H. (1998). Calculated milk production losses associated with elevated somatic cells counts in dairy cows: review and critical discussion. *Veterinary Research* 29: 497–510.

Hristov, K., Parvanov, P., Pepovich, R., and Nikolov, B. (2015). Prevalence of mastitis and dynamics of health status mammary gland during lactation and dry period in goats. *Scientific Works. Series C. Veterinary Medicine* LXI (1): 163–167.

Ilhan, Z., Ekin, H.I., Koltas, S. et al. (2016). Occurrence of fungal agents in mastitis in dairy goats. *Journal of Animal and Plant Science* 29 (3): 4691–4700.

Islam, M.A., Samad, M.A., and Anisur Rahman, A.K.M. (2011). Bacterial pathogens and risk factors associated with mastitis in black Bengal goats in Bangladesh. *Bangladesh Journal of Veterinary Medicine* 9 (2): 155–159.

Kahinda, C.T.M. (2022). Mastitis in small ruminants. In: *Mastitis in Dairy Cattle, Sheep and Goats*, 1e (ed. O.K. Dego). www.intechopen.com/chapters/76529.

Kautz, F.M., Nickerson, S.C., and Ely, L.O. (2014). Use of a staphylococcal vaccine to reduce prevalence of mastitis and lower somatic cell counts in a registered Saanen dairy goat herd. *Research in Veterinary Science* 97 (1): 18–19.

Khalaf, D.D., Soliman, M.M.H., and Mansour, A.S. (2020). Conventional and molecular identification of mycotic mastitis caused by Candida in farm animals. *International Journal of Veterinary Science* 10 (1): 64–68. .

Khan, M.Z. and Khan, A. (2006). Basic facts of mastitis in dairy animals: a review. *Pakistan Veterinary Journal* 26 (4): 204–208.

Kiossis, E., Brozos, C.N., Petridou, E. et al. (2007). Program for the control of subclinical mastitis in dairy Chios breed ewes during lactation. *Small Ruminant Research* 73: 194–199.

Koop, G., Van-Werven, T., Toft, N. et al. (2011). Estimating test characteristics of somatic cell count to detect Staphylococcus aureus-infected dairy goats using latent class analysis. *Journal of Dairy Science* 94 (6): 2902–2911.

Koop, G., Nielen, M., and Werven, T.V. (2012). Diagnostic tools to monitor udder health in dairy goats. *Veterinary Quarterly* 32 (1): 37–44.

Koskinen, M.T., Holopainen, J., Pyörälä, S. et al. (2009). Analytical specificity and sensitivity of a real-time polymerase chain reaction assay for identification of bovine mastitis pathogens. *Journal of Dairy Science* 92: 952–959.

Machado, G.P. (2018). Mastitis in small ruminants. *Animal Husbandry, Dairy and Veterinary Science* 2 (4): 1–9.

Mahlangu, P., Maina, N., and Kagira, J. (2018). Prevalence, risk factors, and antibiogram of bacteria isolated from milk of goats with subclinical mastitis in Thika east subcounty, Kenya. *Journal of Veterinary Medicine* 2018: 3801479. .

Manning, A.I., Vasileiou, N., and Crilly, J.P. (2021). Control of mastitis in dairy sheep and goats. *Livestock* 26 (3): 161–168.

Matuozzo, M., Spagnuolo, M.S., Hussein, H.A. et al. (2020). Novel biomarkers of mastitis in goat milk revealed by MALDI-TOF-MS-based peptide profiling. *Biology* 9 (8): 193.

Mavrogianni, V.S., Menzies, P.I., Fragkou, I.A., and Fthenakis, G.C. (2011). Principles of mastitis treatment in sheep and goats. *Veterinary Clinics of North America: Food Animal Practice* 27 (1): 115–120.

Megersa, B., Tadesse, C., Abunna, F. et al. (2010). Occurrence of mastitis and associated risk factors in lactating goats under pastoral management in Borana, southern Ethiopia. *Tropical Animal Health and Production* 42: 1249–1255.

Menzies, P.I. (2018). Guide to udder health for dairy goats – providing guidance for veterinarians and producers in improving milk quality. *AABP Proceedings* 51 (2): 205–2011.

Menzies, P.I. and Ramanoon, S.Z. (2001). Mastitis of sheep and goats. *Veterinary Clinics of North America: Food Animal Practice* 17 (2): 333–358.

Miglio, A., Moscati, L., Fruganti, G. et al. (2013). Use of milk amyloid A in the diagnosis of subclinical mastitis in dairy ewes. *Journal of Dairy Research* 80: 496–502.

Mohammadian, B. (2011). The effect of subclinical mastitis on lactate dehydrogenase in dairy cows. *International Journal of Animal and Veterinary Advances* 3 (3): 161–163.

Moroni, P., Pisoni, G., Ruffo, G., and Boettcher, P.J. (2005). Risk factors for intramammary infections and relationship with somatic-cell counts in Italian dairy goats. *Preventive Veterinary Medicine* 69 (3–4): 163–173.

Najeeb, M.F., Anjum, A.A., Ahmad, M.U.D. et al. (2013). Bacterial etiology of subclinical mastitis in dairy goats and multiple drug resistance of the isolates. *Journal of Animal and Plant Sciences* 23 (6): 1541–1544.

Oliver, S.P., Gonzalez, R.N., Hogan, J.S. et al. (2004). *Microbiological Procedures for the Diagnosis of Bovine Udder Infection and Determination of Milk Quality*. Verona, WI: National Mastitis Council.

Paape, M.J., Wiggans, G.R., Bannerman, D.D. et al. (2007). Monitoring goat and sheep milk somatic cell counts. *Small Ruminant Research* 68: 114–125.

Park, Y.W. (1991). Interrelationships between somatic cell counts, electrical conductivity, bacteria counts, percent fat and protein in goat milk. *Small Ruminant Research* 5: 367–375.

Paterna, A., Contreras, A., Gómez-Martín, A. et al. (2014). The diagnosis of mastitis and contagious agalactia in dairy goats. *Small Ruminant Research* 121: 36–41.

Paulrud, C.O. (2005). Basic concepts of the bovine teat canal. *Veterinary Research Communications* 29 (3): 215–245.

Persson, Y. and Olofsson, I. (2011). Direct and indirect measurement of somatic cell count as indicator of intramammary infection in dairy goats. *Acta Veterinaria Scandinavica* 53: 15.

Polveiro, R.C., Vidigal, P.M.P., de Oliveira Mendes, T.A. et al. (2022). Distinguishing the milk microbiota of healthy goats and goats diagnosed with subclinical mastitis, clinical mastitis, and gangrenous mastitis. *Frontiers in Microbiology* 13: 918706.

Rudra, P.G. and Dutta, A. (2018). E. coli coliform mastitis in doe and its antibiogram. *Journal of Bacteriology and Mycology* 5 (1): 1059.

Sanchez, J., Montes, P., Jimenez, A., and Andres, S. (2007). Prevention of clinical mastitis with barium selenate in dairy goats from a selenium-deficient area. *Journal of Dairy Science* 90: 2350–2354.

Sar, T.K., Mandal, T.K., Das, S.K. et al. (2006). Pharmacokinetics of ceftriaxone in healthy and mastitic goats with special reference to its interaction with polyherbal drug (Fibrosin®). *International Journal of Applied Research in Veterinary Medicine* 4 (2): 142–154.

Schwaiger, K., Wimmer, M., Huber-Schlenstedt, R. et al. (2012). Hot topic: bovine milk samples yielding negative or nonspecific results in bacterial culturing – the possible role of PCR-single strand conformation polymorphism in mastitis diagnosis. *Journal of Dairy Science* 95: 98–101.

Shearer, J.K. and Harris, B. Jr. (2003). *Mastitis in Dairy Goats*. Institute of Food and Agricultural Sciences, University of Florida.

Stelwagen, K., Carpenter, E., Haigh, B. et al. (2009). Immune components of bovine colostrum and milk. *Journal of Animal Science* 87: 3–9.

Tarazona-Manrique, L.E., Salamanca-Acuña, E.E., Andrade-Becerra, R.J., and Vargas-Abella, J.C. (2022). Determination of risk factors related to prevalence of subclinical mastitis in dairy goats in Boyacá, Colombia. *Revista MVZ Cordoba* 27 (Suppl): e2774. .

Winter, P., Miny, M., Fuchs, K., and Baumgartner, W. (2006). The potential of measuring serum amyloid A in individual ewe milk and in farm bulk milk for monitoring udder health on sheep dairy farms. *Research in Veterinary Science* 81 (3): 321–326.

Yesilmen, S., Isik, N., Ozyurtlu, N. et al. (2017). Investigation on the effectiveness of mastitis vaccine (Startvac®) in sheep and goat gangrenous mastitis cases caused by Staphylococcus aureus. *Dicle Üniversitesi Veteriner Fakültesi Dergisi* 10 (2): 107–114.

Zecconi, A., Hamann, J., Bronzo, V. et al. (2000). Relationship between teat tissue immune defences and intramammary infections. *Advances in Experimental Medicine and Biology* 480: 287–293.

Zigo, F., Vasil', M., Ondrašovičová, S. et al. (2021). Maintaining optimal mammary gland health and prevention of mastitis. *Frontiers in Veterinary Science* 8: 607311.

37

General Preparations for the Newborn Kid

Rohit Kumar, Meesam Raza, and Ankaj Thakur

Department of Livestock Production Management, Dr G.C. Negi College of Veterinary and Animal Sciences, Palampur, India

37.1 Introduction

Welcome to the world of goat keeping! As you embark on this rewarding journey, one of the most exciting experiences you'll encounter is the arrival of a newborn goat kid. These adorable creatures can bring immense joy and fulfillment to your life, but it's crucial to be well prepared to ensure their health, safety, and well-being right from the start.

In this chapter, we will discuss the general preparation required before the arrival of a newborn goat kid. Whether you are a beginner in goat keeping or an experienced goat enthusiast, understanding the steps involved in preparing for a kid's arrival is essential in order to provide them with a solid foundation for a healthy and thriving life. In this chapter, we will cover important topics such as creating a safe and comfortable birthing space, gathering essential supplies for newborn care, and understanding the unique nutritional needs of a newborn goat kid. We will also explore the importance of socialization, vaccinations, and proper record keeping to ensure the kid's long-term health and future growth. While each goat kid is unique and may have individual needs, this chapter aims to provide you with a general foundation for preparing for their arrival. It is important to remember that consulting with a veterinarian and experienced goat keepers in your community can provide valuable guidance tailored to your specific circumstances.

By following the guidelines outlined in this chapter, you will be well equipped to provide a nurturing and supportive environment for your newborn goat kid. Whether you are raising them for companion purposes, dairy production, or show purposes, the proper preparation during this critical stage will create a strong bond between you and your kid, setting the stage for a fulfilling and rewarding journey in goat keeping.

For goat breeders, the breeding season is typically one of the most stressful times of the year. We can prepare to deal with practically any issue a doe or kid may have by putting in a little time and effort in the months before kidding and having the right tools on hand. A comprehensive program for raising goat kids starts before birth because meeting the doe's nutritional demands during her pregnancy is essential to get a healthy newborn kid.

37.2 Care of Newborn Kids

Survival and increased performance of newborn kids significantly improve the goat producer's likelihood of success in the goat industry. The objective of good care and management of newborn kids is to minimize death and enhance health and performance. In most situations, does take care of their kids and minimal attention from owners may be required.

Does with good mothering ability – the capability to care and raise kids successfully – and experience clean their kids by licking immediately after kids are born. Does bleat from time to time to communicate and get the kids' attention. Kids in good health and condition stand up, seek teats, and suckle within half an hour or so after birth. These actions of does and kids develop a maternal bond. Early development of a maternal bond is crucial for the survival and growth of newborn kids. Does keep their kids nearby and protect them from other animals in the herd. They nourish their kids by producing acolostrum and milk. Well-fed does provide sufficient colostrum, which is the only source of nutrients and immunoglobulin for the newborns. After 2–3 days, colostrum gradually changes to normal milk. Milk is the only source of food for young kids

Elements of Reproduction and Reproductive Diseases of Goats, First Edition. Edited by Tanmoy Rana.

until they develop the ability to digest other feedstuffs, which starts by 3–4 weeks of age and completes by 8–9 weeks. Does that have a well-developed udder will produce enough milk for their kids if they are receiving a sufficient quality and quantity of feed.

Although most does in a herd will raise their kids with minimum problems, owners should keep their eyes on newborn kids and their mothers and be prepared to provide support when needed. Common situations when newborn kids may need extra support and vigilance are listed below.

- *Very cold and/or wet weather during kidding*: kids lose body heat very rapidly when in cold or wet environments. As a result, they may become weak and die.
- *Maiden does*: these does do not have experience to take care of newborn kids and may abandon their kids easily, especially to near-term does with strong maternal instincts.
- *Does in poor health*: sick or weak does may show indifference to their newborns and/or may not be able to produce enough colostrum and milk for the kids.
- *Multiple births*: when three or more kids are born, even an experienced doe may not be able to provide enough care and nourishment for all.
- *Weak newborn kids*: they may not be able to stand up and suckle on their own.
- *Does with poor mothering ability*: may not provide enough care and also may abandon their kids.
- *Risk of predators*: when the kidding area is not well protected from predators, newborn kids may be killed or injured.
- *Poor sanitation and hygienic conditions*: under such conditions, there is a high risk of infectious diseases and parasites. Newborn kids, especially those weak or poorly fed, easily succumb to pathogens.
- *Crowded conditions*: aggressive animals in a herd may approach and attack or steal newborn kids. Also, such conditions harbor more pathogens and make the environment stressful compared to less crowded conditions.

37.3 General Preparations to Ensure the Kid's Well-being

37.3.1 Health Check-up Prior to Kidding

Don't forget to perform a thorough health check on does 4–6 weeks prior to kidding, which should cover hoof care, vaccination, lice and worm management (deworming). This will optimize the chances of successful kidding and contribute to overall health of the offspring. Pregnancy toxemia and milk fever are two dangerous, sometimes fatal metabolic illnesses that are more likely to develop in improperly nourished pre- and postkidding does. Therefore, pregnant does should be kept on good and well-balanced nutritional regimes before and after their delivery.

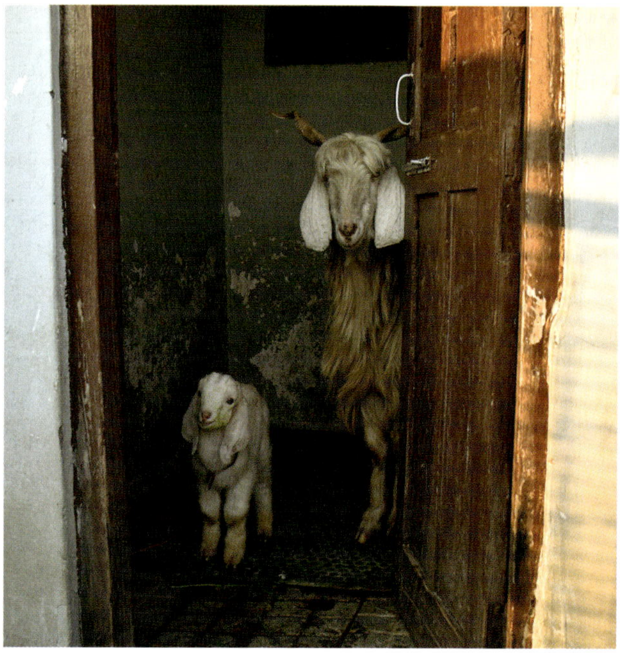

Figure 37.1 Individual kidding pen.

37.3.2 Readying the Facilities

The following facilities should be ready prior to kidding.

37.3.2.1 Provision of a Clean and Cozy Shelter

- The pregnant does should be kept in a separate clean shed or new pasture around their kidding date to reduce the possibility of injuries and illness.
- Individual kidding pens (Figure 37.1) or a large pen for multiple does can be created. For a single doe, a pen about 5 ft by 5 ft will serve the purpose.
- A personalized pen could be helpful for first-time mothers or does with several kids.
- Always be careful not to overstock kidding does.

37.3.2.2 Arrangement of Bedding

- Before bringing the does inside the kidding pen (at least 3–4 weeks before), clean the pens and lay fresh straw for bedding (Figure 37.2).
- Before putting a new doe in the same pen for kidding, replace the bedding.
- Provide adequate weather protection for the does and kids in the pen.
- Clean straw or bedding for the kid's comfort should also be provided. This will also help with insulation and moisture control.

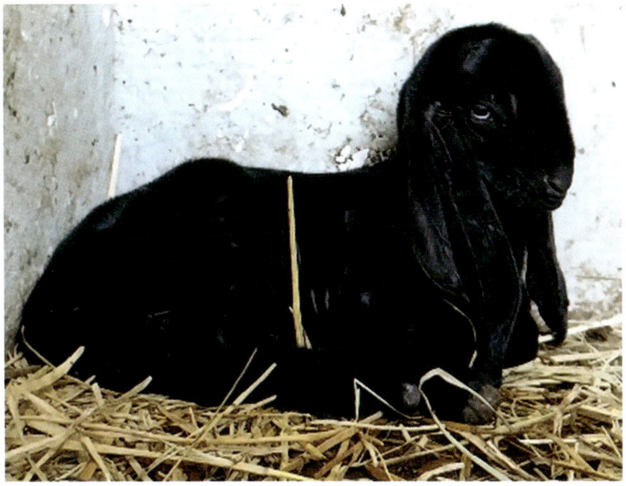

Figure 37.2 Clean straw bedding for a kid.

37.3.2.3 Set Up a Goat Kid Enclosure

Create a secure area for the kid to explore, play, and rest. Make sure there are no sharp edges, loose wires, or dangerous objects that could harm the kid. This set-up will protect kids from the adult flock and also help to encourage socialization among young goat babies, which is essential for friendlier goats. Additionally, the kids will also get protection from predators and harsh weather. Therefore, prepare a warm and dry enclosure for the kids. Ensure it is draft-free, well ventilated, and protected from predators.

The following points should be kept in mind while preparing the enclosure (Figure 37.3).

- To make a goat kid pen, first divide an area inside your goat shelter or barn.
- The walls/fences and doors of this enclosure should be about 1.3 m high and if the goats kept are good jumpers, then these walls/fences may be extended to the ceiling.
- One enclosure with the dimensions of 1.8 m^2 can provide sufficient space for up to 10 kids.

37.3.3 Observing the Signs of Kidding

The gestation period of a goat is 145–152 days (five months). This is a fairly precise time frame, and it is really useful to know from the start. When breeding your goats, keep an eye out for their act of mating and use that to predict your first likely kidding date. If you're not sure when it happened, take the first day of breeding as your "early" date. This duration is critical for you to be prepared for the actual kidding. In situations when you don't know when the breeding has occurred, it is best to start observing the signs of kidding at least 1–3 days prior to kidding.

Figure 37.3 Goat kid enclosure.

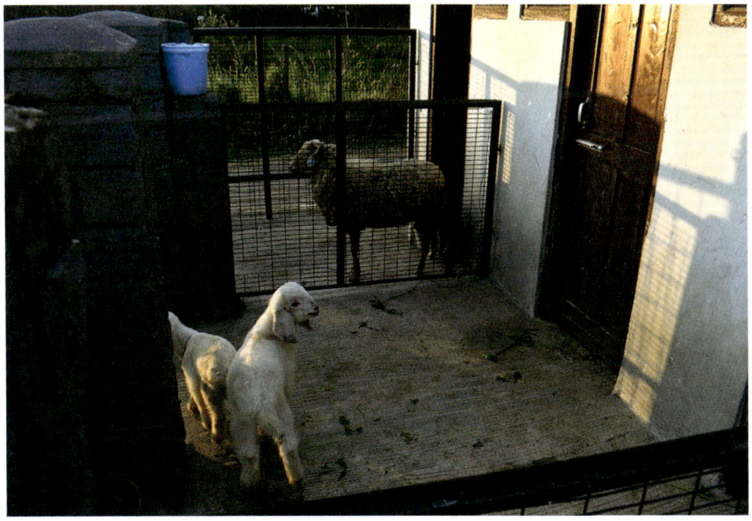

Table 37.1 The process of kidding in goats.

Phases of kidding	Events
Relaxing or opening phase	• Shows typical signs of birth and can last for a few hours
Expulsion phase	• Belly muscles contract to expel the kid or kids and lasts for an average of 30 minutes • In delayed expulsion, the nose and tongue of the kid can turn bluish, which is normal
Expulsion of fetal membranes	• The last delivered kid brings the fetal membrane with it after birth • Sometimes it can take up to 8 hours for fetal membrane expulsion • A small amount of bleeding during kidding should be of no concern

Kidding is completed in three phases (Table 37.1) and the major signs of kidding are as follows.

- Swelling of udder.
- Softening of ligaments (back, belly, and pelvis).
- Swollen vulva.
- Protruding back and pelvic bones.
- Reluctance to eat.
- Staying away from the herd.
- Restlessness.
- Water bag appearance (filled with clear fluid).

37.3.4 Be Prepared with Necessary Materials and Supplies Prior to Kidding

Purchase essential supplies such as feed, hay, water buckets, bedding, kid-safe toys, and grooming brushes. Keep a veterinarian's contact information handy in case of any health concerns. Be prepared to help with kidding. Trim your nails and clean hands with soap and water; use gloves when touching kids or does.

The following kidding supplies must be kept ready.

- Propylene glycol or molasses (for treating pregnancy toxemia)
- Calcium borogluconate (for treating milk fever)
- Dextrose (50%) and antibiotics
- Thermometer, scissors, syringes, and needles
- Bearing retainer (spoon) or prolapse harness
- Rubber gloves, protective sleeves, or latex gloves
- Lubricants, nylon rope, snare, or leg puller
- Towels and rags
- Heat lamp or warming box
- Weak iodine solution (or other disinfectant)
- Frozen colostrum (ewe, doe, or cow)
- Kid feeding tube
- Kid milk replacer
- Nipples
- Disinfected feeding bottle
- Scale and sling
- Injectable vitamin E/selenium
- Ear tags

37.3.5 Things to Bear in Mind While Kidding

The doe should be left alone once the process of kidding is initiated. Normally, the kid should be born 30 minutes after rupture of the water bag. The natural birth position is for the front feet to point downward, with the head resting on the feet.

If the kid's hooves are facing upward, it is in breach posture and may need help. Ninety percent of all goat kiddings occur without human involvement. This means you should not intervene until you feel compelled to. That being said, having equipment on hand in case you are needed is a must for every conscientious goat keeper. It is usual for young or maiden does to take their time. Typically, assistance is needed to rectify the defective position of the legs or neck, or to turn the kid into the correct position for birth. If assistance is required, use aseptic procedures and a "no jewelry" policy. Sometimes the situation deteriorates to the point where a cesarean section is required. Cull does who require regular assistance during kidding.

37.3.6 Things to Do Immediately After Birth

- Check the kid is breathing by cleansing its mouth and nose. In chilly weather, properly dry the kid's ears and tail to avoid freezing. If there is some breathing problem, artificial means of breathing should be adopted.
- After birth the umbilical cord should break on its own. Treat it with antiseptic (tincture of iodine) to protect the umbilicus from infection. If the umbilical cord is intact, it should be severed with a sterile knife/blade about 4–7 cm from the umbilicus. The severed end should be swabbed with tincture iodine.
- Allow the doe to lick her kid; this helps in mother and offspring bonding.
- It is important for kids to drink the first milk from the doe (colostrum) within 30 minutes after birth to gain immunity and expulsion of meconium (first fecal material) during early life. Ensure that the kid consumes enough colostrum during the first 12 hours of life so that the quantity of colostrum around 10–20% of its body weight is consumed between three and 12 hours after birth. If the mother does not have enough colostrum, use fresh colostrum from another doe.
- Kids' birth weight should be recorded.
- An identification number must be given to each kid at an early age.

37.3.7 Establish a Feeding Routine

Consult with a veterinarian or experienced goat breeder to determine the appropriate feeding schedule and type of milk replacer for your kid. Ensure you have the necessary feeding equipment, like bottles or nipple buckets, and an appropriate milk replacer on hand.

The following points should be kept in mind while establishing a feeding routine.

- Ensure that the kid gets enough colostrum in time and later the milk should be fed daily depending upon their body weight (Table 37.2).
- Feeding of kid starter should begin at the age of three weeks to a month old. It should be introduced gradually and the amount should be increased at a rate at which the kids can consume it without upsetting their digestion.
- Milk feeding can be discontinued by the age of 3–4 months or possibly sooner if the kids start consuming grass or hay and concentrate.
- Kids should be weaned at the age of 90 days.

For feeding of kids from three months to one year of age:

- grazing on pasture should be allowed for around eight hours per day
- provide concentrate mixture (protein 16–18%) at 100–200 g/kid/day
- dry fodder should be provided during the night (in summer and rainy months).

Table 37.2 Feeding of goat kids (0–90 days).

Age of kids (d)	Body weight (kg)	Milk (ml)	No. of feedings	Creep feed (g)	Forage, green/day (g)
0–7	1–3	Free choice	With mother	–	–
8–30	3–5	200–350	2–3	Free choice	Free choice
31–60	5–7	300–400	2	Free choice	Free choice
61–90	6–10	200	2	100–150	Free choice

37.3.8 Create a Warm Environment

If the weather is cold, ensure the kid stays warm by using heat lamps, blankets, or a heat pad. Provide a draft-free environment and monitor temperatures regularly.

37.3.9 Plan for Regular Care

Establish a schedule for hoof trimming, vaccinations (Table 37.3), deworming, and general health checks for the kids. Consult with a veterinarian to create a plan based on your kid's specific needs.

37.3.9.1 Hoof Trimming

Hooves should be clipped one to two times per year, depending on growth, nutrition, and climate. Consideration should be given to the time of year. During the wetter seasons of the year, hooves are softer and easier to trim. Furthermore, lameness and the spread of foot-related disorders frequently occur during these wetter periods, and hoof trimming enables early assessment and detection of any potential concerns.

37.3.9.2 Vaccination Schedule

Following a proper vaccination schedule is a mandatory prophylactic measure for kids as well as adults. The colostrum from a doe which was vaccinated during the last trimester of pregnancy will protect to the kids from pulpy kidney (enterotoxemia) and tetanus during the first few weeks. The vaccination schedule in Table 37.3 can be altered as per regional variations and state policy under consultation with a local veterinarian.

37.3.9.3 Deworming Schedule

The best primary strategy for preventing internal parasites is routine deworming. Kids must be at least 60 days (about two months) old when receiving their first deworming. For kids, the deworming schedule in Table 37.4 can be undertaken after birth.

37.3.9.4 General Health Checks

General health check-ups such as routine monitoring for any kind of problem, fecal examinations, and eye examination to rule out FAMACHA scores etc. can help to mitigate serious complications of various common conditions like diarrhea, anemia, worm infestation, etc.

Table 37.3 Vaccination schedule for goats.

	Schedule	
Name of disease	**Primary vaccination**	**Regular vaccination**
Anthrax (Figure 37.6)	At the age of six months for kids	Once annually (in endemic areas only)
Hemorrhagic septicemia	At the age of six months for kids	Once annually (before monsoon)
Enterotoxemia	• Four-month-old kid (if dam was vaccinated) • During the first week (if dam was not vaccinated)	• Before monsoon (preferably in May) • Vaccination booster 15 days (about two weeks) after first vaccination
Black quarter (BQ)	At the age of six months for kids	Once annually (before monsoon)
Peste des petits ruminant (PPR) (Figure 37.7)	At the age of three months and above for kids	Once in three years
Foot and mouth disease (FMD) (Figure 37.4)	At the age of four months and above for kids	Twice in a year (September and March)
Goat pox (Figure 37.5)	At the age of three months and above for kids	Once annually (December)
Contagious caprine pleuropneumonia (CCPP)	At the age of three months and above for kids or lambs	Once annually (January)

Source: Adapted from Tamizhkumaran (2016).

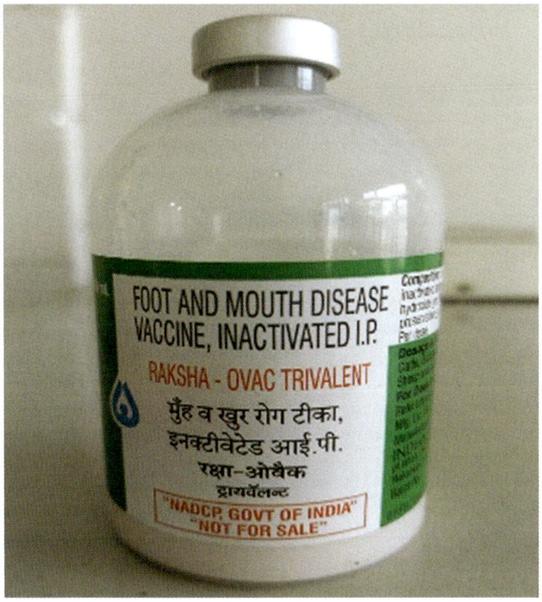

Figure 37.4 FMD vaccine.

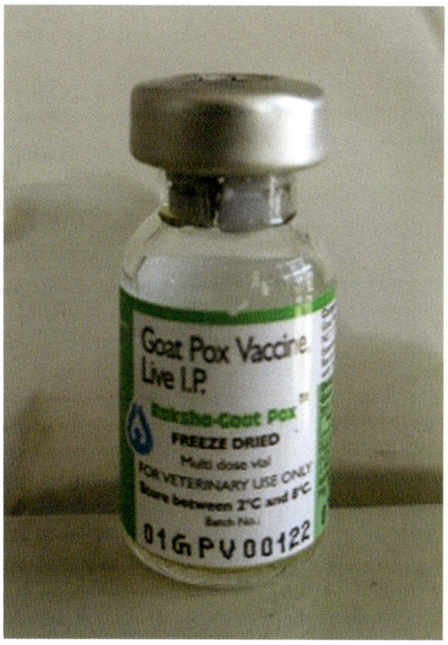

Figure 37.5 Goat pox vaccine.

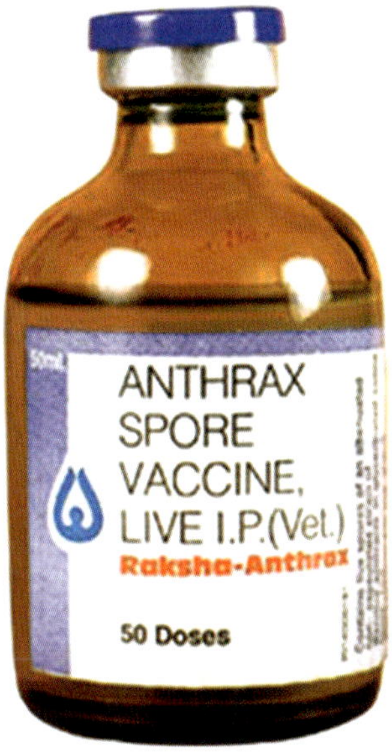

Figure 37.6 Anthrax vaccine.

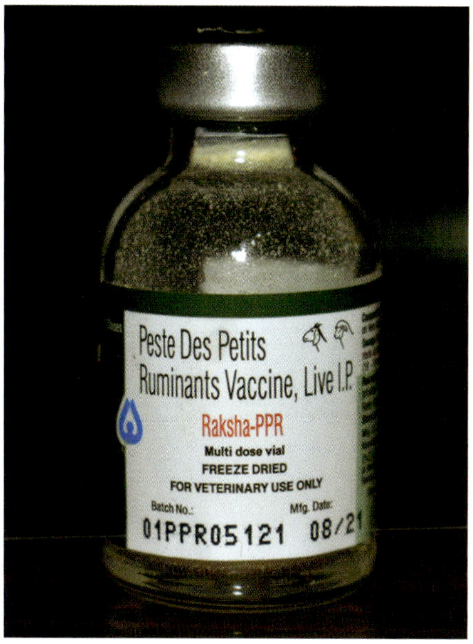

Figure 37.7 PPR vaccine.

Table 37.4 Deworming in goat kids.

Type of drugs	Period of the year	Schedule
Anticoccidial treatment • Sulphamethazine + Trimethoprim	June/July	• In young animals and in cases of diarrhea • Can be added in creep feed from 15th day of age till they obtain their weaning age
Broad-spectrum anthelmintics • Ivermectin • Closantal • Albendazole	–	• Medicines should be administered every two months and should also be rotated to prevent resistance developing
Narrow-spectrum anthelmintics • Praziquantel	April/May	All kids and weaners should be dewormed as per their body weight • At the age of two months and repeat at 4–6 months

Note: Before deworming the flock, a fecal test must be performed.
Source: Adapted from DAHD (2016).

It is important to stay well informed about the specific care requirements of the breed you are raising. Consulting with experienced goat breeders or veterinarians will help you ensure the best care for your newborn kid.

37.4 Conclusion

Preparing for the arrival of a newborn goat kid is crucial to ensure its health and overall well-being. We have emphasized the importance of a clean and safe kidding area, complete with bedding, heat lamps or heating pads, and proper sanitation to prevent the risk of infection. Additionally, it is essential to have necessary supplies readily available, such as clean towels, gloves, iodine solutions for umbilical cord care, and a thermometer. Moreover, preparing for the newborn goat kid involves being knowledgeable about common birthing complications and having a plan in place to address any potential issues. Understanding the signs of labor, assisting with the birthing process when necessary, and being able to recognize and address any complications promptly are essential for the survival and well-being of both the mother and kid. Finally, we have highlighted the significance of creating a warm, clean, and safe environment for the newborn kid immediately after birth. Ensuring that the kid is adequately dried, providing colostrum within the first hours of life, and monitoring its general health and behavior are vital steps in promoting a strong start to life.

Overall, proper preparation for the arrival of a newborn goat kid involves careful planning, attention to detail, and proactive measures to create a healthy and nurturing environment. By following the guidelines and recommendations outlined in this chapter, goat owners can contribute to the successful, thriving, and rewarding experience of raising healthy goat kids.

References

DAHD (2016). General guidelines for biosecurity at Central Sheep Breeding Farm, Hissar. www.dof.gov.in/sites/default/files/2019-12/Biosecurity%20guidelines%20for%20sheep%20and%20goat%20.pdf (accessed 2 January 2024).

Tamizhkumaran, J. (2016). Vaccination schedule for goats. https://vikaspedia.in/agriculture/livestock/sheep-and-goat-farming/vaccination-schedule-for-goats (accessed 2 January 2024).

Further Reading

Anthrax Vaccine. https://indianimmunologicalsltd.tradeindia.com/bacillus-anthracis-vaccine-live--1178654.html (accessed 2 January 2024).

PPR Vaccine. https://m.indiamart.com/proddetail/raksha-ppr-vaccine-22460729612.html (accessed 2 January 2024).

Goats (2019). Newborn goat kids. https://goats.extension.org/newborn-goat-kids (accessed 2 January 2024).

Pritchett, K. (2023). Birthing a goat on the farm. https://hiddenheightsfarms.com/birthing-a-goat-on-the-farm (accessed 2 January 2024).

Sagar, R. (2009). *Commercial Goat Farming*. Lahrauli Khadar, India: Central Institute for Research on Goats.

Team Pashudhan Praharee (2020). Deworming (control of internal parasites) in sheep and goats. www.pashudhanpraharee.com/deworming-control-of-internal-parasites-in-sheep-goats (accessed 2 January 2024).

Weaver, S. (2014). 7 Ways to get your farm ready for baby goats. www.hobbyfarms.com/7-ways-to-get-your-farm-ready-for-baby-goats-3 (accessed 2 January 2024).

38

Feeding of Kids

Rohit Kumar and Meesam Raza

Department of Livestock Production Management, Dr. G.C. Negi College of Veterinary and Animal Sciences, Palampur, India

38.1 Introduction

The nourishment provided during the early stages of a goat kid's life plays a pivotal role in their growth, immunity development, and overall health. It is during these initial weeks and months that goat kids form the foundation for a healthy adulthood. Therefore, it is of the utmost importance to focus on proper nutrition and feeding strategies tailored specifically to their needs.

In this chapter, we will explore the various aspects of goat kid nutrition, including the importance of colostrum, milk replacers, weaning, solid food supplements, and monitoring intakes. By understanding these factors, goat owners can ensure the optimal feeding practices required to raise healthy and thriving goat kids which is crucial not only for their overall well-being but also for the long-term success of the goat-farming venture.

38.2 Colostrum – Gold Standard for Goat Kids

Immediately after birth, goat kids should receive colostrum, which is the nutrient-rich first milk produced by the mother. It is essential for newborn kids' health as it is rich in antibodies, providing them with passive immunity against various diseases. Kids should suckle their mothers to consume colostrum at a minimum rate of 10–20% of their body weight, preferably within 2–3 hours after birth. It is recommended that kids should be fed colostrum within half an hour after their birth.

Colostrum is crucial for growth and resistance to disease in goat kids. Here are several ways in which colostrum aids in their development and immune system support.

- *Passive immunity*: colostrum contains high levels of immunoglobulins, also known as antibodies, which provide essential passive immunity to newborn kids to protect them from various diseases and infections early in their lives when their own immune system is not fully developed. This early protection is crucial in ensuring the kid's survival and reducing the risk of illness.
- *Nutrient-rich*: colostrum is packed with crucial nutrients, including proteins, vitamins, minerals, and fats. These play a vital role in the kid's growth, providing them with energy and building blocks for healthy development.
- *Digestive health*: colostrum contains high levels of lactose and easily digestible fats, promoting the growth of beneficial gut bacteria. This helps establish a healthy gut microbiome in the kid, which is vital for good digestion and absorption of nutrients throughout their lives.
- *Development of vital organs*: the growth factors present in colostrum help in the development and maturation of important organs, such as the gut, liver, and immune system, ensuring proper bodily functions in the future.
- *Prevention of health issues*: adequate colostrum intake has been linked to a lower risk of various health issues in goat kids, including diarrhea, respiratory infections, and general weakness. It strengthens their immune system, reducing the likelihood of illness and improving overall health.

Elements of Reproduction and Reproductive Diseases of Goats, First Edition. Edited by Tanmoy Rana.

- *Long-term benefits*: proper colostrum feeding has been associated with improved growth rates and overall performance of goat kids, leading to better productivity and profitability in the long run.

Remember, it is crucial to provide colostrum to goat kids within the first few hours after birth to maximize these benefits.

38.2.1 Best Practices for Administration of Colostrum

When it comes to the administration of colostrum in goat kids, there are a few best practices to ensure their health and proper development. Here are some guidelines to follow.

- *Timing*: it is crucial to provide colostrum to newborn goat kids as soon as possible after birth. The first 24 hours are the most critical period for absorption of colostrum antibodies.
- *Quality*: use high-quality colostrum from healthy does. The colostrum should be thick and yellowish in color. Avoid using colostrum from goats with a known history of health issues or diseases.
- *Quantity*: provide enough colostrum to the newborn kid. As a general guideline, feed about 10–20% of the kid's body weight in colostrum within the first 24 hours. For smaller kids, consider dividing the colostrum into multiple feedings.
- *Feeding method*: the best way to administer colostrum to goat kids is through tube feeding or bottle feeding. Tube feeding ensures the kid receives the proper amount of colostrum and reduces the risk of aspiration. Use clean equipment to avoid contamination.
- *Hygiene*: maintain proper hygiene during all stages of colostrum administration. Clean the doe's udder and teats before milking and ensure that feeding equipment is thoroughly cleaned and sanitized between uses.
- *Temperature*: warm the colostrum to a temperature of around 102 °F (39 °C) before feeding. This helps ensure better digestion and absorption by the kid's body.
- *Storage*: if you need to store colostrum, do so in a clean, airtight container in the refrigerator or freezer. Colostrum can be stored in the refrigerator for up to 48 hours or frozen for longer periods. Thaw frozen colostrum slowly in warm water, never in a microwave.

Remember that colostrum is vital for the health and immunity of goat kids. If a kid is unable to nurse from its mother, it is crucial to intervene and provide colostrum as soon as possible. It is because the kid's ability to absorb antibodies decreases over time.

38.3 Tube Feeding in Kids

In cases where a doe didn't let her kid nurse, or the newborn kid is too weak, is unable to suck, or is too sick to nurse or take a bottle, tube feeding can be used. A tube feeding kit contains a syringe (60 ml) and a feeding tube (Figure 38.1). This set-up can be used to tube feed a newborn kid that won't nurse or in case a doe doesn't let her kid nurse. Feeding a newborn kid directly with a syringe may look easy but it can lead to aspiration of fluid into the lungs and can cause pneumonia or choking. It might only take one tube feed to wake up and energize a frail kid. If a kid needs to be tube fed more than once, only do so every 2–4 hours and only with a tiny amount. Smaller, more frequent meals are preferable to irregular, substantial meals.

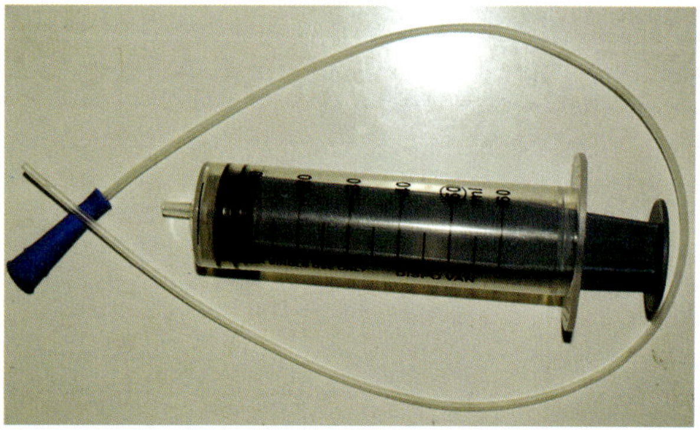

Figure 38.1 Sixty milliliter syringe and feeding tube.

38.3.1 Equipment Required for Tube Feeding

- Feeding tube
- Sixty milliliter syringe with an irrigation tip
- Warm water
- Six milliliter syringe
- A helper

The kid will struggle while tube feeding and you really need to be gentle.

The following steps should be taken to tube feed a kid (Smith 2021)

1) It is necessary to know how far the tube needs to be inserted to get it to the kid's stomach. This can be done by measuring a kid's nose to ear distance and from the ear to the floor of the chest and then adding the two measurements (Figure 38.2). This distance should be marked on the tube with a piece of tape and the tube can be inserted up to this mark.
2) Make sure the kid is securely held so that it is sitting up rather than on its side.
3) Hold the kid's head up straight, lining up the front of the neck with the bottom of the chin.
4) The tube's end should be softened by dipping it in warm water before being inserted into the kid's mouth, across the tongue, and down the throat until it is fully inserted to the length you noted.
5) Use one of the following techniques to check that the tube is placed properly.
   - Check for the milky stomach scent at the tube's end. Naturally, this won't work for newborns who haven't yet consumed any milk.
   - Keep an eye out for little crackles at the tube's end. If you notice breath noises, take out the tube and restart.
   - Dip the tube's tip into a cup of water. You need to try again if it blasts bubbles since you are in the lungs.
6) With a 6 ml syringe, inject around 5 ml of water into the tube to ensure that it runs down the tube. If not, pull it back a little and try again. This procedure aids in ensuring that the tube is not rubbing up against the stomach wall, twisted, or clogged in any manner.
7) Tube feed the kid after making sure the tube is in the right spot and is functional. Fill the syringe with 2–4 oz of the feeding liquid, then screw the syringe onto the tube's end. Don't use the inside of the syringe; if you hold it above the kid, gravity will transfer the fluid to the stomach.
8) After giving the fluids, rinse the tube by filling the syringe with an additional 10 ml of water. Although it is not essential, this procedure helps to prevent the kid from aspirating milk or electrolytes as the tube is being removed.
9) Take the syringe out of the tube's tip. Next, slowly remove the tube while holding the end with your finger. To stop extra fluid from entering the lungs, place your finger over the end. Removing the tube too quickly could result in tissue injury and pain for the kid.
10) After each feeding, sterilize and clean your supplies.

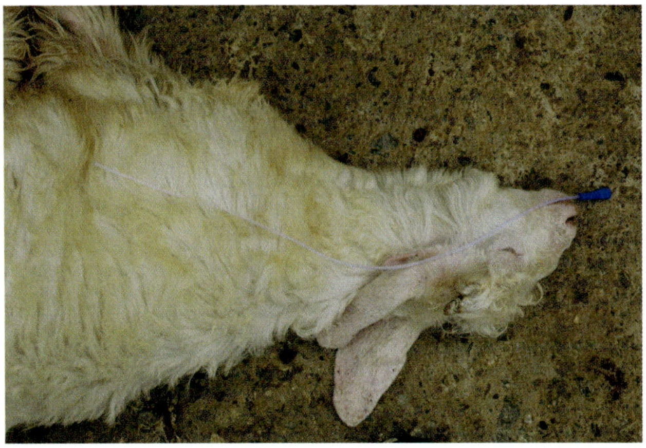

Figure 38.2 Measurements before insertion.

38.4 General Kid Nutrition

After colostrum feeding, goat kids needs sufficient nutrition for proper growth and development of immunity against various diseases. Therefore, we should decide on the food we want to feed them and how. There are many options available, including individual or group feeding, bottle or dam raised, milk or milk substitute. Make a plan and stick to it because their little stomachs don't appreciate change (unless you have a valid reason to change the plan, like switching to a bottle if the mother becomes ill or switching to milk if a kid experiences diarrhea on milk replacer).

Kids suckle for the first eight weeks of their lives at the very least before progressively transitioning to hay and grain. However, they must be consuming solid food well before being weaned. They begin tasting hay and grain as early as the first week. This allows you additional time to choose and acquire a source of solid meals.

38.4.1 Milk Replacers and Dam's Milk

In instances where goat kids are not receiving sufficient milk from their dams or are orphaned, milk replacers are a good alternative (Table 38.1). In addition, saving the milk for human consumption may be an economic necessity. Feeding milk

Table 38.1 Method of feeding milk replacer diet.

Days	Milk replacer (%)	Dam's milk (%)
5–7 d	10	90
Next 5–7 d	25	75
Next 5–7 d	50	50
Next 5–7 d	75	25
Next 5–7 d	90	10
Approximately up to 90 d	100	0

replacer also helps to achieve faster body weight gains. From 2–3 days after birth, kids can be kept on whole milk or milk replacer if they are not nursing with their mother.

Goat milk replacer should have about 20% protein and 20% fat, with the majority of the protein coming from an animal source (whey proteins). To help lower the prevalence of bacterial respiratory and gastrointestinal illnesses, antibiotics are frequently added to milk replacer. It should be enriched with vitamin A (20 000–30 000 IU/kg dry matter), vitamin E (30–40 mg/kg dry matter), and vitamin D (2500–3500 IU/kg dry matter). While mixing the milk replacer, ensure that the powder is properly mixed with the water to make a suspension. Frequent small-quantity feedings will lessen the likelihood of bloat. Some kids may be able to transition to a twice-daily feeding schedule by the third week of life.

Kids should be weaned as soon as possible because milk substitutes are expensive. Feeding milk replacer may be continued till kids are four months old. On milk replacer, it takes a lot of time and money to raise orphaned kids. Keepers should try to graft the orphans onto another dam whenever possible, and should only nurture them on milk replacement if this is not possible. Orphans should ideally drink small amounts of milk several times a day, but this is usually not feasible for most goat farmers.

38.4.2 Bottle-feeding Schedule and Weaning

Establishing an appropriate bottle-feeding schedule is vital to ensure proper nourishment for goat kids (Figure 38.3). In this section, we will discuss the optimal frequency and amount of milk kids should consume at different stages of their growth (Table 38.2). Emphasizing the importance of consistent feeding schedules, we will provide guidelines for gradually reducing bottle feedings as kids grow older. We will also outline the weaning process, including the introduction of solid foods, such as hay, grass, and high-quality grain concentrates, along with strategies for a smooth transition.

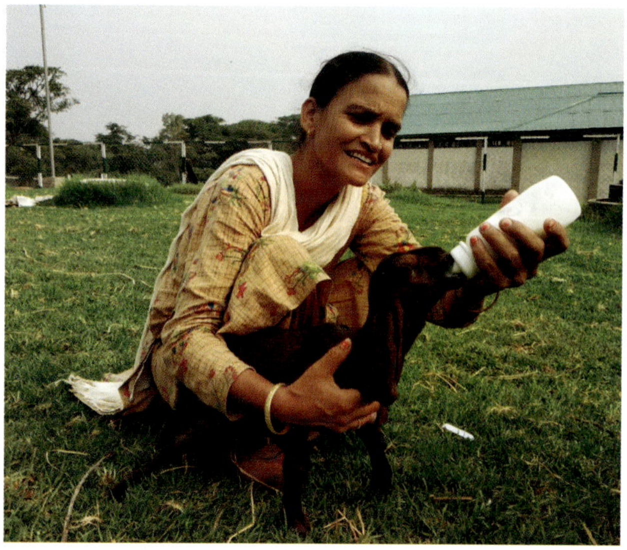

Figure 38.3 Bottle feeding in goat kids.

Milk feeding should be done thrice a day during the first week followed by twice a day. Overfeeding should be checked in kids as it may lead to diarrhea and lead to improper stomach development.

38.4.2.1 Why Bottle Feed Kids?

- Bottle-raised goats are more docile and friendly than dam-raised kids. Kids raised with the dam are frequently more aloof, more difficult to train, and more herd oriented.
- It saves milk for human consumption or sale.
- Goats can contract the infectious virus known as caprine arthritis encephalitis (CAE) which results in painful symptoms like arthritis, pneumonia, and swollen joints. The disease is most frequently passed from dam to kid through colostrum and milk. It may also spread via other bodily fluids. To contain the sickness and prevent it from infecting future generations, many farms remove the kids from the herd and feed replacement milk.

Table 38.2 Feeding of goat kids (0–90 days).

Age of kids (d)	Body weight (kg)	Milk (ml)	No. of feedings (frequency)	Creep feed (g)	Forage, green/day (g)
0–7	1–3	Free choice	With mother	–	–
8–30	3–5	200–350	2–3	Free choice	Free choice
31–60	5–7	300–400	2	Free choice	Free choice
61–90	6–10	200	2	100–150	Free choice

- Bottle feeding is useful when mothers reject their kids.
- Kids may be weak and lack the strength to stand and suckle from their mothers. Until the kid is strong enough to nurse independently, you will need to bottle feed in this situation.

38.4.2.2 Weaning

Weaning is a stressful event for a kid. Kids can be weaned as early as 3–4 weeks, although waiting until 8–12 weeks may yield better outcomes. Weaning can be done as late as six months in kids. Due to labour constraints, weaning should be practiced as early as possible after birth in large herds.

Introduce solid food in small amounts at first, such as hay, grass, and high-quality grain concentrates. Until the kids are completely weaned, gradually reduce the bottle feedings. Good-quality hay must be made available to kids as a free choice during the first two days of the weaning process. The next step is to introduce the weanlings to a concentrate feed given at a rate of about 1% of body weight every day. Prior to being weaned, kids should weigh between 2.5 and three times their birth weight. Kids of most meat- and dairy-producing breeds should weigh at least 9.1–11.4 kg and eat 0.23 kg of a grain containing 16–18% crude protein per day at weaning. Around 60 days (8.5 weeks) old, a typical kid will weigh 2.5–3 times their birth weight and consume 1% of their body weight in solid food. Despite this, weaning one month later (at 90 days), if it is economically viable, may lessen stress and enhance growth, breeding success, and production in the first lactation.

38.4.3 Creep Feeding

The use of additional feed for nursing kids is referred to as creep feeding. A creep feeding program's objectives are to encourage sufficient feed intake with good palatability (as it is competing with milk), and should give all necessary nutrients in a most cost-effective manner. Feeds that has been coarsely ground or pelletized typically increases consumption. Pellet sizes greater than 5–7 mm may cause a decrease in feed intake in goats.

Kids must eat more than 0.23 kg creep feed every day from three weeks of age until weaning if increased performance is to be achieved through creep feeding. The most effective creep meals are often those with low fiber and 16–20% protein. Most creep diets can be improved in performance by adding salt (0.5% of the creep feed), ammonium chloride (0.2 kg/440 kg of feed), and vitamin E. For every 1.8–3.2 kg of feed consumed, creep feeding should typically result in an additional 0.5 kg of growth. The degree of efficiency will vary depending on the specific circumstances, but creep feeding is typically lucrative when feed costs are low and sale prices are high and less profitable when both feed prices and sale prices are high.

A few examples of creep feed mixtures are shown in Table 38.3.

38.4.4 Feeding of Kids Over Three Months to One Year of Age

Kids start nibbling forages such as pasture grasses or hay by the age of two weeks and start consuming grains by four weeks. A good leguminous hay (or fresh green grass) and a creep mixture along with fresh water should be provided at 3–4 weeks of age. They should be allowed to graze for eight hours per day and dry fodder may be provided to them during night hours in summer and rainy seasons. Generally, kids kept on ad lib milk intake have higher growth rate than those kept on limited milk intake. Provision of concentrate supplementation makes up for limited milk intake mainly three weeks after birth.

After the age of four months, provide concentrate mixture (protein 16–18%) 100–200 g/kid/day. Composition of concentrate mixture and feeding schedule for goat kids are provided in Tables 38.4 and 38.5, respectively. Provision of concentrate feed prior to weaning improves weight gain after weaning as it prepares goat kids well to cope with weaning stress. From four months of age up to breeding, they may be fed roughages that will support normal growth by providing sufficient nutrients.

Table 38.3 Compositions of various creep mixtures for goat kids.

Ingredients	Sample 1	Sample 2	Sample 3
Maize grain	60	–	20
Barley/oats grains	–	40	45
Groundnut cake	20	22	20
Fish meal	10	10	10
Molasses	–	20	–
Wheat bran	7	5	2
Mineral mixture	2	2	2
Salt	1	1	1
Calculated digestible crude protein (DCP) %	18	17	17
Calculated DCP %	78	70	75

To one quintal or more of creep mixture, add Aurofac® 150 g, Vitablend/Rovomix® 25 g, and shark liver oil 1 teaspoon per kid/day.
Source: Adapted from Singh (2014).

Table 38.4 Composition of concentrate mixture for growing kids (3–12 months).

Ingredients	Sample 1	Sample 2
Maize	7	30
Ground gram	42	13
Wheat bran	7	30
Crushed groundnut cake	42	20
Molasses	–	5
Mineral mixture	1	1
Salt	1	1

Source: Adapted from Sagar (2009).

Table 38.5 Feeding schedule of growing kids 3–12 months.

Age of kids (mo)	Concentrate feed (g)	Green/day (g)	Dry/day
3	150–200	300–500	Free choice
4	200–250	400–600	Free choice
5	225–275	500–700	Free choice
6	250–300	600–800	Free choice
7	275–325	700–900	Free choice
8	300–350	800–1000	Free choice
9	300–350	900–1200	Free choice
10	300–350	1000–1300	Free choice
11	300–350	1100–1400	Free choice
12	300–350	1200–1500	Free choice

Source: Adapted from Sagar (2009).

38.5 Conclusion

Feeding goat kids is a critical aspect of their rearing, requiring careful attention to their nutritional needs at different stages of growth. By prioritizing colostrum, establishing proper bottle-feeding schedules, gradually introducing solid food, and monitoring their intake, goat owners can foster healthy development and ensure robust kids. Understanding the principles outlined in this chapter will empower goat owners to provide optimal nutrition and set the foundation for happy, thriving goat kids.

References

Sagar, R. (2009). *Commercial Goat Farming*. Lahrauli Khadar, India: Central Institute for Research on Goats.

Singh, R.R. (2014). *Goat Production. Farm Animal Management: Principles and Practices*. Delhi: New India Publishing Agency.

Smith, C.K. (2021). *Raising Goats for Dummies*. Hoboken, NJ: Wiley.

Further Reading

Campbell, B. (2020). Weaning Management for Goat Kids. Ohio State University. https://u.osu.edu/sheep/2022/03/01/weaning-management-for-goat-kids (accessed 2 January 2024).

Government of Assam (2023). Goat Management. https://veterinary.assam.gov.in/sites/default/files/swf_utility_folder/departments/ahvetdir_webcomindia_org_oid_4/portlet/level_1/files/Goat%20Farming%20and%20Management.pdf (accessed 2 January 2024).

McCoard, S.A., Ryrie, J., MacDonald, T. et al. (2021). Impact of casein- versus whey-based lamb milk replacers on growth and health of artificially reared lambs. *New Zealand Journal of Animal Science and Production* 81: 22–28.

Misra, R.P., Sharma, D.K., and Kumar, P. (2009). *Common Scientific Practices for Goat Rearing*. Lahrauli Khadar, India: Central Institute for Research on Goats.

Section 6

Early Diseases of Kids

39

Stillborn, Weak or Dead Kid

Amitava Roy[1] *and Tanmoy Rana*[2]

[1] *Department of Livestock Farm Complex, West Bengal University of Animal & Fishery Sciences, Kolkata, India*
[2] *Department of Veterinary Clinical Complex, West Bengal University of Animal & Fishery Sciences, Kolkata, India*

39.1 Introduction

Neonatal farm animal death causes waste, lowers farm profitability, has negative effects on animal welfare, and frequently lowers farmer morale. Animals are particularly vulnerable on the day of birth; in sheep (Nowak et al. 2000) and goats (Singh et al. 2008), up to 50% of preweaning mortality occurs on this day. The extrauterine environment, which can be chilly or wet and where predators or other animals may attack the young animal, is more demanding for newborns when they leave the warm and safe uterus. There are numerous potential reasons of fetal loss in livestock, including infectious, nutritional, toxic, environmental, and genetic factors. Therefore, it may not come as a surprise that death rates have been extremely resilient to efforts to lower them; reported average mortality estimates for sheep over the last 40 years across numerous nations and systems remain practically unchanged at 15%.

Even though there have been fewer studies on newborn mortality in goats than in sheep, published estimates range from 11.5% to 37% (e.g., Thiruvenkadan and Karunanithi 2007), indicating that the problem is of a similar size in both small ruminant species. Although there is a considerable interfarm variation, some farms are able to significantly lower mortality. For instance, a survey of 22 sheep farms in New Zealand found that mortality ranged from 1.4% to 43.5% of all lambs (Forrest et al. 2006).

The most frequent reasons for miscarriages in sheep and goats will be the subject of this chapter. Good records will make it easier to identify and diagnose abortions. Losses of 1–5% per year can be typical for a particular herd; diligent record keeping and analysis will reveal that a problem is present when it may still be possible to take action. A few animals will always miscarry due to genetic flaws, stress, weather events, and nutritional mistakes, but several managerial and viral factors can lead to significant abortion disasters.

According to Thiruvenkadan and Karunanithi (2007), annual mortality at goat farms in Tamil Nadu, India, ranged from 2.2% to 30.5%. Fragkou et al. (2010) suggested that lamb mortality should be as low as 3%, with an upper tolerable limit of 5% – a figure that is currently not met on many farms based on analysis of lamb mortality related to disease. Although there is a lot of scientific knowledge about neonatal mortality, it does not seem to have significantly decreased lamb or kid losses. There are a number of reasons why this research was not adopted or had an impact: (i) while numerous studies have described the causes of lamb mortality, they have not offered practical, on-farm solutions to address these issues; (ii) experimental studies may not adequately replicate the "real" on-farm environment and, as a result, may not be able to offer pertinent solutions; (iii) scientific investigations have frequently focused on single issues or causal factors, when mortality is a complex interaction of many factors; (iv) the scientific solutions may not have been properly tested.

In this chapter, we will discuss why scientific research on lamb and kid mortality has not had much of an impact and how things can change. We start by talking about the state of science today and any potential solutions it might offer for farming. In the second section, we will look at more real-world uses of this knowledge on industrial farms and how quickly these techniques may be implemented to increase lamb survival.

Elements of Reproduction and Reproductive Diseases of Goats, First Edition. Edited by Tanmoy Rana.

39.2 Biological Variables that Affect Lamb and Kid Survival

The causes of lamb mortality have been well studied. There is general agreement that the following factors contribute to lamb mortality: (i) birth trauma following a challenging or prolonged delivery that causes hypoxia and typically results in stillbirth; (ii) a poor bond between the ewe and lamb that results in starvation and hypothermia in the lamb, usually resulting in death on the day of birth; (iii) infectious disease; and (iv) a number of other relatively minor factors like congenital malformation, predation, and accident.

The proportional prevalence of various causes of death will fluctuate depending on the system. For instance, infectious disease may be more common in housed systems, while deaths from severe injury may be decreased since obstetric assistance is more readily available. Mortality from malnutrition, hypothermia, or predation may be more significant than infectious disease in outdoor lambing systems. Compared to sheep, goats have received less research and the literature that is currently available has a tendency to focus on traditional small-scale or village production environments (such as those found in West and South Africa, India, the Middle East, Central and southern America) rather than larger-scale commercial production environments, which have been the subject of sheep studies.

Although disease-related death (neonatal illnesses, tick-borne or parasitic) appears to be more common, the causes of kid mortality are remarkably similar to those of lambs (Singh et al. 2008). It is unclear whether this is because goat kids are more susceptible to disease or because, in the published studies, they are more exposed to and less likely to have received vaccinations against common infectious diseases that affect small ruminants (like clostridial disease via dam vaccination). There is also a good description of lamb mortality risk factors. Low-birthweight lambs, larger litters, lambs born to inexperienced or young ewes, and male lambs have greater rates of lamb mortality (Sawalha et al. 2007). The rate of lamb survival can be influenced by management factors related to diet, breeding goals, hygienic procedures during lambing, and management interventions. Goats have also been found to have hazards related to birth weight, sex, parity, and litter size, while season of birth is also a substantial risk factor (Singh et al. 2008). Given that the majority of studies are focused on tropical areas, seasonal effects – particularly whether it is the rainy or dry season – are probably primarily connected to nutritional factors, while the presence of parasites and diseases may also be important.

Deep physiological adaptations are needed after expulsion from the uterus at birth, including the establishment of pulmonary respiration, cardiovascular adaptation, loss of thermal insulation and placental nutrient supply, vigorous locomotion and coordination required to express teat-seeking behavior, consumption of colostrum and, as a result, gastrointestinal and metabolic adaptation and the development of neonatal immunity. The main physiological, behavioral, and immunological difficulties that the newborn faces are covered in the section below, along with how nutrition and genetics may affect these interactions.

39.3 Neonatal Survival

39.3.1 Behavior

The ewe searches for a good area to give birth as soon as parturition is imminent (Dwyer and Lawrence 2005). If ewes choose sheltered and protected birth places, this will dictate the microenvironment in which the lamb will be born and may have an impact on the effectiveness of the newborn's thermoregulatory responses. Lambs who die from hypothermia frequently experience wet, windy, and chilly weather (Alexander et al. 1980). The choice of a birth location with elements that will encourage the sheep to stay at the site for an extended amount of time can also affect survival because time spent at the birth site is a crucial factor in preventing separation between ewes and lambs.

According to Poindron et al. (2007), parturient ewes and goats exhibit extremely comparable maternal behaviors. Ewes and goats are particularly drawn to the taste and smell of amniotic fluids during and immediately after birth, and they will lick fluids that have been spilt during the birth process, passing this attraction to the infant. Within the first few hours following delivery, a mother's behavior is characterized by focused licking and grooming of the newborn, numerous low-pitched bleats, and acceptance of the neonate at the udder. Licking or grooming helps to dry the baby and is crucial in the development of a mother's unique scent memory for her own newborns.

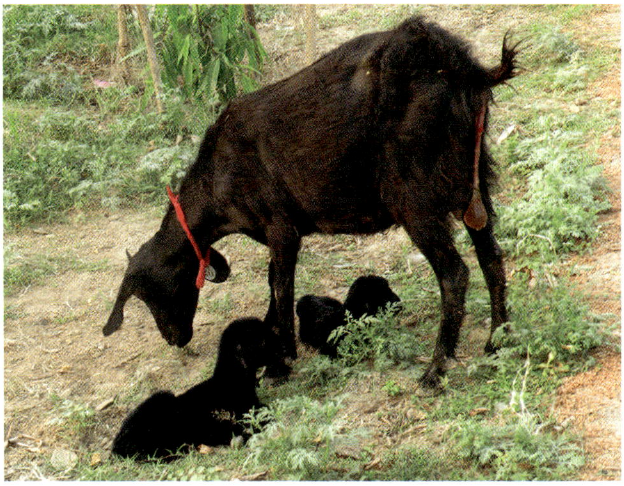

The dam will only limit her maternal care to those offspring with which she has established an exclusive attachment within an hour or two after giving birth. If this attachment is not formed, the mother will not recognize the lamb or kid as her own, and the newborn's attempts to suck from the udder will be rejected. These infants cannot live without human intervention since other lactating mothers will also reject the lamb or kid. After olfactory recognition, mothers learn to recognize their youngster by their distinct visual appearance, followed by their vocalizations (Poindron et al. 2007).

The ewe's maternal behaviors, such as standing up and making the udder more accessible to the teat-seeking lamb, can encourage lamb-sucking responses. Primiparous ewes may have a lower success rate with lambing because inexperienced ewes are initially less inclined to cooperate with attempts to suckle the lambs. The separation of ewe and lamb behavioral effects by embryo transfer (Dwyer and Lawrence 1999) reveals that maternal behavior does not promote increased vigor and vitality in her newborn offspring. However, the behavior of the ewe alone cannot cause the lamb to suckle. According to Hatcher et al. (2010), there is little correlation between maternal attachment scores and lamb survival. According to Brien et al. (2014), there is also little genetic correlation between maternal behavior measures and lamb survival. This suggests that variations in the quantity or quality of maternal behavior expressed may not have a significant impact on lamb survival.

In contrast, a lamb's conduct is very important to survival. Lambs go through a number of behavioral stages at birth that are geared toward standing, udder seeking, and sucking. Standing helps the lamb maintain body temperature by reducing heat loss to the ground. The lamb then uses a series of reflex and synchronized actions to walk down the ewe's body and find the udder. The lamb's likelihood of survival is known to be correlated with the speed at which it performs these behaviors (Dwyer et al. 2003). According to Cloete and Scholtz (1998) and Hergenhan et al. (2014), lambs from sires or lines of sheep with high survival are quicker to stand and suckle than lambs from low survival lines or sires. The lamb receives nutrients from nursing quickly, notably those needed to maintain thermoregulation and immunoglobulins for passive immunity. The formation of the lamb's bond with its mother is also influenced by sucking and colostrum consumption (Goursaud and Nowak 1999).

Many of the risk variables that are linked to higher mortality have an impact on lamb and kid behaviors. Lambs born after a protracted labor, lambs in larger litters, and male as opposed to female lambs show slower behavioral development (Dwyer 2003). According to Dwyer et al. (2003), lamb birth weight shows a U-shaped distribution with lamb vigor at birth, which is related to lamb survival. Numerous studies have shown breed, line, and sire within breed diversity in lamb behavior (Hergenhan et al. 2014). According to research by Matheson et al. (2012), the early vigor or sucking capacity of lambs has a moderate heritability. This finding implies that enhancing lamb vigor by genetic selection may be possible and would increase survival. It is unknown if goat kid behavior has comparable genetic linkages and phenotypic correlates with survival.

39.3.2 Physiology

Temperatures in the birthing environment can drop from 39 °C *in utero* to 10 °C or below. Maintaining a healthy balance between heat production and loss is essential for maintaining body temperature. Body surface area (small lambs have a larger surface area/body weight ratio than large lambs; as a result, they lose heat more quickly and are more susceptible to hypothermia) and coat insulation value (short, fine birth coats have lower insulation value than long, coarse coats) are the key factors influencing heat loss. The insulating value of an amniotic fluid-soaked coat is reduced, but removal of the fluid by the mother's licking or grooming helps the lamb maintain a healthy body temperature.

Within 10 minutes of birth, the lamb starts to produce more heat but there are significant interindividual variances that can lead to hypothermia that cannot be reversed (Dwyer and Morgan 2006). In the most severe situations, where lambs are unable to produce enough heat, hypothermia can be fatal. Nonshivering thermogenesis, which is generally if not entirely attributed to brown adipose tissue, and shivering thermogenesis, which typically occurs under cold conditions, primarily in older, dry lambs, and metabolizes muscle glycogen, are the two main ways by which heat is produced in the neonate. Nutrients, immunoglobulins, and other substances such as enzymes, hormones, growth factors, and neuroendocrine peptides are all found in colostrum.

According to Nowak and Poindron (2006) and Banchero et al. (2015), colostrum contains fat (7–13%), nonimmunoglobulin protein (4–10%), and lactose (2–5%), and has an energy density of 6–7 kJ/ml. Lambs need 50 ml of colostrum per kilogram within the first 18 hours of life at temperatures between 18 °C and 26 °C to make up for lipid energy deficits and prevent hypothermia; from 0 °C to 10 °C, this amount rises to 280 ml per kilogram. A further advantage of colostrum consumption early on is that it raises body temperature by 17% even while energy stores are still full, increasing resistance to hypothermia.

In ideal circumstances, newborns would ingest enough colostrum to satisfy their need for carbohydrates for 14 hours of the first 24 hours of life (Mellor and Cockburn 1986). In order to make up the deficit, glycogen must be used and during the first few days, the liver and muscle stores of glycogen are largely exhausted in lambs. The ewe's ability to produce enough colostrum depends on having enough protein and energy during the final three weeks of pregnancy. In spite of the fact that twin-bearing ewes typically generate more colostrum than single-bearing ewes, they start lactation later and produce less colostrum per lamb (Banchero et al. 2015). As a result, multiple-birth lambs are less advantageous than single-birth lambs due to lower birth weights, fewer energy reserves, and larger surface area/body weight ratios. Inadequate nutrition during pregnancy might impact the viscosity of colostrum, delay the start of lactogenesis, and decrease milk and colostrum production (Banchero et al. 2015).

As a result, delayed suckling may cause energy reserves to be depleted within six hours of birth and lower heat output. After body reserve depletion, inadequate colostrum consumption is the second critical factor impacting infant survival. Due to the stimulation of the hypothalamic-pituitary-adrenal function, which starts the delivery process, late pregnancy is linked to a significant increase in cortisol concentration in the lamb in the last 24–48 hours (Challis and Brooks 1989). Due to the fact that vaginal birth and the accompanying stress hormones are linked to greater newborn alertness, this causes high levels of circulating cortisol, which may be the cause of their vigorous locomotor activity and teat-seeking conduct (Lagercrantz and Slotkin 1986). High plasma cortisol levels in lambs during the first neonatal hours delay premature gut closure, which may improve the absorption of macromolecules (Hough et al. 1990). In the days that follow, cortisol levels drop, thyroid hormone levels rise as thermal efficiency rises, and rectal temperature stabilizes. Triiodothyronine and thyroxine levels rise concurrently with the perinatal rise in cortisol, and this increase persists throughout the early postnatal period. According to Symonds et al. (1995), failure to maintain a high plasma triiodothyronine concentration leads to a decrease in oxygen consumption, hypothermia, and death. Thyroid hormones are known to play a significant role in controlling oxygen consumption.

However, the link between cortisol and survival is complicated. In addition to the protective effects of elevated neonatal cortisol, excessively high levels at birth may be related to difficult parturition and fatal dystocia, whereas an increase in circulating cortisol in the days that follow reflects a state of chronic stress due to insufficient milk supply and is associated with elevated blood glucose to make up for a lack of nutrient intake (Chniter et al. 2013). Increased presuckling body temperature, lower presuckling glucose concentrations, high plasma concentrations of proteins, lipids, and immunoglobulins, and a modest increase in neonatal cortisol concentration are all linked to improved lamb viability beyond 72 hours (Eales et al. 1982; Miller et al. 2010).

In terms of strength and thermoregulation, being larger is advantageous since larger lambs are better at sucking and enduring exposure to cold temperatures. Breed (Slee 1981; Dwyer and Morgan 2006), season of birth (Chniter et al. 2013), diversity within a litter, and prenatal diet can all have an impact on birth weight.

39.3.3 Immune System Efficiency

The epitheliochorial placenta of ruminants prevents the transmission of immunological components from the mother to the fetus. Thus, newborn lambs and children are significantly hypogammaglobulinemic at birth and completely rely on the passive transfer of colostral immunoglobulins acquired by nursing to provide them with immune protection after birth. Since newborn lambs' guts close to immunoglobulin absorption between 24 and 36 hours after birth, passive immunity must be acquired within a relatively short window of time (Hough et al. 1990). Early suckling is necessary for efficient transfer because colostral immunoglobulins also decrease quickly in the hours following birth, nearly disappearing within 24 hours (Al Sabbagh et al. 1995). Low immunoglobulin status 24 hours after delivery is linked to lamb mortality (Kenyon et al. 2005), highlighting the significance of ensuring adequate colostrum intake in newborn small ruminants. The ability of the lamb to consume sufficient amounts of colostrum and the concentration and availability of colostral immunoglobulins from the ewe are two complementary elements that determine adequate colostrum consumption.

According to a division of the sources of variance in lamb serum immunoglobulin, the lamb, the ewe, and the farm, respectively, account for 56%, 36%, and 7% of the variation (Christley et al. 2003). Correlation between ewe colostral immunoglobulin concentrations and lamb serum immunoglobulin concentrations is generally low (McGuire et al. 1983), suggesting that other factors are important in ensuring good immunological protection for the offspring. To achieve proper immune protection, the lamb must exhibit adequate sucking behavior and the dam must cooperate. But increasing maternal immunoglobulin production would also be advantageous. According to data collected on farms, 22% of ewes produced less than 50 g/l of immunoglobulin G at lambing, which is deemed inadequate for a lamb's nutritional demands due to its limited capacity for ingesting. According to Gilbert et al. (1988), there is a significant interanimal variation in the amount of IgG present in colostrum depending on dam age (younger ewes produced more immunoglobulin), litter size, udder health, season of lambing in tropical areas, and late pregnancy feeding. With sire and breed effects observed and a heritability of 0.19 for ewe immunoglobulin concentration in colostrum, there is some evidence that genetic variables may affect maternal colostrum immunoglobulin content (Gilbert et al. 1988).

39.3.4 Influence of Nutrition

To have healthy kids that can flourish in the postnatal environment, the pregnant sheep or goat must receive adequate nutrition. The impact of changes in nutrition, including total and specific nutrient supply, on neonatal lamb survival characteristics has been extensively studied (Rooke et al. 2015). An annual cycle strategy to feeding the sheep has long been recommended because the ewe is a seasonal breeder in temperate regions and pregnancy in these climate zones occurs during winter, when nutrient availability from grazing is limited (Russell 1985). The time when a cow needs the most nutrients is during lactation, which often happens in spring when pasture growth and quality are at their highest. The sheep is able to rebuild body reserves used during gestation and lactation after weaning lambs in mid- to late summer. Consequently, mobilization of adipose tissue balances deficiencies in feed nutritional supply, especially energy, throughout gestation. Thus, undernutrition (UN) is the nutrient imbalance that the pregnant ewe experiences most frequently. Although in tropical places this occurs from the annual cycle of wet and dry rather than day length as in temperate zones, this imbalance is also evident in pregnant goats.

Numerous factors, including maternal UN, might affect newborn lamb mortality. UN could directly lower lamb birth weight and raise mortality risk. Additionally, maternal UN can have a negative impact on a lamb's capacity to regulate its body temperature and neonatal behaviors. UN also affects the sheep's capacity to give birth, leading to the development of the ewe–lamb relationship (Dwyer et al. 2003), as well as the quantity and quality of colostrum the ewe produces. Similar to humans, UN in the final third of pregnancy is linked to reduced maternal care and decreased maternal recognition. The impact of UN on mortality through each of these channels has not been fully explored, however.

In the last third of ovine pregnancy, Rooke et al. (2015) discovered that UN consistently lowered birth weight exclusively, with the reduction in birth weight being related to both the length and severity of UN. Only under specified conditions during the first two-thirds of pregnancy did UN diminish birth weight. These included the severity of UN: between gestational days 0 and 60, feeding only 0.15 of the need lowered birth weight and increased death. In response to an early gestational UN challenge, breeds more acclimated to challenging environments (such as Scottish Blackface) partitioned more resources to the fetus and thus maintained birth weight, whereas birth weight was decreased in breeds bred for fast growth (such as Suffolk). Ewes in better physical shape were better equipped to handle the UN than those in worse physical condition.

However, decreased birth weight simply serves as a risk factor for higher lamb mortality. Only half of the studies (Rooke et al. 2015) where lamb birth weight and mortality were recorded also found an increase in mortality along with a drop in birth weight. The degree of birth weight loss, the physical surroundings, and the quantity and caliber of husbandry will all be contributing factors. It is significant to note that feeding the ewe nutrients in excess of what was necessary for fetus growth and ewe maintenance was not related to better lamb survival; in fact, adverse results were more frequent than favorable ones. Studies that demonstrate a U-shaped link between lamb birth weight and survival lend credence to this. Regarding particular nutrients, the majority of study has concentrated on trace elements and vitamins where insufficiency is a real issue and associated with a higher death rate (for example, deficiencies of copper, cobalt, or iodine). The baseline status of ewes (deficient, marginal, or adequate) before the investigation is typically not adequately described, making it difficult to interpret many studies.

Supplementation increased survival or related metrics for cobalt, selenium, and vitamin E in areas where the status of ewes was marginal (Rooke et al. 2008). Responses where preexperiment ewe status was adequate have been more ambiguous, and there is little proof that providing trace nutrients in excess of what is needed but short of hazardous levels has any advantages (Rooke et al. 2008).

In conclusion, UN is the primary nutritional risk to newborn lamb survival, especially in the final trimester, assuming there are no chronic shortages in trace element and vitamin supplies. Loss of body condition during the first 100 days of pregnancy does not significantly increase the probability of lamb death as long as ewes have sufficient body reserves before mating. If ewes are properly fed during late pregnancy, loss of body condition can be prevented. Ewes housed outside on pasture are presumably more susceptible to acute or chronic udder obstruction, such as from snowfall or a lack of grass growth.

39.4 Early Embryonic Death vs Abortion vs Stillbirth

Early-stage abortions are known as "early embryonic death" and manifest as irregular or recurrent heat cycles; the dam normally does not release any conceptus or fluids before reabsorbing the embryo and its contents. When a fetus dies in the middle or later stages of pregnancy, the fluids can sometimes be reabsorbed, creating a mummy. The deceased mummy can either be "born" at the typical labor period alongside live siblings or can be kept as a singleton indefinitely as long as no infection occurs. In the latter case, the animal will look to be pregnant but not progress further and will not go into heat again unless the mummy is removed.

Deliveries of dead fetuses which would have lived if something unfavorable had not prevented them from drawing their first breath are known as stillbirths. Near-term conditions including ketosis, milk fever, selenium deficiency, dystocia, or numerous viral causes can result in stillbirths.

39.4.1 Infectious Causes of Abortions

Small ruminants can experience abortions for a variety of reasons, although infectious illnesses are typically to blame. When handling animals, especially those that are giving birth or seem sick, precautions should be taken because many of these diseases can be transmitted to people, especially pregnant women. Wear protective gear, use gloves, dispose of contaminated bedding with care, and thoroughly wash your hands. Do not consume dairy products that have not been pasteurized.

39.4.2 Embryonic and Fetal Losses

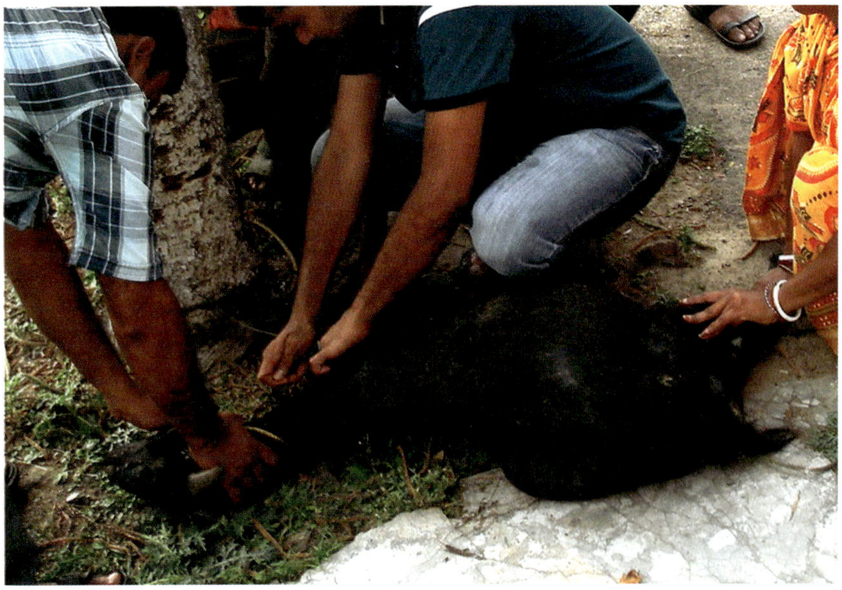

According to Diskin and Morris (2008), embryonic mortality is a cause of reproductive wastage in goats, with levels of 18% for twin ovulations and 40% for triplets. Inadequate nutrition has been linked to these losses as a major contributing factor. Does abort in subsequent pregnancies less frequently. Does have been shown to lose more fetuses when their liveweight is lost by as little as 25 g per day (Urrutia-Morales et al. 2012). In Angora goats, it has been demonstrated that a 2 kg weight reduction (6%) during midpregnancy causes a 17% fetal loss, as opposed to a 2% fetal loss in does receiving their maintenance requirements (McGregor 2016). Extremely high rates of fetal loss, such as 53% of does (Urrutia-Morales et al. 2012) and 70% of does (Mellado et al. 2004), have been linked to nutritional stress during late pregnancy. Limited pasture and the detrimental impacts of social status on food consumption can also cause stress (Pretorius 1970; Urrutia-Morales et al. 2012). While undernutrition during late pregnancy is likely to cause pregnancy toxemia and death of the sheep and fetus (Besier et al. 2010), midpregnancy restriction down to 0.3 times the maintenance needs leads to minor increases in fetal loss in ewes.

According to guidelines that does should have a condition score of >2 at mating (Mellado et al. 2004), a low condition score at mating increases the probability of fetal loss. According to estimates (Mellado et al. 2004), does with a condition score of 3 at mating will lose an estimated 7% of their fetuses, whereas does with a condition score of 2 will lose 20% of their fetuses. This estimate is consistent with prior reports (Shelton and Groff 1984) that show larger fetal losses with lower liveweights.

Early nutrition may also be important because young animals that grow at less than 136 g per day between birth and 25 days of age are more likely to abort as adults (Mellado et al. 2006). Therefore, managing nutrition is a crucial component in preventing fetal losses in pregnancy. Fetal losses are influenced by an interaction between age (parity) and nutrition. According to Mellado et al. (2004), does in their first pregnancy lose more fetuses than adult goats do. Despite the fact that the total rate of fetal loss was just 3.5%, does in parities 2–5 were half as likely to abort as does in their first or more than fifth pregnancy.

Similar to this, Rattner et al. (1994) found that first-parity does experienced 11% fetal loss, compared to 5% in adults. However, rather than age or parity specifically, insufficient growth and nutrition in young does may be the main reason for their greater rates of fetal loss (Shelton and Groff 1984). When compared to mature does, first parity does experience lower fetal losses due to disease (Aldomy et al. 2009). Although certain places have endemic infectious diseases like brucellosis and bluetongue, Australia does not (Givens and Marley 2008). In Norwegian dairy herds that had previously experienced substantial fetal loss (>15%) but were housed, viral reasons were not connected (Engeland et al. 1997). Instead, a pregnancy from the third or later estrus opportunity, more than two fetuses, low socioeconomic standing, and prior fetal loss all pointed to an increased probability of loss by at least twofold. Although this was not noted in a study utilizing dairy breeds (Engeland et al. 1997), polled goats may be more prone to miscarry than those with horns (Mellado et al. 2004). Although a higher rate of fetal loss has been observed for winter-mated does in Israel (Rattner et al. 1994), a Mexican study indicated that does mated during the summer were less likely to abort than those mated in the autumn. These variations may result from varying dietary needs, environmental influences, or genetic variations.

Poor documentation exists regarding the extent of fetal loss in Australian herds (Ferrier and McGregor 2002; McGregor 2016). Although it has been suggested that the breed of buck affects doe conception rate (Jones 2012), this was not confirmed in an experiment (Norton 2004). The kidding rate of crossbred Boer rangeland does, however, was 18% lower than that of rangeland does (62.5% vs 80.4%; Norton 2004). In experimental settings, April-mated Australian rangeland goats had kidding rates of 88–89% (Restall 1992), and stud Boer herds in high-rainfall locations of New South Wales and Queensland have reported conception or kidding rates of 94% (Nogueira et al. 2016). Fetal loss may be a contributory cause, but Victorian farmers have identified decreased doe fertility as a major problem (Ferrier and McGregor 2002). High rates of fetal loss brought on by dietary stress could be a substantial contributor to reproductive wastage in Australian goats. Although this does not seem to be a significant loss in herds that are carefully managed, additional research is required from commercial herds, especially in pastoral areas with lower rainfall where nutritional stress may be more prevalent. According to Brown et al. (2015), walk-over weighing systems may provide a low-cost way to explore variations in liveweight change and their connections to fetal loss.

39.5 General Patterns of Kid Survival from Birth and Post Weaning

Although there is little information on commercial herds in Australia, perinatal loss is a significant cause of reproductive wastage in goats. Mortality to weaning averaged 20%, according to data from 16 050 entries in KIDPLAN (the Australian genetic recording project) (Aldridge et al. 2015). As opposed to the 33.3% ± 23 recorded for three commercial herds in pastoral regions, 14 stud herds in high-rainfall locations reported a death rate (mean s.d.) of kids (0–3 months) of 11.6% ± 9.9

(Nogueira et al. 2016). Mortality to 16 days ranged between 2.9% and 21% under experimental grazing settings (Goodwin and Norton 2004), and between 6.4% and 21% for goats kidding in pens (McGregor 2016). Each component has the potential to affect physiology, behaviors in the mother or offspring, and death-causing mechanisms. According to Sherman (1987), the intensity of the management system, the climate, and nutrition may affect regional variances.

The kid's gender does not seem to have an impact on survival (Snyman 2010) but goat breed may be a factor; for example, Angora kids have poorer survival rates than other meat breeds and hybrids (Norton 2004). Although under experimental conditions the mortality of Boer and Boer-cross kids (10%) was comparable to that of rangeland goats (Norton 2004), it has been demonstrated that the Boer goat has a lower kid survival rate than some other breeds in South Africa (Lehloenya et al. 2005) and the United States (Browning et al. 2011). The disparity across research may be due to different breed comparisons, genetic variations, or environmental factors.

The date of neonate loss is not extensively documented in the research that is currently accessible, although it is evident that significant losses take place during pregnancy (Allan et al. 1991). Although postweaning losses can also be considerable in some circumstances (Rattner et al. 1994; Nogueira et al. 2016), losses at older ages may be augmented by disease under housed conditions (Sherman 1987). The reported death rates from four to 12 months in the survey by Nogueira et al. (2016) were likewise typically lower in the high-rainfall zones (6% ± 5.1) than in the rangeland regions (15.7% ± 17).

39.5.1 Causes of Perinatal Mortality

The main factors that contribute to prenatal mortality in sheep and goats are comparable, and earlier reviews have discussed the factors that contribute to perinatal mortality in lambs and kids in Australia and other countries (Dwyer et al. 2016). Internal reports from the department or veterinary laboratory may contain additional information but accessing these data can be challenging. The absence of data for goats emphasizes the necessity to quantify the causes of death and their relative relevance under the different management regimes so that suitable management measures can be developed. The majority of perinatal deaths in Australian lambs and kids occur due to dystocia or stillbirth (including birth injury) and the starvation–mismothering–exposure (SME) combination, which accounts for around 80% of all perinatal deaths.

Any one of these factors, however, might become more significant in specific locations or years (Refshauge et al. 2016). Predation and weak kids were the two main causes, according to a large South African study by Snyman (2010), however, this study only included kids which were born alive, and the cause of death was only known for 29.8% of those which died. Various causes at various ages were documented in a New Zealand study (Buddle et al. 1988), although a random sampling method was not adopted. With respect to managerial rigor, climate, and exposure to potential risk factors like predators, it is reasonable to anticipate that the relative significance of the various mortality classes will change over time.

39.5.2 Dystocia or Stillbirth

Dystocia refers to both normally born young who are either delivered dead or compromised as a result of a prolonged or challenging delivery as well as neonates in which the mother needs assistance to birth the term fetus. Stillbirth refers to newborns which die during parturition or are born dead. However, terminology in the literature is frequently either not specified or defined differently, so both words are employed in this section to encompass the meaning of the many findings.

There are few studies on the prevalence of dystocia in goats, despite the fact that it is a frequent cause of kid loss. Dystocia has been recognized as a significant cause of loss in Angora goats that are pen-fed (McGregor 2016) as well as grazing rangeland goats (Allan et al. 1992).

Mellado et al. (2006) noted 4.2% stillbirths among dairy breed goats. Rattner et al. (1994) found that triplets had a higher rate of kid stillbirths (15.5%) than singletons or twins (7.1%), and older does had a greater incidence of kid stillbirths (Mellado et al. 2006). However, numerous studies (Kouri et al. 2018) do not include dystocia or stillbirth as a cause of kid loss. The absence of dystocia or stillbirth from reports of intensive trials may be due to the intense surveillance during kidding. On big rangeland holdings, on the other hand, kidding is not seen, so the cause of death is unknown. In sheep, where the association between birth weight and survival is quadratic, a high birth weight is a significant risk factor for dying from dystocia (Geenty et al. 2014). Rattner et al. (1994), Snyman (2010), and Aldridge et al. (2015), reporting on Boer goats on the Australian KIDPLAN database, indicate that the link appears to be curvilinear for goats and that larger weights are not associated with a decrease in survival. However, further research is necessary under commercial management circumstances.

When compared to sheep, goats' propensity for numerous fetuses may lessen the probability of excessive birth weights. According to Lehloenya et al. (2005), there is a substantial correlation between litter size, birth weight, and kid survival. As a result, management methods must be developed to increase the survival of low-birthweight twins and higher-order births.

Another potential strategy to decrease deaths from dystocia is genetic selection. In Boer goats, the heritability of birth weight is 0.53 and the genetic connection between kid survival and good traits is minimal (0.19, standard error not provided; Aldridge et al. 2019). At the greatest birth weights, survival is not currently lowered, but selection for larger birth weights may increase dystocia losses in the future (Aldridge et al. 2015). In contrast, in sheep the genetic association between birth weight and lambing ease was estimated to be −0.56 0.27 and the genetic correlation between birth weight and lamb survival to three days of life was −0.32 0.23 (Brien et al. 2010). According to Brown et al. (2014), the genetic connection between all classes of dystocia and lambing ease (where 1 denotes no assistance during parturition and 5 denotes veterinarian aid) was estimated to be 0.26 ± 0.12. Since this takes into account mortality from all causes, selection for survival directly is more successful than selection for birth weight to promote survival. But in both kids (0.08; Aldridge et al. 2019) and lambs (0.01–0.03; Brien et al. 2014), the heritability of survival is insignificant, necessitating the use of alternative tactics.

Goats have the capacity to wean at high rates; some commercial Australian herds wean at rates of more than 160% per doe. However, there is considerable variety among farms, suggesting room for improvement. It is currently unknown if infertility brought on by out-of-season mating or inadequate buck management significantly contributes to low weaning rates. Clear evidence suggests that intensively managed herds' conception and kidding rates are at predicted levels (>90%) and that the main cause of kid loss in these herds is often perinatal loss. Given the seasonal variations in pasture conditions, inadequate nutrition may be a contributor to both fetal and perinatal kid loss in goats, which may be significant in pastoral areas.

39.6 Conclusion

Weaning rates are high for goats; in fact, some commercial Australian herds wean at rates exceeding 160% per doe. There is nevertheless a good deal of variation among farms, indicating potential for development. It is still uncertain how much low weaning rates are caused by infertility resulting from out-of-season mating or poor buck management. There is ample evidence to support the prediction that the conception and kidding rates of intensively managed herds are at or above 90%, and that postnatal loss is frequently the primary source of kid loss in these herds. Inadequate nutrition may play a role in both postnatal and fetal kid loss in goats, which could be severe in pastoral settings due to seasonal fluctuations in pasture quality.

However, there is not enough information on herds in pastoral areas or in-depth data from commercial nonstud herds to explain the large range in weaning rates between properties or to pinpoint the exact moment and reason for poor performance. While infant death is commonly acknowledged as the most significant cause of loss, this variation is comparable to that observed in commercial sheep flocks. As in sheep, SME and dystocia or stillbirth are typically the leading causes of perinatal kid loss. It is advised to conduct additional research, using sentinel herds if necessary, to more precisely pinpoint the period of reproductive failure on industrial farms throughout the world. There is a need to attempt to quantify the relative relevance of the various postweaning and perinatal loss causes in various geographic locations, as well as the elements contributing to their prevalence. With the help of these data, recommendations for preventing possible kid loss could be made that are specific to the local area.

References

Al Sabbagh, T.A., Swanson, L.V., and Thompson, J.M. (1995). The effect of ewe body condition at lambing on colostral immunoglobulin-G concentration and lamb performance. *Journal of Animal Science* 73: 2860–2864.

Aldomy, F., Hussein, N.O., Sawalha, L. et al. (2009). A national survey of perinatal mortality in sheep and goats in Jordan. *Pakistan Veterinary Journal* 29: 102–106.

Aldridge, M.N., Brown, D.J., and Pitchford, W.S. (2015). Genetic and phenotypic relationships between kid survival and birth weight in Australian meat goats. *Proceedings of the Association for the Advancement of Animal Breeding and Genetics.* 21: 350–353.

Aldridge, M.N., Pitchford, W.S., and Brown, D.J. (2019). Current progress on developing a selection index for Australian meat goats. *Proceedings of the Association for the Advancement of Animal Breeding and Genetics.* 23: 51–54.

Alexander, G., Lynch, J.J., Mottershead, B.E., and Donnelly, J.B. (1980). Reduction in lamb mortality by means of grass wind-breaks: results of a five-year study. *Proceedings of the Australian Society for Animal Production* 13: 329–332.

Allan, C.J., Holst, P.J., and Hinch, G.N. (1991). Behaviour of parturient Australian bush goats. I. Doe behaviour and kid vigour. *Applied Animal Behaviour Science* 32: 55–64.

Allan, C.J., Hinch, G.N., and Holst, P.J. (1992). Comparison of techniques for determination of early post-natal deaths of kids. In: *Fifth International Conference on Goats.* Little Rock, AR: International Goat Association.

Banchero, G.E., Milton, J.T.B., Lindsay, D.R. et al. (2015). Colostrum production in ewes: a review of regulation mechanisms and of energy supply. *Animal* 9: 831–837.

Besier, B., Jacobsen, C., Woodgate, R., and Bell, K. (2010). Sheep health. In: *In: International Sheep and Wool Handbook* (ed. D.J. Cottle), 471–488. Nottingham, UK.: Nottingham University Press.

Brien, F.D., Hebart, M.L., Smith, D.H. et al. (2010). Opportunities for genetic improvement of lamb survival. *Animal Production Science* 50: 1017–1025.

Brien, F.D., Cloete, S.W.P., Fogarty, N.M. et al. (2014). A review of genetic and epigenetic factors affecting lamb survival. *Animal Production Science* 54: 667–693.

Brown, D.J., Jones, R.M., and Hinch, G.N. (2014). Genetic parameters for lamb autopsy traits. *Animal Production Science* 54: 736–744.

Brown, D.J., Savage, D.B., Hinch, G.N., and Hatcher, S. (2015). Monitoring liveweight in sheep is a valuable management strategy: a review of available technologies. *Animal Production Science* 55: 427–436.

Browning, R. Jr., Leite-Browning, M.L., and Byars, M. Jr. (2011). Reproductive and health traits among Boer, Kiko, and Spanish meat goat does under humid, subtropical pasture conditions of the southeastern United States. *Journal of Animal Science* 89: 648–660.

Buddle, B.M., Herceg, M., Ralston, M.J. et al. (1988). A goat mortality study in the southern North Island. *New Zealand Veterinary Journal* 36: 167–170.

Challis, J.R.G. and Brooks, A.N. (1989). Maturation and activation of hypothalamicpituitary adrenal function in fetal sheep. *Endocrine Reviews* 10: 182–204.

Chniter, M., Hammadi, M., Khorchani, T. et al. (2013). Aspects of neonatal physiology have an influence on lambs' early growth and survival in prolific D'man sheep. *Small Ruminant Research* 111: 162–170.

Christley, R.M., Morgan, K.L., Parkin, T.D.H., and French, N.P. (2003). Factors related to the risk of neonatal mortality: birthweight and serum immunoglobulin concentrations in lambs in the UK. *Preventive Veterinary Medicine* 57: 209–226.

Cloete, S.W.P. and Scholtz, A.J. (1998). Lamb survival in relation to lambing and neonatal behaviour in medium wool merino lines divergently selected for multiple rearing ability. *Australian Journal of Experimental Agriculture* 38: 801–811.

Diskin, M.G. and Morris, D.G. (2008). Embryonic and early foetal losses in cattle and other ruminants. *Reproduction in Domestic Animals* 43 (2): 260–267.

Dwyer, C.M. (2003). Behavioural development in the neonatal lamb: effect of maternal and birth-related factors. *Theriogenology* 59: 1027–1050.

Dwyer, C.M. and Lawrence, A.B. (1999). Does the behaviour of the neonate influence the expression of maternal behaviour in sheep? *Behaviour* 136: 367–389.

Dwyer, C.M. and Lawrence, A.B. (2005). A review of the behavioural and physiological adaptations of extensively managed breeds of sheep that favour lamb survival. *Applied Animal Behaviour Science* 92: 235–260.

Dwyer, C.M. and Morgan, C.A. (2006). Maintenance of body temperature in the neonatal lamb: effects of breed, birth-weight, and litter size. *Journal of Animal Science* 84: 1093–1101.

Dwyer, C.M., Lawrence, A.B., Bishop, S.C., and Lewis, M. (2003). Ewe-lamb bonding behaviours at birth are affected by maternal undernutrition in pregnancy. *British Journal of Nutrition* 89: 123–136.

Dwyer, C.M., Conington, J., Corbiere, F. et al. (2016). Invited review: improving neonatal survival in small ruminants: science into practice. *Animal* 10: 449–459.

Eales, F.A., Murray, L., and Small, J. (1982). Effects of feeding ewe colostrum, cow colostrum or ewe milk replacer on plasma glucose in newborn lambs. *Veterinary Record* 11: 451–453.

Engeland, I.V., Waldeland, H., Andresen, Ø., and Tverdal, A. (1997). Foetal loss in dairy goats: an epidemiological study in 515 individual goats. *Animal Reproduction Science* 49: 45–53.

Ferrier, G.R. and McGregor, B.A. (2002). Benchmarks of Victorian commercial goat meat enterprises. *Animal Production in Australia* 24: 65–68.

Forrest, R.H., Hickford, J.G.H., Wynyard, J. et al. (2006). Polymorphism at the ovine β3-adrenergic receptor locus of merino sheep and its association with lamb mortality. *Animal Genetics* 37: 465–468.

Fragkou, I.A., Mavrogianni, V.S., and Fthenakis, G.C. (2010). Diagnostic investigation of cases of deaths of newborn lambs. *Small Ruminant Research* 92: 41–44.

Geenty, K.G., Brien, F.D., Hinch, G.N. et al. (2014). Reproductive performance in the sheep CRC information nucleus using artificial insemination across different sheep-production environments in southern Australia. *Animal Production Science* 54: 715–726.

Gilbert, R.P., Gaskins, C.T., Hillers, J.K. et al. (1988). Genetic and environmental factors affecting immunoglobulin G1 concentration in ewe colostrum and lamb serum. *Journal of Animal Science* 66: 855–863.

Givens, M.D. and Marley, M.S.D. (2008). Infectious causes of embryonic and fetal mortality. *Theriogenology* 70: 270–285.

Goodwin, N. and Norton, B.W. (2004). Improving doe nutrition immediately prior to kidding increases kid survival. *Animal Production in Australia* 25: 251.

Goursaud, A.P. and Nowak, R. (1999). Colostrum mediates the development of mother preference by newborn lambs. *Physiology and Behavior* 67: 49–56.

Hatcher, S., Eppleston, J., Thornberry, K.J., and Watt, B. (2010). High merino weaner survival rates are a function of weaning weight and positive post-weaning growth rates. *Animal Production Science* 50: 465–472.

Hergenhan, R.L., Hinch, G.N., and Ferguson, D.M. (2014). Sire effects on neonatal lamb vigour and following-behaviour. *Animal Production Science* 54: 745–752.

Hough, R.L., McCarthy, F.D., Thatcher, C.D. et al. (1990). Influence of glucocorticoid on macromolecular absorption and passive immunity in neonatal lambs. *Journal of Animal Science* 68: 2459–2464.

Jones, A. (2012). *Rangeland Goat Production in Western NSW*. Orange, NSW, Australia: NSW Department of Primary Industries.

Kenyon, P.R., Stafford, K.J., Morel, P.C.H., and Morris, S.T. (2005). Does sward height grazed by ewes in mid- to late-pregnancy affect indices of colostrum intake by twin and triplet lambs? *New Zealand Veterinary Journal* 53: 336–339.

Kouri, A., Charallah, S., Kouri, F. et al. (2018). Reproductive performances and abortion etiologies of native Bedouin goats in the arid zones of Algeria. *Livestock Research for Rural Development* 30: 7–15.

Lagercrantz, H. and Slotkin, T.A. (1986). The 'stress' of being born. *Scientific American* 254: 100–107.

Lehloenya, K.C., Greyling, J.P.C., and Schwalbach, L.M.J. (2005). Reproductive performance of South African indigenous goats following oestrous synchronisation and AI. *Small Ruminant Research* 57: 115–120.

Matheson, S.M., Bünger, L., and Dwyer, C.M. (2012). Genetic parameters for fitness and neonatal behavior traits in sheep. *Behavior Genetics* 42: 899–911.

McGregor, B.A. (2016). The effects of nutrition and parity on the development and productivity of angora goats: 1. Manipulation of mid pregnancy nutrition on energy intake and maintenance requirement, kid birth weight, kid survival, doe live weight and mohair production. *Small Ruminant Research* 145: 65–75.

McGuire, T.C., Regnier, J., Kellom, T., and Gates, N.L. (1983). Failure in passive transfer of immunoglobulin-G1 to lambs – measurement of immunoglobulin-G1 in ewe colostrum. *American Journal of Veterinary Research* 44: 1064–1067.

Mellado, M., Valdez, R., Lara, L.M., and García, J.E. (2004). Risk factors involved in conception, abortion, and kidding rates of goats under extensive conditions. *Small Ruminant Research* 55: 191–198.

Mellado, M., Valdéz, R., García, J.E. et al. (2006). Factors affecting the reproductive performance of goats under intensive conditions in a hot arid environment. *Small Ruminant Research* 63: 110–118.

Mellor, D.J. and Cockburn, F. (1986). A comparison of energy metabolism in the newborn infant, piglet and lamb. *Quarterly Journal of Experimental Physiology* 71: 361–379.

Miller, D.R., Blache, D., Jackson, R.B. et al. (2010). Metabolic maturity at birth and neonate lamb survival: association among maternal factors, litter size, lamb birth-weight, and plasma metabolic and endocrine factors on survival and behavior. *Journal of Animal Science* 88: 581–593.

Nogueira, D.M., Gummow, B., Gardiner, C.P. et al. (2016). A survey of the meat goat industry in Queensland and New South Wales. 2. Herd management, reproductive performance and animal health. *Animal Production Science* 56: 1533–1544.

Norton, B.W. (2004). *The Role of the Boer Goat in the Development of the Australian Goat Meat Industry*. Sydney, NSW, Australia: Meat & Livestock Australia.

Nowak, R. and Poindron, P. (2006). From birth to colostrum: early steps leading to lamb survival. *Reproduction, Nutrition, Development* 46: 431–446.

Nowak, R., Porter, R.H., Lévy, F. et al. (2000). Role of mother–young interactions in the survival of offspring in domestic mammals. *Reviews of Reproduction* 5: 153–163.

Poindron, P., Levy, F., and Keller, M. (2007). Maternal responsiveness and maternal selectivity in domestic sheep and goats: the two facets of maternal attachment. *Developmental Psychobiology* 49: 54–70.

Pretorius, P.S. (1970). Effect of aggressive behaviour on production and reproduction in the angora. Goat (copra hircus angoraensis). *Agroanimalia* 2: 161–164.

Rattner, D., Riviere, J., and Bearman, J.E. (1994). Factors affecting abortion, stillbirth and kid mortality in the goat and Yaez (goat × ibex). *Small Ruminant Research* 13: 33–40.

Refshauge, G., Brien, F.D., Hinch, G.N., and van de Ven, R. (2016). Neonatal lamb mortality: factors associated with the death of Australian lambs. *Animal Production Science* 56: 726–735.

Restall, B.J. (1992). Seasonal variation in reproductive activity in Australian goats. *Animal Reproduction Science* 27: 305–318.

Rooke, J.A., Dwyer, C.M., and Ashworth, C.J. (2008). The potential for improving physiological, behavioural and immunological responses in the neonatal lamb by trace element and vitamin supplementation of the ewe. *Animal* 2: 514–524.

Rooke, J.A., Arnott, G., Dwyer, C.M., and Rutherford, K.M.D. (2015). The importance of the gestation period for welfare of lambs: maternal stressors and lamb vigour and wellbeing. *Journal of Agricultural Science* 153: 497–519.

Russell, A.J.F. (1985). Nutrition of the pregnant ewe. *In Practice* 7: 23–29.

Sawalha, R.M., Conington, J., Brotherstone, S., and Villanueva, B. (2007). Analyses of lamb survival in Scottish blackface sheep. *Animal* 1: 151–157.

Shelton, M. and Groff, J. (1984). *Improving Reproductive Efficiency in Angora Goats*. San Angelo, TX, USA: Texas Agricultural Experiment Station.

Sherman, D.M. (1987). Causes of kid morbidity and mortality: an overview. In: *Proceedings of the IV International Conference on Goats*, 14–19 July, Brasilia, Brazil., 335–355. Little Rock, AR, USA: International Goat Association.

Singh, M.K., Rai, B., and Sharma, N. (2008). Factors affecting survivability of Jamunapari kids under semi-intensive management system. *Indian Journal of Animal Sciences* 78: 178–181.

Slee, J. (1981). A review of genetic aspects of survival and resistance to cold in newborn lambs. *Livestock Production Science* 8: 419–429.

Snyman, M.A. (2010). Factors affecting pre-weaning kid mortality in south African angora goats. *South African Journal of Animal Science* 40: 54–64.

Symonds, M.E., Bird, J.A., Clarke, L. et al. (1995). Nutrition, temperature and homeostasis during perinatal development. *Experimental Physiology* 80: 907–940.

Thiruvenkadan, A.K. and Karunanithi, K. (2007). Mortality and replacement rate of tellicherry and its crossbred goats in Tamil Nadu. *Indian Journal of Animal Sciences* 77: 590–594.

Urrutia-Morales, J., Meza-Herrera, C.A., Tello-Varela, L. et al. (2012). Effect of nutritional supplementation upon pregnancy rates of goats under semiarid rangelands and exposed to the male effect. *Tropical Animal Health and Production* 44: 1473–1477.

40

Hypothermia and Hypoglycemia

Ankit S. Prajapati[1], *Kashyap Patel*[2], *Prakash M. Chauhan*[3], *and Sarita Devi*[2]

[1] *Veterinary Clinical Complex (Medicine), College of Veterinary Science and Animal Husbandry, Kamdhenu University, Anand, Gujarat, India*
[2] *Department of Medicine, College of Veterinary Science and Animal Husbandry, Kamdhenu University, Sardarkrushinagar, Gujarat, India*
[3] *Department of Clinics, College of Veterinary Science and Animal Husbandry, Kamdhenu University, Sardarkrushinagar, Gujarat, India*

40.1 Introduction

Goat farming is prevalent in marginal farming communities (Nyakwawa et al. 2022). Goats are a primary or additional income source for many families in resource-poor areas (Utaaker et al. 2021). Profitable goat farming depends on kid production. The early days after birth are critical for kids as they are susceptible to many conditions that favor death in the early stages of life. Gastrointestinal and respiratory problems are more common in kids with lower immunity. Apart from these, hypothermia and hypoglycemia are the two important conditions. Very little information is available on hypothermia and hypoglycemia in goat kids. This chapter mainly focuses on the above two aspects.

40.2 Hypothermia

Thermoregulation is one of the brain's vital functions, particularly the hypothalamus. All animals maintain relatively constant body temperatures. In a homeostatic state, physiological and behavioral mechanisms continuously support the body temperature. Heat loss and heat production are two primary functions of the animal body. In order to keep the core body temperature regular, the loss rate is equal to the heat produced by the body. Newborn ruminants are precocial animals with advanced locomotor development that allows them to stand up within the first minutes or hours of life and begin to ingest colostrum. Newborns also have thermoregulatory mechanisms that enable them to maintain or reestablish normothermia, but several factors can affect this (Starck and Ricklefs 1998).

Heat production in the animal body mainly occurs through muscular activity. Continuous muscular movement maintains muscle tone and temperature. Another mechanism is shivering thermogenesis whichoccurs in response to sudden exposure to cold and is a significant contributor to enhance heat production (Hohtola 2004). Nonshivering mechanisms also play a role in temperature regulation, such as the metabolism of brown adipose tissue to prevent low body temperature.

Heat loss from the neonate body happens via four main mechanisms: (i) conduction (transfer of heat between two media that are in direct contact); (ii) convection (transfer of heat between two media at different temperatures); (iii) radiation (absorption/emission of electromagnetic waves); and (iv) evaporation (radiation from the body surface). Heat loss by evaporation of water and by sweating, salivation, and respiration comes under this. Heat regulatory functions of the hypothalamus control the balance between heat gain and heat loss (Figure 40.1).

A low body temperature, known as hypothermia, happens when too much heat is lost or not enough heat is created (Hancock et al. 1996). Newborn goat kids are susceptible to hypothermia which is also considered one of the crucial causes of perinatal mortality in goat kids. A newborn may have severe temperature shifts once they leave the uterus's warm, comfortable environment and enter a cold environment. The wet newborn can lose heat because of the exposed large surface area. It has been suggested that hypothermia accounts for more than 15% of neonatal mortality (Hernandez et al. 2012). Kids with a birth weight of less than 2.5 kg are at risk for hypothermia and are likely to have a higher mortality

Elements of Reproduction and Reproductive Diseases of Goats, First Edition. Edited by Tanmoy Rana.

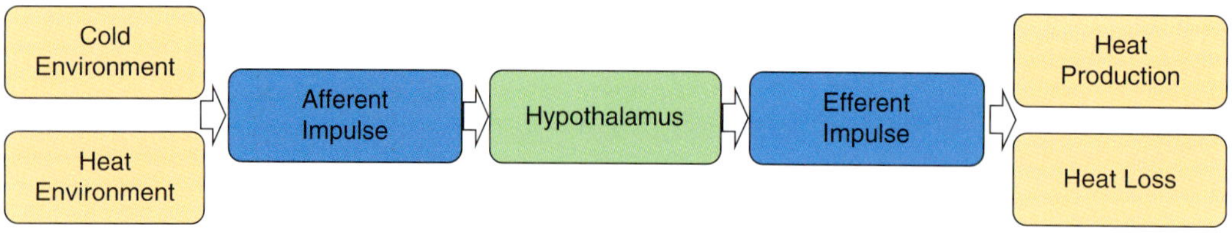

Figure 40.1 Heat homeostasis in goat kids. *Source:* Ankit S. Prajapati.

rate than normal-weight kids (Hart and Delaney 2016). During the first few days of life, kids and lambs are most at risk for hypothermia (Hassan et al. 2020).

Newborn farm animals generally have two ways to generate heat: shivering thermogenesis and nonshivering thermogenesis (Washburn and Streeter 2004). In neonatal goat kids, nonshivering thermogenesis is promoted by brown fat located mainly around the kidneys for heat production before suckling colostrum (Hassan et al. 2020). Hypothermia also occurs, secondary to other conditions such as weakness, shock, enteric diseases, and environmental stress, where a decrease in cardiac output is noticed. Robust, active newborns are often protected by the heat generated during muscle activity and can find food and shelter. Particularly in small or weak newborns, poorly licked off or rejected by their dams, cold, windy weather or tube feeding with cold milk replacer or fluids can cause a fast decrease in core body temperature.

According to a study by Poindron et al. (2003), mother sheep and goats develop an early bond with their neonate based on olfactory recognition. The difference in the early mother–offspring relationship between the two species due to the different behavior of the young is not associated with marked differences in the dynamics or mechanisms controlling the development of recognition of the neonate by its mother.

Climatic conditions also play a vital role in the development of hypothermia which is a primary cause of kid mortality. Cold ambient temperature can change the normal homeothermy of animals, and the body temperature may change transiently. This also leads to the activation and regulation of the immune system against the newly exposed antigens by paying off the metabolic machinery of the animal, thereby compromising growth, production, and reproductive performance (Hassan et al. 2020). Death of the kid may occur in severe cases due to cellular hypoxia (Sanin et al. 2016). Lambs are more prone to hypothermia than kids because brain development occurs faster in kids than lambs (Richardson et al. 2015).

40.2.1 Clinical Signs

Clinical signs of hypothermia are very familiar to all veterinarians. A drop in core body temperature is the main sign of this condition. The entire body, especially the extremities, becomes cold, and the rectal temperature is below 37 °C and may drop to 30 °C in neonates. Clinical symptoms develop when the rectal temperature falls to 98 ° F (36.7 °C) or less. Shivering, droopy ears, lethargy, nonalertness and labored breathing are the essential clinical signs recorded. Panting and respiratory distress are common signs of hypothermia in kids. A compensatory mechanism is normally activated for heat production. However, no further heat is produced in kids with low energy storage, so that hypothermia will persist.

40.2.2 Diagnosis

Diagnosis of hypothermia is mainly based on clinical signs and temperature measurement. Measurement of rectal temperature quickly identifies hypothermia. Mercury or digital thermometers can be used for temperature measurement (Figure 40.2). A goat kid with a very stressed system will not regulate its body temperature and is at higher risk for hypothermia. In these situations, the body temperature is not a reliable tool. Infrared thermography imaging is an emerging technique and can be used to assess temperature in the ruminant neonate (Mota-Rojas et al. 2022).

40.2.3 Treatment

The infant should be treated for hypothermia as soon as possible. Starvation and hypothermia often go hand in hand. Because of the body's low energy stores due to inadequate feed intake, dextrose (20%) should be provided as the instant energy source along with multivitamin injections (Figure 40.3). Fluid administration will provide immediate glucose for utilization by the kid. The fluid should be warmed to room temperature. Body temperature should be continuously monitored until the average temperature is regained.

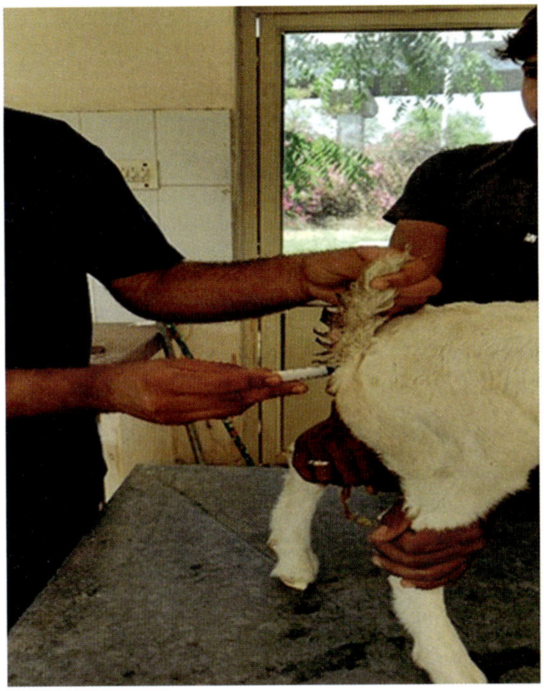

Figure 40.2 Measurement of rectal temperature in a kid. *Source:* Ankit S. Prajapati. (Chapter Contributor)

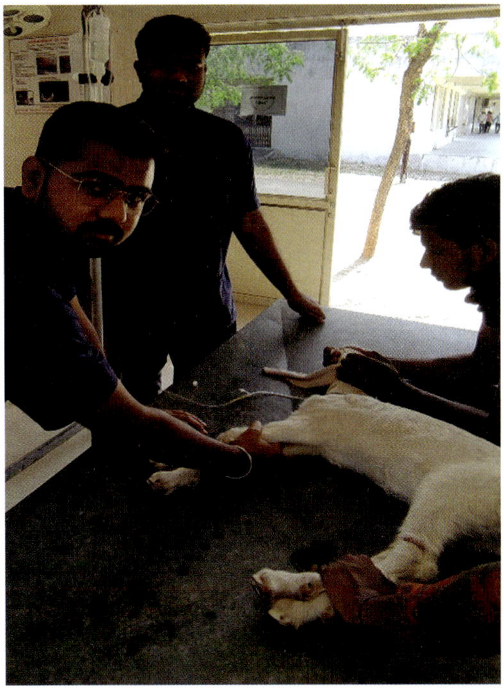

Figure 40.3 Management of hypothermia in the kid by fluid therapy. *Source:* Ankit S. Prajapati. (Chapter Contributor)

A three-day prophylactic cover of antibiotics is advised to prevent any chance of secondary bacterial infection. Intraperitoneal injection of dextrose may be tried. Drugs such as dexamethasone reduce the gradient between skin and body core temperature and can reduce shivering by regulating immune responses (Hammon et al. 2012). Extreme cases may result in muscular weakness and mental depression, respiratory failure, recumbency, and a state of collapse and, eventually, coma and death (Radostits et al. 2011).

A goat kid with hypothermia lacks a sucking reflex and may need to be tube fed colostrum to provide energy to help warm their bodies. A feeding tube can be inserted using a #14 French urethral catheter. This is cautiously introduced into the esophagus and appropriate placement is confirmed by palpation and injecting a few milliliters of water. Kids can be fed 60 ml of colostrum every two hours until they can suck (Hart and Delaney 2016).

40.2.4 Prevention

Prevention of hypothermia includes using a personal pen for a kid. The heat source can be arranged in the pen to provide heat to the affected kid. These heat sources must be placed at a safe distance, along with hot water bottles, blankets, and delivery of warm liquids to protect from wind and cold. If a separate pen is unavailable, a heat box can be prepared manually using a cardboard box. The chances of hypothermia are greater in the summer season due to evaporation. In the summer, proper care and attention should be given to reduce kid mortality.

Apart from genetic and physical abnormalities, the three main life-threatening issues which create a problem in the kid's early days are a kid that cannot feed itself, a dam that cannot or will not feed her kid, and a hypothermic kid.

Colostrum feeding has a significant role in maintaining body temperature and immunity. A kid must be given 10% body weight colostrum during the initial six hours of life. Colostrum is one of the leading energy sources for newborns. Its thermogenic effect is associated with the production of metabolic heat through such processes as the digestion, absorption, and processing of nutrients. Moreover, as a source of lactose, amino acids, and triglycerides, colostrum is an important energy source for heat production via diet-induced thermogenesis and nonshivering thermogenesis (Silva and Bittar 2019).

Milk replacers are used to save milk from the doe for sale and provide similar nutrition for the kid (Figure 40.4). Some milk replacers contain lactose-digesting bacteria or probiotic organisms, which may mitigate digestive upset. Farmers have used cow, sheep, and kid milk replacers to raise kids. Proper management practices include good maternal attention, adequate bedding, especially during winter months, and good balanced maternal nutrition.

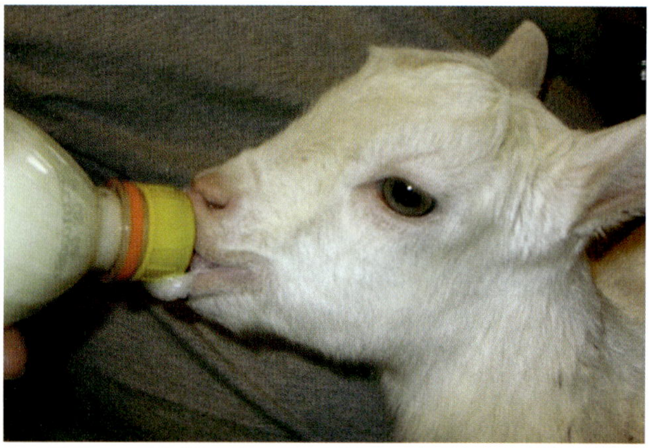

Figure 40.4 Administration of milk replacer. *Source:* Google.

40.3 Hypoglycemia

Hypoglycemia can be defined as a lower glucose level than the standard range (40–60 mg/dl) (Barakat et al. 2007). Hypoglycemia is the most prevalent metabolic abnormality in neonate kids (Straussman and Levitsky 2010). The productivity of goat farms depends upon the survival rate of neonates.

Because of immature anatomical and physiological characteristics, neonates face complex metabolic adjustments in the first few months of extrauterine life (Saddiqi et al. 2011). During this phase, kids are monogastric and glucose is essential for normal physiological functions (Hammon et al. 2013). Efficient postnatal metabolism provides the energy needed for motor activities and enables the neonate to stand and suckle colostrum. Proper colostrum feeding is critical to the health and survival of goat kids (Mellor and Murray 1986). If colostrum feeding is delayed, death occurs due to hypothermia or hypoglycemia. Kids under 24 hours are most at risk but older kids can still be affected (Clair et al. 2019). The morbidity for hypoglycemia is 20–30%, and mortality rates depend upon recognizing and managing the condition (Habibu et al. 2021).

40.3.1 Etiology

Hypoglycemia is chiefly caused by a female goat's inability to supply milk to her young owing to mastitis, teat abnormalities, or mismothering. Large litter sizes result in mismothering, which decreases the doe's interest in later-born kids. Weak kids who cannot suckle due to several congenital abnormalities, contracted tendons, fractures, and swayback conditions are predisposed to hypoglycemia. Inclement weather causes an increase in energy requirement due to thermoregulation, potentially leading to hypoglycemia. Hypothermic kids over five hours will not be able to suckle and will be hypoglycemic. Kids in large litters and those born with lower body weights are predisposed to hypoglycemia due to lower body lipids (Harwood and Mueller 2018).

40.3.2 Pathophysiology

The fetus depends on the maternal metabolism during fetal life, and placental circulation provides glucose and other nutrients. In early postnatal life, glucose is the source of energy for kids. Neonatal glucose concentrations fall once the umbilical cord is clipped because the glucose source is cut off. Glucose concentration reaches a low point within 1–2 hours of birth. Also, insulin concentration decreases while glucagon concentration increases, stimulating gluconeogenesis and glycogenolysis (Edwards and Harding 2021). Gluconeogenesis is crucial in neonatal ruminants, accounting for around 75% of their total glucose requirements (Donkin and Hammon 2005). Inadequate glycogen reserve and a poorly responding endocrine system after birth might impair glucose homeostasis and result in neonatal hypoglycemia (McGowan 1999). Kids with neonatal hypoglycemia depend upon continuous and excessive lipid metabolization, which causes lower levels of blood lipids. Due to this, kids who have survived hypoglycemia show a noticeable drop in their weekly weight growth (Pesantez-Pacheco et al. 2019).

Glucose is an essential metabolic fuel for the brain and in newborns, the proportionately large brain accounts for almost all the total tissue glucose requirements. Thus, low glucose concentrations will likely result in an inadequate brain energy supply. Hypoglycemia associated with asphyxia leads to severe encephalopathy and central nervous system damage. Permanent neuronal damage following hypoglycemia is not fully understood (Straussman and Levitsky 2010).

40.3.3 Clinical Signs

Initially, the kid is normal at birth but then becomes increasingly weak, incoordinated, and unresponsive over 12–24 hours. Clinical signs start when glucose levels are below 35–40 mg/dl. Suckle reflex is absent in weak kids, and less affected kids raise their heads and suckle with poor suck. Decreased muscle tone (hypotonia) may be seen. Incoordination is observed first, and the kid has difficulty getting up and maintaining balance. Apnea, grunting, tachycardia, and tachypnea may occur. Cyanosis of the mucus membrane can be observed. Hypothermia (100–102 °F) is evident in kids with hypoglycemia. Neurological signs like facial cramps, convulsions, and opisthotonos can be observed. Eventually, the kid becomes recumbent and comatose, and death occurs within 24–36 hours. Affected kids become normoglycemic after treatment but cannot gain weight even after adequate feed consumption (Abramowski et al. 2021; Harwood and Mueller 2018).

40.3.4 Diagnosis

Based on clinical signs and a kidding history, a tentative diagnosis can be made. As clinical signs are not specific, estimation of blood glucose level is paramount. Blood glucose estimation can be done using a hand-held glucometer by taking a drop of blood from the ear tip or with the help of serum blood glucose analysis (Marina et al. 2022). Another alternative for blood glucose estimation is enzymatic point-of-care analyzers, which have the same accuracy as laboratory methods. In goat kids with neonatal hypoglycemia, glucose levels may be as low as 20 mg/dl; these levels can remain low for almost 10 days after birth, suggesting proper nutrition (Habibu et al. 2021).

Hypoglycemia should be differentiated from hypothermia, floppy kid syndrome, neonatal septicemia, and various congenital abnormalities.

40.3.5 Management

If a kid can hold its head up and has a suckle reflex, 150–200 ml of colostrum or milk should be given with the help of a stomach tube. If the kid cannot get up and the suckle reflex is absent, then an intraperitoneal dextrose injection is given. For this, 50% dextrose is diluted with sterile water to make a 20% solution. Before use, this solution is warmed to normal body temperature. The kid is held in dorsoventral recumbency, and a solution is injected lateral and caudal to the umbilicus at approximately 25 mm with a 20 G needle. After this solution, an antibiotic is given to prevent infection and the kid is warmed if hypothermia is present. If warmth is given to kids without correcting hypoglycemia, there will be increased cerebral metabolism, leading to convulsions and death (Smith and Sherman 2009). Twins and triplets should be monitored continuously for sufficient milk intake and if this does not occur, they should be fostered. If fostering is impossible, artificial colostrum can be given but it does not provide passive immunization and blood metabolites (Mellado et al. 2008).

Kids should be given adequate colostrum after birth to prevent hypoglycemia. Colostrum feeding improves glucose absorption. Also, it supports maturation of the gastrointestinal tract and increases lactose metabolism (Hammon et al. 2013). Around 50 ml/kg body weight of colostrum should be given four times a day for adequate nutrition and immunity. Dextrose gel with colostrum is a good option for large litter numbers. Kids should not be exposed to inclement weather because it causes hypothermia and higher energy requirements. Adequate nutrition for a doe during pregnancy supports maternal metabolism and provides fetal growth and development. This in turn reduces the chances of hypoglycemia due to higher birth weight of kids (Estrada-Cortes et al. 2009).

Good management practices and nutritional support should be provided to goat kids to minimize the occurrence of hypothermia and hypoglycemia.

References

Abramowski, A., Ward, R., and Hamdan, A.H. (2021). Neonatal hypoglycemia. StatPearls Publishing. www.ncbi.nlm.nih.gov/books/NBK537105/ (accessed 23 December 2024).

Barakat, S.E.M., Al-Bhanasawi, G.E., Elazhari, N.M., and Bakhiet, A.O. (2007). Clinical and serobiochemical studies on naturally occurring pregnancy toxaemia in Shamia goats. *Journal of Animal and Veterinary Advances* 6: 768–772.

Clair, E.S., Russell, R.W., and Van Saun, R.J. (2019). Assessment of goat colostrum quality and passive transfer. *American Association of Bovine Practitioners Conference Proceedings*, Pennsylvania State University (12 September 2019).

Donkin, S.S. and Hammon, H. (2005). Hepatic gluconeogenesis in developing ruminants. *Biology of Growing Animals* 3: 375–390.

Edwards, T. and Harding, J.E. (2021). Clinical aspects of neonatal hypoglycemia: a mini review. *Frontiers in Pediatrics* 8: 562251.

Estrada-Cortes, E., Vera-Avila, H.R., Urrutia-Morales, J. et al. (2009). Nutritional status influences reproductive seasonality in creole goats: 1. Ovarian activity during seasonal reproductive transitions. *Animal Reproduction Science* 116 (3–4): 282–290.

Habibu, B., Umaru Kawu, M., Aluwong, T., and Joan Makun, H. (2021). Postnatal hypoglycemia and blood glucose concentrations in neonatal tropical goat kids. *Veterinary Clinical Pathology* 50 (4): 525–534.

Hammon, H.M., Steinhoff-Wagner, J., Schonhusen, U. et al. (2012). Energy metabolism in the newborn farm animal with emphasis on the calf: endocrine changes and responses to milk-born and systemic hormones. *Domestic Animal Endocrinology* 43 (2): 171–185.

Hammon, H.M., Steinhoff-Wagner, J., Flor, J. et al. (2013). Lactation biology symposium: role of colostrum and colostrum components on glucose metabolism in neonatal calves. *Journal of Animal Science* 91 (2): 685–695.

Hancock, R.D., Coe, A.J., and Silva, F.C. (1996). Perinatal mortality in lambs in southern Brazil. *Tropical Animal Health and Production* 28 (4): 266–272.

Hart, S. and Delaney, C. (2016). Husbandry of dairy animals – goat: replacement management. www.ncbi.nlm.nih.gov/pmc/articles/PMC7157435/ (accessed 4 April 2020).

Harwood, D. and Mueller, K. (2018). *Goat Medicine and Surgery*, 95–96. Boca Raton, FL: CRC Press.

Hassan, N., Shaheen, M., and Bashir, S. (2020). Hypothermia in a lamb: a case report. *Journal of Entomology and Zoology Studies* 8 (6): 1777–1778.

Hernandez, H., Terrazas, A., Poindron, P. et al. (2012). Sensorial and physiological control of maternal behavior in small ruminants: sheep and goats. *Tropical and Subtropical Agroecosystems* 15: 91–102.

Hohtola, E. (2004). Shivering thermogenesis in birds and mammals. In: *Life in the Cold: Evolution, Mechanisms, Adaptation, and Application* (ed. M. Barnes and H.V. Carey), 241–252. ARCUS: Alaska.

Marina, G.C., Matheus, D.V., Isabelle, M.C. et al. (2022). Validation of a portable glucose meter in blood glucose measurement in normoglycemic goats induced to hypoglycemia and hyperglycemia. *Small Ruminant Research* 214: 106741.

McGowan, J.E. (1999). Neonatal hypoglycemia. *Pediatrics in Review* 20 (7): 6–15.

Mellado, M., Pittroff, W., Garcia, J.E., and Mellado, J. (2008). Serum IgG, blood profiles, growth and survival in goat kids supplemented with artificial colostrum on the first day of life. *Tropical Animal Health and Production* 40: 141–145.

Mellor, D.J. and Murray, L. (1986). Making the most of colostrum at lambing. *Veterinary Record* 118 (13): 351–353.

Mota-Rojas, D., Wang, D., Titto, C.G. et al. (2022). Neonatal infrared thermography images in the hypothermic ruminant model: anatomical-morphological-physiological aspects and mechanisms for thermoregulation. *Frontiers in Veterinary Science* 9: 1–17.

Nyakwawa, C., Mulagha-Maganga, A., and Mangisoni, J.H. (2022). Profit inefficiency of goat farming in Malawi: a Bayesian approach. *Heliyon* 8 (11): e11318.

Pesantez-Pacheco, J.L., Heras-Molina, A., Torres-Rovira, L. et al. (2019). Influence of maternal factors (weight, body condition, parity, and pregnancy rank) on plasma metabolites of dairy ewes and their lambs. *Animals* 9 (4): 122.

Poindron, P., Gilling, G., Hernandez, H. et al. (2003). Early recognition of newborn goat kids by their mother: I Nonolfactory discrimination. *Developmental Psychobiology* 43 (2): 82–89.

Radostits, O.M., Gay, C.C., Hinchcliff, K.W., and Constable, P.D. (2011). *Veterinary Medicine: A Textbook of the Diseases of Cattle, Sheep, Pigs, Goats and Horses*, 11e. St Louis, MO: Elsevier Saunders.

Richardson, S.J., Wijayagunaratne, R.C., D'Souza, D.G. et al. (2015). Transport of thyroid hormones via the choroid plexus into the brain: the roles of transthyretin and thyroid hormone transmembrane transporters. *Frontiers in Neuroscience* 9: 66.

Saddiqi, H.A., Nisa, M., Mukhtar, N. et al. (2011). Documentation of physiological parameters and blood profile in newly born Kajli lambs. *Asian-Australasian Journal of Animal Sciences* 24 (7): 912–918.

Sanin, L.Y., Cabrera, A.M.Z., and Morales, A.M.T. (2016). Adaptive responses to thermal stress in mammals. *Revista de Medicina Veterinaria* 31: 121–135.

Silva, F.L.M. and Bittar, C.M.M. (2019). Thermogenesis and some rearing strategies of dairy calves at low temperature – a review. *Journal of Applied Animal Research* 47: 115–122.

Smith, M.C. and Sherman, D.M. (2009). *Goat Medicine*. Hoboken, NJ: Wiley.

Starck, J.M. and Ricklefs, R.E. (1998). *Avian Growth and Development Evolution Within the Altricial Precocial Spectrum*. New York: Oxford University Press.

Straussman, S. and Levitsky, L.L. (2010). Neonatal hypoglycemia. *Current Opinion in Endocrinology, Diabetes and Obesity* 17 (1): 20–24.

Utaaker, K.S., Chaudhary, S., Kifleyohannes, T., and Robertson, L.J. (2021). Global goat! Is the expanding goat population an important reservoir of *cryptosporidium*? *Frontiers in Veterinary Science* 8: 648500.

Washburn, K.E. and Streeter, R.N. (2004). Congenital defects of the ruminant nervous system. *Veterinary Clinics of North America. Food Animal Practice* 20 (2): 413–434.

41

Bacteria and Toxins

Ranjani Rajasekaran[1] *and Saahithya Rajamohan*[2]

[1] *Department of Veterinary Microbiology, Veterinary College and Research Institute, Tamil Nadu Veterinary and Animal Sciences University, Theni, India*
[2] *Department of Veterinary Pathology, Veterinary College and Research Institute, Tamil Nadu Veterinary and Animal Sciences University, Salem, India*

41.1 Introduction

Toxins are defined as small protein or peptide molecules secreted within living cells or organisms. The word *toxin* is derived from the Greek word "toxikon" and was first used by an organic chemist named Ludwig Brieger. Toxins produced by bacteria are called bacterial toxins and are large noninvasive soluble protein antigens that are important determinants of the virulence of a bacterium. The ability of bacteria to secrete a toxin is termed toxigenicity. The toxigenicity of *Corynebacterium diphtheriae* to secrete diphtheria toxin was the first documentation of bacterial toxins in the history of science. Since then, enormous numbers of bacterial toxins have been identified.

Bacterial toxins can be classified broadly into exotoxins and endotoxins. Exotoxins are high molecular weight proteins that are produced by live Gram-positive or Gram-negative bacteria. They are heat-labile, highly antigenic potent toxins, that induce specific activity in the host. The synthesis of exotoxins is determined extrachromosomally. They can be converted readily into toxoids, thereby inducing production of neutralizing antibodies. Endotoxins are lipopolysaccharide complexes, a component of the Gram-negative cell wall, that are released upon death of the bacterium. They are heat-stable, weak antigens that induce generalized nonspecific activity. The synthesis of endotoxins is encoded in the chromosomes. They cannot be converted into toxoids, and hence neutralizing antibodies will not be produced (Quinn et al. 2016). The various effects of exotoxins and endotoxins are depicted schematically in Figure 41.1.

Goats are susceptible to various bacterial pathogens. Bacterial diseases in which toxins are produced as part of the pathogenesis include those caused by *Bacillus anthracis*, *Clostridium* spp., *Corynebacterium pseudotuberculosis*, *Escherichia coli*, *Fusobacterium necrophorum*, *Listeria monocytogenes*, *Mannheimia haemolytica*, *Staphylococcus aureus*, and *Trueperella pyogenes*. The toxins produced by these bacteria and the diseases they cause in goats are provided in Table 41.1.

41.2 *Bacillus anthracis*

Bacillus anthracis is a Gram-positive, nonmotile, aerobic, facultative, spore-forming, rod-shaped bacterium that causes anthrax in goats. Anthrax is a fatal disease in goats, where death occurs in 1–3 days primarily due to shock, renal failure, and anoxia. Transmission of anthrax usually occurs through ingestion of spores in grazing lands where spores are present. Upon entry into the host, they sporulate, localize in tissue and cause infection. Septicemia, hyperthermia, anorexia, and depression are some of the characteristics of anthrax in goats along with hematuria and bloody diarrhea (Quinn et al. 2016).

Bacillus anthracis produces a tripartite toxin that is encoded by the pXO1 plasmid. The toxin consists of three proteins: edema factor (EF), protective antigen (PA), and lethal factor (LF). These three proteins are nontoxic separately. The proteins EF and LF, upon binding with PA, become edema toxin (EdTx) and lethal toxin (LeTx) respectively. The binding of EF or LF with PA occurs at the amino-terminal region of the former (Brossier and Mock 2001).

Edema factor is an 89 kD protein molecule that belongs to the adenylate cyclase family of toxins, which converts intracellular cyclic adenosine monophosphate (cAMP) into adenosine triphosphate (ATP) with the help of the host protein

Elements of Reproduction and Reproductive Diseases of Goats, First Edition. Edited by Tanmoy Rana.

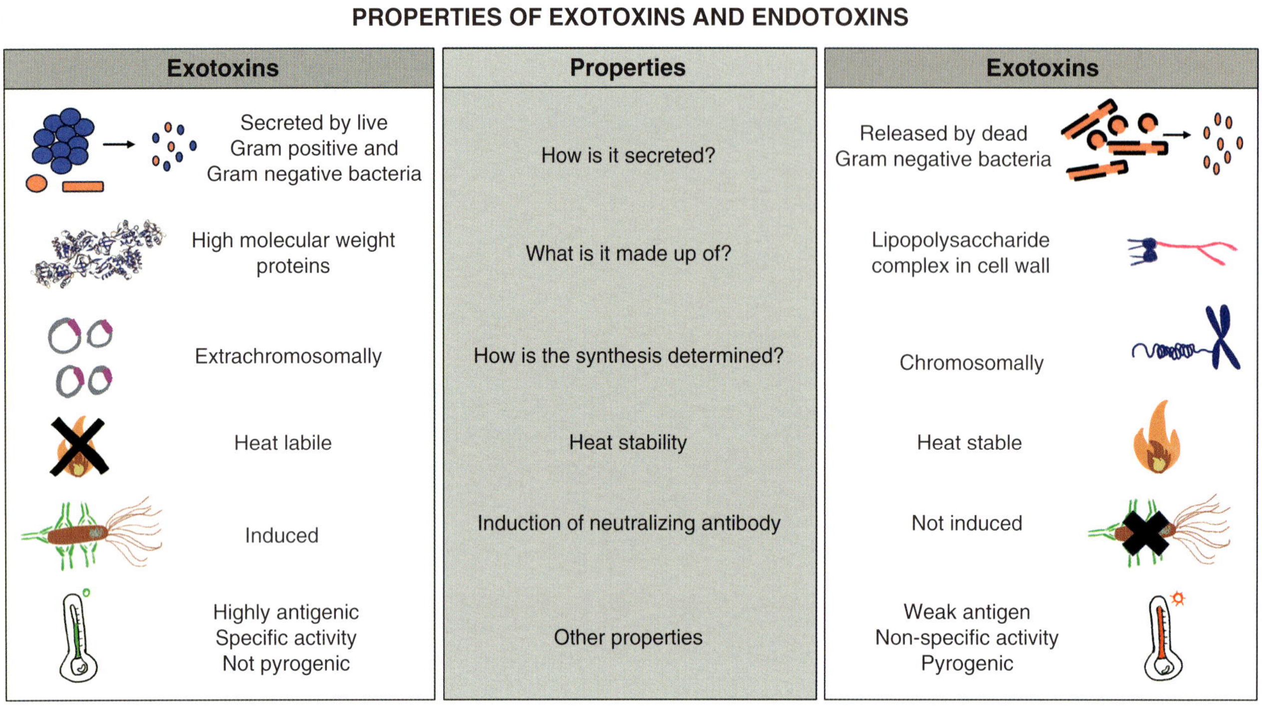

Figure 41.1 Schematic representation of effects of exotoxins and endotoxins. *Source:* Created by Ranjani Rajasekaran using www.biorender.com under academic license.

molecule, calmodulin (Leppla 1982). LF is an 85 kD protein molecule that belongs to the zinc-metalloproteinase family of toxins, which inactivates cellular signaling pathways through proteolysis of mitogen-activated protein (MAP) kinases (Arora and Leppla 1993). PA is an 83 kD protein molecule that attaches to the host cell receptor and initiates the activation of *B. anthracis* toxins (Petosa et al. 1997). The host cell receptors for *B. anthracis* toxins are type I transmembrane proteins, namely ANTXR1 and ANTXR2. PA consists of four functional domains, D1–D4. Domain D1 consists of a proteolytic cleavage site that cleaves D1 into two subdomains, 1a (PA20) and 1b (PA63), by cellular proteases. D2 is structurally identified as a beta-barrel core that helps in pore formation. D3 is a hydrophobic patch that helps in protein–protein interaction, and D4 aids in the attachment of PA to host cell receptors (Petosa et al. 1997).

Upon entry of *B. anthracis* spores into the host, phagocytosis occurs followed by germination of spores, proliferation of the bacteria, and release of vegetative bacilli through cytolysis (Petosa et al. 1997). Inside the phagocytic cell, the vegetative bacilli release the toxin and all the three proteins, EF, PA, and LF, are released. Upon release, D4 of PA attaches to the anthrax toxin receptor (ATR) on the surface of host cell, forming a PA–ATR complex. Following this, PA is cleaved into PA20 and PA63, thereby exposing the site of attachment for EF/LF. Oligomerization of PA63 occurs, leading to ring-shaped heptamers or prepore formation. Following the PA63 prepore formation, EF/LF is attached to the prepore, forming an PA–ATR–EF/LF prepore complex, which enters the cell through receptor-mediated endocytosis. Inside the cell, the pH is low and hence the prepore is converted into a pore. Following this, EF and LF are translocated, leading to edema by converting cAMP into ATP by binding with calmodulin, and LF inactivates MAP kinases, leading to cell death (Brossier and Mock 2001).

In addition to these toxins, a toxin named anthrolysin O (ALO) is secreted by *B. anthracis*. ALO is a cholesterol-dependent cytolysin (CDC) of beta-pore-forming toxin that facilitates the evasion of phagolysosomes of *B. anthracis* by the host cells (Shannon et al. 2003).

41.3 Clostridium Species

41.3.1 *Clostridium perfringens* type C

This is a Gram-positive, anaerobic, nonmotile, spore-forming bacillus that causes enterotoxemia in goats. *Cl. perfringens* is ubiquitously present in the soil and gastrointestinal tract of animals. Transmission occurs through ingestion of contaminated feed or water. The disease presents itself in per-acute form wherein sudden death of goats will be observed.

Table 41.1 Details of toxins produced by bacterial organisms affecting goats.

Organism	Toxin name	Toxin family	Toxin type	Plasmid /gene encoded	Receptor	Disease caused	Effect of toxin
Bacillus anthracis	Edema factor (binds with PA to form EdTx)	Calcium- and calmodulin-dependent adenylate cyclase	Exotoxin	pXO1	Type I transmembrane proteins – ANTXR1 and ANTXR2	Anthrax	Pore formation leads conversion of cAMP into ATP and inactivation of MAP kinases leading to edema and cell death
	Lethal factor (binds with PA to form LeTx)	Zinc-dependent metalloproteinase					
Corynebacterium pseudotuberculosis	Phospholipase D	Phospholipase superfamily	Exotoxin	*pld* gene	Sphingomyelin	Caseous lymphadenitis	Hydrolysis of sphingomyelin leading to vascular leakage
Fusobacterium necrophorum	Leukotoxin and hemolysin	NA	Exotoxin	NA	Polymorphonuclear leukocytes and erythrocytes	Foot abscess	Cytoplasmic condensation and pore-forming activity
Listeria monocytogenes	Listeriolysin O	Cholesterol-dependent or cholesterol binding cytolysin	Exotoxin	*hly* gene	Membrane cholesterol	Listeriosis	Cytolysis by formation of pores in host cell
Mannheimia haemolytica	Leukotoxin	RTX family	Exotoxin	lktA gene	Leukocytes	Pleuropneumonia	Formation of transmembrane pores
Staphylococcus aureus	Hemolysin-α	Pore-forming toxin	Exotoxin	*hla* gene	ADAM10	Mastitis in goats	Cytolysis by formation of pores in host cell
	Hemolysin-β	Nonpore forming		Encoded in lysogenic bacteriophage	NA		Hydrolysis of sphingomyelin leading to irregularity of plasma membrane fluidity
Trueperella pyogenes	Pyolysin	Cholesterol-dependent or cholesterol binding cytolysin	Exotoxin	*plo* gene	Membrane cholesterol	Abscess	Cytolysis by formation of pores in host cell

In some cases, the goats may exhibit tremors and convulsions, and abdominal pain (Quinn et al. 2016). *Cl. perfringens* secretes various toxins including alpha-toxin (hemolytic), beta-toxin (necrotizing), delta-toxin (cytotoxic and hemoltyic), epsilon-toxin, and lambda-toxin. Of these, beta-toxin has been reported to be associated in the pathogenesis of enterotoxemia in goats. Beta-toxin is an oligomerizing pore-forming toxin (PFT) that is encoded as additional toxin genes *cpe* or *tpeL* in large virulence plasmids. It is sensitive to trypsin and proteases. Beta-toxin binds with the ATP-gated P2X7 receptor in the plasma membrane and forms functional pores through which efflux of potassium and influx of calcium, sodium, and chlorine occur. Due to this imbalance, cell swelling occurs which is followed by cell death (Navarro et al. 2018).

41.3.2 *Clostridium tetani*

This is a Gram-positive, motile, spore-forming, strict anaerobic bacillus that is present in soil and gastrointestinal tracts of ruminants. All animals are susceptible and it causes tetanus in goats. *Cl. tetani* gains entry into the body through abrasions, that might be caused during farm management practices such as castration, tail docking, dehorning, and ear tagging. The disease presents in an acute form and shows typical clinical symptoms including rigid limbs, hyperthermia, and lock jaw with a unique saw-horse stance.

Clostridium tetani produces two exotoxins: a neurotoxic tetanospasmin (TeNT) and hemolytic tetanolysin. TeNT is a high molecular weight protein of 150 kD that is encoded in the tetX gene on the PE88 plasmid. Protein translation of the tetX gene yields one protein that is subsequently cleaved into a 100 kD heavy or B-chain and a 50 kD light or A-chain. The A- and B-chains are connected by a disulfide bond. Upon entry of *Cl. tetani* into the host cell, TeNT is released. The B-chain of TeNT establishes a neuro-specific binding to the GT1b polysialogangliosides located in the lipid microdomains of the nerve terminal membranes. Followed binding, endocytosis of TeNT occurs which leads to retrograde axonal transport of the toxin to spinal neurons, after which transcytosis from axon to central nervous system inhibitory interneuron occurs.

Following transcytosis, TeNT is translocated into the cytosol, which is mediated by pH and temperature. In the cytosol, the NADPH-thioredoxin reductase-thioredoxin enzyme acts on the disulfide bond rendering the A- and B-chain free. The A-chain cleaves the Gln76-Phe77 bond of synaptobrevin, which interferes with exocytosis of neurotransmitters from inhibitory interneurons and interferes with release of excitatory neurotransmitters. Interference with the neurotransmitters gamma-aminobutyric acid (GABA) and glycine leads to inhibition of motor neurons and thus to spastic paralysis and tetanic spasm (Winter et al. 1996).

Tetanolysin is a protein of 55 kD molecular weight and belongs to the thiol-activated cytolysin family of toxins that bind with cholesterol and form pores in cytoplasmic membrane, causing efflux and influx of ions and other molecules, leading to physiological imbalance followed by cell death (Billington et al. 2000).

41.3.3 *Clostridium chauvoei*

This is a Gram-positive, motile, spore-forming, anaerobic bacillus that causes blackleg in goats. The toxins produced by this organism include CCtA with cytotoxin activity, alpha-toxin with lethal hemolytic, necrotizing activity, beta-toxin with deoxyribonuclease activity, gamma-toxin with hyaluronidase activity, and delta-toxin with oxygen-labile hemolysin activity (Underwood et al. 2015).

41.3.4 *Clostridium novyi* type A

This Gram-positive, motile, spore-forming, anaerobic bacillus causes bighead in goats but is uncommon. The toxins secreted include alpha-toxin with lethal, necrotizing activity (Underwood et al. 2015).

41.4 *Corynebacterium pseudotuberculosis*

Corynebacterium psedotuberculosis is a Gram-positive, nonmotile, non-spore forming, aerobic, pleomorphic coccobacillus that causes caseous lymphadenitis in goats. The disease is characterized by abscessation of superficial and deep lymph nodes with eroded peripheral lymph nodes of head and neck producing creamy-white or yellowish secretions. The disease can present in a chronic form causing debilitation in goats. *C. pseudotuberculosis* can survive in the environment for a period of six months and hence transmission is possible through ingestion, inhalation, or open wound infection caused during livestock management practices like shearing, castration or docking (Underwood et al. 2015).

Corynebacterium pseudotuberculosis produces phospholipase D (PLD), which is the first exotoxin that was identified to be able to hydrolyse sphingomyelins without activation by diethyl ether and calcium ions (Souček et al. 1971). PLD is a sphingomyelinase which acts on sphingomyelins of the cell membrane of endothelial cells (Jernigan et al. 2015). Endothelial cell membranes are made up of lipids, of which sphingomyelins and ceramides are integral components. Sphingomyelins are sphingolipids that are essential for maintaining cell integrity and ceramides are the backbone of sphingolipids that facilitate physiological vascular leakage (de Chaves and Sipione 2010). The independent function of both these metabolites is essential for maintaining normal physiological function of the cell (Jernigan et al. 2015). Hence, when PLD acts on sphingomyelin and converts it into ceramide phosphate and choline (Carne and Onon 1978), vascular leakage occurs due to abundance of ceramide phosphate. Therefore, phagocytosis of *C. pseudotuberculosis* occurs. However, phagocytic cell membranes are also made of sphingomyelins, so PLD acts on phagocytic cells, which (i) facilitates *C. pseudotuberculosis* to withstand phagocytosis and (ii) helps *C. pseudotuberculosis* to enter the lymphatic system, thus spreading infection lymphatically. Further, PLD is also described as a dermonecrotoxin, hence exotoxin-induced hemolytic crisis has been reported to occur occasionally (Underwood et al. 2015).

41.5 *Escherichia coli*

Escherichia coli is a Gram-negative, facultatively anaerobic, motile, nonspore-forming coccobacillus that causes colibacillosis in goats. *E. coli* can be classified into enterotoxigenic *E. coli* (ETEC), enteropathogenic *E. coli* (EPEC), Shiga toxin-producing *E. coli* (STEC), verotoxigenic *E. coli* (VTEC) and the attaching/effacing *E. coli* (AEEC). Among these pathotypes of *E. coli*, only ETEC, STEC, and VTEC are reported to secrete toxins (Quinn et al. 2016). However, as *E. coli* is a Gram-negative bacterium, the cell wall consists of lipopolysaccharide (LPS), which is an endotoxin that is released upon death of *E. coli*. LPS is a glycolipid component composed of lipid A, the core oligosaccharide, and the O antigen. LPS induces production of proinflammatory cytokines, activates complement, induces release of histamine, and activates the coagulation cascade, thereby causing inflammation, hemorrhage, intravascular coagulation, and septic shock (Underwood et al. 2015).

Enterotoxigenic *E. coli* secretes enterotoxins that are heat labile (LT) and heat stable (ST). LT can be classified as LT-I and LT-II that are encoded by plasmid and chromosome respectively. LT enterotoxin is an oligomer consisting of one A subunit and five B subunits of 88 and 11.5 kD (each) respectively. The B subunits are arranged in a doughnut-like configuration forming a pentamer. This pentamer binds to the intestinal cell membrane and activates the A subunit, which leads to elevated levels of cAMP. This leads to influx of sodium ions and efflux of chloride ions, thus resulting in diarrhea. ST are enterotoxins that are resistant to 100 °C heat for 15 minutes and can be classified into ST-I and ST-II. ST-I stimulates expression of guanyl cyclase that results in production of cyclic guanosine monophosphate (cGMP), causing rapid efflux of fluid, leading to diarrhea. ST-II is smaller in size than ST-I but its mechanism of action is yet to be explored (Quinn et al. 2016).

Escherichia coli secretes cytotoxins that possess the ability to lyze erythrocytes. They have been termed either as Shiga toxin (Stx), relating to their similarity with toxins secreted by *Shigella dysenteriae*, or verotoxin, relating to their cytotoxic activity in vero cells. Shiga toxin is composed of one 33 kD A subunit and five 7.5 kD noncovalently attached B subunits. The B subunit is involved in recognition of and binding with host cell receptor globotriasylceramide (Gb3) found on renal and intestinal epithelial cells, platelets, and erythrocytes, whereas the A subunit is involved in enzymatic activities (Batt 2014). Upon binding of Stx with the Gb3 receptor, the Stx–Gb3 complex is internalized within endosomes and transported to the endoplasmic reticulum (ER) through the Golgi apparatus. In the ER, the A subunit is cleaved by furin-like proteases and the enzymatically active A-1 subunit is released. The A-1 subunit acts on the 28s rRNA within the 60S ribosomal subunit and renders it inactive by removing a single adenine base. This results in inhibition of protein synthesis, eventually resulting in cell death. The depurinated 28s rRNA induces a signal transduction response called the ribotoxic stress response, which elicits various cytokines and chemokines leading to cell apoptosis. Further, the Stx–Gb3 complex induces a unique cytoplasmic signal transduction pathway (Obrig 2010). The inflammatory and apoptotic response induced by Stx results in damage to the epithelial cells.

41.6 *Fusobacterium necrophorum*

Fusobacterium necrophorum is a Gram-negative, obligately anaerobic pleomorphic bacillus causing foot abscess in goats. It is found ubiquitously in the soil, gastrointestinal tract, skin, and hoof of goats. The disease is characterized by a swollen hoof with purulent discharge, and the goat is unable to bear weight on the affected hoof leading to lameness

(Underwood et al. 2015). Transmission occurs primarily in moist and overcrowded environments through direct or indirect contact. The organism enters the host through hoof injuries caused by physical abrasion or larvae bites (Underwood et al. 2015).

This bacterium has been reported to secrete two exotoxins, namely leukotoxin and hemolysin, and one endotoxin, namely lipopolysaccharide. Leukotoxin is a potent exotoxin of high molecular weight (336 000 daltons) that is toxic to ruminant polymorphonuclear leukocytes (PMNs). Due to the killing of PMNs by leukotoxin, phagocytosis of *F. necrophorum* is diminished which facilitates uninterrupted establishment of infection (Tadepalli et al. 2008). In addition, leukotoxin causes cytoplasmic condensation, apoptosis, and degranulation of PMNs, and releases toxic reactive intermediates that cause necrosis. Hemolysins are PFTs that lyze erythrocytes to acquire iron which is essential for the growth of *F. necrophorum* (Nagaraja et al. 2005).

Lipopolysaccharide is present in the bacterial membrane of *F. necrophorum* and interacts with macrophages and neutrophils to elicit a proinflammatory cytokine response and nitric oxide secretion resulting in endotoxic shock. It causes disseminated intravascular coagulation and creates an anaerobic microenvironment which favors foot abscess formation (Nagaraja et al. 2005).

41.7 *Listeria monocytogenes*

Listeria monocytogenes is a Gram-positive, pleomorphic, motile, nonspore-forming, micro-aerophilic coccobacillary bacterium that causes listeriosis in goats, otherwise called circling disease or silage disease. The disease presents mostly in the encephalitic form, wherein neurological symptoms are evinced. Other forms of the disease include the placental form characterized by late abortion and the septicemic form characterized by hepatitis and pneumonia. Transmission of disease occurs through ingestion of contaminated feed or water, through cut wounds in the oral cavity or through inhalation (Underwood et al. 2015).

Listeria monocytogenes secretes an exotoxin named listeriolysin O (LLO), which is classified in the beta-pore-forming toxin family of CDC toxins. The activity of LLO is regulated by pH, which is a distinguishable characteristic among the various other CDC toxins. The structure and mechanism of action of LLO are similar to *Trueperalla pyogenes* pyolysin toxin (see *Trueperalla pyogenes* below).

In addition to facilitating cell death, LLO has been reported to have other intracellular and extracellular roles in the pathogenesis of listeriosis in goats. Intracellularly, it has been reported to inhibit NADPH oxidase in macrophages, thereby avoiding being killed by reactive oxygen species (ROS) during the respiratory burst. Extracellularly, LLO has been reported to cause calcium influx, thereby facilitating easy entry of bacteria into cells (Hamon et al. 2012).

41.8 *Mannheimia haemolytica*

Mannheimia haemolytica is an aerobic, nonmotile, nonspore-forming, bipolar, Gram-negative coccobacillus that causes pleuropneumonia in goats. *M. haemolytica* is an opportunistic pathogen that causes disease when goats are subjected to stressful conditions such as long distance transportation. Hence, the disease caused by *M. haemolytica* is called shipping fever. In addition, *M. haemolytica* can cause disease due to weaning, overcrowding, change in diet and weather. The clinical signs include acute onset of anorexia, dyspnea, high fever, and death. Transmission occurs through direct or indirect contact, through ingestion or inhalation (Underwood et al. 2015).

The toxins secreted by *M. haemolytica* include leukotoxin, cellular LPS endotoxin, and capsular polysaccharide. Leukotoxin is toxic to PMNs of goats and results in fibrin deposition in lungs and on pleural surfaces. Cellular LPS endotoxin causes systemic circulatory failure and shock. Capsular polysaccharide plays a pivotal role in attachment of the bacterium to the alveolar epithelial surface and inhibits phagocytosis of *M. haemolytica*.

Leukotoxin is an exotoxin and a significant virulent determinant of *M. haemolytica* of protein size ranging from 102 to 105 kD belonging to the Repeats in ToXin (RTX) family of toxins. Toxins belonging to this family possess a motif of glycine–aspartic acid nonapeptide repeats in the third carboxy terminal that are highly conserved. This conserved motif can transform into a tertiary conformation to facilitate binding of *M. haemolytica* to target host cells. Further, this motif is involved in calcium binding and inducing leukocyte toxicity, and aids in transportation of bacteria across biological membranes through the tolC-dependent type I secretion system.

The genetic organization of leukotoxin includes upstream genes lktC and lktA and downstream genes lktB and lktD (Highlander et al. 1989). The lktA gene encodes leukotoxin in a biologically inactive protoxin form, which is then converted into a biologically active component through fatty acid acylation by transacylase, that is encoded in the gene lktC. During acylation, lysine residues are added to the fatty acid groups of the active leukotoxin, to increase the hydrophobicity of active leukotoxin, thereby allowing entry of leukotoxin into the host cell to form transmembrane pores. Acylation is critical for increasing intracellular calcium ion concentration, generation of ROS, production of proinflammatory cytokines, and causing cytolysis (Jeyaseelan et al. 2001). lktB and lktD are essential for transporting active leukotoxin from the bacterial cytoplasm into the host environment. The N-terminal region of active leukotoxin is involved in receptor binding and the C-terminal domain consists of glycine- and aspartate-rich repeats, and neutralizing epitopes. The hydrophobic residues of active leukotoxin are attributed to pore formation and calcium binding.

At low concentration, leukotoxin activate neutrophils and macrophages to stimulate respiratory burst and degranulation, and induce proinflammatory cytokine and histamine release. High concentration of leukotoxin leads to transmembrane pore formation, cell swelling, and cell death. Cell death leads to leakage of products of respiratory burst, nitric oxide, lysosomal enzymes, and arachidonic acid metabolites into the lung parenchyma, thus contributing to pulmonary damage through fibrinous and necrotizing bronchopneumonia (Singh et al. 2011).

41.9 *Staphylococcus aureus*

Staphylococcus aureus (*S. aureus*) is a Gram-positive, nonmotile, round commensal bacterium that forms irregular clusters and appears like a bunch of grapes microscopically (Quinn et al. 2016). *S. aureus* is a predominant cause of mastitis in goats among other bacteria such as *Streptococcus* sp., *Pasteurella* sp., and *Escherichia coli*. *S. aureus* enters the udder of goats through teat openings immediately after milking. It can enter teats from an unhygienic environment or from lambs infected with respiratory diseases. Mastitis in goats can occur as the clinical or subclinical form of infection. In clinical mastitis, the udder will be swollen, hot and painful to touch, and the secreted milk will be discolored, clotted in consistency, and scanty. In subclinical mastitis, the udder looks apparently healthy but there is a change in the consistency of milk (Kahinda 2022).

Staphylococcus aureus produces a plethora of toxins that contribute to the establishment of mastitis in goats. These can be broadly classified into the PFTs, exfoliative toxins (ETs), and superantigens (SAgs). The PFTs are further classified into hemolysin-alpha (Hla or alpha-toxin), hemolysin-beta, leukotoxins, and phenol-soluble modulins (PSMs). The toxins of *S. aureus* involved in causing mastitis in goats are primarily Hla and Hlb (Abril et al. 2020). In brief, Hlb damages the mammary epithelium and facilitates adhesion and multiplication of *S. aureus*, whereas Hla intensifies the damage by destruction of mammary cells by apoptosis (Wang et al. 2011).

Hemolysin-alpha is a 33 kD polypeptide that is encoded by the *hla* gene of the monocistronic operon in the genome of *S. aureus* (Gouaux et al. 1994). The target cells of Hla include various epithelial and endothelial cells, red blood cells, leukocytes, T cells, macrophages, monocytes, and platelets, except neutrophils (Kong et al. 2016). Hla binds to these target cells through a cellular receptor called ADAM10, which is a type I transmembrane protein, and a zinc-dependent metalloprotease expressed on the surface of most host cells (Wilke and Wardenburg 2010). Hla is secreted as a water-soluble monomer, which upon binding to target cells through cellular receptors oligomerises to form a prepore. On the prepore lies a toxic substructure called the amino latch, the conformational change of which leads to the formation of a beta-barrel pore (Valeva et al. 1997). The beta-barrel pore resembles the structure of a mushroom and consists of three domains: the extracellular cap domain, stem domain, and rim domain (Tam and Torres 2019). This beta-barrel pore extrudes into the lipid bilayer of cells to form a hydrophilic transmembrane channel.

The formation of a beta-barrel pore results in irreversible osmotic changes including rapid efflux of potassium ions, rapid influx of calcium ions, release of nitric oxide from epithelial and endothelial cells, secretion of proinflammatory cytokines, activation of caspase-1 and nucleotide binding oligomerization domain-like receptor protein 3 (NLRP3) inflammasome, which leads to inflammation and cell death. Further, Hla induces activation of the ADAM10 protease that cleaves epithelial cadherin, a junction protein that is an important epithelial barrier, resulting in easier invasion of *S. aureus* (Oliveira et al. 2018).

Hemolysin-beta is a nonpore-forming hemolysin which is encoded by the lysogenic bacteriophage. The detailed mechanism of action of Hlb is yet to be explored. It hydrolyzes sphingomyelin, lyzes monocytes and erythrocytes, and does not lyze lymphocytes and granulocytes. Upon hydrolyzing sphingomyelin, the plasma membrane lipid bilayer is destabilized, which causes irregularity of plasma membrane fluidity. Hlb has the potential to inhibit expression of interleukin (IL)-8 by endothelial cells, which helps *S. aureus* to evade phagocytosis and induce biofilm formation (Kong et al. 2016).

In goat milk obtained from mastitis-affected goats, Panton–Valentine leukocidin (PVL) of PFTs, staphylococcal enterotoxin (SE), toxic shock syndrome toxin-1 (TSST-1) of SAgs, and ET that specifically cleaves desmoglein 1 (Dsg1) toxins are reported to possess public health implications (Abril et al. 2020).

41.10 *Trueperella pyogenes*

Trueperella pyogenes (*T. pyogenes*) is a Gram-positive, pleomorphic, nonspore-forming, nonmotile, noncapsulated, facultatively anaerobic rod-shaped commensal bacterium that was formerly known as *Arcanobacterium pyogenes*, *Actinomyces pyogenes*, and *Corynebacterium pyogenes* (Rzewuska et al. 2019). *T. pyogenes* is an opportunistic pathogen that is commonly found on the skin of animals and causes abscess formation when there is tissue damage during immunocompromised conditions. However, direct transmission through contact and indirect transmission through fomites are also possible. An abscess is formed in most of the body including skin, regional lymph nodes, mammary glands, lungs, liver, gastrointestinal tract, bone marrow, and even foot. These abscesses develop rapidly and are soft to palpate. The pus in the abscess is greenish-yellow or grayish in color.

Trueperella pyogenes produces only one exotoxin called pyolysin (PLO), belonging to the cholesterol-dependent or cholesterol-binding cytolysins (CDC). PLOs are 51–60 kD single-chain proteins encoded by the *plo* gene and have been detected in almost all strains of *T. pyogenes*. PLOs cause cell death by forming pores in the host cell (Liang et al. 2022); thus, they are classified as PFTs (Jost et al. 1999).

The monomeric structure of PLO consists of four domains, D1–D4, where D1 is the N-terminal and D4 is the C-terminal. D1 is made up of alpha-helix and beta-sheet elements, D2 and D3 are made up of one and five layers of antiparallel beta-sheets respectively, except the central beta-sheet of D3 is flanked on either side with helical layers and short alpha-helices. D4 is the contiguous domain, on the tip of which is a tryptophan-rich region which recognizes the host plasma membrane and binds with cholesterol (Pokrajac et al. 2012).

When PLO is secreted into the extracellular environment of the host, the D4 domain binds to the cholesterol-rich regions of the host plasma membrane. Upon binding, D2 and D3 domains initiate monomeric oligomerization, thereby forming a number of incomplete arc-shaped structures called prepores. During this process, D2 and D3 are separated and D2 is structurally collapsed. The short alpha-helices are then converted into two beta-transmembrane hairpins. Large numbers of these beta-transmembrane hairpins are inserted into the plasma membrane, resulting in the formation of a beta-barrel pore. This pore protrudes above the plasma membrane. Through this pore there is leakage of cellular cytoplasmic components leading eventually to cell death. The free iron and other cytoplasmic molecules present in the host cell are released, which are essential growth factors for multiplication of *T. pyogenes* (Preta et al. 2016). Further, PLO causes upregulation of proinflammatory cytokines IL-1-beta and IL-8, thus having an essential role in inflammation (Zhang et al. 2018).

41.11 Conclusion

In conclusion, bacterial toxins can be classified as exotoxins and endotoxins which are major virulence determinants in certain bacterial diseases. These toxins are responsible for the establishment, manifestation, and progression of disease.

References

Abril, A.G., Villa, T.G., Barros-Velázquez, J. et al. (2020). Staphylococcus aureus exotoxins and their detection in the dairy industry and mastitis. *Toxins* 12 (9): 537.

Arora, N. and Leppla, S.H. (1993). Residues 1-254 of anthrax toxin lethal factor are sufficient to cause cellular uptake of fused polypeptides. *Journal of Biological Chemistry* 268 (5): 3334–3341.

Batt, C.A. (2014). Escherichia coli. In: *Encyclopedia of Food Microbiology*, 2e (ed. C.A. Batt and M.L. Tortorello), 688–694. New York: Academic Press.

Billington, S.J., Jost, B.H., and Songer, J.G. (2000). Thiol-activated cytolysins: structure, function and role in pathogenesis. *FEMS Microbiology Letters* 182 (2): 197–205.

Brossier, F. and Mock, M. (2001). Toxins of bacillus anthracis. *Toxicon* 39 (11): 1747–1755.

Carne, H.R. and Onon, E.O. (1978). Action of Corynebacterium ovis exotoxin on endothelial cells of blood vessels. *Nature* 271 (5642): 246–248.

de Chaves, E.P. and Sipione, S. (2010). Sphingolipids and gangliosides of the nervous system in membrane function and dysfunction. *FEBS Letters* 584 (9): 1748–1759.

Gouaux, J.E., Braha, O., Hobaugh, M.R. et al. (1994). Subunit stoichiometry of staphylococcal alpha-hemolysin in crystals and on membranes: a heptameric transmembrane pore. *Proceedings of the National Academy of Sciences* 91 (26): 12828–12831.

Hamon, M.A., Ribet, D., Stavru, F., and Cossart, P. (2012). Listeriolysin O: the Swiss Army knife of Listeria. *Trends in Microbiology* 20 (8): 360–368.

Highlander, S.K., Chidambaram, M., Engler, M.J., and Weinstock, G.M. (1989). DNA sequence of the Pasteurella haemolytica leukotoxin gene cluster. *DNA* 8 (1): 15–28.

Jernigan, P.L., Makley, A.T., Hoehn, R.S. et al. (2015). The role of sphingolipids in endothelial barrier function. *Biological Chemistry* 396 (6–7): 681–691.

Jeyaseelan, S., Kannan, M.S., Briggs, R.E. et al. (2001). Mannheimia haemolytica leukotoxin activates a nonreceptor tyrosine kinase signaling cascade in bovine leukocytes, which induces biological effects. *Infection and Immunity* 69 (10): 6131–6139.

Jost, B.H., Songer, J.G., and Billington, S.J. (1999). An Arcanobacterium (Actinomyces) pyogenes mutant deficient in production of the pore-forming cytolysin pyolysin has reduced virulence. *Infection and Immunity* 67: 1723–1728.

Kahinda, C.T.M. (2022). Mastitis in small ruminants. In: *Mastitis in Dairy Cattle, Sheep and Goats* (ed. O.K. Dego). IntechOpen http://dx.doi.org/10.5772/intechopen.97585.

Kong, C., Neoh, H.M., and Nathan, S. (2016). Targeting Staphylococcus aureus toxins: a potential form of anti-virulence therapy. *Toxins* 8 (3): 72.

Leppla, S.H. (1982). Anthrax toxin edema factor: a bacterial adenylate cyclase that increases cyclic AMP concentrations of eukaryotic cells. *Proceedings of the National Academy of Sciences* 79 (10): 3162–3166.

Liang, H., Wang, B., Wang, J. et al. (2022). Pyolysin of Trueperella pyogenes induces Pyroptosis and IL-1β release in murine macrophages through potassium/NLRP3/Caspase-1/Gasdermin D pathway. *Frontiers in Immunology* 13: 832458.

Nagaraja, T.G., Narayanan, S.K., Stewart, G.C., and Chengappa, M.M. (2005). Fusobacterium necrophorum infections in animals: pathogenesis and pathogenic mechanisms. *Anaerobe* 11 (4): 239–246.

Navarro, M., McClane, B., and Uzal, F. (2018). Mechanisms of action and cell death associated with Clostridium perfringens toxins. *Toxins* 10 (5): 212.

Obrig, T.G. (2010). Escherichia coli Shiga toxin mechanisms of action in renal disease. *Toxins* 2 (12): 2769–2794.

Oliveira, D., Borges, A., and Simões, M. (2018). Staphylococcus aureus toxins and their molecular activity in infectious diseases. *Toxins* 10 (6): 252.

Petosa, C., Collier, R.J., Klimpel, K.R. et al. (1997). Crystal structure of the anthrax toxin protective antigen. *Nature* 385 (6619): 833–838.

Pokrajac, L., Baik, C., Harris, J.R. et al. (2012). Partial oligomerization of pyolysin induced by a disulfide-tethered mutant. *Biochemistry and Cell Biology* 90: 709–717.

Preta, G., Jankunec, M., Heinrich, F. et al. (2016). Tethered bilayer membranes as a complementary tool for functional and structural studies: the pyolysin case. *Biochimica et Biophysica Acta* 1858: 2070–2080.

Quinn, P.J., Markey, B.K., Leonard, F.C. et al. (2016). *Concise Review of Veterinary Microbiology*, 2e. Oxford: Wiley.

Rzewuska, M., Kwiecień, E., Chrobak-Chmiel, D. et al. (2019). Pathogenicity and virulence of Trueperella pyogenes: a review. *International Journal of Molecular Sciences* 20 (11): 2737.

Singh K., Ritchey J.W., Confer A.W. (2011). Mannheimia haemolytica: bacterial–host interactions in bovine pneumonia. *Vet. Pathol.* 48 (2): 338–348.

Shannon, J.G., Ross, C.L., Koehler, T.M., and Rest, R.F. (2003). Characterization of anthrolysin O, the Bacillus anthracis cholesterol-dependent cytolysin. *Infection and Immunity* 71 (6): 3183–3189.

Souček, A., Michalec, Č., and Součková, A. (1971). Identification and characterization of a new enzyme of the group "phospholipase D" isolated from Corynebacterium ovis. *Biochimica et Biophysica Acta (BBA)-Enzymology* 227 (1): 116–128.

Tadepalli, S., Stewart, G.C., Nagaraja, T.G., and Narayanan, S.K. (2008). Human fusobacterium necrophorum strains have a leukotoxin gene and exhibit leukotoxic activity. *Journal of Medical Microbiology* 57 (2): 225–231.

Tam, K. and Torres, V.J. (2019). Staphylococcus aureus secreted toxins and extracellular enzymes. *Microbiology Spectrum* 7 (2).

Underwood, W.J., Blauwiekel, R., Delano, M.L. et al. (2015). Biology and diseases ruminants (sheep, goats, and cattle). In: *Laboratory Animal Medicine*, 3e (ed. J.G. Fox, L.C. Anderson, G.M. Otto, et al.), 623–694. New York: Academic Press.

Valeva, A., Pongs, J., Bhakdi, S., and Palmer, M. (1997). Staphylococcal α-toxin: the role of the N-terminus in formation of the heptameric pore – a fluorescence study. *Biochimica et Biophysica Acta (BBA)-Biomembranes* 1325 (2): 281–286.

Wang, F., Hongjun, Y., Hong-Bin, H. et al. (2011). Study on the hemolysin phenotype and the genetype distribution of staphyloccocus aureus caused bovine mastitis in Shandong dairy farms. *International Journal of Applied Research in Veterinary Medicine* 9: 416–421.

Wilke, G.A. and Wardenburg, J.B. (2010). Role of a disintegrin and metalloprotease 10 in Staphylococcus aureus α-hemolysin-mediated cellular injury. *Proceedings of the National Academy of Sciences* 107 (30): 13473–13478.

Winter, A., Ulrich, W.P., Wetterich, F. et al. (1996). Gangliosides in phospholipid bilayer membranes: interaction with tetanus toxin. *Chemistry and Physics of Lipids* 81 (1): 21–34.

Zhang, W., Wang, H., Wang, B. et al. (2018). Replacing the 238th aspartic acid with an arginine impaired the oligomerization activity and inflammation-inducing property of pyolysin. *Virulence* 9: 1112–1125.

42

Pneumonia

Shashi Pradhan, Aditya Pratap, Salil Kumar Pathak, and Akanksha Agnihotri

Department of Veterinary Medicine, College of Veterinary Science and Animal Husbandry, Jabalpur, India

42.1 Introduction

Pneumonia is a serious herd concern associated with the lower respiratory tract in small ruminants. In kid herds, pneumonia increases production costs associated with expensive treatments and is hard to cure due to the sequelae of disease. Although pneumonia can occur at any age, it is known to occur more often in kids which experience severe illness soon after encountering the etiological agent and death may occur at any stage depending on the immune defense system.

Medically, pneumonia is defined as an inflammation of one or both lung parenchymas that may be associated with multiple infectious etiologies and also noninfectious causes.

In general, pneumonia is classed as inflammation of the pulmonary parenchyma usually accompanied by inflammation of the bronchioles (lower respiratory tract infection). Pneumonia occurs when infectious and noninfectious agents cause lung inflammation in sheep/kids. The causes of pneumonia include viruses, bacteria, fungi, mycoplasma, parasites, irritating dust and fumes, and aspiration of liquids. Depending on the clinical course, the disease can become acute, chronic, or progressive. Identifying a specific cause of pneumonia is not easy and diagnostic help is needed. Previous studies and case interpretation suggest that pneumonia is the result of a combination of factors. Administrative problems such as overcrowding, inadequate ventilation, and inadequate nutrition can predispose to the action of infectious agents.

Newborn kids are exposed to bacteria from their mother and other kids, but colostrum contains antibodies that help keep them healthy in the early stage of life. Other factors that can lead to pneumonia include unsuitable living conditions such as overcrowding, lack of ventilation, and lack of cleanliness. Stressful travel, sudden separation from mothers, or another disease that damages the lungs (such as the presence of lungworms or viruses) will increase the number of deaths among kids. They tend to lose weight, become lethargic, have a runny nose and rapid breathing, and a moderate fever. The first sign is a loss of interest in nursing. This is more likely to be seen in bottle-fed kids for obvious reasons.

When treating pneumonia in kids, time is of the essence as the lungs can be damaged if not detected and treated early. When this happens, the kid may recover but may be more susceptible to further pneumonia, develop a chronic cough, and not grow as well as it should and becomes susceptible to future bacterial infections.

In India, kid farming is successfully integrated into both traditional and agricultural systems. It has become a valuable asset for farmers and plays an important role in enhancing their socioeconomic status in society. However, pneumonia is a multifactorial disease that primarily affects kids (all age groups).

Sheep and kids are two of the most important sources of animal protein for human consumption in India. Therefore, it is important to know the prevalence of different diseases that cause pneumonia in different rearing environments and geoclimatic conditions that directly or indirectly affect human health too.

Elements of Reproduction and Reproductive Diseases of Goats, First Edition. Edited by Tanmoy Rana.

42.2 Classification of Pneumonia

On the basis of etiology, pneumonia results in the inflammation and consolidation of lung tissue. It can be caused by infectious and noninfectious agents. Common causes of respiratory infection and death in kids/sheep include *Pasteurella multocida* and *Mannheimia haemolytica* (previously known as *Pasteurella haemolytica*). *M. haemolytica* usually inhabits the upper respiratory tract of healthy kids (Brogden et al. 1998).

Primary or secondary bronchopneumonia in sheep and kids is basically caused by *Bibersteinia trehalosi* and *Mycoplasma* spp. Also, *Chlamydia pneumoniae* and *Salmonella* spp. are associated with both forms of bronchopneumonia in sheep and kids.

Chronic, progressive pathological changes in the lungs are frequently associated with the lentiviruses (family Retroviridae). In progressive pneumonia, the entire lung can switch to a gradual process of abnormal cell proliferation. In affected kids, the loss of functional lung tissue results in increased episodes of dyspnea, anorexia leading to weight loss, cough, and more (Ackerman and Brogden 2000).

Pneumonia due to a viral etiology can be acute and progressive in nature. Acute viral infections in a susceptible population can alter the immune defense system in the respiratory tract of small ruminants so that bacteria may invade lung tissue, multiply, and cause severe inflammation. An initial infection with the parainfluenza type 3 virus may predispose an animal to infection with pathogenic *Mannheimia haemolytica*. *Mycoplasma ovipneumoniae* alone generally causes a mild bronchopneumonia in small ruminants. However, it is often isolated along with *M. haemolytica* from sheep and kids with severe pneumonia which strongly suggests that *Mycoplasma* species may predispose a healthy kid's lung to invasion by *M. haemolytica*.

Caseous lymphadenitis due to *Corynebacterium pseudotuberculosis* forms abscesses of the lungs and mediastinal lymph nodes (MLNs). This results in progressive weakening in sheep and kids, with or without obvious clinical signs of respiratory distress.

Parasitic (verminous) pneumonia in kids is mostly due to infection with lungworms including *Dictyocaulus filaria*, *Muellerius capillaris*, and *Protostrongylus rufescens*. Verminous pneumonia affects the caudal lung lobe margins, in contrast to the acute viral and bacterial pneumonias which result in an anteroventral bronchopneumonia. *Dictyocaulus* has a direct life cycle, whereas *Protostrongylus* and *Muellerius* have an indirect life cycle, with various snails and slugs acting as intermediate hosts. Adults of *Dictyocaulus* and *Protostrongylus* inhabit the bronchi but rarely cause clinical symptoms. Adult *Muellerius* lives in alveoli and lung parenchyma and is considered the least pathogenic of the three lungworms. *Muellerius* seems to cause more trouble with kids than with sheep.

Bacterial, viral, and parasitic infections break down tissue defense barriers. Loss of this natural protection increases a kid's susceptibility to secondary infection by *P. multocida* and *M. haemolytica*. Animals whose lungs are already weakened from previous diseases will suffer from leukotoxins and lipopolysaccharides, both potent toxins that, at high levels, promote inflammation and severe lung damage. In kids acute events of pneumonia can occur with low morbidity rates and high mortality rates. Typically, kids that appear healthy die suddenly. Signs of the disease are not yet pronounced and disease is diagnosed only after a significant number of kids die and are inspected for lesions post mortem.

Pasteurella multocida and *M. haemolytica* can lead to significantly decreased growth performance. These two pathogens (agents that cause disease) cause outbreaks of acute pneumonia in kids of all ages. Transportation stress, viral infections (e.g., parainfluenza 3 virus), lung parasites, prior bacterial infections, overcrowded pens, poor housing conditions, sudden environmental changes, and other stressful conditions increase kids' susceptibility to *P. multocida* and *M. haemolytica* pneumonias.

In kids, pneumonic pasteurellosis caused by *M. haemolytica* and *P. multocida* usually affects animals younger than 3–4 months of age with higher mortality rates in kids aged 2–3 weeks. *Pasteurella multocida* and *M. haemolytica* cause bronchopneumonia in kids (Oros et al. 1997). Bronchopneumonia presents with a cranioventral lung distribution and affects sheep and kids of all ages globally. Young animals around the time of weaning are affected particularly severely. It is a common cause of morbidity and death in lambs and kids, especially those that have not received adequate colostrum or in which passive immunity is waning. The disease is mostly encountered in animal units that have recently gone through unwanted transportation stress, weaning, change of diet, or mingling with newly introduced animals from unrelated farms. *Bibersteinia* (formerly *Pasteurella*) *trehalosi* causes septicemia and bronchopneumonia in lambs and has also been reported as a causative agent of bronchopneumonia in calves and kids (Daniel et al. 2006).

Contagious caprine pleuropneumonia (CCPP) is considered one of the most serious and highly contagious kid diseases. This causes severe economic losses in countries involved in kid farming, especially in Africa, Asia and the Middle East. The disease is one of the *Mycoplasma* infections causing significant losses in about 40 countries, with morbidity and mortality rates that can reach 100%, especially in exotic species; 100% morbidity and 80% mortality were recorded in naive and native herds. The total annual cost of CCPP in endemic areas is estimated at about US$507 million, resulting in significant economic losses.

Economic losses arise from both morbidity, mortality, and reduced or lost production, in addition to prevention, control, and treatment costs. CCPP is caused by *Mycoplasma capricolum* subsp. *capripneumoniae*, abbreviated as Mccp, formerly known as *Mycoplasma* biotype F38. These pathogenic bacteria belong to the Mollicutes class, which have no cell wall but a galactan and a small genome (0.58–1.35 Mb). They have limited biosynthetic capacity and cause various infectious diseases in animals.

The four *Mycoplasma* lineages correspond to different geographical regions. *Mycoplasma capricolum* subsp. *capripneumoniae* (Mccp) is classified in the *Mycoplasma mycoides* cluster and has several species and subspecies, namely *Mycoplasma mycoides* subsp. *mycoides* large colony strain (MmmLC), *Mycoplasma mycoides* subsp. *mycoides* small colony strain (MmmSC), *Mycoplasma* sp. Bovine group 7 of the leech (Mbg7), *Mycoplasma capricolum* subsp. *capricolum* (Mcc), and *Mycoplasma mycoides* subsp. *capri* (MMC).

Classification of pneumonia in domestic animals can be further extended on the basis of combination of possible etiologies, distribution of lesions, exudate type, morphological features, and epidemiology.

42.3 Bronchopneumonia

This is the most common type of pneumonia seen in domestic animals. It is always demarcated by cranioventral consolidation of lungs. Causes include bacteria or mycoplasma and even bronchoaspiration pneumonia resulting from accidental aspiration of feed or gastric contents. Route of entry of bacteria is mainly aerogenous (through contaminated air). In their course to the tract, the organisms cause primary injury to the mucosal surface of bronchioles and alveoli. Inflammatory exudate produced by the injury to the mucosa is collected mainly in the bronchial and alveolar lumina and the alveolar interstitium is left unaffected. Lesions and exudates spread through the pores of Kohn to neighboring alveoli. Entire lung lobes are involved by the initiated inflammatory process from one lobule to the next through damaged alveolar walls.

The pulmonary vessels are engorged with blood (active hyperemia) in the early stages. The bronchi, bronchioles, and alveoli show signs of pulmonary edema. If there is a mild to moderate injury to the lung tissue, cytokines may cause rapid neutrophil and alveolar macrophage recruitment. With severe injury to the tissue, chemical mediators produce defined vascular changes and increase vascular permeability which will lead to fibrinous inflammation. Microbial toxins can further aggravate the permeability changes in blood vessels which leads to considerable leakage of plasma fluid and proteins (fibrinogen) into the alveoli. The kid with bronchopneumonia can be identified by observing the filling of alveoli, bronchioles, and small bronchi with excess exudate which also destroys airspaces. As a result, portions of consolidated lung sink to the bottom of the vessel when put in fixative. Replacing air by exudate also changes the texture of the lungs; the lung becomes firmer than normal.

A total of 1350 lungs from adult sheep (888) and kids (462) from slaughtered animals (1050 cases) and collapsed animals (300 cases) were examined for gross abnormalities. Of these, 270 cases (20%) had severe pulmonary involvement, 121 cases in sheep (44.1%) and 149 cases in kids (55.1%); 90 (33.3%) of 270 affected sheep and kid lungs showed lesions of acute bronchopneumonia. Overall, the lungs showed patchy to diffuse, reddish-brown to grayish-red areas of consolidation and hepatosis. The apical portion of the diaphragmatic lobe, the heart, and the ventral cranial part, especially the right lung, were more frequently affected. Sections showed straw-colored fluid in the bronchi and bronchioles, and in other cases the exudate was slimy and frothy. Histopathologically, there was neutrophil infiltration around the bronchi and bronchioles. In 30 cases (11.11%), fibrous bronchopneumonia changes from 270 affected lungs were noted. Dense, coarse patchy to diffuse areas were observed primarily in the cranial-ventral region, particularly involving the right lung. The affected part of the lung was hard and in some cases adhered to the diaphragm. In most cases, there was pleural thickening, and sections showed diffuse, consolidated, and hard areas from the lung focal point. Chronic bronchopneumonia changes were found in 15 (5.55%) cases in 270 affected lungs. Broadly speaking, the lungs on either side of the lobe were tight and hard. The overlying pleura was most often thickened and attached to the diaphragm and chest wall. Fibrous tissue proliferation in foci and diffused manner was seen around bronchi, alveoli, and blood vessels. The pleura also showed thickening with proliferation of fibrous tissue. The alveolar lumen contained macrophages and in one case, edematous fluid. In 10 (3.70%) cases, suppurative bronchopneumonia changes were observed out of 270 affected lungs.

Overall, the purulent lungs were red to gray, firm and pale, with purulent exudate in the bronchi and bronchioles. Abscesses the size of small peas to walnuts were scattered throughout the lung parenchyma. Calcified nodules of various sizes were found in various lobes and even the pectoral wall. Cut section showed thick, semiliquid, yellow-greenish pus in the lung abscess, and a spherical onion-like appearance of the abscess in the mediastinal lymph nodes.

42.4 Interstitial Pneumonia

This is a special type of pneumonia that primarily affects one of the three layers of the alveolar wall (endothelium, basal macrophages, and alveolar epithelium) and the adjacent bronchiolar interstitium. Pneumonia is most difficult to diagnose at autopsy and requires microscopic examination. The etiology is complex. It can occur by aerodynamic injury (by air) to the alveolar epithelium or by hematogenous injury (by blood circulation) to the alveolar capillary endothelium or alveolar basement membrane.

Causes include inhalation of toxic gases, such as smoke. Local production of toxic metabolites by Clara cells, release of free radicals, and infection with pneumotropic viruses can damage the alveolar epithelium. Endothelial damage occurs in sepsis, disseminated intravascular coagulation, migration of circulating larvae, uptake of toxins into the gastrointestinal tract, toxic metabolites produced locally in the lungs, and infection by viruses. Also, inhaled antigens, such as fungal spores, can bind with circulating antibodies and form antigen–antibody complex deposits on the alveolar walls. They cause inflammation and damage the alveolar walls (allergic alveolitis).

As in humans, interstitial pneumonia in domestic animals is classified as acute and chronic. Not all interstitial pneumonia is fatal or progresses to the chronic form. Acute interstitial pneumonia begins with damage to type 1 alveolar cells or the alveolar-capillary epithelium. Injury causes disruption of the air–blood barrier and extravasation of plasma proteins into the alveolar space. Leakage of proteinaceous fluid into the alveolar lumen forms the exudative phase. Occasionally, secreted plasma proteins mix with lipids and pulmonary surfactant constituents to form a membrane that partially adheres to the alveolar and bronchiolar walls. These membranes are called hyaline membranes because they have a hyaline-like appearance. Adjacent to the alveolar lumen, inflammatory exudate and neutrophils accumulate in the alveolar interstitium, causing alveolar wall thickening. The exudation phase is later followed by the proliferative phase which is characterized by hyperplasia of type II alveolar cells that replace lost type I alveolar cells. As a result, the walls of the alveoli thicken.

Acute interstitial pneumonia is often mild, especially when caused by respiratory viruses. In severe cases, animals can die from respiratory failure due to diffuse alveolar damage. Leakage of proteinaceous fluid (exudative phase) into the alveolar spaces causes fatal pulmonary edema. Examples of this lethal form are pulmonary edema in bovines, acute respiratory disease syndrome (ARDS) in all species, and massive lung migration of roundworm larvae in pigs.

If alveolar damage persists, proliferative and infiltrative lesions may progress to a stage called chronic interstitial pneumonia. The typical hallmark is alveolar fibrosis and, in some cases, the accumulation of mononuclear inflammatory cells in the interstitium. Also, there is presence of persistent hyperplastic type II pneumocytes. Lesions are present in the interstitial alveolar walls but epithelial cells, macrophages, and mononuclear cells are usually present in the bronchioles and alveolar lumen. Other changes that may occur include the formation of microscopic granulomas and smooth muscle hyperplasia in airways or blood vessels. Examples of chronic interstitial pneumonia include progressive pneumonia in sheep. In contrast to bronchopneumonia, in which lesions are mostly cranioventral, in acute or chronic interstitial pneumonia lesions are more diffusely distributed, affecting all lung lobes.

Three important gross features of interstitial pneumonia are:

- the absence of lung collapse when the thoracic cavity is opened
- the occasional presence of rib marks on the pleural surface of the lung
- the respiratory tract should be free of exudate unless secondary bacterial pneumonia develops.

Color varies from red to pale gray to a mottled appearance marked with spots of different colors. Pale lungs are due to loss of alveolar capillaries (decrease in blood tissue fraction), especially when fibrosis is present. The texture of lungs when uncomplicated is elastic or rubbery.

The term bronchointerstitial pneumonia was introduced to describe cases in which pulmonary lesions share the microscopic features of both bronchopneumonias and interstitial pneumonia. This is seen in many viral infections where the virus replicates and causes damage in bronchial, bronchiolar, and alveolar cells. Damage to the bronchial and bronchiolar epithelium causes accumulation of neutrophils similar to that in bronchopneumonia and damage to the alveolar walls results in a type II lung similar to that occurring during the proliferative phase of acute interstitial pneumonia.

42.5 Embolic Pneumonia

This condition is characterized by multifocal lesions randomly distributed in all lung lobes and is caused by cessation of septic emboli. The lungs act as a biological filter to circulating particles. Unless they are very large, sterile thrombi are rapidly dissolved by fibrinolysis and dislodged from the vessel without causing damage. However, most types of bacteria in the circulatory system (bacteremia) usually bypass the lungs and end up trapped in the liver, spleen, joints or other organs. To cause pulmonary infection, circulating bacteria must first adhere to the vascular endothelium and escape phagocytosis by intravascular neutrophils. When trapped in pulmonary blood vessels, usually alveolar capillaries, bacteria spread from the interstitium and lung to form an infection focus. Grossly, early lesions are characterized as a 1 mm small white focus surrounded by a distinct red halo.

Embolic pneumonia is usually not fatal in kids until the emboli are accumulated in great numbers. Unresolved acute lesions may form abscesses randomly distributed in all the lobes. It should be differentiated from suppurative bronchopneumonia which has abscesses developing mainly in the cranioventral aspect of the lungs. Early lesions in embolic pneumonia seen during postmortem are always focal compared to the diffus pattern of endothelial damage in endotoxemia or septicemia.

Bacteria commonly isolated from the septicemic pulmonary emboli include *Arcanobacterium (Actinomyces) pyogenes*, *Fusobacterium necrophorum*, *Erysipelothrix rhusiopathiae*, *Streptococcus suis* type 2, *Streptococcus equi*, and *Staphylococcus aureus*.

42.6 Granulomatous Pneumonia

This condition is characterized by the presence of caseating or nondrying granulomas in the lungs. On palpation, the lungs have typical nodular features, with nodules of varying sizes that are usually firm tissue, especially where calcifications have occurred. At autopsy, pulmonary granuloma can be mistaken for a neoplasm. The etiology of granulomatous pneumonia shares some similarities with interstitial and embolic pneumonia. What makes granulomatous pneumonia a separate type is a unique inflammatory response that leads to the formation of granulomas that are easily recognized macroscopically or microscopically, rather than the point of entry or the site of initial injury in the lung which may be aerogenous or hematogenous.

Pathogens can enter the lungs via air or blood. In principle, the causative agents of granulomatous pneumonia are resistant to intracellular killing by phagocytic cells and acute inflammatory responses. As a result, they remain in the affected tissue for a long time. *Cryptococcus neoformans*, *Coccidioides immitis*, *Histoplasma capsulatum*, and *Blastomyces dermatitidis* are the most common organisms in domestic animals with a common air-borne route of infection. From the lungs, the fungus spreads to other organs, especially lymph nodes, liver, and spleen. Several bacterial diseases, such as tuberculosis (*Mycobacterium bovis*) in all species and *Rhodococcus equi* in foals, and inhaling foreign bodies (starch) also cause granulomatous pneumonia. Lesions are caused by deposition of antigen–antibody complexes in the blood vessels of many organs, including the lung, and subsequent vasculitis. Microscopically, granulomas consist of a core of necrotic tissue surrounded by a rim of macrophages (epidermoid cells) and giant cells and an outer layer of connective tissue infiltrated by lymphocytes and plasma cells.

A pneumonia prevalence study based on age, sex, and season will help us understand the epidemiology of pneumonia in kids and help establish pneumonia prevention and control measures. A prevalence survey was carried out in and around Bidar (India) for respiratory diseases, especially in relation to pneumonia in kids. Required information was collected from March 2015 to February 2017 by the Veterinary College Clinical Complex (VCC), Veterinary College, Bidar. Seventy-five animals had pneumonia and the overall prevalence of pneumonia in kids in and around Bidar was increased by20%. The age-dependent determination of pneumonia in this study revealed the highest prevalence in kids of 0–6 months with 36 cases (48.00%), following by 22 in those aged 1–2 years (29.33%) and six in those aged 2 years (8.00%). The results showed that very young kids are highly susceptible to respiratory infections such as pneumonia due to lack of immunity. The prevalence of sex-specific pneumonia in female and male kids was 54 (72.00%) and 21 (28.00%), respectively. The higher prevalence of pneumonia in females may be due to herd composition rather than sex susceptibility to pneumonia in kids.

The seasons were divided into summer (March–June), rainy season (July–October), and winter (November–February). The highest prevalence of disease was seen in winter (161 : 42.93%), followed by the rainy season (143 : 38.13%), and was lowest in summer (71 : 18.93%). A similar pattern was observed for seasonal pneumonia prevalence with the winter season having a higher prevalence of pneumonia in kids (37 : 49.33%), followed by the rainy season (28 : 37.33%), and summer (10 : 13.33%). This may be due to cold stress, where the drop in temperature is sufficient to inhibit defense mechanisms against infection, including mucociliary clearance and leukocyte phagocytic activity during winter. It is also hypothesized that animals will be overcrowded in winter housing and that bacterial infections will spread rapidly from infected to susceptible animals.

42.7 Transmission Routes

Pasteurella can be transmitted in several ways. Possible sources of infection include inhalation of infectious droplets from carrier animals, direct contact with infected animals, and lambs nursing ewes with *Pasteurella* mastitis.

Mycoplasma ovipneumoniae is transmitted primarily through the respiratory tract by direct contact or inhalation of an aerosol. *Mycoplasma* infection causes pulmonary ciliary stasis and exudate production. These factors may predispose infected animals to secondary bacterial infections. In some research studies, *Mycoplasma* infection appeared to limit the severity of *Pasteurella* infection.

A number of reports have suggested a role for the ear mite *Raillietina caprae* in the transmission and maintenance of *Mycoplasma* species in kids. The likelihood of *Mycoplasma* culture-positive earwax is increased in animals harboring ear mites compared to those not infected with ear mites. However, the exact role of ticks in transmission is still unknown.

Several predisposing factors may favor the development of *Mycoplasma pneumoniae*. In addition to stressors, minor viral pathogens play an important role in predisposing animals to pneumonia caused by *Mycoplasma* species. Lambs raised intensively under conditions of poor ventilation and herds of lambs on fattening farms are examples of groups in which *M. pneumoniae* is common. Aged or convalescent animals serve as reservoirs for other animals in the enclosure. Encapsulation of the organism allows it to evade the host's immune system and promotes long-term colonization of the upper respiratory tract. Pneumonia associated with *M. ovipneumoniae* in kids is not common but has been reported occasionally.

Viral pneumonia generally presents with relatively mild disease and clinical manifestations, but may act as a predisposing factor for bacterial pneumonia. A number of viral pathogens have been identified as potential causes of viral pneumonia in sheep and kids.

Contagious caprine pleuropneumonia infections are transmitted primarily through inhalation of infected aerosols. Direct contact with an infected flock or sharing the same space is the main source of contamination for susceptible animals. Persistence in the environment and in animals may be related to environmental friendliness, pathogen concentration, breed, herd density or animal immunity. The duration of infection is highly variable but recent reports suggest a short duration in the environment (hours to days) and a longer duration in infected animals. Also, frequent outbreaks of CCPP in Pashmina kids have been observed in Changthang, Ladakh, India, especially during the long winter months October to May (Yatoo et al. 2018).

This susceptibility due to seasonal variation is variable among different breeds of kids (EFSA 2017), with exotic breeds being more prone to clinical disease while native ones become infected only under adverse stress conditions.

42.8 Clinical Signs

In some cases of *Pasteurella* infection, clinical manifestations may be sudden death or lacrimation, including tachypnea, cough, and increased lung sounds. Affected animals may become isolated from the herd. The typical course of the disease lasts from 12 hours to three days and full recovery usually takes 14–20 days. Chronic infections in lambs and kids can lead to reduced lung capacity, weight gain, and reduced feed conversion.

In *Mycoplasma pneumoniae*, clinical manifestations are usually seen in mild disease. Typical manifestations are chronic cough and exertional dyspnea. *M. pneumoniae* reduces productivity in affected animals, even when only mild clinical signs are present. Overall, *M. pneumoniae* is associated with high morbidity but low mortality, consistent with the nonprogressive and asymptomatic nature of the infection.

Clinical respiratory illness occurs concomitantly with herd problems of septic arthritis, infertility or abortion as these are common signs of systemic *Chlamydia* infection. Clinical signs associated with parainfluenza type 3 infections are frequent coughing, serous nasal discharge, and occasional ocular discharge. Fever is rare. Clinically evident disease is more common in animals under one year of age. Clinical symptoms of adenovirus infection include fever, anorexia, sneezing, and serous nasal discharge. Autopsy findings included atelectasis and hyperemia, mainly in the cranioventral portion of the lungs. Histopathological lesions included desquamation of terminal bronchioles and alveolar epithelial cells and focal desquamation.

Contagious caprine pleuropneumonia is characterized by clinical signs of airway involvement, exacerbated by *Mycoplasma*-induced systemic serofibrinous and inflammatory cascades, resulting in affected lower respiratory tract (including lungs), pleura, pleural cavity and associated organs (heart), and sometimes upper airways (Young and Griffith 1985). It can also rarely affect the eyes, joints, breasts, liver, and kidneys. The disease can be hyperacute, acute, or chronic. Hyperacute and acute forms usually occur when fully susceptible flocks are exposed to the pathogen, whereas chronic forms occur in endemic affected areas. In the hyperacute form, death usually occurs suddenly within 24–72 hours

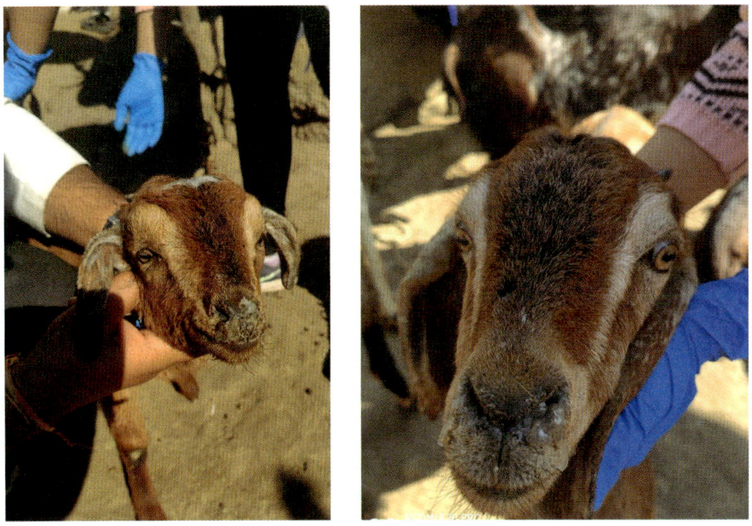

Figure 42.1 Nasal discharge in kids.

and, by definition, without prior surveillance. Respiratory signs, high fever (41–44 °C), cough, runny nose, lying down, chest pain, poor physical condition, severe morbidity (up to 100%) and mortality (80–100%) are common. Organ symptoms include difficulty breathing with grunting and snoring due to inflammatory lesions or exudates. Cough is generally painful, moist, and productive aggravated by physical activity. Continuous nasal discharge may be observed, initially with a serous, fibrous, straw-colored exudate followed by mucous or purulent, rust-colored exudate (Figure 42.1).

42.9 Diagnosis

Adequate sampling is an important aspect for accurate diagnosis of disease. Sample size, type, and preparation will vary depending on availability, facility, and local feasibility. As many samples as possible should be collected using standard procedures in a sterile environment. Nasal swabs, pleural effusions, and lung samples (from dissected animals) are collected from kids showing typical signs of CCPP (Iqbal Yatoo et al. 2019). Blood or serum samples are essential for serology, feces, exudates, blood and tissue culture or isolation and gene/DNA-based research. After adequate cleansing of the nostrils, nasal swabs are collected and placed in a universal transport medium. Lung specimens are aseptically obtained from the interface between the affected and unaffected areas at necropsy and placed in sterile, single-use plastic bags. Pleural fluid is collected with a sterile syringe.

Thoracocentesis or bronchoalveolar lavage (BAL) is also recommended to minimize contamination. Thoracocentesis is usually performed in the seventh intercostal space of the left chest or the sixth intercostal space of the right chest and the needle/cannula is held cranially to avoid damaging the intercostal vessels or nerves at the caudal end of the ribs. As a rule, the hair is cut and the skin is numbed with local anesthesia after proper disinfection. Another preferred method is inferior intrathoracic puncture using a large-bore needle and ultrasonographic guidance. About 10 ml of pleural effusion is sufficient. Hepatized lung (pulmonary) tissue samples are also suitable. A 3 cm^2 section should be taken from diseased lung tissue that approximates normal, healthy tissue.

Diagnosis may include microbiological, biochemical, serological, and genetic-based identification after provisional clinical diagnosis. Microbiological methods include culture, isolation, and identification. Although these are more common, they are considered the standard method for detecting Mccp. However, microbiological diagnosis of CCPP is considered challenging for two main reasons: first, due to the very poor growth of Mccp *in vitro*, and second, due to the usual contamination of samples with other proliferative mycoplasmas. In addition, Mccp's precision and special requirements make diagnostics even more problematic. Therefore, it is necessary to resort to other diagnostic methods. All of these tests focus on the growth and metabolic properties of Mccp, such as its ability to ferment glucose, digest casein and serum and reduce tetrazolium, or its immunogenic potential, such as its surface antigens, which are glycolipids and proteins (based on research as shown by complement fixation test [CFT] or enzyme-linked immunosorbent assay [ELISA]).

A preliminary diagnosis of *Pasteurella* infection can be made based on a history of stress, the presence of clinical signs of acute bronchopneumonia, and corresponding gross lesions observed at autopsy. Typical autopsy findings are pneumonia with foci of acute fibrinous purulent bronchopneumonia, coagulative necrosis, and fibrous pleuritis. A preliminary diagnosis is confirmed when *M. haemolytica* or *Bibersteinia trehalosi* is isolated from tissue. A diagnosis of *Mycoplasma* infection can be made based on characteristic findings at autopsy. Such findings include consolidation of the cranial lung lobes and occasionally consolidation of the leading edge of the caudal lobe. Integrated areas appear gray to reddish brown with red atelectasis. Firm and consistent grayish-white nodules are also seen on the cut surface. There are also signs of pleurisy. Histopathological features are of cuff-type interstitial pneumonia with nodular lymphoid hyperplasia and mononuclear lymphocyte coating around bronchioles and vessels. Exudate composed mainly of macrophages and some neutrophils is observed in the alveoli. *Mycoplasma* infections are characterized by the presence of nodular hyaline "scars" on the bronchial walls. However, in a recent study, these autopsy findings were present in only 60% of cases and the remaining 40% of cases did not exhibit these pathological features.

Organism culture is an important diagnostic technique. When submitting specimens for *Mycoplasma*, it is important to request this testing from a diagnostic laboratory as routine bacterial cultures do not grow this organism. Serological studies can be performed to screen antibodies using ELISA, but crossreactivity is a potential problem. A sterile swab can be taken from the kid's ear to test for the presence of a potential carrier condition. These swabs may undergo routine *Mycoplasma* culture or novel PCR-based techniques with higher sensitivity and negative predictive value for carrier status. Clinical experience (especially with *Pneumocystic jiroveci* pneumonia [PJP]) suggests that *Mycoplasma* cultures are most effective when inoculated with multiple types of *Mycoplasma* media simultaneously, as different media types grow differently. The clinical presentation is typically that of acute fulminant fibrous pleural pneumonitis without polyarthritis or mastitis. If there is clinical suspicion of this disease process, the appropriate state health authority should be contacted for further diagnostic information.

Diagnosis of chlamydial infection involves identification of the organism on stained swabs, immunofluorescence on fixed tissue sections, Gimenez staining, and yolk sac inoculation and isolation. Antibody titers using ELISA or CFT and real-time quantitative PCR assays are now commercially available and can provide faster and more reproducible results. Available research data indicate that PCR assays and ELISAs are significantly more sensitive than the CFT. Autopsy findings include consolidation of the cranial lung lobes with interstitial changes. Histopathological examination shows intracytoplasmic elementary bodies of alveolar macrophages. Edematous septa and thickened bronchioles are also observed. When the lungs are compressed, a cloudy exudate is seen.

Diagnosis of lungworm infection requires a stool Behrman test. Treatment of lungworm infections is rarely indicated but goats with such infections often harbor other nematodes that cause parasitic gastroenteritis and limit production.

Diagnosis can be made by viral isolation, but infection must last less than one week for the virus to have a reasonable chance of isolating the virus. Vaccination with a live intranasal vaccine against PI3 can be attempted to reduce disease incidence in flocks and flocks where PI3 infection is a problem. An unlicensed live intranasal vaccine for cattle is available for use in sheep and kids. Diagnosis of adenovirus infection is based on either virus isolation or paired serology.

42.9.1 Postmortem Lesions

One case was tentatively diagnosed as pneumonic pasteurellosis and the kid was treated with broad-spectrum antibiotics, nonsteroidal antiinflammatory drugs (NSAIDs), and fluid therapy. The prognosis in this case was poor and the kid died the day after admission.

Necropsy findings in this kid were consolidation of the left and right cranial lateral lung lobes. Bubbles were also seen along the cut surfaces of the trachea, bronchi, and lungs. In addition, the presence of straw-colored pericardial fluid was observed. Based on clinical manifestations, necropsy findings, and bacteriological results, this case was finally diagnosed as pneumonic pasteurellosis (Al-Kawari and Al-Shammari 2019).

In another study, 93 kid lung samples were collected from a slaughterhouse in northern Diyala state and carefully examined. The prevalence of disease was 43% (40/93). Overall, the lungs showed a variety of lesions. Histopathological changes were grouped into five categories: (i) interstitial lung disease 10%, (ii) fibrin bronchopneumonia 20%, (iii) bronchopneumonia 30%, (iv) purulent pneumonia 25%, and (v) hemorrhagic pneumonia 15%. Bronchopneumonia was manifested by the presence of exudate in the alveoli, hemorrhage, vascular obstruction, and hyperplasia of bronchial lymphoid tissue. Pyogenic pneumonia shows the presence of inflammatory cells, particularly neutrophils, in the bronchiolar lumen and alveoli and occasionally an increase in red blood cells in the alveoli of the lungs, in addition to neutrophil-mediated inflammatory cells with infiltration and few leukocytes. Fibrin showed the presence of intraalveolar hemorrhage (H&E, 10×), while showing fibrinous pneumonia: thickening of the alveolar walls by inflammatory cells (neutrophils) (H&E, 40×). Endothelial injury was characterized by numerous inter- and intraalveolar neutrophils, parenchymal sclerosis, lymphoid tissue hyperplasia, and desquamation of the bronchial epithelium (Singh et al. 2017).

Hemorrhagic pneumonia is characterized by bleeding in the alveoli, bronchiole, and alveolar septa. Interstitial pneumonia is characterized by thickening of interalveolar septa due to proliferation of fibrous connective tissue and accumulation of macrophages, hemorrhage in alveoli and round bronchi, reactive cells, severe vascular obstruction, and inflammation of the bronchial lumen. Lung abscesses showed the presence of inflammatory cells, especially neutrophils, and few mononuclear cells were seen in the lung tissue.

42.10 Treatment

Pasteurella therapy consists of long-acting oxytetracyclines. Sulfonamides can be administered orally or added to the drinking water, but inconsistent dosages can occur via the latter method. Various other antibiotics have been reported to be effective in treating pasteurellosis, including ceftiofur, tulathromycin, and florfenicol. Low levels of antibiotic resistance have been observed in *Pasteurella* and *Mannheimia* species. Due to anecdotal reports of lethal toxicity, tilmicosin should be avoided in kids. Culture and susceptibility testing of transtracheal lavage samples or material obtained at necropsy can be used to guide antibiotic selection in herd outbreaks or chronic cases or in high-value animals.

Treatment of *Mycoplasma* infections includes the use of oxytetracycline, tilmicosin, and florfenicol. *Chlamydophila* infections can usually be treated with tetracycline antibiotics but long-term treatment may be required. Tetracycline can also be used to slow or reduce the spread of disease during outbreaks.

The antibiotics most commonly used to treat pneumonia in ruminants are macrolides and quinolones. Beta-lactams and florfenicol are also commonly used. Procaine penicillin, amoxicillin, ampicillin, oxytetracycline, erythromycin, tylocin, enrofloxacin, and newer molecules such as ceftiofur, tulathromycin, and florfenicol are antibiotics commonly used to treat pneumonia in kids (Berge et al. 2006).

Quinolone antibiotics are commonly used for pneumonia due to their broad activity spectrum and high lung tissue penetration. The quinolone antibiotic marbofloxacin (MR) has been shown to be effective in the treatment of infectious kid pleuropneumonia (Kacar et al. 2018). Marbofloxacin treatment for *M. haemolytica* and *Mycoplasma* spp. is 2-3 mg/kg for three consecutive days or two doses three days apart. Single doses of MR at higher dose rates have been reported to be effective in treating respiratory disease in cattle (Grandemange et al. 2012). Pharmacokinetic evaluation of MR in kids showed favorable tissue distribution and clearance when administered intravenously or intramuscularly. However, the efficacy of MR in kid pneumonia has not been reported so far.

Macrolide antibiotics are preferred for the treatment of pneumonia because they can reach high concentrations in lung tissue (DeDonder et al. 2016). Gamithromycin is a macrolide antibiotic approved for the treatment and control of bovine respiratory disease, *M. hemolytica*, *P. multocida*, and *Mycoplasma bovis* (Apley and Coetzee 2013; Baggott et al. 2011). Gamithromycin has been used successfully for herd-wide antibiotic treatment of leg rot in sheep caused by *Dichelobacter nodosus*.

Tylosin is the drug of preference for Mccp but is not normally available within the regions in which CCPP is widespread. The use of oxytetracycline in CCPP has been validated but long-term use can predispose to facet effects (teratogenicity in kid kids).

42.11 Prevention and Control

As with many kid health issues, management is important to prevent pneumonia. Make sure the kid has adequate shelter and can escape the elements if necessary. Avoid overcrowding and other stressors. Make sure they have a good diet with plenty of minerals and fresh water. When a kid gets sick, isolate it from other kids. This serves two purposes: to prevent other kids from getting sick and to prevent others from bullying sick kids. (One caveat here: if you have a small number of kids that have never been separated, you may find it too taxing to separate sick kids from their families.)

Vaccination has become an important aspect of CCPP prevention and control in countries where CCPP is widespread. This is because large numbers of kids are infected and the native population increases the risk of outbreaks. However, vaccines are not available in most of these countries and only laboratory-based studies are being conducted in some. Vaccines are essential to overcome ineffectiveness. The development of vaccines from local isolates, specific species, subspecies or strains and their potent antigens should be investigated for better and highly specific immune responses. Many attempts in this direction have also been made around the world, but only a few have been successful. First, MacOwan and Minette (1978) initiated a vaccine trial against this disease using the high-passage *Mycoplasma* strain F38 to study its impact on disease progression. This was followed by research which developed an inactivated saponin-adjuvanted vaccine whose efficacy was demonstrated under field conditions (Litamoi et al. 1989). However, the major drawback of these vaccines has been their production costs. This is due to the austere nature of Mccp, which requires abundant and expensive media, is slow to grow and requires large amounts of vaccine to ensure a large amount of media for its supply.

Systematic vaccination of the entire herd is recommended. The FDA has approved the Colorado Serum Company's *M. haemolytica–P. multocida* bacterin vaccine was approved. The product label provides vaccination recommendations for young kids up to six months of age. This vaccine can cause temporary lameness in some kids.

Improve management practices by providing housing with optimal sanitation and air quality. Minimize shipping stress. Isolate new animals before introducing them into an existing herd. Administer trace elements such as Cu, Se, and Zn to improve immune function. Adding pharmacological amounts of vitamin E to the diet (e.g., >1000 IU per animal per day) may also be beneficial. Provide and supplement with good-quality hay and water. Talk to your veterinarian to prescribe and administer decongestants and antihistamines to reduce congestion in the lungs. Keep sick kids in a dry, well-ventilated area away from other animals (Duff and Galyean, 2007).

Prevention of pasteurellosis is desirable given the economic costs of treatment, loss, and reduced weight gain in survivors. Avoiding or mitigating known stressors such as heat, overcrowding, adverse weather conditions, poor ventilation, handling, nutritional problems, transportation, and mixing are major considerations for disease prevention. Including metaphylactic antimicrobial treatment, primarily with tetracyclines, during the months with the highest incidence of pasteurellosis is common practice. Vaccination programs to prevent respiratory virus infections are expected to reduce the incidence of respiratory pasteurellosis by avoiding the initial injury that allows colonization.

Intranasal recombinant vaccine protected lambs infected with *P. multocida*. However, this vaccine is not commercially available.

The only means of controlling and preventing progressive pneumonia in small ruminants is serological testing and elimination of positive animals. Due to the long latency period and long time to seroconversion, it may be appropriate to retest the animals once or twice a year. In addition to testing and culling approaches, it was previously recommended to keep kids and lambs separate from seropositive dams. Recent studies have shown that seroconversion is more common when young animals enter breeding herds. Some producers feed kids with colostrum or heat-treated colostrum from seronegative animals and milk replacers. Cow's milk from seronegative animals or heat-treated milk are the primary sources.

References

Ackermann, M.R. and Brogden, K.A. (2000). Responses of the ruminant respiratory tract to Mannheimia (Pasteurella) haemolytica. *Microbes and Infection* 2 (9): 1079–1088.

Al-Kawari, M. and Al-Shammari, S. (2019). Post mortem features of kid pneumonia in Northern of Diyala province-converted. *Plant Archives* 10 (5): 569.

Apley, M.D. and Coetzee, J.F. (2013). Antimicrobial drug use in cattle. In: *Antimicrobial Therapy in Veterinary Medicine* (ed. S. Giguere, J. Prescott, and P. Dowling), 495–518. Oxford: Wiley.

Baggott, D., Casartelli, A., Fraisse, F. et al. (2011). Demonstration of the metaphylactic use of gamithromycin against bacterial pathogens associated with bovine respiratory disease in a multicentre farm trial. *Veterinary Record* 168 (9): 241.

Berge, A.C., Sischo, W.M., and Craigmill, A.L. (2006). Antimicrobial susceptibility patterns of respiratory tract pathogens from sheep and kids. *Journal of the American Veterinary Medical Association* 229 (8): 1279–1281.

Brogden, K.A., Lehmkuhl, H.D., and Cutlip, R.C. (1998). Pasteurella haemolytica complicated respiratory infections in sheep and kids. *Veterinary Research* 29 (3-4): 233–254.

Daniel, J.A., Held, J.E., Brake, D.G. et al. (2006). Evaluation of the prevalence and onset of lung lesions and their impact on growth of lambs. *American Journal of Veterinary Research* 67 (5): 890–894.

DeDonder, K.D., Apley, M.D., Li, M. et al. (2016). Pharmacokinetics and pharmacodynamics of gamithromycin in pulmonary epithelial lining fluid in naturally occurring bovine respiratory disease in multisource commingled feedlot cattle. *Journal of Veterinary Pharmacology and Therapeutics* 39 (2): 157–166.

Duff, G.C. and Galyean, M.L. (2007). Recent advances in management of highly stressed newly received feedlot cattle. *Journal of Animal Science* 85: 823–840.

EFSA Panel on Animal Health and Welfare (2017). Assessment of listing and categorisation of animal diseases within the framework of the Animal Health Law (Regulation (EU) No 2016/429): bluetongue. *EFSA Journal* 15 (8): e04957.

Grandemange, E., Fournel, S., Giboin, H., and Woehrle, F. (2012). Efficacy of a single injection of marbofloxacin in the treatment of bovine respiratory disease. *Revue de Médecine Vétérinaire* 163 (6): 287–294.

Iqbal Yatoo, M., Raffiq Parray, O., Tauseef Bashir, S. et al. (2019). Contagious caprine pleuropneumonia – a comprehensive review. *Veterinary Quarterly* 39 (1): 1–25.

Jesse Abdullah, F.F., Tijjani, A., Adamu, L. et al. (2014). Pneumonic pasteurellosis in a kid. *Iranian Journal of Veterinary Medicine* 8 (4): 293–296.

Kacar, Y., Batmaz, H., Yilmaz, O.E., and Mecitoglu, Z. (2018). Comparing clinical effects of marbofloxacin and gamithromycin in kid kids with pneumonia. *Journal of the South African Veterinary Association* 89 (0): e1–e5.

Litamoi, J.K., Lijodi, F.K., and Nandokha, E. (1989). Contagious caprine pleuropneumonia: some observations in a field vaccination trial using inactivated Mycoplasma strain F38. *Tropical Animal Health and Production* 21 (2): 146–150.

MacOwan, K.J. and Minette, J.E. (1978). The effect of high passage Mycoplasma strain F38 on the course of contagious caprine pleuropneumonia (CCPP). *Tropical Animal Health and Production* 10 (1): 31–35.

Merck & Company (2006). *Pasteurellosis of Sheep and Kids: Introduction. Merck Manual*. Whitehouse Station, NJ: Merck & Company.

Oros, J., Fernandez, A., Rodriguez, J.L., and Poveda, J.B. (1997). Bacteria associated with enzootic pneumonia in kids. *Zentralblatt für Veterinärmedizin. Reihe B/Journal of Veterinary Medicine, Series B* 44 (2): 99–104.

Ramirez-Romero, R. and Brogden, K.A. (2000). The potential role of the Arthus and Shwartzman reactions in the pathogenesis of pneumonic pasteurellosis. *Inflammation Research* 49 (3): 98–101.

Singh, R., Kumar, P., Sahoo, M. et al. (2017). Spontaneously occurring lung lesions in sheep and kids. *Indian Journal of Veterinary Pathology* 41: 18–24.

Yatoo, M.I., Parray, O.R., Mir, M.S. et al. (2018). Mycoplasmosis in small ruminants in India: a review. *Journal of Experimental Biology* 6 (2): 264–281.

Young, J.D. Jr. and Griffith, J.W. (1985). Spontaneous Pasteurella pneumonia in adult laboratory kids complicated by superinfection with corynebacterium pseudotuberculosis and Muellerius capillaris. *Laboratory Animal Science* 35 (4): 409–411.

43

Scours (Diarrhea)

Ranjani Rajasekaran[1], Hridya Susan Varughese[2], Saahithya Rajamohan[3], and Krishnan Padmanath[4]

[1] *Department of Veterinary Microbiology, Veterinary College and Research Institute, Tamil Nadu Veterinary and Animal Sciences University, Theni, India*
[2] *Department of Veterinary Microbiology, Veterinary College, Karnataka Veterinary Animal and Fisheries Sciences University, Hebbal, India*
[3] *Department of Veterinary Pathology, Veterinary College and Research Institute, Tamil Nadu Veterinary and Animal Sciences University, Salem, India*
[4] *Veterinary Clinical Complex, Veterinary College and Research Institute, Tamil Nadu Veterinary and Animal Sciences University, Theni, India*

43.1 Introduction

Diarrhea in livestock is defined as an increased frequency, fluidity, or volume of fecal excretion that is caused by environmental stress, nutritional status or infectious agents. Diarrhea in livestock is commonly referred as "scours," a word derived from Old Norse (the North Germanic language of medieval Norway, Iceland, Denmark, and Sweden) – *skyra* meaning "rush in" or *skur* which means "storm, shower, shower of missiles."

Scours or diarrhea is a multifactorial condition specific to goat kids and lambs. It is characterized by pasty white to watery brown feces in goat kids of 1–3 months of age, culminating in severe dehydration and death. The earliest mention of scours in lambs and kids was in 1837 (Hare and Glynn 1927), wherein suckling lambs had diarrhea and the source of infection was traced back to milk and inflammation of the mucous membrane of the small intestine. The history of scours in small ruminants is not as well described as scours in calves, and it is paralleled with navel ill. It was initially referred to as "blood pens" describing blood in the stomach (Hare and Glynn 1927) concurrent with "white scour" in calves. It has also been described as "bacillary dysentery," due to the multiple pathogens involved, "lamb dysentery" that is analogous to "navel ill" of calves (Hare and Glynn 1927) or neonatal diarrhea complex.

43.2 Etiology

Scours can be caused by either infectious (Figure 43.1) or noninfectious agents (Figure 43.2) in goat kids and the etiology varies among the three growth stages of goat kids, which is less than four weeks old, 4–12 weeks old, and 12 weeks old to less than a year (Thompson 1985).

In kids less than four weeks old, infectious causes for occurrence of scours involve agents of bacterial (*Escherichia coli*, *Salmonella* sp., *Clostridium perfringens* types B and C, and *Campylobacter* sp.), viral (rotavirus and adenovirus), protozoal (*Cryptosporidium* sp., *Eimeria* sp. and *Giardia* sp.) and parasitic (*Strongyloides papillosa*) origin. In kids between 4 and 12 weeks of age, infectious agents are of bacterial (*Clostridium perfringens* type D, *Salmonella* sp. and *Yersinia* sp.), protozoal (*Eimeria* sp. and *Giardia* sp.) and parasitic (*Teladorsagia* sp. and *Trichostrongylus* sp.) origin (Matthews 2016). In kids between 12 weeks and less than a year, bacteria (*Clostridium perfringens* type D and *Salmonella* sp.), protozoa (*Eimeria* sp.), and parasites (*Teladorsagia* sp., *Trichostrongylus* sp., and rumen fluke) have been reported to cause scours (Matthews 2016).

Noninfectious etiology includes nutritional mismanagement, faulty animal husbandry practices, and stress-related factors (Shabana et al. 2017; Abdou et al. 2021). As far as scours are concerned, multietiological patterns of infection are more common than a single source of infection.

Elements of Reproduction and Reproductive Diseases of Goats, First Edition. Edited by Tanmoy Rana.

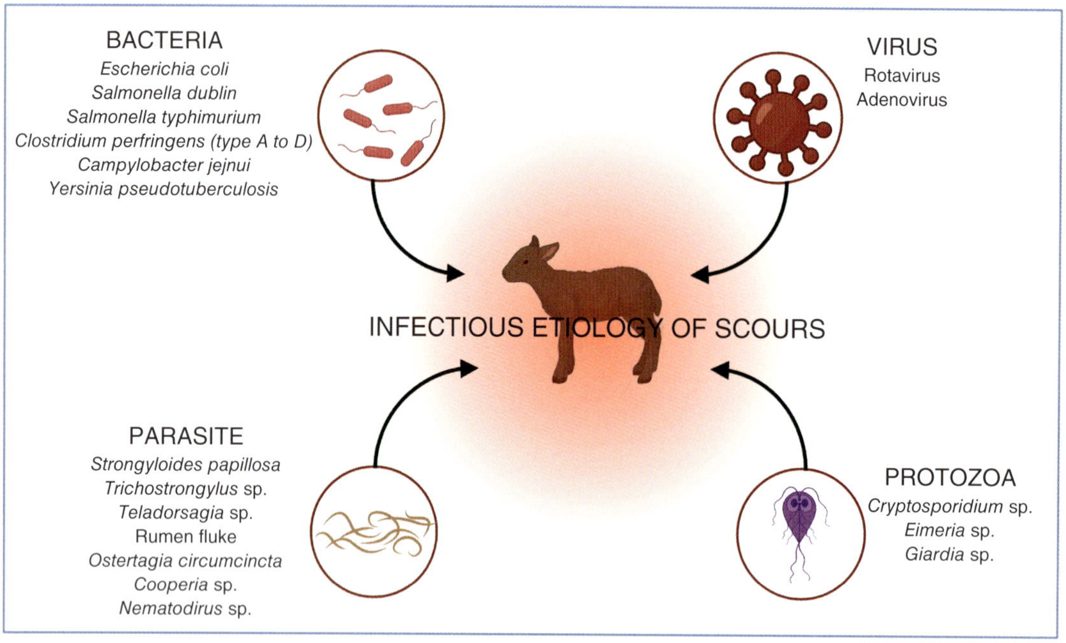

Figure 43.1 Schematic representation of scours caused by infectious etiology. *Source:* Created by Ranjani Rajasekaran using www.biorender.com under academic license.

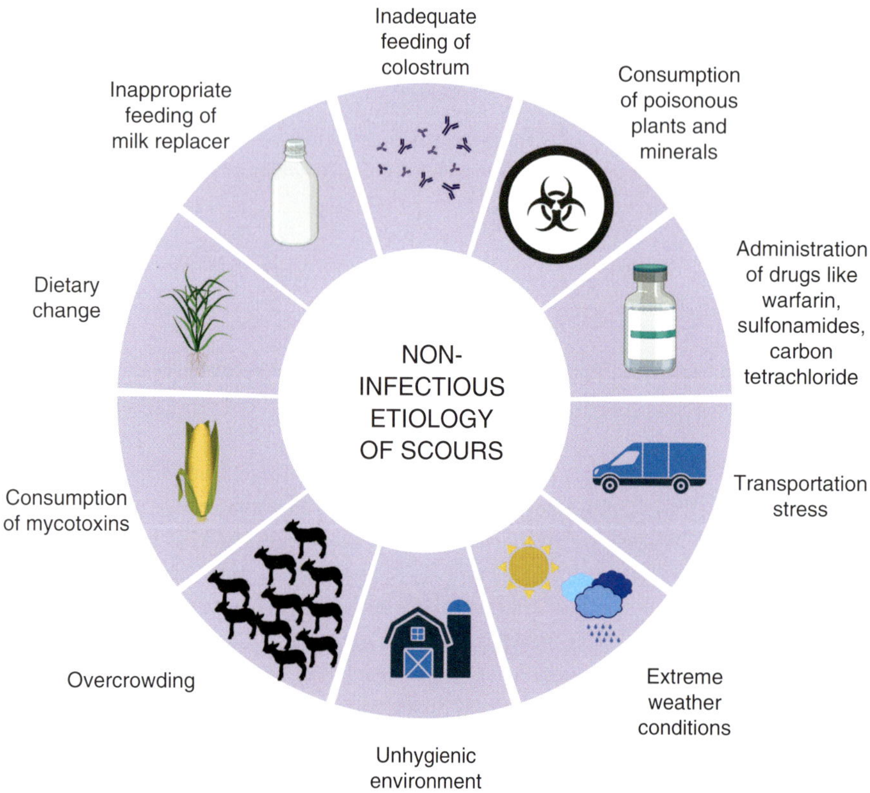

Figure 43.2 Schematic representation of scours caused by noninfectious etiology. *Source:* Created by Ranjani Rajasekaran using www.biorender.com under academic license.

43.3 Infectious Agents Causing Scours

43.3.1 Bacteria

Bacterial agents that cause scours in goat kids include *Escherichia coli*, *Salmonella dublin*, *Salmonella typhimurium*, *Clostridium perfringes* (types A–D), *Campylobacter jejuni*, and *Yersinia pseudotuberculosis*.

43.3.1.1 *Escherichia coli*

Scours caused by *E. coli* is an opportunistic occurrence in goat kids that occurs mainly due to compromised sanitary status of the environment or farm. The occurrence of scours in goat kids is most common at 1–4 days of age. The major pathotypes of *E. coli* that are significant causes of scours in goat kids include enterotoxigenic *E. coli* (ETEC), enteropathogenic *E. coli* (EPEC), Shiga toxin-producing *E. coli* (STEC), verotoxigenic *E. coli* (VTEC), and the attaching/effacing *E. coli* (AEEC) (Quinn et al. 2011; Osman et al. 2013).

- *ETEC*: strains including K99 and F41 produce heat-stable enterotoxin which is nonantigenic. However, these strains of ETEC have fimbrial adhesins that facilitate colonization, which induces hypersecretion, leading to scours, and reduces absorption of fluid in the intestine, leading to dehydration.
- *EPEC*: does not produce toxins but possesses virulence factors adhesin and intimin that facilitate colonization, leading to destruction of microvilli which causes malabsorption and maldigestion of intestinal content, leading to diarrhea.
- *STEC*: has been reported in the intestinal contents of healthy goats. However, scours in goats mediated by STEC has been recorded in outbreaks pertaining to hemorrhagic diarrhea (Matthews 2016).
- *VTEC*: been reported in the intestinal contents of healthy goat kids. The occurrence of scours in goat kids due to VTEC has only been reported once; VTEC serotype O103:H2 was attributed to diarrheic goats (Duhamel et al. 1992).
- *AEEC*: are those *E. coli* that can cause attaching/effacing lesions in intestinal epithelial cells. *E. coli* classified as AEEC predominantly belongs to the EPEC group. AEEC produces a virulence factor called intimin that facilitates intimate bacterial adhesion to enterocytes (de la Fuente et al. 2002).

Among these pathotypes, STEC and AEEC have been reported to affect older goats also.

- *Transmission and pathogenesis*: the main route of transmission is feco–oral where susceptible goat kids ingest the *E. coli*-laden feces of the infected animal. By and large, *E. coli* are commensals of the goat alimentary tract but all these pathotypes of *E. coli*, upon gaining entry to the gastrointestinal tract, adhere to the intestinal epithelium and cause damage by either producing toxins or adhering strongly to the intestinal epithelial cells.
- *Clinical signs*: profuse, watery yellowish scours along with dehydration, followed by death.
- *Diagnosis*: based on clinical signs, identification of history of feeding inadequate colostrum during the first 36 hours of life, and laboratory diagnosis. Laboratory diagnosis involves isolation of *E. coli* from feces of infected animals in MacConkey agar or eosin methylene blue (EMB) agar, IMViC test, and demonstration of fimbrial antigens and enterotoxins. On MacConkey agar, bright pink colonies are produced due to lactose fermentation and in EMB agar, colonies with a metallic sheen are produced if *E. coli* is present. the IMViC test provides a quick presumptive diagnosis, wherein the presence of *E. coli* produces in an unique result – indole and methyl red positive and Voges–Proskauer and citrate negative. Demonstration of fimbrial antigens can be carried out via the latex agglutination test, enzyme-linked immunosorbent assay (ELISA), slide agglutination test, fluorescent antibody technique or polymerase chain reaction (PCR). Demonstration of enterotoxins through oxoid tests in cell culture supernatant of filtrates or through ELISA using monoclonal antibodies can be done (Quinn et al. 2011).
- *Treatment*: oral antibiotics such as neomycin or spectinomycin along with supportive fluid therapy to reverse the dehydrated status of the goat kid. Parenteral antibiotics are not required as bacteremia does not occur.
- *Prevention*: ensuring adequate ingestion of colostrum by goat kids during the first few hours of life decreasse the incidence of scours. Ensuring provision of a clean environment for goat kids immediately after birth is necessary. Vaccination of pregnant does seven and three weeks before kidding with *E. coli* multivalent sheep vaccine has been reported to induce passive immunity in goat kids.
- *Zoonotic potential*: goat kids are subclinical carriers or reservoirs of STEC O157 strain, VTEC, and AEEC, which serve as potential sources of zoonotic occurrence of *E. coli*-related life-threatening disease in human beings (Table 43.1).

Table 43.1 List of infectious pathogens of scours with zoonotic potential.

Pathogen	Details	Remarks
Bacteria	STEC O157 strain, VTEC, and AEEC of *E. coli*	Organism shed in feces. Goat kids are subclinical carriers
	Salmonella typhimurium and *S. dublin*	Organism shed in feces and milk
	Campylobacter jejuni	Organism shed in feces
Virus	Betacoronavirus (Coronaviridae)	Organism shed in feces. No zoonotic potential reported so far
Protozoa	*Giardia* sp.	Organism shed in feces

43.3.1.2 *Salmonella* Species

Most of the serotypes of *Salmonella* sp. can cause scours in goat kids. However, *Salmonella typhimuirum and S. dublin* are regarded as the most important causes of scours in goat kids (Matthews 2016).

- *Transmission and pathogenesis*: transmission occurs either through direct ingestion of excreta of infected goats/other domestic animals/wild animals/birds/human beings or through infected feed or water. Infection through exposure to contaminated material via the upper respiratory tract and conjunctiva has also been reported. Upon ingestion, *Salmonella* attaches to the intestinal epithelial cells or mucosal cells through fimbrial attachment. Once adhesion is firmly established, *Salmonella* enters the lamina propria of intestinal cells, which stimulates an inflammatory response, and/or are engulfed by macrophages or neutrophils. Engulfment leads to uninhibited entry of the organism into the lymphatic system, which leads to bacteremia or septicemia. Further, following fimbrial attachment, a bridge-like structure between *Salmonella* and intestinal epithelial cells is formed with the help of the type III secretion system (TTSS), through which various virulence factors are transferred into the intestinal epithelial cells (Quinn et al. 2011). Apart from inducing the immune response and causing influx of inflammatory cells, this also activates the secretory pathway which causes fluid ion imbalance. Thus, the inflammatory response induced by the host immune system primarily mediates scours in goat kids.
- *Clinical signs*: profuse watery yellow-colored scours with increase in body temperature, dehydration, inappetence, and lethargy are the primary clinical signs. Unlike calves, blood is not observed in scours in goat kids. Peracute death can be observed in goat kids of less than one week of age. In kids of more than 10 days old, scours will be observed. In older goats, diarrhea will occur concurrently with abortion during late gestation.
- *Diagnosis*: based on clinical signs, gross lesions, and histopathological changes. Isolation of the organism from feces, milk, mesenteric lymph nodes, heart, blood, or spleen can be done on MacConkey agar or brilliant green agar (BGA). On MacConkey agar, pale colonies will be produced due to lack of lactose fermentation except *S. typhimurium*. On BGA, red colonies are produced due to alkaline reaction. On XLD medium, red colonies are produced with a black center due to production of hydrogen sulfide by most of the *Salmonella* sp. On triple sugar iron agar slope, presence of *Salmonella* sp. shows an alkaline slant/acid but with superimposed black color due to the production of hydrogen sulfide. Agglutination tests, ELISA, and complement fixation test (CFT) can be performed to detect antibody responses to scours caused by *Salmonella* infection (Quinn et al. 1999).
- *Treatment*: supportive therapy to alleviate dehydration in goat kids and administration of antibiotics based on the antibiotic sensitivity test are essential.
- *Prevention*: proper hygienic measures pertaining to environment, feed, and water must be followed. Overcrowding of animals should be avoided. Proper quarantine and isolation protocols must be followed when moving animals from one place to another.
- *Zoonotic potential*: *Salmonella* is of zoonotic importance and can be transmitted from infected goats to human beings through milk or feces (Table 43.1). Hence, humans should be made aware of the risk. Infected goats have been reported to shed *Salmonella* in their feces and hence are carriers. It is important to note that even healthy goats shed *Salmonella* in their feces.

43.3.1.3 *Clostridium perfringens* Type A–D

Enteropathogenic and enterotoxemia-producing clostridia include *Clostridium perfringens* (A–D), *Cl. difficile*, *Cl. colinum*, *Cl. piliforme*, and *Cl. spiroforme*. Among these clostridial species, *Cl. perfringens* type A, B, C, and D have been reported to cause scours in goat species. *Cl. perfringens* produces a range of major (alpha, beta, epsilon, iota) and various minor toxins (hemolysins, collagenase, perfringolysin O, beta-2 toxin, hyaluronidase). All the strains of *Cl. perfringens* produce an enterotoxin, which causes enteric implications including scours.

Clostridium perfringens type A is a commensal pathogen that is generally present in the intestinal flora of goats. It produces two major toxins, alpha and beta, both of which have been reported to cause scours in five-week-old kids. *Cl. perfringens* type B produces three major toxins, alpha, beta and epsilon, of which epsilon toxin possesses the ability to increase intestinal and capillary permeability. This toxin is a prototoxin and needs to be activated by proteolytic enzymes to induce activity. *Cl. perfringens* type C produces alpha, beta, and enterotoxin. *Cl. perfringens* type D produces alpha and epsilon toxins.

By and large, *Cl. perfringens* causes disease in adult goats but types A and B have been reported to cause scours in goat kids.

- *Transmission and pathogenesis*: *Cl. perfringens* is present in the normal intestinal flora of animals and humans and hence is widely distributed in soil. Thus, ingestion of *Cl. perfringens* occurs normally. However, certain animal husbandry practices, such as overfeeding, providing high-protein feed, and change in feeding frequency causing impairment in digestion, lead to production of toxins which cause scours.
- *Clinical signs*: acute and profuse scours along with abdominal pain, dehydration, and loss of appetite are the major clinical signs. Due to dehydration and continuous excessive loss of fluid, death ensues.
- *Diagnosis*: Gram staining of intestinal contents of a freshly dead animal showing large numbers of fat Gram-positive rods can be considered positive for *Cl. perfringens* infection. Demonstration of toxin by intravenous inoculation of suspected clarified ileal contents in mice leads to death within 10–12 hours; specific antisera in ELISA can also be used. A glycosuria test will be positive.
- *Treatment*: administration of antitoxins will be effective along with general supportive therapy for dehydration.
- *Prevention*: continuous monitoring and proper animal husbandry practices are the primary methods of prevention of scours caused by *Cl. perfringens*. Vaccination of pregnant does during late gestation confers passive immunity to kids at birth.

43.3.1.4 *Campylobacter* Species

Among the *Campylobacter* sp. of bacteria, *C. jejuni* causes scours in goat kids. *C. jejuni* is a commensal organism found in the intestinal tracts of birds, which can contaminate water bodies, feed, and feed storage units of farms. It produces an adhesin factor, a cytotoxin, and a heat-labile toxin (Quinn et al. 2011).

- *Transmission and pathogenesis*: the common route of transmission is feco–oral. Upon ingestion, *C. jejuni* adheres to the epithelial cells. With the help of adhesin factors, it enters the cell, multiplies within the membrane-bound compartment, and is released by exocytosis.
- *Clinical signs*: enteritis and scours are the major clinical symptoms in goat kids.
- *Diagnosis*: *C. jejuni* can be visualized directly in wet mounts of feces under dark-field or phase contrast microscopy, where characteristic corkscrew darting motility can be observed. Isolation of *C. jejuni* may not be confirmatory, as they are present as commensals in intestinal flora. Agglutinating antibody titer of more than fourfold can confirm the involvement of *C. jejuni* in causing scours in goat kids (Quinn 1994).
- *Treatment*: supportive rehydration therapy is helpful.
- *Prevention*: general hygienic measures should be followed in farms.
- *Zoonotic potential*: *C. jejuni* is a zoonotic pathogen that causes gastroenteritis in humans through contaminated food material.

43.3.1.5 *Yersinia* Species

Among the *Yersinia* sp. of bacteria, *Y. pseudotuberculosis* causes scours in goat kids of 1–6 months old. Domestic animals, wild mammals, and rodents are carriers of *Y. pseudotuberculosis*, and birds are the amplifier host.

- *Transmission and pathogenesis*: *Y. pseudotuberculosis* is shed in the feces of carrier animals, and ingestion of feed or water contaminated with *Y. pseudotuberculosis*-laden feces leads to infection. Upon ingestion, *Y. pseudotuberculosis* adheres to the mucosal cells with the help of adhesins and invasins. It then enters the mucosal layer of the intestine and is engulfed into macrophages, from where it is transported to mesenteric lymph nodes (Brubaker 1991), thereby causing bacteremia. Replication in the lymph nodes leads to neutrophil infiltration, and hemorrhagic or necrotic lesions. Subclinical infection of *Y. pseudotuberculosis* is common in goat kids and the clinical condition is favored by extreme weather conditions, transportation stress, weaning or poor nutrition (Quinn et al. 2011).
- *Clinical signs*: profuse watery scours that is sometimes hemorrhagic can be observed. Watery luminal small and large intestine contents, mucosal hyperemia, and enlarged mesenteric lymph nodes can be observed during postmortem.

- *Diagnosis*: isolation of *Y. pseudotuberculosis* in blood agar or MacConkey agar can be done. Histological examination of intestinal lesions shows clusters of microabscesses. Molecular techniques like PCR can be done to confirm the presence of *Y. pseudotuberculosis* (Bogdanovich et al. 2003).
- *Treatment*: supportive fluid therapy along with broad-spectrum antibiotic is essential.

43.3.2 Viruses

Rotavirus, coronavirus, adenovirus, astrovirus, bunyavirus, calicivirus, and picornavirus have been reported as viral agents that cause diarrhea in sheep and goats (Martella et al. 2015). Of these, astrovirus and calicivirus have been reported only in sheep and not in goats. Bunyavirus, picornavirus, and coronavirus have been reported only in adult goats.

Bunyaviruses, including Nairobi sheep disease virus, Rift Valley fever virus, and Schmallenberg virus that are vector-borne viral diseases transmitted by ticks, mosquitoes, and biting midges respectively, cause severe hemorrhagic diarrhea leading to death in adult goats and abortion in pregnant does (Daubney and Hudson 1931; Weinbren et al. 1958; Tarlinton et al. 2012). Rift Valley fever virus transmitted by *Aedes* and *Culex* mosquitoes causes hyperacute scours in kids less than seven days old with a mortality rate higher than 70% (Martella et al. 2015).

Of the picornaviruses, bovine enterovirus E (Gür et al. 2008) and bovine kobuvirus (Lee et al. 2012) have been reported in the feces of adult goats.

Documentation of diarrhea caused by the betacoronavirus (BCoV) genus of the Coronaviridae family is less frequent in adult goats. There are very few reports of coronavirus-mediated scours in goat kids (Eisa and Mohamed 2004). It is also important to note that adult goats are subclinical carriers of BCoV, shedding the virus in their feces (Table 43.1), which needs to be addressed given the vast host range and ability of BCoVs to be zoonotic (Han et al. 2006).

Only rotavirus and adenovirus have been reported as common viral agents causing scours in goat kids. Scours due to viral agents can also occur as a coinfection with other bacterial or protozoal organisms (Uzzau et al. 2001).

43.3.2.1 Rotavirus

Rotaviruses belong to the Reoviridae family of viruses that are nonenveloped, consisting of a double- or triple-layered capsid along with a segmented RNA genome. Based on a major capsid protein named VP6, rotaviruses are classified into seven antigenically distinct serogroups – A–G (Alam et al. 2007). All these serogroups are species specific and among them, group B rotaviruses cause scours in goat kids.

- *Transmission and pathogenesis*: infected animals shed virus through feces, hence the major route of transmission is feco–oral. Infection of goat kids by rotavirus is influenced by age of infection, maternally derived immunity and immunity conferred by colostrum, overcrowding, time of exposure, and presence of other enteric bacterial and viral pathogens. In addition, enteric infection by rotavirus also depends on the virulence and amount of ingestion of the rotavirus. Upon ingestion, the virus passes to the intestine through the stomach, surviving the gastric acidity, and infects the enterocytes in the tip of the villi in the small intestine. The enterocytes are damaged and their replacement is slower in goat kids, thereby leading to malabsorption of feed and thus scours. Further, the damaged enterocytes fail to absorb lactose so the undigested lactose serves as a niche for proliferation of bacteria. Due to an osmotic effect, there is retention of luminal fluid along with malabsorption of fluid leading to scours (Ramig 2004).
- *Clinical signs*: light-colored pasty semisolid scours, along with anorexia, dehydration, and depression are seen. Goat kids usually recover in four days with or without supportive therapy. However, coinfection with *E. coli*, *Salmonella* and *Cryptosporidium* may lead to severe scours and death (Quinn et al. 2011).
- *Diagnosis*: suitable samples for diagnosis include faces and intestinal contents. Virus particles can be demonstrated via negative electron microscopy. Viral antigens can be demonstrated with specific antisera through ELISA or latex agglutination tests, or in smears from intestinal contents via immunofluorescence. Sodium dodecyl sulfate-polyacrylamide gel electrophoresis (SDS-PAGE) can also be used for demonstration of viral antigens.
- *Treatment*: fluid replacement therapy along with antibiotics is the mode of treatment.
- *Control*: adequate ingestion of colostrum provides local immunity in the intestine by producing protective antibodies. Vaccination of pregnant does against rotavirus confers passive immunity to goat kids upon birth (Quinn et al. 2011).

43.3.2.2 Adenovirus

Adenoviruses are nonenveloped viruses with a double-stranded DNA genome. The genera affecting sheep and goats are categorized as *Mastadenovirus*, comprising ovine adenovirus D species, and *Atadenovirus*, comprising ovine adenovirus

A and B species. Although adenovirus commonly affects sheep, it is important to note that similar clinical signs are also manifested in goats. The serotypes identified under these adenovirus species include ovine adenovirus 1–7, goat adenovirus 1, and bovine adenovirus 2 (Martella et al. 2015). Among these, ovine adenovirus serotypes 2 and 5 have been reported to cause scours in goat kids (Olson et al. 2004). Further, adenovirus has been isolated from sheep and goats affected with peste des petits ruminants (PPR) disease (Gibbs et al. 1977).

- *Transmission*: adenovirus causes both enteric and respiratory forms of disease and hence transmission is primarily through the feco–oral route or through inhalation of respiratory secretions. It affects 2–12-week-old goat kids and is usually hyperacute, leading to death (DeBey et al. 2001).
- *Clinical signs*: acute, watery yellowish diarrhea leading to death within 4–5 hours.
- *Diagnosis*: serum virus neutralization tests can be done to identify the serotype. Histopathological examination of intestine may reveal inclusion bodies (Gibbs et al. 1977).
- *Treatment*: general supportive therapy with administration of broad-spectrum antibiotics.
- *Prevention*: good hygienic practices, proper quarantine and isolation protocols, limitation of movement of farm workers and animals around the farm, proper sanitization of equipment to avoid infection through fomites, and feeding adequate colostrum immediately after birth (Gibbs et al. 1977).

43.3.3 Protozoa

43.3.3.1 *Cryptosporidium* Species

Cryptosporidium parvum, the cause of cryptosporidiosis, is a protozoan parasite that causes scours in goat kids aged 5–10 days. The life cycle of *C. parvum* involves production of oocysts consisting of sporozoites in the intestine of infected animals, which when passed through feces are immediately infective to other susceptible animals. Upon ingestion, they adhere to the epithelial cells of the distal small intestine, cecum, and colon and cause villous atrophy leading to malabsorption and thus diarrhea. Yellowish watery diarrhea, along with dehydration, and anorexia leading to death can be observed (Pavlovic et al. 2010). Fecal smears can be examined for the presence of bluish circular oocysts with reddish granules with the help of methanol fixation and Giemsa staining. Fluorescent antibody tests and ELISA can be done.

Treatment is targeted toward reducing the secretion and excretion of oocysts in infected goat kids within 24 hours of infection with the help of halofuginone, paromomycin, and decoquinate along with necessary supportive therapy. Administration of adequate amounts of colostrum helps to confer local immunity.

If cryptosporidiosis infection occurs on the farm, it should be completely disinfected with ammonia and formalin (Majeed et al. 2018).

43.3.3.2 *Eimeria* Species

Eimeria sp. are protozoa that cause scours in goat kids aged 1–4 months, leading to blood- or mucus-tinged watery diarrhea. Infection during the initial days of life may confer immunity to coccidiosis. Administration of coccidiostats is an effective treatment.

43.3.3.3 *Giardia* Species

Giardia sp. are protozoa that cause scours in goat kids, especially aged 2–4 weeks. Transmission is via the feco–oral route and upon ingestion, the agent damages the microvilli of the duodenum and proximal jejunum, causing malabsorption, lactose indigestion, fluid retention, and excessive luminal fluid accumulation leading to diarrhea. Giemsa-stained wet fecal smears can be examined for binucleated, pear-shaped central bodied, motile flagellates. Treatment involves administration of fenbendazole.

Giardia is a zoonotic pathogen and hence giardiasis in goat kids must be managed with meticulous personnel care (Table 43.1).

43.3.4 Parasites

Scours induced by gastrointestinal (GI) parasitism primarily involves *Strongyloides papillosa*, *Trichostrongylus* sp. (bankrupt or hair worm), *Teladorsagia* sp., rumen fluke, *Ostertagia circumcincta* (medium or brown stomach worm), *Cooperia* sp. (small intestinal worm), and *Nematodirus* sp. (threadneck worm). GI worms develop in and destroy the gastric glands of the abomasum, change the abomasal pH, affect feed absorption, and lead to diarrhea. Growth is hindered in kids infected with GI worms due to lack of nutrient absorption. Care must be taken to achieve good pasture, grazing, and animal management, and administration of anthelmintics.

43.4 Noninfectious Agents Causing Scours

Noninfectious agents causing scours involve nutritional mismanagement such as dietary changes, inappropriate feeding practices, consumption of poisonous plants (aconite, bluebell, box, buckthorn, dog's mercury, irises, rhododendron, spurges, and wild arum), minerals (copper, fluorides, arsenicals, barium, chromium, mercury, zinc, selenium, molybdenum, lead), mycotoxins, and certain drugs (sulfonamides, carbon tetrachloride, copper sulfate, and warfarin), mycotoxins, poor-quality milk replacers, inadequate feeding of colostrum, faulty animal husbandry practices such as overcrowding, unhygienic environments, and stress-related factors such as transportation, improper handling, weaning, and extreme weather conditions (Matthews 2016).

43.5 Conclusion

In conclusion, scours in goat kids can occur due to various pathogenic and nonpathogenic causes. The transmission and pathogenesis of scours caused by infectious pathogens are depicted schematically in Figure 43.3. Management of scours may not be possible as death ensues quickly in goat kids; hence, it is highly important to prevent and control the incidence of scours.

For control purposes, general hygienic practices after kidding should be followed such as isolating affected kids and moving them to a clean pen and ensuring that does give birth in a clean area. After birth, kids should not be allowed to become chilled or starved and should receive colostrum in early life. Bedding should be clean and dry and all equipment should be cleaned and disinfected between uses. Kids should be offered access to hay and grain ration to initiate good rumen development and a normal flora, and to avoid subsequent weaning shock. Feed kids in trays or buckets outside the pen to avoid fecal contamination of feedstuffs, and practice excellent sanitation and remove manure promptly.

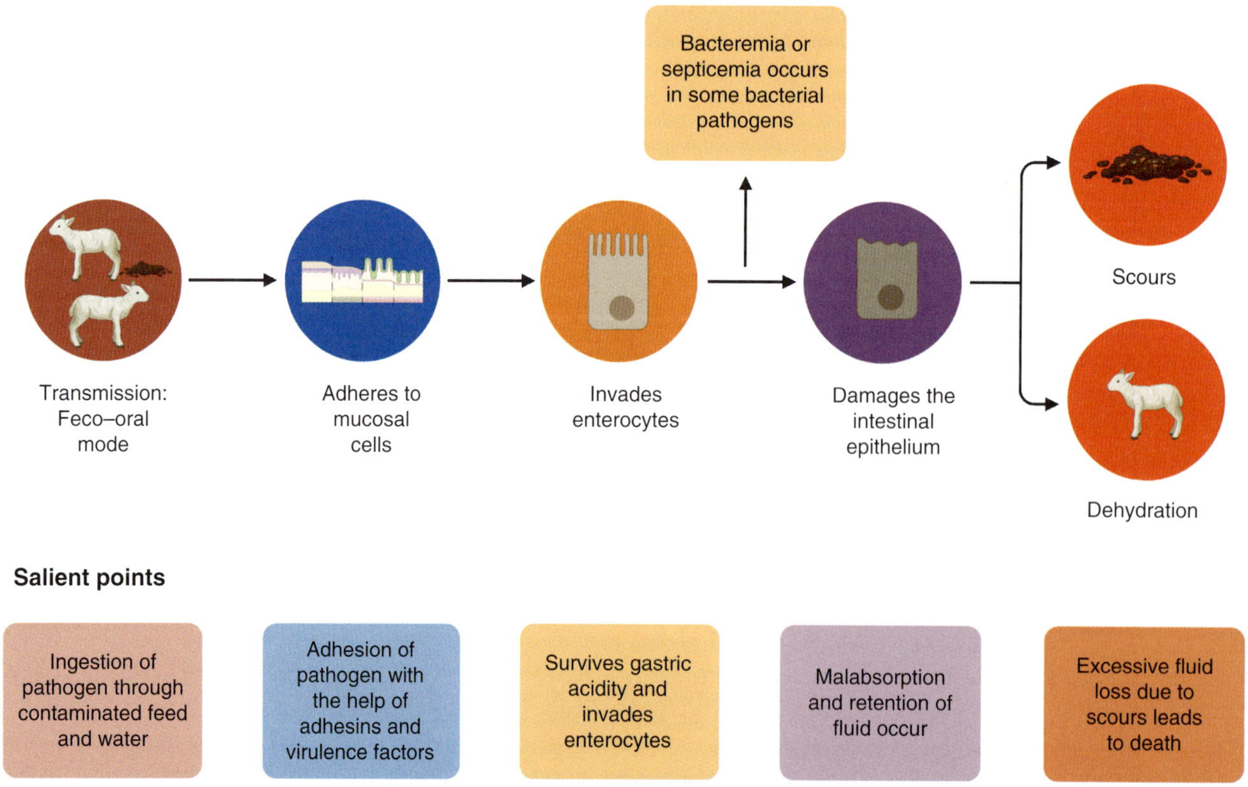

Figure 43.3 General transmission and pathogenesis of infectious pathogens causing scours. *Source:* Created by Ranjani Rajasekaran using www.biorender.com under academic license.

References

Abdou, N.E., Majeed, Q.A.H., El-Azazy, O.M.E. et al. (2021). Risk factors of diarrhea in small ruminants in Kuwait. *Iranian Journal of Veterinary Research* 22 (2): 146.

Alam, M.M., Kobayashi, N., Ishino, M. et al. (2007). Genetic analysis of an ADRV-N-like novel rotavirus strain B219 detected in a sporadic case of adult diarrhea in Bangladesh. *Archives of Virology* 152: 199–208.

Bogdanovich, T.M., Carniel, E., Fukushima, H., and Skurnik, M. (2003). Genetic (sero) typing of Yersinia pseudotuberculosis. *Advances in Experimental Medicine and Biology* 529: 337–340.

Brubaker, R.R. (1991). Factors promoting acute and chronic diseases caused by Yersiniae. *Clinical Microbiological Reviews* 4: 309–324.

Daubney, R. and Hudson, J.R. (1931). Enzootic hepatitis or Rift Valley fever. An un-described virus disease of sheep, cattle and man from East Africa. *Journal of Pathology and Bacteriology* 34: 545–579.

DeBey, B.M., Lehmkuhl, H.D., Chard-Bergstrom, C., and Hobbs, L.A. (2001). Ovine adenovirus serotype 7-associated mortality in lambs in the United States. *Veterinary Pathology* 38: 644–648.

Duhamel, G.E., Moxley, R.A., Maddox, C.W., and Erickson, E.D. (1992). Enteric infection of a goat with enterohemorrhagic Escherichia coli (0103, H2). *Journal of Veterinary Diagnostic Investigation* 4 (2): 197–200.

Eisa, M. and Mohamed, A. (2004). Role of enteric pathogens in enteritis in lambs, goat kids and children and their zoonotic importance. *Veterinary Medical Journal – Giza* 52: 41–59.

de la Fuente, R., García, S., Orden, J.A. et al. (2002). Prevalence and characteristics of attaching and effacing strains of Escherichia coli isolated from diarrheic and healthy sheep and goats. *American Journal of Veterinary Research* 63 (2): 262–266.

Gibbs, E.P.J., Taylor, W.P., and Lawman, M.J.P. (1977). The isolation of adenoviruses from goats affected with peste des petits ruminants in Nigeria. *Research in Veterinary Science* 23 (3): 331–335.

Gür, S., Yapkiç, O., and Yilmaz, A. (2008). Serological survey of bovine enterovirus type 1 in different mammalian species in Turkey. *Zoonoses and Public Health* 55 (2): 106–111.

Han, M.G., Cheon, D.S., Zhang, X., and Saif, L.J. (2006). Cross-protection against a human enteric coronavirus and a virulent bovine enteric coronavirus in gnotobiotic calves. *Journal of Virology* 80 (24): 12350–12356.

Hare, T. and Glynn, E. (1927). Observations on lamb dysentery. *Journal of Pathology and Bacteriology* 30 (2): 473–502.

Lee, M.H., Jeoung, H.Y., Lim, J.A. et al. (2012). Kobuvirus in south Korean black goats. *Virus Genes* 45: 186–189.

Majeed, Q.A., El-Azazy, O.M., Abdou, N.E.M. et al. (2018). Epidemiological observations on cryptosporidiosis and molecular characterization of cryptosporidium spp. in sheep and goats in Kuwait. *Parasitology Research* 117: 1631–1636.

Martella, V., Decaro, N., and Buonavoglia, C. (2015). Enteric viral infections in lambs or kids. *Veterinary Microbiology* 181 (1–2): 154–160.

Matthews, J. (2016). Diarrhoea. In: *Diseases of the Goat*, 4e, 208–227. Chichester, UK: Wiley.

Olson, E.J., Haskell, S.R., Frank, R.K. et al. (2004). Isolation of an adenovirus and an adeno-associated virus from goat kids with enteritis. *Journal of Veterinary Diagnostic Investigation* 16 (5): 461–464.

Osman, K.M., Mustafa, A.M., Elhariri, M., and Abdelhamed, G.S. (2013). The distribution of Escherichia coli serovars, virulence genes, gene association and combinations and virulence genes encoding serotypes in pathogenic E. coli recovered from diarrhoeic calves, sheep and goat. *Transboundary and Emerging Diseases* 60 (1): 69–78.

Pavlović, I., Ivanović, S., Žujović, M., and Tomić, Z. (2010). Goat cryptosporidiosis and its importance at goat production pathology. *Biotechnology in Animal Husbandry 26* (3-4): 187–192.

Quinn, P.J. (1994). *Clinical Veterinary Microbiology*. Prescott, AZ: Wolfe.

Quinn, P.J., Carter, M.E., Markey, B.K., and Carter, G. (1999). *Clinical Veterinary Microbiology*, 226–234. London: Mosby Yearbook Europe Ltd.

Quinn, P.J., Markey, B.K., Leonard, F.C. et al. (2011). *Veterinary Microbiology and Microbial Disease*. Hoboken, NJ: Wiley.

Ramig, R.F. (2004). Pathogenesis of intestinal and systemic rotavirus infection. *Journal of Virology* 78: 10213–10220.

Shabana, I.I., Bouqellah, N.A., and Zaraket, H. (2017). Investigation of viral and bacterial enteropathogens of diarrheic sheep and goats in Medina, Saudi Arabia. *Tropical Biomedicine* 34 (4): 944–955.

Tarlinton, R., Daly, J., Dunham, S., and Kydd, J. (2012). The challenge of Schmallenberg virus emergence in Europe. *Veterinary Journal* 194: 10–18.

Thompson, K.G. (1985). Enteric diseases of goats. *Proceedings of the Course in Goat Husbandry and Medicine*, Massey University New Zealand, 78–85.

Uzzau, S., Leori, G.S., Petruzzi, V. et al. (2001). Salmonella enterica serovar-host specificity does not correlate with the magnitude of intestinal invasion in sheep. *Infectious Immunology* 69: 3092–3099.

Weinbren, M.P., Gourlay, R.N., Lumsden, W.H.R., and Weinbren, B.M. (1958). An epizootic of Nairobi sheep disease in Uganda. *Journal of Comparative Pathology and Therapeutics* 68: 174–187.

44

Navel and Joint Ill

Saahithya Rajamohan[1], *Ranjani Rajasekaran*[2], *Padmanath Krishnan*[3], *and Richard Jagatheesan Pitchai Navlon*[4]

[1] Department of Veterinary Pathology, Veterinary College and Research Institute, Tamil Nadu Veterinary and Animal Sciences University, Salem, India
[2] Department of Veterinary Microbiology, Veterinary College and Research Institute, Tamil Nadu Veterinary and Animal Sciences University, Theni, India
[3] Veterinary Clinical Complex, Veterinary College and Research Institute, Tamil Nadu Veterinary and Animal Sciences University, Theni, India
[4] Veterinary College and Research Institute, Tamil Nadu Veterinary and Animal Sciences University, Theni, India

44.1 Introduction

Navel ill and joint ill frequently affect newborn goat kids. The conditions are life-threatening, leading to death if prompt treatment is not provided. Navel ill is an acute localized inflammation and infection of the external umbilicus. Joint ill refers to the condition of polyarthritis. Both conditions occur either singly or in combination and usually begin with poor management of the herd. Various bacterial etiological agents are reported to be the causative agents. Affected kids present with pyrexia, swollen umbilicus, and painful joints. Early treatment with antibiotics can help, preventing untoward economic losses. However, prevention of this condition mainly relies on careful management practices being followed in the herd.

This chapter reviews navel ill and joint ill affecting goat kids with an emphasis on etiopathogenesis, clinical signs, diagnosis, treatment, and control.

44.2 Navel Ill

In young goat kids, navel ill is usually referred to as omphalophlebitis, omphaloarteritis or omphalitis. It is defined as infection of the umbilicus in young animals.

44.2.1 Etiopathogenesis

Multiple etiological agents have been suggested as the causative factors for omphalitis. These agents are mostly of bacterial origin, among which the most frequently encountered is *Trueperella* (formerly *Corynebacterium*) *pyogenes*. Other organisms associated with this condition include *Escherichia coli*, *Enterococcus* spp., *Proteus* spp., *Streptococcus* spp., and *Staphylococcus* spp. and they are all considered to be environmental contaminants.

Underwood et al. (2015) reported that *Trueperella pyogenes* occurs in conjunction with *E. coli* in kids, causing acute localized inflammation and infection of the external umbilicus. Also, most cases occur within the first three months of age or in the neonatal stage with painful enlargement of the umbilicus. As a result, purulent discharges may be noticed from the umbilicus. In cases of ascending infection, the urachus is involved which would be followed by cystitis. Septicemia, peritonitis, septic arthritis, meningitis, patent urachus, urachal abscesses, umbilical hernias, osteomyelitis, and endocarditis are the various sequelae reported. The organism can be identified by bacteriological culture.

Elements of Reproduction and Reproductive Diseases of Goats, First Edition. Edited by Tanmoy Rana.

44.2.2 Clinical Signs

Underwood et al. (2015) reported that goat kids usually evince clinical signs of dullness, pyrexia, enlargement of the umbilicus resulting in severe pain and varying degrees of anorexia. In severe cases, purulent discharges may be noticed draining from the umbilicus. In addition, if the urachus is involved, cystitis may develop, resulting in clinical signs of dysuria, stranguria, and hematuria.

Other frequently observed sequelae include septicemia, pneumonia, peritonitis, joint ill, patent urachus and urachal abscesses, umbilical hernias, meningitis, osteomyelitis, uveitis, endocarditis, and diarrhea as mentioned in the reports by Underwood et al. (2015).

Abdullah et al. (2015) reported a single case of omphalitis in a two-month-old goat kid with resultant septicemia wherein the kid exhibited clinical signs including lethargy, lateral recumbency, pale mucous membranes, and dehydration. Also, there was hypothermia, bradycardia, and a shallow respiratory rate.

44.2.3 Diagnosis

The foremost aspect of diagnosis is observation of clinical signs and priority should be given to animals in their first week of life or within three months of birth. Clinical signs of fever of unknown origin in kids which fail to thrive are characteristic. The etiological agents can be narrowed down by conventional bacteriological culture and identification methods carried out as per standard procedure. As per Underwood et al. (2015), the differential diagnosis should be made from an umbilical hernia which should be neither infected nor painful to touch and can be reduced.

44.2.4 Treatment and Control

Treatment modalities include debridement, drainage of the affected area in severe cases, and administration of systemic antimicrobial therapy. In kids which respond to treatment, omphalitis can be treated with broad-spectrum antibiotics such as ampicillin, ceftiofur, and florfenicol for a period of 10–14 days as reported by Underwood et al. (2015). In cases of umbilical abscessation, it should be surgically opened and flushed with iodine solutions frequently. If there is no systemic involvement, the prognosis is good. However, Scott et al. (2011) have reported that the prognosis is grave if the case is coupled with peritoneal infection.

In a report by Ribeiro et al. (2015), they have stated that the most effective antibiotics against *Trueperella pyogenes* were florfenicol (99.1%), cefoperazone (96.0%), cephalexin (95.0%), and ceftiofur (94.8%). In addition, a high rate of resistance was observed against trimethoprim-sulfamethoxazole (49.3%), followed by norfloxacin (10.9%) and tetracycline (9.2%). This study was conducted in a retrospective manner from 2002 to 2012 in domestic animals from infections caused by *T. pyogenes*, including omphalitis.

Prevention and control measures by means of proper hygienic husbandry practices should be followed. Day-to-day management of proper hygienic conditions in the barn must be undertaken. Pregnant goats should be provided with clean birthing environments. Ensuring clean hands while delivering the newborn and dipping the umbilicus with a 7% iodine solution will be helpful. It is also essential that the newborn kid is able to access colostrum from the dam in order to provide adequate immunity (Thedford 1983).

44.3 Joint Ill

Joint ill is also called bacterial polyarthritis. The condition usually occurs in young kids under three months of age.

44.3.1 Etiopathogenesis

Similar to navel ill, joint ill is caused by several etiological agents of bacterial origin, either occurring singly or in combination. They include hemolytic *Streptococcus* spp. and *Staphylococcus* spp., *Trueperella* spp. and *Escherichia coli*, which are environmental contaminants. In addition, *Streptococcus dysgalactiae* (Blanchard and Fiser 1994), *Pasteurella multocida* (Bhomik and Dalapati 1995), and *Klebsiella pneumoniae* (Bernabé et al. 1998) have been reported as causative agents of joint ill in goat kids. Guss (1977) and Vaissaire et al. (1985) have indicated *Erysipelothrix rhusiopathiae* as a causative agent in polyarthritis in goat kids. However, as per Eamens et al. (1988), documented cases due to the above etiological agent are scarce. Similarly, chlamydial organisms have been indicated in polyarthritis. It is well established in lambs but documentation in goats is lacking (Nietfeld 2001). DaMassa et al. (1992) and Matthews (2016) have reported the etiology of *Mycoplasma* spp. in goat kids under six months of age in Europe, Australia, and the United States. It includes *M. capricolum*, *M. mycoides* subsp. *capri*, *M. putrifaciens*, and *Mycoplasma agalactiae*.

Infection occurs through the umbilical cord immediately after birth, as a result of bacteremia due to enteroinvasion, or via the upper respiratory tract and or tonsil. It also occurs secondary to bacteremia after localization in joints which further produces a destructive inflammatory response. Underlying immunodeficiencies can predispose to the development of bacterial polyarthritis.

Potential sources of infection with streptococci include teats, milk and vagina of the dam, and *S. dysgalactiae* can survive on dry straw for up to 42 days as reported by Matthews (2016). For *Mycoplasma* spp.-mediated arthritis in goat kids, milk tends to be the primary mode of transmission directly from feeding or suckling and indirectly from milk-contaminated buckets or via hands or milk-contaminated clothing as reported by Agnello et al. (2012).

Chlamydophila pecorum (formerly *Chlamydia psittaci*) has been reported to cause polyarthritis in young goats in parts of Europe and the United States (Matthews 2016).

44.3.2 Predisposing Factors

The various predisposing factors of joint ill are illustrated in Figure 44.1. Bernabé et al. (1998) reported that the factors that predispose goats to bacteremia include kidding in contaminated environments, poor sanitation in housing, the development of omphalophlebitis after failure to disinfect the navel at birth and, most importantly, when the kid is devoid of colostrum after birth leading to failure in passive transfer of immunity from the dam. Also, these authors indicated that navel infection is not a prerequisite for bacteremia and polyarthritis; they reported an outbreak due to *Klebsiella pneumoniae* in a farm where disinfection of navel was routinely carried out. They postulated that infection might have spread via the intestinal route due to feeding of artificial colostrum to the goat kids.

44.3.3 Clinical Signs

The affected goat kids usually are pyrexic (range 39.4–40.6 °C). There may be pain and swelling in one or more joints, especially carpus, shoulder, hock and stifle, with moderate to nonweight-bearing lameness. In some cases, there is severe lameness with minimal swelling of joint. In more chronically affected cases, the affected joint will be stiff or ankylosed.

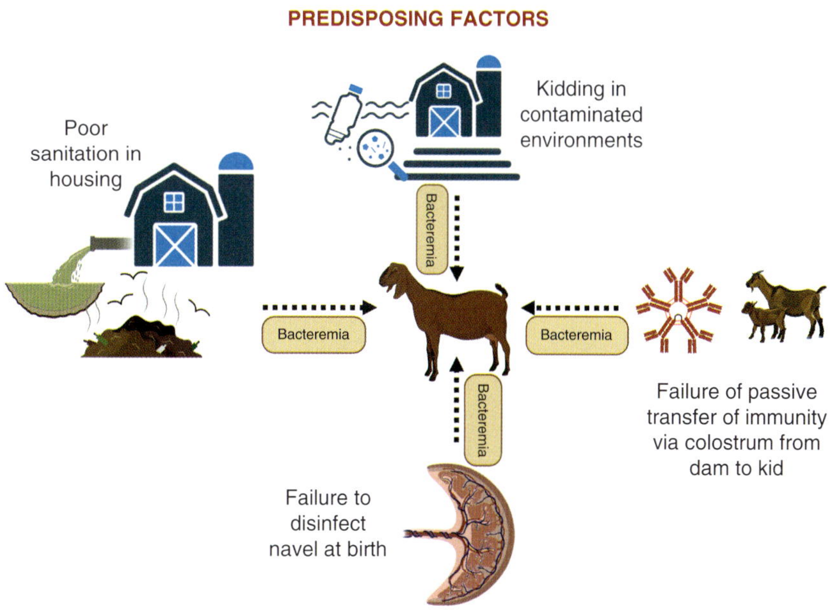

Figure 44.1 Schematic representation of the predisposing factors of joint ill in goat kids. *Source:* Created by Saahithya Rajamohan using www.biorender.com.

Involvement of the atlantooccipital joint can produce sudden-onset tetraparesis and recumbency. Concurrently, the umbilicus is often inflamed.

As per reports by Agnello et al. (2012), in mycoplasmal arthritis clinical signs involve acutely swollen joints and pyrexia with or without pneumonia.

In *Chlamydophila pecorum*, Matthews (2016) stated that the clinical signs in goat kids involve polyarthritis and stiffness of joints and the condition develops as an acute febrile illness. The joint fluid may not be purulent in appearance. Also, the elevation in white blood cells is mainly due to a rise in mononuclear cells.

44.3.4 Diagnosis

Early diagnosis is required in cases of joint ill as the condition may worsen within a couple of days and provision of the required treatment may not be possible. Culturing and identification of bacteria from the joint fluid (or umbilical swabs) is the preferred method. Routine bacteriological culture and identification methods need to carried out to identify the causative agent.

Synovial fluid from infected joints is usually thick and cloudy due to an increased total protein concentration (normal <3 g/l). Cytological examination of the fluid reveals pleocytosis almost entirely of neutrophils. However, in chronically affected kids, there is little joint effusion and performing an arthrocentesis often yields more blood than joint fluid.

According to Nayak and Bhowmik (1990) and Bhomik and Dalapati (1995), clinical pathology may indicate neutrophilic leukocytosis or leukopenia (in the case of Gram-negative sepsis). Diagnosis by arthrocentesis indicates turbid and flocculent synovial fluid with increased total protein concentration and elevated cell counts consisting primarily of neutrophils in cytology. Estimation of serum immunoglobulin levels might help in an advanced diagnostic setting. Immunoglobulin levels are often low, indicating failure of passive transfer of colostral antibody to the kid.

At necropsy, gross examination of the joint cavities reveals serofibrinous or purulent synovial fluid. The synovium may be inflamed with erosion of the cartilage. Evidence of infection may also be present in other organ systems, mainly lungs, gastrointestinal tract, and central nervous system. Microscopically, there is hyperplasia of the synovial villi.

In joint ill due to *Mycoplasma* spp., necropsy findings include purulent or fibropurulent arthritis with hemorrhagic erosions of articular surfaces (East 1996; Filioussis et al. 2011; Matthews 2016). In a diagnostic setting, the agent can be diagnosed by serological techniques such as the complement fixation test. PCR testing is also available for the detection and differentiation of *Mycoplasma* species. However, some closely related species may be misdiagnosed. At the field level, isolation of the organism from joint fluid in *Mycoplasma* medium can be performed. However, long-term surveillance by culturing milk is necessary to detect infected does.

In cases due to *Chlamydophila pecorum*, on necropsy, fibrinous arthritis occurs without any changes to the cartilage. In such cases, smears can be taken from the joint exudate and can be stained by Giemsa stain in which the chlamydial organisms stain purple. In order to characterize an organism, isolation of *Chlamydia* in embryonating yolk sacs can be done to characterize the organism (Matthews 2016).

44.3.5 Treatment and Control

In affected cases, treatment is likely to be successful only if given early by administering broad-spectrum antibiotics both parenterally and intraarticularly. It is also important to note that the selection of antibiotic should be based on culture and sensitivity testing. Matthews (2016) reported that injection of high doses of parenteral antibiotics for a week may be curative if combined with proper nursing, but the response to treatment is often poor as progressive and degenerative changes occur within the infected joints (Smith and Sherman 2009).

For streptococcal-mediated polyarthritis, administration of procaine penicillin at a dose rate of 44 000 IU/kg (every 24 hours for minimum of five days) is the antibiotic of choice. It can be administered at 36–48 hours of age which could be effective in preventing an outbreak (East 1996; Filioussis et al. 2011; Matthews 2016).

Cases of acute septic arthritis require joint lavage with saline and antibiotic solutions combined with systemic and local antimicrobial treatment. Lavage should be repeated daily whenever needed. To relieve pain, NSAIDs, flunixin, meloxicam or ketoprofen should be administered IV for three consecutive days. The purpose of joint lavage is to remove the inflammatory exudate, thereby reducing damage to the joint surfaces and eliminating infection. Also, proper management practices like good nursing, provision of a soft bed, and frequent massaging of the affected joints. Animals that survive may remain unthrifty.

In cases where the umbilicus is also affected, treatment of the cord with 7% tincture of iodine or administration of an antibiotic spray as soon as possible after birth is is required. Also, the site of infection must be checked regularly for signs of inflammation.

In goat kids affected by *Mycoplasma*, no antibiotics are effective. Although tylosin, 10–50 mg/kg every eight hours, and other antibiotics like tetracyclines, florfenicol, and enrofloxacin have been used to improve the clinical condition, recovered animals often become asymptomatic carriers (Filioussis et al. 2011; Matthews 2016).

The most important control measure is provision of a clean environment at the time of kidding. It has been reported that the bacteria can persist for several weeks in straw in deep-bedded pens. Also, addition of new straw to a poorly maintained pen will not prevent infection and all kidding pens should be cleaned out completely between kiddings.

In *Mycoplasma*-mediated infections, strict quarantine and screening are recommended to prevent introduction of the organism into the herd. Adequate colostrum (300 ml within six hours of birth) must be given to kids in order to prevent them from developing an immunocompromised state. However, once the organism has been introduced into the herd, managing the infection is very difficult due to the chronicity and ability to develop a carrier state. In such cases, culturing of each doe's first colostrum for *Mycoplasma* is essential. Adult carriers should be identified and culled if economically feasible. The kids should be reared on pasteurized colostrum or milk replacers (East 1996; Filioussis et al. 2011; Matthews 2016).

44.4 Conclusion

Due to the occurrence of multiple bacterial organisms as etiological agents in this condition, following a careful management plan and excellent husbandry practices is essential as this will minimize the loss of kids. Maintenance of strict hygiene in the kidding environment, following closed herd practices, training farm workers in taking care of the kids immediately after birth and ensuring adequate provision of colostrum to the newborn will help in managing the condition. In addition, administration of specific antibiotics to affected goat kids will help to treat the condition at the early stages. Antibiotic administration to the doe 24–48 hours prior to kidding will prove beneficial and strengthen herd resistance.

References

Abdullah, F.F.J., Abba, Y., Tijjani, A. et al. (2015). Septicemia associated with omphalitis in a goat kid. *International Journal of Livestock Research* 5 (4): 113.

Agnello, S., Chetta, M., Vicari, D. et al. (2012). Severe outbreak of polyarthritis in kids caused by *Mycoplasma mycoides* subspecies *capri* in Sicily. *Veterinary Record* 170 (16): 416.

Bernabé, A., Contreras, A., Gomez, M.A. et al. (1998). Polyarthritis in kids associated with *Klebsiella pneumoniae*. *Veterinary Record* 142 (3): 64–66.

Bhomik, M.K. and Dalapati, M.R. (1995). Infectious arthritis in goats caused by *Pasteurella multocida*. *Indian Journal of Veterinary Pathology* 19 (1): 26–29.

Blanchard, P.C. and Fiser, K.M. (1994). Streptococcus dysgalactiae polyarthritis in dairy goats. *Journal of the American Veterinary Medical Association* 205: 739–739.

DaMassa, A.J., Wakenell, P.S., and Brooks, D.L. (1992). Mycoplasmas of goats and sheep. *Journal of Veterinary Diagnostic Investigation* 4: 101–113.

Eamens, G.J., Turner, M.J., and Catt, R.E. (1988). Serotypes of *Erysipelothrix rhusiopathiae* in Australian pigs, small ruminants, poultry, and captive wild birds and animals. *Australian Veterinary Journal* 65 (8): 249–252.

East, N.E. (1996). *Mycoplasma mycoides* polyarthritis of goats. In: *Large Animal Internal Medicine*, 2e (ed. B.P. Smith), 1277–1278. St Louis, MO: Mosby.

Filioussis, G., Giadinis, N.D., Petridou, E.J. et al. (2011). Congenital polyarthritis in goat kids attributed to *Mycoplasma agalactiae*. *Veterinary Record* 169 (14): 364.

Guss, S.B. (1977). *Management and Diseases of Dairy Goats*. Arizona, USA: Dairy Goat Journal Publishing Corporation.

Matthews, J. (e.) (2016). Lameness in kids. In: *Diseases of the Goat*, 105–114. Oxford, UK: Wiley-Blackwell.

Nayak, N.C. and Bhowmik, M.K. (1990). Caprine bacterial arthritis: physical, biochemical and cytologic properties of synovial fluid. *Indian Veterinary Journal* 67 (11): 1016–1020.

Nietfeld, J.C. (2001). Chlamydial infections in small ruminants. *Veterinary Clinics of North America: Food Animal Practice* 17 (2): 301–314.

Ribeiro, M.G., Risseti, R.M., Bolaños, C.A.D. et al. (2015). Trueperella pyogenes multispecies infections in domestic animals: a retrospective study of 144 cases (2002 to 2012). *Veterinary Quarterly* 35 (2): 82–87.

Scott, P., Penny, C., and Macrae, A. (2011). *Cattle Medicine*, 1e. London: Manson/Veterinary Press.

Smith, M.C. and Sherman, D.M. (2009). *Goat Medicine*. Wiley.

Thedford, T.R. (1983). *Goat Health Handbook*. Morrilton, AR: Winrock International.

Underwood, W.J., Blauwiekel, R., Delano, M.L. et al. (2015). Biology and diseases of ruminants (sheep, goats, and cattle). In: *Laboratory Animal Medicine* (ed. J. Fox, L. Anderson, G. Otto, et al.), 623–694. New York: Academic Press.

Vaissaire, J., Desmettre, P., Paille, G. et al. (1985). Erysipelothrix rhusiopathiae: agent du rouget, dans les différentes espèces animales. *Bulletin de l'Académie Vétérinaire de France* 138 (3): 259–265.

Section 7

Late Diseases of Kids

45

Coccidiosis

Bhupamani Das[1], Sirigireddy Sivajothi[2], Husen R. Parsani[1], and Abhinav N. Suthar[3]

[1] Department of Clinics, College of Veterinary Science and Animal Husbandry, Kamdhenu University, Sardarkrushinagar, Gujarat, India
[2] Department of Veterinary Parasitology, College of Veterinary Science, Sri Venkateswara Veterinary University, Proddatur, Andhra Pradesh, India
[3] Department of Veterinary Medicine, College of Veterinary Science & Animal Husbandry, Kamdhenu University, Sardarkrushinagar, India

45.1 Introduction

Small ruminants have a significant role in domestication (Walker and Hudson 2014). Sheep and goats are important livestock that have a big impact on the economies and food security of developing nations. In the livestock industry, particularly in developing nations, goats play a significant role by supporting incomes and sustainable agriculture, and providing nutritional security (Namutosi et al. 2019).

Numerous health issues are common in small ruminants (Pezzanite et al. 2022). Ruminant animals can contract internal parasites (or endoparasites), including protozoans (coccidians) from a variety of taxonomic groupings. For a very long time, parasites had a big impact on domestic ruminant output and health. In tropical and subtropical areas of the world, parasitic infection is a significant barrier to the health and productivity of livestock. They are to blame for livestock's significant illness, weight loss, poor reproductive health, and probable mortality (Grzybek et al. 2016). A stronger resistance to infection is seen in adult animals when it comes to parasites (such as coccidians), thanks in large part to acquired immunity.

The apicomplexan disease known as small ruminant coccidiosis, which can result in severe enteritis and/or typhlocolitis, is caused by various species of the genus *Eimeria* (Hermosilla et al. 2016). According to Khor et al. (2018), coccidiosis caused by *Eimeria* spp. can result in significant financial losses for a small ruminant business. According to Majeed et al. (2020), the primary cause of infection is consumption of tainted food and water. Warm and humid weather has a beneficial impact on the prevalence rate of coccidiosis, making it more common during the rainy season (Mohammed et al. 2021). Coccidiosis is one of the major issues that frequently results in kid fatalities. Unicellular protozoans of the *Eimeria* genus are the cause of the intestinal disorder. Since intensive animal husbandry practices raise the risk of coccidiosis, it is an issue with confined animals.

Although 16 *Eimeria* species in goats and 15 species in sheep have been described separately up to this point, the majority of them may not cause severe clinical manifestations or have the same level of pathogenicity (Table 45.1). In actuality, just a few species were responsible for disease epidemics. Coccidia are highly host specific, meaning that species of coccidia that affect sheep do not affect goats.

45.1.1 Historical Background

The microscopic size of coccidians and difficulties encountered when interpreting the different stages of their development explain the complexity of the history. Antony van Leewenhock, in 1674, was the first to observe oocysts of protozoan parasites in the bile of rabbits. The name "coccidium" appeared for the first time in 1879 in the writings of Leuckart. Its life cycle, with alternating sexual and asexual phases, was later clarified due to the hard work of researchers like Balbiani, Eimer, and Kauffman. Its classification in the twentieth century was complicated by the worldwide distribution of Apicomplexa and the diversity of its species (Clark and Colwell 1974).

Elements of Reproduction and Reproductive Diseases of Goats, First Edition. Edited by Tanmoy Rana.

Table 45.1 Valid *Eimeria* species in goats.

Pathogenicity	*Eimeria* species	References
High	*E. ninakohlyakimovae*	Jolley and Bardsley (2006)
	E. caprina	
Moderate	–	
Low	*E. alijevi*	
	E. arloingi	
	E. aspheronica	
Other species	*E. caprovina*	
	E. hirci	
	E. jolchijevi	
	E. christenseni	
	E. kocharli	

45.1.2 Economic Importance

In intensive breeding conditions, coccidiosis can become an infection of great economic importance. On the other hand, subclinical coccidiosis is probably not of major importance in comparison with other infections. Fitzgerald (1980) estimated global annual losses of up to US$723 million. He calculated that losses to sheep and goats worldwide could reach $140 million. Animal mortality, the expense of treating specific animal groups (for example, with feed additives), the symptomatic treatment of animals with diarrhea, the affected animals' increased susceptibility to secondary diseases, and decreased animal productivity all create losses. In addition to the acute impacts, long-term impacts in terms of reduced feed conversion ratio, a lower final body weight gain, and a lower lifetime reproduction potential have been proposed (Lassen and Ostergaard 2012); however, long-term research is mostly lacking for ruminants. Because more animals are affected and the long-term impacts of decreased intestinal integrity are significant, it is expected, interestingly, that subclinical coccidiosis may result in larger output losses than clinical coccidiosis.

45.2 Classification

Eimeria has been classified as follows.

- Kingdom: Protista
- Phylum: Apicomplexa
- Class: Sporozoa
- Order: Eucoccidiorida
- Suborder: Eimeriorina
- Family: Eimeriidae
- Genus: *Eimeria*

45.3 Epidemiology and Immunology

Coccidiosis should always be regarded as a herd disease rather than a problem in individual animals. Once *Eimeria* species are present in a herd, they spread widely within a few life cycles of the parasite. Older animals develop partial immunity to the infection so they excrete only a small number of oocysts on reinfection. Younger animals are naive up to their first infection, leading to a considerable multiplication of the parasite and excretion of high numbers of oocysts, further contaminating the environment for the next naive animals. During primary infections, ruminants can shed more than a million oocysts per gram of feces (Bangoura and Daugschies 2007).

It is widely assumed that adult animals play a minor role in the epidemiology of the disease, and the major problem on commercial farms is transmission within the young animal population (Daugschies and Najdrowski 2005).

However, kids can acquire a primary infection from their mothers (Carrau et al. 2018). Transmission is most efficient on farms with high stocking densities and a concentration of young animals. It occurs by the feco–oral route within a group, and can also be introduced into a susceptible herd by contaminated boots, tools, tires, or feed. Most clinical cases of coccidiosis are observed in animals younger than 12 months of age. Although all farms may be affected by coccidial infections, operations such as feedlots and other intensive production settings are at highest risk of coccidiosis owing to the facilitated transmission.

Eimeria oocysts have a high survival potential in the environment. They can remain viable and infectious for at least one year and withstand many adverse environmental influences because of their thick wall. Few chemical and physical stressors are capable of inactivating *Eimeria* oocysts. They are resistant to freezing, extreme pH changes, and low oxygen availability. However, direct exposure to ultraviolet light over several hours and extreme dryness are detrimental to oocysts. Therefore, good environmental hygiene and exposure of the premises to direct sunlight can be of great benefit in minimizing problems with coccidiosis. By contrast, covered areas that are wet and contaminated by feces provide optimal conditions for transmission. High temperatures (about 39 °C) over longer time periods can prevent oocyst sporulation. In natural conditions where oocysts are commonly covered in feces and the nights are much cooler than 39 °C, this leaves many environmental oocysts unaffected for long enough to infect another host animal.

The global prevalence of coccidia is high; infections are common in all ruminants and most infections involve multiple species. A study from England indicated a prevalence of 98% in goats, with pathogenic species being most common in the examined goat kids (Norton 1986). Numerous authors have reported heavy excretion of oocysts by kids aged between two and four months (tens of thousands of oocysts per gram of feces, OPG), that is to say, a short time after weaning, and a rapid decrease of the excretion of oocysts (to some thousands) with age (Agyei et al. 2004; Chartier 1991; Faizal and Rajapakse 2001; Jalila et al. 1998; Koudela and Bokova 1998; Ruiz et al. 2006; Yvore et al. 1981). Certain authors have interpreted a minor increase in the excretion of oocysts in older goats (over seven years) as a relative weakness of the immune system. Similarly, Ruiz et al. (2006) found greater oocyst counts in adult goats on the island of Gran Canaria during the hot season. An attempt to immunize kids with a heterologous infection of sheep origin (*E. ovinoidalis*) was unsuccessful (Chartier et al. 1994).

Although *Eimeria* species are highly host specific and not transmissible between different livestock species, they may be transmitted between defined wildlife and domestic animals, each serving as a potential reservoir to infect the other. Immunity occurs after primary infection. The immunity is strictly *Eimeria* species specific as infections with one *Eimeria* species do not crossprotect against later infections with another species. This implies that goats can be prone to coccidiosis several times in their life, mostly as young animals.

The acquired immunity is largely based on a T helper cell 1 (Th1) cellular immune response. A detectable humoral response with formation of specific antibodies also occurs but contributes little to immunoprotection (Rose and Wakelin 1990). The immunity is partial; it is protective against clinical coccidiosis but does not completely suppress parasite replication on reinfection. Thus animals may be reinfected and shed oocysts transiently throughout their life, although excreted parasite numbers are much lower because the immune system controls the parasite infection to a major extent.

45.4 Life Cycle and Mode of Transmission

The life cycle of coccidiosis in goats is shown in Figure 45.1. The feco–oral pathway is the mode of coccidiosis transmission from animal to animal. The oocysts are transported via feces that contaminate feed, water, or soil (Figure 45.2). Both symptomatic and subclinical versions of the disease exist.

Clinical coccidiosis is a highly lethal condition that is mostly influenced by the species of *Eimeria*, the age of the infected animal, the quantity of oocysts consumed, the presence of other illnesses, and management techniques. The risk of sickness is also significantly influenced by overcrowding and poor sanitation. Sporulated oocyst consumption marks the beginning of the life cycle. Unsporulated oocysts are excreted in the feces of infected goats. The oocyst is not infectious when it is first passed; it has to go through sporulation. Moisture, oxygen, and heat are necessary for sporulation which typically occurs outside the host in the environment. Oocysts have a thick wall, which accounts for their high level of environmental resistance and resistance to common disinfectants. The only environmental conditions that can destroy the sporulated oocysts are extreme desiccation or direct sunshine. A sporulated oocyst can actually live for a year or longer if it is protected from the sun.

Goats are infected by the ingestion of a sporulated oocyst. Following ingestion, under the influence of bile, trypsin, and carbon dioxide, the outer wall of the oocyst excysts. Once swallowed, a single oocyst releases eight sporozoites that move through the intestines. Invading sporozoites cause schizogony by penetrating the lacteals or tiny intestine villi lining cells.

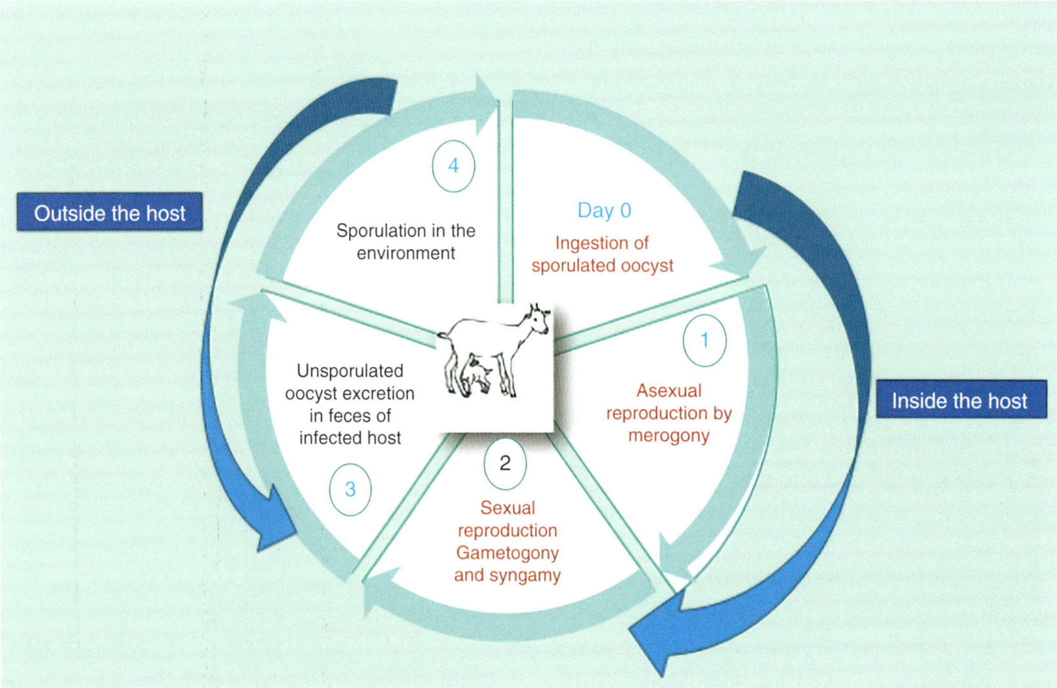

Figure 45.1 Life cycle of goat coccidiosis. *Source:* Courtesy of Bhupamani Das.

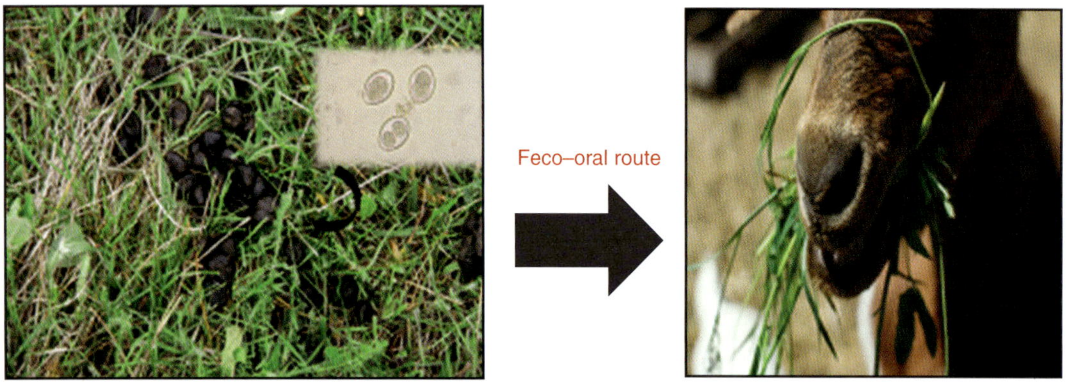
Feco–oral route
Grass contaminated with sporulated oocysts of *Eimeria* spp.
Goat takes up the infection while feeding

Figure 45.2 Transmission pattern of coccidian occysts in goats. *Source:* Courtesy of Bhupamani Das (chapter contributor).

They finish their life cycle in around 14 days. Along with causing the parasites to multiply inside epithelial cells, this condition also impairs food absorption, damages the mucosa's integrity, and worsens productive parameters. The risk of developing secondary infections, which are diseases caused by pathogens which take advantage of the tissue weakening, is considerably increased by this loss of integrity.

Schizogony is used by each trophozoite to create 100 or more first-generation sporozoites from a first-generation schizont. In the epithelial cells of the gut wall, first-generation merozoites spread out and enter other parts of the intestine. Both second-generation schizonts and second-generation merozoites are then produced. The merozoites can multiply up to a million-fold in just 10–14 days. The intestine's walls are covered in merozoites by this point in the infection, particularly second-generation merozoites. Some of the merozoites from the second generation start the schizogony of the third generation. All of the third-generation merozoites and the remaining second-generation merozoites will develop into gametocytes that are specific for each sex and release micro- (male) and macro- (female) gamonts as they mature. The macrogamete is fertilized by hundreds of released microgametes.

With the development of the oocyst wall, the resulting zygote matures into an oocyst. The oocysts escape their cells, enter the intestinal lumen, and then expel themselves with feces. The cycle restarts when oocysts are shed in the feces. Intestinal cells are thus invaded and then destroyed at each stage, resulting in repeated harm to the intestine. The gut lining becomes inflamed as a result of intestinal injury. Epithelial cells and intestinal mucosal capillaries are destroyed as a result of the growth of nonsexual stages, particularly second-generation merozoites, which also cause anemia and hypoproteinemia. The animal loses blood, water, and protein and is less effective in absorbing nutrients. It becomes very unwell and could even die if enough harm is done (Bangoura and Bardsley 2020).

45.5 Pathogenesis

Young stock – either nursing or weaned kids, 1–6 months of age – are at greatest risk for coccidiosis (Figure 45.3). The most common clinical signs are diarrhea and poor growth rate. Coccidiosis is often seen along with other concurrent diseases, most often pneumonia and soremouth (orf) as a herd/flock problem. Fighting more than one disease causes stress to the kids and is often fatal. Other stresses include overcrowding, intensive grazing situations or weather stresses (cold, heat, high humidity), weaning, transportation, and malnourishment.

In the pathogenesis of intestinal lesions during infections with pathogenic *Eimeria* species, two major elements are involved. On the one hand, the parasite causes direct damage arising from mucosal host cell destruction during its multiplication. On the other hand, the immune system contributes to the local damage and dysfunction by a severe inflammatory response with attraction of immune cell populations (Khodakaram-Tafti and Hashemnia 2017). In other words, pathological changes frequently last longer than the duration of the patent period and observable parasite excretion (Gregory 1990).

Prolonged tissue repair is evident after parasitic development is complete and before normal intestine function is substantially recovered. The direct harm caused by parasite multiplication and infection is typically at its peak in late schizogony and even more so in gamogony. This is caused by the parasite's fast rate of multiplication during its first schizogony, which causes infection of an exponentially growing number of intestinal cells during subsequent multiplication rounds (Friend and Stockdale 1980). Therefore, the majority of the harm occurs in infected animals just before oocyst excretion begins.

Why some *Eimeria* species cause major harm, inflammation, and clinical disease while others are significantly less pathogenic or even lack detectable pathogenicity is still not fully understood. Furthermore, it is believed that species-specific virulence factors contribute to the pathogenesis of coccidiosis; however, compared to chickens, ruminants have not yet been the subject of a great deal of research in this area. Proteins like cathepsins and rhoptry proteins, which are involved in host cell invasion, remodeling, and metabolic regulation, are possible virulence factors. Although little is known about this issue, their existence, structure, and function might be crucial for the harm produced, similar to other coccidian genera (Weilhammer and Rasley 2011).

Depending on the *Eimeria* species, the developmental phases' specific intestinal locations and the degree of damage vary (Table 45.2). Hemorrhagic enteritis is a hallmark of early infections with *E. ninakohlyakimovae* or *E. caprina* in young goats (Taylor and Catchpole 1994). Polyps in the small intestine are sometimes caused by *E. arloingi* infections (Gregory and Norton 1986), while white nodules in the mucosa that are visible from the serosal surface are often caused

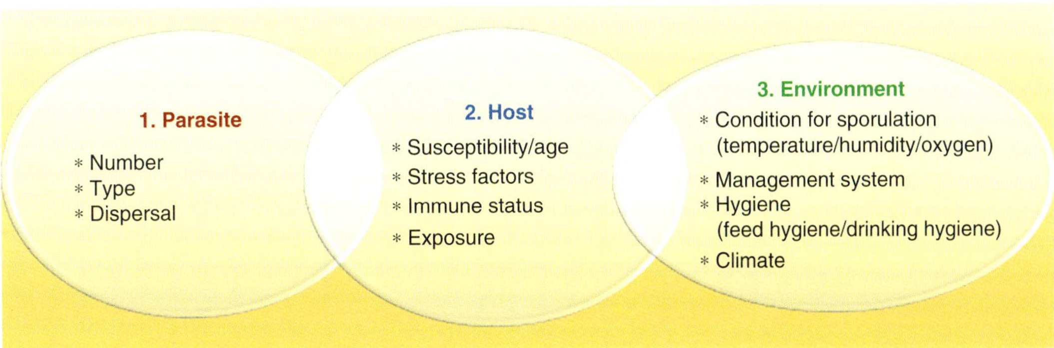

Figure 45.3 Contributory factors in the development of coccidiosis. *Source:* Courtesy of Bhupamani Das (chapter contributor).

Table 45.2 Merogony, gametogony, prepatent and patent period of different species of goat coccidia.

Species	Meronts	Gamonts	Prepatent period	Patent period	Reference
E. ninakohlyakimovae	Ileum, cecum, proximal colon	Ileum, cecum, proximal colon	10–17	4–10	Bangoura and Bardsley (2020)
E. caprina	ND	Colon, cecum, rectum	21	7	
E. arloingi	Jejunum, mesenteric lymph node	Small intestine, proximal third of colon	21	ND	
E. christenseni	Small intestine	ND	21–24	ND	

ND, not described.
No data available for *E. aijevi*, *E. aspheronica*, *E. caprovina*, *E. hirci*, *E. jolchijevi*, and *E. kocharli*.

by *E. apsheronica* stages (Kanyari 1990). Coinfections with other intestinal pathogens have been shown to worsen the disease and the clinical result in cattle and sheep. Additionally, compared to infection with a single pathogen, illness brought on by coinfection with bovine parvovirus is substantially more severe. It has been demonstrated that *Nematodirus* (thread-necked strongyle) infections in sheep significantly worsen *Eimeria*-induced enteritis, and vice versa (Catchpole and Harris 1989).

45.6 Clinical Signs

Whether an *Eimeria* infection develops into subclinical or clinical coccidiosis may depend on factors such as infection pressure, the species involved, management system, hygiene status, and nutrition of both kid and adult goat.

Acute signs of coccidiosis include different degrees of yellow to dark watery diarrhea (± blood and/or intestinal tissue), pale mucous membranes, abdominal pain, anorexia, emaciation, and dehydration (Figure 45.4). Loss of fluid and nutrients usually leads to reduced body condition score and weight loss (Bangoura and Bardsley 2020). Recovery time is largely dependent on the severity of the intestinal damage, and epithelialization of lost crypt epithelium will particularly affect the recovery time. Acute coccidiosis in goats may cause increased hematocrit (HCT) due to diarrhea and fluid loss, and decreased levels of electrolytes, such as sodium, chloride, and potassium. Loss of electrolytes is commonly seen in animals with malabsorptive diarrhea. The loss of body weight associated with coccidiosis is mainly due to loss of nutrients as a result of parasite-induced mucosal lesions and, to a lesser degree, to alterations of intestinal digestion and absorption of nutrients.

(a) (b)

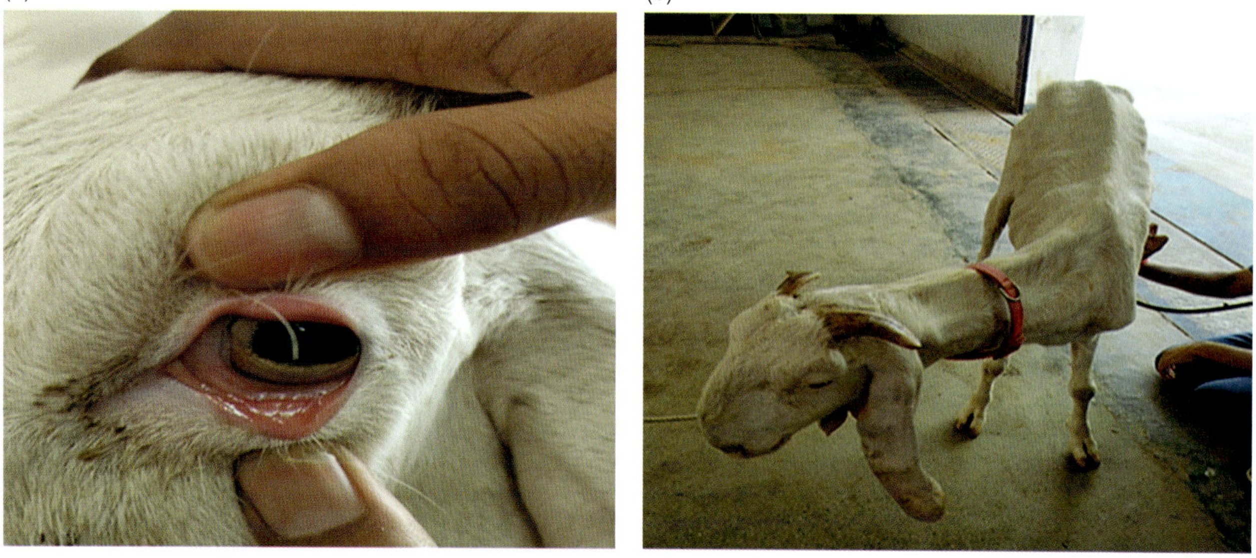

Figure 45.4 (a) Pale congested mucous membrane. (b) Poor body weight in a goat affected with coccidiosis. *Source:* Courtesy of Bhupamani Das (chapter contributor).

Subclinical coccidiosis may also lead to reduced growth, uneven kid size, and higher food conversion ratio. Symptoms vary from loss of pellet formation to weight loss, anorexia and diarrhea (with or without blood), lowered feed intake, poor absorption of nutrients, and dehydration. Treatment of subclinically infected kids has been shown to increase the average growth rate and improve feed conversion rates, compared with untreated controls.

Numerous investigations in small ruminants have demonstrated the impact of anticoccidial therapies on animal growth during and after weaning (Foreyt 1990). In French settings, for example, prophylactic diclazuril injection in weaned animals cut the mean fattening period by 5–8 days and enhanced the feed conversion rate by 7–16% (Alzieu et al. 1999). Furthermore, the level of oocyst excretion at three months old is inversely connected to growth in kids until the age of six months (Chartier et al. 1992). Similarly, mean or maximum oocyst counts and body weight in animals have an inverse association (Reeg et al. 2005).

45.7 Postmortem Lesions

Goats with severe illness, dehydration, emaciation, and poor physical condition often die. On postmortem, the intestinal mucosa thickens and petechiates, yet mucosal scrapings show masses of gamonts and oocysts. Giant meronts, which appear as little white spots in the small intestine mucosa, are rarely harmful unless present in large numbers. Aside from second-generation schizonts, the gamonts are the most pathogenic stage. A dehydrated carcase, inflammation, hemorrhage, and thickness of the upper and lower large intestines with denuded mucosa are some of the gross appearances found during postmortem inspection. In the small intestine, *E. arlongi* results in the development of polyps (Figure 45.5) and mucosal hyperplasia. Inflammatory cells can be seen histologically in the lamina propria and submucosa, and villous epithelium has sloughed off. Abomasitis caused by *E. gilruthi* includes edema, hemorrhage, and elevated nodules of the abomasal mucosa. Histologically, the organisms are surrounded by a necrotic region in the nodules.

45.8 Diagnosis

Diagnosis is based on history, clinical signs (severe diarrhea in young animals), postmortem findings (inflammation, hyperemia, and thickening of cecum with masses of gamonts and oocysts in scrapings) supported by oocyst counts (Figure 45.6) and speciation to identify pathogenic species. In small ruminants, sudden mortality around the weaning period should also suggest coccidiosis. All the stress factors should be looked for. A poor growth rate in an appropriate epidemiological setting should suggest a diagnosis of subclinical coccidiosis (Figure 45.7).

Coproscopic investigations should be quantitative and allow the identification of the most harmful *Eimeria* species present in feces (McMaster's technique with NaCl or $MgSO_4$, for example, with an extra flotation cover glass) (Yvoré et al. 1987). The morphological

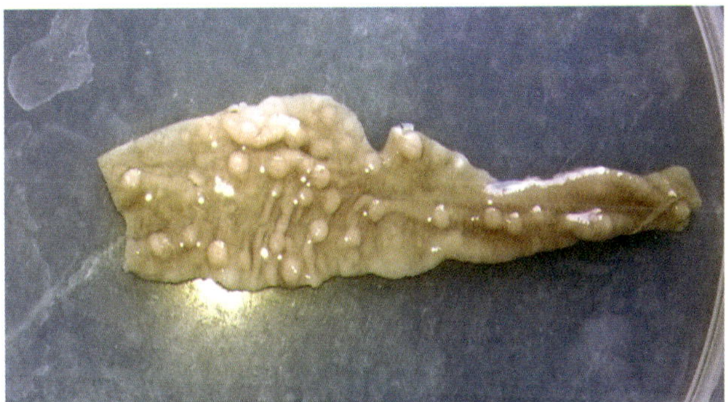

Figure 45.5 White nodules in intestinal mucosa in a goat affected with coccidiosis. *Source:* Courtesy of Bhupamani Das (chapter contributor).

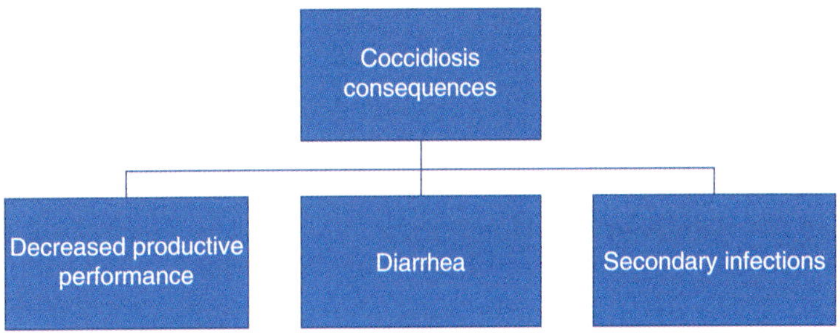

Figure 45.6 Consequences of coccidiosis. *Source:* Courtesy of Bhupamani Das (chapter contributor).

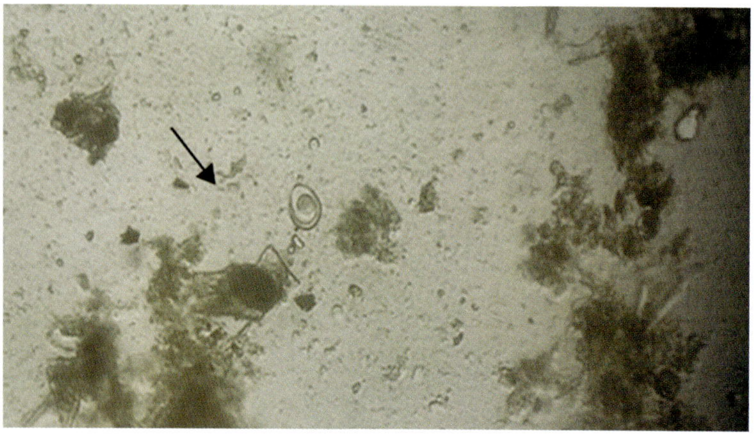

Figure 45.7 Unsporulated oocyst of *Eimeria* spp. in a goat. *Source:* Courtesy of Sivajyoti (chapter contributor).

characteristics of the oocysts can be used to identify *Eimeria* species, most typically after sporulation (fecal matter at room temperature for 2–3 days, or after dilution in 2% bichromate potassium and incubation at 25 °C). The size, form, and presence of distinctive components (polar cap, micropyle, color, aspect of the oocyst wall, oocystal and sporocystal residues, etc.) are used to diagnose the oocyst (Eckert et al. 1995). There are significant differences in excretion between individual animals and between *Eimeria* species. Furthermore, diarrhea may precede oocyst shedding at the individual level, and oocyst output may be significant without any clinical symptoms (Wright and Coop 2007). A total of 7–10 individual samples are required to accurately estimate the average excretion of a group of animals. Otherwise, a collection of fresh fecal matter on the ground (approximately 50 tiny samples combined into one homogeneous mass from which five analyses can be performed) allows the average level of excretion to be determined (Chartier 1991).

Despite the overall link between clinical coccidiosis and excessive oocyst excretion, determining a clear-cut threshold for coproscopical readings is problematic. The threshold value for clinical coccidiosis in small ruminants, according to Yvoré et al. (1987), might be about 50 000–100 000 OPG regardless of the *Eimeria* species involved. However, determining the percentages of harmful species for each host is critical information because some less pathogenic species can be excreted in relatively high numbers without generating any overt clinical consequence (Yvoré et al. 1985).

45.8.1 Molecular Methods

Diagnostic molecular methods such as PCR may be used for quantification as well as for speciation of *Eimeria* spp. By using species-specific primer sets, various species can be differentiated. Furthermore, DNA-based techniques can be used to characterize the genetic diversity of *Eimeria* spp., which is important in, for example, the development of recombinant vaccines. However, molecular methods also have major challenges, such as removal of the oocyst and sporocyst wall in order to obtain the nucleic acids. Some commercial DNA extraction kits may be used to extract DNA directly from feces, but the amount of DNA in the sample may be relatively small and/or the fecal input so large that the method has less sensitivity than some established techniques such as McMaster. In addition, mixed infections may be difficult to detect, as amplification of DNA from the most abundant species may mask more minor species.

45.8.2 Serological Methods

Serological methods (ELISA and Western blot) have been developed for the detection of antibodies to several ruminant *Eimeria* spp. However, antibody titers may remain high even after clearance of the infection, and young animals fed colostrum have maternal antibodies that may interfere with the serological results. In addition, there might also be a problem with crossreaction between species. Such methods are therefore primarily useful for epidemiological and experimental studies, but not for routine diagnosis.

45.9 Differential Diagnosis

Coccidiosis should be differentiated from other diseases such as cryptosporidiosis, collibacillosis, enterotoxemia, salmonellosis, viral enteritis, and dietary diarrhea in cases of diarrhea and abdominal pain. In cases of abdominal pain without diarrhea, abomasal bloat and other intestinal accidents may be suspected. In peracute cases, death due to coccidiosis should be differentiated from enterotoxemia, bacterial septicemia, nematodiasis, and paramphistomosis for kids of 2–5 months old (Levine 1985; Radostits et al. 2007).

45.10 Treatment

Several methods of treatment are available and licensed in different EU countries. There are differences in the ways products are used. However, choosing a therapeutic agent depends on the stage of infestation, efficacy, ease of administration, and expense (Andrews 2013). All severely affected kids should be moved to a separate enclosure or a different pasture. Indoor kids should be given plenty of clean bedding on a regular basis, and feed and water troughs should be elevated to avoid contamination. Outside, any feeding and watering places should be located on well-drained terrain to avoid fecal contamination. The stocking density should be reduced.

Most countries have few or no licensed therapies for goats, although products licensed for cattle and sheep are frequently used. Because water and feed intake is frequently reduced in sick kids, it is recommended to treat by drenching rather than placing any medicine in the drinking water or feed. To feed sick kids, electrolyte and nutritional solutions may be required. Toltrazuril (20 mg/kg, PO, once) and diclazuril (1 mg/kg, PO, once) have been used satisfactorily but doses may need to be repeated. When ponazuril (10 mg/kg, PO, once), a derivative of diclazuril, was administered experimentally in goat offspring, it lowered oocyst numbers. It is not currently licensed in goats, although it is advised for equine protozoal myeloencephalitis. Decoquinate (1 mg/kg, PO, every 24 hours for 28 days) can be used as a therapy for sheep and is approved in several countries. Individual dosing may be required. Sulfadimethoxine (55 mg/kg, PO or in drinking water, for the first day, then 27.5 mg/kg for three days) can be useful in the early stages of acute infection, although it is an off-label use in the United States and certain other countries. Extra-label sulfadimidine (sulfamethazine) treatment for coccidia in goats is 100 mg/kg, PO, every 24 hours for seven days. Potentiated sulfonamides have been administered either intravenously or orally. The use of amprolium oral solution (50 mg/kg, PO, every 24 hours for five days) has been reported. It is not labeled for goats in the United States. It is believed that resistance has evolved where it is used on some goat farms. It may be necessary to supplement amprolium with thiamine (vitamin B_1).

The same broad principles should be followed in kids and goats under the "cascade" system. However, the veterinary surgeon prescribing must specify the withdrawal time, which must be at least equivalent to the required minimum withdrawal period. All parturition pens must be maintained clean and dry, with all bedding rapidly removed to prevent oocysts from sporulating. Water and feed troughs and bowls for all animals should be elevated and kept clean and clear of feces; the area around troughs should be as dry as possible. Separate rotational grazing pastures for young animals is recommended.

Despite appropriate management, preventive treatments in feed or by drench may be required. It is generally recommended that such preventive therapies be carried out roughly a week to 10 days before the onset of symptoms. The issue with this advice is anticipating this period, so if the infestation is minor or nonexistent, therapy will have little effect. Diclazuril and toltrazuril are administered orally for therapy. However, the rate of decoquinate inclusion in feed is cut in half (833 g of premix/tonne of feed for a recommended concentration of 50 mg/kg feed). If feed intake is limited (less than 500 g/50 kg bw), decoquinate levels should be increased to provide a goal intake of 0.5 mg/kg bw. Whatever is done, care should be taken to maintain clean and dry environments, good-quality feed, and moderate stocking densities.

45.10.1 Advantages and Disadvantages of Chemical Control

Coccidiosis disease in small ruminants is chemically controlled with treatments such as coccidiostats and coccidioicides, which reduce the parasite burdens of treated animals. They also indirectly reinforce natural defenses but this does not allow for the long-term elimination of coccidia from a herd because the disease persists due to continuous reinfection of treated animals and infection of healthy animals (Keeton and Navarre 2018).

Anticoccidial medications operate by preventing growth and reproduction of coccidian parasites. The benefits of utilizing this type of chemical control are speed and dosage, as demonstrated by the studies detailed below. Mundt et al. (2005) discovered that therapy with toltrazuril (15 mg/kg bw orally, delivered in a single dosage) suppressed coccidiosis in calves housed in varied settings in a trial conducted in Germany using cattle naturally infected with *E. bovis* and *E. zuernii*. In another study, Mundt et al. (2007) studied the efficacy of toltrazuril (15 mg/kg bw) and diclazuril (1 mg/kg bw) in a single oral dose and found that toltrazuril was more effective than diclazuril because the animals treated with toltrazuril had fewer excreted oocysts and also the duration of the excretion period was significantly reduced compared to the animals treated with diclazuril and the control group. The disadvantage of the previously described use of chemical products to control coccidiosis in ruminants is the resistance to these products that may develop (Stephan et al. 1997). Another very important factor is the residues of these chemical products that build up in the soil (Cruz et al. 2004) and the damage to beneficial organisms (beetles and mites) described with the use of antiparasitic drugs, mainly anthelmintics (Quintero-Elena et al. 2022).

In general, other recommendations to control coccidiosis infection are to carry out proper treatment and avoid mixing animals of different ages, thus controlling infection in affected animals. Feeding troughs and drinking troughs must be placed on a base to avoid contamination with feces. During grazing, kids should be prevented from ingesting dirty and stagnant water, and finally, overcrowding of animals in housing should be avoided.

45.10.2 Alternative Treatment Options

Because of the widespread and indiscriminate use of chemical treatments to prevent coccidiosis in small ruminants, environmentally friendly alternatives have been investigated. The use of these natural chemicals provides organic farmers with some choices for mitigating the consequences of coccidia. Conventional farmers may wish to investigate these natural options as well, because excessive use of conventional substances may result in resistance.

Among these possibilities are ethnoveterinary medicine, medicinal herbs such as *Artemisia annua* (secondary metabolites), and tannins derived from "Quebracho" against *Eimeria* spp. and gastrointestinal worms in small ruminants. Clinical indications of coccidiosis were reduced in animals fed the former plant, and body condition and weight were improved compared to animals not fed this plant (Acharya et al. 2020). Another type of sustainable alternative is the use of edible mushrooms (*Lentinula edodes* and *Ganoderma lucidum*), secondary metabolites such as fatty acids (linoleic acid), and antioxidants. An example is the secondary metabolite curcumin which is present in the medicinal plant *Curcuma longa*, tht could reduce the severity of an infection of the upper and middle part of the small intestine caused by *E. acervulina* and *E. maxima* pathogens (Quiroz-Castañeda and Dantán-González 2015). Essential oils are another possibility, notably in formulations or diets to reduce coccidiosis (Quiroz-Castañeda and Dantán-González 2015).

The herb *Sericea lespedeza* has been demonstrated to be useful in the treatment of barber pole worm and coccidia. *Sericea* pellets (similar to lucerne pellets) can be a helpful strategy in this instance. One distinction between utilizing sericea to treat cocci and barber pole worm is that *Sericea*'s effects last longer for managing coccidiosis, whereas the barber pole worm "recovers" once the host animal no longer has access to the *Sericea*. To maximize the favorable effects and minimize the negative long-term effects, such as a potential mineral shortage, *Sericea lespedeza* should be fed from two weeks before weaning to four weeks after weaning (Coffey 2014). Using pine bark alongside *Sericea* appears to be significantly more effective.

In some cases, oregano oil may be beneficial in the treatment of coccidiosis. Oregano oil functions in the same way as ionophores such as monensin (Schivera 2009).

45.11 Prevention

Coccidiosis prevention is significantly less expensive than treatment, as is the case with other illnesses. This is because the majority of the harm has been done by the time clinical symptoms start to show (Figure 45.8).

45.11.1 Good Hygiene

Good husbandry practices, particularly sanitation, are the first line of defense. It is crucial that livestock are maintained in hygienic circumstances since coccidiosis is spread through manure. Industry recommendations should be followed when stocking pens. Pens must be dried off and kept clean. It is important to keep feces out of feeders and to use designs that reduce fecal contamination. A good technique to reduce fecal contamination is with fence line feeders.

45.11.2 Good Nutrition

All animals need a healthy diet to sustain high levels of immunity. Colostrum must be consumed in sufficient quantities by goat kids to strengthen the immune system. All animals should always be fed balanced rations with the correct proportions of energy, protein, vitamins, and minerals. Rotating pasture will reduce exposure to infectious oocysts in broad production systems.

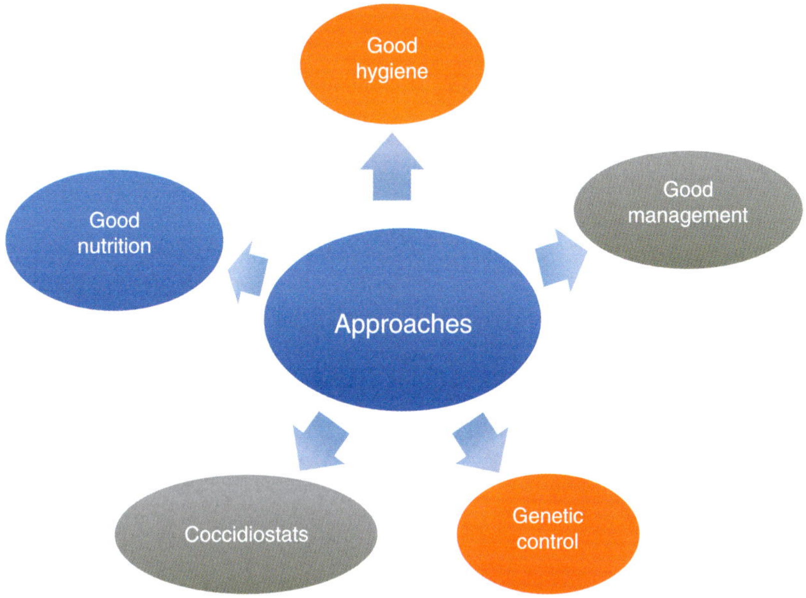

Figure 45.8 An integrated approach to the management of coccidiosis. *Source:* Courtesy of Bhupamani Das.

45.11.3 Management Practices

Kidding should always occur on pastures that are clean and have good drainage. Avoid grazing close to ponds and in low-lying areas. It could be beneficial to shift feeders and water troughs because animals frequently urinate close to them. Low stocking levels will significantly reduce the likelihood of coccidiosis on pasture. Coccidiosis outbreaks are frequently linked to the stress of shipping and transportation. Animals that have just been weaned ought not to be shipped. Kids/goats should be handled gently when being loaded. They should not be packed too tightly in trucks and trailers. Animals should not be handled or transported in the hottest part of the day.

45.11.4 Genetic Control

Specific data suggest that specific breeds and individuals are more resistant to coccidia infections and that heritabilities are similar to nematode (worm) resistance. Genetic selection of animals better able to resist *Eimeria* infections could be an alternative method of control. This may save considerable cost and limit the use of drugs in goat production systems.

45.11.5 Using Coccidiostats

There is no vaccine for coccidiosis in goats but it can be prevented by adding coccidiostats to feed, minerals, water, and milk replacer. Two coccidiostats have been approved for use in goats. The ionophore antibiotic lasalocid (Bovatec®) can be given to sheep kept in enclosures. The coccidiostat decoquinate (Deccox®) can also be used.

45.12 Conclusion

Although coccidiosis is a widely known and diagnosed disease, our understanding of many of its fundamental components is lacking. Therefore, even if management may be partially to blame for the apparent increase in the incidence of clinical symptoms, it cannot account for the entire rise. Additionally, when in-depth analyses are done, it is frequently found that the farm has issues in addition to coccidiosis. More research is needed to fully comprehend how coccidial infections interact with other disorders. Given how pervasive coccidial infestations are in goats, it appears that practically all recent research has been concentrated on the creation of novel therapies, leaving the underlying issues unresolved.

References

Acharya, M., Burke, J.M., Miller, J.E. et al. (2020). Quebracho tannins aid in the control of *Eimeria* spp. and gastrointestinal nematodes in lambs and goat kids. *Veterinary Parasitology* 288: 109295.

Agyei, A.D., Odonkor, M., and Osei-Somuah, A. (2004). Concurrence of Eimeria and helminth parasitic infections in West African Dwarf kids in Ghana. *Small Ruminant Research* 51: 29–35.

Alzieu, J.P., Mage, C., Maes, L., and De Muelenaere, C. (1999). Economic benefits of prophylaxis with diclazuril against subclinical coccidiosis in lambs reared indoors. *Veterinary Record* 144: 442–444.

Andrews, A.H. (2013). Some aspects of coccidiosis in sheep and goats. *Small Ruminant Research* 110 (2–3): 93–95.

Bangoura, B. and Bardsley, K.D. (2020). Ruminant coccidiosis. *Veterinary Clinics of North America: Food Animal Practice* 36 (1): 187–203.

Bangoura, B. and Daugschies, A. (2007). Parasitological and clinical parameters of experimental *Eimeria zuernii* infection in calves and influence on weight gain and haemogram. *Parasitology Research* 100 (6): 1331.

Carrau, T., Silva, L.M.R., Pérez, D. et al. (2018). Associated risk factors influencing ovine Eimeria infections in southern Spain. *Veterinary Parasitology* 263: 54–58.

Catchpole, J. and Harris, T.J. (1989). Interaction between coccidia and *Nematodirus battus* in lambs on pasture. *Veterinary Record* 124 (23): 603–605.

Chartier, C. (1991). Assessment of mean oocyst count in groups of kids: litter, individual randomized and non-randomized faecal samplings. *Veterinary Parasitology* 40: 187–195.

Chartier, C., Pellet, M.P., and Pors, I. (1992). Effects of toltrazuril on oocyst discharge and growth in kids with naturally-acquired coccidial infections. *Small Ruminant Research* 8: 171–177.

Chartier, C., Yvoré, P., Pors, I., and Mancassola, R. (1994). Absence of protection against *Eimeria ninakohlyakimovae* after primo-infection with *E ovinoidalis* in new-born kids. *Veterinary Research* 25: 66–70.

Clark, G.W. and Colwell, D.A. (1974). *Eimeria dalli* sp. n. (protozoa: Eimeridae) from Dall sheep *Ovis dalli*. *Journal of Protozoology* 21: 197–199.

Cruz, A.B., Barra, J.E., del Castillo, R.F., and Gutiérrez, C. (2004). La calidad del suelo y sus indicadores. *Ecosistemas: Revista Cietifica y Tecnica de Ecologia y Medio Ambiente* 13 (2).

Daugschies, A. and Najdrowski, M. (2005). Eimeriosis in cattle: current understanding. *Journal of Veterinary Medicine Series B* 52 (10): 417–427.

Eckert, J., Braun, R., Shirley, M.W., and Coudert, P. (1995). *Guidelines on Techniques in Coccidiosis Research*, 103–117. Brussels: European Commission.

Faizal, A.C.M. and Rajapakse, R.P.V.J. (2001). Prevalence of coccidia and gastrointestinal nematode infections in cross bred goats in the dry areas of Sri Lanka. *Small Ruminant Research* 40: 233–238.

Fitzgerald, P.R. (1980). The economic impact of coccidiosis in domestic animals [USA]. *Advances in Veterinary Science and Comparative Medicine* 24: 121–143.

Foreyt, W.J. (1990). Coccidiosis and cryptosporidiosis in sheep and goats. *Veterinary Clinics of North America: Food Animal Practice* 6 (3): 655–670.

Friend, S.C. and Stockdale, P.H. (1980). Experimental *Eimeria bovis* infection in calves: a histopathological study. *Canadian Journal of Companion Medicine* 44 (2): 129–140.

Gregory, M.W. (1990). Pathology of coccidial infections. In: *Coccidiosis of Man and Domestic Animals* (ed. P.L. Long), 240. Boca Raton, FL: CRC Press.

Gregory, M.W. and Norton, C.C. (1986). Caprine coccidiosis. *Goat Veterinary Journal* 7: 32–34.

Grzybek, M., Kukula-Koch, W., Strachecka, A. et al. (2016). Evaluation of anthelmintic activity and composition of pumpkin (*Cucurbita pepo* L.) seed extracts – in vitro and in vivo studies. *International Journal of Molecular Sciences* 17 (9): 1–21.

Hermosilla, C., Silva, L.M., Taubert, A. et al. (2016). Fatal Eimeria Gilruthi-induced abomasal coccidiosis. *Journal of Veterinary Medical Research* 3: 1–5.

Jalila, A., Dorny, P., Sani, R. et al. (1998). Coccidial infections of goats in Selangor, peninsular Malaysia. *Veterinary Parasitology* 74: 165–172.

Jolley, W.R. and Bardsley, K.D. (2006). Ruminant coccidiosis. *Veterinary Clinics of North America. Food Animal Practice* 22 (3): 613–621.

Kanyari, P.W. (1990). *Eimeria apsheronica* in the goat: endogenous development and host cellular response. *International Journal of Parasitology* 20 (5): 625–630.

Keeton, S.T.N. and Navarre, C.B. (2018). Coccidiosis in large and small ruminants. *Veterinary Clinics of North America: Food Animal Practice* 34 (1): 201–208.

Khodakaram-Tafti, A. and Hashemnia, M. (2017). An overview of intestinal coccidiosis in sheep and goats. *Revue de Médecine Vétérinaire* 168: 9–20.

Khor, S.K., Isa, J.M.A.T., Mazukhi, Z. et al. (2018). A survey of gastrointestinal parasitic infection on small ruminant farms in Seberang Perai Selatan district, Penang, Malaysia. *Malaysian Journal of Veterinary Research* 9: 15–21.

Koudela, B. and Bokova, A. (1998). Coccidiosis in goats in the Czech Republic. *Veterinary Parasitology* 76: 261–267.

Lassen, B. and Ostergaard, S. (2012). Estimation of the economical effects of Eimeria infections in Estonian dairy herds using a stochastic model. *Preventive Veterinary Medicine* 106 (3–4): 258–265.

Levine, N.D. (1985). *Veterinary Protozoology*, 1e, 131–221. Ames, IA: Iowa State University.

Coffey, L. (2014). Coccidiosis: symptoms, prevention, and treatment in sheep, goats, and calves. https://attra.ncat.org/publication/coccidiosis-symptoms-prevention-and-treatment-in-sheep-goats-and-calves/#:~:text=Coccidia%20are%20protozoa%20that%20cause,healthier%20animals%20that%20grow%20faster (accessed 7 October 2023).

Majeed, N.M., A'aiz, N.N., and Niemah, A.J. (2020). Molecular study to detect the Eimeria species in sheep in Al-Diwaniyah province, Iraq. *Iraqi Journal of Veterinary Sciences* 34 (2): 377–381.

Mohammed, N.H., Alobaidii, W.A., and Hasan, M.H. (2021). Coccidiosis in sheep and goats (review). *Assiut Veterinary Medical Journal* 67 (171): 33–39.

Mundt, H.C., Bangoura, B., Mengel, H. et al. (2005). Control of clinical coccidiosis of calves due to *Eimeria bovis* and *Eimeria zuernii* with toltrazuril under field conditions. *Parasitology Research* 97: S134–S142.

Mundt, H.C., Rödder, F., Mengel, H. et al. (2007). Control of coccidiosis due to *Eimeria bovis* and *Eimeria zuernii* in calves with toltrazuril under field conditions in comparison with diclazuril and untreated controls. *Parasitology Research* 101: 93–104.

Namutosi, W., Higenyi, J., Kizito, E., and Omodo, M. (2019). Prevalence and risk factors of gastrointestinal parasite infection in goats in Sironko district, Eastern Uganda. *Uganda Journal of Agricultural Sciences* 19 (1): 1–14.

Norton, C.C. (1986). Coccidia of the domestic goat *Capra hircus*, with notes on *Eimeria ovinoidalis* and *E. bakuensis* (syn. *E. ovina*) from the sheep *Ovis aries*. *Parasitology* 92 (2): 279–289.

Pezzanite, L., Neary, M., Hutchens, T., and Scharko, P. (2022). Common diseases and health problems in sheep and goats. www.extension.purdue.edu/extmedia/as/as-595-commondiseases.pdf (accessed 2 January 2024).

Quintero-Elena, Z.J., Aguilar-Marcelino, L., Castañeda-Ramírez, G.S. et al. (2022). In vitro and micro-plot predatory activity of the mite *Caloglyphus mycophagus* against populations of nematode larvae of agricultural importance. *Biological Control* 165: 104813.

Quiroz-Castañeda, R.E. and Dantán-González, E. (2015). Control of avian coccidiosis: future and present natural alternatives. *BioMed Research International* 2015: 430610.

Radostits, O., Blood, C., Hinchclif, K., and Constable, P. (2007). *Veterinary Medicine: A Text Book of Disease of Cattle, Horse, Sheep, Pig and Goat*, 1498–1506. London: Saunders.

Reeg, K.J., Gauly, M., Bauer, C. et al. (2005). Coccidial infections in housed lambs: oocyst excretion, antibody levels and genetic influences on the infection. *Veterinary Parasitology* 127: 209–219.

Rose, M.E. and Wakelin, D. (1990). Immunity to coccidiosis. In: *Coccidiosis of Man and Domestic Animals* (ed. P.L. Long), 191. Boca Raton, FL: CRC Press.

Ruiz, A., González, J.F., Rodríguez, E. et al. (2006). Influence of climatic and management factors on Eimeria infections in goats from semi-arid zones. *Journal of Veterinary Medicine Series B: Infectious Diseases and Veterinary Public Health* 53: 399–402.

Schivera, D. (2009). Oregano Oil for Internal Parasite Control in Sheep, Goats, and Beef Cattle. Sustainable Agriculture Research and Education (SARE) final report. https://projects.sare.org/sare_project/one08-088/ (accessed 2 January 2024).

Stephan, B., Rommel, M., Daugschies, A., and Haberkorn, A. (1997). Studies of resistance to anticoccidials in Eimeria field isolates and pure Eimeria strains. *Veterinary Parasitology* 69 (1–2): 19–29.

Taylor, M.A. and Catchpole, J. (1994). Coccidiosis of domestic ruminants. *Applied Parasitology* 35 (2): 73–86.

Walker, E.L. and Hudson, M.D. (2014). Species of meat animals | sheep and goats. In: *Encyclopedia of Meat Sciences*, 2e (ed. M. Dikeman and C. Devine), 374–379. New York: Academic Press.

Weilhammer, D.R. and Rasley, A. (2011). Genetic approaches for understanding virulence in *Toxoplasma gondii*. *Briefings in Functional Genomics* 10 (6): 365–373.

Wright, S.E. and Coop, R.L. (2007). Cryptosporidiosis and coccidiosis. In: *Diseases of Sheep*, 4e (ed. I. Aitken), 179–185. Oxford, UK: Blackwell Publishing.

Yvore, P., Esnault, A., and Guillimin, P. (1981). Kid coccidiosis bred in goat-farms – importance of choosing the moment of treatment. *Revue de Médecine Vétérinaire* 132 (3): 205–208.

Yvoré, P., Esnault, A., and Naciri, M. (1985). La coccidiose caprine: effets de contaminations mono ou multispécifiques. *Revue de Médecine Vétérinaire* 161 (4): 347–351.

Yvoré, P., Esnault, A., Mage, C. et al. (1987). Intérêt et interprétation de la coproscopie dans la coccidiose des petits ruminants. *Le Point Vétérinaire: Revue D'enseignement Post-universite et de Formation Permanente* 19 (103): 43–48.

46

White Muscle Disease

Somu Yogeshpriya[1], *Amitava Roy*[2], *and Tanmoy Rana*[3]

[1] *Department of Veterinary Medicine, Veterinary College and Research Institute, Chennai, India*
[2] *Department of Livestock Farm Complex, West Bengal University of Animal & Fishery Sciences, Kolkata, India*
[3] *Department of Veterinary Clinical Complex, West Bengal University of Animal & Fishery Sciences, Kolkata, India*

46.1 Introduction

Nutritional myodegeneration, also known as white muscle disease, is a condition that can affect young ruminant animals such as lambs and kids (Steiss 1985). It results from a lack of vitamin E and/or selenium in the diet. The body's antioxidant defense system and healthy muscle function both depend on selenium, a vital trace element. Vitamin E is an additional antioxidant that aids in preventing oxidative harm to cell membranes (Abdelrahman and Kincaid 1992).

Both nutrient deficiencies have the potential to cause muscular deterioration, weakness, and ultimately death (Abutarbush and Radostits 2003). The illness is known as white muscle disease because the loss of pigmentation causes the affected muscles to look pale or white.

Including enough selenium and vitamin E in the food can help prevent white muscle disease. This can be done by giving the animals fortified feed, supplements, or injections, or by making sure they have access to grass or pasture that has enough of these nutrients (Abutarbush and Radostits 2003). Treatment for an animal with the illness may include vitamin E and selenium supplements, as well as supportive care to treat any muscle weakness or other symptoms (Bain et al. 1998). Infected foals frequently have markedly elevated muscle enzyme levels and low glutathione peroxidase activities. If selenium is given to foals with the subacute form of the disease early on, they may survive; however, mortality rates ranging from 30% to 45% have been recorded, even for this form of the illness (Lofstedt 1997).

46.2 Pathophysiology

A deficiency in the trace element selenium and/or vitamin E in the diet contributes to the pathophysiology of white muscle disease. Important antioxidants that help shield cells from oxidative harm include selenium and vitamin E.

Lambs that are lacking in these nutrients experience a breakdown in their body's antioxidant defense system, which raises the risk of free radicals causing oxidative harm to cells, including muscle cells (Bain et al. 1998). This oxidative harm causes muscle cell death and degeneration, giving the affected muscles their recognizable white or pale look.

Multiple muscle groups, including those necessary for breathing, standing, and walking, can be affected by the disease, which can cause respiratory distress, weakness, and mobility problems (Stewart et al. 2012). Animals with the condition may become seriously disabled and even die if it is not treated right away.

It is thought that both nutrients are crucial for normal muscle function and regeneration, despite the fact that the exact mechanisms that lead selenium and vitamin E deficiencies to cause white muscle disease are not yet fully understood. Selenium is required for the synthesis of selenoproteins, which function as antioxidants and support the integrity of muscle cell membranes (Stewart et al. 2012). On the other hand, the fat-soluble nutrient vitamin E has the ability to neutralise free radicals and protect cell membranes from oxidative damage.

Elements of Reproduction and Reproductive Diseases of Goats, First Edition. Edited by Tanmoy Rana.

One of the main processes by which white muscle disease in lambs develops is oxidative damage. Free radicals, also known as reactive oxygen species, damage cells and tissues when they are created in large quantities. This is referred to as oxidative damage (Abutarbush and Radostits 2003). Oxidative damage specifically impacts the muscle cells in the instance of white muscle disease. Important antioxidants that help shield cells from oxidative harm include selenium and vitamin E (Mass et al. 1984).

In addition to oxidative damage, other factors such as impaired immune function, inflammation, and energy metabolism may also play a role in the development of white muscle disease. However, the precise mechanisms by which these factors contribute to the disease are not yet fully understood (Semenenko et al. 2021).

46.3 Additional Factors Contributing White Muscle Disease

There are several additional factors and mechanisms that may contribute to the development of white muscle disease in lambs and kids.

46.3.1 Genetic Factors

Some breeds of sheep and goats may be more susceptible to selenium and vitamin E deficiency, and therefore more prone to developing white muscle disease (Koyuncu and Yerlikaya 2007; Abdelrahman and Kincaid 1992). However, the susceptibility of a particular breed can vary depending on several factors, including the genetic make-up of the animals, the nutritional status of the soil and forage, and management practices (Koyuncu and Yerlikaya 2007).

Breeds that have been reported to be more susceptible to white muscle disease include:

- Boer goats
- Suffolk sheep
- Hampshire sheep
- Southdown sheep.

However, it is important to note that susceptibility can vary within breeds, and that proper management and supplementation practices can help to prevent and treat the condition regardless of breed (Abutarbush and Radostits 2003).

46.3.2 Soil Composition

Depending on the environment and other variables, the selenium content of soil can differ significantly. Selenium deficiency in grazing animals can result from plants in selenium-poor soil having reduced selenium content.

By influencing the amount of selenium in the diet, soil composition can have an impact on the onset of white muscle disease in sheep (Mass et al. 1984). Lambs, like other animals, require trace quantities of the essential mineral selenium for healthy physiological performance.

While grazing creatures like lambs get their selenium from the plants they eat, plants get their selenium from the soil. As a result, the plants that lambs eat will be low in selenium in regions with low soil levels (Koyuncu and Yerlikaya 2007). This may eventually result in a selenium deficiency in the calves, which may aid in the growth of white muscle disease.

46.3.3 Interactions with Other Nutrients

Menzies et al. (2003) reported that the interactions between selenium and vitamin E and other nutrients in the diet, such as sulfur, copper, and iron, can affect their absorption and utilization. In addition, selenium absorption and utilization in the body can be affected by other minerals in the soil, such as copper and zinc. Selenium deficiency in sheep can be enhanced by nutrient deficiencies or imbalances in the soil (Menzies et al. 2003).

In order to avoid deficiencies and lower the risk of white muscle disease, it is crucial to check the soil composition in regions where lambs are raised and to supplement the diet of the animals with selenium and other nutrients as necessary (Semenenko et al. 2021).

46.3.4 Stress

Environmental stressors can raise the metabolic need for antioxidants and aggravate an existing selenium or vitamin E deficiency. These stressors include extreme temperatures, high altitudes, and high stocking densities (Stewart et al. 2012).

Environmental stressors can raise the metabolic demand for antioxidants like selenium and vitamin E, which are crucial for shielding cells from oxidative damage (Koyuncu and Yerlikaya 2007). Free radicals can harm cells and tissues, including muscle cells, through oxidative injury.

Stress can also impact the immune system and boost the creation of cytokines that promote inflammation (Yavuzer and Bengisu 2023). This can result in long-lasting inflammation, which can aggravate the harm from oxidative stress and aid in the emergence of white muscle disease.

Stress can also affect how well nutrients are absorbed and used by the body. For instance, the body may prioritize using nutrients for vital processes like immune system maintenance during times of stress, which can cause a lack of other nutrients like selenium and vitamin E.

In order to prevent and treat white muscle disease in lambs, stress reduction and appropriate nutrition are crucial. This can be achieved by using the right management techniques, such as giving the animals enough room, reducing environmental stressors, and making sure their diets are balanced and contain enough vital minerals (Semenenko et al. 2021).

46.3.5 Infectious Diseases

Some infectious illnesses, like coccidiosis, can prevent the body from absorbing and using selenium and/or vitamin E, which can result in a deficiency.

Lambs and other ruminants are susceptible to the parasitic disease coccidiosis, which affects the gastrointestinal system. Oocysts, which are shed in the feces of sick animals, are consumed and lead to the disease (Abdelrahman and Kincaid 1992). In addition to causing diarrhea, weight loss, and reduced feed intake, coccidiosis can also result in a nutrient deficiency, including a lack of selenium and vitamin E.

If the animal's diet already lacks these vitamins and minerals, the additional demand may make the situation worse and hasten the onset of white muscle disease. Additionally, coccidiosis can result in GI tract inflammation, which can raise levels of oxidative stress and proinflammatory cytokines (Semenenko et al. 2021). This may lead to a further rise in the metabolic need for antioxidants and a consequent nutritional deficit.

In addition, some drugs used to treat coccidiosis, such as sulfa medicines, can prevent the body from absorbing nutrients (Yavuzer and Bengisu 2023). This may worsen any deficiencies already present and raise the possibility of developing white muscle disease.

Therefore, preventing and managing coccidiosis is an important aspect of preventing white muscle disease in lambs (Rodriguez et al. 2018). This can be achieved through appropriate management practices such as keeping the environment clean and dry, minimizing stress, and providing proper nutrition (Koyuncu and Yerlikaya 2007).

46.3.6 Management Practices

Improper feeding, grazing, or supplementation practices can also contribute to a deficiency of selenium and/or vitamin E in kids.

46.4 Clinical Signs

The clinical signs of white muscle disease can vary depending on the severity of the deficiency and the muscles affected, but commonly include:

- muscle weakness or stiffness, which can result in a stiff gait or reluctance to move or get up, especially after periods of rest or inactivity
- difficulty breathing or rapid breathing due to respiratory muscle weakness
- rapid heart rate or weak pulse
- reduced appetite or weight loss
- muscle tremors or twitching, especially in the hind legs
- overall poor growth and development in young animals.

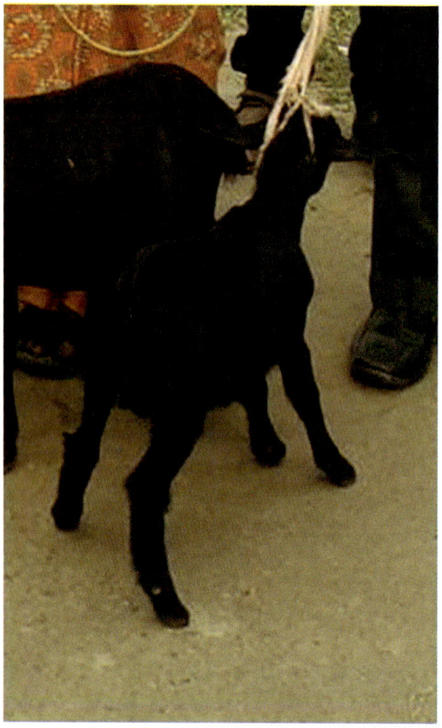

Figure 46.1 Difficulty in standing.

White muscle illness can cause kids to become recumbent, unable to stand or move (Figures 46.1 and 46.2), and they may eventually die from respiratory or cardiac failure.

Important antioxidants that defend cells from oxidative harm include selenium and vitamin E. A lack of these nutrients can lead to oxidative stress, which harms muscle cells and reduces their ability to operate (Rodriguez et al. 2018). The length and severity of the deficiency will determine the breadth and severity of the muscle damage.

The skeletal and cardiac muscles are most frequently affected in kids with white muscle disease. Cardiovascular muscles pump blood throughout the body, while skeletal muscles are in charge of mobility and posture (Stewart et al. 2012). Therefore, white muscle malfunction is reflected in these muscles' dysfunctional symptoms.

White muscle disease frequently manifests as muscle stiffness or weakness because the affected muscles may not be able to contract correctly (Figure 46.3). A stiff gait or reluctance to move may arise from this. The animal may also have difficulty standing or getting up, particularly after rest or inactivity (Semenenko et al. 2021). Respiratory distress or an accelerated pulse rate may result from a muscle disorder that also affects the breathing and heart muscles (Rodriguez et al. 2018). The energy requirements of muscle repair and recovery may lead to reduced appetite or weight reduction (Figure 46.4). Due to the aging of nerve and muscle tissue, there may be muscle tremors or twitching, particularly in the hind legs (Rodriguez et al. 2018).

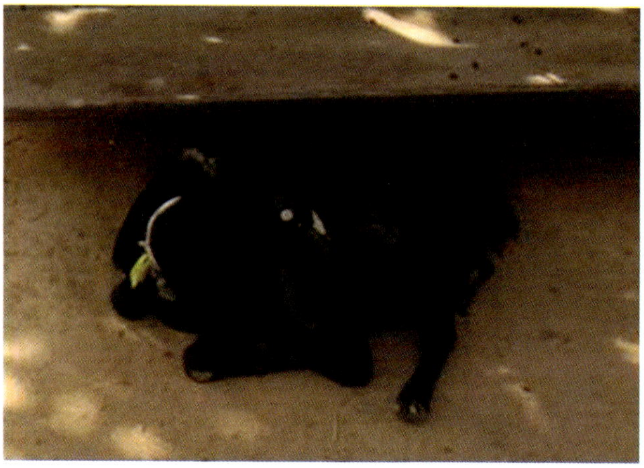

Figure 46.2 Reluctance to move or stand.

46.5 Diagnosis

Diagnosis of white muscle disease typically involves a combination of clinical evaluation, history, and diagnostic tests (Radostits et al. 2000).

46.5.1 History

Obtain a detailed history from the owner or caretaker of the animal. This includes information about the animal's age, breed, diet, management practices, and any recent changes in behavior, appetite, or exercise habits (Menzies et al. 2004). The veterinarian should also ask if there are any other animals in the herd or flock that are exhibiting similar signs.

46.5.2 Physical Examination

Conduct a thorough physical examination of the animal, including assessment of gait, muscle tone, and respiratory function. Look for signs of muscle weakness, stiffness, or tremors, as well as respiratory distress or abnormal heart sounds. Palpate the muscles and joints to check for pain, swelling, or inflammation (Semenenko et al. 2021).

46.5.3 Blood Tests

Perform blood tests to assess levels of selenium and vitamin E, as well as markers of muscle damage such as creatine kinase or lactate dehydrogenase (Yavuzer and Bengisu 2023). Elevated levels of these markers can indicate muscle damage and help confirm a diagnosis of white muscle disease.

46.5.4 Muscle Biopsy or Imaging

Consider muscle biopsy or imaging studies, such as ultrasound or radiography, to assess the extent of muscle damage and identify any underlying structural abnormalities or lesions (Menzies et al. 2004).

46.5.5 Genetic Testing

In certain breeds of sheep and goats, genetic testing may be recommended to identify mutations or polymorphisms that may affect the absorption or utilization of selenium and vitamin E (Yavuzer and Bengisu 2023).

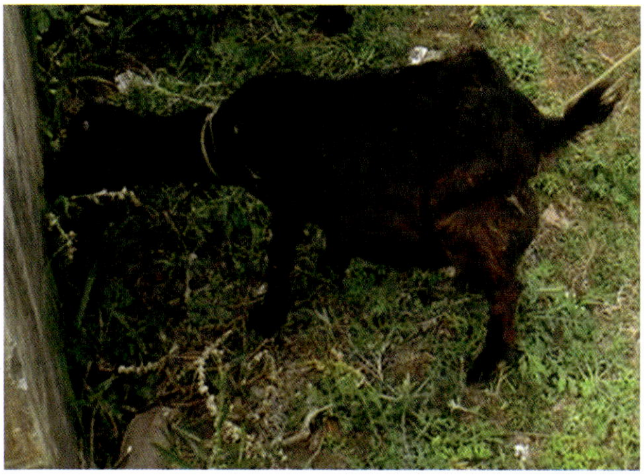

Figure 46.3 Muscle stiffness.

46.5.6 Response to Treatment

Monitor the animal's response to treatment, which typically involves supplementation with selenium and/or vitamin E (Abutarbush and Radostits 2003). Look for improvements in muscle tone, gait, and respiratory function, as well as changes in blood test results.

> The diagnostic approach to white muscle disease will depend on the clinical signs and history of the affected animal, as well as the availability of diagnostic testing and the expertise of the veterinarian. Early diagnosis is important in order to initiate appropriate treatment and prevent further muscle damage.

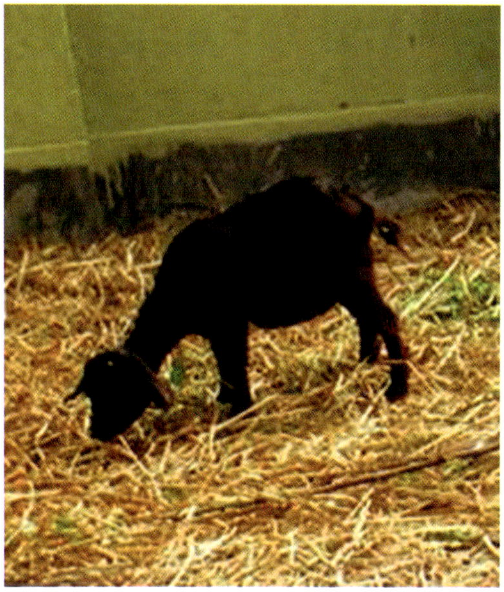

Figure 46.4 Poor growth in young animals.

46.6 Prevention

Prevention of white muscle disease involves ensuring adequate intake of selenium and vitamin E, which are essential nutrients for muscle function and protection against oxidative damage (Menzies et al. 2004). Strategies for preventing white muscle disease are discussed below.

46.6.1 Balanced Diet

Provide a balanced diet that contains adequate levels of selenium and vitamin E. This may involve supplementing with commercial feeds, mineral blocks, or injectable formulations (Figure 46.5).

46.6.2 Soil Testing

Test the soil in pastures or fields where animals graze to ensure that selenium levels are adequate. If soil levels are low, consider supplementing with selenium-enriched fertilizers or providing selenium-rich salt licks (Ochirov and Orobets 2012).

46.6.3 Water Testing

Test the water supply to ensure that it does not contain high levels of minerals or contaminants that may interfere with selenium absorption.

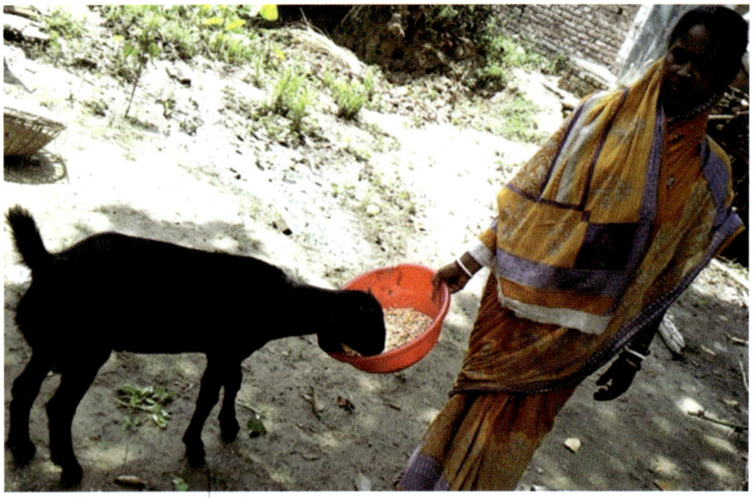

Figure 46.5 Feeding a balanced diet.

46.6.4 Genetic Selection

In breeds of sheep and goats that are known to be more susceptible to white muscle disease, select animals with better genetics for selenium and vitamin E metabolism (Tan et al. 2002).

46.6.5 Routine Monitoring

Monitor animals regularly for signs of muscle weakness, tremors, or respiratory distress (Ochirov and Orobets 2012). Early detection can help prevent further muscle damage and improve treatment outcomes.

46.6.6 Supplementation

Provide regular supplementation with selenium and/or vitamin E, especially during periods of high demand such as pregnancy, lactation, or growth (Figure 46.6). This may involve oral or injectable formulations, depending on the animal's needs (Yavuzer and Bengisu 2023).

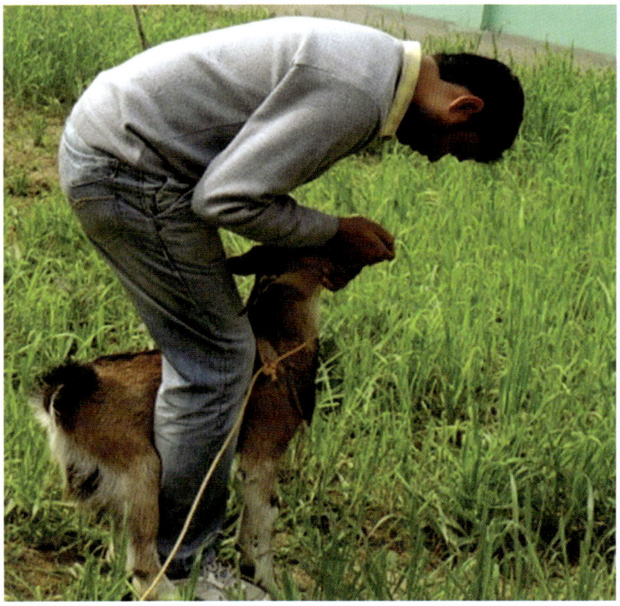

Figure 46.6 Supplementation of selenium and/or vitamin E.

> Prevention of white muscle disease requires a multifaceted approach that includes careful management of diet, genetics, and environmental factors. Regular monitoring and early intervention are key to maintaining optimal muscle health and preventing the development of white muscle disease.

46.7 Control

Control of white muscle disease involves several measures aimed at minimizing the risk of developing the condition and managing affected animals.

46.7.1 Supplementation

Provide regular supplementation with selenium and vitamin E to all animals in the herd or flock, especially during periods of high demand such as pregnancy, lactation, or growth. This may involve oral or injectable formulations, depending on the animal's needs (Ochirov and Orobets 2012).

46.7.2 Environmental Management

Test the soil and water supply regularly to ensure adequate levels of selenium and minimize exposure to contaminants or minerals that may interfere with selenium absorption (Ochirov and Orobets 2012). Manage pastures and fields to reduce exposure to stressors such as overcrowding, poor nutrition, or exposure to toxins.

46.7.3 Genetic Selection

Select animals with better genetics for selenium and vitamin E metabolism. In breeds that are more susceptible to white muscle disease, choose animals that have been screened for mutations or polymorphisms that affect selenium and vitamin E absorption and utilization (Menzies et al. 2004).

46.7.4 Early Detection

Monitor animals regularly for signs of muscle weakness, tremors, or respiratory distress. Early detection can help prevent further muscle damage and improve treatment outcomes.

46.7.5 Treatment

Provide appropriate treatment to animals that are diagnosed with white muscle disease (Bain et al. 1998). This typically involves supplementation with selenium and/or vitamin E, as well as supportive care such as fluid therapy or pain management.

46.7.6 Biosecurity Measures

Implement biosecurity measures such as quarantine, isolation, and disinfection to prevent the spread of infectious diseases that may contribute to the development of white muscle disease.

46.8 Conclusion

Control of white muscle disease requires a proactive and integrated approach that involves careful management of diet, genetics, environment, and animal health. Regular monitoring and early intervention are essential to maintain optimal muscle health and prevent the development of white muscle disease.

References

Abdelrahman, M.M. and Kincaid, R.L. (1992). Effects of concurrent deficiencies of phosphorus and copper in growing lambs on the concentration of minerals in tissues. *Small Ruminant Research* 9: 229–241.

Abutarbush, S.M. and Radostits, O.M. (2003). Congenital nutritional muscular dystrophy in a beef calf. *Canadian Veterinary Journal* 44 (9): 738–739.

Bain, M., Edwards, J., Suttle, N. et al. (1998). Seasonal fluctuations in serum tocopherol concentrations in bovine and ovine samples submitted to veterinary investigation centres. *Proceedings of Sheep Veterinary Society* 22: 63–67.

Koyuncu, M. and Yerlikaya, H. (2007). Effect of selenium-vitamin E injections of ewes on reproduction and growth of their lambs. *South African Journal of Animal Science* 37: 233–236.

Lofstedt, J. (1997). White muscle disease of foals. *Veterinary Clinics of North America. Equine Practice* 13: 169–185.

Mass, J., Bulgin, M.S., Anderson, B.C. et al. (1984). Nutritional myodegeneration associated with vitamin E deficiency and normal selenium status in lambs. *Journal of the American Veterinary Medical Association* 184: 201–204.

Menzies, P.I., Boermans, H., Hoff, B. et al. (2003). Survey of the status of copper, interacting minerals and vitamin E levels in the livers of Ontario sheep. *Canadian Veterinary Journal* 44: 898–906.

Menzies, P., Langs, L., Boermans, H. et al. (2004). Myopathy and hepatic lipidosis in weaned lambs due to vitamin E deficiency. *Canadian Veterinary Journal* 45 (3): 244–247.

Ochirov, D.S. and Orobets, V.A. (2012). Indicators of micronutrient status of sheep. *Bulletin of Veterinary Medicine* 4: 89–90.

Radostits, O.M., Gay, C.C., Blood, D.C., and Hinchcliff, K.C. (2000). *Veterinary Medicine*, 9e, 1515–1533. London: WB Saunders.

Rodriguez, A.M., Schild, C.O., Cantón, G.J. et al. (2018). White muscle disease in three selenium deficient beef and dairy calves in Argentina and Uruguay. *Ciência Rural* 48: 5.

Semenenko, M.P., Grin, V.A., Kuzminova, E.V. et al. (2021). Pharmacological therapy of white muscle disease in lambs with selenium preparations in a comparative aspect. *IOP Conference Series: Earth and Environmental Science* 677: 042020.

Steiss, J.E. (1985). Effect of disulfiram in experimentally induced vitamin E deficiency myopathy in lambs. *American Journal of Veterinary Research* 46: 2141–2144.

Stewart, W.C., Bobe, G., Vorachek, W.R. et al. (2012). Organic and inorganic selenium: II. Transfer efficiency from ewes to lambs. *Journal of Animal Science* 90: 577–584.

Tan, J., Zhu, W., Wang, W. et al. (2002). Selenium in soil and endemic diseases in China. *Science of the Total Environment* 284: 227–235.

Yavuzer, U. and Bengisu, G. (2023). Effect of selenium on the reproductive performance of ewes and white muscle disease in lambs. *Indian Journal of Animal Research* 48 (3): 248–250.

47

Enterotoxemia

Saahithya Rajamohan[1] and Ranjani Rajasekaran[2]

[1] Department of Veterinary Pathology, Veterinary College and Research Institute, Tamil Nadu Veterinary and Animal Sciences University, Salem, India
[2] Department of Veterinary Microbiology, Veterinary College and Research Institute, Tamil Nadu Veterinary and Animal Sciences University, Theni, India

47.1 Introduction

Enterotoxemia (ET) in goats is caused by *Clostridium perfringens* type D and is reported to be common in this species with a high case fatality rate (Blood et al. 1983; Uzal and Kelly 1996; Veschi et al. 2008). However, the disease is poorly understood in goats (Uzal and Kelly 1996; Smith and Sherman 2011). The disease condition is primarily due to absorption of toxins from the intestinal epithelium into the bloodstream resulting in toxemia (Popoff 1998). *Clostridium* spp. occur as part of the normal intestinal microflora and the diseased state occurs when this is disrupted or altered due to various stressors.

Hill and Smith (2013) have described that *Clostridium* spp. produce more than 20 extracellular toxins and hydrolytic enzymes. These toxins can be subdivided into types A–G, of which type D produces epsilon-toxin (ETX) which is of prime importance in the goat population (Mohiuddin et al. 2020). ETX in goats causes enterocolitis by altering water and ion transport in the intestines (Bokori-Brown et al. 2011; Alves et al. 2014; Uzal et al. 2015). Specific typing of this toxin is essential in confirmative disease diagnosis. ET can be controlled with vaccines and management practices but the available vaccines provide short-lived protective titers in goats necessitating frequent booster doses.

Most of the per-acute and acute cases progress very rapidly before a diagnostic intervention is possible. In cases in which a presumptive diagnosis has been arrived at, the disease can be treated with administration of antitoxins and electrolyte fluids to alleviate the symptoms produced by the underlying state of toxemia.

This chapter discusses enterotoxemia in goats with special emphasis on epidemiological aspects, pathogenesis, clinical signs, diagnosis, treatment, and control.

47.2 Etiology

The genus *Clostridium* includes various significant human and animal pathogens. *Clostridium perfringens* is a Gram-positive, rod-shaped, nonmotile, spore-forming and toxin-producing anaerobe. The genus is classified into several species on the basis of mode and site of action of the potent exotoxin. *Clostridium perfringens* is normally part of the resident microflora of the gastrointestinal tract in animals and humans (Cato 1986).

Owing to the presence of four lethal toxins, namely alpha, beta, epsilon, and iota, *C. perfringens* is classified into five toxigenic types from A to E. Type A produces alpha toxin, type B produces alpha, beta and epsilon toxins, type C produces alpha and beta toxins, type D produces alpha and epsilon toxins, and type E produces alpha and iota toxins (Jolivet-Reynaud et al. 1988; Hatheway 1990). Moreover, *C. perfringens* type F and G have been discovered (Rood et al. 2018). The virulence of the bacterium is mediated by its toxins which in turn have lethal properties (McDonel 1986; Hatheway 1990; Renu et al. 2022).

Elements of Reproduction and Reproductive Diseases of Goats, First Edition. Edited by Tanmoy Rana.

Da Costa et al. (2013), Rood et al. (2018), and Fu et al. (2022) have reported that the strains are now categorized into seven toxin types (A–G) and their six major toxins are named as alpha (CPA), beta (CPB), epsilon (ETX), iota (ITX), enterotoxin (CPE), and enteritis B-like toxin (NetB).

Several authors have reported that multiple bacteriological media could be exploited for culturing the organism in laboratory conditions. It is usually cultured at 37 °C anaerobically using cooked meat medium (Fernandez-Miyakawa et al. 2007), Duncan–Strong sporulation medium (Duncan and Strong 1968), fluid thioglycolate medium (FTG) (Willardsen et al. 1979), tryptic soy broth (TSB) (Wang et al. 2019), tryptose-sulfite-cycloserine (TSC) agar (Hauschild et al. 1974), and tryptic soy agar (TSA) with egg yolk emulsion or 5% sheep blood (Goldstein et al. 2012). *C. perfringens* grows in TSC agar as black colonies, reducing nitrates to nitrites, producing acid and gas from lactose and liquefying gelatin within 48 hours (Rhodehamel and Harmon 2001).

47.3 Epidemiology

Enterotoxemia in goats is highly prevalent worldwide as a common and important disease of goats with high rates of mortality and causing severe economic losses to farmers. Within India, cases have been reported from Kashmir by Nazki et al. (2017) with prevalence of toxinotypes A and D. In goat kids, occurrence of toxinotype D (46.16%) was higher than that of toxinotype A (15.38%) (Nazki et al. 2017). In Tamil Nadu, nine ET outbreaks in sheep and goats were identified by active surveillance and five by passive surveillance from June 1997 to May 2009 in seven agroclimatic zones by Selvaraju (2014). They reported that the outbreaks were more prevalent when the monthly mean maximum and minimum temperatures ranged were 29.1–31.0 °C and 19.1–21.0 °C respectively. Also, outbreaks were more common with monthly total rainfall ranging from 101 to 200 mm, which in turn indicated excess supply of lush green pasture and fodder contamination with soil during moderate levels of rainfall.

Karthik et al. (2017) recorded a 15.7% (n = 19) incidence of ET in Tellicherry goats in an organized farm in Tamil Nadu. In a recent study by Singh (2017), incidences of ET in goat kids were found to be 15.13% (n = 238) and 27.38% (n = 84) from samples collected from diarrheic fecal and intestinal loops respectively. Further, Gangwar and Pawaiya (2018) reported the incidence to be 16.07% (n = 168) and 22.75% (n = 189) from diarrheic fecal and intestinal loop samples respectively in adult goats.

On the global front, ET in goats was reported from Patagonia, Argentina, in 44 Angora goats by Uzal et al. (1994). The authors established the definitive diagnosis of ET by demonstration of epsilon toxin in the intestinal contents and stated that the underlying parasitic etiology was due to coccidiosis which increased the permeability of the intestinal mucosa. Several authors have reported the incidence of cases from Australia (Oxer 1956), Brazil (Miyashiro et al. 2007), Canada (Blackwell and Butler 1992), Germany (Scharfe and Elze 1995), Britain (Shanks 1949), Greece (Tarlatzis et al. 1963), France (Delahaye 1975), Iran (Brooks and Entessar 1957), South Africa (Van Tonder 1975), Sri Lanka (Wanasinghe 1973), Switzerland (Von Rotz et al. 1984), and the United States (Boughton and Hardy 1941; Guss 1977). Recently, Hussain et al. (2022) reported the occurrence in descriptive and nondescriptive goats in Pakistan with a 76.11% case fatality rate (types A and D), among which the deaths caused by type D were more prevalent.

47.4 Economic Impact

Enterotoxemia results in heavy economic losses to the goat-farming community all over the world. Singh and Prasad (2008) analyzed economic losses due to various important diseases in goats by computational methods for a 15-year period in India. They revealed that ET had a high case fatality rate of 38.4% with incidence of 4.7% and deaths accounting for 10.9%. Enterotoxemia in goats accounts for 6.1% (16.2 lakhs) out of the total annual average loss due to all diseases in goats of Rs. 264.8 lakhs. This was an increasing trend in the economic losses over the 15-year period under study.

Al-Assaf (2012) estimated the economic losses due to ET in small ruminants in Jordan for the period 2004–2005 in which mortality rate due to ET accounted for 32.79% and 29.67% in 2004 and 2005 respectively. These losses incurred by goat farmers were indicated in terms of marketing failure due to animal rejection during sale. Also, in terms of financial losses, reduction in the value of germplasm, milk, and meat was indicated.

Therefore, once diagnosis is established in a herd, excessive feeding of carbohydrates must be stopped immediately and a booster dose should be given to previously vaccinated animals. Nonvaccinated animals must receive two doses of vaccine at 2–3-week intervals as reported by Smith and Sherman (2011).

47.5 Pathogenesis

This chapter gives an overall outline of the underlying pathogenesis of ET in goats (Figure 47.1) without delving into the molecular and genetic aspects.

Older reports indicated poor understanding of the pathogenesis of ET in goats. However, over time, various diagnostic tests and research studies have allowed a better understanding. The organisms tend to be a normal commensal of the digestive tract (McClane et al. 2006). Pawaiya et al. (2020) opined that under normal circumstances, they are present in low numbers in the gut without producing intestinal epithelial damage. The normal gut peristalsis tends to wash out the small amount of toxins produced. In addition, the host GI microenvironment poses barriers to bacterial proliferation and colonization including competition with other commensals, inhibition of proliferation by production of secondary bile acids, deoxycholate (Sorg and Sonenshein 2008) and inhibition of growth and toxin production by *Lactobacillus* spp. (Guo et al. 2017).

Pawaiya et al. (2020) added that certain virulence factors and environmental conditions favor bacterial proliferation and colonization. They stated that sialidases (NanI, NanH, NanJ) secreted by organisms are highly important in the initial establishment of infection as they alter host cell surface and promote bacterial attachment (Li et al. 2011, 2016).

Based on the report of Pawaiya et al. (2020), when the animal ingests carbohydrate-rich feeds suddenly or in cases of excessive feeding, more undigested starch passes to the intestine. This in turn serves as a nutrient substrate for rapid proliferation of the organism and reduced motility of the intestine. This is the important predisposing factor for the subsequent production of epsilon toxin by the bacterium. In order to exert its toxic effects, the epsilon toxin in its protoxin form will be converted by intestinal trypsin and lambda protease of *C. perfringens* to a more active form. This results in an increase in GI permeability, thus facilitating its own absorption, and is then transported to several target organs, including brain, lungs, and kidney (Bullen 1970; Uzal et al. 2016). Based on *in vitro* findings by Uzal et al. (2016), it was postulated that the absence of glucose in the small intestine, due to failure of starch digestion, can stimulate ETX production by *C. perfringens* type D. Also, Li et al. (2011) reported that the sialidases enhance ETX binding and cytotoxicity.

In goats, apart from the intestine, the kidney is one of the target organs of epsilon toxin. The so-called "pulpy kidney" lesion has diagnostic significance in ovine ET whereas renal lesions are not considered a valid diagnostic point in caprine ET (Uzal and Songer 2008). The brain is also a prime target of epsilon toxin (Bokori-Brown et al. 2011). ETX initially binds to endothelial cells of the blood–brain barrier, resulting in cell swelling, vacuolation, and necrosis of affected vascular endothelial cells with rupture of perivascular astrocyte processes (Finnie 1984; Uzal 2004; Soler-Jover et al. 2007). This results in leakage of fluid and proteins and hypoxia of the neural parenchyma (Stiles et al. 2013; Garcia et al. 2015).

47.6 Clinical Signs

Naturally occurring ET in goats has four forms: peracute, acute, subacute, and chronic (Ayers 1984). For all the four forms of ET, diarrhea is the cardinal clinical sign (Sumithra et al. 2013). In peracute cases, pyrexia of 40.5 °C has been recorded in goats by Shanks (1949) and Smith and Sherman (2011). The clinical signs are summarized in Table 47.1.

47.6.1 Peracute Form

Enterotoxemia is a common feature in young kids and the clinical course is less than 24 hours. They are often found dead without exhibiting any clinical signs (Shanks 1949; Blackwell et al. 1991; Blackwell and Butler 1992). If clinical signs are evident, there is fever rising to 40.5 °C, incidence of severe shock, terminal convulsions, coma, and death within hours of onset (Baxendell 1988; Smith and Sherman 2011). Recovery is rare in this form (Smith and Sherman 2011).

47.6.2 Acute Form

This form is commonly observed in adult goats (Smith and Sherman 2011). The clinical course lasts for 4–24 hours (Ayers 1984). It is characterized by abdominal discomfort, diarrhea resulting in severe shock with cold extremities, opisthotonus, and intermittent convulsions. The diarrheic feces will be yellow-green and pasty in consistency in the initial stages but watery to mucoid admixed with shreds of bowel mucosa and blood in later stages (Baxendell 1988). The underlying

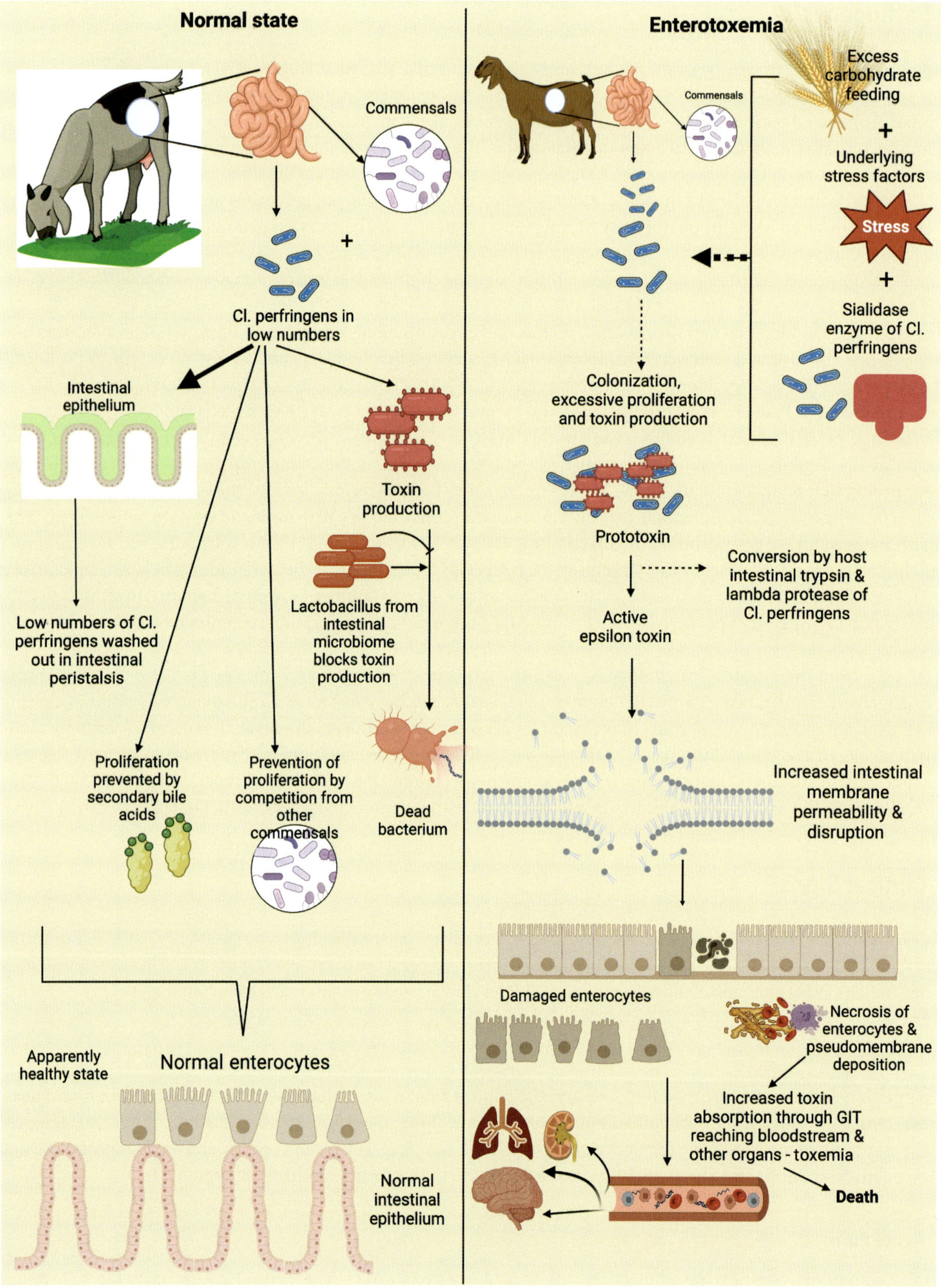

Figure 47.1 Simplified diagrammatic representation of the pathogenesis of enterotoxemia in goats. *Source:* Created by Dr Saahithya Rajamohan using www.biorender.com.

Table 47.1 Clinical signs in goats affected by enterotoxemia.

Stage of the disease	Age group affected	Clinical signs/features	References
Peracute form (less than 24 hours)	Young goat kids	• Found dead without exhibiting any clinical signs • Pyrexia (40.5 °C) • Shock • Terminal convulsions • Coma and death	Shanks (1949), Blackwell et al. (1991), Blackwell and Butler (1992), Baxendell (1988), Smith and Sherman (2011)
Acute form (4–24 hours)	Adult goats	• Dehydration • Acidosis • Abdominal discomfort • Diarrhea – yellow-green and pasty at initial stages and watery to mucoid admixed with shreds of bowel mucosa and blood in later stages • Shock • Cold extremities • Opisthotonus • Intermittent convulsions	Ayers (1984), Blackwell et al. (1991), Blood et al. (1983), Uzal and Kelly (1996), Uzal (2004)
Subacute form (several days or weeks)	Older goat kids and adults	• Dullness • Anorexia • Severe intermittent diarrhea • Presence of epithelial shreds in the feces	
Chronic form (several weeks)	Adult goats	• Dullness • Anorexia • Abdominal discomfort • Profuse watery diarrhea containing blood and mucus • Progressive emaciation/weakness • Agalactia in milking does	

systemic effects involve dehydration and acidosis (Smith and Sherman 2011). The outcome may be recovery or death (Baxendell 1988; Blackwell et al. 1991).

47.6.3 Subacute Form

This is a common manifestation in older kids and adults. Ayers (1984) reported that the course of the disease may last several days or weeks. They recorded clinical signs of anorexia and severe diarrhea which was intermittent. In addition, there were epithelial shreds in the feces. In this form, the animals might recover on administration of appropriate treatment.

47.6.4 Chronic Form

This is usually observed in adults (Smith and Sherman 2011) and characterized by intermittent illness lasting several weeks (Ayers 1984). The clinical signs include profuse, watery diarrhea (often containing blood and mucus), dullness, anorexia, abdominal discomfort, progressive emaciation/weakness (Shanks 1949), and agalactia in milking does (Blackwell and Butler 1992). This form may terminate in either death or recovery of the animal (Blood et al. 1983).

47.7 Diagnosis

The confirmative diagnosis of ET can be done primarily by the detection of epsilon toxin in intestinal fluid, tissue, and culture supernatants (Pawaiya et al. 2020). Several other diagnostic tests for detection are elucidated below.

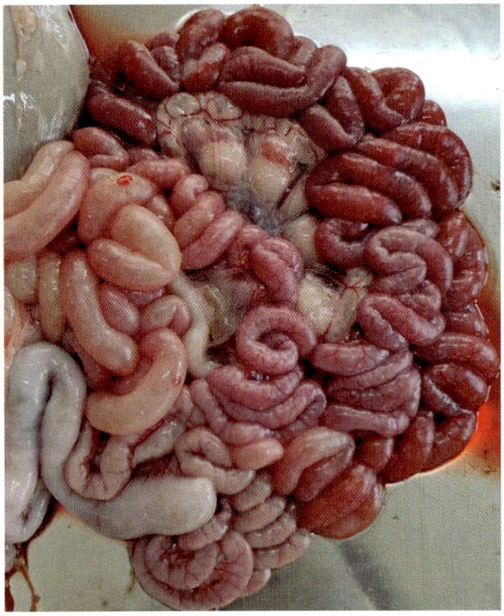

Figure 47.2 A four-month-old goat kid affected by enterotoxemia revealing severe congestion and hemorrhage of the intestinal serosa along the jejunum, ileum, and colon. *Source:* Dr Saahithya Rajamohan (chapter contributor).

47.7.1 Pathomorphological Findings

In the peracute form of the disease in goats, an excess of straw-colored pericardial fluid rich in protein, interstitial lung edema, and subendocardial hemorrhages are usually seen which are suggestive of the disease as reported by Uzal (2004).

In the chronic form, Blackwell and Butler (1992) and Uzal (2004) have recorded fibrinohemorrhagic enterocolitis and pulmonary edema as consistent lesions in goats. The prominent lesion of so-called "pulpy kidney" is considered to be only suggestive of ET in goats which should be carefully differentiated from animals whose carcases indicate normal autolysis. Gross changes may be entirely absent in a few cases of caprine *C. perfringens* type D ET (Blackwell et al. 1983). In certain goat cases which were found to be positive for ET, we have observed severe congestion of the intestinal serosa, especially of the jejunum, ileum, and colon with hemorrhages in the mucosal layer (unpublished data) (Figure 47.2).

47.7.2 Histopathological Findings

In goats, subacute and chronic cases of ET are characterized by fibrinonecrotic colitis with pseudomembrane formation as recorded by Smith and Sherman (1994). However, this lesion cannot be used to establish a definitive diagnosis of ET. Uzal (2004) reported the most striking histopathological changes as severe congestion, hemorrhage, and necrosis in the colonic epithelium and villi of duodenum and ileum.

Miyashiro et al. (2007) reported the histopathological findings of necrotizing enteritis in the small intestine, hemorrhagic foci in the renal parenchyma, and coagulation necrosis in the cortex and medulla. There was intense hyperemia, degeneration, and centrilobular necrosis of the liver. The lungs revealed severe pulmonary edema and congestion. In the brain, extensive areas of hyperemia were observed in the cerebellum and cerebral cortex with intense perivascular and perineuronal edema.

Uzal et al. (1997a) and Barker et al. (1993) observed that changes in the brain are not considered to be a common feature of caprine ET, although cerebral edema may be observed in peracute and acute cases. Reports by Uzal et al. (1997a) and Uzal (2004) observed perivascular edema and degeneration of white matter in three cases of naturally occurring acute ET in goats. Recently, Ortega et al. (2019) reported the characteristic histopathological finding in brain with intramural vascular edema in ET-affected goats.

47.7.3 Farm Level – Simple and Ancillary Tests

At farm level, diagnosis can be arrived at taking into account the characteristic clinical history of sudden death without premonitory signs and from necropsy findings. The important diagnostic criterion at necropsy tends to be the acute hemorrhagic colitis with hemorrhagic intestinal contents. The ideal sample of choice for diagnosis following a necropsy would be a ligated intestinal loop collected from the location showing lesions of hemorrhages and enterocolitis (Pawaiya et al. 2020).

Smears from intestinal mucosa can be retrieved during postmortem examination and stained by Gram staining which can also be used as a diagnostic method to establish the presence of any of the *C. perfringens* in goats. Gram smears would reveal predominantly larger amounts of Gram-positive bacilli with rounded ends though other bacterial forms can be seen (Carter 1984).

For bacteriological and culture examination, samples should be collected from fresh carcases. The ligated intestinal loop should be kept at 4 °C for proper transport and its stability can be further enhanced by addition of one drop of chloroform in 10 ml of intestinal content (Constable et al. 2017).

Uzal (2004) opined that the most useful pen-side test involves urinalysis for the presence of glucose which would strongly suggest an ET origin. However, the author reported this finding to be inconsistent in goats with type D ET. Later, Uzal and

Kelly (1998) performed experimental ET in a flock of 15 goats. High levels of glycosuria were found in nine animals in which urine glucose was measured. They established that glycosuria is a useful indicator of the possibility of type D ET but its absence does not rule out the possibility.

47.7.4 Diagnosis Through Complex Laboratory Tests

These tests involve the isolation of *C. perfringens* from the feces or gut lumen (Uzal and Kelly 1996) and identification of epsilon toxin or the gene expressing epsilon toxin in *C. perfringens* cultures from feces (Uzal and Songer 2008).

Bacteriological tests are performed mainly through isolation and culturing of *C. perfringens* from gut contents of goats. Several culture media have been indicated, the most widely used being Robertson's cooked meat media, thioglycolate media, reinforced clostridial media, tryptose sulfite cycloserine agar, and TSC-egg yolk agar as mentioned by Kotsanas et al. (2010), Javed et al. (2012), and Gangwar and Pawaiya (2018). The organism produces gas in Robertson's cooked meat media as reported by Gangwar and Pawaiya (2018) and Kumar (2019). Kotsanas et al. (2010) observed the occurrence of black colonies with opaque halos in TSC-egg yolk agar. Although various culture characteristics have been described by different authors, this method is questionable as this organism is a normal inhabitant of the intestine in goats. In such cases, Uzal (2004) described that a bacterial count of 10^4–10^7 CFU/g of fecal sample is considered normal in goats (Uzal 2004). However, reports on the quantification of normal levels of these organisms in intestinal content are not available.

Detection of toxin genes by PCR, multiplex PCR, and real-time PCR can be performed. Detection of epsilon toxin-encoding gene (ETX) is most relevant and helpful in the diagnosis of ET (Uzal et al. 1997b). Kalender et al. (2005) and Mohiuddin et al. (2016) have reported the use of multiplex PCR-based toxinotyping for *C. perfringens* strains from the feces. Toxin gene detection using real-time PCR in other species has been reported by various authors (Alwan et al. 2016; Mizher et al. 2016).

The most accepted criterion in establishing a definitive diagnosis of ET in goats is detection of its toxins in intestinal contents as reported by Uzal (2004). This can be performed by various complex diagnostic techniques involving immunohistochemistry, mouse neutralization tests, enzyme-linked immunosorbent assay (ELISA), latex agglutination test (LAT), indirect hemagglutination test (IHT), indirect hemagglutination inhibition test (IHIT), and mass spectrometry techniques (Naylor et al. 1987).

Naylor et al. (1987) detected the presence of epsilon toxin in samples collected from animals by the mouse neutralization test. They reported that this test could be utilized as a comparative test for other diagnostic aids and for testing the potency of clostridial vaccines.

Naylor et al. (1987) ascertained that the ELISA was a valid test for epsilon toxin detection from samples obtained from gut contents. Among various variations in this technique, El Idrissi and Ward (1992) reported 94.6% specificity and 97.4% sensitivity for sandwich ELISA. Recently, Ortega et al. (2019) devised a monoclonal antibody-based capture ELISA for the identification of epsilon toxin in samples collected from both small and large intestinal contents in affected goats.

For qualitative detection of the epsilon toxin in intestinal contents, Martin and Naylor (1994) and Tahir et al. (2013) utilized the LAT; this is a rapid and simple test which could serve as a potential field test owing to its cost-effectiveness. Further, Goekce et al. (2007) found that this technique detected toxins in 58.46% of intestinal contents, providing a sensitivity and specificity of 96.5% and 95.2% respectively, which were similarly observed by Martin and Naylor (1994) and Pawaiya et al. (2020).

Tahir et al. (2013) effectively utilized the IHT and IHIT to measure serum antibody titer against adjuvanted toxoid vaccines. They collected samples from the blood and intestinal contents of ET-affected goats. They detected antiepsilon toxin antibodies from the sera and epsilon toxin from the intestinal contents of ET-affected animals (Pawaiya et al. 2020).

Highly specialized techniques requiring heavy investment are also available for diagnosis. These include mass spectrometry techniques involving liquid chromatography mass spectrometry, matrix-assisted laser desorption ionization-time of flight (MALDI-TOF) and ultra-performance liquid chromatography-mass spectrometry. They are used to detect and quantify epsilon toxins in different biological samples from animals (Seyer et al. 2012; Alam et al. 2012; Dupré et al. 2015). However, they have their own cost limits.

All the above tests mainly depend upon culture methods and serological assays. However, these tests may not be feasible under field conditions. In those conditions, immunohistochemistry is used to detect the presence of clostridial toxins in tissues. Miyakawa et al. (2007) detected the CPE toxin from the ileal mucosa of goat. Similarly, Uzal et al. (2008) demonstrated the CPB2 in small and large intestines of goats positive for ET.

47.8 Treatment and Control

Devising treatment protocols in ET-affected goats at peracute and acute stages of the disease is ineffective, because disease progression is rapid even before a diagnosis can be made. As per reports by Ayers (1984), in subacute and chronic cases, antitoxin along with oral doses of tetracycline at the rate of 11–22 mg/kg bodyweight will prove useful in treating the disease. Reports by Guss (1977), Baxendell (1988), and Smith and Sherman (2011) stated that administration of epsilon antitoxin in affected cases resulted in clinical improvement. Also, management of acutely affected animals in a warm, dry pen and administration with intravenous fluid therapy of mixed electrolyte solutions, including bicarbonate, were suggested by Smith and Sherman (2011). These authors also recommended the administration of nonsteroidal antiinflammatory drugs, such as flunixin meglumine, together with oral sulfonamides, parenteral antibiotics, and oral adsorbents. Smith and Sherman (2011) suggested the administration of the above supportive therapies in order to alleviate dehydration, acidosis, and toxemic state.

Recently, nanoparticle-based delivery systems have been studied under *in vivo* conditions for treatment of ET in sheep and goats. However, this is still under research conditions and extensive analysis is needed (Xu et al. 2023).

For control of ET in goats, proper vaccination strategies and management practices are essential. According to Blackwell et al. (1983), there is no specific vaccine available for goats and so vaccines for sheep are used. According to reports by Uzal and Kelly (1996), after primary double immunization, a booster dose is recommended every three or four months. Smith and Sherman (2011) added that vaccination 2–3 weeks before parturition is required to increase the protective effect of colostrum in pregnant does. In case of kids, the first dose is to be given at 4–6 weeks of age. Further, administration of vaccines limited to types C and D with or without tetanus toxoid is generally preferred (Smith and Sherman 2011). Naz et al. (2012) reported that single administration of enterotoxemia-cum-lamb dysentery vaccine in goats produced an antibody titer of 2.64 and the booster dose produced 12.12 titer. Uzal and Kelly (1998) reported that parenteral vaccination with epsilon toxoid could protect goats against both systemic and intestinal effects of ET.

47.9 Conclusion

Enterotoxemia still poses a severe threat and massive economic losses to the goat-farming community. Future research could be directed more toward development of cost-effective and less time-consuming diagnostic aids with higher sensitivity and specificity for accurate and prompt detection of ET in goats as this would be highly beneficial to the low margin income farmers whose sole means of generating income is goat rearing. Moreover, studies on disease forecasting methods region wise through computational methods could benefit the creation of control strategies. Development of specific vaccines for prevention in goats will be required for devising management strategies at herd level. Better awareness and understanding of feeding management strategies by livestock owners would help to reduce incidence at farm or household level.

References

Alam, S.I., Kumar, B., and Kamboj, D.V. (2012). Multiplex detection of protein toxins using MALDI-TOF-TOF tandem mass spectrometry: application in unambiguous toxin detection from bioaerosol. *Analytical Chemistry* 84 (23): 10500–10507.

Al-Assaf, A. (2012). Economic implications of small ruminant diseases in the northern area of Jordan. *Journal of Food, Agriculture and Environment* 10 (1): 323–326.

Alves, G.G., de Ávila, R.A.M., Chávez-Olórtegui, C.D., and Lobato, F.C.F. (2014). Clostridium perfringens epsilon toxin: the third most potent bacterial toxin known. *Anaerobe* 30: 102–107.

Alwan, J.A., Al-zaidy, A.A., and Abbas, K.H. (2016). Real-time PCR for direct detection of Clostridium perfringens from horse with enterocolitis infection. *Kufa Journal for Veterinary Medical Sciences* 7 (1).

Ayers, J.L. (1984). Enterotoxemia. In: *Extension Goat Handbook* (ed. G.F.W. Haenlein and D.L. Ace), G-10. Washington, DC: USDA.

Barker, I.K., Van Dreumel, A.A., and Palmer, N. (1993). The alimentary system. In: *Pathology of Domestic Animals*, 4e, vol. 2 (ed. K.F. Jubb, P.C. Kennedy, and N. Palmer). San Diego, CA: Academic Press.

Baxendell, S.A. (1988). *The Diagnosis of the Diseases of Goats*. Sydney, Australia: Post-Graduate Committee in Veterinary Science.

Blackwell, T.E. and Butler, D.G. (1992). Clinical signs, treatment, and postmortem lesions in dairy goats with enterotoxemia: 13 cases (1979–1982). *Journal of the American Veterinary Medical Association* 200 (2): 214–217.

Blackwell, T.E., Butler, D.G., and Bell, J.A. (1983). Enterotoxemia in the goat: the humoral response and local tissue reaction following vaccination with two different bacterin-toxoids. *Canadian Journal of Comparative Medicine* 47 (2): 127.

Blackwell, T.E., Butler, D.G., Prescott, J.F., and Wilcock, B.P. (1991). Differences in signs and lesions in sheep and goats with enterotoxemia induced by intraduodenal infusion of Clostridium perfringens type D. *American Journal of Veterinary Research* 52 (7): 1147–1152.

Blood, D.C., Radostits, O.M., and Henderson, J.A. (1983). *Veterinary Medicine. A Textbook of the Diseases of Cattle, Sheep, Goats and Horses*, 6e. London: Baillière Tindall.

Bokori-Brown, M., Savva, C.G., Fernandes da Costa, S.P. et al. (2011). Molecular basis of toxicity of Clostridium perfringens epsilon toxin. *FEBS Journal* 278 (23): 4589–4601.

Boughton, I.B. and Hardy, W.T. (1941). Infectious entero-toxemia (milk colic) of lambs and kids. *Texas Agricultural Experiment Station* 598: 5–20.

Brooks, M.E. and Entessar, F. (1957). Anomalous Clostridium welchii type B strains isolated in Iran. *British Veterinary Journal* 113 (12): 506–508.

Bullen, J.J. (1970). Role of toxins in host–parasite relationships. *Microbial Toxins* 1: 233–276.

Carter, G.R. (1984). *Diagnostic Procedures in Veterinary Microbiology*, 4e. Springfield, IL: Charles C. Thomas.

Cato, E.P. (1986). Genus clostridium. In: *Bergey's Manual of Systematic Bacteriology* (ed. D. Bergey, P. Sneath, and J. Holt), 1141–1200. Baltimore, MD: Williams & Wilkins.

Constable, P.D., Hinchcliff, K.W., Done, S.H., and Grunberg, W. (2017). *Veterinary Medicine. A Textbook of the Diseases of Cattle, Horse, Sheep, Pigs and Goats*, 11e. St Louis, MO: Saunders Elsevier.

da Costa, S.P.F., Mot, D., Bokori-Brown, M. et al. (2013). Protection against avian necrotic enteritis after immunisation with NetB genetic or formaldehyde toxoids. *Vaccine* 31 (37): 4003–4008.

Delahaye, J. (1975). *Maladies, Prevention, Traitements* (ed. L.C.E. Qnittet). Paris: La Maison Rustique.

Duncan, C.L. and Strong, D.H. (1968). Improved medium for sporulation of Clostridium perfringens. *Applied Microbiology* 16 (1): 82–89.

Dupré, M., Gilquin, B., Fenaille, F. et al. (2015). Multiplex quantification of protein toxins in human biofluids and food matrices using immunoextraction and high-resolution targeted mass spectrometry. *Analytical Chemistry* 87 (16): 8473–8480.

El Idrissi, A.H. and Ward, G.E. (1992). Evaluation of enzyme-linked immunosorbent assay for diagnosis of Clostridium perfringens enterotoxemias. *Veterinary Microbiology* 31 (4): 389–396.

Fernandez-Miyakawa, M.E., Marcellino, R., and Uzal, F.A. (2007). Clostridium perfringens type A toxin production in 3 commonly used culture media. *Journal of Veterinary Diagnostic Investigation* 19 (2): 184–186.

Finnie, J.W. (1984). Histopathological changes in the brain of mice given Clostridium perfringens type D epsilon toxin. *Journal of Comparative Pathology* 94 (3): 363–370.

Fu, Y., Alenezi, T., and Sun, X. (2022). Clostridium perfringens-induced necrotic diseases: an overview. *Immuno* 2 (2): 387–407.

Gangwar, N.K. and Pawaiya, R.V.S. (2018). Molecular pathology and transcriptional profiling of enterotoxaemia in post-weaned goats. *Indian Journal of Veterinary Pathology* 42 (2): 153.

Garcia, J.P., Giannitti, F., Finnie, J.W. et al. (2015). Comparative neuropathology of ovine enterotoxemia produced by Clostridium perfringens type D wild-type strain CN1020 and its genetically modified derivatives. *Veterinary Pathology* 52 (3): 465–475.

Goekce, H.I., Genç, O., Soezmen, M., and Gökçe, G. (2007). Determination of Clostridium perfringens toxin-types in sheep with suspected enterotoxemia in Kars Province, Turkey. *Turkish Journal of Veterinary and Animal Sciences* 31 (5): 355–360.

Goldstein, M.R., Kruth, S.A., Bersenas, A.M. et al. (2012). Detection and characterization of Clostridium perfringens in the feces of healthy and diarrheic dogs. *Canadian Journal of Veterinary Research* 76 (3): 161–165.

Guo, S., Liu, D., Zhang, B. et al. (2017). Two Lactobacillus species inhibit the growth and α-toxin production of Clostridium perfringens and induced proinflammatory factors in chicken intestinal epithelial cells in vitro. *Frontiers in Microbiology* 8: 2081.

Guss, S.B. (1977). *Management and Diseases of Dairy Goats*. Wisconsin, USA: Dairy Goat Journal Publishing Corporation.

Hatheway, C.L. (1990). Toxigenic clostridia. *Clinical Microbiology Reviews* 3: 66–98.

Hauschild, A.H.W., Hilsheimer, R., and Griffith, D.W. (1974). Enumeration of fecal Clostridium perfringens spores in egg yolk-free tryptose-sulfite-cycloserine agar. *Applied Microbiology* 27 (3): 527–530.

Hill, K.K. and Smith, T.J. (2013). Genetic diversity within Clostridium botulinum serotypes, botulinum neurotoxin gene clusters and toxin subtypes. *Botulinum Neurotoxins* 364: 1–20.

Hussain, R., Guangbin, Z., Abbas, R.Z. et al. (2022). Clostridium perfringens types A and D involved in peracute deaths in goats kept in Cholistan ecosystem during winter season. *Frontiers in Veterinary Science* 9: 849856.

Javed, S., Rafeeq, M., Tariq, M.M. et al. (2012). Study on in-vitro biochemical growth characterization and assessment of hemolytic toxin of Clostridium perfringens type B and D. *Pakistan Journal of Zoology* 44 (6): 1575–1580.

Jolivet-Reynaud, C., Moreau, H., and Alouf, J.E. (1988). Purification of alpha toxin from clostridium perfringens: phospholipase C. In: *Methods in Enzymology*, vol. 165, 91–94. New York: Academic Press.

Kalender, H., Ertas, H.B., Cetinkaya, B. et al. (2005). Typing of isolates of Clostridium perfringens from healthy and diseased sheep by multiplex PCR. *Veterinarni Medicina-Praha* 50 (10): 439.

Karthik, K., Manimaran, K., Bharathi, R., and Shoba, K. (2017). Report of enterotoxaemia in goat kids. *Advances in Animal and Veterinary Science* 5: 289–292.

Kotsanas, D., Carson, J.A., Awad, M.M. et al. (2010). Novel use of tryptose sulfite cycloserine egg yolk agar for isolation of Clostridium perfringens during an outbreak of necrotizing enterocolitis in a neonatal unit. *Journal of Clinical Microbiology* 48 (11): 4263–4265.

Kumar, R. (2019). Pathology and transcriptional response of enterotoxaemia in goats. MVSc thesis. Indian Veterinary Research Institute (IVRI).

Li, J., Sayeed, S., Robertson, S. et al. (2011). Sialidases affect the host cell adherence and epsilon toxin-induced cytotoxicity of Clostridium perfringens type D strain CN3718. *PLoS Pathogens* 7 (12): e1002429.

Li, J., Uzal, F.A., and McClane, B.A. (2016). Clostridium perfringens sialidases: potential contributors to intestinal pathogenesis and therapeutic targets. *Toxins* 8 (11): 341.

Martin, P.K. and Naylor, R.D. (1994). A latex agglutination test for the qualitative detection of Clostridium perfringens epsilon toxin. *Research in Veterinary Science* 56 (2): 259–261.

McClane, B.A., Uzal, F.A., Miyakawa, M.F. et al. (2006). The enterotoxic clostridia. *Prokaryotes* 4: 698–752.

McDonel, J.L. (1986). Toxins of Clostridium perfringens types a, B, C, D and E. In: *Pharmacology of Bacterial Toxins*, 477–517. Oxford: Pergamon Press.

Miyakawa, M.E.F., Saputo, J., Leger, J.S. et al. (2007). Necrotizing enterocolitis and death in a goat kid associated with enterotoxin (CPE)-producing Clostridium perfringens type a. *Canadian Veterinary Journal* 48 (12): 1266.

Miyashiro, S., Nassar, A.F.C., Del Fava, C. et al. (2007). Clostridium perfringens types A and D associated with enterotoxemia in an 18-month-old goat. *Journal of Venomous Animals and Toxins Including Tropical Diseases* 13: 885–893.

Mizher, B.M., Sadeq, J.N., and Esmaeel, J.R. (2016). Direct detection of Clostridium perfringens based alpha toxin gene from sheep and cattle by real time PCR technique. *Basrah Journal of Veterinary Research* 15 (2): 1–9.

Mohiuddin, M., Iqbal, Z., and Rahman, S.U. (2016). Prevalence of Clostridium perfringens β2-toxin in sheep and goat population in Punjab, Pakistan. *Thai Journal of Veterinary Medicine* 46 (3): 491–496.

Mohiuddin, M., Iqbal, Z., Siddique, A. et al. (2020). Prevalence, genotypic and phenotypic characterization and antibiotic resistance profile of Clostridium perfringens type A and D isolated from feces of sheep (Ovis aries) and goats (Capra hircus) in Punjab, Pakistan. *Toxins* 12 (10): 657.

Naylor, R.D., Martin, P.K., and Sharpe, R.T. (1987). Detection of Clostridium perfringens epsilon toxin by ELISA. *Research in Veterinary Science* 42 (2): 255–256.

Naz, S., Ghuman, M.A., Anjum, A.A. et al. (2012). Comparison of immune responses following the administration of enterotoxaemia vaccine in sheep and goats. *Journal of Veterinary and Animal Sciences* 2: 89–94.

Nazki, S., Wani, S.A., Parveen, R. et al. (2017). Isolation, molecular characterization and prevalence of Clostridium perfringens in sheep and goats of Kashmir Himalayas, India. *Veterinary World* 10 (12): 1501.

Ortega, J., Verdes, J.M., Morrell, E.L. et al. (2019). Intramural vascular edema in the brain of goats with Clostridium perfringens type D enterotoxemia. *Veterinary Pathology* 56 (3): 452–459.

Oxer, D.T. (1956). Enterotoxaemia in goats. *Australian Veterinary Journal* 32 (3): 62–66.

Pawaiya, R.S., Gururaj, K., Gangwar, N.K. et al. (2020). The challenges of diagnosis and control of enterotoxaemia caused by Clostridium perfringens in small ruminants. *Advances in Microbiology* 10 (5): 238–273.

Popoff, M.R. (1998). Interactions between bacterial toxins and intestinal cells lecture presented to the 3iemes Journees des rencontres en Toxinologie (Societe pour l'Etude des Toxines), Paris, 7–8 Decembre, 1995. *Toxicon* 36 (4): 665–685.

Renu, H.D., Mathur, M., Boyal, P.K. et al. (2022). Molecular identification of *Clostridium perfringens* from intestine of sheep. *Pharma Innovation Journal* 11: 1173–1174.

Rhodehamel, E.J. and Harmon, S.M. (2001). *Clostridium perfringens*. In: *Bacteriological Analytical Manual (BAM)*. Silver Spring, MD: Food and Drug Administration.

Rood, J.I., Adams, V., Lacey, J. et al. (2018). Expansion of the Clostridium perfringens toxin-based typing scheme. *Anaerobe* 53: 5–10.

Scharfe, S. and Elze, K. (1995). Enzootic occurrence of lamb dysentery in two herds of goats. *Praktische Tierarzt* 76: 769–774.

Selvaraju, G. (2014). Forecasting of enterotoxaemia outbreak in small ruminants. *International Journal of Agriculture Innovations and Research* 3 (1): 86–89.

Seyer, A., Fenaille, F., Féraudet-Tarisse, C. et al. (2012). Rapid quantification of clostridial epsilon toxin in complex food and biological matrixes by immunopurification and ultraperformance liquid chromatography-tandem mass spectrometry. *Analytical Chemistry* 84 (11): 5103–5109.

Shanks, P.L. (1949). Enterotoxaemia in goats. *Veterinary Record* 61: 262–264.

Singh, B. and Prasad, S. (2008). Modelling of economic losses due to some important diseases in goats in India. *Agricultural Economics Research Review* 21: 297–302.

Singh, D.D., Pawaiya, R.V.S., Gururaj, K. et al. (2017). Pathological studies on spontaneous cases of enterotoxaemia in goat kids at organized and unorganized farms. *Indian Journal of Veterinary Pathology* 41: 245.

Smith, M.C. and Sherman, D.M. (1994). *Goat Medicine*. Philadelphia, PA: Lea and Febiger.

Smith, M.C. and Sherman, D.M. (2011). *Goat Medicine*, 2e. Hoboken, NJ: Wiley Blackwell.

Soler-Jover, A., Dorca, J., Popoff, M.R. et al. (2007). Distribution of Clostridium perfringens epsilon toxin in the brains of acutely intoxicated mice and its effect upon glial cells. *Toxicon* 50 (4): 530–540.

Sorg, J.A. and Sonenshein, A.L. (2008). Bile salts and glycine as cogerminants for Clostridium difficile spores. *Journal of Bacteriology* 190 (7): 2505–2512.

Stiles, B.G., Barth, G., Barth, H., and Popoff, M.R. (2013). Clostridium perfringens epsilon toxin: a malevolent molecule for animals and man? *Toxins* 5 (11): 2138–2160.

Sumithra, T.G., Chaturvedi, V.K., Siju, S.J. et al. (2013). Enterotoxaemia in goats – a review of current knowledge. *Small Ruminant Research* 114 (1): 1–9.

Tahir, M.F., Mahmood, M.S., and Iftikhar, H. (2013). Preparation and comparative evaluation of different adjuvanted toxoid vaccines against enterotoxaemia. *Pakistan Journal of Agricultural Sciences* 50 (2): 293–297.

Tarlatzis, C.B., Frangopoulos, A., and Stoforos, E. (1963). Gangrenous mastitis of ewes and goats and the identification of the causative agent Clostridium perfringens type C. *Hellenike Kteniatrikes Hetaireias Deltion* 50: 88–95.

Uzal, F.A. (2004). Diagnosis of Clostridium perfringens intestinal infections in sheep and goats. *Anaerobe* 10 (2): 135–143.

Uzal, F.A. and Kelly, W.R. (1996). Enterotoxaemia in goats. *Veterinary Research Communications* 20: 481–492.

Uzal, F.A. and Kelly, W.R. (1998). Experimental Clostridium perfringens type D enterotoxemia in goats. *Veterinary Pathology* 35 (2): 132–140.

Uzal, F.A. and Songer, J.G. (2008). Diagnosis of Clostridium perfringens intestinal infections in sheep and goats. *Journal of Veterinary Diagnostic Investigation* 20 (3): 253–265.

Uzal, F.A., Pasini, M.I., Olaechea, F.V. et al. (1994). An outbreak of enterotoxaemia caused by Clostridium perfringens type D in goats in Patagonia. *Veterinary Record* 135: 279–279.

Uzal, F.A., Glastonbury, J.R.W., Kelly, W.R., and Thomas, R. (1997a). Caprine enterotoxaemia associated with cerebral microangiopathy. *Veterinary Record* 141 (9): 224–226.

Uzal, F.A., Plumb, J.J., Blackall, L.L., and Kelly, W.R. (1997b). PCR detection of Clostridium perfringens producing different toxins in faeces of goats. *Letters in Applied Microbiology* 25 (5): 339–344.

Uzal, F.A., Fisher, D.J., Saputo, J. et al. (2008). Ulcerative enterocolitis in two goats associated with enterotoxin-and beta2 toxin-positive clostridium perfringens type D. *Journal of Veterinary Diagnostic Investigation* 20 (5): 668–672.

Uzal, F.A., McClane, B.A., Cheung, J.K. et al. (2015). Animal models to study the pathogenesis of human and animal Clostridium perfringens infections. *Veterinary Microbiology* 179 (1–2): 23–33.

Uzal, F.A., Giannitti, F., Finnie, J.W., and García, J.P. (2016). Diseases produced by Clostridium perfringens type D. In: *Clostridial Diseases of Animals* (ed. F. Uzal, J. Songer, J. Prescott, and M. Popoff), 157–172. Ames, IA: Wiley Blackwell.

Van Tonder, E.M. (1975). Notes on some disease problems in Angora goats in South Africa. *Veterinary Medical Review* 1: 109–138.

Veschi, J.L.A., Bruzzone, O.A., Losada-Eaton, D.M. et al. (2008). Naturally acquired antibodies against Clostridium perfringens epsilon toxin in goats. *Veterinary Immunology and Immunopathology* 125 (1–2): 198–202.

Von Rotz, A., Corboz, L., and Waldvogel, A. (1984). Clostridium perfringens type D enterotoxemia of goats in Switzerland. Pathologico-anatomical and bacteriological studies. *Schweizer Archiv für Tierheilkunde* 126 (7): 359–364.

Wanasinghe, D.D. (1973). Outbreak of enterotoxaemia due to Clostridium welchii type D in goats. *Ceylon Veterinary Journal* 21: 6245.

Wang, H., Latorre, J.D., Bansal, M. et al. (2019). Microbial metabolite deoxycholic acid controls Clostridium perfringens-induced chicken necrotic enteritis through attenuating inflammatory cyclooxygenase signaling. *Scientific Reports* 9 (1): 1–12.
Willardsen, R.R., Busta, F.F., and Allen, C.E. (1979). Growth of Clostridium perfringens in three different beef media and fluid thioglycollate medium at static and constantly rising temperatures. *Journal of Food Protection* 42 (2): 144–148.
Xu, J., Li, D., Kang, L. et al. (2023). New insights into membrane-camouflaged nanoparticles for the treatment of ETX intoxication. www.researchsquare.com/article/rs-2592879/v1 (accessed 2 December 2023).

48

Acidosis

Ankit S. Prajapati[1], Prakash M. Chauhan[2], Abhinav N. Suthar[3], and Bhupamani Das[2]

[1] *Veterinary Clinical Complex (Medicine), College of Veterinary Science and Animal Husbandry, Kamdhenu University, Anand, Gujarat, India*
[2] *Department of Clinics, College of Veterinary Science and Animal Husbandry, Kamdhenu University, Sardarkrushinagar, Gujarat, India*
[3] *Department of Medicine, College of Veterinary Science and Animal Husbandry, Kamdhenu University, Sardarkrushinagar, India*

48.1 Introduction

Goat farming is a major source of income for the marginal farmer community. Production and reproduction are the prime objectives of goat farming. Many diseases affect the health of doe and kid in the initial days of life. Economic goat farming depends on preventing certain conditions in caprines, ultimately leading to a profitable income through goat rearing (Brahma et al. 2020).

Digestive disorders are not well understood and are multifactorial. A kid's stomach is also not fully developed for optimum utilization of nutrients. Acidosis is important in terms of kid mortality. During the periparturient period, acid–base balance is vulnerable in both doe and kid (Gomez et al. 2020). Acid–base balance is vital in maintaining normal physiological status. The nutritional status of the doe also predisposes the kid to develop acidosis in the initial days of life. Acidosis can affect all breeds of goats and kids.

Many factors contribute to the development of acidosis. Maternal ketoacidosis has been linked to metabolic and acid–base fetal anomalies in sheep and alterations in fetoplacental unit perfusion (Gomez et al. 2015). Moreover, the anatomical and functional development of the stomach in kids plays an essential role in acidosis (Krause et al. 2013).

Acidosis is also called lactic acidosis, toxic indigestion, grain engorgement, grain overload, and D-lactic acidosis. Acidosis has two types: metabolic acidosis and respiratory acidosis. The increase in hydrogen ion concentration in the systemic circulation, which results in an unusually low serum bicarbonate level, defines metabolic acidosis. To reduce morbidity and mortality, metabolic acidosis needs to be treated (Arul et al. 2019). Ruminal acidosis is lethal in severe conditions and the goat may die within 24 hours if untreated (Weaver et al. 2021). Ventilation problems and carbon dioxide build-up are the usual causes of respiratory acidity. The primary disturbance is an elevated arterial partial pressure of carbon dioxide (pCO_2) and a decreased ratio of arterial bicarbonate to arterial pCO_2, which results in a decline in the pH of the blood (Gallo de Moraes and Surani 2019). Weaning newborns from the doe is another factor requiring attention in managing acidosis.

This chapter discusses the lack of knowledge on acidosis, especially in kids, and provides general guidelines for treating the condition.

48.2 Subacute Ruminal Acidosis

Subacute ruminal acidosis (SARA) negatively impacts the dairy industry by decreasing dry matter intake, milk production, and profitability, and increasing culling rate and mortality (McCann et al. 2016). Subacute ruminal acidosis is commonly defined as a recurring prolonged period of depression of the ruminal pH below normal (Li et al. 2014). In this condition, excessive accumulation of volatile fatty acids (VFAs) will occur without persistent lactic acid

Elements of Reproduction and Reproductive Diseases of Goats, First Edition. Edited by Tanmoy Rana.

accumulation. SARA can be exhibited in goats through indigestion or suspended feed intake, watery to semisolid feces with bubbles, hoof abnormalities, laminitis, and excessive tail twitching (Lettat et al. 2010). Unexplained diarrhea is consistent in all cases of SARA (He et al. 2022). SARA is associated with other metabolic diseases such as rumenitis, fat milk depression, laminitis, liver abscesses, and a shift in the shape and abundance of the ruminal microbiome (Elmhadi et al. 2022). The perianal region is stained with feces, and fiber or undigested materials will be present in feces, especially in adult goats (Hernandez et al. 2014). A history of carbohydrate ingestion and clinical signs can quickly diagnose SARA.

Subacute ruminal acidosis can be managed by removing the causative agents and providing oral buffer solutions and probiotics. Daily water intake is essential management practice for preventing SARA in kids and adult goats. Reduced water consumption leads to reduced forage intake, leaving goats to eat more grain, contributing to the potential for SARA. Heat stress is also a possible factor contributing to SARA. SARA will reduce milk production in lactating goats and, simultaneously, perinatal losses in kids (Dong et al. 2013).

48.3 Etiology

The condition is more commonly known as "grain overload" but wheat, grains, apples, grapes, sugar beets, and potatoes have also been linked. Acidosis in the newborn kid is affected by several etiological agents. An abnormally acidic environment, rumen acidosis, within ruminants' stomach arises from excessive consumption of highly digestible carbohydrates (Braun et al. 1992). Cereal grains like oats, wheat, and barley, particularly fine ground, are common feedstuffs causing complications (He et al. 2022).

Rumen acidosis is most commonly seen in goats on forage-based diets which abruptly acquire access to a significant quantity of highly fermentable concentrates. It may also happen if the feeding of concentrates is raised significantly or access is temporarily prohibited before being restored. Ration mixing error is also crucial for developing digestive tract disorders in goats. Accidental ingestion of human leftovers with high carbohydrate concentration could be a prime cause of acidosis in goat kids.

Acidosis will lead to disturbed acid–base homeostasis and subsequent complications. The traditional Henderson–Hasselbalch approach to acid–base balance indicates that general causes of nonrespiratory (metabolic) acidosis can be divided into three categories based on pathogenesis: excessive loss of base (bicarbonate), accumulation of endogenous or exogenous acid, and combination of both of the above processes. Lactic acid accumulation in the rumen and circulation is a principal cause of acidosis. Of the two isomers of lactate, i.e., D and L, D lactate plays a significant role in developing acidosis (Gianesella et al. 2010). The exact role of D lactate in SARA is not well defined in caprines because many factors drive the catabolism and transformation mechanism (Tremblay et al. 1991). Environmental factors like heat stress and overcrowding influence kid health (Figure 48.1).

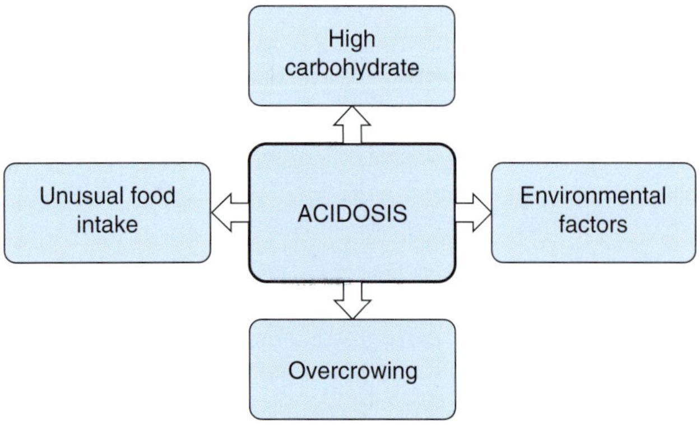

Figure 48.1 Etiology of acidosis in the goat. *Source:* Ankit S. Prajapati.

48.4 Predisposing Factors

48.4.1 Anatomy and Physiology

The development of juvenile ruminant rumens is critical to host health and nutrition. One of the essential functions of the ruminal microbial ecology in ruminants is to produce different enzymes that break down plant polymers and ferment the released sugars into VFAs (Krause et al. 2013). VFAs (primarily butyrate and propionate) are chemical stimulants for the growth of the rumen epithelium and papillae, stimulating structural development and absorption activity and supplying energy to the host. Furthermore, the rumen epithelium acts as a barrier between the host and the rumen environment, and epithelial cells are central to identifying the rumen microbiota (Molinari and Goicoechea 1993).

When a goat kid is born, its rumen, reticulum, and omasum are all extremely small. Instead of ingesting solid meals, the kid gets its nutrition from milk which travels directly to the abomasum via the esophageal groove. When a kid swallows, a flap of skin at the rumen's entrance folds over to form a groove, bypassing the rumen and sending the milk directly to the abomasum to be digested by stomach acid. As a kid grows older, it attempts to swallow roughage. The rumen becomes active and expands. At the same time, the microorganism population also increases. The reticulum and omasum also grow in response to dietary changes. When the kid becomes an adult, roughage is its primary source of nutrition and its rumen is much bigger than its abomasum. The anatomical, functional, and microbial aspects create an integrated system, and it is essential to study them together for a better understanding of the process of rumen development (Jiao et al. 2015; Abdelsattar et al. 2021).

48.4.2 Diet Management

Dietary management is the prime method of acidosis prevention. Misfeeding of highly fermentable carbs, inadequate fiber feeding, bad management techniques, or a combination of the three is a crucial aspect to look for (Taghipoor et al. 2020). Goats and kids are primarily reared in a free-range system and have a history of ingesting large amounts of highly fermentable carbohydrates such as wheat grain, stale chapattis, roti, stale rice, mangoes, bananas, vegetable waste, ceremonial waste, vegetable market waste, hotel waste, feed with an excessive amount of jowar grains, corn, and wheat flour. These goats develop ruminal acidosis, resulting in heavy economic losses due to high morbidity.

Notably, kids below three years of age require special attention in diet management.

48.4.3 Weaning

The development of microflora and its role in the metabolization of lactic acid are essential. Weaning newborn kids has some effect on the development of rumen flora. Newborn kids are usually separated from their dams after birth and fed on milk replacers. This lack of contact with adult animals may hinder the rumen's microbiological and physiological development (Palma-Hidalgo et al. 2021). Weaning ruminants in natural conditions is a progressive process between six and nine months of age. It is characterized by a drop in the frequency of suckling, with an increase in the frequency and amount of solid feed intake and the development of more complex social interactions. Early weaning of kids may lead to a higher occurrence of acidosis.

48.5 Pathogenesis

Three forms of acidosis have been reported in goats: mild, moderate, and severe. The condition's form and severity mainly depend on carbohydrate ingestion quantity (Bayne and Edmondson 2021). When highly fermented carbohydrate is eaten by a kid or goat, it will lead to the proliferation of *Streptococcus bovis* in the rumen within 4–6 hours. *S. bovis* is the most prominent bacterium in the rumen and plays an important role in acidosis (Chen et al. 2016). *S. bovis* starts producing lactic acid in the rumen, reducing the rumen pH below 5.5. The digestive microflora will also be disturbed (Chen et al. 2021). Simultaneously, histamine release occurs, leading to laminitis in kids. Metabolism of the carbohydrate leads to excessive production of VFAs in the rumen (Aslan et al. 1995).

The low rumen pH allows *Lactobacillus* bacteria to grow, further degrading the carbohydrate and producing more lactic acid. Two isomers of lactic acid are reported: D lactate and L lactate (Bleul et al. 2006). Rumen osmolality is also noticeable along with lactic acid production. Because of this, fluids from the circulation drain into the rumen and dehydration occurs. Lactic acid will further decrease the rumen motility in adult goats, and thereby gas production will occur. Lactic acid circulates in the blood and L lactate is rapidly metabolized and D lactate is slowly metabolized (Dunlop 1972). Hence, this condition is also called D-lactic acidosis. Lower ruminal pH also favors the growth of other harmful organisms like *Mucor* and *Rhizopus* (Fliegerova et al. 2021).

The general causes of nonrespiratory (metabolic) acidosis can be divided into two categories: strong ion acidosis due to a decrease in solid cation concentration (hyponatremia) or an increase in intense anion concentration (hyperchloremia, hyper L-lactatemia, hyper D-lactatemia, ketoacidosis), and nonvolatile buffer ion acidosis due to an increase in albumin, globulin, and phosphate concentration. Metabolic acidosis without dehydration, probably due to hyper-D-lactatemia, has been described in neonatal goat kids (Tremblay et al. 1991).

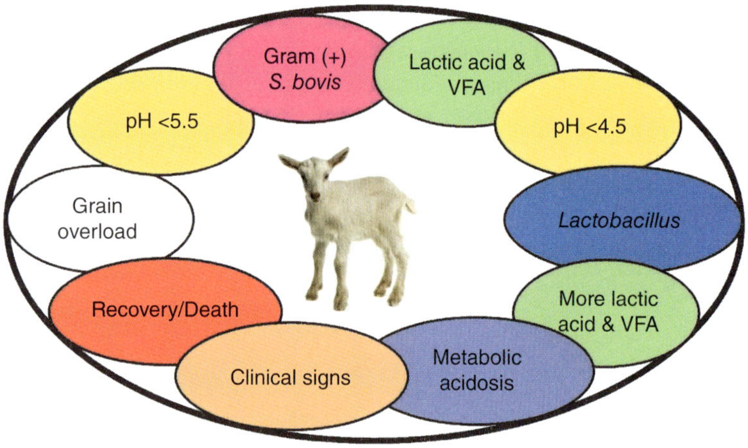

Figure 48.2 Pathogenesis of acidosis. *Source:* Ankit S. Prajapati (chapter contributor).

Metabolic acidosis occurs in the newborn if parturition is prolonged and difficult (Andrade et al. 2019). It is also common in shock with peripheral circulatory failure and anaerobic oxidation. Dehydration, impaired tissue perfusion, and an overwhelming delivery of inflammatory mediators and endotoxins to the liver can result in increased liver and muscle enzymes, depending on the severity of the disease. A decrease in renal excretion of acid in renal insufficiency or renal failure also contributes to metabolic acidosis. The illustration of pathogenesis is shown in Figure 48.2.

Respiratory acidosis occurs when there is retention of CO_2 in the blood due to interference with a regular respiratory exchange. Thus pneumonia, severe pulmonary emphysema, depression of the respiratory center, and left-sided heart failure may all be accompanied by respiratory acidosis.

48.6 Clinical Signs

Clinical signs are an essential aspect of any disease condition. Because severe acidemia inhibits cellular and organ function, it is linked with an elevated risk of death in severely sick animals. In the mild form of acidosis, no obvious clinical signs are evident. However, restlessness and a reduction in feed intake can be observed.

Clinical signs appear within 12–36 hours in moderate and severe acidosis. Clinical signs including temperature, heart rate, mucous membrane condition, rumen motility, rumen consistency, oral cavity examination, rectal examination, abdomen contour, and venous stasis test are significant physical examination features (Bleul et al. 2006). The rectal temperature is slightly lower in most cases but not as low as in hypothermia. A secondary bacterial infection might sometimes affect this trait, and an elevation in temperature may be noticed (Underwood et al. 2015). The heart rate is another vital parameter and is above average per minute in the affected kid. The mucous membrane is normal to congested, depending upon the condition. Rumen motility and consistency are vital signs for acidosis in adult ruminants but are not reliable indicators in kids. Abdominal contour is a sure sign of involvement of the gastrointestinal tract. Enlargement of the abdomen, particularly on the left side, is noted. Physical examination of the left paralumbar fossa gives a better idea regarding the consistency and contour of the abdomen.

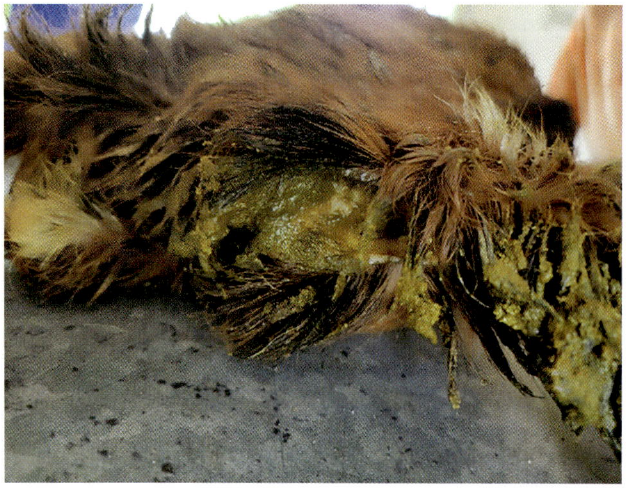

Figure 48.3 Kid with diarrhea. *Source:* Ankit S. Prajapati (chapter contributor).

Other reported clinical signs may include lack of appetite, bloat, absence of rumination (chewing cud), dehydration, watery feces, depressed mentation, incoordination, collapse, and in severe cases death (Braun et al. 1992). Inappetence to anorexia may be seen depending upon the severity of acidosis. Diarrhea will be noticed which is a good prognostic indicator for kid survival (Figure 48.3). The absence of feces is a poor indicator in acidosis cases.

Teeth grinding is seen in almost one-quarter of acidosis cases in goats and sheep. Shallow respiration, staggering gait, drunken behavior, incoordination, dullness, depression, and sternal recumbency are other signs to look for. Visual impairment is noted in severe cases. Lactic acidosis has been attributed to hematological alterations such as increased erythrocytes, leukocytes, hemoglobin content, and packed cell volume.

In comparison, biochemical changes include decreased total protein, hyperglycemia, hyponatremia, hyperkalemia, hypocalcemia, and increased AST, ALT, urea nitrogen, creatinine level, and serum lactic acid (Cao et al. 1987; Trefz et al. 2017). Dehydration status can be assessed by muzzle examination, skinfold test, sunken eyeballs, urine output, and by measuring the packed cell volume (PCV). Prognosis is poor to grave in kids with absence of feces, heart rate more than 100/minute, lateral recumbency with reduced reflexes, dilated pupil, and oral respiration (Figure 48.4).

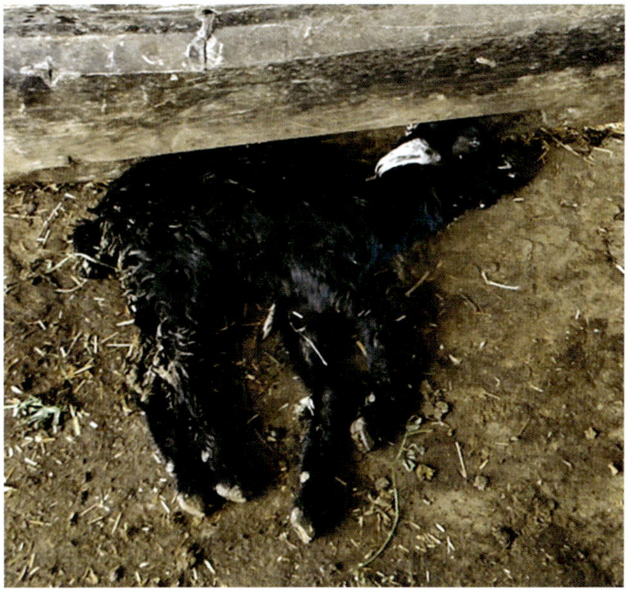

Figure 48.4 Death of kid due to severe acidosis. *Source:* Ankit S. Prajapati (chapter contributor).

48.7 Diagnosis

The diagnosis is usually apparent based on history, clinical signs, and rumen fluid examination (David et al. 2000). History of ingesting unusual food and involvement of multiple animals simultaneously indicate acidosis. Assessment of rumen fluid should be carried out in suspected cases of ruminal acidosis. Rumen fluid can be collected using a stomach tube of appropriate size or probang with fluid collection assembly. A mouth gauge should be used during the procedure to avoid injury, particularly in adult goats. Rumen fluid is milky colored and foul smelling with an acidic odor, and has a lower pH (below 5.5). Commercially available pH paper can be used but for precise measurement, a pH meter can be considered. Direct examination of protozoal motility immediately after fluid collection can be done under a microscope and helps to determine severity. Commercial microscopes are available at low cost to evaluate prozotoa under field conditions. Protozoa numbers and types are markedly reduced with poor to no motility.

In most cases, methylene blue reduction time is prolonged significantly (>9 minutes). The Gram staining method is most helpful in differentiating positive and negative bacteria. The average 60:40 ratio of Gram-negative to Gram-positive bacteria is altered with a predominance of Gram-positive rods (*Lactobacillus* spp.). Rumen lactic acid concentration is increased (Braun et al. 1992).

Clinicopathological laboratory data include hemoconcentration with increased PCV (up to 50–60%) and total protein, prerenal azotemia, and metabolic acidosis, characterized as low blood pH, low blood bicarbonate concentration, and negative base excess. Blood lactate and inorganic phosphorus levels will increase (Bleul et al. 2006). Hypocalcemia may be evident in some cases due to malabsorption. Renal compensation produces acidic urine after 12 hours, increasing urine-specific gravity (Cao et al. 1987). The urine pH will change toward acidic and urine will become concentrated. Changes in the leukogram and acute-phase proteins reflect an acute inflammatory response, ranging from normal to a degenerative left shift and increases in haptoglobin, ceruloplasmin, and reduced albumin concentration (Minuti et al. 2014).

Acidosis must be differentiated from simple indigestion, peritonitis, septicemia, and enterotoxemia.

48.8 Treatment

Therapeutic management is crucial to any disease condition (Kinde and Asfaw 2021). Removal of the causative agent will help and rumen emptying by stomach tube can be tried. Correction of ruminal and systemic acidosis is a prime goal in treatment by restoring fluid and electrolyte loss. Fluid therapy should be given according to the hydration status of the kid (Figure 48.5). Systemic acidosis can be managed by administering 5% sodium bicarbonate intravenously diluted in normal

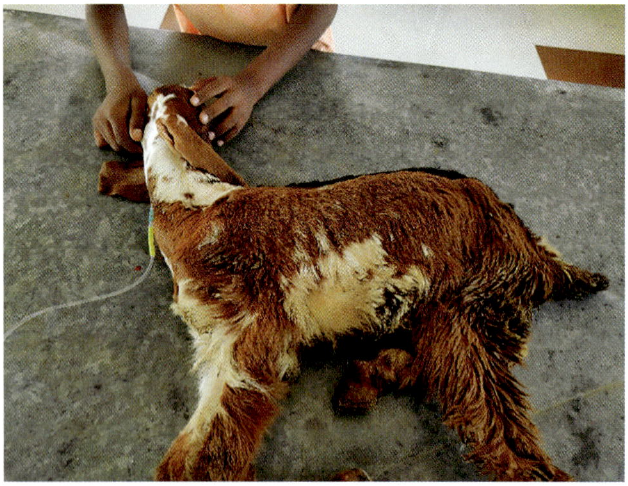

Figure 48.5 Therapeutic management of acidosis by fluid administration in kids. *Source:* Ankit S. Prajapati (chapter contributor).

saline over 30 minutes. Rumen lavage can be tried. In severe cases, warm water is pumped until the left paralumbar fossa is distended, and the rumen is allowed to empty by gravitational force. Alkalinizing agents like magnesium oxide can be used orally to correct ruminal acidosis.

Buffers such as magnesium hydroxide are often desirable to increase rumen pH and provide a proper environment for survival of normal rumen microflora. Antihistaminic preparation should be given to combat the histamine release. B-complex and supportive therapy should be done to support vital activities during and after treatment. Oral antibiotics, such as penicillin and thiamine (vitamin B_1), can be given to minimize secondary bacterial infection. Antacids should be tried in severe cases of acidosis. Beneficial bacteria in the digestive tract will be reduced in an acidic environment so kids should receive oral probiotics to keep the tract healthy. Cud transplantation with rumen fluid collected from a healthy donor can be used effectively in adult goats.

Diagnosis of acidosis is easy for the clinician but high mortality is noted in acidosis cases, due to underdosing of sodium bicarbonate. So, a reasonable dose rate must be calculated to avoid the kid's death. As a rule of thumb, 1 ml sodium bicarbonate per kilogram body weight should be given in moderate acidosis, and 2–3 ml sodium bicarbonate per kilogram body weight in severe acidosis.

48.9 Complications

Acidosis in a kid can be fatal. Acidosis in kids sometimes leads to further complications, which might cause treatment failure. Since ruminal acidosis can be fatal and is associated with other common diseases, including enterotoxemia (overeating disease), B_1 deficiency (polio), urinary tract calculi, laminitis, and liver abscesses, preventing this condition is critical to reducing losses. Floppy kid syndrome is one of the possible complications in which muscle weakness and depression are evident, along with acidosis.

48.10 Preventive Measures

Prevention is better than cure. Keeping rumen development in mind, a concentrate diet must be introduced slowly and gradually. This will allow the rumen microflora to adjust to the new environment, reducing the incidence of acidosis. Dietary modifications from a lower fermentable energy concentration to a greater one should be made gradually, preferably over 2–3 weeks. Young kids can be supplemented with whole-shelled corn feed labeled for goats at 0.5–1% of body weight per day (14–12 lb of corn per head per day for a 50 lb animal). If goats are fed a high-concentrate diet, grain feedings should be divided into three or more daily meals. Human leftovers must be kept away from the kid population to avoid the chance of accidentally ingesting carbohydrates. Overcrowding should be minimized to prevent cases of respiratory acidosis. Any stress and overfeeding should be reduced with proper water consumption to prevent acidosis in kids.

48.11 Conclusion

Improper feeding practices cause acidosis. It is suggested that animals should avoid unnecessary or accidental feeding of immature leaves, paddy grains, cabbage, leafy vegetables, boiled rice, and ceremonial waste. The treatment employed for ruminal acidosis in goats is very effective. Buffer supplementation should be provided to kids as per requirement. Future studies should focus on microbial changes in the kid rumen for better understanding and reduced acidosis occurrence. Animal welfare and production are improved by preventing ruminal acidosis.

References

Abdelsattar, M., Zhuang, Y., Cui, K. et al. (2021). Predicting the digestive tract development and growth performance of goat kids using sigmoidal models. *Animals* 11 (3): 757.

Andrade, I.M., Simoes, P.B.A., Lamas, L.P. et al. (2019). Blood lactate, pH, base excess and pCO_2 as prognostic indicators in caesarean-born kids from goats with pregnancy toxaemia. *Irish Veterinary Journal* 72: 10.

Arul, G.S., Singh, M., Ali, A.M., and Gee, O.J. (2019). Damage control surgery in neonates: lessons learned from the battlefield. *Journal of Pediatric Surgery* 54 (10): 2069–2074.

Aslan, V., Thamsborg, S.M., Jorgensen, R.J., and Basse, A. (1995). Induced acute ruminal acidosis in goats treated with yeast (Saccharomyces cerevisiae) and bicarbonate. *Acta Veterinaria Scandinavica* 36 (1): 65–77.

Bayne, J.E. and Edmondson, M.A. (2021). Diseases of the gastrointestinal system. *Sheep, Goat, and Cervid Medicine* 63–96.

Bleul, U., Schwantag, S., Stocker, H. et al. (2006). Floppy kid syndrome caused by D-lactic acidosis in goat kids. *Journal of Veterinary Internal Medicine* 20 (4): 1003–1008.

Brahma, J., Sarma, M., Scientist, J. et al. (2020). Rumen acidosis in goats under agro-climatic conditions of Assam. *Journal of Entomology and Zoology Studies* 8 (2): 1631–1633.

Braun, U., Rihs, T., and Schefer, U. (1992). Ruminal lactic acidosis in sheep and goats. *Veterinary Record* 130 (16): 343–349.

Cao, G.R., English, P.B., Filippich, L.J., and Inglis, S. (1987). Experimentally induced lactic acidosis in the goat. *Australian Veterinary Journal* 64 (12): 367–370.

Chen, L., Luo, Y., Wang, H. et al. (2016). Effects of glucose and starch on lactate production by newly isolated Streptococcus bovis S1 from Saanen goats. *Applied and Environmental Microbiology* 82 (19): 5982–5989.

Chen, X., Su, X., Li, J. et al. (2021). Real-time monitoring of ruminal microbiota reveals their roles in dairy goats during subacute ruminal acidosis. *NPJ Biofilms and Microbiomes* 7 (1): 45.

David, C., Jeff, W., Tyler, S., and Stehman, M. (2000). Diagnosis of enteric disease in small ruminants. *Veterinary Clinics of North America: Food Animal Practice* 16 (1): 87–115.

Dong, H., Wang, S., Jia, Y. et al. (2013). Long-term effects of subacute ruminal acidosis (SARA) on milk quality and hepatic gene expression in lactating goats fed a high-concentrate diet. *PLoS One* 8 (12): 82850.

Dunlop, R.H. (1972). Pathogenesis of ruminant lactic acidosis. *Advances in Veterinary Science and Comparative Medicine* 16: 259–302.

Elmhadi, M.E., Ali, D.K., Khogali, M.K., and Wang, H. (2022). Subacute ruminal acidosis in dairy herds: microbiological and nutritional causes, consequences, and prevention strategies. *Animal Nutrition (Zhongguo xu mu shou yi xue hui)* 10: 148–155.

Fliegerova, K.O., Podmirseg, S.M., Vinzelj, J. et al. (2021). The effect of a high-grain diet on the rumen microbiome of goats with a special focus on anaerobic fungi. *Microorganisms* 9 (1): 157.

Gallo de Moraes, A. and Surani, S. (2019). Effects of diabetic ketoacidosis in the respiratory system. *World Journal of Diabetes* 10 (1): 16–22.

Gianesella, M., Morgante, M., Cannizzo, C. et al. (2010). Subacute ruminal acidosis and evaluation of blood gas analysis in dairy cow. *Veterinary Medicine International* 2010: 392371.

Gomez, D.E., Kuthiala, S., Liu, H.L. et al. (2015). Effect of maternal ketoacidosis on the ovine fetus. *Canadian Veterinary Journal* 56 (8): 863–866.

Gomez, D.E., Bedford, S., Darby, S. et al. (2020). Acid–base disorders in sick goats and their association with mortality: a simplified strong ion difference approach. *Journal of Veterinary Internal Medicine* 34 (6): 2776–2786.

He, B., Fan, Y., and Wang, H. (2022). Lactate uptake in the rumen and its contributions to subacute rumen acidosis of goats induced by high-grain diets. *Frontiers in Veterinary Science* 9: 964027.

Hernandez, J., Benedito, J.L., Abuelo, A., and Castillo, C. (2014). Ruminal acidosis in feedlot: from aetiology to prevention. *Scientific World Journal* 2014: 702572.

Jiao, J., Li, X., Beauchemin, K.A. et al. (2015). Rumen development process in goats as affected by supplemental feeding v. grazing: age-related anatomic development, functional achievement and microbial colonisation. *British Journal of Nutrition* 113 (6): 888–900.

Kinde, M.Z. and Asfaw, E. (2021). Assessment of ruminal disorders and their therapeutic management at three veterinary clinics in Gondar town, North Western Ethiopia: a retrospective study. *Veterinary Medicine* 12: 7–13.

Krause, D.O., Nagaraja, T.G., Wright, A.D., and Callaway, T.R. (2013). Board-invited review: rumen microbiology: leading the way in microbial ecology. *Journal of Animal Science* 91 (1): 331–341.

Lettat, A., Nozière, P., Silberberg, M. et al. (2010). Experimental feed induction of ruminal lactic, propionic, or butyric acidosis in sheep. *Journal of Animal Science* 88 (9): 3041–3046.

Li, F., Cao, Y., Liu, N. et al. (2014). Subacute ruminal acidosis challenge changed in situ degradability of feedstuffs in dairy goats. *Journal of Dairy Science* 97 (8): 5101–5109.

McCann, J.C., Luan, S., Cardoso, F.C. et al. (2016). Induction of subacute ruminal acidosis affects the ruminal microbiome and epithelium. *Frontiers in Microbiology* 7: 701.

Minuti, A., Ahmed, S., Trevisi, E. et al. (2014). Experimental acute rumen acidosis in sheep: consequences on clinical, rumen, and gastrointestinal permeability conditions and blood chemistry. *Journal of Animal Science* 92 (9): 3966–3977.

Molinari, E. and Goicoechea, O. (1993). Anatomía del desarrollo del tracto digestivo y forma corporal externa durante el período embrionario en el caprino (Capra hircus) [Anatomy of the development of the digestive tract and shape of the external body during the embryonic period of the goat (Capra hircus)]. *Anatomia, Histologia, Embryologia* 22 (2): 123–143.

Palma-Hidalgo, J.M., Yaiez-Ruiz, D.R., Jimenez, E. et al. (2021). Presence of adult companion goats favors the rumen microbial and functional development in artificially reared kids. *Frontiers in Veterinary Science* 8: 706592.

Taghipoor, M., Delattre, M., and Giger-Reverdin, S. (2020). A novel modelling approach to quantify the response of dairy goats to a high-concentrate diet. *Scientific Reports* 10 (1): 20376.

Trefz, F.M., Lorenz, I., Lorch, A., and Constable, P.D. (2017). Clinical signs, profound acidemia, hypoglycemia, and hypernatremia are predictive of mortality in 1,400 critically ill neonatal calves with diarrhea. *PLoS One* 12 (8): 0182938.

Tremblay, R.R., Butler, D.G., Allen, J.W., and Hoffman, A.M. (1991). Metabolic acidosis without dehydration in seven goat kids. *Canadian Veterinary Journal* 32 (5): 308–310.

Underwood, W.J., Blauwiekel, R., Delano, M.L. et al. (2015). Biology and diseases of ruminants (sheep, goats, and cattle). *Laboratory Animal Medicine* 623–694.

Weaver, L.F., Boileau, M.J., Gilliam, L.L., and Taylor, J.D. (2021). Characterizing short- and long-term morbidity and mortality of goat kids born to does with pregnancy toxemia. *Journal of Veterinary Internal Medicine* 35 (2): 1155–1163.

49

Urolithiasis

Antonio Carlos Lopes Câmara[1] and Benito Soto-Blanco[2]

[1] *Large Animal Veterinary Teaching Hospital, Universidade de Brasília, Brasília, Brazil*
[2] *Department of Veterinary Clinics and Surgery, Veterinary School, Universidade Federal de Minas Gerais, Belo Horizonte, Brazil*

49.1 Introduction

Urolithiasis is characterized by the deposition of uroliths (also known as calculi or stones) in the urinary tract. This condition is named obstructive urolithiasis in cases of obstruction of urine flow through the urethra by uroliths. Obstructive urolithiasis is the most frequent condition affecting goats' urinary tract. Usually, the etiology is linked to inadequate management practices (Dória et al. 2007; Riet-Correa et al. 2008; Janke et al. 2009; Matthews 2016; Constable et al. 2017; Harwood and Mueller 2018; Stewart and Shipley 2021; Sickinger and Windhorst 2022). Goats raised as pets are at the highest risk for developing urolithiasis because the owners typically are not well instructed about adequate management, including correct feeding, age at castration, and general husbandry practices (Scully 2021).

49.2 Etiology

Uroliths are formed of several pure or mixed compounds, mainly magnesium calcium phosphate, struvite (magnesium ammonium phosphate), magnesium potassium phosphate, calcium phosphate (apatite), and calcium carbonate (Sun et al. 2010a,b; Jones et al. 2017). Obstructive urolithiasis is a condition that affects almost exclusively males. This difference is due to the anatomical conformation of the male urethra, which favors the deposition of uroliths (Constable et al. 2017; Scully 2021; Jones et al. 2012, 2015). The deposits of uroliths that obstruct the urethra usually occur in the distal sigmoid flexure and ischial curvature (Ewoldt et al. 2008; Guimarães et al. 2012; Riedi et al. 2018). Obstructive urolithiasis has the highest frequency in castrated males, especially those castrated early. Testosterone levels influence the development of the male urethra. Goats castrated before complete maturation of the urethra present a reduced urethral diameter due to insufficient testosterone-stimulated development (Scully 2021; Videla and van Amstel 2016). One case of urolithiasis due to hereditary xanthinuria occurred in a goat that presented xanthine dehydrogenase and molybdenum cofactor sulfurase variants at exome sequencing (Vail et al. 2019).

Several dietary factors can contribute to urolith formation and predispose the goat to obstructive urolithiasis. The most critical is the high content of calcium (Ca), magnesium (Mg), and phosphorus (P) in the diet, notably if the Ca:P ratio is altered (Matthews 2016; Constable et al. 2017; Harwood and Mueller 2018; Sickinger and Windhorst 2022; Scully 2021). These diets increase serum levels of phosphates with consequent increased urinary elimination. Diets with Ca:P ratios of 1.5:1 to 2:1 are less likely to predispose to urolithiasis. On the other hand, decreasing the Ca:P ratio increases the risk of this condition. When feeding for long periods with rations with Ca:P ratio of 1:1 to 0.5:1, the formation of uroliths is increased. Grains and their byproducts are mainly responsible for the occurrence of urolithiasis in confined goats due to their content of about 0.02–0.1% Ca and 0.2–0.4% P (Riet-Correa et al. 2008). The consumption of alfalfa-based diets predisposes goats to calcium carbonate urolithiasis due to a Ca:P ratio higher than 3:1 (Jones et al. 2018).

The amount of food ingested daily and the feeding period are important risk factors for urolithiasis. The formation of uroliths in the urine begins after the animals ingest feed equivalent to 1.5% of their live weight. Urolithiasis is frequent

Elements of Reproduction and Reproductive Diseases of Goats, First Edition. Edited by Tanmoy Rana.

when they ingest 2.5% of their live weight for longer than two months. Concentrated foods with high concentrations of Mg increase the risk of urolithiasis (Sacco and Lopes 2011; Pan et al. 2011; Ferreira et al. 2015). Administration of mineral supplements containing P and Mg to concentrate-fed goats further increases the risk of urolithiasis (Riet-Correa et al. 2008; Sun et al. 2010b; Wang et al. 2009; Riet-Correa 2010). It has been observed in sheep that feeding large amounts of feed, administered at once, causes a momentary reduction in the volume of urine and an increase in the concentration and excretion of Ca, favoring the formation of uroliths (Riet-Correa et al. 2008). It is possible that this effect could also occur in goats.

Nondietary factors predisposing to urolith formation include urine stasis, increased density, pH, mineral excretion, desquamated epithelial cells, mucoproteins, and urinary tract infections (Matthews 2016; Jones et al. 2012). Urine density may be augmented due to increased renal reabsorption of water in response to reduced water consumption, dehydration, or high environmental temperatures. This change in urine density results in a higher concentration of P, which predisposes to the precipitation of phosphates. Alkaline urine also favors the formation of phosphate precipitates. Increased concentrations of urinary mucoproteins may favor urolith formation because they form the organic matrix for depositing minerals. This increased urinary mucoprotein may occur after feeding goats with pelleted concentrates. Goats grassing pastures with excessive content of oxalate, silica, or calcium may also develop urolithiasis. Another factor that predisposes urolith formation is increased epithelial desquamation, as observed in cases of vitamin A deficiency (Riet-Correa et al. 2008; Matthews 2016; Scully 2021; Lemos and Silveira 2008).

Goats of African breeds usually have more chance of developing calcium carbonate uroliths than Anglo-Nubian, Nubian, and Toggenburg breeds. Animals older than one year are more likely to form calcium carbonate uroliths, but younger animals can be affected by other types of uroliths (Nwaokorie et al. 2015).

49.3 Clinical Signs

The first clinical signs of urolithiasis are nonspecific, including isolation from the flock, inappetence or anorexia, apathy, intermittent recumbency with restlessness, tachycardia, tachypnea, dehydration, congested ocular mucosa, hyperthermia, and rumen hypomotility or atony. Affected animals will then adopt a micturition posture with a broad base and stretched hindlimbs as a sign of abdominal discomfort (Constable et al. 2017; Harwood and Mueller 2018; Scully 2021; Riedi et al. 2018). The clinical signs of pain that may be observed are hitting the abdomen, curving the back, jerking, moaning, bruxism, vocalization, penile foreskin sensitivity to the touch, and rapid movements with tail lifting (Scully 2021; Guimarães et al. 2012; Riedi et al. 2018; Videla and van Amstel 2016). Other clinical signs that goats may show are repeated contractions of the abdomen at micturition, movements of the preputial foreskin, and spasmodic contractions of the penis. Efforts to urinate despite the obstruction may result in production of a tiny amount of reddish urine (due to hematuria) and, in some cases, rectal prolapse (Scully 2021; Maciel et al. 2017). In some goats, the distended urinary bladder can be determined by palpation of the abdomen (Videla and van Amstel 2016). The advanced stage of obstructive urolithiasis may present no abdominal discomfort (Riedi et al. 2018) that can lead to rupture of the urethra or bladder (Guimarães et al. 2012; Kannan and Lawrence 2010).

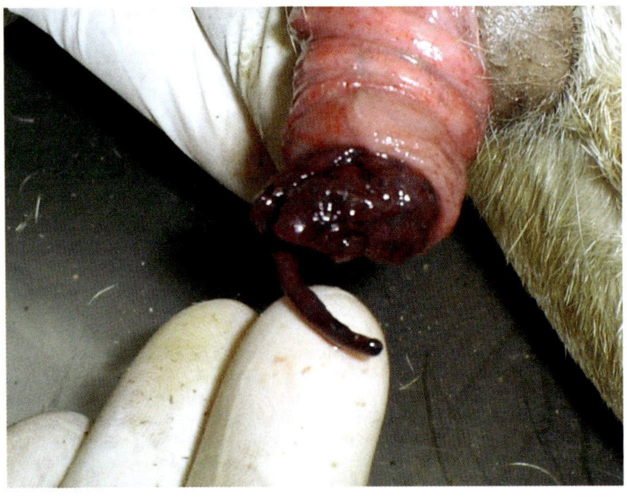

Figure 49.1 Penis showing necrosis of the urethral process and glans due to obstructive urolithiasis. *Source:* Rana (book author).

When possible, the penis should be exteriorized during a physical examination. Several methods can be used to exteriorize the penis. After placing the goat in a sitting position, mechanically or with sedation, infuse 3 ml of 2% lidocaine solution in the preputial orifice to desensitize the penis foreskin and glans. In order to expose the preputial mucosa, the sigmoid flexure is pushed cranially and the preputial skin is pulled caudally (Guimarães et al. 2012; Videla and van Amstel 2016). In cases involving the urethral process or the glans, congestion, cyanosis, or necrosis are usually seen (Figure 49.1) (Guimarães et al. 2012).

Sedation may be required in some cases for manipulation of the penis. For these cases, the administration of diazepam (0.1–0.3 mg/kg, intravenously) provides an anxiolytic effect with urethral relaxation. Alternatively, acepromazine (0.05–0.1 mg/kg intravenously) or xylazine (0.05–0.1 mg/kg intravenously) can be administered, but they may cause hypotension as a side-effect. Furthermore, xylazine is contraindicated in cases of obstruction because of its diuretic effect (Videla and van Amstel 2016).

49.4 Diagnosis

Clinicians make a presumptive diagnosis by combining clinical signs with epidemiological data, including goat management and feeding practices. The first clinical signs should be differentiated from constipation in the early stages (Constable et al. 2017; Harwood and Mueller 2018; Scully 2021) because treatment initiated before complete urethral obstruction improves recovery (Riedi et al. 2018). The obstruction can be visualized by imaging tests, surgery, or necropsy to confirm the diagnosis. Clinical severity and prognosis can be assessed by serum urea and creatinine levels.

49.4.1 Diagnostic Tests

As many cases of urolithiasis lead to urethritis, cystitis, and acute kidney infection, hematological examination frequently reveals leukocytosis with neutrophilia and hyperfibrinogenemia (Guimarães et al. 2012). Serum levels of urea and creatinine are commonly elevated, primarily due to urinary obstruction (Guimarães et al. 2012; Riedi et al. 2018; George et al. 2007). Increased serum activities of gamma-glutamyl transferase (GGT) are associated with hepatic lipolysis after prolonged anorexia. Serum activities of creatine kinase (CK) can also be increased due to increased muscle activity, frequent abdominal contractions, cellulitis, and necrosis in cases of urethral rupture. Other serum biochemical changes that may be observed include hyperphosphatemia, hypocalcemia, hypermagnesemia, hyponatremia, and hypochloremia (Riedi et al. 2018; Maciel et al. 2017; George et al. 2007).

Urine may be collected for urinalysis by urethral process resection, cystocentesis, or laparotomy. The main physicochemical changes are hematuria (reddish color), cloudy appearance, increased density, proteinuria, glycosuria, and aciduria (Guimarães et al. 2012). Inspection of urine sediment shows an increased number of erythrocytes, leukocytes, epithelial cells, bacteria, crystals, and mucus (Maciel et al. 2017). Hemorrhages due to lesions on the urinary tract mucosa caused by uroliths are responsible for hematuria and the cloudy appearance of urine (Lemos and Silveira 2008). Proteinuria and aciduria can be attributed to diets with protein-rich grains or concomitant glomerulonephritis, pyelonephritis, interstitial nephritis, or hydronephrosis (Riet-Correa et al. 2008; Guimarães et al. 2012).

Imaging tests, such as urethral endoscopy (Halland et al. 2002), ultrasonography (Scully 2021; Videla and van Amstel 2016; Tharwat 2021), radiography (Kannan and Lawrence 2010; Palmer et al. 1998; Kinsley et al. 2013), and computed tomography (Stieger-Vanegas et al. 2022), can verify the presence of uroliths in the urethra, ureter, urinary bladder, or kidneys, helping to define diagnosis and prognosis. Transabdominal ultrasound with a 3.5 or 5 MHz transducer can be used for evaluating the urethra, bladder, and kidneys, to search for uroliths, and for identification of free fluid in the abdomen (Scully 2021; Videla and van Amstel 2016; Tharwat 2021). The urinary bladder wall, under ultrasonographic examination, appears as a hyperechoic circle; edema in this structure is seen as an enlarged white line (Riedi et al. 2018). The right kidney can show hydroureters and hydronephrosis, characterized by dilation and fluid accumulation in the renal pelvis. These changes can be caused by continuous urinary pressure for 5–7 days (Scully 2021).

Contrast radiography can be performed by retrograde urethrography, cyst urethrography, excretory urography, and urethrocystography via tube cystotomy. This imaging test helps diagnose obstructive urolithiasis in goats (Palmer et al. 1998). Plain radiography, a test less expensive than contrast radiography, can also provide information for the surgical approach and prognosis by locating the obstruction and determining the extent of urethral obstruction. However, this test only detects radiopaque uroliths (calcium carbonate, calcium oxalate, and silicate) (Riedi et al. 2018; Kannan and Lawrence 2010; Kinsley et al. 2013). Urinary bladder rupture may also be identified by radiography (Kannan and Lawrence 2010).

Multidetector computed tomography is an accurate and noninvasive method for diagnosing urolithiasis in goats. The main findings are the presence of uroliths in the urinary bladder and urethra; all kinds of uroliths can be detected. An intact urinary bladder may be observed containing large amounts of urine but in cases of bladder rupture, uroliths are found freely within the abdomen. One or both kidneys may be enlarged with abnormal architecture, and ureters may be distended (Stieger-Vanegas et al. 2022). Unfortunately, computed tomography is not usually available for use in goats because of its high cost.

49.5 Pathology

The most frequent finding at necroscopy examination is diffuse necrotic or hemorrhagic urethritis that may be restricted to the site of obstruction or expanded along the entire length of the urethra after the obstruction. Other common findings are purulent or necrotizing urethritis, urethral rupture, and hydroureters (Guimarães et al. 2012; Riedi et al. 2018; Lemos and Silveira 2008). The most frequent sites of obstruction are the urethral process and distal sigmoid flexure (Scully 2021) (Figure 49.2). Edema and cellulitis with an accumulation of urine may be observed in cases with rupture of the urethra; some cases also present subcutaneous necrosis (Guimarães et al. 2012).

The bladder may show uroliths (Figure 49.3), diffuse hemorrhagic cystitis, purulent cystitis, necrotic foci, and rupture of the ventral wall with hemorrhagic areas in the serosa and adherence to the pelvic cavity. Usually, the uroliths are observed as sand-like sediment but may appear as well-formed stones. Changes observed in the kidneys include pyelonephritis, diffuse nephritis, uroliths in the renal pelvis (Figure 49.4), hydronephrosis, renal abscesses, hemorrhage, and renal rupture.

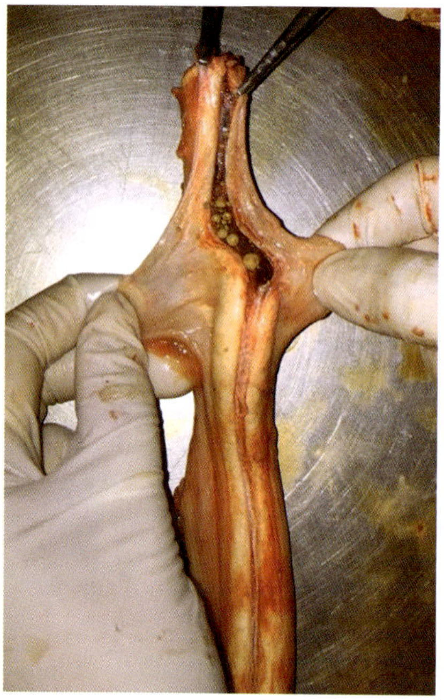

Figure 49.2 Urethra obstructed by uroliths at the sigmoid flexure showing necrotizing urethritis. *Source:* Rana (book author).

49.6 Treatment

The therapy of urolithiasis should start immediately. Treating goats before complete urethral obstruction improves recovery (Riedi et al. 2018). Treating cases of obstructive urolithiasis should start by restoring urinary flow as soon as possible. Supportive measures include the correction of metabolic imbalances using intravenous fluids (Van Metre and Fubini 2006). With adequate treatment, goats with serum potassium <5.2 mEq/l are more likely to survive (Ewoldt et al. 2006).

Struvite uroliths can be dissolved in an acidic solution, whereas Ca uroliths (such as Ca carbonate and apatite) are less likely to dissolve (Videla and van Amstel 2016). In a study evolving 25 goats with obstructive urolithiasis, 20 had the urethral obstruction reverted by ultrasound-guided cystocentesis followed by percutaneous infusion of 50–250 ml Walpole's solution, a buffered acetic acid solution of pH 4.5. However, this method is not a definitive treatment because six of these 20 goats presented a recurrence of the obstruction (Janke et al. 2009).

Obstruction caused by struvite uroliths can be treated by cystocentesis with acidic bladder lavage (Janke et al. 2009), cystostomy with percutaneous Foley

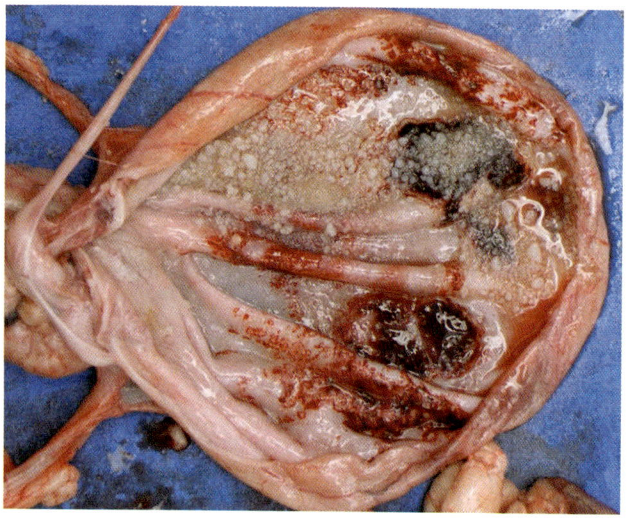

Figure 49.3 Abundant uroliths and hemorrhagic cystitis with necrotic foci in a urinary bladder. *Source:* Rana (book author).

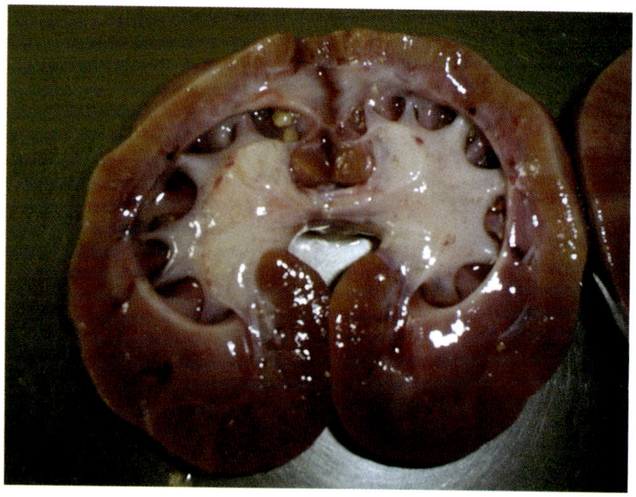

Figure 49.4 Kidney presenting uroliths in the renal pelvis, hydronephrosis, and diffuse nephritis due to urolithiasis. *Source:* Rana (book author).

tube placement (Fazili et al. 2010; Chigerwe et al. 2016, 2017), laparoscopy (Videla and van Amstel 2016), or laparotomy followed by normograde hydropulsion with acid solution (Dória et al. 2007; Ewoldt et al. 2008; Videla and van Amstel 2016; Fazili et al. 2010; Carvalho et al. 2015). Angiographic catheters can be used for retrograde bladder catheterization (Reppert et al. 2016). Endoscopic-guided laser lithotripsy can be used to break up obstructing uroliths that are further removed by urethral flushing (Halland et al. 2002).

The most successful method for treating obstructive urolithiasis is percutaneous laparoscopic or laparotomy tube cystotomy (Guimarães et al. 2012; Riedi et al. 2018; Rakestraw et al. 1995; Streeter et al. 2002; Pearce et al. 2003; Fortier et al. 2004) that can be combined with urethrotomy (Jacobs and Fecteau 2019; Applegate et al. 2020). This method extends a life and allows bucks to recover their reproductive function. Its limitations are the need for 2–3 weeks of hospitalization for the adequate clearance and recovery of urethral patency (Ewoldt et al. 2008), which limits this treatment to high-cost animals or pets (Scully 2021), and the occurrence of recurrences (Jacobs and Fecteau 2019). Furthermore, this procedure has a high risk of complications and death (Gamsjäger and Chigerwe 2021; Kretsch and Chigerwe 2021).

Cases of obstructive urolithiasis caused by Ca carbonate or apatite uroliths present superior recovery by other surgical procedures, including perineal or prepubic urethrostomy (Ewoldt et al. 2008; Videla and van Amstel 2016; Stone et al. 1997), bladder marsupialization (May et al. 1998; Hunter et al. 2012), laser urethroscopy, lithotripsy (Videla and van Amstel 2016), and vesicopreputial anastomosis (Cypher et al. 2017). Prepubic and perineal urethrostomy are indicated for emergencies, especially in meat goats that will be slaughtered within a few weeks because stenosis can occur in 45–78% of cases in up to eight months (Videla and van Amstel 2016). Modified proximal perineal urethrostomy has a lower risk of stenosis than prepubic and perineal urethrostomy (Tobias and van Amstel 2013; Oman et al. 2019). Even though it is a straightforward surgical technique, bladder marsupialization can lead to ascending urinary tract infections and skin irritation due to urine leakage (Ewoldt et al. 2008; Videla and van Amstel 2016; May et al. 2002). Vesicopreputial anastomosis is an alternative technique to redirect urine flow in cases where other techniques to restore urination have not been successful. In addition, this technique has the advantage over bladder marsupialization of not causing skin lesions by urine (Cypher et al. 2017). Penile amputation and prescrotal urethrotomy are alternative surgical techniques, but are not often used (Videla and van Amstel 2016).

49.7 Prevention

Confined goats are most affected by urolithiasis but a balanced diet can prevent this condition. The supplementation with Ca of feeds rich in grains or bran should aim to achieve a Ca:P ratio of at least 1.5:1. Usually, the inclusion of 1–1.5% of calcium carbonate to grains or byproducts is enough to obtain an appropriate Ca:P ratio. However, the ideal is that a nutritionist formulates a balanced diet. The recommended concentrations of P and Mg in goat feed are 0.5% and 0.3%, respectively. Dietary supplementation with mineral salt for goats fed grains and bran is discouraged due to a predisposition to urolithiasis, aside from fibrous osteodystrophy and copper intoxication (Riet-Correa et al. 2008).

Acidification of the urine can prevent the precipitation of phosphate. This acidification can be accomplished by incorporating up to 2.25% ammonium chloride into the feed (Riet-Correa et al. 2008; Videla and van Amstel 2016; Van Metre et al. 1996; Mavangira et al. 2010; Sprake et al. 2012). Feeding goats also obtained urinary acidification with an increased volume of urine with a diet of an anionic ratio of 0 mEq/100 g of dry matter (Stratton-Phelps and House 2004; Jones et al. 2009; Do Nguyen et al. 2022). The oral administration of methionine (200 mg/kg/day) also reduces urinary pH (Grissett et al. 2012). The inclusion of 1–4% of sodium chloride in the feed of confined goats can increase water consumption, which helps to prevent the generation of uroliths (Riet-Correa et al. 2008; Van Metre and Fubini 2006; Sprake et al. 2012).

Goats should not be castrated before complete maturation of the urethra because the development of this tube is dependent on testosterone and the underdeveloped urethra has a reduced diameter, increasing the risk of obstructive urolithiasis (Videla and van Amstel 2016).

References

Applegate, T.J., Barrell, E.A., Hassel, D.M. et al. (2020). Combined tube cystostomy and urethrotomy for the treatment of urethral obstruction due to urolithiasis in goats. *Veterinary Surgery* 49 (2): 373–379.

Carvalho, J.S., Menezes, R.V., de Lima, E.B. et al. (2015). Tratamento da urolitíase obstrutiva em pequenos ruminantes utilizando a técnica de cistostomia com colocação de sonda de Foley: relato de caso. *Scientia Plena* 11 (4): 046114.

Chigerwe, M., Heller, M.C., Balcomb, C.C., and Angelos, J.A. (2016). Use of a percutaneous transabdominal catheter for management of obstructive urolithiasis in goats, sheep, and potbellied pigs: 69 cases (2000–2014). *Journal of the American Veterinary Medical Association* 248 (11): 1287–1290.

Chigerwe, M., Mavangira, V., Byrne, B.A., and Angelos, J.A. (2017). Antibiotic resistance patterns of bacteria isolated from indwelling Foley catheters following tube cystostomy in goats with obstructive urolithiasis. *Journal of Veterinary Diagnostic Investigation* 29 (3): 316–320.

Constable, P.D., Hinchcliff, K.W., Done, S.H., and Grünberg, W. (2017). *Veterinary Medicine: A Textbook of the Diseases of Cattle, Sheep, Pigs and Goat*, 11e. St Louis, MO: Elsevier.

Cypher, E.E., van Amstel, S.R., Videla, R. et al. (2017). Vesicopreputial anastomosis for the treatment of obstructive urolithiasis in goats. *Veterinary Surgery* 46 (2): 281–288.

Do Nguyen, D.K., Semsirmboon, S., Chaiyabutr, N., and Thammacharoen, S. (2022). Effects of low dietary cation and anion difference on blood gas, renal electrolyte, and acid excretions in goats in tropical conditions. *Animals* 12 (23): 3444.

Dória, R.G.S., Canola, P.A., Dias, D.P.M. et al. (2007). Técnicas cirúrgicas para urolitíase obstrutiva em pequenos ruminantes: relato de casos. *Arquivo Brasileiro de Medicina Veterinária e Zootecnia* 59 (6): 1425–1432.

Ewoldt, J.M., Anderson, D.E., Miesner, M.D., and Saville, W.J. (2006). Short- and long-term outcome and factors predicting survival after surgical tube cystostomy for treatment of obstructive urolithiasis in small ruminants. *Veterinary Surgery* 35 (5): 417–422.

Ewoldt, J.M., Jones, M.L., and Miesner, M.D. (2008). Surgery of obstructive urolithiasis in ruminants. *Veterinary Clinics of North America: Food Animal Practice* 24 (3): 455–465.

Fazili, M.R., Malik, H.U., Bhattacharyya, H.K. et al. (2010). Minimally invasive surgical tube cystotomy for treating obstructive urolithiasis in small ruminants with an intact urinary bladder. *Veterinary Record* 166 (17): 528–531.

Ferreira, D.O.L., Santarosa, B.P., Chiacchio, S.B., and Gonçalves, R.C. (2015). Urolitíase obstrutiva em ovinos. *Veterinaria e Zootecnia* 22 (2): 183–197.

Fortier, L.A., Gregg, A.J., Erb, H.N., and Fubini, S.L. (2004). Caprine obstructive urolithiasis: requirement for 2nd surgical intervention and mortality after percutaneous tube cystostomy, surgical tube cystostomy, or urinary bladder marsupialization. *Veterinary Surgery* 33 (6): 661–667.

Gamsjäger, L. and Chigerwe, M. (2021). Risk factors for, frequency, and type of complications after temporary tube cystostomy in goats, sheep, and pigs. *Veterinary Surgery* 50 (2): 283–293.

George, J.W., Hird, D.W., and George, L.W. (2007). Serum biochemical abnormalities in goats with uroliths: 107 cases (1992–2003). *Journal of the American Veterinary Medical Association* 230 (1): 101–106.

Grissett, G., Fleming, S., and Neizman, K. (2012). Evaluation of orally supplemented D, L-methionine as a urine acidified for small ruminants. *Journal of Veterinary Internal Medicine* 26 (3): 760.

Guimarães, J.A., Mendonça, C.L., Guaraná, E.L.S. et al. (2012). Estudo retrospectivo da urolitíase obstrutiva em ovinos: análise de 66 casos. *Pesquisa Veterinaria Brasileira* 32 (9): 824–830.

Halland, S.K., House, J.K., and George, L.W. (2002). Urethroscopy and laser lithotripsy for the diagnosis and treatment of obstructive urolithiasis in goats and pot-bellied pigs. *Journal of the American Veterinary Medical Association* 220 (12): 1831–1834.

Harwood, D. and Mueller, K. (2018). *Goat Medicine and Surgery*. Boca Raton, FL: CRC Press.

Hunter, B.G., Huber, M.J., and Riddick, T.L. (2012). Laparoscopic-assisted urinary bladder marsupialization in a goat that developed recurrent urethral obstruction following perineal urethrostomy. *Journal of the American Veterinary Medical Association* 241 (6): 778–781.

Jacobs, C.C. and Fecteau, M.E. (2019). Urethrotomy in combination with or after temporary tube cystostomy for treatment of obstructive urolithiasis in male goats. *Veterinary Surgery* 48 (3): 315–320.

Janke, J.J., Osterstock, J.B., Washburn, K.E. et al. (2009). Use of Walpole's solution for treatment of goats with urolithiasis: 25 cases (2001–2006). *Journal of the American Veterinary Medical Association* 234 (2): 249–252.

Jones, M.L., Streeter, R.N., and Goad, C.L. (2009). Use of dietary cation anion difference for control of urolithiasis risk factors in goats. *American Journal of Veterinary Research* 70 (1): 149–155.

Jones, M., Miesner, M.D., Baird, A., and Pugh, D.G. (2012). Diseases of the urinary system. In: *Sheep and Goat Medicine* (ed. D.G. Pugh and A.N. Baird), 325–360. Maryland Height, MO: Elsevier.

Jones, M.L., Roussel, A.J., and Ramsey, W.S. (2015). Development of a zinc implant-based model for urolithiasis in goats. *Small Ruminant Research* 127: 97–101.

Jones, M.L., Gibbons, P.M., Roussel, A.J., and Dominguez, B.J. (2017). Mineral composition of uroliths obtained from sheep and goats with obstructive urolithiasis. *Journal of Veterinary Internal Medicine* 31 (4): 1202–1208.

Jones, M.L., Dominguez, B.J., and Deveau, M.A. (2018). An experimental model for calcium carbonate urolithiasis in goats. *Journal of Veterinary Internal Medicine* 32 (3): 1268–1273.

Kannan, K.V.A. and Lawrence, K.E. (2010). Obstructive urolithiasis in a Saanen goat in New Zealand, resulting in a ruptured bladder. *New Zealand Veterinary Journal* 58 (5): 269–271.

Kinsley, M.A., Semevolos, S., Parker, J.E. et al. (2013). Use of plain radiography in the diagnosis, surgical management, and postoperative treatment of obstructive urolithiasis in 25 goats and 2 sheep. *Veterinary Surgery* 42 (6): 663–668.

Kretsch, C.M. and Chigerwe, M. (2021). Assessment of preoperative and postoperative l-lactatemia and clinical outcomes in goats undergoing tube cystostomy: a retrospective study of 34 cases (2015–2020). *Journal of Veterinary Internal Medicine* 35 (6): 2926–2932.

Lemos, R.A.A. and Silveira, A.C. (2008). Urolitíase e ruptura da bexiga. In: *Doenças de Impacto Econômico em Bovinos de Corte* (ed. R.A.A. Lemos and C.R.B. Leal), 337–346. Campo Grande, Brazil: Editora UFMS.

Maciel, T.A., Ramos, I.A., Silva, R.J. et al. (2017). Clinical and biochemical profile of obstructive urolithiasis in sheep. *Acta Scientiae Veterinariae* 45: 1515.

Matthews, J. (2016). *Diseases of the Goat*, 4e. Oxford, UK: Wiley-Blackwell.

Mavangira, V., Cornish, J.M., and Angelos, J.A. (2010). Effect of ammonium chloride supplementation on urine pH and urinary fractional excretion of electrolytes in goats. *Journal of the American Veterinary Medical Association* 237 (11): 1299–1304.

May, K.A., Moll, H.D., Wallace, L.M. et al. (1998). Urinary bladder marsupialization for treatment of obstructive urolithiasis in male goats. *Veterinary Surgery* 27 (6): 583–588.

May, K.A., Moll, H.D., Duncan, R.B. et al. (2002). Experimental evaluation of urinary bladder marsupialization in male goats. *Veterinary Surgery* 31: 251–258.

Nwaokorie, E.E., Osborne, C.A., Lulich, J.P. et al. (2015). Risk factors for calcium carbonate urolithiasis in goats. *Journal of the American Veterinary Medical Association* 247 (3): 293–299.

Oman, R.E., Reppert, E.J., Streeter, R.N., and Jones, M. (2019). Outcome and complications in goats treated by perineal urethrostomy for obstructive urolithiasis: 25 cases (2010–2017). *Journal of Veterinary Internal Medicine* 33 (1): 292–296.

Palmer, J.L., Dykes, N.L., Love, K., and Fubini, S.L. (1998). Contrast radiography of the lower urinary tract in the management of obstructive urolithiasis in small ruminants and swine. *Veterinary Radiology and Ultrasound* 39 (3): 175–180.

Pan, X.L., Wen, Z.S., Zou, X.T. et al. (2011). Chemical composition and microstructure of uroliths associated with the feeding of high-level cottonseed meal diet to sheep. *Research in Veterinary Science* 91 (3): 405–411.

Pearce, S.G., Dearo, A.C., Howard, B.E., and Brisson, B.A. (2003). Management of obstructive urolithiasis and concurrent urethral rupture in a goat. *Australian Veterinary Journal* 81 (5): 268–270.

Rakestraw, P.C., Fubini, S.L., Gilbert, R.O., and Ward, J.O. (1995). Tube cystostomy for treatment of obstructive urolithiasis in small ruminants. *Veterinary Surgery* 24 (6): 498–505.

Reppert, E.J., Streeter, R.N., Simpson, K.M., and Taylor, J.D. (2016). Retrograde catheterization of the urinary bladder in healthy male goats by use of angiographic catheters. *American Journal of Veterinary Research* 77 (11): 1295–1299.

Riedi, A.K., Knubben-Schweizer, G., and Meylan, M. (2018). Clinical findings and diagnostic procedures in 270 small ruminants with obstructive urolithiasis. *Journal of Veterinary Internal Medicine* 32 (3): 1274–1282.

Riet-Correa, F. (2010). Suplementação mineral em pequenos ruminantes. In: *Deficiências Minerais em Animais de Produção* (ed. C.H. Tokarnia, P.V. Peixoto, J.D. Barbosa, et al.), 172–187. Rio de Janeiro, Brazil: Helianthus.

Riet-Correa, F., Simões, S.D.V., and Vasconcelos, J.S. (2008). Urolitíase em ovinos e caprinos. *Pesquisa Veterinaria Brasileira* 28 (6): 319–322.

Sacco, S.R. and Lopes, R.S. (2011). Urolitíase: estudo comparativo em bovinos Guzerá oriundos de propriedades com e sem o problema. *Pesquisa Veterinaria Brasileira* 31 (3): 206–212.

Scully, C.M. (2021). Management of urologic conditions in small ruminants. *Veterinary Clinics of North America: Food Animal Practice* 37 (1): 93–104.

Sickinger, M. and Windhorst, A. (2022). A systematic review on urolithiasis in small ruminants according to nutrition-dependent prevalence and outcome after surgery. *Veterinary World* 15 (3): 809–817.

Sprake, P., Roussel, A.J., Stewart, R., and Bissett, W.T. (2012). The effect of ammonium chloride treatment as a long term preventative approach for urolithiasis in goats and a comparison of continuous and pulse dosing regimes. *Journal of Veterinary Internal Medicine* 26 (3): 760.

Stewart, J.L. and Shipley, C.F. (2021). Management of reproductive diseases in male small ruminants. *he Veterinary Clinics of North America: Food Animal Practice* 37 (1): 105–123.

Stieger-Vanegas, S.M., Caldwell, L., Vanegas, J.A. et al. (2022). Clinical utility of abdominal multidetector CT in 85 goats with suspected abdominal disease. *Veterinary Radiology and Ultrasound* 63 (4): 403–413.

Stone, W.C., Bjorling, D.E., Trostle, S.S. et al. (1997). Prepubic urethrostomy for relief of urethral obstruction in a sheep and a goat. *Journal of the American Veterinary Medical Association* 210 (7): 939–941.

Stratton-Phelps, M. and House, J.K. (2004). Effect of a commercial anion dietary supplement on acid–base balance, urine volume, and urinary ion excretion in male goats fed oat or grass hay diets. *American Journal of Veterinary Research* 65 (10): 1391–1397.

Streeter, R.N., Washburn, K.E., and McCauley, C.T. (2002). Percutaneous tube cystostomy and vesicular irrigation for treatment of obstructive urolithiasis in a goat. *Journal of the American Veterinary Medical Association* 221 (4): 546–549.

Sun, W.D., Zhang, K.C., Wang, J.Y., and Wang, X.L. (2010a). The chemical composition and ultrastructure of uroliths in Boer goats. *Veterinary Journal* 186 (1): 70–75.

Sun, W.D., Wang, J.Y., Zhang, K.C., and Wang, X.L. (2010b). Study on precipitation of struvite and struvite-K crystal in goats during onset of urolithiasis. *Research in Veterinary Science* 88 (3): 461–466.

Tharwat, M. (2021). Clinical, ultrasonographic, and postmortem findings in sheep and goats with urinary tract disorders. *Veterinary World* 14 (7): 1879–1887.

Tobias, K.M. and van Amstel, S.R. (2013). Modified proximal perineal urethrostomy technique for treatment of urethral stricture in goats. *Veterinary Surgery* 42 (4): 455–462.

Vail, K.J., Tate, N.M., Likavec, T. et al. (2019). Hereditary xanthinuria in a goat. *Journal of Veterinary Internal Medicine* 33 (2): 1009–1014.

Van Metre, D.C. and Fubini, S.L. (2006). Ovine and caprine urolithiasis: another piece of the puzzle. *Veterinary Surgery* 35 (5): 413–416.

Van Metre, D.C., House, J.K., Smith, B.P. et al. (1996). Obstructive urolithiasis in ruminants: surgical management and prevention. *Compendium on Continuing Education for the Practicing Veterinarian* 18 (Suppl. 10): 275–289.

Videla, R. and van Amstel, S. (2016). Urolithiasis. *Veterinary Clinics of North America: Food Animal Practice* 32 (3): 687–700.

Wang, J.Y., Sun, W.D., and Wang, X.L. (2009). Comparison of effect of high intake of magnesium with high intake of phosphorus and potassium on urolithiasis in goats fed with cottonseed meal diet. *Research in Veterinary Science* 87 (1): 79–84.

50

Polioencephalomalacia

Benito Soto-Blanco[1] *and Antonio Carlos Lopes Câmara*[2]

[1] *Department of Veterinary Clinics and Surgery, Veterinary School, Universidade Federal de Minas Gerais, Belo Horizonte, Brazil*
[2] *Large Animal Veterinary Teaching Hospital, Universidade de Brasília, Brasília, Brazil*

50.1 Introduction

Polioencephalomalacia (PEM), or cerebrocortical necrosis, is a metabolic disease that causes neurological disturbances. It occurs in goats of all ages but young animals are most often affected. Several factors have been suggested as responsible for PEM, but this disease is mainly attributed to thiamine (vitamin B_1) deficiency or excessive sulfur intake (Smith and Sherman 2009; Matthews 2016; Harwood and Mueller 2018).

50.2 Etiology

The main causes of PEM in ruminants are summarized in Table 50.1. PEM in goats has been linked to thiamine deficiency or excessive sulfur intake. Causes associated with PEM in cattle are excessive salt consumption with or without water deprivation, bovine herpesvirus infection, and lead poisoning (Cebra and Cebra 2004; Sant'Ana and Barros 2010; Cebra et al. 2015). In sheep, PEM is also observed in cases of peracute poisoning by *Phalaris* spp. (Bourke et al. 2003, 2005).

50.2.1 Thiamine Deficiency

Polioencephalomalacia was earlier exclusively attributed to thiamine deficiency. Thiamine is an essential nutrient produced by ruminal microbiota in amounts almost reaching the ruminants' requirements. Nevertheless, young ruminants without a fully functional rumen depend on the ingestion of dietary thiamine (Cebra and Cebra 2004; Rammell and Hill 1986; Assis et al. 2020). Thiamine participates in cellular energy metabolism as a cofactor of pyruvate dehydrogenase and alpha-ketoglutarate dehydrogenase (Pan et al. 2018; Tylicki et al. 2018; Hrubša et al. 2022).

The main factor that may impair thiamine production by microbiota is ruminal lactic acidosis due to the consumption of high-grain or carbohydrate-rich diets. Reduced ruminal pH decreases the population of thiamine-producing bacteria and favors the proliferation of thiaminase-producing bacteria, including *Clostridium sporogenes*, *Bacillus aneurinolyticus*, and *Bacillus thiaminolyticus* (Smith and Sherman 2009; Cebra et al. 2015; Assis et al. 2020; Pan et al. 2018; Chigerwe and Aleman 2016; Constable et al. 2017). Thiamine deficiency may also result from the ingestion of plants that contain thiaminase, usually pteridophyte plants such as bracken (*Pteridium* spp.), nardoo (*Marsilea drummondii*), poison rock or mulga (*Cheilanthes sieberi*) ferns, horsetail (*Equisetum* spp.) (Cebra and Cebra 2004; Cebra et al. 2015; Meyer 1989; Kul et al. 2006), and prostrate pigweed (*Amaranthus blitoides*) (Ramos et al. 2005) (Table 50.2). Kochia (*Bassia* [*Kochia*] *scoparia*), another plant responsible for PEM in cattle, is suspected of containing a nonidentified compound that antagonizes thiamine (Dickie and James 1983), which possibly is thiaminase because this plant belongs to the same family as prostrate pigweed (Amaranthaceae). However, PEM due to the consumption of thiaminase-containing plants has not yet been described in goats.

Elements of Reproduction and Reproductive Diseases of Goats, First Edition. Edited by Tanmoy Rana.

Table 50.1 Main causes of polioencephalomalacia in ruminants.

Thiamine deficiency
Excessive sulfur intake
Lead poisoning
Salt poisoning/water deprivation
Petroleum poisoning

Table 50.2 Some thiaminase-containing plant species (Cebra and Cebra 2004; Cebra et al. 2015; Meyer 1989; Kul et al. 2006; Ramos et al. 2005).

Common name	Scientific name
Bracken fern	*Pteridium* spp.
Horsetail	*Equisetum* spp.
Nardoo fern	*Marsilea drummondii*
Poison rock or mulga fern	*Cheilanthes sieberi*
Prostrate pigweed	*Amaranthus blitoides*

Table 50.3 Some thiamine antagonists (Tylicki et al. 2018; Hrubša et al. 2022; Giacomini et al. 2017; Vora et al. 2020; Linklater et al. 1977; Gastaldi et al. 1988).

Amprolium
Fedratinib
Hydroxychloroquine
Levamisole
Metformin
Methylxanthines (caffeine, theophylline, and theobromine)
Penicillamine ethanolamine
Sulfonamides
Trimethoprim
Verapamil

In cattle, consuming carcase fragments containing thiaminase-producing clostridia might also result in thiamine deficiency (Sant'Ana and Barros 2010; Cebra et al. 2015). Another cause of deficiency of thiamine is the use of inadequate milk replacers containing insufficient amounts of this vitamin, which can lead to PEM in goat kids (Cebra and Cebra 2004).

Amprolium, sulfonamides, trimethoprim, and other coccidiocides and coccidiostats are suspected of causing PEM in goats (Loew and Dunlop 1972; Lonkar and Prasad 1994; Allen et al. 2013) because they are thiamine antagonists (Tylicki et al. 2018; Giacomini et al. 2017; Vora et al. 2020) (Table 50.3). The occurrence of PEM in two flocks of sheep was associated with administration of the anthelmintics levamisole hydrochloride and thiabendazole (Linklater et al. 1977); levamisole is a thiamine antagonist (Gastaldi et al. 1988). Other compounds are also thiamine antagonists, including verapamil, metformin, hydroxychloroquine, fedratinib, penicillamine ethanolamine (Vora et al. 2020), and methylxanthines (caffeine, theophylline, and theobromine) (Hrubša et al. 2022). These antagonists decrease the intestinal uptake of thiamine by THTR1 and THTR2 transporters of the enterocytes (Tylicki et al. 2018; Hrubša et al. 2022; Giacomini et al. 2017; Vora et al. 2020).

It has been hypothesized that the energy metabolism of brain neurons is compromised in cases of thiamine deficiency. The reduced availability of thiamine would affect the synthesis of thiamine diphosphate-dependent enzyme transketolase, an enzyme that participates in the pentose phosphate pathway, affecting the energy production in nervous tissue (Cebra et al. 2015; Pan et al. 2018; Tylicki et al. 2018; Hrubša et al. 2022). Moreover, thiamine deficiency reduces neurotransmitter synthesis (Hrubša et al. 2022) and induces neuronal degeneration and death by endoplasmic reticulum stress, oxidative stress, and autophagy (Liu et al. 2017; Wang et al. 2017; Lonsdale 2019).

50.2.2 Excessive Sulfur Intake

Most cases of PEM have been attributed to excessive sulfur intake from food and water. Sulfur-rich dietary ingredients include molasses, gypsum, some forages, urine acidifiers, distiller's grains (byproducts of the ethanol industry), and plants of the Brassicaceae family (Table 50.4) (Cebra and Cebra 2004; Cebra et al. 2015; Constable et al. 2017; Olkowski 1997; Niles et al. 2000; McKenzie et al. 2009; Drewnoski et al. 2014; Amat et al. 2017). Water may also contain sulfur at toxic levels (Beke and Hironaka 1991; Haydock 2003). Beef cattle can tolerate up to 0.39% of dietary sulfur (Castro et al. 2022), but the amount of sulfur tolerated by goats is still unknown. The sulfur source possibly influences sulfur toxicity (Amat et al. 2017; Neville et al. 2010). Feed intake is not affected by high consumption of sulfur (Niles et al. 2002). Probably, excessive sulfur intake does not result in thiamine deficiency since no reduction in total thiamine levels was observed in the blood or brain of several sulfur-induced PEM animals (Giacomini et al. 2017; Gould et al. 1991, 1997; Hamlen et al. 1993; Amat et al. 2013). Nevertheless, dietary supplementation with thiamine may decrease the severity of brain lesions of sulfur-induced PEM (Rousseaux et al. 1991; Olkowski et al. 1992).

Physiologically, sulfates in the rumen are reduced into sulfide (HS^-) ions by assimilatory sulfo-reducing ruminal bacteria for further synthesis of sulfur-containing amino acids such as methionine and cysteine. Sulfates may also be used by dissimilatory sulfo-reducing ruminal bacteria for anaerobic energy production, also releasing sulfide ions. When the pH of the ruminal fluid is reduced, sulfide ions form hydrogen sulfide (H_2S) that is primarily absorbed by the ruminal epithelium or the lungs after inhalation of the eructed gas. After reaching the blood, H_2S is transported to the liver, where hepatocytes detoxify it by conversion into sulfate. Excessive concentrations of H_2S can overwhelm the hepatic detoxification capacity, allowing nondetoxified H_2S to reach the systemic bloodstream. In the central nervous system, H_2S damages neurons due to the inhibition of cytochrome c oxidase, impairing energy production by oxidative phosphorylation (Cebra and Cebra 2004; Cebra et al. 2015; Assis et al. 2020; Constable et al. 2017; Drewnoski et al. 2014; Amat et al. 2017; Gould 2000). Two other thiamine-dependent enzymes, alpha-ketoglutarate dehydrogenase and pyruvate dehydrogenase, have their activities inhibited in the cerebral cortex after sulfur-induced PEM, impairing the cellular energy metabolism in brain neurons (Amat et al. 2017). H_2S was also found to bind to hemoglobin, reducing the blood transport of oxygen (Bulgin et al. 1996).

50.2.3 Other Causes

Other causes of PEM reported in goats include petroleum (crude oil) poisoning (Batista et al. 2013; Câmara et al. 2018), consumption of *Hovenia dulcis* (Colodel et al. 1998), and closantel overdose (Sakhaee and Derakhshanfar 2010). The ingestion of residual petroleum probably results in sulfur toxicosis, even though salt and lead poisoning may also occur (Batista et al. 2013; Câmara et al. 2018). One outbreak of PEM was observed in goats that ingested the fruits of the Japanese or oriental raisin tree (*Hovenia dulcis*) for five days (Colodel et al. 1998). The administration of an overdose of the anthelmintic closantel was linked to the development of PEM in a goat, possibly due to some interference with neuronal metabolism (Sakhaee and Derakhshanfar 2010). Closantel overdose in goats was also responsible for status spongiosis of the cerebrum and cerebellum, optic neuropathy, and retinopathy (Sakhaee and Derakhshanfar 2010; Ecco et al. 2006; van der Lugt and Venter 2007).

Table 50.4 Some sulfur-rich dietary ingredients (Cebra and Cebra 2004; Cebra et al. 2015; Constable et al. 2017; Olkowski 1997; Niles et al. 2000; McKenzie et al. 2009; Drewnoski et al. 2014; Amat et al. 2017).

Distiller's grains (byproducts of the ethanol industry)
Gypsum
Molasses
Plants of the family Brassicaceae
Some forages
Urine acidifiers

50.3 Clinical Signs

Clinical manifestations of PEM are variable. The first clinical signs may include apathy, separation from the flock, loss of appetite, and diarrhea. Goats presenting severe ruminal acidosis may show a lack of rumen movements. The gas eliminated by eructation may have a similar smell to a rotten egg due to sulfite. Clinical signs of neurological damage develop gradually and include excitability, circling or staggering gait, ataxia, frequent vocalization, head pressing, stargazing (upward lift of the head and neck, staring at the sky), fixed and dilated pupils, apparent blindness, and muscle trembling (Smith and Sherman 2009; Matthews 2016; Harwood and Mueller 2018; Constable et al. 2017; Câmara et al. 2018; Sakhaee and Derakhshanfar 2010; Maxwell 1980; Newsholme and O'Neill 1985; Lima et al. 2005; Sivaraman et al. 2016; Deepa 2020). The blindness can last 2–3 weeks. The electrodiagnostic visual testing of one goat kid and one lamb presenting with PEM revealed altered visual-evoked potential but the electroretinogram results were as expected (Strain et al. 1990).

In advanced cases, clinical signs that may be observed include nystagmus, lateral recumbency with opisthotonos, strabismus, muscle rigidity, odontoprisis (bruxism), and convulsions (Smith and Sherman 2009; Matthews 2016; Harwood and Mueller 2018; Constable et al. 2017; Câmara et al. 2018; Sakhaee and Derakhshanfar 2010; Newsholme and O'Neill 1985; Lima et al. 2005; Sivaraman et al. 2016; Deepa 2020). PEM is one of the main causes of convulsions in goats (Chigerwe and Aleman 2016). Goats may die 1–3 days after manifestation of the initial clinical manifestations (Smith and Sherman 2009; Matthews 2016; Constable et al. 2017; Câmara et al. 2018; Sakhaee and Derakhshanfar 2010; Lima et al. 2005; Sivaraman et al. 2016).

50.4 Pathology

The usual gross finding observed at necropsy in severe cases of PEM is the grayish-yellow or yellow coloration of the cerebrum (Smith and Sherman 2009; Matthews 2016; Sant'Ana and Barros 2010; Câmara et al. 2018; Lima et al. 2005; Smith 1979; Matayoshi et al. 2012). The typical PEM macroscopic change is malacia (softening due to loss) of the neocortex's gray matter, mainly in areas supplied by the middle and caudal cerebral arteries (Finnie et al. 2022). The cut surface of the affected areas of the cerebral cortex shows fluorescence on examination under ultraviolet light. The occurrence of cerebral edema is evidenced by flattened cerebral gyri that may be associated with partial herniation of the cerebellum through the foramen magnum (Smith and Sherman 2009; Matthews 2016; Sant'Ana and Barros 2010; Câmara et al. 2018; Newsholme and O'Neill 1985; Lima et al. 2005; Matayoshi et al. 2012; Andrie et al. 2018).

The characteristic microscopic finding is pseudo-laminar necrosis affecting neurons from more than one cortical segment of the telencephalon. Other lesions observed in the cerebrum are edematous vascular endothelium, thick basement membrane, and diffuse macrophage infiltration (Sant'Ana and Barros 2010; Câmara et al. 2018; Smith 1979; Matayoshi et al. 2012; Andrie et al. 2018). These changes are usually accompanied by spongiosis (Sant'Ana and Barros 2010; Câmara et al. 2018). Damaged neurons in an area of pseudo-laminar cerebrocortical necrosis show increased affinity with eosin in routine hematoxylin and eosin-stained fragments, which is why they are known as eosinophilic, acidophilic, pink, or red neurons. In sheep, these red neurons were found to present amyloid precursor protein (APP) immunolabeling. As this protein is known to have a protective effect on neurons, upregulated expression of APP could be a neuroprotective response (Finnie et al. 2022).

50.5 Diagnosis

The presumptive diagnosis is based on the clinical signs of blindness, opisthotonos, nystagmus, strabismus, extensor rigidity, and convulsions. The response to thiamine treatment is vital for conditions caused by thiamine deficiency. The rumen fluid changes are relevant to identify ruminal lactic acidosis (Smith and Sherman 2009; Chigerwe and Aleman 2016; Constable et al. 2017; Sivaraman et al. 2016). A common finding in the CSF analysis is a slight increase in protein levels and mononuclear pleocytosis (Smith and Sherman 2009; Matthews 2016; Câmara et al. 2018); usually, the mononuclear cells present vacuoles (Cebra and Cebra 2004). Excessive sulfur intake and toxicosis can be diagnosed by increased concentrations of H_2S in the rumen gas cap (Smith and Sherman 2009). At necropsy, fluorescence of the cerebral cortex observed under ultraviolet light is a good indicator of PEM that can be tested on the farm (Edwin and Jackman 1981; Markson and Wells 1982; Jackman and Edwin 1983).

Deficiency of thiamine may be demonstrated by direct measurement of thiamine or thiamine diphosphate levels in the blood, brain, and liver of goats with PEM. Nevertheless, blood thiamine levels in live animals may remain unaffected. Thiamine deficiency can be estimated indirectly by the erythrocyte transketolase assay, which is determined using heparinized blood (Smith and Sherman 2009; Matthews 2016; Cebra and Cebra 2004; Cebra et al. 2015; Rammell and Hill 1986; Horino et al. 1994; Smith 1979; Spicer and Horton 1981; Thomas et al. 1987; Ramos et al. 2006). Furthermore, pyruvate and lactate serum levels are frequently increased (Spicer and Horton 1981; Ramos et al. 2006). Thiaminase activity may be measured in the rumen content and feces (Smith and Sherman 2009; Matthews 2016; Cebra and Cebra 2004; Cebra et al. 2015; Spicer and Horton 1981; Edwin and Jackman 1973).

The definitive diagnosis is achieved on pathological examination that reveals the specific PEM. The differential diagnoses should include enterotoxemia caused by *Clostridium perfringens* type D, pregnancy toxemia, tetanus, caprine arthritis encephalitis, meningoencephalitis, lead poisoning, and salt poisoning (Smith and Sherman 2009; Constable et al. 2017; Maxwell 1980).

50.5.1 Ancillary Diagnostic Tests

Hematological exams typically do not demonstrate significant changes (Sivaraman et al. 2016; Sharma et al. 2021). Hyperglycemia and glucosuria are found in some goats (Matthews 2016). CSF analysis may reveal a slight increase in protein levels and mononuclear pleocytosis (Smith and Sherman 2009; Matthews 2016; Câmara et al. 2018); vacuoles are usually observed in CSF mononuclear cells (Cebra and Cebra 2004). The rumen fluid analysis of goats that presented ruminal lactic acidosis may show decreased ruminal pH and microbial activity (Smith and Sherman 2009; Chigerwe and Aleman 2016; Sivaraman et al. 2016).

Excessive sulfur intake and toxicosis can be indicated by increased concentrations of H_2S in the rumen gas cap (Smith and Sherman 2009; Cebra et al. 2015; Castro et al. 2022). For this assay, H_2S concentrations should be measured in unaffected goats from the flock because the reference range values are unavailable (Smith and Sherman 2009). One limitation of this assay is that ruminal synthesis of H_2S may be reduced in anorexic animals (Cebra et al. 2015).

The electroencephalographic (EEG) examination of sheep with PEM showed continuous high-amplitude slow waves and long-lasting spindles (Itabisashi et al. 1990; Horino et al. 1994). EEG was not performed in goats but it is expected that similar results would be found.

In PEM, radiographic evaluation of the brain is not adequate. On the other hand, magnetic resonance imaging (MRI) is helpful for the diagnosis of PEM. Bilaterally symmetrical lesions characterize MRI findings in the gray matter of the forebrain and cerebellar cortex (Schenk et al. 2007; Ertelt et al. 2016). Even though it has practical usefulness for identifying PEM, MRI is not usually available for use in goats because of the high cost.

50.6 Treatment

Thiamine has been recommended for treating PEM, irrespective of cause (Smith and Sherman 2009; Matthews 2016; Sivaraman et al. 2016; Low et al. 1996). However, responsiveness to thiamine treatment of animals with sulfur toxicosis is variable (Chigerwe and Aleman 2016; Deepa 2020). The usual form is thiamine hydrochloride, 10 mg/kg in 5% dextrose-normal saline or other isotonic fluid, administered intravenously. The administration of thiamine should be repeated four times every six hours, intramuscularly or subcutaneously (Smith and Sherman 2009; Matthews 2016; Sivaraman et al. 2016; Deepa 2020; Sharma et al. 2013, 2021). Thiamine should be supplemented in the diet (50 mg/kg of feed) for 2–3 weeks (Constable et al. 2017) to prevent the disease in asymptomatic animals of the flock.

Dexamethasone (1.0–2.0 mg/kg, intramuscularly or subcutaneously) is indicated for treating brain edema and inflammation. Goats with seizures can be treated with anticonvulsants, such as diazepam (0.5–1.5 mg/kg) (Smith and Sherman 2009; Matthews 2016; Sivaraman et al. 2016).

The efficacy of treatment varies according to the extent and severity of the brain damage. Clinical improvement of goats with mild brain damage may occur within 6–8 hours, with complete recovery in up to three days. The recovery of goats with moderate PEM may take nine days. On the other hand, PEM may be irreversible in severely affected goats (Smith and Sherman 2009; Matthews 2016; Sivaraman et al. 2016).

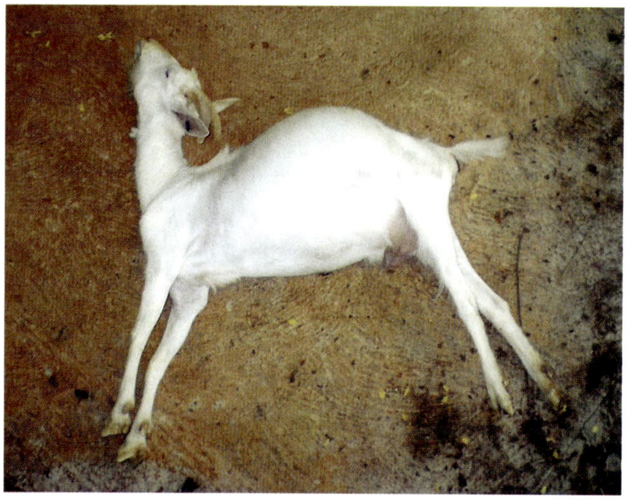

Figure 50.1 Goat that died due to polioencephalomalacia showing typical position.

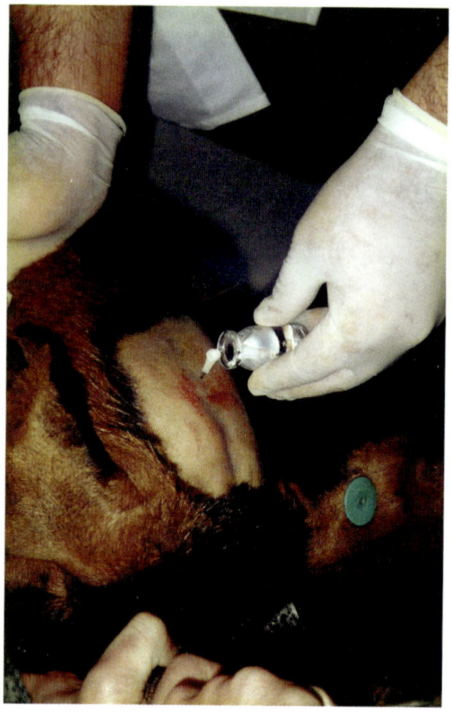

Figure 50.2 Collection of cerebrospinal fluid from the cerebellomedullary cistern in a goat suspected of PEM.

50.7 Prevention

Prevention measures vary according to the cause. An adequate adaptation is a need for high-grain or carbohydrate-rich diets aiming to avoid ruminal lactic acidosis (Cebra and Cebra 2004; Constable et al. 2017). The diet of goats should contain thiamine levels of 1.5–4.5 mg/kg of feed.

The total dietary sulfur in the feed and water must be determined to avoid excessive intake (Constable et al. 2017). Beef cattle require 0.15% of dietary sulfur (on a dry matter basis) in feed and drinking water, but they can tolerate up to 0.39% of dietary sulfur (Castro et al. 2022). However, the amount of sulfur tolerated by goats is still unknown. Copper, zinc, and molybdenum may form insoluble complexes with sulfur (Cebra and Cebra 2004). In fact, dietary supplementation with copper improved the thiamine status of cattle with high sulfur intake (Gooneratne et al. 1989).

Goats dosed with antihelminthic drugs or amprolium should be monitored to detect any sign of neurological disturbance. Determining the erythrocyte transketolase activity and estimating the thiaminase content in feces may help identify susceptible animals at periods of greater risk (Figures 50.1 and 50.2) (Ramos et al. 2003; Meena 2022).

References

Allen, A.L., Goupil, B.A., and Valentine, B.A. (2013). A retrospective study of brain lesions in goats submitted to three veterinary diagnostic laboratories. *Journal of Veterinary Diagnostic Investigation* 25 (4): 482–489.

Amat, S., McKinnon, J.J., Olkowski, A.A. et al. (2013). Understanding the role of sulfur-thiamine interaction in the pathogenesis of sulfur-induced polioencephalomalacia in beef cattle. *Research in Veterinary Science* 95 (3): 1081–1087.

Amat, S., Hendrick, S., Moshynskyy, I., and Simko, E. (2017). Reduced activities of thiamine-dependent and cytochrome c oxidase enzymes in cerebral cortex of cattle affected by sulfur-induced polioencephalomalacia. *Canadian Journal of Veterinary Research* 81 (4): 242–248.

Andrie, K.M., Kirejczyk, S.G.M., and Brown, C.C. (2018). Pathology in practice. *Journal of the American Veterinary Medical Association* 252 (9): 1067–1070.

Assis, J.R., Assis, A.C.M., Nunes, D., and Carlos, A.B. (2020). Nutritional and food aspects related to polioencephalomalacy in ruminant. *Scientific Electronic Archives* 13 (4): 96–104.

Batista, J.S., Câmara, A.C.L., Almeida, R.D. et al. (2013). Poisoning by crude oil in sheep and goats. *Revue de Médecine Vétérinaire* 164 (11): 517–520.

Beke, G.J. and Hironaka, R. (1991). Toxicity to beef cattle of sulfur in saline well water: a case study. *Science of the Total Environment* 101 (3): 281–290.

Bourke, C.A., Rendell, D., and Colegate, S.M. (2003). Clinical observations and differentiation of the peracute *Phalaris aquatica* poisoning syndrome in sheep known as 'polioencephalomalacia-like sudden death'. *Australian Veterinary Journal* 81 (11): 698–700.

Bourke, C.A., Colegate, S.M., Rendell, D. et al. (2005). Peracute ammonia toxicity: a consideration in the pathogenesis of *Phalaris aquatica* 'Polioencephalomalacia-like sudden death' poisoning of sheep and cattle. *Australian Veterinary Journal* 83 (3): 168–171.

Bulgin, M.S., Lincoln, S.D., and Mather, G. (1996). Elemental sulfur toxicosis in a flock of sheep. *Journal of the American Veterinary Medical Association* 208 (7): 1063–1065.

Câmara, A.C.L., Batista, J.S., and Soto-Blanco, B. (2018). Polioencephalomalacia in ruminants from the semi-arid region of Rio Grande do Norte, Brazil. *Semina: Ciencias Agrarias* 39 (1): 231–240.

Castro, D.J., Cerón-Cucchi, M.E., Ortiz-Chura, A. et al. (2022). Ruminal effects of excessive dietary sulphur in feedlot cattle. *Journal of Animal Physiology and Animal Nutrition* 106 (5): 978–987.

Cebra, C.K. and Cebra, M.L. (2004). Altered mentation caused by polioencephalomalacia, hypernatremia, and lead poisoning. *Veterinary Clinics of North America: Food Animal Practice* 20 (2): 287–302.

Cebra, C., Loneragan, G.H., and Gould, D.H. (2015). Polioencephalomalacia (cerebrocortical necrosis). In: *Large Animal Internal Medicine*, 5e (ed. B.P. Smith), 954–956. St Louis, MO: Elsevier.

Chigerwe, M. and Aleman, M. (2016). Seizure disorders in goats and sheep. *Journal of Veterinary Internal Medicine* 30 (5): 1752–1757.

Colodel, E.M., Loretti, A.P., Cruz, F.C.E., and Driemeier, D. (1998). Polioencefalomalacia em caprinos associada à ingestão dos frutos de Hovenia dulcis (uva-do-Japão). *Boletim do Laboratório Regional de Diagnóstico (Pelotas)* 25: 35–42.

Constable, P.D., Hinchcliff, K.W., Done, S.H., and Grünberg, W. (2017). *Veterinary Medicine: A Textbook of the Diseases of Cattle, Sheep, Pigs and Goat*, 11e. St Louis, MO: Elsevier.

Deepa, K. (2020). Polioencephalomalacia in goats – a study of 24 cases. *International Journal of Advanced Research in Biological Sciences* 7 (5): 61–63.

Dickie, C.W. and James, L.F. (1983). Kochia scoparia poisoning in cattle. *Journal of the American Veterinary Medical Association* 183 (7): 765–768.

Drewnoski, M.E., Pogge, D.J., and Hansen, S.L. (2014). High-sulfur in beef cattle diets: a review. *Journal of Animal Science* 92 (9): 3763–3780.

Ecco, R., de Barros, C.S., Graça, D.L., and Gava, A. (2006). Closantel toxicosis in kid goats. *Veterinary Record* 159 (17): 564–566.

Edwin, E.E. and Jackman, R. (1973). Ruminal thiaminase and tissue thiamine in cerebrocortical necrosis. *Veterinary Record* 92 (24): 640–641.

Edwin, E.E. and Jackman, R. (1981). Nature of the autofluorescent material in cerebrocortical necrosis. *Journal of Neurochemistry* 37 (4): 1054–1056.

Ertelt, K., Oevermann, A., Precht, C. et al. (2016). Magnetic resonance imaging findings in small ruminants with brain disease. *Veterinary Radiology & Ultrasound* 57 (2): 162–169.

Finnie, J.W., Jerrett, I.V., and Manavis, J. (2022). Red neurons in ovine polioencephalomalacia (cerebrocortical necrosis) are strongly amyloid precursor protein immunopositive. *Veterinary Research Communications* 46 (1): 289–293.

Gastaldi, G., Casirola, D., Patrini, C. et al. (1988). Intestinal transport of thiamin and thiamin monophosphate in rat everted jejunal sacs: a comparative study using some potential inhibitors. *Archives Internationales de Physiologie et de Biochimie* 96 (5): 223–230.

Giacomini, M.M., Hao, J., Liang, X. et al. (2017). Interaction of 2,4-diaminopyrimidine-containing drugs including fedratinib and trimethoprim with thiamine transporters. *Drug Metabolism and Disposition* 45 (1): 76–85.

Gooneratne, S.R., Olkowski, A.A., Klemmer, R.G. et al. (1989). High sulfur related thiamine deficiency in cattle: a field study. *Canadian Veterinary Journal* 30 (2): 139–146.

Gould, D.H. (2000). Update on sulfur-related polioencephalomalacia. *Veterinary Clinics of North America: Food Animal Practice* 16 (3): 481–496.

Gould, D.H., McAllister, M.M., Savage, J.C., and Hamar, D.W. (1991). High sulfide concentrations in rumen fluid associated with nutritionally induced polioencephalomalacia in calves. *American Journal of Veterinary Research* 52 (7): 1164–1169.

Gould, D.H., Cummings, B.A., and Hamar, D.W. (1997). In vivo indicators of pathologic ruminal sulfide production in steers with diet-induced polioencephalomalacia. *Journal of Veterinary Diagnostic Investigation* 9 (1): 72–76.

Hamlen, H., Clark, E., and Janzen, E. (1993). Polioencephalomalacia in cattle consuming water with elevated sodium sulfate levels: a herd investigation. *Canadian Veterinary Journal* 34 (3): 153–158.

Harwood, D. and Mueller, K. (2018). *Goat Medicine and Surgery*. Boca Raton, FL: CRC Press.

Haydock, D. (2003). Sulfur-induced polioencephalomalacia in a herd of rotationally grazed beef cattle. *Canadian Veterinary Journal* 44 (10): 828–829.
Horino, R., Itabisashi, T., and Hirano, K. (1994). Biochemical and pathological findings on sheep and calves dying of experimental cerebrocortical necrosis. *Journal of Veterinary Medical Science* 56 (3): 481–485.
Hrubša, M., Siatka, T., Nejmanová, I. et al. (2022). Biological properties of vitamins of the B-complex, part 1: vitamins B1, B2, B3, and B5. *Nutrients* 14 (3): 484.
Itabisashi, T., Horino, R., Hirano, K., and Maeda, M. (1990). Electroencephalographic observation on sheep and cattle with experimental cerebrocortical necrosis. *Journal of Veterinary Medical Science* 52 (3): 551–558.
Jackman, R. and Edwin, E.E. (1983). Cerebral autofluorescence and thiamine deficiency in cerebrocortical necrosis. *Veterinary Record* 112 (23): 548–550.
Kul, O., Karahan, S., Basalan, M., and Kabakci, N. (2006). Polioencephalomalacia in cattle: a consequence of prolonged feeding barley malt sprouts. *Journal of Veterinary Medicine. A, Physiology, Pathology, Clinical Medicine* 53 (3): 123–128.
Lima, E.F., Riet-Correa, F., Tabosa, I.M. et al. (2005). Polioencefalomalacia em caprinos e ovinos na região semi-árida do Nordeste do Brasil. *Pesquisa Veterinaria Brasileira* 25 (1): 9–14.
Linklater, K.A., Dyson, D.A., and Morgan, K.T. (1977). Faecal thiaminase in clinically normal sheep associated with outbreaks of polioencephalomalacia. *Research in Veterinary Science* 22 (3): 308–312.
Liu, D., Ke, Z., and Luo, J. (2017). Thiamine deficiency and neurodegeneration: the interplay among oxidative stress, endoplasmic reticulum stress, and autophagy. *Molecular Neurobiology* 54 (7): 5440–5448.
Loew, F.M. and Dunlop, R.H. (1972). Induction of thiamine inadequacy and polioencephalomalacia in adult sheep with amprolium. *American Journal of Veterinary Research* 33 (11): 2195–2205.
Lonkar, O.S. and Prasad, M.C. (1994). Pathology of amprolium-induced cerebrocortical necrosis in goats. *Small Ruminant Research* 13 (1): 85–92.
Lonsdale, D. (2019). Thiamin and protein folding. *Medical Hypotheses* 129: 109252.
Low, J.C., Scott, P.R., Howie, F. et al. (1996). Sulphur-induced polioencephalomalacia in lambs. *Veterinary Record* 138 (14): 327–329.
van der Lugt, J.J. and Venter, I. (2007). Myelin vacuolation, optic neuropathy and retinal degeneration after closantel overdosage in sheep and in a goat. *Journal of Comparative Pathology* 136 (2–3): 87–95.
Markson, L.M. and Wells, G.A. (1982). Evaluation of autofluorescence as an aid to diagnosis of cerebrocortical necrosis. *Veterinary Record* 111 (15): 338–340.
Matayoshi, M., Tsuha, O., Shimoji, S. et al. (2012). Occurrence of cerebrocortical necrosis in a goat in Okinawa prefecture, Japan. *Journal of Veterinary Medical Science* 74 (9): 1199–1201.
Matthews, J. (2016). *Diseases of the Goat*, 4e. Oxford, UK: Wiley-Blackwell.
Maxwell, J.A. (1980). Polioencephalomalacia in a goat. *Australian Veterinary Journal* 56 (7): 352.
McKenzie, R.A., Carmichael, A.M., Schibrowski, M.L. et al. (2009). Sulfur-associated polioencephalomalacia in cattle grazing plants in the family Brassicaceae. *Australian Veterinary Journal* 87 (1): 27–32.
Meena, Y.K. (2022). Polioencephalomalacia in goats. *epashupalan* 2 (3): 6–8.
Meyer, P. (1989). Thiaminase activities and thiamine content of *Pteridium aquilinum*, *Equisetum ramosissimum*, *Malva parviflora*, *Pennisetum clandestinum* and *Medicago sativa*. *Onderstepoort Journal of Veterinary Research* 56 (2): 145–146.
Neville, B.W., Schauer, C.S., Karges, K. et al. (2010). Effect of thiamine concentration on animal health, feedlot performance, carcass characteristics, and ruminal hydrogen sulfide concentrations in lambs fed diets based on 60% distillers dried grains plus solubles. *Journal of Animal Science* 88 (7): 2444–2455.
Newsholme, S.J. and O'Neill, T.P. (1985). An outbreak of cerebrocortical necrosis (polioencephalomalacia) in goats. *Journal of the South African Veterinary Association* 56 (1): 37–38.
Niles, G.A., Morgan, S.E., and Edwards, W.C. (2000). Sulfur-induced polioencephalomalacia in stocker calves. *Veterinary and Human Toxicology* 42 (5): 290–291.
Niles, G.A., Morgan, S., Edwards, W.C., and Lalman, D. (2002). Effects of dietary sulfur concentrations on the incidence and pathology of polioencephalomalicia in weaned beef calves. *Veterinary and Human Toxicology* 44 (2): 70–72.
Olkowski, A.A. (1997). Neurotoxicity and secondary metabolic problems associated with low to moderate levels of exposure to excess dietary sulphur in ruminants: a review. *Veterinary and Human Toxicology* 39 (6): 355–360.
Olkowski, A.A., Gooneratne, S.R., Rousseaux, C.G., and Christensen, D.A. (1992). Role of thiamine status in sulphur induced polioencephalomalacia in sheep. *Research in Veterinary Science* 52 (1): 78–85.

Pan, X., Nan, X., Yang, L. et al. (2018). Thiamine status, metabolism and application in dairy cows: a review. *British Journal of Nutrition* 120 (5): 491–499.
Rammell, C.G. and Hill, J.H. (1986). A review of thiamine deficiency and its diagnosis, especially in ruminants. *New Zealand Veterinary Journal* 34 (12): 202–204.
Ramos, J.J., Marca, C., Loste, A. et al. (2003). Biochemical changes in apparently normal sheep from flocks affected by polioencephalomalacia. *Veterinary Research Communications* 27 (2): 111–124.
Ramos, J.J., Ferrer, L.M., García, L. et al. (2005). Polioencephalomalacia in adult sheep grazing pastures with prostrate pigweed. *Canadian Veterinary Journal* 46 (1): 59–61.
Ramos, J.J., Marca, C., Ferrer, L.M. et al. (2006). Faecal thiaminase, plasma lactate and pyruvate concentrations and erythrocyte transketolase activity changes in apparently normal replacement ewes after the initiation to the pasture. *Research in Veterinary Science* 80 (1): 11–16.
Rousseaux, C.G., Olkowski, A.A., Chauvet, A. et al. (1991). Ovine polioencephalomalacia associated with dietary sulphur intake. *Zentralblatt für Veterinärmedizin. Reihe A* 38 (3): 229–239.
Sakhaee, E. and Derakhshanfar, A. (2010). Polioencephalomalacia associated with closantel overdosage in a goat. *Journal of the South African Veterinary Association* 81 (2): 116–117.
Sant'Ana, F.J.F. and Barros, C.S.L. (2010). Polioencephalomalacia in ruminants in Brazil. *Brazilian Journal of Veterinary Pathology* 3 (1): 70–79.
Schenk, H.C., Ganter, M., Seehusen, F. et al. (2007). Magnetic resonance imaging findings in metabolic and toxic disorders of 3 small ruminants. *Journal of Veterinary Internal Medicine* 21 (4): 865–871.
Sharma, N., Kumar, A., Kumar, R. et al. (2013). Thiamine responsive polioencephalomalacia in a kid. *Veterinary Practitioner* 14 (2): 325–356.
Sharma, N., Kumar, A., Singh, M.K. et al. (2021). Clinical management of polioencephalomalacia in goats – a retrospective study of 18 cases. *Veterinary Practitioner* 22 (2): 52–54.
Sivaraman, S., Vijayakumar, G., Venkatesakumar, E., and Ponnuswamy, K.K. (2016). Clinical management of polioencephalomalacia in goats – a retrospective study of 18 cases. *Indian Veterinary Journal* 93 (5): 70–72.
Smith, M.C. (1979). Polioencephalomalacia in goats. *Journal of the American Veterinary Medical Association* 174 (12): 1328–1332.
Smith, M.C. and Sherman, D.M. (2009). *Goat Medicine*, 2e. Ames, IA: Wiley-Blackwell.
Spicer, E.M. and Horton, B.J. (1981). Biochemistry of natural and amprolium-induced polioencephalomalacia in sheep. *Australian Veterinary Journal* 57 (5): 230–235.
Strain, G.M., Claxton, M.S., Olcott, B.M., and Turnquist, S.E. (1990). Visual-evoked potentials and electroretinograms in ruminants with thiamine-responsive polioencephalomalacia or suspected listeriosis. *American Journal of Veterinary Research* 51 (10): 1513–1517.
Thomas, K.W., Turner, D.L., and Spicer, E.M. (1987). Thiamine, thiaminase and transketolase levels in goats with and without polioencephalomalacia. *Australian Veterinary Journal* 64 (4): 126–127.
Tylicki, A., Łotowski, Z., Siemieniuk, M., and Ratkiewicz, A. (2018). Thiamine and selected thiamine antivitamins – biological activity and methods of synthesis. *Bioscience Reports* 38 (1): BSR20171148.
Vora, B., Green, E.A.E., Khuri, N. et al. (2020). Drug–nutrient interactions: discovering prescription drug inhibitors of the thiamine transporter ThTR-2 (SLC19A3). *American Journal of Clinical Nutrition* 111 (1): 110–121.
Wang, X., Xu, M., Frank, J.A. et al. (2017). Thiamine deficiency induces endoplasmic reticulum stress and oxidative stress in human neurons derived from induced pluripotent stem cells. *Toxicology and Applied Pharmacology* 320: 26–31.

51

Salmonellosis

Anil Kumar[1], Pardeep Sharma[2], Bhoomika Sirsant[3], Sonam Bhatt[1], and Tanmoy Rana[4]

[1] Department of Veterinary Medicine, Bihar Veterinary College, Bihar Animal Sciences University, Patna, India
[2] Department of Veterinary Medicine, Dr G.C. Negi College of Veterinary and Animal Sciences, CSK HPKV Palampur, India
[3] Department of Veterinary Public Health and Epidemiology, Bihar Veterinary College, Bihar Animal Sciences University, Patna, India
[4] Department of Veterinary Clinical Complex, West Bengal University of Animal and Fishery Sciences, Kolkata, India

51.1 Introduction

The *Salmonella* genus of bacteria was named in honor of veterinarian Daniel Elmer Salmon and Mr Theobald Smith, who discovered *Bacillus cholerasuis*, later known as *Salmonella enterica* serovar Cholerasuis, in 1885 while looking for the origins of the cholera prevalent in hogs (Chlebicz and Slizewska 2018; Fàbrega and Vila 2013).

Salmonella is a member of the Enterobacteriaceae family and is a Gram-negative, rod-shaped, facultative anaerobe, flagellated bacterium. Different serotypes (serovars) are classified based on the presence of *Salmonella* spp. lipopolysaccharide (O), flagellar protein (H), and possibly capsular antigen (Vi) (Pal et al. 2020). There are more than 2500 different *Salmonella* serovars in the world (Adem et al. 2022). However, only a small number of these serovars produce clinical disease in animals, and many only affect certain specific species. Based on genomic relatedness and biochemical reactions (Brenner et al. 2000), *S. enterica* and *S. bongori* species are the only two that constitute the genus *Salmonella*. The six subspecies of *S. enterica* are *S. enterica* subsp. *enterica* (I), *S. enterica* subsp. *salamae* (II), *S. enterica* subsp. *arizonae* (IIIa), *S. enterica* subsp. *diarizonae* (IIIb), *S. enterica* subsp. *houtenae* (IV), and *S. enterica* subsp. *indica* (VI). *S. bongori* is also referred to as subsp. V. The majority of *Salmonella* organisms that infect people and domestic animals are members of *S. enterica* subsp. *enterica* (I) because *S. bongori* as well as subspecies II, IIIa, IIIb, IV, and VI are found principally in cold-blooded vertebrates and in the environment (Fàbrega and Vila 2013).

Salmonellosis causes significant economic losses in animal husbandry. This can be attributed to the costs associated with diagnosing and treating diseases, cleaning and disinfection costs, and management and prevention costs. In addition, the emergence of antimicrobial resistance can increase morbidity, mortality, and costs associated with treating the disease (Pal et al. 2020).

51.2 Etiology

Salmonellosis is an infectious disease of animals that causes severe damage to livestock and serious public health problems worldwide. One of the most serious bacterial zoonotic diseases, salmonellosis is caused by *Salmonella* bacteria that can affect humans, animals, and poultry species. It is the most prevalent diseases in small ruminants. The species that cause typhoid fever and produce salmonellosis in humans can be separated from nontyphoidal species, which are believed to account for 85% of human cases through contaminated food. In sheep and goats the most common serovars causing disease are *S. typhimurium*, *S. dublin*, *S. anatum*, *S. enterica* subsp. *diarizonae* 61:(k):1,5,(7), and *S. montevideo* (No authors listed 2017).

Elements of Reproduction and Reproductive Diseases of Goats, First Edition. Edited by Tanmoy Rana.

51.3 Distribution

Salmonella species are prevalent in a wide range globally, including India. Salmonellosis has been detected in all countries, but nontyphoid infections appear to be most prevalent in areas where livestock production, especially poultry and pigs, is intensively practiced (Jajere 2019). Among the *Salmonella* species, S. *enteritidis* is the most prevalent followed by *S. typhimurium*, and both are worldwide in distribution. Food of animal origin is the most important source of nontyphoid salmonellosis, but little information is available from developing countries (Acha and Szyfres 2001).

In Bangladesh, the prevalence of *Salmonella* spp. was 12.76% (6/47) on fecal samples. Based on biochemical testing and serotyping (slide agglutination test), *S. typhimurium*, *S. enteritidis*, *S. brandenburg*, *S. salford*, *S. newbrunswick*, *S. newport*, and *S. dublin* were found (Saha et al. 2013). In Egypt (Giza governorate), the prevalence of *Salmonella* was 3.86% (20/518) in diarrheic sheep and goats, and the *Salmonella* spp. strains revealed a wide range of recovered serovars (*S. mississippi*, *S. durham*, *S. enteritidis*, *S. ferruch*, *S. paratyphi* A, *S. allerton*, *S. bonariensis*, *S. kottbus,* and *S. stanleyville*) (Farouk et al. 2021). In Iraq (Baghdad governorate), 300 fecal samples i.e., 100 diarrheal people, 100 sheep, and 100 goats, were examined. The highest prevalence rate was observed in sheep at 11% (33/300), followed by human feces at 10% (30/300) and goat feces at 5% (15/300), and the isolates recovered were *S. typhimurium* and *S. enteritidis* in goats (Ibrahem and Abdul-Kareem 2022). Goats slaughtered for chevon yielded 17.6% (35/204) *Salmonella* in Bareilly, India (Chandra et al. 2006).

The study of *Salmonella* serovars in sheep and goats and their probable zoonotic risk to humans in the Suez Canal area of Egypt revealed 23.3% in sheep feces, 7% in goat feces, and 13% in human feces (Hawwas et al. 2022). In the Sylhet district of Bangladesh, a total of 220 goat feces samples were collected, of which 27 (12.27%) were positive for *Salmonella* by conventional culture methods and 20 (9.09%) by biochemical and PCR techniques (Sabur et al. 2021).

Salmonella causes significant mortality in kids and even has the potential to lead to abortion in adult female goats (Arruda et al. 2004; Saha et al. 2013). This infection may lead to problems of producing goats and goat meat (chevon), as well as the areas where it will undoubtedly affect the health and body condition of goats. Poor market value is caused by the low quality and quantity of chevon (Arruda et al. 2004).

51.4 Transmission

Infection with *Salmonella* is common in goats. The gastrointestinal tracts of birds and other animals are the first source of infection. Apparently healthy animals can become subclinical carriers and act as a reservoir for the pathogen by persistently shedding *Salmonella* in their feces.

Salmonella is predominantly enteric, widely distributed in the environment and commonly found in agricultural wastewater (farm effluents), human sewage, and any material subject to fecal contamination (Pal et al. 2020). Transmission routes for *Salmonella* are determined by their diversity and origins (Figure 51.1). Foods of animal origin and their products are the most common vehicles of *Salmonella* in humans. It is transmitted mainly through contaminated food and characterized clinically by septicemia and enteritis.

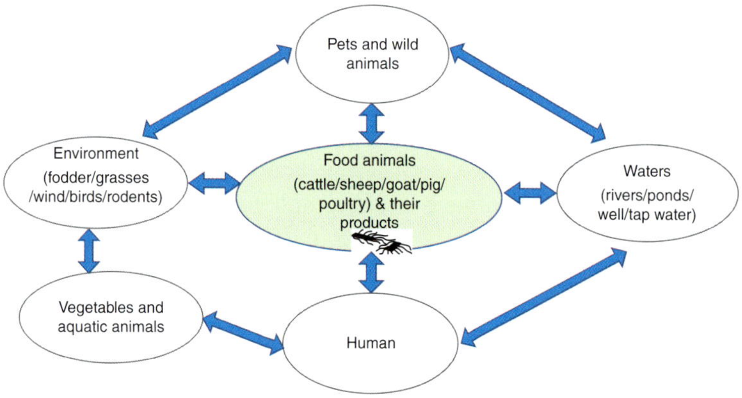

Figure 51.1 Diversity and source of transmission routes of *Salmonella*.

Infections are also acquired through direct or indirect animal contact in homes, veterinary clinics, zoological gardens, farm environments and other public, professional or private settings.

Salmonella contamination of livestock compound feeds is discussed in the literature (Sharma and Sharma 2015), and moving materials from one location to another, placing materials in catchment pits, and other human interventions create large amounts of dust that can carry *Salmonella* (Sharma et al. 2020). Contamination can also occur via biological vectors (Pellegrini et al. 2015). Due to the zoonotic nature of *Salmonella*, feed-to-food transmission is quite possible, and *Salmonella* prevalence in feed pellets was recorded with two major species, *S. enteritidis* and *S. typhimurium*. *Salmonella* contamination has been identified in feed pellets and mash collected from feed mills, which can serve as a source of transmission to people through the food supply chain (Sharma et al. 2020).

Salmonellosis in humans and animals is an infectious and food-borne disease. Although *Salmonella* can cause disease in animals, they are usually asymptomatic carriers (Duffy et al. 2009). Animals that are clinically affected may shed *Salmonella* more frequently than animals that appear healthy, but both may continue to do so for extended periods of time. *Salmonella* infection in goats can affect both sexes at any age and throughout any season. It occurs more frequently in winter and spring and is often associated with parturition periods and animal housing, but can occur at any time of year.

Stress and high stocking density are important factors that can lead to disease outbreaks, especially when animals from different sources are mixed (No authors listed 2017). Severe weather, such as flooding, can also drive animals into small areas of potentially contaminated pasture. Other stressors include long-term periods of no feeding, long transport times, gathering, shearing, dystocia, large variations in temperature and humidity during the day, or cold, damp, windy weather (No authors listed 2017). In carrier animals, stress reduces resistance and allows *Salmonella* to multiply more rapidly. If stocking densities are high, fecal contamination of feed, water, bedding, and skin can lead to disease outbreaks.

Salmonella causes diarrhea and systemic infections in humans. Those most susceptible to salmonellosis are young children, the elderly, people with weakened immune systems, or those taking proton pump inhibitors (World Organisation for Animal Health 2022). In general, human *Salmonella* infections range from self-limiting to life-threatening illnesses that cause death in children, the elderly, and immune compromised individuals (Abuaita et al. 2021). In addition to established routes of food poisoning, humans can also become infected through interaction with live animals or environments contaminated with animal feces, followed by accidental ingestion of the bacteria (Cummings et al. 2012). In addition, animal gut microbiota and associated pathogens in the animal's gut or feces can contaminate carcases and readily transfer to meat, organ surfaces, wool, and skin during meat processing. Additionally, this may occur indirectly through human hands and equipment in the slaughterhouse (Thomas et al. 2020).

51.5 Clinical Signs of Salmonellosis in Goats and Humans

The course of infection, clinical manifestations, necropsy findings, and epidemiological patterns vary according to the serotype and animal species involved (World Organisation for Animal Health 2022). Three age patterns of salmonellosis have been identified in goats: one-week-old neonatal sepsis, preweaning enteritis in kids aged 2–8 weeks, and enteritis/sepsis in adult goats. The prognosis is grave in the first case, poor in the second, and guarded in the third (Smith and Sherman 2009).

Salmonella infections most commonly cause enteritis and diarrhea in humans and animals. Bacteria can also enter the body and cause septicemia. This invasion causes fever, often accompanied by enteritis. Affected animals become lethargic with drooping ears, arched back, separation from the herd, refusal to eat, and diarrhea. Affected feeder goats may exhibit yellowish to greenish-brown diarrhea. This is often indistinguishable from diarrhea caused by other organisms (Demirbilek 2022). Tachycardia, tachypnea, and a subnormal rectal temperature are common when septic or endotoxic shock occurs. Death may occur after 1–5 days of illness. There can also be a chronic form of the disease in adults, characterized by symptoms that are similar but less severe, followed by recovery and sporadic episodes of diarrhea. These animals may experience anemia and tend to lose weight over time (Smith and Sherman 2009). Rarely there are reports of fibrinous casts or bloody diarrhea in goats as is frequently reported in cattle and sheep (Smith and Sherman 2009).

Differential diagnoses in adult small ruminants include coccidiosis, gastrointestinal nematosis, Johne disease, enterotoxemia, and ruminal acidosis. In neonates, viral or cryptic enteritis, coccidiosis, and enterotoxigenic *Escherichia coli* (ETEC) are important differential diagnoses. For septicemia caused by *Salmonella*, colisepticemia, type D enterotoxemia, and in kids *Mycoplasma* septicemia should be considered (Van Metre et al. 2000). Clinical symptoms in goats experimentally infected with *S. typhimurium* consisted of dyspnea, anorexia, pyrexia, progressive weakness, and diarrhea. Important hemato-biochemical findings included leukocytosis, neutrophilia, decreased packed cell volume (PCV), total erythrocyte count (TEC), and albumin/globulin ratio (Sharma et al. 2001).

Severity and clinical manifestations of *Salmonella* infection in small ruminants vary by age group and serotype (Hoelzer et al. 2011; Uzzau et al. 2001). Very young, old, or immune-compromised animals can be severely affected by diarrhea-related dehydration, develop sepsis, and even die. Survivors may have temporary diarrhea but most recover completely. Each recovering animal may be a carrier for a different period of time. This organism may occur in small numbers in the intestinal mucosa and regional lymph nodes, especially in lymphatic areas, and its persistence in animals can lead to recurrent infections (Demirbilek 2022). Less commonly, *Salmonella* can cause abortion, arthritis, respiratory disease, and meningitis (No authors listed 2017).

Reproductive disorders are also reported due to *Salmonella* infection in goats (Smith and Sherman 2009). *S. enterica* subsp. *diarizonae* 61:(k):1,5,(7) as a cause of caprine abortion has been reported (Schnydrig et al. 2018). *Salmonella abortusovis* affects sheep and causes abortions and stillbirths in pregnant ewes and neonatal deaths. It is adapted to sheep and considered to be host specific, but a few reports of its presence in goats are recorded. Typhoid fever and gastroenteritis are two of the most prevalent clinical manifestations of the illness. Unlike other Salmonella species, *S. abortusovis* does not appear to pose a significant threat to human health (Spickler 2017).

51.6 Diagnosis

Diagnosis of salmonellosis is based on isolation of the pathogen from tissues obtained aseptically at necropsy or from animal feces, milk, blood, rectal swabs, or environmental samples (Pal et al. 2020). If reproductive organs are infected or abortion occurs, it is essential to culture vaginal swabs, placenta, and fetal stomach contents (Demirbilek 2022). In cases of septicemia, due to the increasing incidence of *Salmonella* antibiotic resistance, blood cultures may be attempted prior to antibiotic therapy and antibiotic susceptibility testing of isolates will be required (Smith and Sherman 2009).

Numerous methods are used worldwide to isolate and detect *Salmonella*. The best culture technique and media used for a given diagnostic situation will depend on many factors, including *Salmonella* serotype, specimen source and type, animal species of origin, microbiologist experience, and availability of selective enrichment and plating media (World Organisation for Animal Health 2022). Isolation and identification of *Salmonella* should be done according to the International Organization for Standardization protocol (ISO-6579:2002/AMD:2017) and serotyped using a slide agglutination test following the Kauffmann–White scheme (Chamlakhorn et al. 2021).

A variety of techniques can be used to identify the organism, such as preenrichment to resuscitate sublethally damaged salmonellae, enrichment media containing inhibitory compounds to prevent competing organisms, and selective agars to distinguish salmonellae from other enterobacteria. To allow for reliable verification of an isolated strain, various biochemical, serological, and molecular tests can be applied to pure cultures. Culture is the gold standard diagnostic method for *Salmonella*. The somatic (O), flagellar (H), and virulence (Vi) antigens of the organism can be recognized by special typing sera. The serovar can be detected using the antigenic formulae in the Kauffman–White scheme. In order to confirm the full serological identity of the isolate and, where appropriate, the phage type and genotype of the strain, many laboratories require that isolates be sent to a reference laboratory (OIE 2008). The selective media most commonly used against *Salmonella* are SS agar, bismuth sulfite agar (Figure 51.2), hectoene enteric-coated medium (HE), brilliant green agar (Figure 51.3), and xylose-lisinedeoxycholate agar (XLD). All these media contain both selective and discriminatory components and are commercially available.

Salmonella detection from primary animal production must be done using the modified semisolid Rappaport–Vassiliadis (MSRV) agar-based method, which has been validated for fecal, food, feed, and environmental samples. *Salmonella* detection from food or feeding materials is optional.

The standard procedure starts with preenrichment in buffered peptone water, followed by mandatory selective enrichment on MSRV agar for samples of primary production, while for food and feedstuffs the recommended selective enrichment is Müller–Kauffmann tetrathionate broth (MKTTn), Rappaport–Vassiliadis-soya (RVS) broth, or MSRV. Finally, isolation is done on XLD agar. It has been demonstrated that MSRV agar is a highly reliable method for detecting motile salmonellae. Quantification methods can also be used to detect *Salmonella*. Direct plating can be used to count *Salmonella* from infected tissues, but most probable number (MPN) techniques are required for samples from feces, feed, or the environment. ISO,2012 (ISO/TS 6579-2:2012) has described and listed a miniaturized MPN method.

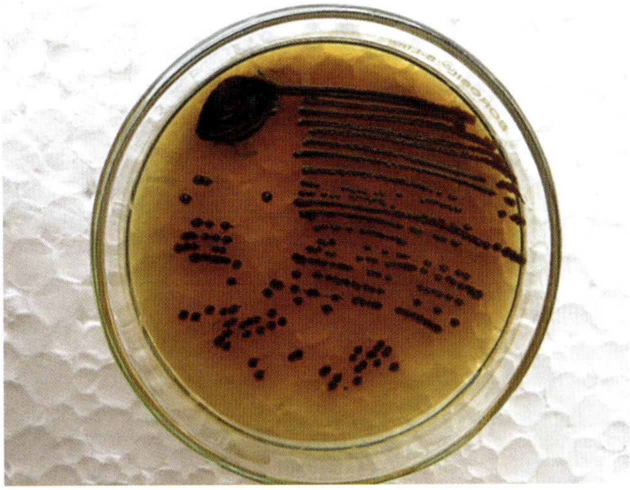

Figure 51.2 Black-centered colonies of *Salmonella* spp. on bismuth sulfite agar.

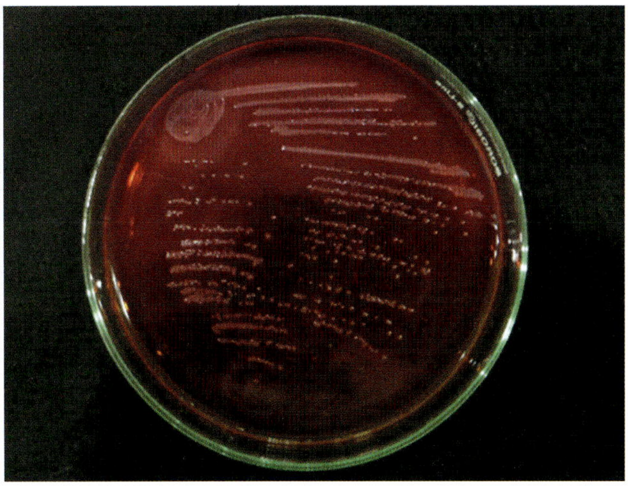

Figure 51.3 Small, round, smooth-edged, pink colonies of *Salmonella* spp. on brilliant green agar.

Direct hybridization (DNA probe) and amplification (PCR) methods are the two major techniques of the molecular assays used for the detection of *Salmonella* pathogens (Lee et al. 2015). Additionally, quantitative real-time PCR techniques have been created (World Organisation for Animal Health 2022). *Salmonella* can also be identified quickly and accurately using MALDI-TOF (Dieckmann and Malorny 2011). The slide agglutination test can be used for rapid detection of *Salmonella* in field cases (Saha et al. 2013).

51.7 Treatment

Antimicrobial agents are valuable tools for treating infectious diseases and for keeping animals healthy and productive. However, antibiotic resistance is becoming more common worldwide and poses a serious and costly problem for animal health, thus limiting therapeutic options in both humans and animals, so antibiotic selection should be done very carefully.

The disease is generally self-limited and usually does not require specific treatment. Animals with severe diarrhea may require rehydration, sometimes with intravenous fluids. In newborn kids with septicemia glucose supplementation is also recommended. If the newborn is hypogammaglobulinemic, whole-blood or preferably plasma transfusion is desirable. Parenterally administered nonsteroidal antiinflammatory drugs (flunixin meglumine) can be helpful (Smith and Sherman 2009).

Antibiotics are not recommended for uncomplicated cases and should be used only if the infection is spreading or is very likely to spread from the intestine into the bloodstream and other organs. However, for systemic infections in animals and humans with septicemia, antibiotic therapy is warranted and should be based on susceptibility of the cultured bacteria (Adem et al. 2022).

Ciprofloxacin, gentamicin, and neomycin are the most effective antibiotics for the majority of *Salmonella* isolates in goats (Sabur et al. 2021), while they are moderately sensitive to oxytetracyline, streptomycin, and amoxicillin, less sensitive to sulfamethoxazole and resistant to penicillin-G (Saha et al. 2013). Caprine *Salmonella* isolates are also frequently susceptible to cephalothin, the aminoglycosides gentamicin and kanamycin, and trimethoprim sulfonamide combinations. Gentamicin 1 mg/kg, IM/SC eight hourly is effective. Chloramphenicol every 12 hours at a dose of 10 mg/kg IV is a proven drug in most goat isolates of *Salmonella* (Smith and Sherman 2009). Additionally, supportive treatment with intravenous fluids is necessary for patients with anorexia, depression, and significant dehydration. Individual patients can be treated aggressively after acid–base and electrolyte evaluation (Pal et al. 2020). Silver nanoparticles can effectively fight multidrug-resistant (MDR) *Salmonella* spp. *in vitro* and *in vivo* without adverse effects (Farouk et al. 2020).

51.8 Prevention and Control

Salmonellosis is diagnosed based on both clinical symptoms and pathogen isolation from infected animals' feces, blood, or tissues. To prevent infection spread, affected animals should be segregated. A disease control strategy should take into account the fact that certain *Salmonella* serotypes are amenable to vaccination, which may lessen the severity of clinical symptoms. *Salmonella* carrier introduction must be avoided at all costs. Only trade with trusted sources and avoid markets and dealers, and also keep new stock away from the main herd for one month.

Everyone should be aware of the risks associated with handling infectious animals and the value of maintaining good personal hygiene. Hence, good hygiene practices and personal protective clothing are crucial to prevent occupational infections. It is necessary to implement a stringent farm management program. People should not eat or drink in areas where animal feces are present. Before eating, drinking, or smoking, properly wash and dry the hands. Between farm visits, thoroughly disinfect and wash protective clothing and equipment. *Salmonella* thrives in pools of water, which can infect or contaminate animals, pets, and motor vehicles. Movement of people must be restricted as they may spread infection between farms. Control of rodents and wild birds can reduce infection as they may carry *Salmonella* and other pathogens back into previously disinfected areas and between farms (No authors listed 2017).

Feed and water supplies must be protected from fecal contamination. Contaminated buildings must be vigorously cleaned and disinfected.

References

Abuaita, B.H., Lawrence, A.E., Berger, R.P. et al. (2021). Comparative transcriptional profiling of the early host response to infection by typhoidal and non-typhoidal *Salmonella* serovars in human intestinal organoids. *PLoS Pathogens* 17: e1009987.

Acha, P.N. and Szyfres, B. (2001). *Zoonoses and Communicable Disease Common to Man and Animals*, 3e, 233–245. New York: World Health Organization.

Adem, J., Ame, M.M., Ali, A., and Mokeria, E. (2022). Review of the zoonotic importance of salmonellosis and associated risk factors. *Open Journal of Veterinary Medicine* 7 (2): 62–69.

Arruda, S.G.B., Biscontini, T.M.B., and Stamford, T.L.M. (2004). Microbiological characterization of goat meat subjected to different forms of management. *Hygiene Alimentar* 18: 58–62.

Brenner, F.W., Villar, R.G., Angulo, F.J. et al. (2000). Salmonella nomenclature. *Journal of Clinical Microbiology* 38: 2465–2467.

Chamlakhorn, W., Phuektes, P., Khang-Air, S., and Angkititrakul, S. (2021). Prevalence, genetic characterization, and antimicrobial resistance of Salmonella isolated from meat goats in the northeastern region of Thailand. *Veterinary Integrative Sciences* 19 (3): 363–378.

Chandra, M., Singh, B.R., Shankar, H. et al. (2006). Study on prevalence of *Salmonella* infection in goats. *Small Ruminant Research* 65 (1–2): 24–30.

Chlebicz, A. and Slizewska, K.S. (2018). Campylobacteriosis, salmonellosis, yersiniosis, and listeriosis as zoonotic foodborne diseases: a review. *International Journal of Environmental Research and Public Health* 15: 863.

Cummings, K.J., Warnick, L.D., Gröhn, Y.T. et al. (2012). Clinical features of human salmonellosis caused by bovine-associated subtypes in New York. *Foodborne Pathogens and Disease* 9: 796–802.

Demirbilek, S.K. (2022). Salmonellosis in animals. In: *Salmonella – A Re-emerging Pathogen* (ed. M. Mascellino). Intechopen http://dx.doi.org/10.5772/intechopen.72192.

Dieckmann, R. and Malorny, B. (2011). Rapid screening of epidemiologically important *Salmonella enterica* subsp. enterica serovars by whole-cell matrix-assisted laser desorption ionization-time of flight mass spectrometry. *Applied and Environmental Microbiology* 77: 4136–4146.

Duffy, L., Barlow, R., Fegan, N., and Vanderlinde, P. (2009). Prevalence and serotypes of Salmonella associated with goats at two Australian abattoirs. *Letters in Applied Microbiology* 48: 193–197.

Fàbrega, A. and Vila, J. (2013). Salmonella enterica serovar typhimurium skills to succeed in the host: virulence and regulation. *Clinical Microbiology Reviews* 26: 308–341.

Farouk, M.M., El-Molla, A., Salib, F.A. et al. (2020). The role of silver nanoparticles in a treatment approach for multidrug-resistant salmonella species isolates. *International Journal of Nanomedicine* 15: 6993–7011.

Farouk, M.M., El-Molla, A., Salib, F.A., and Soliman, Y.A. (2021). Epidemiology of *Salmonella* species in diarrheic sheep and goats. *Pakistan Journal of Zoology* 54: 381–389.

Hawwas, H.A.E., Aboueisha, A.M., Fadel, H.M., and El-Mahallawy, H.S. (2022). *Salmonella* serovars in sheep and goats and their probable zoonotic potential to humans in Suez Canal Area, Egypt. *Acta Veterinaria Scandinavica* 64 (1): 17.

Hoelzer, K., Moreno Switt, A.I., and Wiedmann, M. (2011). Animal contact as a source of human non-typhoidal salmonellosis. *Veterinary Research* 42: 34.

Ibrahem, H.A. and Abdul-Kareem, I.Q. (2022). Molecular detection of *Salmonella* spp. isolated from diarrheic human, sheep and goats in Baghdad governorate by multiplex PCR. *Annals of Forest Research* 65 (1): 6168–6181.

Jajere, S.M. (2019). A review of *Salmonella enterica* with particular focus on the pathogenicity and virulence factors, host specificity and antimicrobial resistance including multidrug resistance. *Veterinary World* 12: 504.

Lee, K., Runyon, M., Herrman, T.J. et al. (2015). Review of Salmonella detection and identification methods: aspects of rapid emergency response and food safety. *Food Control* 47: 264–276.

No authors listed (2017). Salmonella investigations in ruminants. *Veterinary Record* 181: 366–367.

Office International des Epizooties (OIE) (2008). Chapter 2.9.9. Salmonellosis. In: *Manual of Diagnostic Tests and Vaccines for Terrestrial Animals*. Paris: World Organisation for Animal Health.

Pal, M., Teashal, B.M., Gizaw, F. et al. (2020). Animals and food of animal origin as a potential source of Salmonellosis: a review of the epidemiology, laboratory diagnosis, economic impact and public health significance. *American Journal of Microbiological Research* 8 (2): 48–56.

Pellegrini, D.D.C.P., Paim, D.S., Lima, G.J.M.M. et al. (2015). Distribution of *Salmonella* clonal groups in four Brazilian feed mills. *Food Control* 47: 672–678.

Sabur, M.A., Das, M.R., Uddin, M.B. et al. (2021). Molecular detection and antibiotic sensitivity of salmonella species isolated from goat feces in Sylhet district of Bangladesh. *World's Veterinary Journal* 11 (3): 395–401.

Saha, G.K., Paul, A.K., Abdussamad et al. (2013). Epidemiological investigation and antibiotic sensitivity of salmonellosis in goats at selected areas of Bangladesh. *Journal of Animal Reproduction and Biotechnology* 28 (4): 337–342.

Schnydrig, P., Overesch, G., Regli, W. et al. (2018). *Salmonella enterica* subspecies diarizonae serovar 61: (k):1,5,(7) as cause of caprine abortion. *Small Ruminant Research* 166: 78–82.

Sharma, V. and Sharma, S. (2015). Potential hazards in animal feeds: safety and regulation. *Indian Journal of Animal Nutrition* 32: 242–262.

Sharma, A.K., Tripathi, B.N., Verma, J.C., and Parihar, N.S. (2001). Experimental *Salmonella enterica* subspecies *enterica* serovar *Typhimurium* infection in Indian goats: clinical, serological, bacteriological and pathological studies. *Small Ruminant Research* 42 (2): 125–134.

Sharma, V., Sharma, S., Verma, A. et al. (2020). Feed safety evaluation for prevalence of zoonotic *Salmonella* spp. in animal feed. *Indian Journal of Animal Sciences* 90 (1): 17–21.

Smith, M.C. and Sherman, D.M. (2009). *Goat Medicine*, 2e, 412–416. Ames, IA: Wiley-Blackwell.

Spickler, A.R. (2017). *Salmonella* Abortusovis. www.cfsph.iastate.edu/Factsheets/pdfs/salmonella_abortusovis.pdf (accessed 20 November 2023).

Thomas, K.M., de Glanville, W.A., Barker, G.C. et al. (2020). Prevalence of *Campylobacter* and *Salmonella* in African food animals and meat: a systematic review and meta-analysis. *International Journal of Food Microbiology* 315: 108382.

Uzzau, S., Leori, G.S., Petruzzi, V. et al. (2001). Salmonella enterica serovar-host specificity does not correlate with the magnitude of intestinal invasion in sheep. *Infection and Immunity* 69 (5): 3092–3099.

Van Metre, D.C., Tyler, J.W., and Stehman, S.M. (2000). Diagnosis of enteric disease in small ruminants. *Veterinary Clinics of North America: Food Animal Practice* 16 (1): 87–115.

World Organisation for Animal Health (2022). Chapter 3.10.7. Salmonellosis. In: *Manual of Diagnostic Tests and Vaccines for Terrestrial Animals*., 1–19. Paris: World Organisation for Animal Health.

52

Rectal Prolapse in Kids

Priyanka Duggal and Ram Niwas

Department of Veterinary Surgery and Radiology, College of Veterinary Sciences, Lala Lajpat Rai University of Veterinary and Animal Sciences, Hisar, India

52.1 Introduction

Goat farming in India is generally practiced by either a marginal farmer, who has a very small area of land, or a landless laborer, due to the much lower risk and initial investment compared with other forms of farming. Goats are appropriately referred to as "the poor man's cow" because they promise a decent return on investment (Pashudhan Praharee 2022). According to a recent livestock census (2019), the total goat population in India is 148.88 million which is about 27.80% of the total livestock population followed by buffalo, sheep, and pigs. The demand for goat milk has increased recently because of its medicinal property, encouraging more and more farmers to invest in goat farming in India. This led to a 10.14% increase in the goat population since the previous livestock census in 2012 (Department of Animal Husbandry and Dairying 2012).

Many disease conditions have a deleterious effect on production which directly or indirectly affects the health of the goat and rectal prolapse is one of them. Rectal prolapse in goats is a complicated health condition and accounts for nearly 12% of the digestive disorders in goats. Numerous factors, including sex, age, food, coughing, and chronic scours, are believed to be contributing causes.

The term "rectal prolapse" refers to the protrusion of one or more layers of the rectum through the anal orifice (Figure 52.1). The typical diagnostic sign is an elongated, cylindrical mass that is bright red in color, which can be treated nonsurgically if detected early enough and treated promptly. Over time, the exposed tissue becomes dry and cracked, aggravating the pain which leads to further irritation, straining, and exacerbation of the prolapse.

52.2 Prevalence and Etiology

All domestic animal species are susceptible to rectal prolapse but pigs are more likely to experience it than cows, cattle, sheep, goats, or other species. Sheep and goats have many common diseases due to their proximity in anatomical and physiological features (Agrawal et al. 2014), but there is still a distinct nature of each species that makes some disorders more prevalent in one species than the other. Congenital anomalies are more prevalent in goats than sheep (Farghali et al. 2020) and sheep are more commonly affected by rectal prolapse than goats, primarily because of the practice of short tail docking in exhibition lambs. In one study, the incidence of rectal prolapse was significantly higher in sheep with short tail dock (7.8%) than medium dock (4.0%) or long dock (1.8%) (Hartnack and Jones 2017).

Rectal prolapse in goats is typically caused by a combination of many factors, including sex, age, food, coughing, and chronic scours. Rectal prolapses are more common in females than males. Internal fat is more likely to be stored in the female pelvic region and this affects the hind stomach and rectal tissue when a goat coughs or strains. Therefore, regardless of other risk factors, the majority of prolapsing animals are female. A fatty doe is most prone to rectal prolapse.

Rectal prolapse is most often observed as a consequence of some other disease condition or disorder that increases intraabdominal pressure, intrapelvic pressure or abdominal straining. Multiple fetuses during gestation increase intraabdominal pressure which ultimately strains the pelvic muscles and weakens the rectal support tissue inside the pelvic region

Elements of Reproduction and Reproductive Diseases of Goats, First Edition. Edited by Tanmoy Rana.

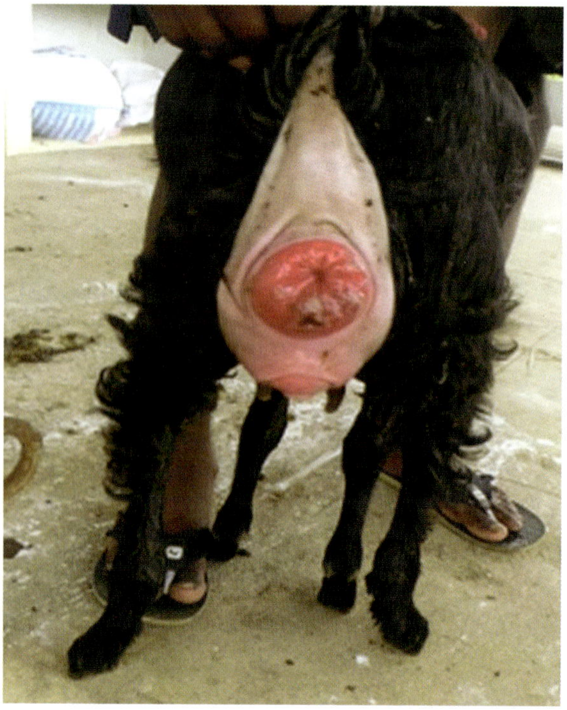

Figure 52.1 Rectal prolapse in a goat. *Source:* Arulkumar et al. (2022).

(Anderson and Miesner 2008). Riding behavior, chronic coughing, enteritis (coccidia, Salmonella), chronic diarrhea (Radostits et al. 2009), and persistent tenesmus associated with intestinal, anorectal or urogenital disease (Arulkumar et al. 2022), such as dyschezia, dysuria, urinary tract obstruction in males and vaginal prolapse in females, are some of the factors that increases intrapelvic pressure (Roberts 1986). Gastrointestinal parasitic load, especially coccidiosis, may cause diarrhea and be associated with increased incidence of rectal prolapse. Kids are most susceptible to coccidiosis at approximately 1–4 months of age, although younger animals may become infected.

Other risk factors for rectal and/or vaginal prolapse include denervation of the pelvic region, intoxication with estrogenic feeds like barseem (*Trifolium alexandrinum*), feeds that contain estrogen as a growth promoter and zearalenone, and alkaloids like *Atropa belladonna* (Koekkoek 2014). Zearalenone is a mycotoxin which activates the estrogen receptors in the body. This hyperestrogenic effect of zearalenone and anticholinergic effect of *Atropa belladonna* causes relaxation of rectal smooth muscles which eventually leads to rectal prolapse (Fink-Gremmels and Malekinejad 2007).

Reduced calcium intake can result in decreased serum calcium concentrations, particularly in animals that are pregnant with multiple fetuses and have increased calcium requirements, which most often occurs during late gestation. Additionally, there is a higher risk of hypocalcemia in the three weeks before delivery when the fetal skeleton is mineralizing, especially when many fetuses present. The physiological responses of hypocalcemia include ruminal stasis, secondary bloat, constipation, anus relaxation, and loss of anal reflex. These effects are in addition to atony of skeletal and smooth muscle. Additionally, it may be inferred that rectal prolapse in advanced pregnancy may be caused by many fetuses and concurrent hypocalcemia.

Rectal prolapse in goats has also been observed to be associated with spastic paresis (Koekkoek 2014). Prolapsed ileocolic intussusception resembles rectal prolapse so these must be differentiated. To distinguish rectal prolapse from prolapsed ileocolic intussusception, a probe such as a finger or blunt object is inserted between the prolapsed mass and the inner rectal wall. The fornix makes it impossible to place the probe in cases of rectal prolapse.

52.3 Classification of Rectal Prolapse

Many classifications of rectal prolapse have been proposed by researchers based on severity and the tissue involved. In 2004, Chakrabarti classified rectal prolapse as incomplete, in which only a portion of the circumference of the rectum is everted, or complete, in which all rectal layers are protruded circumferentially (Chakrabarti 2004). Based on the tissue involved, rectal prolapse is classified into four types as shown in Table 52.1

Table 52.1 Classification of rectal prolapse based on rectal tissue involved.

Classification	Tissue involved
Class I	Tearing of the mucosa and submucosa
Class II	Tearing of the muscular layers
Class III	Tearing of the mucosa, submucosa, and muscular layers
Class IV	Full-thickness tear, mucosa through serosa

Table 52.2 Classification of rectal prolapse based on rectal layer involved.

Classification	Tissue layer involved
Grade I	Small amount of rectal mucosa
Grade II	All layers of rectum
Grade III	All layers of rectum along with intussusception of large colon
Grade IV	All layers of rectum and intussusception of large colon that is constricted by the action of the anal sphincter

Source: Adapted from Haskell (2004).

Classification of rectal prolapse based on the anatomical structures involved is shown in Table 52.2. A Grade I prolapse is of mild and intermittent type which is easy to replace as only a small amount of rectal mucosa is everted. Grade II prolapses include all layers of the rectum and may also be intermittent. Grade III and Grade IV prolapses are large due to involvement of all layers of the rectum and large colon. In Grade IV prolapses, the contents are squeezed by the action of the anal sphincter, causing great pain to the animal.

52.4 Pathophysiology

When a rectal prolapse occurs, venous and lymphatic return is compromised, and swelling and edema develop quickly. The straining response is heightened, exacerbating the prolapse. Although rectal prolapses are rarely considered as emergencies, they should be treated as soon as possible as any partial or intermittent prolapse can cause rectal mucosal damage and irritation from outside stress and persistent tenesmus which ultimately lead to complete prolapse (Arthur et al. 1996; Kumar et al. 2020).

52.5 Treatment

General management of rectal prolapse includes the elimination of predisposing factors, soothing of the irritated mucosa, elimination of straining, and resolving the prolapse. Rectal prolapse can be treated either surgically or nonsurgically based on the grade/class of prolapse.

52.5.1 Nonsurgical Treatment

Nonsurgical treatment is often possible for Grade I and II prolapses as most of these prolapses may be manually corrected with gentle massage and the placement of a purse-string suture (Figure 52.2) that enables feces to flow normally. The purse string is frequently made with umbilical tape. The majority of the suture should be hidden beneath the skin and a slip knot should be placed so that the size of the lumen can be modified.

The injection of counterirritants around the rectum either alone or in conjunction with anal purse-string suturing is a quick and inexpensive treatment in recurrent prolapses. Here an irritating material (typically iodine based) is injected in a line into the pelvis along the serosal surface of the rectum to induce scar tissue development, attaching the rectum into the pelvis and preventing recurrent prolapse. The clinician inserts an

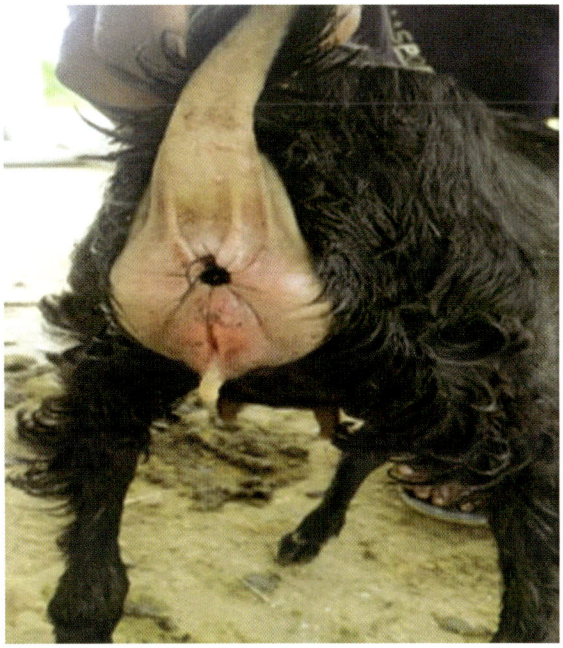

Figure 52.2 Retention of prolapsed mass with purse-string sutures. *Source:* Arulkumar et al. (2022).

18 gauge needle (5 cm) deeply into the skin around the anus at 12, 3, and 9 o'clock. An injection at the 6 o'clock position should be avoided because swelling around the urethra can result in obstruction. In all of these techniques, a caudal epidural anesthetic (2% lidocaine, 0.5 ml/45 kg) is recommended to decrease straining and ease pain from the procedures. An epidural anesthetic using a combination of 2% xylazine (0.1mg/kg) and 2% lignocaine (2 mg/kg) provides faster onset and longer duration of analgesia than either agent used alone.

Other approach is an alcohol epidural that may prevent straining for extended periods. Either isopropyl alcohol or ethanol can be used. This type of anesthesia can be permanent and therefore should be used only for animals intended for slaughter. Because of the potential for some loss of sciatic nerve function, the clinician should perform a test injection of a local anesthetic (2% lidocaine) before using alcohol.

52.5.2 Surgical Treatment

Surgical resection is indicated in cases with recurrent prolapse if nonsurgical treatment is unsuccessful. Amputation is a typical surgical procedure that leads to immediate reduction of the prolapsed mass. It is indicated in Grade III and IV rectal prolapse where the exteriorized prolapsed mass is not viable enough to be replaced by purse-string sutures alone.

Surgical management of prolapse includes caudal epidural anesthesia which is given at the lumbosacral intervertebral space (L6–S1) with the goat in sternal recumbency under aseptic conditions. Lidocaine 2% 2–5 mg/kg is used to provide total anesthesia and loss of motor function to the pelvic organs and hindlimbs (Ismail 2016). Epidural anesthesia temporarily eliminates straining, allowing tissue evaluation, facilitating repositioning, and allowing surgical intervention. The hindquarter may be elevated after washing the prolapsed mass with a 1:1000 potassium permanganate solution or mild antiseptic and applying lubricant. The tissue is evaluated for necrosis, trauma, and tear.

The condition of the prolapsed tissue plays a crucial role in choosing the treatment protocol. The color of the mucosa, degree of edema, necrotic tissue, and presence and depth of erosions are parameters used to decide whether the tissue is salvageable. Treatment options include replacement and purse-string sutures, submucosal resection, or amputation. After achieving epidural anesthesia, an appropriate size of rubber or plastic tube with offset holes is placed into the prolapsed rectum and two Steinman pins or long (6 in.) needles are passed through the holes to form an X in the healthy part of the rectum. This helps in identifying the anatomy of the rectal layers during the procedure. The nonviable part is then resected out and the healthy part is sutured with absorbable suture material.

In market animals, nonsurgical amputation is commonly used and can be achieved by introducing a plastic tube into the lumen and an elastrator band proximal to the prolapse in healthy tissue. This results in ischemic necrosis of the prolapse's distal part, as well as scarring at the band level, leading to anastomosis. When the tissue sloughs, the rigid tube keeps a lumen open for feces. Once the tissue has sloughed, the tube and band will be removed, and the rectum will shrink.

In Grade I, replacement and then purse string is applied for retention of the prolapse until resolution of the condition. Alternatively, it may be retained *in situ* with an improvised prolapse retainer. This technique requires a 5 or 10 ml disposable syringe whose plunger has been removed and the needle end is cut to provide a wider diameter. Smoothing of the cut end is done to prevent trauma and rectal wall irritation. Two holes are then drilled in the wings of the syringe for anchoring. After repositioning the rectal prolapse, this modulated syringe is inserted after lubrication with lubricant. Two stay sutures are then applied through the predrilled holes at the anocutaneous junction. These sutures and the prolapse retainer may be removed after a week or after resolution of the condition. Caudal epidural anesthesia may be repeated if the goat shows straining.

In all Grade II, III, and IV prolapses that are recurrent or resistant to replacement, resection and anastomosis is preferred. If the prolapsed mucosa is necrotic, ulcerated, or damaged but the underlying tissue is healthy, submucosal resection is the recommended approach. This method involves removing the damaged mucosa while preserving the healthy underlying tissue.

After caudal epidural anesthesia, the mucosa is cleaned and edema is reduced by temporary topical application of a hyperosmotic solution. To control movement of the prolapse during surgery, a piece of flexible tubing of suitable diameter is introduced into the lumen of the prolapse and crosspin fixation is done. For this procedure, two 1.5 in., 22 gauge needles are inserted at a 90° angle to one another, at the anal orifice, across the prolapse, and through the tubing. On either side of the area where the tissue is to be removed, two circular incisions are made into the mucosa. The circular incisions are then connected by a longitudinal incision at the same depth as the circular incision. The affected tissue layer is removed from the healthy submucosal plane by blunt dissection. Hemorrhage may be controlled by ligature of individual blood vessels.

Four simple interrupted sutures are placed equidistant around the diameter of the prolapse to align the healthy mucosa. Monofilament absorbable material of sizes 2-0 to 3-0 with a taper-point swaged needle is used. Then a circumferential simple continuous pattern is applied for end-to-end apposition of both circular incisions involving mucosa. The above-mentioned suture patterns and tubing act as a place holder and prevent the occurrence of a purse-string effect at the suture site that might reduce the lumen and cause postoperative stricture development.

Several benefits of this method over amputation have been mentioned, including quicker healing, reduced risk of peritonitis or a perirectal abscess as the serosal lining is not exposed, less postoperative straining, a minimally constricted lumen, and preservation of healthy tissue. Additionally, the risk of postoperative hemorrhage is reduced because the main blood supply is not transected.

For Grade IV, amputation may be the only option when the prolapsed tissue is significantly compromised. Although numerous amputation procedures have been published, a stair-stepped approach reduces the likelihood of stricture development. The preoperative procedures, such as epidural anesthesia, tubing insertion, and needle fixation, are the same as those mentioned for submucosal resection. In this technique, a circumferential incision is made just cranial to the necrotic tissue. All tissues except the inner mucosa and parts of the inner submucosa are incised. With blunt dissection, a plane is created toward the caudal aspect of the prolapse within the inner submucosa between the inner and outer segments. The outer segment is moved forward, while the inner section is amputated 2–3 cm more distally if the length of the prolapsed mass permits.

52.6 Aftercare and Complications

The crosspins should be removed after rectal amputation and mucosal excision, and a regular purse-string suture may be applied and removed within one week. For the first few days following surgery, lidocaine jelly can be used topically. Before and after surgery, analgesics and antimicrobials should be used, and steps should be taken to soften the feces. This could include administering mineral oil or magnesium hydroxide, or increasing the legume or grain portion of the diet slightly. Owners should monitor animals for general demeanor, appetite, abdominal contour, and fecal passage. Animals with increases in abdominal size, reductions in appetite, or evidence of constipation should be evaluated. Stricture development, perirectal abscess, dehiscence, peritonitis, or evisceration of the intestine after dehiscence are all possible postoperative complications.

52.7 Conclusion

Rectal prolapse in kids is a complicated problem which is a consequence of many disease conditions. Elimination of the underlying cause, early diagnosis, and successful management through surgical and nonsurgical methods are critical factors in restoring health.

References

Agrawal, A.R., Karim, S.A., Kumar, R. et al. (2014). Sheep and goat production: basic differences, impact on climate and molecular tools for rumen microbiome study. *International Journal of Current Microbiology and Applied Sciences* 3 (1): 684–706.

Anderson, D.E. and Miesner, M.D. (2008). Rectal prolapse. *Veterinary Clinics of North America: Food Animal Practice* 24: 403–408.

Arthur, G.H., Noakes, D.E., Peterson, H., and Parkinson, T.J. (1996). *Veterinary Reproduction and Obstetrics*, 7e. London: WB Saunders.

Arulkumar, S., Arunkumar, R., Ragulraj, S., and Priyadharsini, R. (2022). Correction and management of rectal prolapse in indigenous goat: a case report. *Pharma Innovation Journal* 8: 698–699.

Chakrabarti Amalendu, *Text Book of Clinical Veterinary Medicine*. Kalyani Publishers, New Delhi, 2004, 233.

Department of Animal Husbandry & Dairying (2012). Livestock census. https://dahd.nic.in/documents/statistics/livestock-census (accessed 20 November 2023).

Farghali, H.A.M.A., Ali, K.K., and Shamaa, A.A.E. (2020). Incidence of the most common surgical affections among sheep and goats admitted to a referral hospital in the State of Kuwait. *Advances in Animal and Veterinary Sciences* 8 (s2): 41–57.

Fink-Gremmels, J. and Malekinejad, H. (2007). Clinical effects and biochemical mechanisms associated with exposure to the mycoestrogen zearalenone. *Animal Feed Science and Technology* 137 (3): 326–341.

Hartnack, A. and Jones, M. (2017). Surgery of the sheep and goat digestive system. In: *Farm Animal Surgery*, 2e (ed. S. Fubini and N. Ducharme), 561–567. St Louis, MO: Elsevier.

Haskell, S.R. (2004). Surgery of the sheep and goat digestive system. In: *Farm Animal Surgery* (ed. S. Fubini and N (e. Ducharme), 521–526. St Louis, MO: Saunders.

Ismail, Z.B. (2016). Epidural analgesia in sheep and goats: a review of recent literature. *Bulletin of University of Agricultural Sciences and Veterinary Medicine* 73 (2): 197–202.

Koekkoek, L.M. (2014). Spastic paresis and rectal/vaginal prolapse in Dutch dairy goats. Master's thesis. Utrecht University.

Kumar, R., Diwakar, R.P., Ramakant, S.H., and Alam, K. (2020). A rare case of antepartum rectal prolapse in a goat and its management: a case report. *Journal of Entomology and Zoology Studies* 8 (2): 1285–1287.

Pashudhan Praharee (2022). Goat farming. www.pashudhanpraharee.com/goat-farming (accessed 20 November 2023).

Radostits, O.M., Gay, C.C., Hinchcliff, K.W., and Constable, P.D. (2009). *Veterinary Medicine: A Textbook of the Diseases of Cattle, Horses, Sheep, Pigs and Goats*, 10e. Philadelphia, PA: W.B. Saunders.

Roberts, S.J. (1986). Injuries and diseases of the puperal period. In: *Veterinary Obstetrics and Genital Diseases*, 3e, 364. Woodstock, VT: Roberts SJ publisher.

53

Copper Deficiency

Abhishek Pathak[1], Kritika Dhial[1], Varun Asediya[2], and Amaan Ghaazi[1]

[1] Apollo College of Veterinary Medicine, Jaipur, Rajasthan, India
[2] Animal Nutrition Research Station, Anand Agricultural University, Anand, Gujarat, India

53.1 Introduction

Copper is a trace mineral that plays a vital role in many aspects of goat health, especially reproduction. However, copper deficiency is a common and serious problem that affects goats worldwide. It can impair their fertility, pregnancy outcomes, offspring survival, and overall well-being. Copper acts as a cofactor for various enzymes and proteins that regulate reproductive functions at the hormonal, cellular, and molecular levels.

Copper deficiency can be caused by inadequate dietary intake of copper or by interference of copper absorption by other minerals or substances in the diet or environment (Figure 53.1). Copper deficiency can also vary depending on the breed, age, sex, and physiological status of the goat, as well as the environmental and nutritional factors that influence copper availability.

The signs and diagnosis of copper deficiency can be challenging, as they may vary depending on the severity and duration of the deficiency and may overlap with other conditions or diseases (Zatta and Frank 2007). Some general signs that indicate possible copper deficiency in goats are poor growth rate; rough or faded hair coat; hair loss around eyes or tail; anemia; diarrhea; lameness; swayback or paralysis in kids; reduced milk yield or quality; reduced fertility or conception rate; increased abortion or stillbirth rate; increased neonatal mortality or morbidity; and increased susceptibility to infections or diseases (Gooneratne et al. 1989).

The methods of copper supplementation and management depend on the cause and extent of the deficiency, as well as the availability and suitability of different sources of copper for goats. Some common methods include providing free-choice minerals that contain adequate amounts of copper, feeding commercial feeds fortified with copper, administering oral or injectable copper supplements, or using copper oxide wire particles (COWP) as a bolus (Martins 2011).

Therefore, it is important for goat owners, veterinarians, researchers, and anyone interested in goat health to understand the role of copper in goat physiology, the signs and diagnosis of copper deficiency, and the methods of copper supplementation and management. This chapter provides an overview of these topics.

53.2 Effects of Copper Deficiency on Goat Reproductive Performance

Copper acts as a cofactor for various enzymes and proteins that regulate reproductive functions at the hormonal, cellular, and molecular levels. For example, copper is involved in the synthesis of steroid hormones (such as estrogen, progesterone, and testosterone), which control the reproductive cycle, behavior, and development of goats (Khalifa et al. 2013). It is also involved in the formation and maintenance of connective tissue (such as collagen and elastin), which is essential for the integrity and function of the reproductive organs (such as the uterus, cervix, placenta, and mammary glands) (Karamanos et al. 2021). Moreover, copper is involved in the protection of reproductive tissues from oxidative stress, which is caused by an imbalance between the production and removal of reactive oxygen species (ROS). ROS are molecules that can damage

Elements of Reproduction and Reproductive Diseases of Goats, First Edition. Edited by Tanmoy Rana.

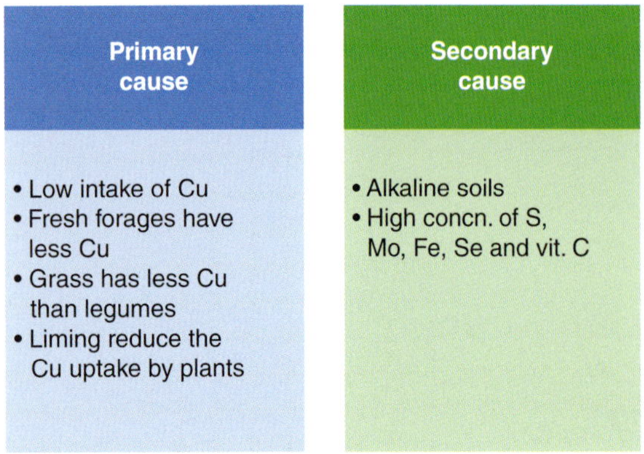

Figure 53.1 Common causes of copper deficiency.

DNA, proteins, lipids, and other cellular components if not neutralized by antioxidant enzymes (such as superoxide dismutase [SOD] and glutathione peroxidase [GPX]), which also require copper as a cofactor (Lushchak 2014).

The effects of copper deficiency on reproductive performance vary depending on the severity and duration of the deficiency, the age and sex of the animal, the breed and genetic background of the animal, and the environmental and nutritional factors that influence copper availability. However, some general signs that indicate possible copper deficiency in goats are poor growth rate; rough or faded hair coat; hair loss around eyes or tail; anemia; diarrhea; lameness; swayback or paralysis in kids; reduced milk yield or quality; reduced fertility or conception rate; increased abortion or stillbirth rate; increased neonatal mortality or morbidity; and increased susceptibility to infections or diseases (Table 53.1).

53.2.1 Ovaries

The ovaries are the female reproductive organs that produce and release eggs (oocytes) and secrete sex hormones (estrogen and progesterone). The ovaries are composed of two main types of cells: follicular cells, which surround and nourish the developing oocytes, and interstitial cells, which produce and secrete hormones. The development and maturation of the oocytes and follicles are regulated by a complex interplay of hormones from the hypothalamus, pituitary gland, and the ovaries themselves.

Copper is involved in several aspects of ovarian function, such as follicle development, ovulation, hormone synthesis, and antioxidant defense. Copper deficiency can impair these functions by affecting the activity and expression of various enzymes and proteins that require copper as a cofactor or a structural component. For example, copper deficiency can affect the following processes.

- *Follicle development*: copper is involved in the synthesis of cytochrome P450 aromatase (CYP19A1), which converts testosterone to estrogen in the follicular cells. Estrogen is essential for the growth and maturation of the follicles and oocytes. Copper deficiency can reduce the expression and activity of CYP19A1, leading to decreased estrogen production and impaired follicle development (Soni et al. 2018).
- *Ovulation*: copper is involved in the synthesis of lysyl oxidase (LOX), which crosslinks collagen and elastin fibers in the ovarian stroma. Collagen and elastin are important for the structural integrity and elasticity of the ovary, which are required for ovulation. Copper deficiency can impair the activity of LOX, leading to reduced collagen and elastin crosslinking and impaired ovulation (Papachroni et al. 2010).
- *Hormone synthesis*: copper is involved in the synthesis of cytochrome P450 17-alpha-hydroxylase/17,20-lyase (CYP17A1), which converts progesterone to androgens in the interstitial cells. Androgens are precursors for estrogen synthesis in the follicular cells. Copper deficiency can reduce the expression and activity of CYP17A1, leading to decreased androgen production and reduced estrogen synthesis (Acién and Acién 2020).

Table 53.1 Effects of copper deficiency on goat reproductive performance.

Aspect of reproduction	Effects of copper deficiency
Ovaries	Decreased follicle development, reduced ovulation, and cycle irregularities
Testes	Reduced sperm production, lower sperm motility and quality, abnormal sperm morphology
Hormones	Altered levels of estradiol, progesterone, and gonadotropins, disrupted estrous cycle
Conception	Decreased conception rate, increased embryo mortality
Pregnancy	Increased risk of pregnancy loss, small litter size, premature birth, increased fetal malformations
Offspring survival	Decreased survival rate of kids due to weak immune system, anemia, and skeletal deformities

- *Antioxidant defense*: copper is involved in the synthesis of SOD, which scavenges ROS in the ovarian cells. ROS are generated during normal metabolic processes or under stress conditions, such as inflammation or infection. ROS can damage DNA, proteins, lipids, and other cellular components if not neutralized by antioxidant enzymes or molecules. Copper deficiency can reduce the expression and activity of SOD, leading to increased oxidative stress and damage in the ovarian cells (da Silva et al. 2014).

53.2.2 Testes

The testes are the male reproductive organs that produce and release sperm and secrete sex hormones (testosterone and inhibin). The testes are composed of two main types of cells: germ cells, which undergo spermatogenesis to produce sperm, and Leydig cells, which produce and secrete testosterone. The development and maturation of the sperm and the testes are regulated by a complex interplay of hormones from the hypothalamus, the pituitary gland, and the testes themselves.

Copper is involved in several aspects of testicular function, such as spermatogenesis, hormone synthesis, and antioxidant defense. Copper deficiency can impair these functions by affecting the activity and expression of various enzymes and proteins that require copper as a cofactor or a structural component. For example, copper deficiency can affect the following processes.

- *Spermatogenesis*: copper is involved in the synthesis of SPO11, DMC1, and RAD51, which mediate homologous recombination and repair of DNA breaks during meiosis. Meiosis is a specialized type of cell division that produces haploid gametes (sperm or eggs) from diploid cells. Copper deficiency can impair the expression and function of these proteins, leading to reduced recombination and increased DNA damage during meiosis, resulting in impaired spermatogenesis (Huang and Roig 2023).
- *Hormone synthesis*: copper is involved in the synthesis of cytochrome P450 17-alpha-hydroxylase/17,20-lyase (CYP17A1), which converts progesterone to androgens in the Leydig cells. Androgens are essential for the development and maintenance of male secondary sexual characteristics and reproductive behavior. Copper deficiency can reduce the expression and activity of CYP17A1, leading to decreased androgen production and reduced testosterone levels (Ye et al. 2011).
- *Antioxidant defense*: copper is involved in the synthesis of SOD, which scavenges ROS in the testicular cells. ROS are generated during normal metabolic processes or under stress conditions, such as inflammation or infection. ROS can damage DNA, proteins, lipids, and other cellular components if not neutralized by antioxidant enzymes or molecules. Copper deficiency can reduce the expression and activity of SOD, leading to increased oxidative stress and damage in the testicular cells (Baskaran et al. 2021).

The effects of copper deficiency on testicular function can result in reduced fertility and reproductive performance in male goats. For instance, copper deficiency can cause reduced sperm production, lower sperm motility and quality, abnormal sperm morphology, reduced libido, infertility, or reduced male offspring ratio.

53.2.3 Hormones

The effects of copper deficiency on hormonal function can result in reduced fertility and reproductive performance in goats. For instance, copper deficiency can cause irregular estrous cycles, reduced libido, infertility, abortion, or dystocia in females, and reduced sperm production, lower sperm motility and quality, abnormal sperm morphology, reduced libido, infertility, or reduced male offspring ratio in males.

Hormones are chemical messengers that regulate various physiological processes in the body, including reproduction. Hormones are produced and secreted by various endocrine glands, such as the hypothalamus, pituitary gland, ovaries, testes, adrenal glands, and thyroid gland. Hormones act on specific target cells that have receptors for them and elicit specific responses. Hormones can also interact with each other and modulate their effects.

Copper is involved in the synthesis and metabolism of several hormones that regulate reproductive functions in goats, such as estrogen, progesterone, testosterone, gonadotropins, and thyroid hormones. Copper deficiency can impair the production and secretion of these hormones, leading to hormonal imbalance and disrupted reproductive cycle. For example, copper deficiency can affect the following processes.

- *Estrogen synthesis*: copper is involved in the synthesis of cytochrome P450 aromatase (CYP19A1), which converts testosterone to estrogen in the ovarian follicular cells and other tissues. Estrogen is essential for the growth and maturation of the follicles and oocytes, as well as for the development and maintenance of female secondary sexual characteristics and reproductive behavior. Copper deficiency can reduce the expression and activity of CYP19A1, leading to decreased estrogen production and reduced fertility (Hammes and Levin 2019).
- *Progesterone synthesis*: copper is involved in the synthesis of cytochrome P450 11-beta-hydroxylase (CYP11B1), which converts 11-deoxycortisol to cortisol in the adrenal cortex. Cortisol is a glucocorticoid hormone that regulates stress response and metabolism. Cortisol can also inhibit the synthesis of progesterone in the corpus luteum, which is a temporary endocrine structure that forms after ovulation and secretes progesterone. Progesterone is essential for the implantation and maintenance of pregnancy, as well as for the inhibition of estrus during gestation. Copper deficiency can increase the expression and activity of CYP11B1, leading to increased cortisol production and reduced progesterone synthesis.
- *Testosterone synthesis*: copper is involved in the synthesis of cytochrome P450 17-alpha-hydroxylase/17,20-lyase (CYP17A1), which converts progesterone to androgens in the testicular Leydig cells and other tissues. Androgens are essential for the development and maintenance of male secondary sexual characteristics and reproductive behavior. Copper deficiency can reduce the expression and activity of CYP17A1, leading to decreased androgen production and reduced testosterone levels (Naamneh Elzenaty et al. 2022).
- *Gonadotropin synthesis*: copper is involved in the synthesis of gonadotropin-releasing hormone (GnRH) in the hypothalamus and gonadotropins (follicle-stimulating hormone [FSH] and luteinizing hormone [LH]) in the pituitary gland. GnRH stimulates the release of FSH and LH from the pituitary gland, which in turn stimulate the growth and maturation of the follicles in the ovaries and the production and release of estrogen and progesterone in females and testosterone in males. Copper deficiency can reduce the expression and activity of GnRH and gonadotropins, leading to reduced stimulation and feedback of the reproductive axis (Szeliga et al. 2022).
- *Thyroid hormone synthesis*: copper is involved in the synthesis of thyroid hormones (thyroxine [T4] and triiodothyronine [T3]) in the thyroid gland. Thyroid hormones regulate metabolism, growth, development, and thermoregulation. They can also affect reproductive functions by modulating gonadotropin secretion and steroidogenesis. Copper deficiency can impair the activity of thyroid peroxidase (TPO), which catalyzes the iodination of thyroglobulin to form T4 and T3. Copper deficiency can also impair the activity of deiodinases (DIO1, DIO2, DIO3), which convert T4 to T3 or reverse T3 (rT3) in peripheral tissues. T3 is more biologically active than T4 or rT3. Copper deficiency can result in reduced thyroid hormone production or conversion, leading to hypothyroidism or subclinical hypothyroidism (Citterio et al. 2019).

53.2.4 Conception

Conception is the process of fertilization of an egg by sperm, resulting in the formation of a zygote. Conception depends on several factors, such as the quality and quantity of gametes (sperm and egg), the timing and frequency of mating, the viability and transport of gametes in the reproductive tract, the recognition and fusion of gametes, and the activation and development of the zygote.

Copper is involved in several aspects of conception, such as gamete maturation, gamete transport, gamete recognition, gamete fusion, and zygote activation. Copper deficiency can impair these aspects by affecting the activity and expression of various enzymes and proteins that require copper as a cofactor or a structural component. For example, copper deficiency can affect the following processes.

- *Gamete maturation*: copper is involved in the synthesis of SPO11, DMC1, and RAD51, which mediate homologous recombination and repair of DNA breaks during meiosis in both male and female gametes. Copper deficiency can impair the expression and function of these proteins, leading to reduced recombination and increased DNA damage during meiosis, resulting in impaired gamete maturation (De Storme and Geelen 2014).
- *Gamete transport*: copper is involved in the synthesis of LOX, which crosslinks collagen and elastin fibers in the reproductive tract. Collagen and elastin are important for the structural integrity and elasticity of the reproductive tract, which are required for the transport of gametes from the site of production to the site of fertilization. Copper deficiency can impair the activity of LOX, leading to reduced collagen and elastin crosslinking and impaired gamete transport (Hayashi et al. 2004).
- *Gamete recognition*: copper is involved in the synthesis and function of ZP1, ZP2, and ZP3, which form the zona pellucida that surrounds oocytes and mediates sperm binding. The zona pellucida is a glycoprotein layer that protects the oocyte

from polyspermy and ensures species-specific fertilization. Copper deficiency can impair the expression and function of these proteins, leading to reduced zona pellucida formation and impaired gamete recognition (Egge et al. 2015).

- *Gamete fusion*: copper is involved in the synthesis and function of PLCZ1, which triggers oocyte activation and calcium oscillations after sperm penetration. Oocyte activation is a series of events that initiate embryonic development after fertilization. Calcium oscillations are periodic changes in intracellular calcium concentration that regulate various cellular processes during oocyte activation. Copper deficiency can impair the expression and function of PLCZ1, leading to reduced oocyte activation and calcium oscillations (Meng et al. 2020).
- *Zygote activation*: copper is involved in the synthesis and function of several enzymes that regulate gene expression, DNA methylation, histone modification, and chromatin remodeling in the zygote. These processes are essential for the establishment and maintenance of the epigenetic state and the developmental potential of the zygote. Copper deficiency can impair the expression and function of these enzymes, leading to altered gene expression, DNA methylation, histone modification, and chromatin remodeling in the zygote (Li and Zhang 2014).

53.2.5 Pregnancy

Pregnancy is the period of gestation that lasts from conception to parturition. It involves several physiological changes and adaptations in the maternal and fetal systems, such as hormonal regulation, placental development, fetal growth, and immune modulation. Pregnancy also requires adequate nutrition and energy supply for the maintenance and development of the mother and fetus.

Copper is involved in several aspects of pregnancy, such as placental function, fetal development, immune function, and oxidative stress. Copper deficiency can impair these aspects by affecting the activity and expression of various enzymes and proteins that require copper as a cofactor or a structural component. For example, copper deficiency can affect the following processes.

- *Placental function*: copper is involved in the synthesis of LOX, which crosslinks collagen and elastin fibers in the placental tissue. Collagen and elastin are important for the structural integrity and elasticity of the placenta, which is essential for the exchange of nutrients, gases, and wastes between the maternal and fetal blood. Copper deficiency can impair the activity of LOX, leading to reduced collagen and elastin crosslinking and impaired placental function (Rucker et al. 2002).
- *Fetal development*: copper is involved in the synthesis of several enzymes and proteins that regulate fetal growth and development, such as cytochrome c oxidase (COX), SOD, vascular endothelial growth factor (VEGF), and thyroid hormones. Copper deficiency can impair the expression and function of these enzymes and proteins, leading to reduced fetal growth and development (Ruiz et al. 2021).
- *Immune function*: copper is involved in the synthesis of several enzymes and proteins that regulate immune function and inflammation, such as ceruloplasmin (CP), SOD, cytokines, and chemokines. Copper deficiency can impair the expression and function of these enzymes and proteins, leading to reduced immune response and increased inflammation (Pereira et al. 2016).
- *Oxidative stress*: copper is involved in the synthesis of several enzymes and proteins that protect against oxidative stress, such as SOD, GPX, catalase (CAT), and metallothionein (MT). Copper deficiency can impair the expression and function of these enzymes and proteins, leading to increased oxidative stress and damage (Sanchez et al. 2005) (Table 53.2).

53.3 Signs and Diagnosis of Copper Deficiency in Goats

One of the most common and visible signs of copper deficiency in goats is the change in coat color and quality. Copper is involved in the synthesis of melanin, the pigment that gives color to the hair and skin. Copper deficiency can cause the coat to fade, lose its luster, and become rough and brittle. The coat color may also change from black to brown, red to yellow, or cream to white, depending on the original color and the severity of the deficiency. Hair loss may be more pronounced in certain areas, such as the tail tip (fish tail), the face (especially around the eyes or the bridge of the nose), or the legs. Some goats may also not shed their winter coat promptly, resulting in a wooly appearance (Bhat et al. 2019).

Another sign of copper deficiency in goats is anemia, characterized by low levels of red blood cells or hemoglobin in the blood. Copper is involved in the synthesis of hemoglobin, the protein that carries oxygen in the blood. Copper deficiency

Table 53.2 Mechanisms and effects of copper deficiency on goat reproductive performance.

Mechanism	Effect of copper deficiency
Oxidative stress	Reduced synthesis of SOD leading to increased oxidative damage to reproductive tissues. This can result in lipid peroxidation, DNA damage, and protein oxidation, which can lead to apoptosis, tissue injury, and reduced reproductive performance
Hormonal imbalance	Disruption of estrogen, progesterone, and testosterone synthesis and metabolism, resulting in reduced fertility. Copper is essential for the activity of several enzymes involved in steroid[a] hormone synthesis and metabolism. Copper deficiency can alter the balance of these hormones, negatively impacting the reproductive system by affecting follicular growth, ovulation, implantation, and maintenance of pregnancy
Reduced blood flow	Impaired synthesis of enzymes that regulate blood vessel function and vasodilation, leading to reduced blood flow to reproductive tissues and negatively impacting fertility. Copper is involved in the synthesis of enzymes that regulate vascular function and blood flow[b] to reproductive tissues. Copper deficiency can impair the synthesis of these enzymes, resulting in reduced blood flow to the reproductive system, negatively impacting fertility
Increased inflammation	Reduced synthesis of enzymes that regulate immune function and inflammation, leading to increased inflammation and negatively impacting reproductive performance. Copper is involved in the synthesis of several enzymes that regulate immune function and inflammation.[c] Copper deficiency can impair the synthesis of these enzymes, resulting in increased inflammation and negatively impacting the reproductive system
Impaired gamete development	Impaired gamete maturation and reduced sperm and egg quality, resulting in reduced fertility. Copper is involved in the synthesis and function of several enzymes that regulate gamete development and maturation. Copper deficiency can impair the synthesis and function of these enzymes, resulting in impaired gamete development, reduced sperm and egg quality, and reduced fertility
Abnormal fetal development	Reduced copper availability for fetal growth and development, resulting in fetal abnormalities and reduced birth weight. Copper is essential for fetal growth and development, and copper deficiency can negatively impact fetal development, resulting in abnormal growth, malformations, and reduced birth weight
Altered gene expression	Altered gene expression patterns in reproductive tissues, resulting in impaired reproductive function. Copper is involved in the regulation of gene expression[d] in reproductive tissues, and copper deficiency can alter gene expression patterns, resulting in impaired reproductive function
Reduced enzyme activity	Reduced synthesis and function of several enzymes involved in reproductive processes, resulting in impaired reproductive function. Copper deficiency can impair the synthesis and function of these enzymes, resulting in impaired reproductive function
Altered energy metabolism	Altered energy metabolism in reproductive tissues, leading to reduced fertility. Copper is involved in the regulation of energy metabolism in reproductive tissues, and copper deficiency can alter energy metabolism, resulting in reduced fertility
Impaired immune function	Impaired immune function and increased susceptibility to reproductive infections, resulting in reduced fertility. Copper is involved in the regulation of immune function, and copper deficiency can impair immune function, resulting in increased susceptibility to reproductive infections and reduced fertility
Neural dysfunction	Impaired development and function of the nervous system, including impaired reproductive function. Copper is involved in the development and function of the nervous system, and copper deficiency can impair the development and function of the nervous system, resulting in impaired reproductive function

[a] Enzymes involved in steroid hormone synthesis and metabolism that require copper are:

- cytochrome P450 aromatase (CYP19A1), which converts testosterone to estrogen
- cytochrome P450 17-alpha-hydroxylase/17,20-lyase (CYP17A1), which converts progesterone to androgens
- cytochrome P450 11-beta-hydroxylase (CYP11B1), which converts 11-deoxycortisol to cortisol.

[b] Enzymes that regulate blood vessel function and vasodilation that require copper are:

- COX, involved in cellular energy production and oxygen utilization
- lysyl oxidase, involved in the crosslinking of collagen and elastin in the blood vessel walls
- multi-copper oxidases or ferroxidases, involved in iron metabolism and transport
- vascular endothelial growth factor (VEGF), involved in angiogenesis and blood vessel repair.

[c] Enzymes that regulate immune function and inflammation that require copper are:

- ceruloplasmin, which has antioxidant and antiinflammatory properties and modulates iron metabolism
- superoxide dismutase (SOD), which scavenges reactive oxygen species and protects against oxidative stress.

[d] Some of the genes that require copper involvement for gamete development are:

- SPO11, which initiates meiotic recombination by creating double-strand breaks in DNA and requires copper as a cofactor
- DMC1 and RAD51, which mediate homologous recombination and repair of DNA breaks and contain copper-binding motifs
- ZP1, ZP2, and ZP3, which form the zona pellucida that surrounds oocytes and mediates sperm binding and contains copper-dependent crosslinks
- PLCZ1, which triggers oocyte activation and calcium oscillations and has a copper-binding domain.

can impair the production and function of hemoglobin, leading to reduced oxygen delivery to the tissues and organs. Anemia can cause weakness, lethargy, pale mucous membranes, increased heart rate and respiratory rate, and reduced tolerance to exercise or stress (Jones and Allison 2007).

Copper deficiency can also affect the skeletal system of goats, causing abnormal bone growth and increased bone fragility. Copper is involved in the formation and maintenance of connective tissue, such as collagen and elastin, which are important for the strength and elasticity of bones, cartilage, tendons, and ligaments. Copper deficiency can impair the crosslinking of collagen and elastin fibers, leading to reduced bone density and increased risk of fractures. It can also affect the development and mineralization of bones in growing kids, resulting in skeletal deformities such as bowed legs, enlarged joints, or spinal curvature (Gambling and McArdle 2004).

Copper deficiency can also affect the immune system of goats, making them more susceptible to infections and parasites. Copper is involved in the regulation of immune function and inflammation, as well as in the synthesis of antioxidant enzymes that protect against oxidative stress. Copper deficiency can impair these processes, leading to reduced immune response and increased inflammation. This can make goats more prone to bacterial, viral, fungal, or protozoal infections, such as pneumonia, mastitis, foot rot, coccidiosis, or cryptosporidiosis. Copper deficiency can also make goats more vulnerable to parasitic infestations, such as gastrointestinal worms or external parasites (lice or mites) (Hoste et al. 2008).

Methods for diagnosis of copper deficiency are shown in Figure 53.2.

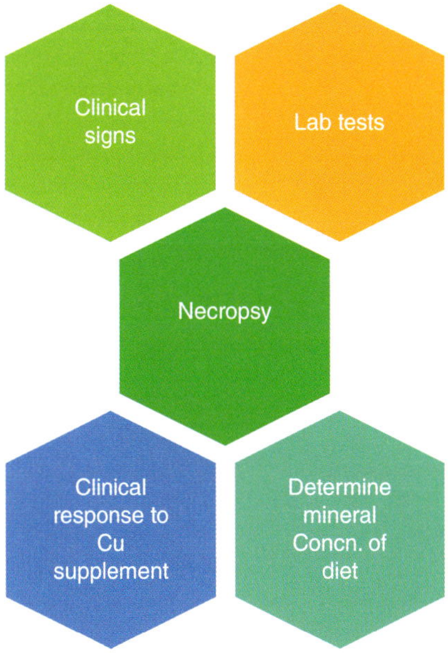

Figure 53.2 Diagnosis of copper deficiency.

53.3.1 Laboratory Tests for Copper Deficiency in Goats

The most common tests are blood (serum or plasma), liver (biopsy or necropsy), or hair analysis. Each test has its advantages and disadvantages, depending on the availability, cost, accuracy, and interpretation. The most reliable indicator of copper status in goats is liver copper concentration, which can be measured by biopsy or necropsy. However, this test is invasive, expensive, and not widely available. The blood (serum or plasma) copper concentration is more accessible and less invasive but it is not very sensitive or specific, as it can be influenced by various factors, such as diet, stress, infection, or inflammation. The hair copper concentration is also easy and inexpensive to measure, but it is not very accurate or consistent as it can be affected by external contamination, coat color, or seasonal variation (Table 53.3).

53.3.2 Factors That Influence the Diagnosis of Copper Deficiency in Goats

The diagnosis of copper deficiency can be influenced by various factors that affect the copper requirements and metabolism of goats, as well as their response to copper supplementation or treatment.

- *Breed*: different breeds of goats may have different susceptibility to copper deficiency or toxicity, depending on their genetic make-up and adaptation to their environment. For example, breeds such as Angora, cashmere, pygmy, or Boer goats may have higher copper requirements than other breeds, such as dairy goats. Some breeds, such as Alpine or Saanen goats, may have lower tolerance to copper than other breeds, such as Nubian or Toggenburg goats.
- *Coat color*: the coat color of goats may also affect their copper status and diagnosis. Generally, darker-colored goats tend to have higher copper requirements and lower copper tolerance than lighter-colored goats. This is because darker pigments require more copper for their synthesis and metabolism than lighter pigments. Therefore, darker-colored goats may be more prone to copper deficiency or toxicity than lighter-colored goats.
- *Age*: the age of goats may also influence their copper status and diagnosis. Younger goats tend to have higher copper requirements and lower copper tolerance than older goats. This is because they have higher growth rates and metabolic rates than older goats. Therefore, younger goats may be more susceptible to copper deficiency or toxicity than older goats.
- *Diet*: the diet of goats may also affect their copper status and diagnosis. The diet can influence copper intake and absorption as well as the interaction of copper with other minerals in the digestive tract. For example, high levels of iron, sulfur,

Table 53.3 Laboratory tests for copper deficiency in goats.

Technology	Advantages	Disadvantages
Liver biopsy or necropsy	Most reliable indicator; provides quantitative data	Invasive, expensive, requires specialized equipment and expertise
Blood (serum or plasma) analysis	Easy to collect, less invasive	Less sensitive and specific; influenced by various factors
Hair analysis	Easy and inexpensive	Not very accurate or consistent; affected by external contamination and other factors
Ultrasound	Noninvasive, real-time results	Requires specialized equipment and expertise
X-ray fluorescence (XRF) spectroscopy	Fast, nondestructive, can analyze multiple samples	Requires specialized equipment and expertise
Genomic and proteomic analysis	Improves understanding of molecular mechanisms	Expensive, time-consuming, requires specialized expertise and equipment

Other techniques that can be used to assess copper status in goats include:

- inductively coupled plasma mass spectrometry (ICP-MS): measures trace elements in various tissues, including copper
- atomic absorption spectroscopy (AAS): measures the amount of copper in a sample by analyzing its absorption of light at a specific wavelength
- copper stable isotope analysis: measures the ratio of stable isotopes of copper in a sample, which can provide information on copper metabolism and sources of copper in the diet.

molybdenum, or zinc in the diet can reduce the availability and absorption of copper by forming insoluble complexes or competing for binding sites. Low levels of protein or energy in the diet can also impair the utilization and retention of copper by affecting liver function or metabolic rate.

- *Season*: the season of the year may also affect the copper status and diagnosis of goats. The season can affect the quality and quantity of forage available for grazing, as well as the environmental conditions and stress levels of goats. For example, during winter or drought periods, the forage may have lower levels of copper or higher levels of antagonistic minerals than during spring or summer. Cold or dry weather may also increase the energy expenditure and water loss of goats, which can affect their copper metabolism and balance.

53.4 Copper Supplementation and Management

Copper supplementation and management are essential to prevent and treat copper deficiency in goats. Copper supplementation can be done by using various sources, forms, doses, frequencies, and methods of administration, depending on the type and severity of copper deficiency (Figure 53.3). Copper status can be monitored and evaluated by measuring the copper levels in blood, liver, hair, or milk samples. Other factors that influence copper status in goats, such as diet, environment, genetics, interactions with other minerals or drugs, and stress, should also be managed appropriately.

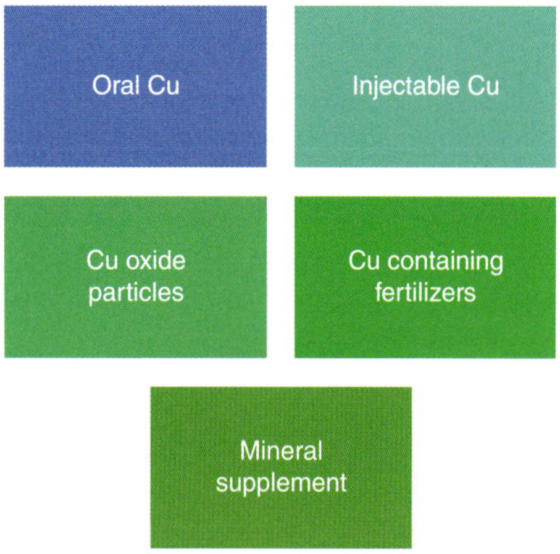

Figure 53.3 Treatment of copper deficiency.

Common sources of copper supplementation for goats include copper sulfate, copper oxide, copper proteinate, and copper boluses. Copper sulfate is a soluble form of copper that can be added to water or feed. Copper oxide is an insoluble form of copper that can be mixed with feed or given as a bolus. Copper proteinate is a chelated form of copper that is bound to amino acids and can be added to feed. Copper boluses are capsules that contain copper oxide particles and are given orally to goats (Table 53.4).

The optimal form, dose, frequency, and method of copper supplementation for goats depend on several factors, such as the type and severity of copper deficiency, the availability and cost of copper sources, the palatability and stability of copper sources, interactions with other minerals or

Table 53.4 Recommended copper supplementation for goats.

Age/stage of production	Copper supplementation
Growing kids	10–20 mg copper/kg of DMI
Lactating does	20–30 mg copper/kg of DMI
Bucks	8–12 mg copper/kg of DMI
Breeding does	10–20 mg copper/kg of DMI

DMI, dry matter intake.

drugs, and individual variation among goats. Generally, soluble forms of copper (such as copper sulfate) are more readily absorbed than insoluble forms (such as copper oxide), but they are also more prone to interactions with other minerals (such as iron, sulfur, molybdenum, and zinc) that can reduce their bioavailability. Chelated forms of copper (such as copper proteinate) are more stable and less affected by interactions with other minerals but are also more expensive than other forms. Copper boluses are convenient and effective ways to deliver a large dose of copper to goats at once or at long intervals (such as every 3–6 months), but they may cause irritation or damage to the gastrointestinal tract if not administered properly.

53.5 Conclusion

This chapter has discussed the importance of copper for goat health, especially reproduction. It has explained how copper deficiency can impair the reproductive performance of goats by affecting their hormonal, cellular, and molecular functions. It has also described the signs and diagnosis of copper deficiency, as well as the factors that can cause or contribute to it. Finally, it has suggested some methods of copper supplementation and management to prevent or treat copper deficiency in goats.

Copper deficiency is a common and serious problem that affects goats worldwide. It can have negative consequences for their fertility, pregnancy outcomes, offspring survival, and overall well-being. Therefore, it is essential for goat owners, veterinarians, researchers, and anyone interested in goat health to understand the role of copper in goat physiology and to monitor and maintain adequate copper levels in their animals. By doing so, we can improve the health and productivity of goats and contribute to the sustainability and profitability of farms.

References

Acién, P. and Acién, M. (2020). Disorders of sex development: classification, review, and impact on fertility. *Journal of Clinical Medicine* 9 (11): 3555.

Baskaran, S., Finelli, R., Agarwal, A., and Henkel, R. (2021). Reactive oxygen species in male reproduction: a boon or a bane? *Andrologia* 53 (1).

Bhat, B., Singh, A., Iqbal, Z. et al. (2019). Comparative transcriptome analysis reveals the genetic basis of coat color variation in Pashmina goat. *Scientific Reports* 9 (1): 1–9.

Citterio, C.E., Targovnik, H.M., and Arvan, P. (2019). The role of thyroglobulin in thyroid hormonogenesis. *Nature Reviews Endocrinology* 15 (6): 323–338.

De Storme, N. and Geelen, D. (2014). The impact of environmental stress on male reproductive development in plants: biological processes and molecular mechanisms. *Plant, Cell and Environment* 37 (1): 1–18.

Egge, N., Muthusubramanian, A., and Cornwall, G.A. (2015). Amyloid properties of the mouse egg zona pellucida. *PLoS One* 10 (6): 1–19.

Gambling, L. and McArdle, H.J. (2004). Iron, copper and fetal development. *Proceedings of the Nutrition Society* 63 (4): 553–562.

Gooneratne, S.R., Buckley, W.T., and Christensen, D.A. (1989). Review of copper deficiency and metabolism in ruminants. *Canadian Journal of Animal Science* 69 (4): 819–845.

Hammes, S.R. and Levin, E.R. (2019). Impact of estrogens in males and androgens in females. *Journal of Clinical Investigation* 129 (5): 1818–1826.

Hayashi, K., Fong, K.S.K., Mercier, F. et al. (2004). Comparative immunocytochemical localization of lysyl oxidase (LOX) and the lysyl oxidase-like (LOXL) proteins: changes in the expression of LOXL during development and growth of mouse tissues. *Journal of Molecular Histology* 35 (8–9): 845–855.

Hoste, H., Torres-Acosta, J.F.J., and Aguilar-Caballero, A.J. (2008). Nutrition-parasite interactions in goats: is immunoregulation involved in the control of gastrointestinal nematodes? *Parasite Immunology* 30 (2): 79–88.

Huang, Y. and Roig, I. (2023). Genetic control of meiosis surveillance mechanisms in mammals. *Frontiers in Cell and Developmental Biology* 11 (February): 1–22.

Jones, M.L. and Allison, R.W. (2007). Evaluation of the ruminant complete blood cell count. *Veterinary Clinics of North America: Food Animal Practice* 23 (3): 377–402.

Karamanos, N.K., Theocharis, A.D., Piperigkou, Z. et al. (2021). A guide to the composition and functions of the extracellular matrix. *FEBS Journal* 288 (24): 6850–6912.

Khalifa, E.I., Ahmed, M.E., Hafez, Y.H. et al. (2013). Age at puberty and fertility of Rahmani sheep fed on biological inoculated corn silage. *Annals of Agricultural Sciences* 58 (2): 163–172.

Li, E. and Zhang, Y. (2014). DNA methylation in mammals. *Cold Spring Harbor Perspectives in Biology* 6 (5): a019133.

Lushchak, V.I. (2014). Free radicals, reactive oxygen species, oxidative stress and its classification. *Chemico-Biological Interactions* 224 (December 2015): 164–175.

Martins, M.D.S. (2011). Use of condensed tannins supplementation and inorganic copper as deworming agents in naturally infected ewes and lambs. Master's thesis, Louisiana State University.

Meng, X., Melo, P., Jones, C. et al. (2020). Use of phospholipase C zeta analysis to identify candidates for artificial oocyte activation: a case series of clinical pregnancies and a proposed algorithm for patient management. *Fertility and Sterility* 114 (1): 163–174.

Naamneh Elzenaty, R., du Toit, T., and Flück, C.E. (2022). Basics of androgen synthesis and action. *Best Practice and Research: Clinical Endocrinology and Metabolism* 36 (4): 101665.

Papachroni, K.K., Piperi, C., Levidou, G. et al. (2010). Lysyl oxidase interacts with AGE signalling to modulate collagen synthesis in polycystic ovarian tissue. *Journal of Cellular and Molecular Medicine* 14 (10): 2460–2469.

Pereira, T.C.B., Campos, M.M., and Bogo, M.R. (2016). Copper toxicology, oxidative stress and inflammation using zebrafish as experimental model. *Journal of Applied Toxicology* 36 (7): 876–885.

Rucker, R., Last, J., Armstrong, L., and Samimi, A. (2002). Lysyl hydroxylase. In: *Handbook of Food Enzymology* (ed. J. Whitaker, A. Voragen, and D. Wong), 245–267. Oxford: Taylor & Francis.

Ruiz, L.M., Libedinsky, A., and Elorza, A.A. (2021). Role of copper on mitochondrial function and metabolism. *Frontiers in Molecular Biosciences* 8 (August): 1–17.

Sanchez, W., Palluel, O., Meunier, L. et al. (2005). Copper-induced oxidative stress in three-spined stickleback: relationship with hepatic metal levels. *Environmental Toxicology and Pharmacology* 19 (1): 177–183.

da Silva, F.M., Marques, A., and Chaveiro, A. (2014). Reactive oxygen species: a double-edged sword in reproduction. *Open Veterinary Science Journal* 4 (1): 127–133.

Soni, R.K., Gupta, P.S.P., Nandi, S. et al. (2018). Effect of in vitro copper supplementation on granulosa cell estradiol synthesis and associated genes. *Indian Journal of Animal Research* 52 (5): 652–657.

Szeliga, A., Rudnicka, E., Maciejewska-Jeske, M. et al. (2022). Neuroendocrine determinants of polycystic ovary syndrome. *International Journal of Environmental Research and Public Health* 19 (5): 1–13.

Ye, L., Su, Z.J., and Ge, R.S. (2011). Inhibitors of testosterone biosynthetic and metabolic activation enzymes. *Molecules* 16 (12): 9983–10001.

Zatta, P. and Frank, A. (2007). Copper deficiency and neurological disorders in man and animals. *Brain Research Reviews* 54 (1): 19–33.

Index

Page numbers followed by *f* and *t* indicate figures and tables.

Elements of Reproduction and Reproductive Diseases of Goats, First Edition. Edited by Tanmoy Rana.

b

O

r

S